Practical Rheumatology

John H Klippel
National Institute of Arthritis and
Musculoskeletal and Skin Diseases
National Institutes of Health
Bethesda, USA

Paul A Dieppe
Rheumatology Unit
Bristol University
Bristol, UK

Peter M Brooks
Department of Medicine
The University of New South Wales
St Vincent's Hospital
Sydney, Australia

Simon Carette
Départment de Rhumatologie
Centre Hospitalier
De L'Université Laval
Quebec, Canada

Jan Dequeker
Division of Rheumatology
Department of Internal Medicine
University Hospitals KU Leuven
Belgium

Lynn H Gerber
Department of Rehabilitation Medicine
Clinical Center
National Institutes of Health
Bethesda, USA

Brian L Hazleman
Rheumatology Research Unit
Addenbrooke's Hospital
Cambridge, UK

Andrew CS Keat
Department of Rheumatology
Charing Cross & Westminster Medical School
London, UK

Robert P Kimberly
Department of Medicine
Hospital for Special Surgery
Cornell University Medical College
New York, USA

Matthew H Liang
Department of Medicine
Department of Rheumatology
and Immunology
Brigham & Women's Hospital
Boston, USA

Ravinder N Maini
Kennedy Institute of Rheumatology
London, UK

Leo van de Putte
Department of Rheumatology
University Hospital Nijmegen
Nijmegen, The Netherlands

Roger D Sturrock
Centre for Rheumatic Diseases
Royal Infirmary
Glasgow, UK

Murray B Urowitz
Department of Medicine
University of Toronto
Wellesley Hospital
Toronto, Canada

Frank A Wollheim
Department of Rheumatology
Lund University Hospital
Lund, Sweden

Nathan J Zvaifler
Division of Rheumatic Diseases
University of California at San Diego
San Diego, USA

M Mosby

London Baltimore Barcelona Bogotá Boston Buenos Aires Caracas Carlsbad, CA Chicago Madrid Mexico City Milan Naples, FL New York Philadelphia St. Louis Seoul Singapore Sydney Taipei Tokyo Toronto Wiesbaden

A CIP catalogue record for this book is available from the British Library.

ISBN: 07234 2429 2

For full details of Times Mirror International Publishers Limited titles please write to:

Times Mirror International Publishers Limited
Lynton House
7–12 Tavistock Square
London WC1H 9LB
UK

Typeset in Times, legends set in Univers.
Reproduced by Mandarin Offset Ltd, Hong Kong.
Printed and bound by Grafos S.A. Arte Sobre Papel, Barcelona, Spain.

***Practical Rheumatology* Team**

Project Manager Alison Taylor

Developmental Editor Alison Whitehouse

Layout and Illustration Marie McNestry, Richard Prime

Production Jane Tozer

Index Lawrence Errington

Publisher Fiona Foley

***Rheumatology* 1st edition Team**

Project Managers: David Cooke, Michael Smith, Lucy Hamilton, Alison Whitehouse

Designer: Judith Gauge

Design and Illustration: Judith Gauge, Richard Prime, Jenni Miller, Mark Willey, Chris Read, Tim Read, Lynda Payne, Anne-Marie Woodruff, Dereck Johnson

Linework: Lee Smith

Editorial Assistant: Chris Downs

Production: Adam Phillips, Jane Tozer, Susan Bishop

Index: Nina Boyd

Publisher: Fiona Foley

Drug Notice
The contributors, the editors, and the publishers have made every effort to ensure the accuracy and appropriateness of the drug dosages presented in this textbook. The medications described do not necessarily have specific approval by the Food and Drug Administration for use in the diseases and dosages for which they are recommended. The package insert for each drug should be consulted for use and dosage as approved by the FDA. Because standards for usage change, it is advisable to keep abreast of revised recommendations, particularly those concerning new drugs.

Every effort has been made to contact holders of copyright to obtain permission to reproduce copyright material. However, if any have been inadvertently overlooked, the publishers will be pleased to make the necessary arrangements at the first opportunity.

PREFACE

Disorders of the musculoskeletal system account for a high proportion of patient visits to internists, primary care and general physicians. The task of sorting out the cause of the complaints, developing a plan of therapy and recognizing those patients in need of referral to a specialist is difficult and requires a good working knowledge of the common rheumatic diseases and their management. *Practical Rheumatology* has been specifically developed to help with this need. In addition to chapters on the clinical features and management of common types of arthritis, it features sections on common symptoms, signs and presentations of regional disorders, including back and neck pain, as well as periarticular problems and generalized joint pain. *Practical Rheumatology* also aims to fulfil its name and provide practical advice of direct use at the bedside. To this end it includes a large number of 'Practical Problems' – clinical vignettes addressing common clinical issues – as well as a chapter on periarticular and intra-articular injection techniques. The book is highly illustrated throughout, providing a valuable atlas of clinical signs and radiographic features of the rheumatic diseases, and the numerous artworks and illustrations aid in both the understanding of these disorders and in how to manage them.

Practical Rheumatology is a direct derivative of the much larger text reference book, *Rheumatology*, designed for specialists and trainees with a special commitment to musculoskeletal disorders. *Rheumatology* contains 1766 pages and covers the scientific background to the rheumatic diseases and antirheumatic therapy, as well as many chapters on bone disorders and the less common forms of arthritis. The more clinically oriented chapters of *Rheumatology* and those concerned with common disorders have been included in *Practical Rheumatology* and supplemented by a small number of new Practical Problems as well as a new introductory chapter and section on injection techniques, resulting in a book of only 432 pages which we believe will answer the needs of a primary care physician or generalist.

Rheumatology was commissioned and edited by a team of 16 Section Editors, each of whom have therefore made a major contribution to this derivative text *Practical Rheumatology*. This book belongs as much to them as it does to us.

We also owe a huge debt of gratitude to the publisher Fiona Foley, development editor Alison Whitehouse and the excellent team of editors, illustrators, designers and producers who have been responsible for both books.

John H Klippel
Paul A Dieppe

CONTENTS

RHEUMATOID ARTHRITIS

ANKYLOSING SPONDYLITIS

PSORIATIC ARTHRITIS

GOUT AND PSEUDOGOUT

INFECTION AND REACTIVE ARTHRITIS

CONNECTIVE TISSUE DISORDERS

CONTRIBUTING AUTHORS

MICHA ABELES
Associate Professor of Medicine, Associate Director, Multipurpose Arthritis Center, Department of Medicine, University of Connecticut Health Center, Farmington, Connecticut, USA

MARK H ARNOLD
Department of Rheumatology, Royal North Shore Hospital, St Leonard's, New South Wales, Australia

JAMES E BALOW
Clinical Director, National Institutes of Diabetes and Digestive and Kidney Disease, National Institutes of Health, Bethesda, Maryland, USA

MAURICE A BARRY
Consultant Rheumatologist, Department of Rheumatology, James Connolly Memorial Hospital, Dublin, Eire

WERNER F BARTH
Professor of Medicine, George Washington University, Chairman, Section of Rheumatology, Washington Hospital Center, Washington DC, USA

DAVID G BORENSTEIN
Medical Director, The Spine Center, Associate Director for Education and Research, Division of Rheumatology, Professor of Medicine, George Washington University Medical Center, Washington DC, USA

PETER BROOKS
Department of Medicine, The University of New South Wales, St Vincent's Hospital, Sydney, Australia

SIMON CARETTE
Dẻpartement de Rheumatologie, Centre Hospitalier, De L'Université Laval, Quebec, Canada

JOSEPH M CASH
Staff Physician, Department of Rheumatic and Immunologic Disease, The Cleveland Clinic Foundation, Cleveland, Ohio, USA

ARNOLD CATS
Professor of Rheumatology, Emeritus, Depsrtment of Rheumatology, University Hospital, Leiden, Netherlands

KUNTAL CHAKRAVARTY
Consultant Rheumatologist, Warrington Hospital NHS Trust, Warrington, Cheshire, UK

MICHAEL D CHARD
Consultant Rheumatologist, Worthing Hospital, Worthing, West Sussex, UK

MARC D COHEN
Assistant Professor of Medicine, Mayo Medical School, Mayo Jacksonville, Jacksonville, Florida, USA

MICHAEL G COHEN
Former Director of Rheumatology, Princess Alexandra Hospital, Brisbane, Queensland, Australia

DOYT L CONN
John Finn Minnesota Arthritis Foundation Professor of Medicine, Mayo Medical School, Mayo Clinic, Rochester, Minnesota, USA

CYRUS COOPER
MRC Clinical Scientist, Consultant Rheumatologist, MRC Environmental Epidemiology Unit, Southampton General Hospital, Southampton, Hampshire, UK

PAUL CREAMER
Senior Registrar, Rheumatology Unit, Bristol Royal Infirmary, Bristol, Avon, UK

MARTA L CUÈLLAR
Research Fellow in Rheumatology, Louisiana State School of Medicine, New Orleans Department of Medicine, New Orleans, Louisiana, USA

JANET CUSHNAGHAN
Chartered Physiotherapist and Clinical Research Assistant, Rheumatology Unit, Bristol Royal Infirmary, Bristol, UK

SEAMUS E DALTON
Specialist in Rehabilitation and Sports Medicine, Director of Sports Medicine, North Sydney Orthopaedic and Sports Medicine Centre , Crows Nest, New South Wales, Australia

RICHARD O DAY
Professor of Clinical Pharmacology, University of New South Wales, Director of Clinical Pharmacology, St Vincent's Hospital, Darlinghurst, New South Wales, Australia

PAUL A DIEPPE
ARC Professor of Rheumatology, Bristol University Rheumatology Unit, Bristol, UK

ALLAN ST J DIXON
Consultant, Royal National Hospital for Rheumatic Diseases, Bath, Avon, UK

MICHAEL DOHERTY
Reader in Rheumatology, University of Nottingham Medical School, Rheumatology Unit, City Hospital, Nottingham, Nottinghamshire, UK

BRYAN T EMMERSON
Professor and Head, Department of Medicine, University of Queensland, Princess Alexandra Hospital, Brisbane, Queensland, Australia

LUIS R ESPINOZA
Professor and Chief, Section of Rheumatology, Louisiana State School of Medicine, New Orleans Department of Medicine, New Orleans, Louisiana, USA

JOHN A FAIRCLOUGH
Consultant Orthopaedic Surgeon, Cardiff Royal Infirmary, Cardiff, UK

ADEL G FAM
Professor of Medicine, Head, Division of Rheumatology, Sunnybrook Health Science Center, University of Toronto, Toronto, Ontario, Canada

DAVID L GEORGE
Assistant Professor of Medicine, Temple Medical School, Associate Director of Medicine, Reading Hospital and Medical Center, West Reading, Pennsylvania, USA

DAFNA D GLADMAN
Professor of Medicine, University of Toronto, Rheumatic Disease Unit, The Wellesley Hospital, Toronto, Ontario, Canada

DUNCAN A GORDON
Professor of Medicine, University of Toronto, President of the Panamerican League Against Rheumatism, Editor of the Journal of Rheumatology, Senior Rheumatologist, The Toronto Hospital Arthritis Centre, Toronto, Ontario, Canada

GEOFFREY P GRAHAM
Consultant Orthopaedic Surgeon, Cardiff Royal Infirmary, Cardiff, UK

GERALD D GROFF
Associate Professor of Clinical Medicine, College of Physicians and Surgeons, Columbia University, Attending Physician, Mary Imogen Bassett Hospital, Cooperstown, New York, USA

IAN HASLOCK
Visiting Professor in Clinical Bioengineering, University of Durham, Consultant Rheumatologist, South Cleveland Hospital, Middlesborough, Cleveland, UK

DAVID E HASTINGS
Professor of Surgery, University of Toronto, Chief, Division of Orthpaedics, Surgeon-in-Chief, The Wellesley Hospital, Toronto, Ontario, Canada

BRIAN L HAZELMAN
Consultant Physician, Department of Rheumatology, Addenbrooke's Hospital, Director of Rheumatology Research Unit, Cambridge, UK

SVEN ÅKE HEDSTRÖM
Director, Department of Infectious Diseases, Halmstad Hospital, Halmstad, Sweden

PHILIP S HELLIWELL
School of Medicine, Rheumatology & Rehabilitation Research Unit, University of Leeds, Leeds, Yorkshire, UK

DAVID B HELLMANN
Deputy Director, Department of Medicine, Johns Hopkins University School of Medicine, Baltimore, Maryland, USA

PASCEL HILLIQUIN
Senior Assistant, Department of Rheumatology, Hôpital Cochin, Paris, France

RODNEY A HUGHES
Senior Registrar, Department of Rheumatology, Charing Cross Hospital, London, UK

SHEPARD HURWITZ
Univeristy of Rochester, Rochester, New York, USA

LAWRENCE J KAGEN
Professor of Medicine, Hospital for Special Surgery, New York, New York, USA

JOACHIM R KALDEN
Professor of Internal Medicine, Head of Department of Internal Medicine III, Institute for Clinical Immunology and Rheumatology, University Erlangen-Nürnberg, Erlangen, Germany

ANDREW CS KEAT
Department of Rheumatology, Charing Cross & Westminster Medical School, London, UK

MUHAMMAD ASIM KHAN
Professor of Medicine, Case Western Reserve University, Director, Division of Rheumatology, MetroHealth Medical Center, Cleveland, Ohio, USA

JOHN H KLIPPEL
Clinical Director, National Institute of Arthritis and Musculoskeletal and Skin Diseases, National Institutes of Health, Bethesda, Maryland, USA

MATTHEW H LIANG
Department of Medicine, Division of Rheumatology, Brigham & Women's Hospital, Boston, Massachusetts, USA

LARS LIDGREN
Professor and Chairman, Department of Orthopedic Surgery, University Hospital of Lund, Lund, Sweden

ROBERT W LIGHTFOOT JR
Professor of Medicine, Director, Internal Medicine Residency Program, Associate Chairman for Education, Director, Division of Rheumatology, University of Kentucky, Lexington, Kentucky, USA

GEOFFREY O LITTLEJOHN
Clinical Associate Professor, Monash University, Director Rheumatology, Monash Medical Centre, Melbourne, Victoria, Australia

JOHN A MATHEWS
Consultant and Clinical Director, Department of Rheumatology, St Thomas's Hospital, London, UK

ERIC L MATTESON
Assistant Professor of Medicine, Mayo Medical School, Mayo Clinic, Rochester, Minnesota, USA

BERNARD MAZIÈRES
Professor of Rheumatology, Head of Department of Rheumatology, University Hospital Rangueil, Toulouse, France

CONOR McCARTHY
Research Fellow, Department of Internal Medicine, Division of Rheumatology, University of Michigan Medical Center, Ann Arbor, Michigan, USA

THOMAS A MEDSGER JR
Deptartment of Medicine/Rheumatology, University of Pittsburgh School of Medicine, Pittsburgh, Pennsylvania, USA

CHARLES-JÖEL MENKES
Professor of Rheumatology, Head of Department of Rheumatology, Hôpital Cochin, Paris, France

HERMAN MIELANTS
Professor of Rheumatology, Department of Rheumatology, University Hospital, Gent, Belgium

HARALAMPOS M MOUTSOPOULOS
Director, Department of Pathophysiology, School of Medicine, National University of Athens, Athens, Greece

CHRISTOPHER NEEDS
Consultant Rheumatologist, Royal North Shore Hospital, St Leonard's, New South Wales, Australia

CHESTER V ODDIS
Assistant Professor of Medicine, Department of Medicine, Division of Rheumatology and Clinical Immunology, University of Pittsburgh School of Medicine, Pittsburgh, Pennsylvania, USA

DANIEL W RAHN
Vice Dean for Clinical Affairs, School of Medicine, Medical College of Georgia, Augusta, Georgia, USA

IAN F ROWE
Consultant Rheumatologist, Droitwich Centre for Rheumatic Diseases, Highfield Hospital, Droitwich, West Midlands, UK

ANTHONY S RUSSELL
Professor of Medicine, Rheumatic Disease Unit, University of Alberta, Edmonton, Alberta, Canada

LESLIE SCHRIEBER
Associate Professor, Department of Rheumatology, Royal North Shore Hospital, St Leonards, New South Wales , Australia

DAVID L SCOTT
Reader in Rheumatology, Kings's College Hospital, Denmark Hill, London, UK

JAMES R SEIBOLD
WH Conzen Chair of Clinical Pharmacology, Director, Clinical Research Center, UMDNJ-Robert Wood Johnson Medical School, New Brunswick, New Jersey, USA

HARRY SPIERA
Clinical Professor of Medicine, Chief, Division of Rheumatology, Mount Sinai Medical Center, New York, New York, USA

VIRGINIA D STEEN
Associate Professor of Medicine, Department of Medicine/ Rheumatology, Georgetown University, Washington, DC, USA

ROGER D STURROCK
McLeod/ARC Professor of Rheumatology, Centre for Rheumatic Diseases, Royal Infirmary, Glasgow, UK

AULI TOIVANEN
Professor of Medicine, Head of Department of Medicine, Turku University, Turku, Finland

ALAN G TYNDALL
Professor and Head, Department of Rheumatology, University of Basel, Basel, Switzerland

ATHANASIOS G TZIOUFAS
Fellow in Rheumatology, Department of Pathophysiology, School of Medicine, National University of Athens, Athens, Greece

MURRAY B UROWITZ
Department of Medicine, University of Toronto, Wellesley Hospital, Toronto, Ontario, Canada

ERIC M VEYS
Head of Rheumatology Department, University Hospital, Gent, Belgium

JOHN R WARD
Professor of Medicine, University of Utah School of Medicine, Salt Lake City, Utah, USA

MICHAEL H WEISMAN
Professor of Medicine, University of California School of Medicine, University of California, San Diego, California, USA

ROBERT L WORTMANN
Professor and Chairman, Department of Medicine, East Carolina University School of Medicine, Greenville, North Carolina, USA

VERNA WRIGHT
ARC Professor of Rheumatology, Rheumatology and Rehabilitation Research Unit, The School of Medicine, University of Leeds, Leeds, Yorkshire, UK

HASAN YAZICI
Professor and Chief, Division of Rheumatology, Department of Medicine, Cerrahpasa Medical Faculty, University of Istanbul, Istanbul, Turkey

NEVILLE D YEOMANS
Professor of Medicine, Department of Medicine, The University of Melbourne, Western Hospital, Melbourne, Australia

INTRODUCTION

1

DISORDERS OF THE MUSCULOSKELETAL SYSTEM

Paul A Dieppe
& John H Klippel

Disorders of the musculoskeletal system are common. They range from mild regional problems such as 'tennis elbow' or 'trigger finger', to severe life-threatening, multisystem disorders such as systemic lupus erythematosus or vasculitis. Most rheumatic diseases are thought to be *initiated* by the interaction of complex genetic predispositions with a variety of environmental factors, including trauma and infection. Their *pathogenesis* involves disturbances of connective tissue turnover, changes in immune function, inflammation, crystal deposition and many other disease processes. The many possible *outcomes* of a rheumatic disease include pain, physical disability and psychosocial problems. Rheumatology is therefore an exciting subspecialty of medicine, which must encompass multidisciplinary areas of medical science, as well as the art of managing patients with chronic disease.

CLASSIFICATION OF THE RHEUMATIC DISEASES

The World Health Organization has divided disorders of the musculoskeletal system into four main classes: back pain, periarticular disorders, osteoarthritis and inflammatory arthropathies. In addition disorders of bone have become an increasingly important aspect of rheumatology. These categories can be further subdivided to include the main categories of rheumatic disorders (Fig. 1.1).

A PRAGMATIC CLASSIFICATION OF THE MAJOR MUSCULOSKELETAL DISORDERS	
1. Back Pain Can be subdivided into a number of clinical categories	Mechanical (including periarticular problems around the spine) Inflammatory (e.g. ankylosing spondylitis) Neurogenic (involving irritation of nerve roots or spinal cord) 'Sinister' (infection or neoplasm) Other types/causes of back pain
2. Periarticular Also called 'soft tissue' or regional disorders	Bursitis, tendon problems and enthesopathies Regional pain syndromes Generalized non-articular pain syndromes such as fibromyalgia
3. Osteoarthritis	Idiopathic and secondary forms of OA and related diseases
4. Inflammatory Covers many different classes of disease	Rheumatoid arthritis Juvenile chronic arthritis Seronegative spondyloarthropathies Diffuse connective tissue disorders Crystal-related arthropathies Infectious arthritis
5. Bone diseases Includes developmental and acquired skeletal abnormalities	Metabolic, endocrine and other systemic arthropathies Osteopenia (osteoporosis and osteomalacia) Osteonecrosis Paget's disease Other forms of bone disease

Fig. 1.1 A pragmatic classification of the major musculoskeletal disorders.

FREQUENCY OF THE MAJOR RHEUMATIC DISEASES

A rough guide to the frequency of the rheumatic diseases is provided in Figure 1.2. Back pain and periarticular disorders are extremely common, both affecting well over 20% of the population. The major bone disorder is osteoporosis, which is very common in elderly females. Radiographic evidence of osteoarthritis is present in a large proportion of the older population, but the overall prevalence of significant hip or knee disease is nearer 5%. Inflammatory arthropathies are less common but more severe, and affect about 2% of the population. All forms of rheumatic disease rise in prevalence with increasing age. This is due to the fact that most of musculoskeletal disorders have little effect on life expectancy, as well as the higher incidence of some disorders in older people.

THE ETIOPATHOGENESIS OF RHEUMATIC DISEASES

A few rheumatic diseases result purely from a single genetic, or isolated environmental factor, but in the majority of cases there is a complex interaction between multiple causes (Fig. 1.3) and a variety of different risk factors can be delineated, some of which (obesity and osteoarthritis for example) are potentially treatable. Age and gender both have a major effect on the structure and function of the musculoskeletal system and on disease susceptibility and expres-

PREVALENCE ESTIMATES FOR SELECTED RHEUMATIC DISORDERS	
Disorder	**Prevalence (%)**
Back pain and periarticular disorders (both)	> 20
Osteoporosis	
Spine, hip or wrist fracture	c. 5
Osteoarthritis	
Radiographic (all sites)	25
Knee disease	3.8
Hip disease	1.3
Inflammatory arthropathies	
Rheumatoid arthritis	1.0
Crystal arthropathies	1.0
Ankylosing spondylitis	0.1
Psoriatic arthritis	0.1
Arthritis in children (<16 years)	0.06
Systemic lupus erythematosus	0.02

Fig. 1.2 Prevalence estimates for selected rheumatic disorders.

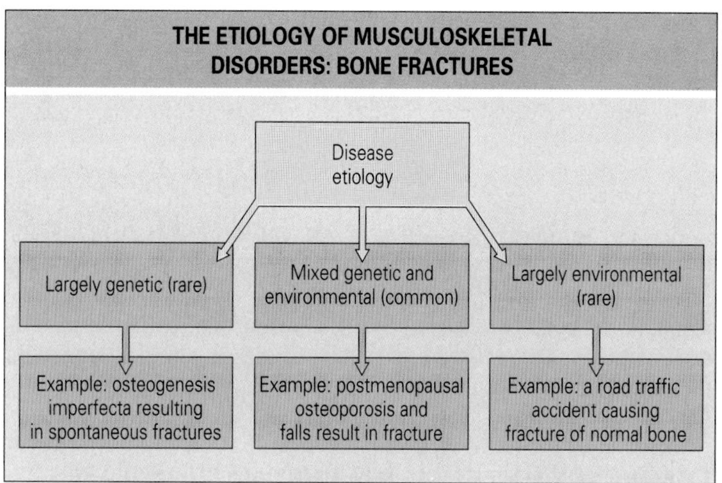

Fig. 1.3 The etiology of rheumatic diseases is usually a mixture of genetic and environmental factors. Bone fractures are an example.

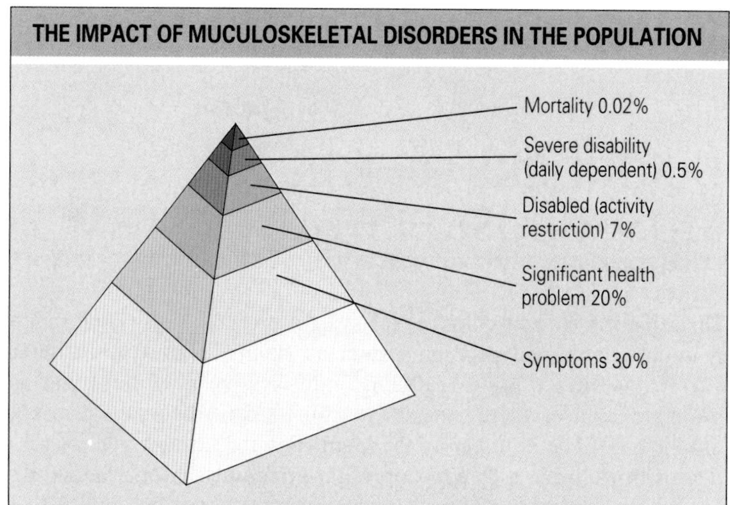

Fig. 1.4 A summary of the impact of musculoskeletal disorders in the population.

sion, while trauma, and other exposures may initiate damage. Key processes in the pathogenesis of bone and joint damage include immune-driven inflammatory reactions in the synovial tissues, immune complex deposition along endothelial surfaces, and alterations in the normal balance of synthesis and degradation of connective tissues. Cytokines and growth factors appear to play a key role in many of these processes, and new preventive and therapeutic strategies are being developed through our increasing understanding of immunological function and connective tissue turnover.

IMPACT OF RHEUMATIC DISEASE

A summary of the impact of the rheumatic diseases is given in Figure 1.4. The overall prevalence is very high (30% with some symptoms), but mortality is low (0.02%). The main impact is through the very high prevalence of disability, which is usually combined with pain. Rheumatic diseases also cause a huge economic burden, and have been estimated to cost the US about 1% of its GNP through a combination of lost wages and health costs.

TREATMENT OF RHEUMATIC DISEASES

Good management of the rheumatic diseases involves the co-ordination of several different modalities of care (Fig. 1.5). Specific, effective therapy is available for some disorders, such as gout, and recent advances in our understanding of disease processes in rheumatology are resulting in the introduction of exciting new drugs and biologic agents which may control many of the inflammatory arthropathies. However, in many diseases there is, as yet, no totally effective way of halting or controlling the progression of the disease. In these instances, and where a disease has caused severe joint damage, a multidisciplinary approach to care is needed, with modalities such as patient education (including the empowerment of self-help) and physical and occupational therapy being of paramount importance. It is also necessary to use a framework that extends beyond the narrow medical approach to many illnesses. One such framework is shown in Figure 1.6, which emphasizes the interaction of rheumatic diseases with psychosocial factors.

MODALITIES OF TREATMENT FOR RHEUMATIC DISORDERS

- **Patient education,** including self empowerment and joint protection techniques
- **Physical therapies,** including exercise therapy, manipulation and hydrotherapy
- **Occupational therapy,** including the use of aids and appliances
- **Drug therapy,** including both disease-modifying and symptomatic therapy
- **Surgery,** including joint replacement

Fig. 1.5 Modalities of treatment for rheumatic disorders.

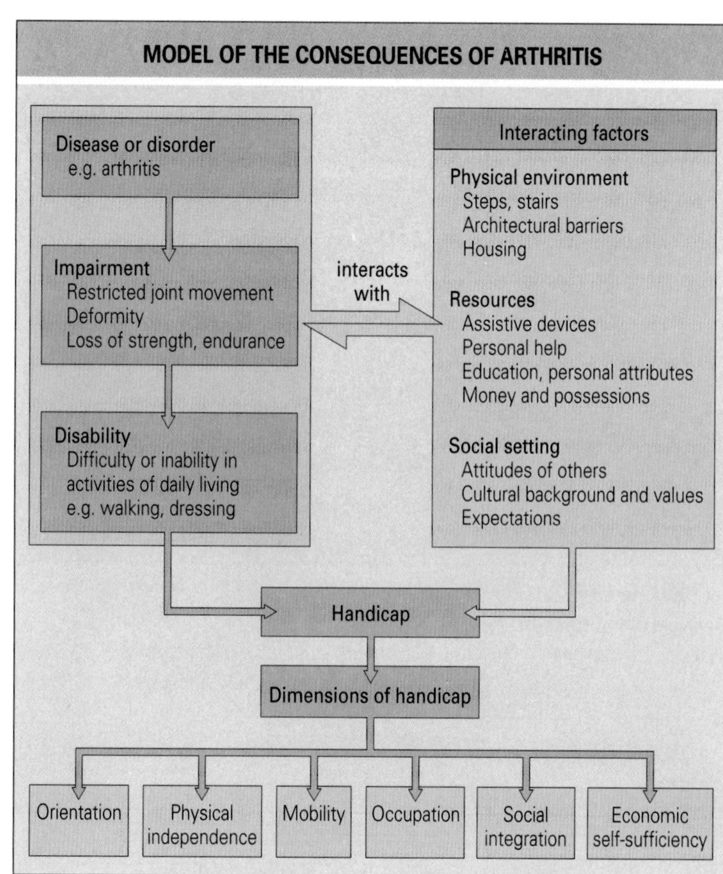

Fig. 1.6 A framework for approaching the consequences of rheumatic disorders.

SIGNS AND SYMPTOMS

2

EVALUATION OF MUSCULOSKELETAL SYMPTOMS

Matthew H Liang & Roger D Sturrock

INTRODUCTION

The key to the initial evaluation of musculoskeletal complaints is to take a careful history, to examine the joints carefully in order to identify the anatomic structure(s) involved, and to recognize synovitis and joint instability. Nothing else is as productive as a thorough history and physical examination, not even laboratory tests and imaging techniques.

HISTORY

The goals of the history are to find clues as to whether the pain is inflammatory or noninflammatory, determine how and when the pain started and what makes the pain worse or better, establish its temporal pattern and confirm whether or not there are constitutional symptoms. Such symptoms as fever or weight loss would suggest that the joint complaints are part of a systemic illness [1].

Some clinical presentations of musculoskeletal diseases are distinctive and narrow the diagnostic possibilities so effectively that their diagnostic approach is discussed separately in subsequent chapters. These include the patient with joint and muscle symptoms; with fever or constitutional symptoms; with rash; with respiratory symptoms; or with renal signs or symptoms.

Arthralgia implies pain originating from or around the joint but not necessarily that the pain comes from within the joint itself. Pain originating from joint structures should be improved by resting the joint and made worse by stretching the joint or by weight bearing. Stiffness after prolonged immobility ('gelling') suggests inflammatory joint disease or synovitis. This symptom probably results from a combination of altered viscosity of inflammatory joint fluid and pericapsular inflammation. Stiffness alone is nonspecific and not very sensitive, being present in older individuals and patients with hypothyroidism, Parkinson's disease, and disorders with only a minor component of inflammation. Clinically significant gelling lasts more than 30 minutes. Patients with florid synovitis can describe little or no gelling or gelling which lasts all day. In inflammatory disease the length of gelling is roughly proportional to the severity of the inflammation and may shorten as the patient improves. When asking about morning stiffness, ask the patient for their usual time of awakening and the time of maximum mobility during the day. The time between these two points is the duration of morning stiffness and is more reliable than a casual question such as, "How much stiffness do you have?".

Night pain is a cardinal symptom. Pain that wakes the patient can be neurogenic, vascular or infectious, result from crystalline disease (gout, pseudogout) or arise from severe structural joint damage. Tendinitis and bursitis can also wake a patient. Synovitis without structural damage rarely wakes a patient. Neurogenic pain is described in vague terms ("I can't describe it.") or as numbness, an extremity 'falling asleep', shooting pain, or pins and needles, etc. Pain that comes from vascular insufficiency is brought on by use and relieved by rest within seconds. Symptoms caused by peripheral vascular disease may sound like those of spinal stenosis (so-called pseudoclaudication), but in the latter, pain brought on by walking is usually bilateral and usually does not radiate below the knee. Cessation of walking and flexion of the spine improve the symptoms slowly.

Giving Way or Locking

A complaint of 'giving way' at the knee or hip needs to be clarified as either giving way that occurs without warning with an unstable knee or muscle weakness, or giving way resulting from pain (which may occur with meniscus tears and loose bodies within the joint). Locking is the inability to take a joint smoothly through its complete range of motion because of an internal derangement (loose body, torn cartilage or meniscus) or an extra-articular soft tissue block such as a tendon nodule seen in trigger finger.

Weakness, Cramping and Aching

Four common types of weakness are described by patients. The first is generalized, painless weakness and easy fatigability, as may occur with disuse atrophy, deconditioning that occurs after systemic illness, or myasthenia. Secondly, there is painless loss of power in a specific muscle group from complete denervation and nerve root damage (polio) and/or localized muscle atrophy. The third type of weakness is that associated with paresthesias which occur in compressive neuropathies or radiculopathies, such as in carpal tunnel or sciatica. Finally, weakness may also be associated with pain or cramping and suggests inflammatory muscle disease or a metabolic muscle disorder.

Cramping, spasms, muscle pain, aching or myalgias may not be distinguishable by history alone. Cramping is a commonly experienced symptom. The prototype is nocturnal cramps, an intense pain of the calf or intrinsic foot muscles relieved by stretching the muscle, time, and heat or massage. Spasm or cramping of the musculature crossing a joint forces the joint into flexion. Cramping of the intrinsic muscles of the feet forces the toes into plantar flexion. Spasm of paraspinous muscles of the low back causes secondary scoliosis, and spasm of the sternomastoid muscles is a feature of cervical torticollis. Cramping is acute and is over once the muscle is relaxed. On the other hand, muscle pain, myalgias and aching are less intense, usually do not wake the patient from sleep and occur with use and at rest. Common examples of myalgias include that seen with bacterial or viral sepsis and the achiness that occurs after prolonged exertion. Cramping in a peripheral muscle is almost always benign and self-limiting. Cramping of multiple muscles, muscles of the abdomen or upper extremity and cramping induced by strenuous exercise implies a primary muscle disease or a metabolic-toxic myopathy. Regional cramping and muscle pain may also be caused by arterial insufficiency, which is suggested by a history of symptoms that are brought on by repetitive use and promptly cease with subsidence of activity. Weakness, malaise and tiredness are nonspecific symptoms and these terms are frequently used interchangeably by patients.

Weakness implies loss of power or endurance in which the individual has difficulty initiating and maintaining a functional activity requiring strength. When a patient has weakness or decreased endurance of one extremity there may be a neurologic lesion, local muscle atrophy, a disrupted musculoskeletal unit, such as a disrupted tendon or muscle (viz., rotator cuff tear), or a locally painful lesion.

Review of Systems

Other organ systems involved in systemic rheumatic diseases should be screened by a review of systems. For example, constititional symptoms, pleurisy, chest pain, Raynaud's phenomenon, conjunctivitis or iritis, nasopharyngeal ulceration, skin rash, hair loss, diarrhea, urethral or vaginal discharge, and paresthesias. One needs to have a high index of suspicion for infection when a patient is immunosuppressed or on steroids. High dose steroids can mask pain, blunt fever and help a patient look surprisingly well in both joint infection and septicemia.

PHYSICAL EXAMINATION

The history, the physical examination and time are the three most important and useful 'tests' in the diagnosis and management of musculoskeletal disorders. Examination of the musculoskeletal system follows the sequence *'look', 'feel'* and *'move.'*

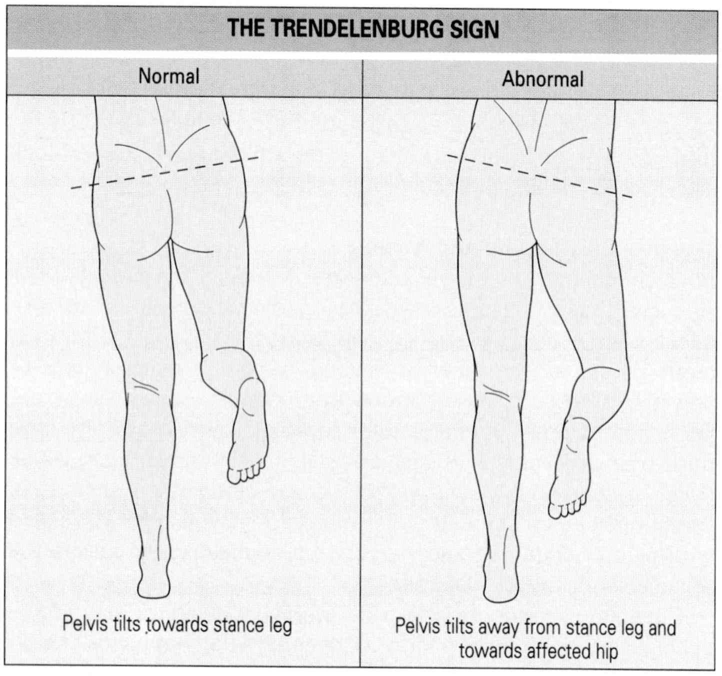

THE TRENDELENBURG SIGN

Normal — Pelvis tilts towards stance leg

Abnormal — Pelvis tilts away from stance leg and towards affected hip

Fig. 2.1 The Trendelenburg sign. Normally the pelvis tilts towards the stance leg because of adequate abductor muscle power. In a positive test the pelvis tilts away from the stance leg.

The purpose of the examination is to identify the anatomical site of the pain and determine whether or not it is due to an inflammatory process. The cardinal signs of an intra-articular problem are an effusion, warmth, diminished range of movement in all directions of joint motion, and pain or swelling over the joint capsule.

Point tenderness over the anatomical site of a bursa indicates a bursitis or a tear in a muscle or tendon. Tendinitis, on the other hand, is suggested by linear swelling of the tendon sheath, warmth, tenderness over the course of the tendon, and occasionally an audible or palpable rub. Stretching the tendon should reproduce the pain. Muscle pain is diffuse and not well localized either by the patient or the examiner.

The gait and posture should be observed and any obvious deformity noted. Some easily recognizable abnormal gaits are as follows.

- **The Trendelenburg gait.** This is a characteristic 'dipping' gait which is due to weakness of the gluteus medius muscle. This muscle normally pulls the iliac crest and the greater trochanter towards each other when the patient is standing on the 'good' leg, thus elevating the pelvis on the opposite side (Fig. 2.1). With disorders of the hip, such as congenital dislocation, osteoarthritis or failed arthroplasty, weak gluteals will result in the pelvis dropping below the horizontal when standing on the normal leg. If both hips are affected then the patient will have a characteristic 'waddling' gait.
- **The antalgic gait**. Pain in the leg will result in the patient 'hurrying' to take weight off the painful limb in order to take more weight on the other leg.
- **Neurological disorders.** Examples of gait abnormalities resulting from neurological disorders are the 'high stepping' gait of a foot drop, the 'hestinant' gait of Parkinsonism, the 'wide based' gait of a cerebellar ataxia and the 'scissors' gait of a spastic diplegia.

Upper Limb

Examine the hands carefully; these are the patient's 'calling card'. Much information about the patient can be derived from inspection of the nails, the muscles of the hands, the skin and the distribution of joint involvement by arthritis (Fig. 2.2). The presence of abnormal

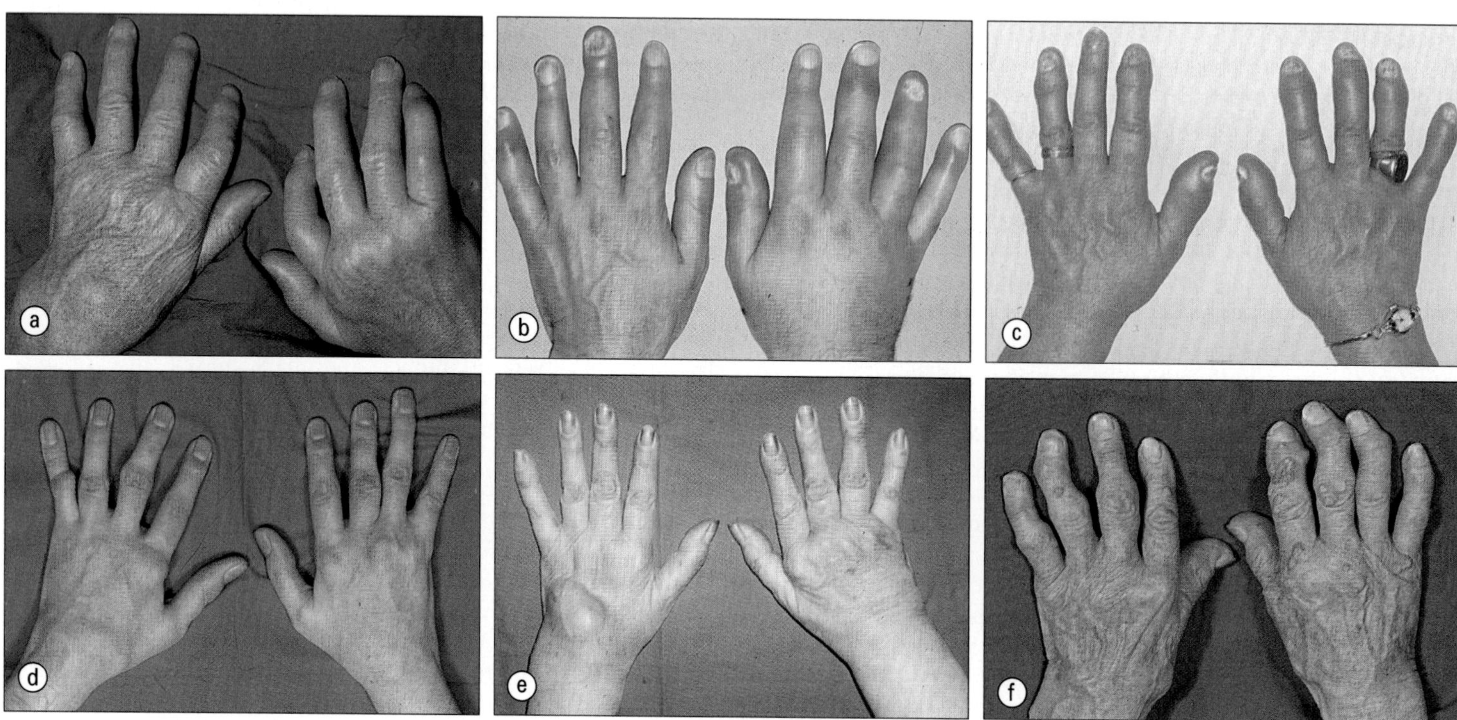

Fig. 2.2 Involvement of small joints of the hand by arthritis. Rheumatoid arthritis (a). Psoriatic arthritis (b) & (c). Juvenile chronic arthritis (d). Rheumatoid arthritis (e). Osteoarthritis (f).

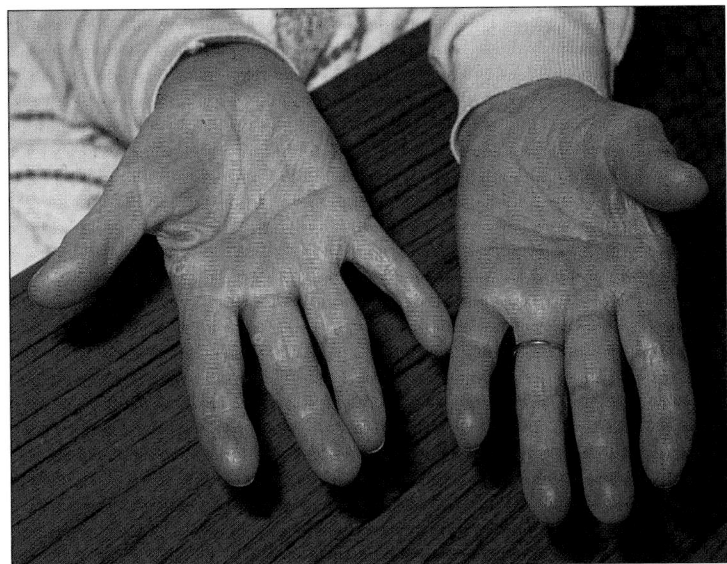

Fig. 2.3 The appearance of the hands in advanced carpal tunnel syndrome.

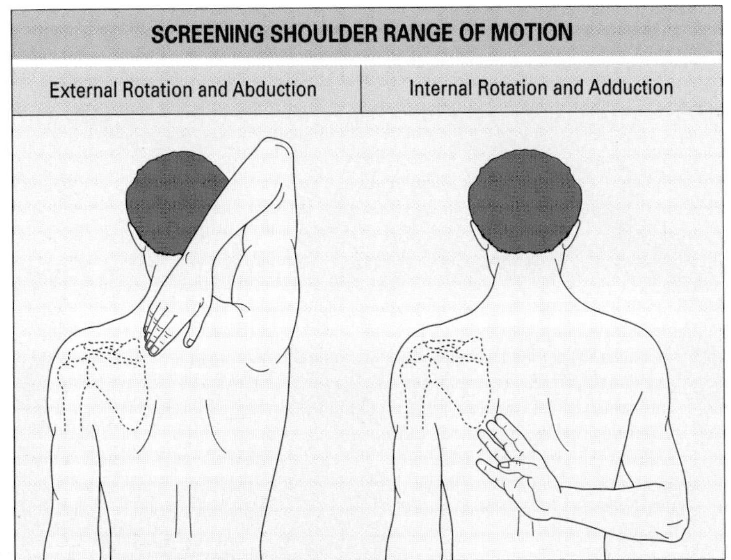

Fig. 2.4 Screening shoulder range of motion. External rotation and abduction and internal rotation and adduction should be assessed.

sensation and muscle weakness and/or wasting are clues to the existence of a local nerve entrapment (e.g., carpal tunnel syndrome) (Fig. 2.3) or a regional problem (e.g., cervical spondylosis). The functionally critical range of motion for the fingers can be quickly checked by having the patient attempt a tight fist, an 'O' with their thumb and index finger, and a lateral pinch.

Look for flexion deformities of the elbow or hyperextension. Nodules over the extensor surface of the joint and psoriatic patches may give the diagnosis. Examine the radiohumeral joint, which is involved in pronation and supination, as well as the radio-ulna joints. Both are very superficial and readily palpable.

Movements of the shoulder joint may be tested by asking the patient to put their hands behind the neck and behind the back. These movements test external rotation and abduction, and internal rotation and adduction, respectively (Fig. 2.4). Any difficulty should lead to a more detailed examination of the shoulder.

Lower Limb

As previously mentioned, the patient's gait may give a clue to the presence of a hip, knee or foot problem. Wasting of the gluteal muscles will point to a long-standing hip problem. The 'true' and 'apparent' leg lengths can be measured (Fig. 2.5) to differentiate abduction or adduction deformities of the hip from real shortening of the leg. The examination of hip movements is illustrated in Figure 2.6. Quadriceps wasting is an important sign of knee arthritis and a valgus or varus deformity should be noted. Synovial thickening and moderate to large effusions of the knee obliterate the distinct concavities on each side of the patella. A small effusion may not be obvious to inspection but can be elicited as the bulge sign. For this to be demonstrated, the patient is examined supine with the leg extended and the muscles relaxed. The medial and lateral aspects of knee are stroked to express the synovial fluid into the suprapatellar pouch. The examiner then presses and strokes the lateral aspect of the knee, eliciting a distinct fluid wave or bulge on the medial aspect. An examination of the feet may reveal signs of structural deformity (pes planus), arthritis or a sausage digit, which may be the only abnormal signs in a patient complaining of generalized stiffness in inflammatory joint disease.

The Spine

Observe active and passive movements of the cervical spine [2]. Looking over the shoulder and nodding backwards and forwards occurs at the atlanto-occipital joint, flexion takes place at the lower cervical vertebrae and lateral flexion at the mid cervical region. With the patient standing, look for deformities of the thoracolumbar spine. A scoliosis may be exaggerated by forward flexion. Movements of flexion, extension and lateral flexion should be noted. Abnormalities of posture may give a clue to the underlying diagnosis, for example the characteristic 'stoop' of ankylosing spondylitis (Fig. 2.7). Remember that lateral flexion is often impaired early in inflammatory spinal disease such as ankylosing spondylitis. Movements of the lumbar spine can be measured in a simple fashion using Schober's test. (Fig. 2.8). Rotation of the spine must be tested for by fixing the pelvis or when the subject is seated. Percussion of the vertebral processes will reproduce pain over a local problem such as a spinal abscess. Decreased chest expansion may result from disease of the costovertebral joints and can be measured by placing a tape measure at the level of the nipple line in men and just above it in women and measuring the circumference between full expiration and full inspiration. Variable with age and general physical condition, it should be at least 5–6cm in young adults.

Range of Motion

The difference between the active and passive ranges of motion has clinical significance. Normally the active range of movement is less than the passive range. The patient is asked to imitate the examiner's taking the joint through an active range of motion. If there is no limitation or pain (look at the face) the joint need not be examined, except to look for subtle signs of inflammation when the suspicion is high. Limitation of active range of motion may be due to pain, weakness or mechanical block. The patient should then be taken through a passive range of motion. If the passive range is normal and the active

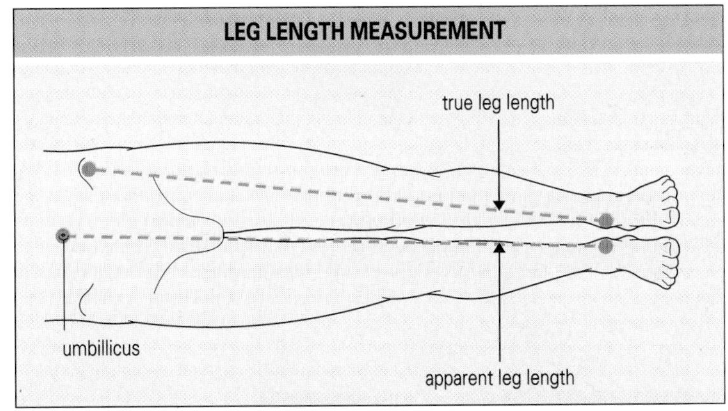

Fig. 2.5 Leg length measurement. True leg length is the distance from the anterior superior iliac spine to the medial malleolus. Apparent leg length is the distance from the umbilicus to the medial malleolus.

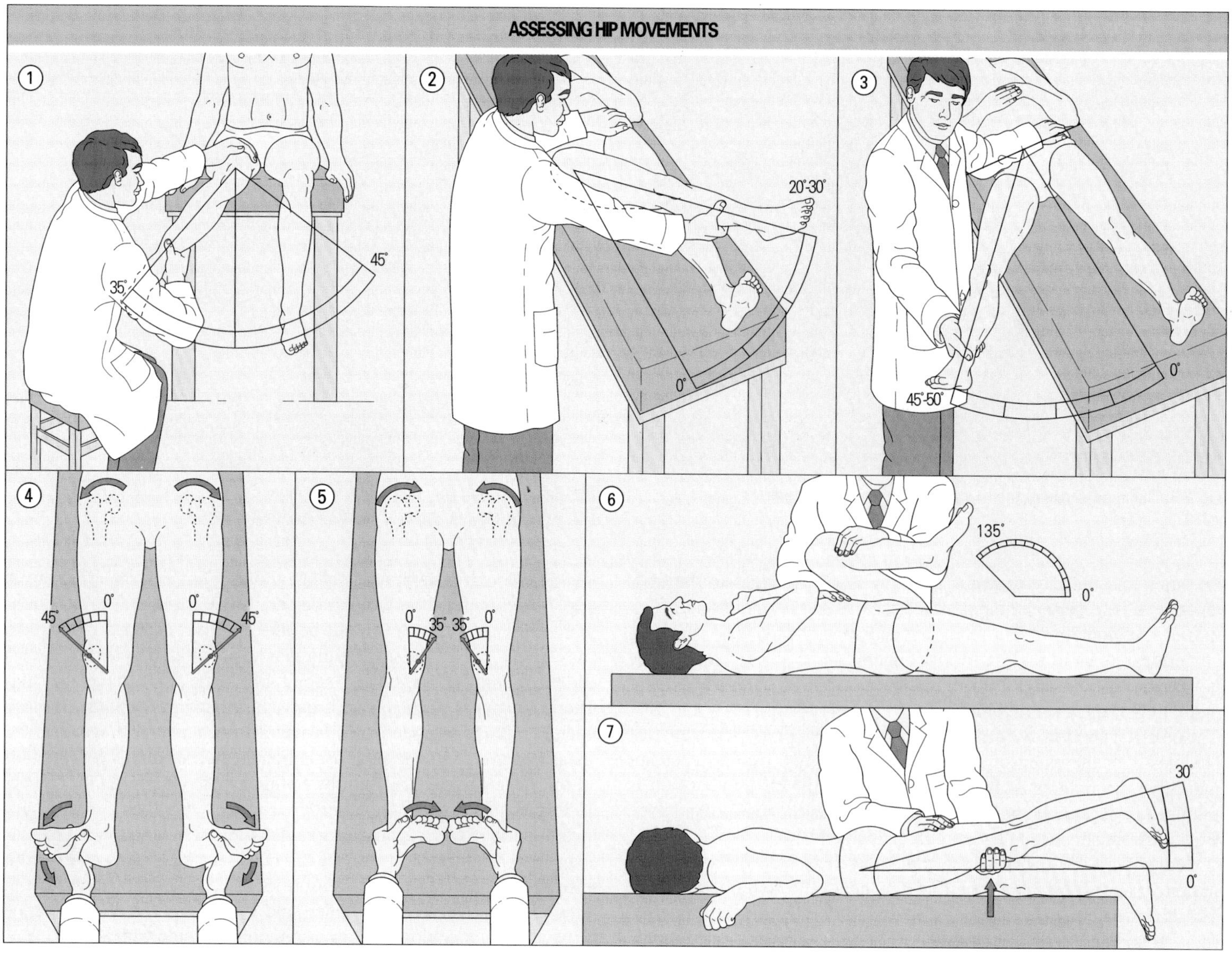

ASSESSING HIP MOVEMENTS

Fig. 2.6 Assessing hip movements. Internal and external rotation in the flexed position (1), adduction (2), abduction (3), external rotation (4), internal rotation (5), flexion (6) and extension (7). The normal range is indicated for each movement.

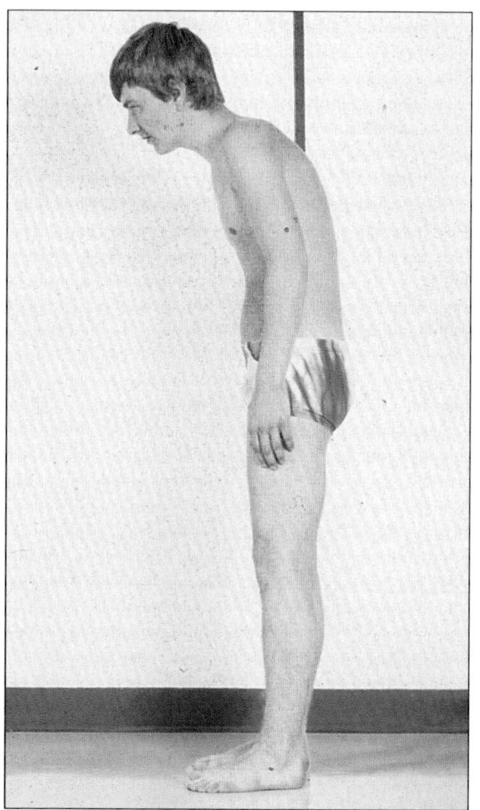

Fig. 2.7 The characteristic posture of a patient with ankylosing spondylitis.

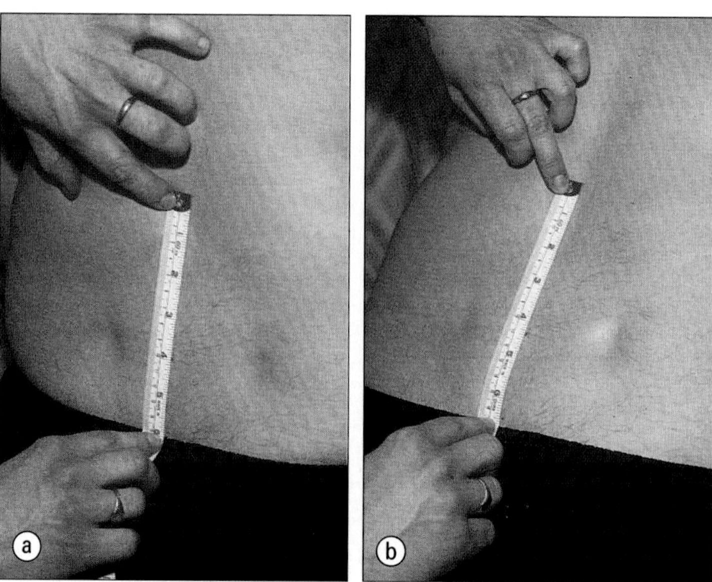

Fig. 2.8 Macrae's modification of Schober's test. This is a measure of lumbar spine anterior flexion. With the patient standing erect, make a mark on the imaginary line joining the posterior superior iliac spines. Make another mark 10cm above the first. Ask the patient to bend forward. With the spine in fullest flexion, measure the distance between the two marks. The normal distance is greater than 15cm.

range limited, suspect a muscle or neurological problem; myopathy, torn ligament or muscle, or neuropathy. If the active range equals the passive range suspect a soft tissue or mechanical block such as in a frozen shoulder or synovitis. Another useful clue is the 'end-feel' at the extreme of the range of motion. The distinction is made between a 'hard' end-feel versus a 'soft' end-feel. The hard end-feel is abrupt, firm and suggests a structural block such as osteoarthritis. More effort by the examiner to overcome the block fails and results in pain. In contrast, a soft end-feel is the feel of an automobile clutch: the range is limited but can be overcome with additional force although this may initiate pain. The soft end-feel is the typical feel of synovitis without significant structural damage.

The problem of differentiating between edema, cellulitis and synovitis arises frequently. Synovitis has signs of inflammation (dolor, calor, rubor, tumor) over the visible, palpable areas of the joint capsule. The swelling does not usually extend beyond the confines of the anatomical joint space; when it does this suggests either a joint rupture or tendinitis as well. Rubor, a sign of classic inflammation, is not common in synovitis except in crystalline disease or joint infection. Cellulitis, in contrast, has diffuse, warm and red swelling with or without a margin between the normal and the inflamed skin, occasionally with lymphangitis and regional lymphadenopathy. Edema on the other hand is swelling that goes beyond the confines of the joint margin and is frequently associated with pitting without redness or local warmth. Edema, cellulitis and synovitis may coexist in a given patient, and synovitis may need to be confirmed by aspirating the joint. There is usually an area of the joint space which can be entered without passing through potentially infected skin. One would not attempt aspiration in this situation without prior antibiotic coverage if there is any question of overlying cellulitis.

DIFFERENTIAL DIAGNOSIS OF MONOARTHRITIS
Infection
Bacterial, viral, fungal, Lyme
Inflammatory arthritis
Crystalline RA/JCA Spondyloarthropathy Plant thorn synovitis Palindromic Paraneoplastic Intermittent hydrarthrosis
Bone/cartilage disorder
Osteoarthritis Osteonecrosis Loose body Tumor
Traumatic
Fracture Internal derangement Hemarthrosis

Fig. 2.9 Differential diagnosis of monoarthritis.

PATTERNS OF DIAGNOSTIC SIGNIFICANCE

Monoarthritis

A patient who complains of a single painful joint presents a broad differential (Fig. 2.9) that includes extra-articular conditions, such as overuse syndromes, and arthritis such as monoarticular rheumatoid arthritis (RA) or Reiter's syndrome.

The patient's age is key. A young sexually active person may have gonococcal arthritis or a reactive arthritis. Monoarticular complaints in prepubertal patients require careful evaluation for traumatic conditions, congenital defects such as a slipped capital epiphysis, and hip dysplasia. The patient's age orders the probabilities of the differential and helps rule out specific diseases. For example, one rarely thinks of crystal-induced arthritides, intermittent hydrarthrosis or gonococcal arthritis in prepubertal patients. Like age, sex is useful for ordering diagnostic possibilities within the differential diagnostic list, but it is not enough to rule out certain conditions. For example, gout and Reiter's syndrome are less common, but can occur, in females. The degree of pain and the circumstances with which it occurs are very helpful clues to diagnosis. Severe pain at rest narrows the differential but implies infection until proven otherwise, or possibly crystal-induced synovitis (gout and pseudogout). Mild to moderate pain is seen in inflammatory monoarthritides, hemarthrosis, tendinitis and ligamentous strains.

The duration of the complaint may be helpful. For example, pain that has been present for weeks is not gout but could be chronic tophaceous gout. It is also unlikely to be a bacterial infectious arthritis but could be tuberculosis or a fungal arthritis.

Monoarthritis is infection until proven otherwise

Only a culture of the synovial fluid can definitively rule out infection. Gout may have associated fever but this should not be greater than 38.3°C, or 38.8°C with polyarticular gout. In any case a joint aspiration is still mandatory. The workup of acute monoarthritis even without fever usually requires aspiration of the joint. There are exceptions, and joint aspiration should be done when there is any doubt. The exceptions include those patients with little to moderate pain who have few signs or symptoms of inflammation, i.e., small effusions that are not particularly warm, and patients for whom pain is not very severe and is related primarily to use of the joint rather than pain with rest.

In classic podagra (inflammation of the first metatarsophalangeal joint) (Fig. 2.10) without any unusual features, some clinicians might opt to treat the patient for gout and follow them closely, i.e. over the next 48–72 hours, since the incidence of infection in this joint is low. Atypical features necessitating joint aspiration of the first MTP joint include: age less than 40 years; systemic symptoms; temperature greater than 38.3°C; evidence for a primary source of infection or local breakdown of skin barriers; joint previously damaged with inflammatory arthritis; prior joint surgery; immunosuppressive therapy; and concurrent disease associated with impaired immunity (diabetes, HIV, etc.).

Technique of joint aspiration

Some general principles should be kept in mind. The size of the needle to be used depends on the size of the joint (25 gauge for small joints; 22 gauge for moderate sized to large joints).

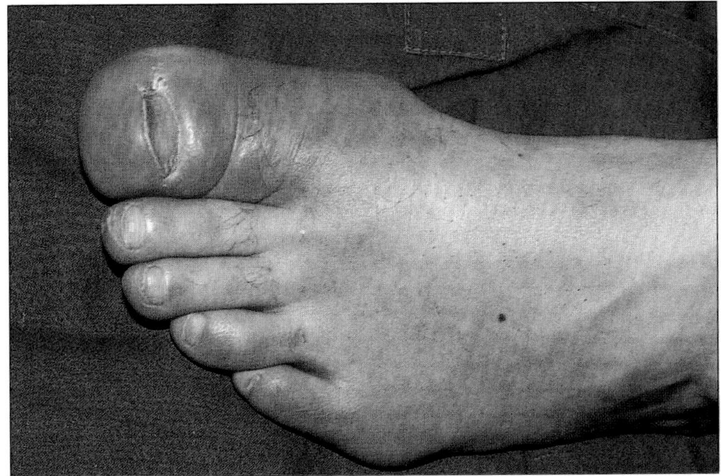

Fig. 2.10 The classical appearance of podagra.

A 22-gauge needle may suffice when joint fluid is aspirated, but a chronic effusion which is likely to have viscous material is difficult to aspirate with needles less than an 18 gauge.

The joint should be placed in the position which accommodates the largest volume of fluid (see Chapter 10). Wrists, metacarpophalangeal joints, interphalangeal joints and knees should be in slight flexion, others in a neutral position. Enter the joint to avoid the neurovascular bundle, tendons and ligaments. If one cannot identify the tendons around the joint with confidence, do not attempt injection.

Although the procedure is carried out under sterile conditions, only one glove need be kept sterile to palpate the landmarks, and this only if the anatomy is not well appreciated. Prior to cleansing the area, press the needle cover (which usually has a dimple) firmly against the skin to mark the spot. Standard preparation includes betadine followed by alcohol to dryness. Some rheumatologists do not use local xylocaine anesthesia unless the patient is apprehensive, or a child, or when a needle larger than 22 gauge is used, or when biopsy or irrigation is contemplated. To make the injection as tolerable as possible one should wait for the alcohol to dry, stretch the skin firmly, and insert the needle perpendicular to the surface of the skin. To anesthetize skin, an intradermal wheal with xylocaine 1% without epinephrine, ethyl chloride spray, or ice may be used. Don't neglect the value of distraction during the procedure; talk to the patient.

The examination of synovial fluid is a skill not generally available in routine laboratories and it's important that a physician examines fresh fluid to optimize the chance of identifying diagnostic elements [3,4]. Fresh fluid is particularly important for crystal identification and especially pseudogout crystals.

Polyarthralgias

Polyarthralgia (joint pains without clinical synovitis) is a common but nonspecific symptom. Patients may report multiple joint symptoms and have in fact unrelated regional musculoskeletal syndromes. Others present with polyarthralgias and forget they have had polyarthritis or polyarthralgias in the past, which would expand the possibilities considerably. If the examination reveals signs of inflammation or synovitis, the approach outlined below under *Polyarthritis* should be followed. With duration of symptoms under 6 weeks, benign conditions such as postviral arthralgias and myalgias and post-exertional syndromes are common, a limited evaluation and follow-up is the most efficient. A complete evaluation should be carried out in older patients, those with constitutional symptoms or symptoms referable to other organ systems, and patients with symptoms lasting more than 6 weeks. Patients with benign arthralgias and no functional impairment or objective findings on repeated clinical examination or laboratory evaluation are a puzzling group who should not be over treated or managed as if they had a disease. Some patients have fears of crippling illness or having a serious unrecognized disease. In these cases, it is best to address their concerns directly.

Polyarthritis

Polyarthritis is inflammation of four or more joints and is distinct from polyarthralgias in which there are multiple joint complaints without obvious inflammation. Acute polyarthritis is a major diagnostic challenge as it includes almost every disease of importance in rheumatology and some that are potentially life-threatening and associated with a high morbidity. Acute arthritis of less than 6 weeks' duration cannot be diagnosed with certainty but can be benign, for example postviral arthritis. A complete history and physical and diagnostic evaluation are necessary to identify other organ system involvement.

Polyarthritis may have three major patterns: additive, migratory and intermittent. In additive arthritis, joints become progressively involved, with more joints becoming affected with time. In migratory arthritis, joints become symptomatic and then subside, and different ones become involved. In intermittent arthritis the signs and symptoms come and go.

These patterns may coexist in the same patient, but when one dominates, the clinical presentation may suggest a specific diagnosis. For instance, an additive pattern is seen in patients with RA, systemic lupus erythematosus (SLE) and psoriatic arthritis; migratory arthralgias and arthritis are typical of patients with gonococcal sepsis, acute rheumatic fever and the arthritis associated with bacterial endocarditis. Intermittent arthritis is typically seen in gout before it becomes tophaceous gout, in pseudogout, and in familial Mediterranean fever.

Which joints are involved and the pattern of involvement can help narrow the diagnostic possibilities. Peripheral and axial joints (Fig.2.11) are targeted by different rheumatic diseases. For instance, RA typically gives symmetrical synovitis of the small joints of the hands, and wrists (excluding the distal interphalangeal joints), elbow, knee, ankle, and feet. DIP involvement without synovitis is osteoarthritis; with synovitis it is psoriatic arthritis. Asymmetric synovitis of knees and the ankle with inflammatory back symptoms and enthesitis (such as bilateral epicondylitis, Achilles tendonitis and bilateral plantar fasciitis) suggests the spondyloarthropathies. Metacarpophalangeal (MCP) involvement without synovitis suggests hemochromatosis. Pattern recognition in polyarthritis is helpful but not diagnostic, since there is considerable overlap between the major causes of inflammatory polyarthritis. The pace of the evaluation depends on whether the patient is ill. The detailed review of systems looking for other organ involvement may help to establish that the arthritis is part of a systemic disease. In multisystem disease, heart, lung, kidney, and brain involvement usually have more functional

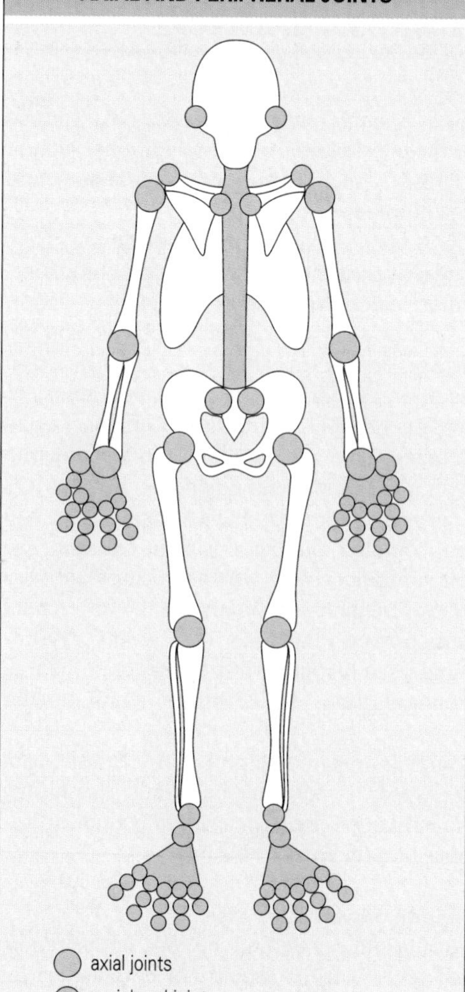

Fig. 2.11 Axial and peripheral joints.

EVALUATION IN MULTISYSTEM DISEASES
Electrocardiogram
Chest radiograph
Liver function tests
Complete blood count, differential
Erythrocyte sedimentation rate
Urine analysis
Creatinine
Creatine phosphokinase
Stool occult blood

Fig. 2.12 Evaluation in multisystem disease.

consequences than joint involvement symptoms. Laboratory tests and radiographs should be dictated by signs or symptoms (Fig. 2.12), but some early organ system involvement can only be suspected by a laboratory survey (lung, kidney, hematologic, heart, liver). A complete blood count, measurement of erythrocyte sedimentation rate, tests of renal and hepatic function, urinalysis, and rheumatoid factor and antinuclear antibody tests comprise the minimum evaluation, and other testing should be dictated by clinical suspicion. Chronically symptomatic joints should be radiographed and it is important to remember that in inflammatory joint disease, for example RA, radiographic changes may be seen in the feet before they appear in the hands. If there is a fever, potential sources should be cultured.

LOW BACK PAIN - RED FLAGS	
Clinical data	**Diagnostic significance**
Pain not relieved by supine position with hips flexed	Infection, osseous lesion, ? compliance
Pain worse with walking	Spinal stenosis
Pain worse with hyperextension of the spine and improved by flexing the spine	Spinal stenosis
Pain (stiffness) worse in morning	Spondylitis, epiphysitis
Acute, severe pain without precipitants	Abdominal aneurysm, compression fracture, spinal vascular accident, ruptured viscus, herniated disc
Pain increased by cough, sneeze or Valsalva	Nerve root compression
Pain described as numbness, stinging or tingling	Nerve root compression
Fever, weight loss	Infection, tumor
Pain greater than 2 months	Metabolic bone disease, herniated disc, compensation, psychological, tumor
Bilateral radiation	Tumor, central herniation, spondylitis
First onset under 30 years old or over 50	Tumor, metabolic disease, epiphysitis
Synovitis	Spondyloarthropathy
Midline deformities (palpable step, midline hair)	Structural defect, tumor (dermoid, epidermoid)
Neuromotor deficit or asymmetry	Nerve root compression
Progressive neuromotor deficit	Central herniation, myelopathy, tropical paraparesis
Bilateral neurological deficits	Tumor, spinal vascular accident
Nerve-root level above LI	Tumor
Positive Babinski's, clonus	Myelopathy, tropical paraparesis

Fig. 2.13 Low back pain — red flags.

BACK PAIN

Most acute low back pain is self-limited and related to postural problems or strain and is not related to a systemic rheumatic illness. The practical task is to sort out the benign and self-limited cases of back pain from the serious or chronic cases, and to recognize when the pain is a symptom of other problems. Radiographic examinations of the lumbosacral spine, the major expense in an uncritical approach to the diagnosis of low back pain, are insensitive and nonspecific. Many spinal lesions, including disease of the disc, which may cause back pain, are not detected by radiography. Radiographic findings of osteophytes, narrowed disc space, lumbarization, sacralization, mild scoliosis, facet arthrosis, subluxation and spina bifida occulta are found equally in symptomatic and asymptomatic individuals. Magnetic resonance imaging (MRI) and computerized axial tomography (CAT) are far more useful in imaging all the structures of the spine but are also more costly and sensitive to anatomical changes of unproven significance. However, where they are easily available they have nearly replaced myelography. Both are useful when epidural tumor, spinal stenosis, early osteomyelitis or fracture are strongly suspected. When the history and physical examination are compatible with a benign disease, radiographs have limited clinical utility. Radiographs of the spine are indicated in the following situations.

- Unimproved or worsening symptoms. Symptoms lasting longer than a month with treatment.
- New onset of back pain without antecedent trauma under the age of 15 years or over 50 years of age.
- Back pain after significant trauma.
- Severe back pain.
- History or physical examination suggestive of sacroiliitis.
- Pain not significantly relieved by bedrest.
- Previous vertebral fracture, surgery.
- An anxious person who will not be reassured by clinical examination alone.
- Spinal deformity or mass.
- Known malignancy (thyroid, kidney, breast, prostate).
- Constitutional symptoms (fever, weight loss).

If a lumbar nerve root is compressed, the earliest clinical sign is loss or diminution of deep tendon reflexes. After 3–6 weeks of compression, objective muscle wasting or diminished strength may be evident. Neurophysiological studies are helpful in establishing the baseline, measuring change and documenting whether the denervation is acute or chronic. For most cases, if surgical intervention is not a possibility, the electromyelograph provides little additional information beyond that of the examination and the patient's symptoms. To separate those patients with mechanical causes from all the others and to not miss causes of back pain which require prompt treatment, therefore, can be done by a directed history and examination [5] in order to identify atypical clinical features ('Red Flags' – Fig. 2.13) which suggest diagnoses other than mechanical causes. If the history and physical examination are typical for a mechanical origin, conservative treatment is indicated. The patient should be followed to ensure adequate pain control and seen again after 3 weeks to ensure resolution of the problem and to reinforce back care instructions and specific exercise therapy.

The individual should be asked to point to the symptomatic area and to where the pain radiates or spreads. A history of the onset, duration and tempo of the symptoms suggests the diagnostic possibilities. If the pain started suddenly, the cause is likely to be a tear of the muscles, ligaments or disc, or a fracture. If the pain started gradually and is chronic or subacute, chronic low back pain, tumor, metabolic bone disease and spondylitis are possibilities. Is the pain getting worse? Is it because the attacks are more frequent, more severe and more prolonged, or is it because the patient has lost tolerance?

Disc disease occurs usually between L3 and S1 and is unilateral. When pain originates above the L3 level or is bilateral, infection, tumor, or spondylitis should be considered. When biomechanical causes of low back pain recur or flare, the pattern usually repeats itself. If the pattern changes or the pain is worsening, think of tumor.

Nerve root compression is suggested when pain comes on rapidly in the distribution of the sensory dermatome of that nerve root. Dorsal nerve root pain is sharp, lancinating and accompanied by paresthesias and numbness. Paresthesias or numbness felt over the lateral border of the foot suggest an S1 lesion, while those over the dorsal surface of the foot suggest an L5 lesion. Increasing tension on the nerve roots by Valsalva, coughing, sneezing, and straining while defecating exacerbate the pain. In contrast, pain in deep structures, such as ligaments, fascia and muscles, is vaguely localized, aching in character, radiates widely, and is generally slow in onset and long in duration.

What activities make the pain worse or better? Mechanical pain arising from elements of the spine is almost always aggravated by movement and relieved by rest. Pain referred to the back from the gastrointestinal tract, female reproductive system, and other structures in the abdomen is unaltered by spinal movement. Occasionally a person with disc disease finds the pain worse in bed, but may actually be sleeping prone, hyperextending their spine and exacerbating the pain. In contrast, inflammatory back pain, ankylosing spondylitis and Scheuermann's disease cause pain or stiffness which is worse after prolonged inactivity and improved by activity.

In an emotionally stable person, pain out of proportion to physical findings for which the person cannot find a comfortable position suggests an infected disc (discitis) or an epidural abscess. Pain is modified by a host of environmental and psychological factors, but pain which interferes with work, recreation or sleep or which occurs in a person who 'never has pain' is important.

In some persons the back pain complaint is a proxy for depression or an excuse for not coping. For a manual worker in a strenuous job, recurrent back pain can be a disaster financially if it prevents him from being employable, and his symptoms may be exaggerated far out of proportion to his actual organic problem. Likewise, the continued necessity to claim symptoms for disability benefits may make continued back pain an economic 'necessity.'

Watch the person as they disrobe for the examination, in order to note painful movements, and in the standing position, to look for exaggerated lordosis or flattening of the normal lordosis. The latter is seen in anklylosing spondylitis and with muscle spasm. Lumbar lordosis is increased in pregnancy or obesity in order to preserve the body's center of gravity.

With the patient standing with feet about a foot apart, inspect the back for a pelvic tilt, which may be due to a leg length discrepancy, scoliosis, or muscle spasm. Note the presence of scoliosis. Fixed scoliosis due to structural problems differs from secondary scoliosis due to muscle spasm, painful splinting or leg-length discrepancy, which disappears on recumbency. Spasm of the glutei or sacrospinalis muscles will make these muscles more prominent when compared with the normal side. A midline dimple or tufts of hair (Faun's beard) indicate a pilonidal cyst, spina bifida occulta, or a dermoid.

The range and rhythm of spinal movements are tested. In forward flexion, the normal lumbar lordosis flattens and flexes until the spine is a smooth curve from sacrum to occiput. Foward bending assesses the mobility of the back, the hamstrings and the hips. Functional or nonstructural scoliosis disappears on flexion, whereas structural scoliosis is exaggerated on bending. A prolapsed intervertebral disc with nerve root irritation results in marked limitation of forward flexion without lumbar movement. Such persons will frequently show deviation of the trunk toward the painful side on forward flexion, but extension and rotation are relatively smooth and symmetrical. In spondylolisthesis, an abnormal step in the lower lumbar spine may be palpated, which disappears in flexion. With the individual standing, the strength of the gastrocnemius is tested by having him stand on tiptoe. Fatigability or asymmetric rising suggests either a lesion of S1 nerve root or weak quadriceps. The dorsiflexors of the ankle are assessed by having the person walk on his heels; difficulty with this maneuver points to an L5 nerve root compression. Peroneal nerve damage may also cause impaired heel walk; so if there is difficulty, check the strength of eversion of the foot, which is solely a peroneal nerve function. Some persons with sciatica will have pain when the ankle dorsiflexors are used with the knee extended and give the impression of weakness when none exists. Sensation is checked in the sitting position. Areas of sensory innervation are variable. Testing the autonomous areas is an efficient way to elicit hypesthesia. The S1 root innervates the sole and lateral border of the foot, and its autonomous area is the area just behind the lateral malleolus and the bottom of the little toe. The L5 root receives sensation from the dorsum of the foot and the anterior aspect of the lower leg, and its autonomous area is the first interdigital space and the lateral calf below the level of the patella. The L4 nerve root innervates the anteromedial thigh and its autonomous sensory zone is a triangle with its apex over the patella and its base above the patella proximally. When sensory and motor signs conflict, make the diagnosis based on the more reliable motor signs rather than the sensory deficits. Stretching of the nerve roots (straight leg raising) may be performed in a sitting position. The patient is instructed to sit with his legs dangling over the side of the bed. One leg is fixed by the examiner and the affected limb is extended passively at the knee. In sciatica, no resistance or pain is noted until the lumbar lordosis is flattened (when the knee has extended 45°), at which point the patient compensates by leaning backward, frequently grabbing on to the table to prevent lurching backward. In sciatica the individual is unable to sit erect with both knees extended but must either flex the knee of the affected extremity or lean backward to avoid the pain associated with nerve root stretching. When no sciatica exists, the patient has no difficulty in sitting erect with the affected knee fully extended.

DIFFUSE ACHES AND PAINS

The majority of patients who have diffuse aches and pains have a benign self-limited syndrome associated with various infectious diseases, primarily viral, and those patients who have soft tissue syndromes (Fig. 2.14) but some systemic rheumatic or serious conditions can also present with aches and pains [6].

A history, physical examination and limited laboratory evaluation suffice to sort out such complaints (Fig. 2.15). The history is directed towards identifying precipitating factors, such as a prodromal illness or associated constitutional symptoms or repetitive tasks. Some associated symptoms in the patient with diffuse aches and pains are red flags for systemic or metabolic diseases (Fig. 2.16). Gelling or morning stiffness lasting longer than 30 minutes is such a symptom and can be seen in polymyalgia rheumatica, RA, SLE, and some inflammatory muscle diseases. Diffuse aches and pains without localizing physical findings may also occur in the myopathies associated with endocrine disorders and metabolic bone disease (particularly osteomalacia).

When the patient has diffuse aches without systemic symptoms or abnormal laboratory evaluation, fibrositis may be the diagnosis. The typical patient is otherwise healthy and complains of sleep disturbance and diffuse aches and pains which do not correspond to any specific anatomic site and has as the only physical finding tender

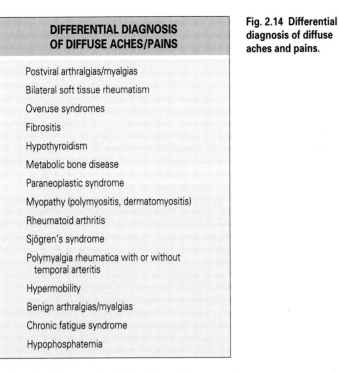

DIFFERENTIAL DIAGNOSIS OF DIFFUSE ACHES/PAINS
Postviral arthralgias/myalgias
Bilateral soft tissue rheumatism
Overuse syndromes
Fibrositis
Hypothyroidism
Metabolic bone disease
Paraneoplastic syndrome
Myopathy (polymyositis, dermatomyositis)
Rheumatoid arthritis
Sjögren's syndrome
Polymyalgia rheumatica with or without temporal arteritis
Hypermobility
Benign arthralgias/myalgias
Chronic fatigue syndrome
Hypophosphatemia

Fig. 2.14 Differential diagnosis of diffuse aches and pains.

points in characteristic locations. These patients are a tremendous challenge and require the patience of Job to treat. Although no physical dysfunction is evident, patients may have a persistent course for many years.

An important inflammatory disease in the elderly patient with aches and pains is polymyalgia rheumatica (PMR) and/or giant cell arteritis (GCA) with PMR (see Chapter 39). This should always be considered in a patient over the age of 50 years who develops aches and pains of the shoulder and hip girdle muscles. It is a myalgia *without* findings of muscle tenderness or weakness. Occasionally synovitis of small joints may be seen, which makes it difficult to differentiate it from an inflammatory polyarthritis. By definition, an elevated Westergren ESR greater than 50mm/hour, and usually over 70mm/hour, is part of the syndrome. A condition of unknown cause, the symptoms and the ESR are dramatically sensitive to low-dose corticosteroids (i.e., prednisone under 20mg/day); the symptoms usually improve within 24–48 hours and the ESR within a week of starting corticosteroids. However, once an elevated ESR is identified in a patient with aches and pains, other systemic diseases need to be considered; for example, early RA, SLE, polymyositis, vasculitis, myeloma and paraneoplastic syndrome.

PMR overlaps with GCA in about 10–30% of cases, but unless the patient has abnormalities of the temporal arteries or its branches, such as redness, nodularity or pain, or has headache, visual disturbance, ischemia or claudication of the masseter muscles or tongue, or systemic symptoms, the general recommendation is to *not* biopsy the temporal arteries. Careful examination of the temporal artery can be useful in targeting an artery for biopsy and for making a presumptive diagnosis of GCA. A clinically reddened and tender artery occurs in less than 10% of the cases now seen. The findings of a potentially involved artery are the lack of a pulse, tenderness, nodularity or a cord. Both branches and both sides should be palpated through their course as skip lesions occur. If GCA is suspected, prednisone should be started and a biopsy of the temporal artery obtained. Blindness, the major complication, can occur with devastating rapidity. Once an eye is involved the contralateral eye is also at considerable risk.

DIFFUSE ACHES AND PAINS – RED FLAGS	
Clinical feature	**Significance**
Age > 50 years	PMR, paraneoplastic syndrome
Constitutional symptoms	Inflammatory disease Vasculitis, sepsis, malignancy
Weakness	Myopathy, endocrinopathy
Gelling	Inflammatory rheumatic disorder
New headache Claudication Visual symptoms Tender, nodular, thickened or reddened temporal artery	Temporal arteritis
Bilateral symptoms	Systemic or metabolic cause

Fig. 2.16 Diffuse aches and pains — red flags.

LABORATORY EVALUATION OF DIFFUSE ACHES AND PAINS
Complete blood count
Westergren ESR
Thyroid function tests (T4 or TSH)
CPK or aldolase (if weakness)
Ca, PO_4

Fig. 2.15 Laboratory evaluation of patients with diffuse aches and pains.

CRAMPS, WEAKNESS AND MYALGIAS

The most common complaints referable to the muscles are cramps, weakness, myalgias and, occasionally, isolated muscle enzyme elevation. These problems (Fig. 2.17) can be sorted out effectively by a good history and an exam looking for signs of abnormal muscle function and being alert to atypical features (Fig. 2.18).

Patients can be sorted out by pursuing the following.

- Are symptoms periodic, constant, or progressive?
- Are symptoms proximal, distal or general?

MUSCLE SYNDROMES
Generalized weakness: subacute or chronic
Usually with atrophy Progressive muscular dystrophy Duchenne type Facioscapulohumeral type Limb girdle types Polymyositis Inclusion body myositis Endocrine myopathies Chronic, slowly progressive polymyopathies, (ie central core disease, glycogen storage disease)
Episodic weakness
Familial (hypokalemic) periodic paralysis Normokalemic or hyperkalemic familial periodic paralysis Acute thyrotoxic myopathy
Exertional stiffness or cramps or spasms
Leg cramps Metabolic defects of muscle metabolism McArdle's Phosphofructokinase deficiency Carnitine palmitoyl transferase deficiency Debranching enzyme deficiency Myoadenylate deaminase deficiency Defects of electron transport Congenital myotonia, paramyotonia congenita, and myotonic dystrophy Hypothyroidism with pseudomyotonia

Fig. 2.17 Muscle syndromes.

WEAKNESS, MUSCLE PAIN, MUSCLE CRAMPS – RED FLAGS	
History	Potential implication
Constitutional or extramuscular symptoms	Infection Inflammatory muscle disease Paraneoplastic syndrome
Menstrual irregularity Change in libido, body hair	Endocrinopathy
Medication use	? Drug-induced myopathy
Abrupt onset	Internal derangement Neurovascular
Severe pain Exercise-induced Generalized weakness Dark, red urine	Neurogenic Metabolic Metabolic, primary muscle disorder Rhabdomyolysis
Physical exam	
Stigmata of Cushing's, Addison's Hypothyroidism Neurovascular deficit	 Endocrinopathy Neurologic or vascular etiology

Fig. 2.18 Weakness, muscle pain and muscle cramps – red flags.

- Are symptoms use-related?
- Is it weakness or is it asthenia or general lassitude?

Constant weakness and loss of muscle power unchanged from day to day, week to week, and within a day suggest a neurologic cause, such as peripheral neuropathy, cord lesion or stroke. In the patient who complains of constant weakness without objective findings of weakness, a functional cause should be sought. Weakness from primary muscle disorders or from metabolic causes, i.e. myasthenia gravis, are variable and often related to ambient temperature (heat makes almost all forms of myopathies worse) or to repeated use of the specific muscles. The location and distribution of weakness can suggest specific syndromes. An asymmetric peripheral weakness is usually neurological. Symmetric proximal weakness is typical of both primary and secondary myopathies. Symmetric proximal and distal myopathy is seen in inclusion body myositis.

Bulbar weakness involving muscles of the eye and swallowing is suggestive of myasthenia. When asymmetric bulbar musculature is involved, think about cranial neuropathies and brain stem lesions. Weakness that is symmetric, distal and bulbar suggests amyotrophic lateral sclerosis.

The regional distribution of cramps can be diagnostic. Nearly all benign cramps are asymmetric and distal (the common nocturnal calf cramp or foot cramp).

Cramps in other muscle groups (abdominal or upper arm) in the absence of overuse or unusual use suggests primary or secondary myopathy. Cramps in specific muscle groups after strenuous exercise suggests myopathies with specific enzyme deficiencies usually involving the oxidative phosphorylation of ATP. These include McArdle's, phosphofructokinase deficiency, carnitine palmitoyl transferase deficiency, myoadenylate deaminase deficiency and problems with electron transport in the cytochrome oxidase pathway of muscle metabolism. As one might imagine, these are exceedingly rare, even in referral practices. However, since some may be treatable by dietary manipulations, the possibility must be kept in mind.

A screening test for induced cramps after ischemic exercise may help in selecting patients for further evaluation. In this test, a sample of blood for serum lactate and pyruvate is drawn from the antecubital fossa after exercising the forearm by squeezing a rolled towel repetitively with a blood pressure cuff pumped over 200mmHg systolic pressure for 3 minutes or until cramping occurs. The cuff is released to 20mmHg for 1 minute and blood taken. The cuff is deflated for another minute and then a second sample is drawn by reinflating the cuff to 20mmHg. A third sample is drawn after deflating the cuff for another minute. A normal response shows at least a three-fold rise in blood lactate between the pre-exercise and any one of the post-exercise values. A sharp fall is seen in normal individuals in the 3-minute post-exercise sample. An abnormal response can identify patients with potential metabolic myopathies and excludes people with myositis and other forms of myopathies.

True loss of muscle power needs to be distinguished from asthenia and easy fatigability. Weakness comes from loss of muscle power, but patients who have generalized weakness may interpret this symptom as not feeling well (asthenia) or as decreased stamina or endurance or fatigability. In a given individual the history may not be decisive and the issue is best resolved by formal muscle testing. People with primary myopathies have fatigability of strength; repetitive use of the muscle groups should induce fatigability. Some muscle disorders are distinguished by an abnormal reaction to repetitive electrical stimulation or repetitive use in which paradoxically the contractions become more intense after repetition. These are the myotonias (congenital myotonia, myotonia dystrophica and paramyotonia).

In a paraneoplastic neuromuscular condition, the Eaton–Lambert syndrome, repetitive electrical stimulation results in increased contractions, and clinically repetitive use does not fatigue the patient as in muscle disorders.

Muscle strength examination is subjective and the clinician who needs to follow muscle strength accurately should attempt to quantitate muscle strength more finely. Maneuvers to quantitate strength include isometric strength measurement, measurement of grip strength and using a weak muscle in some standardized activity to see how many repetitions a patient can do (e.g., the number of times one can get up from a chair in 30 seconds). Respiratory muscles might be investigated by pulmonary function testing.

Tenderness on palpation of muscles is unusual even in inflammatory myopathies (polymyositis, dermatomyositis). Rather, patients complain of muscle pain and myalgias at rest and with use of the muscles. Muscle tenderness on palpation should make one think of *Trichinella* infections of the muscle (myonecrosis), or rhabdomyolysis and compartment syndromes.

Fasciculations or muscle twitches during rest combined with muscle weakness and atrophy usually signifies motor neuron disease (amyotrophic lateral sclerosis, progressive bulbar palsy) but may also be seen in other disorders of the gray matter of the spinal cord, including syringomyelia or tumor, lesions of the anterior horn, ruptured disc, or in peripheral neuropathy. Widespread fasciculations occur after poisoning with pesticides containing organophosphates, severe dehydration (such as after vigorous exercise or running) or overdoses of neostigmine. Fasciculation, or a rippling or twitching sensation of the muscles in which no actual movements are observable and there is no weakness, atrophy or muscle enzyme elevation, is a common benign symptom (without a diagnosis) and needs no evaluation other than a good examination and follow-up. Closely allied is the syndrome of benign fasciculations in which fasciculations may be seen sporadically but without weakness or atrophy. Myokymia is a less common form of benign fasciculation in which there are repeated twitches giving the appearance of rippling muscles; it is diagnosed by electromyopathy.

Laboratory Evaluation

Incisive laboratory evaluation of patients with muscle weakness or cramps (Fig. 2.19) can be done inexpensively and is dictated by the clinical situation. If a patient has a mild nonprogressive weakness and has no constitutional symptoms, an outpatient evaluation includes: thyroid function tests, creatine phosphokinase (CPK), aldolase, sodium, potassium, calcium, phosphate, magnesium, hemoglobin, differential, and sedimentation rate (Fig. 2.20).

Urinary myoglobin and creatine are useful, as are antibodies thought to be more specific for myositis. For patients in whom the

LABORATORY EVALUATION OF PATIENTS WITH WEAKNESS OR CRAMPS
Creatine phosphokinase
Aldolase
24-hour urine for creatinine
Myoglobin
Thyroid function tests (TSH, T4)
Na, K
Ca, PO_4
Magnesium
Complete blood count, differential
Westergren ESR

Fig. 2.19 Laboratory evaluation of patients with weakness or cramps.

FACTORS THAT INFLUENCE THE ERYTHROCYTE SEDIMENTATION RATE	
Increase	Decrease
Anemia	Sickle cell disease
Hypercholesterolemia	Anisocytosis
Female sex	Spherocytosis
Pregnancy	Acanthocytosis
High room temperature	Microcytosis
Inflammatory disease	Polycythemia
Chronic renal failure	Bile salts
Obesity	Clotting of blood samples
Heparin	Greater than 2 hour delay in running test
Tissue damage (myocardial infarction,? stroke)	Low room temperature
	Hypofibrinogenemia
	Congestive heart failure
	Cachexia

Fig. 2.20 Factors that influence ESR [9].

neurologic and a muscular component are difficult to separate, or who have a focal asymmetric fixed lesion, an EMG done by a skilled examiner guided by specific clinical information can help identify whether the symptoms are due to a neuropathy or a primary muscle disorder. It is also useful to locate an involved muscle for biopsy to confirm the diagnosis of myositis. Be careful not to biopsy a site which has been recently studied by needle electromyography because the needle puncture induces an artifactual infiltrate of cells.

MUSCULOSKELETAL COMPLAINTS IN YOUNG PATIENTS

Spontaneous complaints of joint or musculoskeletal complaints in young patients are usually due to trauma, but special features should be kept in mind. The history that is so helpful in sorting out complaints in adults is less helpful in young patients. Although not always true, complaints in young subjects are usually minimized or attributed to trivial causes. Arthritis may present as a limp, delayed growth and development (failure to achieve normal developmental milestones), local growth disturbance, or a systemic febrile illness. A variety of important diagnoses occur with greater frequency in youth and can lead to disability and pain. These diagnoses include osteochondritis, primary bone tumors, growth disturbances, and spontaneous infectious arthritis.

The physician must try to make a diagnosis before attributing complaints to growing pains. When the symptoms and/or signs are confusing or conflicting, one should ask about the functional consequences of the symptoms or how the family reacts when the youth complains. Signs or symptoms that don't make sense may be a sign of school or family stress, or sometimes behavior learned from parents or siblings or used by the child to get attention.

On physical examination, if the patient has constitutional symptoms, or looks sick, a full physical examination is required. If one can find clear evidence of a soft tissue lesion, tendinitis, bursitis, or localized muscle tenderness, further evaluation is usually not needed. However, if joint inflammation is present or the symptom cannot be produced or explained, a radiograph is mandatory. Radiographs are useful because congenital disorders, growth disturbances and tumors occur at a greater frequency in the young and may present with vague symptoms and a normal physical exam. Trauma severe enough to result in soft tissue swelling may be forceful enough to cause a fracture to the epiphyseal plate or a slipped epiphysis, both of which may lead to future problems if not treated properly.

The term 'growing pains' is used most accurately as description rather than as diagnosis and is a diagnosis of exclusion. True growing pains are typically seen in children under 8 years of age in whom there is leg pain between joints that is not associated with growth spurts, aspirin-responsive symptoms or with a family history of the same.

LABORATORY EVALUATION STRATEGY

The laboratory evaluation of patients with arthritis and musculoskeletal symptoms can be extremely informative, although it is rarely definitive or decisive for initial treatment. Measurement of serum uric acid will not diagnose gout and never rules out the possibility of infection. Twenty percent of patients with acute gout have a normal serum uric acid. A normal white blood cell count does not rule out an infectious arthritis. In patients with early RA the rheumatoid factor may be negative, and many other conditions and normal patients may have a positive rheumatoid factor.

Diagnostic tests should change treatment, i.e. make a diagnosis for specific rather than symptomatic treatment, or help in prognosticating or defining response to treatment. Diagnostic testing for undifferentiated rheumatic complaints is most useful when there is strong clinical suspicion suggested by a constellation of signs and symptoms, or in establishing prognosis in limited circumstances (e.g. HLA-B27 in reactive arthritis suggesting an increased risk of sacroiliitis and spondylitis) and in systemic illnesses for defining the extent of disease or other organ systems that may be involved.

Four basic characteristics of diagnostic tests are useful in judging their usefulness in the evaluation of patients [7]. These are sensitivity, specificity, predictive value positive, and predictive value negative.

Sensitivity is the likelihood of a positive test result in a person with a disease. This is also termed the true positive rate of a diagnostic test. Specificity is the likelihood of a negative test in a patient without disease and is the true negative rate of a test. The predictive value positive of a test is the probability of a disease if the test is positive; likewise the predictive value negative of a test is the probability of a disease being absent if the test is negative. It is possible to calculate these characteristics by Bayes' theorem (see Fig. 2.21) if the incidence of the disease in the population is known [8] but the pretest probability of a disease in a given population is frequently not known. However, the relationship is such that the chances of a test being diagnostic of a condition in a given patient is greater when the condition is very common in the population.

Therefore, a patient with polyarthritis seen by a physician whose patients are not selected by referral is more likely to have viral

INTERPRETATION OF DIAGNOSTIC TESTS

	Disease	Non-disease		
Test+ (abnormal)	True + a	False + c	Predictive value positive	$= \frac{a}{a+c}$
Test− (normal)	False − b	True − d	Predictive value negative	$= \frac{d}{b+d}$

Specificity (true negative rate) = $\frac{d}{c+d}$

False positive rate = $\frac{c}{c+d}$

Sensitivity (true positve rate) = $\frac{a}{a+b}$

False negative rate = $\frac{b}{a+b}$

Sensitivity

Sensitivity is the percentage of positive results in patients known to have the disease. A test with a **sensitivity** of 100% gives positive results in all patients with the disease: it is never falsely negative. A test with a sensitivity of 90% has a **true positive rate** of 90%, and a **false negative rate** of 10%.

Specificity

Specificity is the percentage of true negative results in patients known to be free of the disease. A test with a specificity of 100% gives negative results in all subjects who are free from the disease: it is never falsely positive. A test with a specificity of 90% has a **false positive rate** of 10%

Predictive value

While tests are usually described in terms of **sensitivity** and **specificity**, the clinician is more interested in the **predictive value** of a test or the probability that the patient has a disease given a positive test (**predictive value positive**). If the test is negative, what is the probability that this patient does not have the disease (**predictive value negative**)?. Predictive value is also called **posterior** (or **post-test**) probability.

Another way to state these relationships is that the initial estimate of probability of disease is the prior probability, and the revised estimate using the posterior or post-test probability is the added information of the test.

Predictive values are critically dependent on the frequency of disease in the population (prevalence), whereas sensitivity and specificity are independent of disease frequency. Prevalence is also called prior (or pre-test) probability.

Bayes' theorem relating sensitivity, specificity, and predictive value

One can determine the predictive value (positive or negative) of a test if one knows its sensitivity and specificity, and the prevalence of disease in the population. One way of doing it would be to fill out the 2×2 table illustrated and perform the necessary computations.

Bayes' theorem or formula allows one to compute the predictive value. The expression can be written in many different ways. One version is:

$$\text{Predictive value positive} = \frac{\text{(Sensitivity) (Prevalence of disease)}}{\text{(Sens) (Prev)+(1−specificity) (1−Prev)}}$$

Assumptions of Bayes' theorem

Conditional probabilities of findings given a diagnostic hypothesis are independent.

A patient's clinical condition corresponds to one and only one disease from among a given set of diseases.

The central lesson from this probablistic approach is that if the pretest probability of a disease is extremely low, a positive test result will rarely confirm a diagnosis unless the test is highly specific. When the likelihood of a disease is extremely high, a negative test usually does not exclude the presence of disease unless the test is highly sensitive.

Fig. 2.21 Interpretation of diagnostic tests.

arthritis than RA. Patients who are seen in a primary care setting will frequently have less classical disease, milder disease and disease of a better prognosis than those seen in referral or hospital-based setting. Immunochemical tests have been found useful for some rheumatic conditions. Generally speaking, there are few serologic tests in rheumatic conditions that are absolutely diagnostic.

Laboratory tests are also needed to screen for organ involvement and in 'staging' in systemic rheumatic illnesses such as SLE and vasculitis which may affect organ systems not clinically apparent or symptomatic.

Radioimaging also has a role in assessing disease activity and evaluating the organ-specific response to therapy.

Acute Phase Reactants

Acute phase reactants are plasma proteins manufactured in the liver which usually increase following inflammation or tissue necrosis and appear to parallel chronic inflammation. They form a heterogeneous group comprising: coagulation proteins, such as fibrinogen and prothrombin; transport proteins, such as haptoglobin, transferrin and ceruloplasm; complement components, such as C3 and C4; protease inhibitors; and miscellaneous proteins, such as albumin, fibronectin, and serum amyloid-A related protein. Factors and conditions with abnormalities of the ESR are given in Figure 2.20 [9].

The two most commonly used acute phase reactants in the evaluation of rheumatic diseases are the erythrocyte sedimentation rate (ESR) and the C-reactive protein (CRP). The CRP level responds more rapidly than the ESR to changes in inflammatory activity and thus would be a more sensitive measure of inflammation. However, the ESR takes only 1 hour and simple equipment whereas the CRP is assayed by radioimmunodiffusion and takes a day to provide an answer.

Although the ESR is commonly used as a screening test for inflammatory disease, the data suggest that the ESR is not useful in distinguishing inflammatory arthritis from other causes of joint symptoms. In a population survey of 13,002 Scandinavian women, 30% reported joint symptoms in the preceding year [10]. In a subgroup with at least four symptoms or physical signs of RA, only 50% had an ESR that exceeded 30mm/hour. Fourteen percent of the women with osteoarthritis had an ESR greater than 30mm/hour compared to 50% of women with RA. Therefore, a normal ESR is scant evidence against the diagnosis of RA and probably of any inflammatory arthritis. An elevated ESR and CRP may be present in the absence of disease. The ESR increases with age and anemia and is higher in women than in men. The upper limit of normal for an ESR adjusted for age can be estimated for men by dividing age by two and for women by taking the age plus ten divided by two. Both the CRP and ESR are elevated in pregnancy, following trauma and in any situation leading to the release of the cytokines IL-1 and IL-6.

The ESR is needed for the diagnosis of temporal arteritis and polymyalgia rheumatica by definition. It is thought that perhaps some 10% of patients with GCA/PMR may have a normal ESR and still have the disease [11].

In pseudogout, the ESR is not at all helpful and a normal ESR does not reduce the probability of pseudogout enough to preclude other tests such as synovial fluid analysis. The ESR can be normal in patients with certain types of vascular inflammation such as primary CNS angiitis, Henoch-Schönlein purpura, lymphomatoid granulomatosis, and thromboangitis obliterans [12].

The ESR is useful for monitoring the disease activity of patients with RA and PMR/GCA but less useful in patients with SLE and spondyloarthropathies.

Immunological Tests

Serum protein electrophoresis or immunoelectrophoresis are not useful for the routine evaluation of individuals with rheumatic conditions. The primary value of protein electrophoresis is in the identification of a monoclonal protein, which occurs in multiple myeloma, some lymphoproliferative disorders, macroglobulinemia, cryoglobulinemia, and occasionally otherwise uncomplicated rheumatic disease. When such an abnormality is identified, immunoelectrophoresis is used to characterize the abnormal proteins. Elevated gammaglobulin levels can be seen in RA, SLE, chronic hepatitis and other states characterized by immune hyperactivity. The absence of a globulin band usually indicates a congenital deficiency or an acquired immunoglobulin deficiency and these individuals may have manifestations of connective tissue disease [13].

Many rheumatic diseases are thought to be the result of abnormalities of the immune sytem and have abnormalities of cellular and humoral immunity. The number of T-helper and B cells may be abnormal. Humoral abnormalities include high titers of autoantibodies and circulating immune complexes, cryoglobulins, and absent or depressed complement proteins.

Human lymphocytes can be subdivided on the basis of their function into T cells, T-helper cells, T-suppressor/cytotoxic cells, natural killer (NK) cells, B cells and plasma cells. The functional activity of these lymphocytes corresponds to specific cell surface antigens, and T- and B-cell subsets can be identified using monoclonal antibodies that react with the surface antigens. Enumerating lymphocyte phenotype or cell types is expensive and of limited clinical usefulness at present. The most clear cut application is in the diagnosis of AIDS, where a reduced T-helper to T-suppressor ratio may be found [14].

Intradermal skin tests may be used to evaluate cellular immunity and hypersensitivity to antigens or specific antigen. A positive skin test reaction indicates previous exposure to an antigen, T-cell competency and an intact inflammatory response. The inability to react to a battery of common skin antigens is termed anergy and is seen in patients with sarcoid, active infection or immune deficient states. Delayed hypersensitivity skin testing has little value in the diagnosis of defective cellular immunity during the first year of life.

Autoantibodies

Autoantibodies, which are immunoglobulins directed against autologous intracellular, cell surface or extracellular antigens, are seen in a number of rheumatic illnesses. The intracellular antigens include nuclear components (antinuclear antibodies, or ANA) and cytoplasmic components (anticytoplasmic antibodies). Antibodies to cell surface antigens react with a variety of antigens, including HLA molecules. Other antibodies may react with plasma components such as coagulation factors (i.e., lupus anticoagulant).

Autoantibodies are detected by a variety of techniques, including indirect immunofluorescence, enzyme immunocytochemistry, passive hemagglutination, latex particle agglutination, immunodiffusion, counterimmunoelectrophoresis (CIE), and radioimmunoassay (RIA) and enzyme-linked immunosorbant assay (ELISA). When autoantibodies are directed against cellular or insoluble extracellular components, indirect immunofluorescence is the method most widely used to screen body fluids for the presence of these antibodies. Autoantibodies directed against soluble components, such as coagulation factors, DNA, nuclear protein and components of complement are assayed by immunodiffusion, CIE, RIA, or ELISA.

The sensitivity of techniques varies considerably and at present there is no standardization of either the assay method or the units in which they are reported[15]. Therefore, comparison from one lab to another is problematic. Autoantibodies are present in the normal population, albeit in low titer, and the presence of an autoantibody does not make a disease. Many individuals have been made into rheumatic disease patients by indiscriminate shotgun testing. Figure 2.22 summarizes the autoantibodies that occur in rheumatic conditions.

Rheumatoid factors are antibodies directed against the patient's gammaglobulins. These autoantibodies appear to be synthesized in response to immunoglobulins that have been confirmationally altered after reaction with an antigen. The most common rheumatoid factor is an IgM antibody to IgG. Techniques to detect rheumatoid factor include agglutination of antibody sensitized sheep red blood cells, latex agglutination, and hemagglutination.

A low level of rheumatoid factor can be found in some normal individuals. On the other hand, increased levels are seen in many diseases characterized by persistent immune complex formation and in many chronic inflammatory disorders (Fig. 2.23) [16]. The level of rheumatoid factor has some significance and the higher the level the more suggestive it is of RA. High titer rheumatoid factors in patients with RA is associated with extra-articular features, severe disease and the presence of rheumatoid nodules.

Complement

The complement cascade is a series of over 20 biologically active proteins and inhibitors that comprise 2–3% of the total plasma protein concentration. Complement activated by the classic pathway is responsible for the lysis of cells coated with antibody directed against cell surface antigens. The alternative pathway for complement activation can cause cell lysis in the absence of cell bound antibody.

Complement may be assayed by techniques which measure the presence of the component or its function. Functional assays identify enzymatically active complement and depend on the measurement of hemolysis of antibody coated red blood cells. The best screening test for a complement abnormality is the CH50, which is a functional assay of the entire classical pathway. A low titer would suggest the need to assay individual components.

Clinically, the physician is usually looking for low complement levels, which are associated with several immune-complex-mediated diseases, such as SLE, bacterial endocarditis, severe rheumatoid arthritis, and mixed cryoglobulinemia [17]. Monitoring the complement levels can also be used to assess disease activity; this may be particularly useful in SLE nephritis. In comparison, complement levels are normal in most other rhematic diseases.

A low CH50 is most often due to increased complement activation by immune complexes. If, however, the rate of utilization does not exceed the ability to synthesize new complement proteins, then the complement level may remain normal despite active disease.

Hypocomplementemia is occasionally due to genetic deficiencies of complement components. In this setting, the CH50 will be low, but the different complement proteins will be normal except for the one that is missing. The most common genetic deficiencies are heterozygous C4, heterozygous C2, and several homozygous disorders. Patients with C1 and C2 deficiencies often have autoimmune disease. In comparison, patients with homozygous C3, C5, C7 or C8 have recurrent pyogenic infections.

Immune Complexes

Circulating immune complexes consisting of an antigen, an antibody and complement components are believed to play an important role in the pathogenesis of systemic rheumatic diseases, such as SLE and vasculitis. But they also exist in a variety of other conditions, and in low titer in some normal individuals. Methods to detect immune complexes depend on physical or biological properties of the molecular complex or properties of cell-surface receptors. Some assays appear to have greater sensitivity than others for the detection of immune complexes. High concentrations of circulating immune complexes can be seen in active systemic rheumatic diseases, vasculitis, infectious diseases, and some malignancies. In most of these conditions a clear cut pathogenetic role for the complexes has not been established.

IMAGING TECHNIQUES IN THE INITIAL EVALUATION

Radiographs

Radiographs for a new joint complaint are only helpful in certain situations. Plain radiographs show bone best, and changes in soft tissue

AUTOANTIBODIES IN RHEUMATIC DISEASE				
	Autoantibody	Antigen specificity	ANA pattern	Disease associations
Nucleic acids	Anti-DNP	Deoxyribonucleoprotein	Homogeneous/ peripheral	SLE, drug-induced LE
	Anti-DNA	Deoxyribonucleic acid	Homogeneous/ peripheral	SLE, but also in other diseases
	Double-stranded DNA			SLE, SLE nephritis
	Single-stranded DNA			SLE, drug-induced SLE, RA, Sjögren's
	Anti-RNA	Ribonucleic acid	?	SLE
	Anti-nucleolar	4–6s RNA, U3RNP	Nucleolar	Systemic sclerosis, SLE
Histones	Anti-histone		Homogeneous/ peripheral	SLE, drug-induced LE
	Anti-histone (H3)		Large speckles	SLE
Non-histone nuclear proteins	Anti-Sm (Anti-ENA)	Smith	Speckle	SLE
	Anti-nRNP (Anti-ENA)	Ribonucleoprotein (UIRNP)	Speckle	SLE MCTD
	Anti-SS-A/Ro		Speckle (weak)	Sjögren's syndrome SLE Subacute cutaneous LE Neonatal lupus
	Anti-SS-B/La/Ha		Fine speckle	Sjögren's syndrome SLE
	Anti-MA-1	MA-1	?	SLE
	Anti-Sc-70	Scleroderma 70	Speckle	Systemic sclerosis
	Anti-PCNA	Proliferating cell nuclear antigen	Variable speckle	SLE
Cytoplasmic	Anti-centriole	Centriole	Large speckles	Systemic sclerosis
	Anti-Golgi	Golgi	Perinuclear strands	SLE
	Anti-mitochondria	Mitochondria	Irregular granules	SLE Primary biliary cirrhosis
	Anti-ribosomal	Ribosomes/ ribonucleoprotein	Fine speckles	SLE
	Anti-vimentin	Vimentin	Large fibrils	RA, Sjögren's syndrome
	ANCA (antineutrophilic cytoplasmic antibody)	Serine proteinase and myeloperoxidase		Wegener's, Polyarteritis nodosa, Glomerulonephritis
Other	Anti-centromere	Chromosomal centromere	Discrete speckles	Systemic sclerosis Raynaud's
	Anti-nuclear matrix	Nuclear matrix	Irregular speckles	MCTD,SLE
	Anti-Mi-1	Mi-1	?	Polymyositis (adult)
	Anti-Jo-1	Jo-1	Cytoplasm?	Polymyositis
	Anti-Ku	Ku	?	Polymyositis (adult)
	Anti-systems, A,B,C	Su (systems A,B,C)	?	Polymyositis (adult)
	Anti-PM-1 (Pm-Scl)	PM-1 (Pm-Scl)	?	Polymyositis/ systemic sclerosis overlap
	Anti-RANA	RANA	Speckles	RA

Fig. 2.22 Autoantibodies in rheumatic disease.

RHEUMATOID FACTORS IN DISEASE STATES AND NORMALS	
Controls	Percentage positive for rheumatoid factor
Rheumatoid arthritis Sjögren's syndrome	50–85
Subacute bacterial endocarditis Systemic lupus erythematosus Leprosy Liver disease	25–50
Juvenile chronic arthritis Pulmonary diseases Tuberculosis	10–25
Ankylosing spondylitis Rheumatic fever Osteoarthritis Psoriatic arthritis Gout	5–10
Normals	<5

Fig. 2.23 Rheumatoid factors in disease states and normals.

less well. The findings in bone that are useful in diagnosis of early rheumatic symptoms are erosions, such as occur in RA, fractures, avascular necrosis, osteopenia, cartilage space narrowing and calcification, calcification of spinal ligaments, periostitis (diffuse idiopathic skeletal hyperostosis or DISH) and rare conditons such as bone tumors. It takes 6 months of rheumatoid synovitis to create an erosion visible by conventional radiography [18] and therefore a radiograph in early disease is not useful. In a patient who has had multiple acute attacks of arthritis in the same joint, a radiograph may occasionally demonstrate a typical gouty erosion. Radiographs are not helpful for the early diagnosis of osteomyelitis or septic joints because in the initial stages they are usually normal.

CT Scanning

CT scanning is particularly useful for visualizing the spine and for assessing the integrity of the intervertebral discs. Contrast enhancement may be used to determine spinal cord compression or epidural fibrosis [19]. However, images of the small joints of the hands and feet are difficult to interpret and expose the patient to large doses of radiation.

Magnetic Resonance Imaging

MRI is now used extensively to image joints and soft tissues that may be affected by rheumatic diseases. The introduction of more powerful magnets has allowed high definition of soft tissues and the detection of early bony erosions [20]. Enhancement of the MRI images can be obtained using gadolinium-DPTA and gadopentetate dimeglumine [21,22], which may allow the detection of early synovitis and enable disease progression to be monitored. Long term follow-up studies are still required to determine the value of this exciting technique in following disease progression and the effects of treatment.

New techniques in imaging

Attempts have been made to develop objective measures of joint inflammation that are capable of detecting inflammatory synovitis/ cartilage damage before changes are seen on routine radiography. These techniques include, microfocal radiography,isotope scanning and thermography

.

Microfocal radiography

This technique uses enhanced resolution and fine-grain film, which enables erosions to be seen at an early stage, prior to their detection by conventional radiography [23]. However, the current apparatus is bulky and is unlikely to be available outside specialized centers.

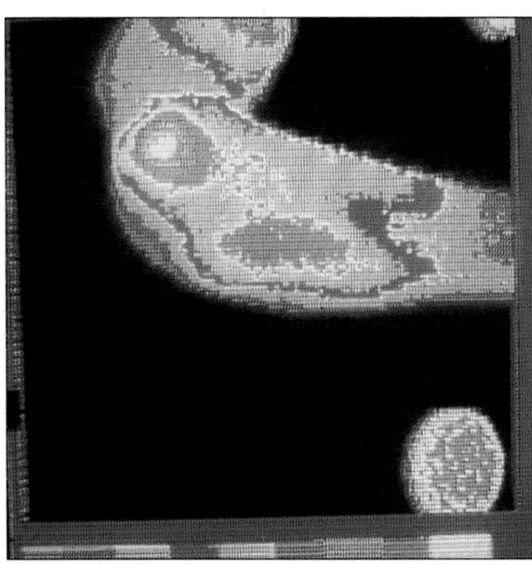

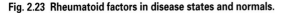

Fig. 2.24 An infrared thermographic pattern in lateral epicondylitis showing a localized 'hot spot'.

Thermography

Infrared thermography has been used to detect increased heat loss from the skin surface over an inflamed joint. The intensity of the infrared radiation measured is a reflection of increased blood flow in tissues near to the skin surface with heat being conducted to the skin surface and subsequently being detected as radiant heat. This is an indirect assessment of the inflammatory response in, for example, RA. It is possible to scan over an area of interest and produce an image (Fig. 2.24) which can be quantified by computer analysis to generate a thermographic index. Some centers using this technique have demonstrated changes in heat radiation which mirror clinical changes occurring during therapy with second line drugs for RA such as methotrexate and D-penicillamine [24] . Infrared thermography is also capable of detecting abnormal heat patterns in soft tissue conditions such as tennis elbow and algodystrophy [25]. The major disadvantage of this technique is the need for a temperature controlled environment – a problem that may be overcome by microwave thermography in the future [26].

Isotope scanning

Technetium pertechnetate in isotope form (^{99m}Tc) has been used as a measure of blood flow in inflamed joints and shows increased uptake in RA [27]. Bone seeking preparations such as diphosphonates labelled with ^{99m}Tc also localize over areas of inflammation where there is increased bone turnover and can show increased uptake in early inflammatory joint disease (Fig. 2.25) and OA when standard radiographs are normal [28]. However, these assessments are time consuming and require 2–4 hours of patient time for each examination. Recently ^{125}I serum amyloid A protein has been used to visualize amyloid deposits in juvenile chronic arthritis [29]. Polyclonal IgG labelled with ^{99m}Tc has been reported to detect joint inflammation in RA [30] and to reflect active inflammation with a reduced joint uptake in patients with inactive disease.

FUNCTIONAL ASSESSMENT

The evaluation is not complete without an evaluation of how the symptoms affect the person's functioning at work, play and home activities. Function is the final common pathway of all forms of arthritis and musculoskeletal conditons, and along with pain is the principal concern of patients.

Function is a complex phenomenon. Dysfunction arises when there is a discrepancy between ability and need. This is dependent on whether there is an actual or perceived need to do something, and the patient's expectations, motivation and support system. Function

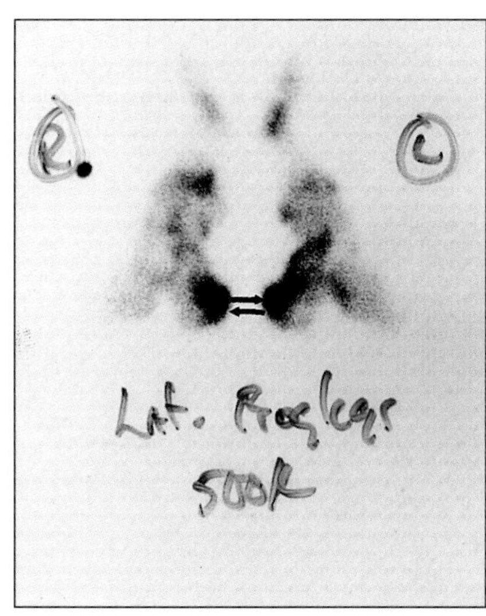

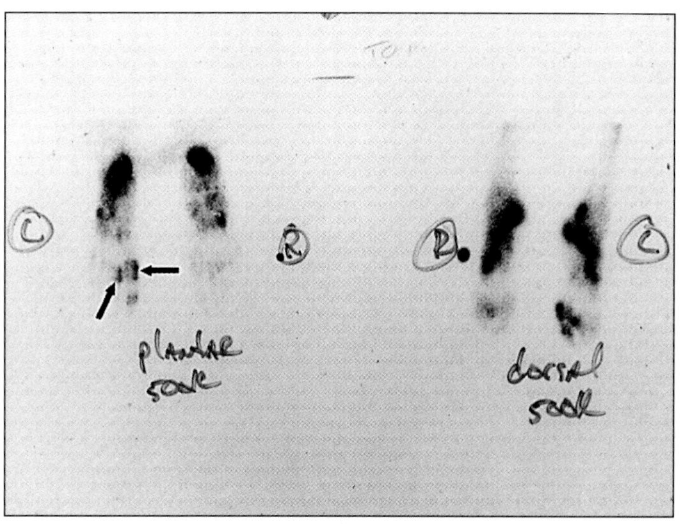

Fig. 2.25 ^{99m}Technetium scan of both feet in a patient with Reiter's disease. Though conventional radiographs were normal, this scan demonstrates increased uptake.

changes over the life of a person's development, both in terms of capability and desire or need. The age of an individual has a major influence on function. In children and adolescents, rapid change and maturation of cognitive, behavioral, emotional and psychological function is the rule, whereas in adult life these aspects are stable but life circumstances are changing. Thus, an assessment needs to examine abilty with a consideration of need, motivation and environmental determinants.

The techniques for measuring function are as varied as their application. Approaches to measuring physical function range from measures that emphasize impairment (demonstrable anatomic damage or physiologic state), such as articular indices and grip strength measurement, those that assess more complex function (complex integrated ability to perform tasks of daily life, self-care, recreation or work) rated by the physician, such as the ACR Functional Classes, to self-administered questionnaires such as the Health Assessment Questionnaire (HAQ) [31, 32].

One cannot use questionnaires to make etiologic diagnosis of the functional problem to guide therapy, although they are useful to screen for problems. Self-reported function can overestimate or underestimate a patient's ability. All self-reported methods probably have floors and ceilings by which the patient with early impairment or with advanced disease cannot be rated accurately or with sensitivity. For example, hand function may be assessed by a question on difficulty with fastening buttons or doing zippers, but the physician may need to detect more subtle changes which might be more appropriately obtained from measurement of grip and pinch strength and standardized dexterity measures.

In patient care, screening for problems can be carried out with a simple history (Fig. 2.26). When a patient's priorities can be discussed and when the doctor and patient develop a congruent notion of how progress or success should be measured, patient satisfaction and results can be improved significantly. The history of functional ability should always be supplemented with an examination. Signs of synovitis are most useful in the assessment of disease activity and range of motion for potential functional problems. Most individuals with arthritis can perform tasks of daily living, albeit with discomfort or impaired efficiency. This is possible because people adapt to and revise their goals within the context of their pain and limited joint motion. When contractures or joint deformity progress beyond a certain range for a given joint, an impairment becomes a functional deficit (Fig. 2.27). However, an individual may not always perceive it as a problem.

Social and emotional functioning include mood, coping skills and one's ability to participate in social roles, and cover the spectrum of human feelings which make up the human condition. Problems in these areas can be suspected when the person's complaints are out of proportion to objective signs of disease.

When problems in these areas are suspected, a psychological history should be pursued to the degree and pace set by the patient. The quality of social supports, interpersonal relationships and financial resources available are the common areas involved. Obtaining the history may not lead to any intervention, but making it a legitimate area of discussion and showing concern is tremendously meaningful to the patient and their family.

QUESTIONS IN SCREENING FOR FUNCTIONAL LIMITATION

- How does your condition affect you?
- What's the most difficult thing for you to do?
- What do you need to do that you can't do or have difficulty doing?
- What do you want to do that you can't do or have difficulty doing?
- During a typical day what limitations do you have to overcome?
- Do you have trouble sleeping and/or bathing?

Fig. 2.26 Questions in screening for functional limitation.

CRITICAL RANGES OF MOTION WHICH SUBSERVE FUNCTION

Joint	Critical range
Temporomandibular	2.5cm of jaw opening
Shoulder	Flexion 45° Abduction 90° External rotation 20°
Elbow	70–80° Flexion
Wrist	5–10° dorsiflexion 10–15° supination
MCP	Flexion greater than 30°
PIP	Flexion greater than 30°
DIP	Flexion greater than 30°
CMC	Internal rotation greater than 30°
Hip	0° extension to 30° flexion
Knee	Neutral to 60° flexion
Ankle	20° plantar flexion to 10° dorsiflexion

Fig. 2.27 Critical ranges of joint motion which subserve function. Data from Gerber, LG [33].

A functional deficit in a patient is a symptom, not an etiologic diagnosis, and should be approached in the same manner as any other abnormal sign or symptom, so that one will not miss treatable disease. Every complex activity has multiple determinants which include cognitive, psychological, neurologic (proprioceptive and perceptual), motor and articular components. The physician must sort through the possibilities and develop a treatment strategy by assessing the capacity of each system and identifying what is the most limiting and what is treatable.

REFERENCES

1. Polley HF, Hunder GG. Rheumatological interviewing and physical examination of the joints, 2E. Philadelphia: WB Saunders; 1978.
2. Hoppenfeld S. Physical examination of the spine and extremities. New York: Appleton-Century-Crafts; 1976.
3. Kerolus G, Clayburne G, Schumacher HR, Jr. Is it mandatory to examine synovial fluids promptly after arthrocentesis? Arthritis Rheum. 1989; **32**:271–8.
4. Mochan BS, Kant JA. Reproducibility of synovial fluid analyses: A study among four laboratories. Arthritis Rheum. 1986;**29**:770–4, .
5. Liang MH, Katz JN. Clinical evaluation of patients with a suspected spine problem. In: Frymoyer J (ed). The adult spine: principles and practice. New York: Raven Press; 1991;223–39.
6. Sheon RP, Moskowitz RW, Goldberg V, eds. Soft tissue rheumatic pain: Recognition. Management. Prevention, 2E. Philadelphia: Lea & Febiger; 1987.
7. ARA Glossary Committee, Dictionary of the rheumatic diseases: Vol II: Diagnostic testing. New York: Contact Associates; 1985.
8. McNeil BJ, Keeler E, Adelstein SJ. Primer on certain elements of medical decision making. N Engl J Med. 1975;**293**:211–5.
9. Sox HC Jr, Liang MH. The erythrocyte sedimention rate: guidlines for rational use. Ann Intern Med. 1986;**104**:515–23.
10. Rafnsson V, Bengtsson C, Lurie M. Erythrocyte sedimentation rate in women with different manifestations of joint disease. Scand J Med. 1982;**11**:87–95.
11. Healey LA, Wilske KR. The systemic manifestations of temporal arteritis. New York: Grune & Stratton; 1978:120.
12. Cupps TR, Fauci AS. The vasculitides. Philadelphia:WB Saunders; 1981:21
13. Hong R. Associations of the skeletal and immune systems. Am J Med. Genet. 1989;**34**:55–9
14. Laurence J. T-cell subsets in Health, infectious disease, and idiopathic CD4+ T Lymphocytopenia. Ann Intern Med. 1993;**119**:55–62.
15. Tan EM. Antinuclear antibodies: Diagnostic markers for autoimmune disease and probes for cell biology. Adv Immunol. 1989;**44**:93.
16. Shmerling RH, Delbanco TL. The Rheumatoid Factor:an analysis of clinical utility. Am J med. 1991;**91**:528–34.
17. Schur PH. Complement studies of sera and other biological fluids. Hum Pathol. 1983;**14**:338.
18. Gennant HK. Methods of assessing radiographic changes in rheumatoid arthritis. Am J Med. 1983;**9**:581–600.
19. Murphy MD, Quale JL, Martin NL, Bramble JM, Cook LT, Dwyer SJ. Computed radiography in musculoskeletal imaging - state of the art. Am J Roentgenol. 1992;**158**:119–27.
20. Rominger MB, Bernreuter WK, Kenney PJ, Morgan SL, Blackburn WD, Alarcon GS. MR imaging of the hands in early rheumatoid arthritis - Preliminary results. Radiographics. 1993;**13**:37–46.
21. Reiser MF, Bongartz GP, Erlemann R, et al. Gadolinium-DTPA in rheumatoid arthritis and related diseases – first results with dynamic magnetic imaging. Skeletal Radiol. 1989;**18**:591–7.

22. Whitten CG, Moore TE, Yuh WTC, Kathol MH, Renfrew DL, Walker CW. The use of intravenous gadopentetate dimeglumine in magnetic resonance imaging of synovial lesions. Skeletal Radiol. 1992;**21**:215–18.
23. Chikanza IC, Clarke GS, Grahame R, Bucklandwright JC. Quantitative microfocal radiography (MFR) detects the onset of erosion. Br J Rheumatol. 1992;**31**:96.
24. Devereaux MD, Parr GR, Thomas DPP, Hazelman BL. Disease activity indexes in rheumatoid arthritis – a prospective, comparative study with thermography. Ann Rheum Dis. 1985;**44**:434–7.
25. Thomas D, Siahamis G, Marion M, Boyle C. Computerized infrared thermography and isotopic bone scanning in tennis elbow. Ann Rheum Dis. 1992;**51**:103–7.
26. Fraser S, Land D, Sturrock RD. Microwave thermography - an index of inflammatory joint disease. Br J Rheum. 1987;**26**:37–9.
27. Boerbooms AM, Buys WC. Rapid assessment of Tc-99m pertechnetate of the knee joint as a parameter of inflammatory activity. Arthritis Rheum. 1978;**21**:348.
28. Rosenthall L. Nuclear medicine techniques in arthritis.Rheum Dis Clin North Am. 1991;**17**:585–97.
29. Hawkins PN, Lavender JP, Pepys MB. Evaluation of systemic amyloidosis by scintigraphy with 123I-labeled serum amyloid P component. N Engl J Med. 1990;**8**:508–13
30. Breedveld FC, Vankroonenburgh MJPG, Camps JAJ, Feitsma HIJ, Markusse HM, Pauwels EKJ. Imaging of inflammatory arthritis with technetium-99M-labelled IGG. J Nucl Med. 1989;**30**:2017–21.
31. Liang MH, Jette AJ. Measuring functional ability in chronic arthritis: A critical review. Arthritis Rheum. 1981;**24**:80-6.
32. Liang MH, Katz JN. Measurement of outcome in rheumatoid arthritis. In: Scott DL, ed. The course and outcome of rheumatoid arthritis. Balliere's Clinical Practice; 1992:23–7.
33. Gerber LH. Rehabilitation of patients with rheumatic diseases. In: Kelley WH, Harris T, Ruddy S, Sledge CB (eds). Textbook of rheumatology. 3E. Philadelphia: WB Saunders; 1990: 1904–18

3

ARTHRITIS WITH SKIN AND NAIL CHANGES

David L George

INTRODUCTION

The diagnosis of rheumatic diseases is commonly based on pattern recognition. The skin is the most accessible organ and often provides valuable diagnostic clues that may lead to a specific diagnosis or limit the list of possibilities [1–3]. For example, a diagnosis of psoriatic arthritis might be based upon the presence of distal interphalangeal (DIP) joint synovitis, erythematous scaling plaques over extensor surfaces and nail pitting. Conversely, unrelated skin lesions may occasionally mislead the clinician. For example, incorrect diagnosis of systemic lupus erythematosus (SLE) might be made in a patient with a symmetric polyarthritis who manifests the facial rash of acne rosacea.

Pattern recognition of skin lesions is based upon the type, configuration (Fig. 3.1), distribution, and evolution of the lesions. Selective laboratory techniques may further assist diagnosis. This chapter focuses on the cutaneous diseases most relevant in patients with rheumatic complaints (Fig. 3.2) and emphasizes characteristic features that will allow the physician to distinguish those cutaneous lesions commonly associated with musculoskeletal syndromes from entities with which they are commonly confused.

EXANTHEMS

An exanthem is a diffuse rash with fever and systemic symptoms which is usually due to a viral or primary immunologic illness, but bacterial infections must be excluded.

SLE, dermatomyositis, Lyme disease and rheumatic fever may have characteristic cutaneous lesions in association with acute systemic disease and are discussed in later chapters. Characteristic exanthems are also seen in Still's disease and Kawasaki disease (see Fig. 3.3).

IMPORTANT DERMATOLOGIC TERMS	
Macule	Flat lesion differentiated from surrounding skin by its color
Papule/nodule	Raised solid lesion less than/greater than 1cm in diameter, respectively
Vesicle/bulla	Raised fluid filled lesion less than/greater than 0.5cm, respectively
Pustule	Vesicle filled with purulent exudate
Wheal (urticaria)	Pale erythematous papule or plaque resulting from upper dermal edema.
Ulcer	Lesion resulting from destruction of the epidermis and at least the upper dermis
Petechia/purpura	Intradermal hemorrhage less than/greater than 3mm in diameter, respectively
Desquamation (scaling)	Abnormal shedding or accumulation of the stratum corneum
Sclerosis	Hardening or induration of the skin
Pathergy (Koebnerization)	Induction of skin lesion in location of minor trauma

Fig. 3.1 Important dermatologic terms.

The patient with Still's disease develops discrete pink to salmon colored macules or slightly elevated papules several millimeters in size on the trunk and extremities, although lesions may occur on the face and rarely on the palms and soles [4,5]. The lesions are maximal during episodes of fever and are prominent in areas of minor skin

TYPES OF CUTANEOUS LESIONS OBSERVED IN RHEUMATIC DISORDERS

Disorder (Lesion type)	Macules/ papules	Papulonodular	Vesicular/bullous	Pustular	Ulcerating	Petechia/purpura
Primary immune disease						
Systemic lupus erythematosus	•	•	•		•	•
Scleroderma		•			•	
Dermatomyositis	•	•			•	•
Rheumatoid arthritis		•			•	•
Still's disease	•					
Sjögren's syndrome					•	•
Erythema nodosum		•				
Pyoderma gangrenosum		•		•	•	
Sarcoid	•	•				
Inflammatory bowel disease	•	•	•	•	•	•
Psoriatic arthritis	•			•		
Reiter's syndrome	•			•		
Behçet's disease	•	•	•	•	•	•
Multicentric reticulohistiocytosis		•				
Serum sickness	•					•
Neutrophilic dermatoses	•	•	•	•	•	
Kawasaki disease	•		•	•		
Necrotizing venulitis	•	•	•		•	•
Polyarteritis nodosa	•	•			•	•
Wegener's granulomatosus	•	•	•		•	•
Lymphomatoid granulomatosis	•	•			•	
Infections						
Neisserial infections	•	•	•	•		•
Rheumatic fever	•	•				
Subacute bacterial endocarditis		•				•
Hydradenitis suppurative/ acne conglobata		•		•		
Syphilis	•	•		•	•	
Lyme disease	•		•			
Rickettsial infections	•					•
Viral infections	•		•	•		•
Fungal infections			•		•	
Mycobacterial infections	•	•			•	
Other conditions						
Diabetes mellitus		•	•		•	
Thyroid disease	•	•				
Hyperlipidema (Type II)		•				
Crystal Disease		•				
Neoplasms	•	•			•	•

Fig. 3.2 Types of lesions observed in diseases with rheumatic expression [1–3].

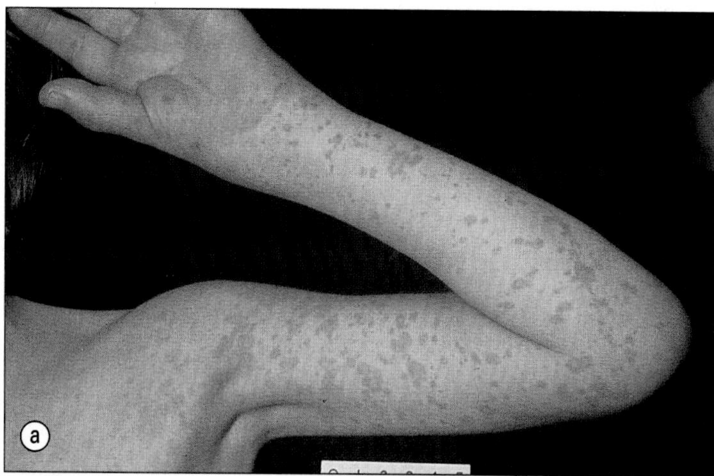

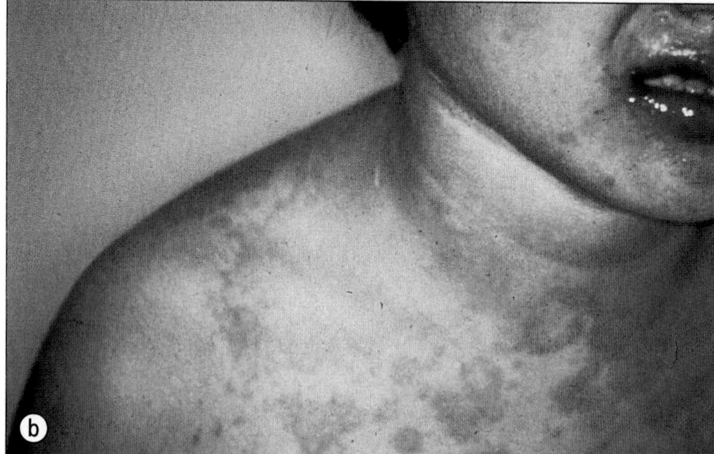

Fig. 3.3 Exanthems: Still's rash (a); Kawasaki disease (b).

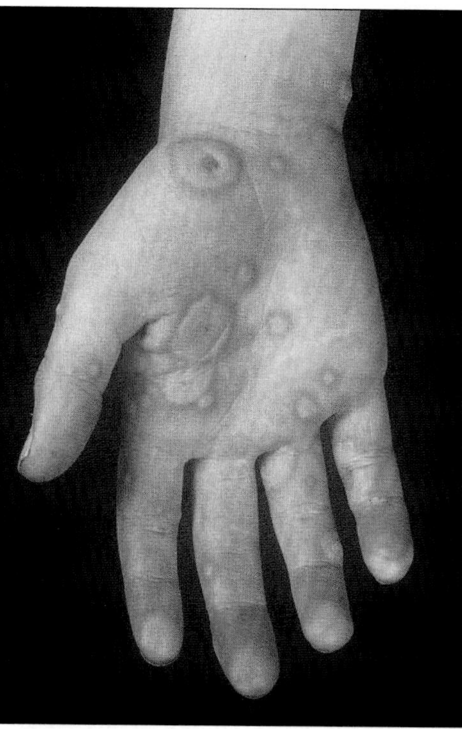

Fig. 3.4 Erythema multiforme. Reproduced, with permission, from Dermatology in Practice, Anthony du Vivier, London, Gower, 1990.

trauma or by stretching the skin (Köebner phenomenon). Still's lesions are irregular in shape and have no associated purpura or vesicles. They are asymptomatic or only mildly pruritic. The lesions do not spread, and last only minutes to hours. When the rash recurs, lesions are in new locations. No enanthem accompanies the rash. Such a rash in the presence of quotidian fever, diffuse palpable lymphadenopathy, and polyarthritis is diagnostic of Still's disease.

Kawasaki disease presents with a polymorphous rash (morbilliform, scarlatiniform, pustular or erythema-multiforme-like rash), which is notable for early erythema of the palms and soles with desquamation days later, along with scarlet-fever-like oral mucosal changes, including strawberry tongue and dry red fissured lips, and conjunctival congestion. The polymorphous rash is often prominent in the diaper area. Such a rash in the setting of prolonged fever, pronounced lymphadenopathy, and polyarthralgias or arthritis in a child would strongly favor the diagnosis of Kawasaki disease.

Bacterial infections with exanthems include acute and chronic meningococcemia. A nonspecific measles-like eruption may antedate the petechial and purpuric lesions of acute meningococcemia. This diagnosis should be considered in a child or young adult who presents with prostration, fever, and morbilliform rash. Early polyarthralgia or polyarthritis during the bacteremic phase has been observed, and reactive pauciarthritis may occur days later [6]. Periodic fever, maculopapular skin rash, and arthritis may occur with chronic meningococcemia [7]. Lesions are often distributed near involved joints or over areas of pressure. They are variable in appearance but are most often macules or papules that later develop central hemorrhage. Petechiae, pustules, and erythema-nodosum-like lesions may also be seen.

Rocky Mountain spotted fever, a rickettsial disease, may have a maculopapular eruption before becoming purpuric. Diagnosis is aided by a characteristic evolution that begins in the distal parts of extremities and spreads centrally. This infection is often associated with arthralgias and myalgias, and rarely with severe muscle weakness, but not generally with arthritis [8,9]. Secondary syphilis should be considered in the sexually active patient with fever and diffuse maculopapular eruption, especially that involving palms and soles [10]. Toxic shock syndrome may express a scarlatiniform eruption similar to Kawasaki disease, and also a reactive arthropathy accompanied by fever and hypotension secondary to toxin-producing staphylococcal infection [11]. *Streptobacillus moniliformis* infection manifests a nonspecific diffuse maculopapular eruption with arthritis of large joints that occurs within a few days to 1 week after a bite from an infected rat or ingestion of contaminated rat excretions [12].

Viral infections [13,14] and drug reactions are the illnesses most commonly confused with Still's disease. Some viral rashes have a characteristic pattern and course. Rubella rash classically begins on the face and spreads rapidly to the neck, arms, trunk and legs, and resolves in the same order. The rash is of short duration, only 2–3 days, and arthritis usually develops as the rash fades. Human parvovirus B19 infection (erythema infectiosum) may be associated with a similar rash; the slapped cheek appearance and a lace-like body rash are more common in children than in adults [15]. Hepatitis B virus may commonly be associated with polyarthritis and rash but, in addition to erythematous papules, urticarial lesions are commonly observed. The presence of an enanthem, petechiae or vesicles, and localized lymphadenopathy may also suggest a viral illness, although mononucleosis, cytomegalovirus infection, and acute HIV infection [16] may be associated with diffuse lymphadenopathy and diffuse maculopapular rash. Arthralgias rather than frank arthritis are usually seen with these illnesses.

Drug eruptions usually develop almost simultaneously over the entire body, although the intensity may increase with time. The initial appearance may be in the flexure creases before becoming generalized [17]. Fever generally resolves within 3 days of stopping the drug. Erythema multiforme [18] may result from drug allergy or infection. The skin findings are characterized by round erythematous lesions which are symmetrically distributed, involving the palms, soles and oral mucosa. The presence of target lesions is helpful diagnostically (Fig. 3.4). The milder form of the disease, erythema multiforme minor, may be associated with fever and polyarthralgias. High fever and polyarthritis are common in erythema multiforme major (Stevens–Johnson syndrome), and this illness must be distinguished from Kawasaki disease. Inspection of the oral mucosa may help in this clinical differential diagnosis [19]. (See *Oral Lesions.*)

Rare disorders with rash, fever, and arthritis include familial Mediterranean fever [20], in which a characteristic erysipelas-like rash may exist on the lower extremity in conjunction with an acute monoarthritis and fever. Angio-immunoblastic lymphadenopathy [21] should be considered in the adult with fever, generalized morbilliform rash, polyarthritis and diffuse lymphadenopathy.

PAPULOSQUAMOUS LESIONS

Rheumatic diseases notable for papulosquamous lesions include psoriatic arthritis, Reiter's syndrome, and lupus erythematosus (subacute and discoid). Scale formation in patients with inflammatory cutaneous papules or plaques results from accumulation of the stratum corneum.

The characteristic lesions of psoriasis are sharply demarcated inflammatory plaques with a silvery scale most commonly present on extensor surfaces of the elbows and knees as well as the scalp, ears and presacral area (Fig. 3.5). Nail abnormalities are common. Pustular psoriasis results from a greater collection of neutrophils and therefore differs histologically from usual psoriasis only in a quantitative way [22]. The lesions of keratodermia blennorrhagica (Fig. 3.6) and pustular psoriasis are histologically identical, but Reiter's patients usually have lesions restricted to the palms and soles and are identified by other clinical characteristics, such as conjunctivitis and urethritis.

Scale formation is also a prominent feature of discoid lupus (Fig. 3.7) and the papulosquamous variety of subacute cutaneous lupus erythematosus (SCLE). In addition to an adherent scale, characteristic features of discoid lesions include follicular plugging, hyper- or hypopigmentation, atrophy (loss of skin markings), sclerosis, and telangiectasia. Lesions are most common on the face (but sparing the nasolabial folds), scalp, neck and ears. Lesions may occur elsewhere in the body only if also present above the neck [23]. Lesions of SCLE do not reveal signs of follicular plugging, pigmentary change or scarring and are distributed primarily on the shoulders, the extensor surface of the forearm and the upper back and upper chest. The face and scalp are generally spared and lesions below the waist are very rare. In the papulosquamous form of SCLE, papules may commonly enlarge and coalesce, leading to a reticulate pattern. Histopathologic studies are diagnostic, although immunofluorescence is not routinely positive in SCLE [23].

Lichen planus and pityriasis rosea may be confused with papulosquamous rashes due to rheumatic disease but have features which allow their differentiation. Lichen planus is a pruritic eruption with violet colored, polygonal, flat-topped lesions with thin white scales often present on flexor aspects of the wrists and ankles, the presacral area, glans penis and mucous membranes. Pityriasis rosea is manifested by erythematous papules with thin scaly borders following truncal lines of cleavage (Christmas tree pattern). The initial lesion, or herald spot, is larger than subsequent lesions. Lichen planus may occur secondary to gold or D-penicillamine therapy, and pityriasis rosea may be seen secondary to gold or antimalarial drug therapy [24]. Other systemic diseases with papulosquamous skin rash are T cell lymphoma [25] and secondary syphilis. The latter may appear as red-brown papules with thin scale, often present on the palms and soles and accompanied by annular plaques on the face, non-scarring alopecia and condyloma lata. Arthralgias are much more common than frank arthritis in secondary syphilis [10].

ANNULAR LESIONS

Three rheumatic illnesses, rheumatic fever, SCLE and Lyme disease, are suggested by characteristic annular or arciform skin lesions in which the central portion has a distinctive appearance compared with the border.

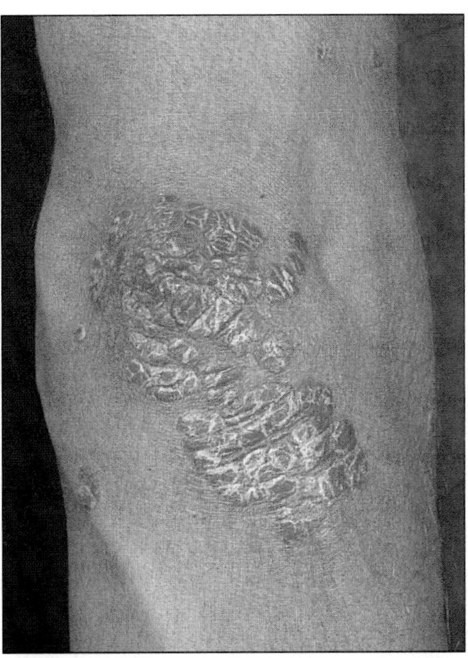

Fig. 3.5 Psoriatic plaque with characteristic silver scale. Reproduced, with permission, from Clinical Atlas of Dermatology, 2E, Anthony du Vivier, London, Gower, 1992.

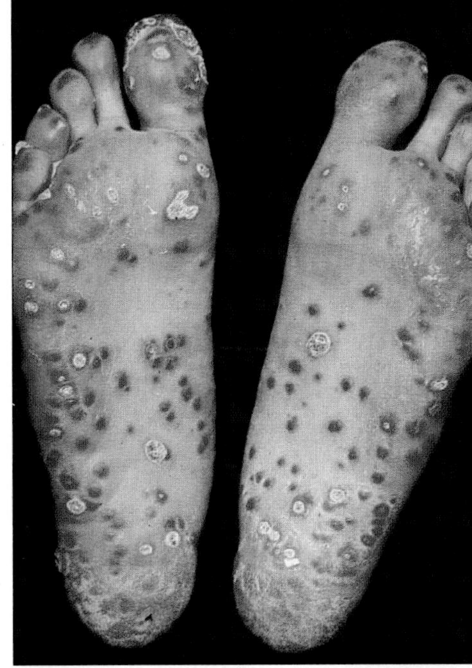

Fig. 3.6 Keratodermia blennorrhagica on the soles. Courtesy of Dr Stephen Wiener.

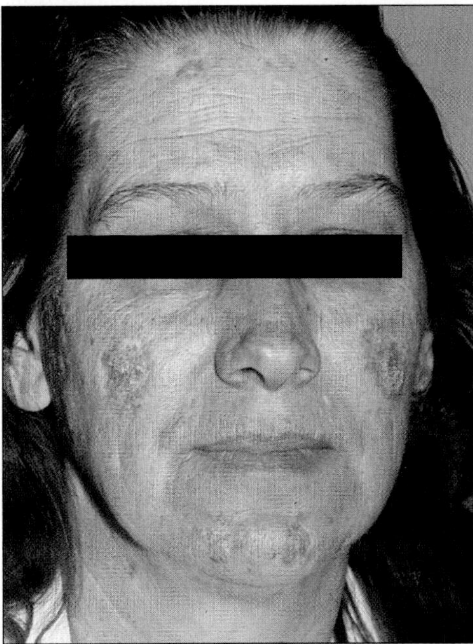

Fig. 3.7 Discoid lupus. Courtesy of Dr Stephen Wiener.

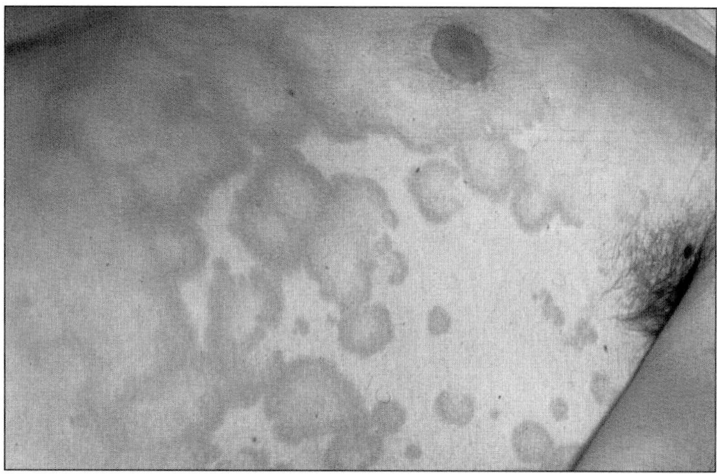

Fig. 3.8 Erythema marginatum. Reproduced from the Revised Clinical Slide Collection on the Rheumatic Diseases, 1981. Used by permission of the American College of Rheumatology. This is also the source of Figs. 3.3b and 3.16a.

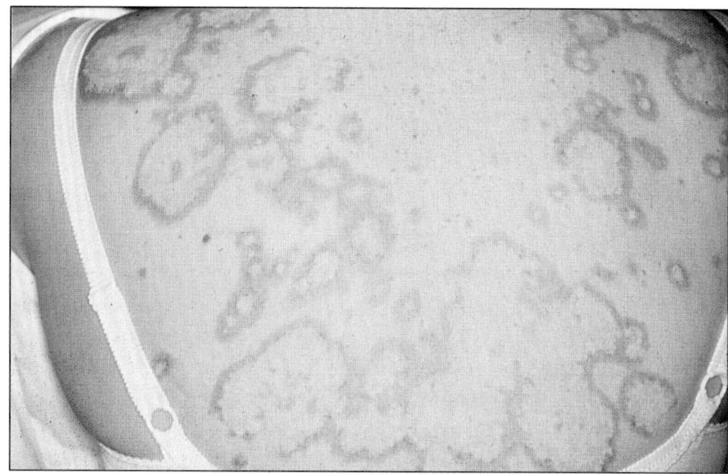

Fig. 3.9 Annular variety of subacute cutaneous lupus. Reproduced, with permission, from Sontheimer RD, et al. Ann Int Med. 1982: 664–71.

In rheumatic fever, migratory polyarthritis may be accompanied by erythema marginatum, an annular eruption with a round or serpiginous border which may be flat or slightly raised and is usually present on the trunk or proximal extremities (Fig. 3.8). Lesions migrate rapidly over a period of hours. The rash typically develops in crops lasting hours to several days [26].

The annular variety of SCLE (Fig. 3.9) is nonmigratory and has the same distribution as the papulosquamous variety. A form of primary cutaneous annular erythema, erythema annulare centrifigum, may occur in association with chloroquine therapy [19].

The primary lesion of erythema chronicum migrans (ECM), which is nearly pathognomonic of acute Lyme disease [27] is at the site of the tick bite, most often the axillae, groin, thigh, or buttocks (Fig. 3.10). The primary lesion migrates outward, much more slowly than that of erythema marginatum, and reaches an average size of 15cm. The central area may reveal blue discoloration, vesicles, purpura, necrosis, or ulceration. A target lesion may form. Secondary lesions are smaller, migrate less, and have less indurated centers. ECM spares the palms, soles and oral mucosa and commonly accompanies constitutional symptoms, headache and arthralgias. Recurrent ECM may be coincident with pauciarthritis.

Other distinctive annular lesions include elastosis perforans serpiginosa, which is seen as a side effect of D-penicillamine therapy and in congenital disorders of collagen, pseudoxanthoma elasticum, Marfan's syndrome, Ehlers-Danlos syndrome type IV and osteogenesis imperfecta [28]. Multiple concentric waves of erythematous rash resembling wood grain might suggest a diagnosis of erythema gyratum repens (Fig. 3.11), which is commonly associated with an underlying malignancy. Annular rashes may be observed in cutaneous granuloma annulare, cutaneous T cell lymphoma, secondary syphilis, sarcoid, erythema multiforme and psoriasis [28], and the clinical picture and histopathology are distinctive.

FACIAL LESIONS

In a patient with polyarthritis, dermatitis involving the face prompts consideration of a diagnosis of SLE. As discussed, discoid lupus has a virtually diagnostic appearance and distribution. Facial erythematous plaques and papules that might be confused with early discoid lesions include benign lymphocytic infiltration of Jessner and polymorphic light eruption [23]. Unlike discoid lupus, these lesions have no follicular plugging or scar. Seborrheic dermatitis is characterized by yellow greasy scale and involves the nasolabial folds (unlike discoid lupus), the eyebrows and hair line. Acne rosacea also involves the nasolabial folds and has pustules (Fig. 3.12). Tinea faciei, a dermatophyte infection that involves the face, can mimic or coexist with discoid lesions [29] but lacks follicular plugging, telangiectasia, and central atrophy [23].

Unfortunately, the histology of discoid skin lesions may be similar to that of polymorphic light eruption, Jessner's, seborrheic dermatitis,

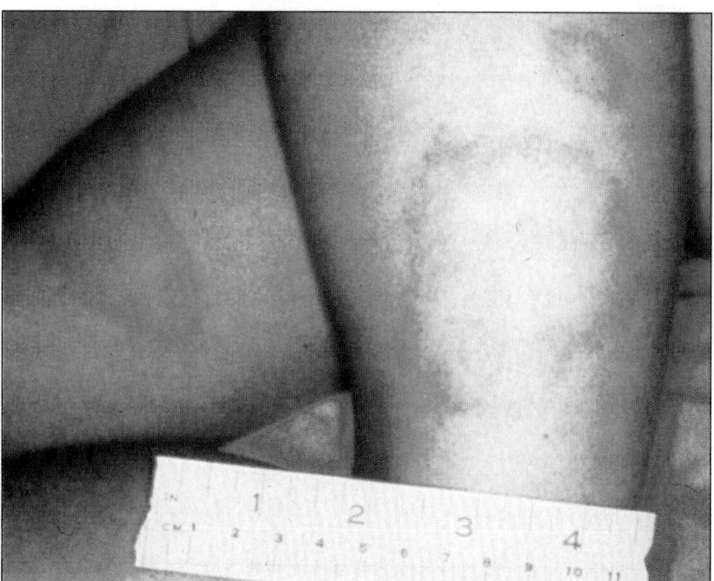

Fig. 3.10 Erythema chronicum migrans. Courtesy of Dr Kenneth DeBenedictus.

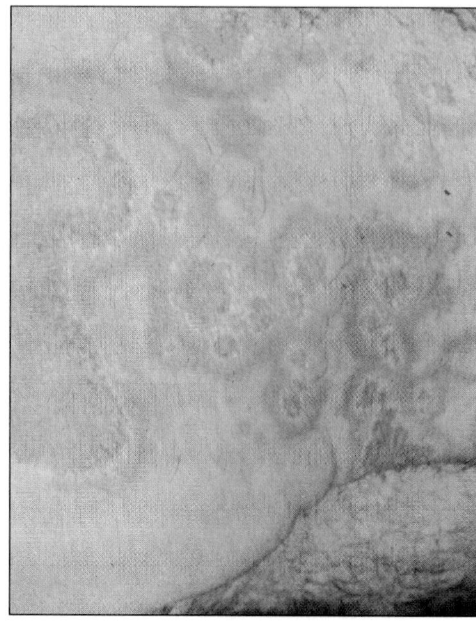

Fig. 3.11 Erythema gyratum. Courtesy of Dr Stephen Wiener.

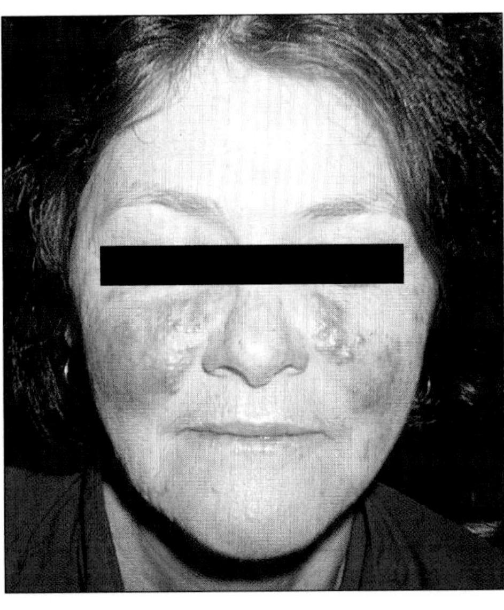

Fig. 3.12 Acne rosacea. Courtesy of Dr Stephen Wiener.

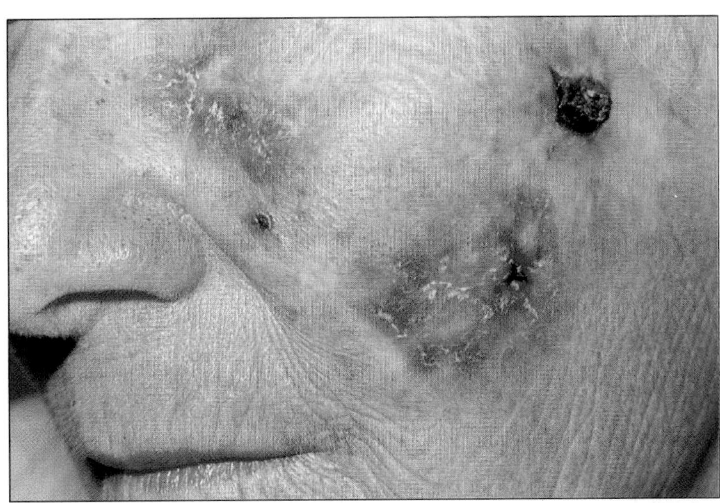

Fig. 3.13 Lupus vulgaris. Reproduced, with permission, from Clinical Atlas of Dermatology, Anthony du Vivier, London, Gower, 1986.

and acne rosacea. When there is any question, immunopathologic studies should be done. Immunofluorescent deposits at the dermal–epidermal junction occur in polymorphous light eruption, porphyria, rosacea, and lichen planus, but the immunofluorescence patterns of these diseases can be distinguished from discoid lupus [30]. However, in the first 2 months of rash immunofluorescence studies of discoid lesions are often negative.

Cutaneous tuberculosis may produce a facial lesion, lupus vulgaris, that may be mistaken for discoid lupus (Fig. 3.13). Lupus vulgaris begins as a solitary papule or nodule and slowly extends, leaving central scarring and atrophy. Smooth yellow-brown nodules may be seen in the periphery (apple jelly appearance) by the technique of diascopy [31]. Cutaneous sarcoid is pleomorphic and its purplish plaques and papules, without scale or atrophy, may be present in a distribution similar to that of discoid lupus. Lupus pernio is a form of chronic sarcoid lesion that may be present either as small nodules on the nose or nodules or plaques upon the cheeks and ears (Fig. 3.14). These lesions are often associated with asymptomatic bone cysts, progressive pulmonary fibrosis and upper respiratory involvement [32]. Accompanying chronic polyarthritis is rare. Both lupus vulgaris and sarcoidosis may be easily diagnosed by skin biopsy.

Acute lupus eruptions must be distinguished from other types of photosensitive dermatitis. The malar rash of acute lupus may be flat (malar blush) or slightly raised (butterfly eruption) [33]. There is no atrophy or sclerosis and little scale. Nasolabial folds are not involved. This rash may resolve over hours or it may persist for days. The facial rash of acute lupus may be more widespread than the malar area. The chin is often involved but the area below the chin is spared. A heliotrope eruption similar to that of dermatomyositis may be observed. Features of dermatomyositis rash [34] (Fig. 3.15) that might allow discrimination from lupus include occasional nasolabial fold involvement, erythema over the interphalangeal joints rather than the extensor surface of skin between phalangeal joints (see Fig. 3.16), erythema following the course of extensor tendons, and scaling and fissuring of lateral aspects of the fingers (mechanics hands). The presence of papules with erythema over the interphalangeal joints, Gottron's papules, is pathognomonic for dermatomyositis.

Early acne rosacea and carcinoid may reveal episodic malar erythema secondary to vascular dilation that may be confused with the

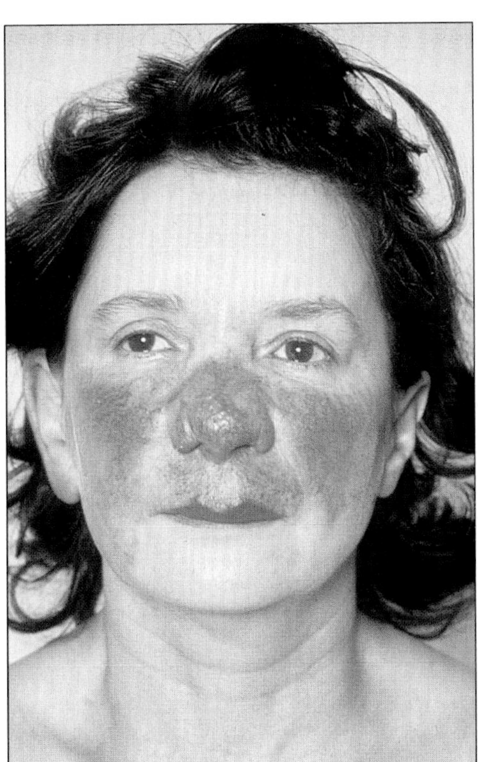

Fig. 3.14 Lupus pernio. Reproduced, with permission, from Clinical Atlas of Dermatology, Anthony du Vivier, London, Gower, 1986.

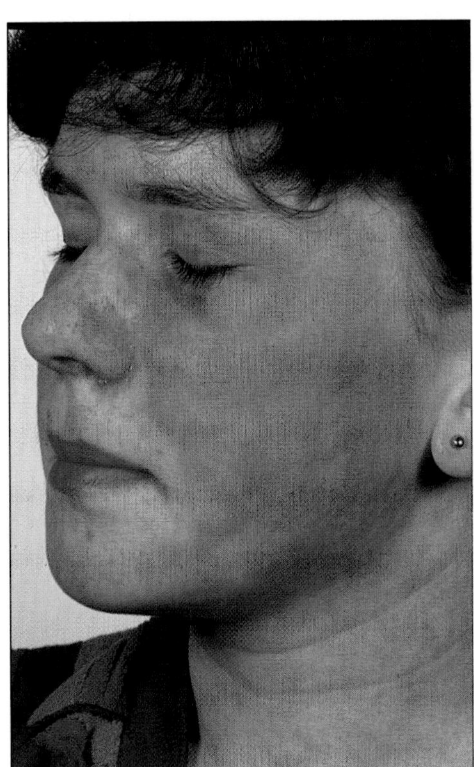

Fig. 3.15 Dermatomyositis. Reproduced, with permission, from Clinical Atlas of Dermatology, 2E, Anthony du Vivier, London, Gower, 1992.

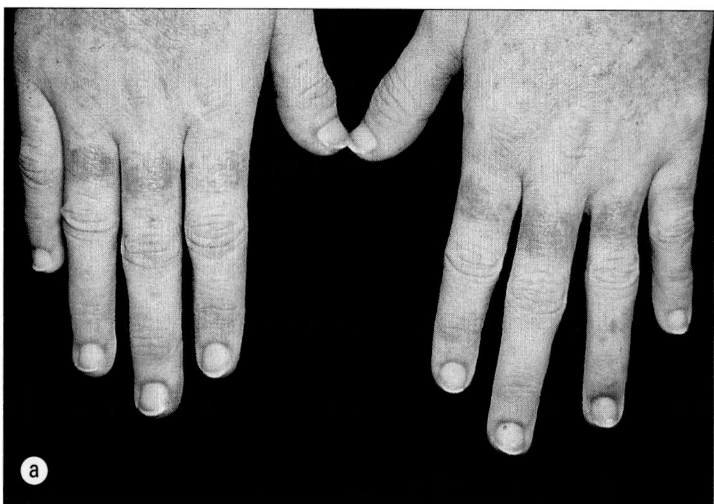

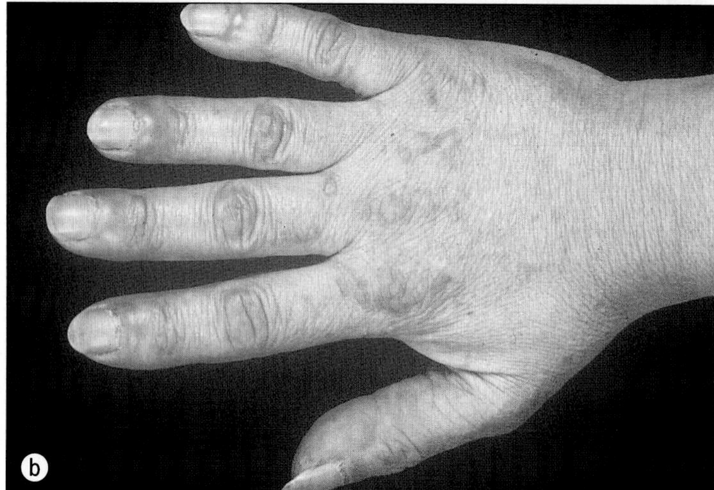

Fig. 3.16 Acute lupus (a); Dermatomyositis (b). Reproduced, with permission, from Dermatology in Practice, Anthony du Vivier, London, Gower, 1990.

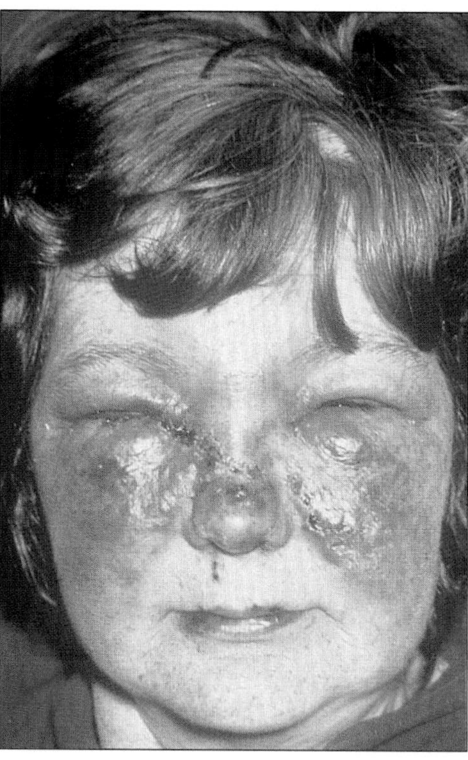

Fig. 3.17 Erysipelas. Reproduced, with permission, from Infectious Diseases, 2E, W Edmund Farrar et al., London, Gower, 1991.

malar blush of acute lupus. Rarely, erysipelas may present as an acute inflammation with a butterfly distribution (Fig. 3.17).

PHOTOSENSITIVE SKIN RASH

Photosensitive cutaneous eruptions are common in systemic and discoid lupus erythematosus and may be observed in dermatomyositis patients. There may sometimes be confusion about patients presenting with other photosensitive eruptions such as photoallergic or phototoxic drug eruptions, polymorphic light eruption, porphyrias, and nutritional deficiency (pellagra). In addition, a number of genetic deficiency states, for example Bloom's syndrome and xeroderma pigmentosum [35], may be associated with photosensitive reactions.

Photoallergic or phototoxic drug eruptions occur with sulfa drugs, thiazides, phenothiazines, tetracycline, and piroxicam. The reaction with piroxicam often occurs within several days of the first exposure [36,37].

Polymorphic light eruption is a relatively common disorder occurring in as many as 10% of the population [37]. Its appearance includes papules, plaques, hemorrhagic lesions and vesicles, although in any individual one type of lesion predominates. Lesions occur hours to days after sun exposure and are often preceded and accompanied by pruritus, a feature atypical for lupus. Unlike discoid lupus lesions the polymorphous light eruptions do not have telangiectases, follicular plugging or atrophy and do not involve the scalp, ear or covered areas [38]. Serum antinuclear antibody (ANA) and anti-Ro antibody are routinely negative in this disorder.

Some porphyrias, such as porphyria cutanea tarda, may express skin lesions in photosensitive areas, particularly vesicular or bullous lesions and skin fragility (Fig. 3.18), which will be followed later by skin sclerosis [39]. Antimalarial drugs may precipitate acute toxic hepatitis in patients with porphyria cutanea tarda.

Pellagra or niacin deficiency may be associated with a photosensitive eruption accompanied by gastrointestinal and psychological disturbances. Such patients routinely have glossitis, mucosal erythematous patches and ulcers prior to onset of the skin lesions [40].

URTICARIA

Diseases that might be considered in the setting of urticaria and arthritis include hepatitis B infection [41], serum sickness [42], primary urticarial vasculitis, mononucleosis, and C1q complement deficiency [43].

Leukocytoclastic vasculitis is the pathologic process in a small number of patients with urticaria (urticarial vasculitis). Such urticaria is more likely to be associated with symptoms of burning or pain, rather than pruritis, tends to resolve more slowly (generally in not less than 4 hours and up to about 72 hours), and may have a purpuric component. Secondary skin changes of pigmentation, scaling or purpura may be found after resolution of the urticaria.

Arthralgias may be observed in chronic urticaria resulting from processes other than leukocytoclastic vasculitis, but arthritis generally suggests underlying vasculitis [44]. The erythrocyte sedimentation rate is nearly always elevated in patients with urticarial vasculitis, and early components of complement are depressed in about 50% of cases of primary urticarial vasculitis [45].

NODULAR LESIONS

The character and distribution of cutaneous and subcutaneous nodules are critical in the evaluation of patients with diseases such as rheumatoid arthritis (RA), rheumatic fever, crystal deposition diseases, atypical infections, panniculitis, vasculitis and malignancy. Rheumatoid nodules [46] are firm, nontender, flesh colored subcutaneous lesions about 0.5–4cm in diameter which may be movable or fixed to periosteum or deep fascia. They are observed most commonly over areas of pressure and are found in about 20% of

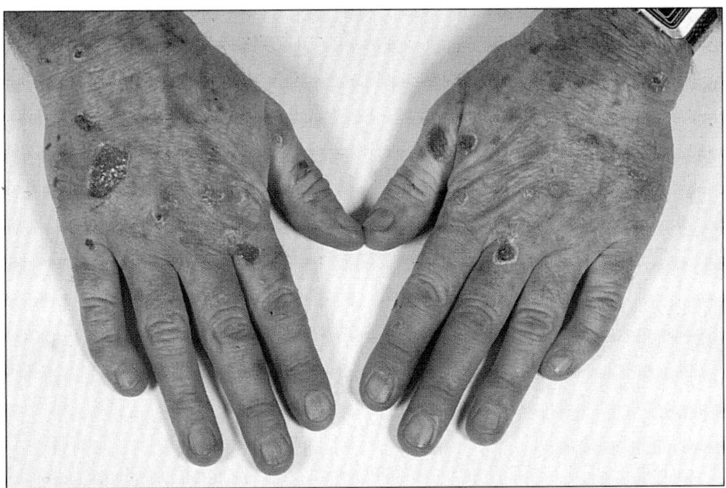

Fig. 3.18 Porphyria cutanea tarda. Reproduced, with permission, from Clinical Atlas of Dermatology, 2E, Anthony du Vivier, London, Gower, 1992.

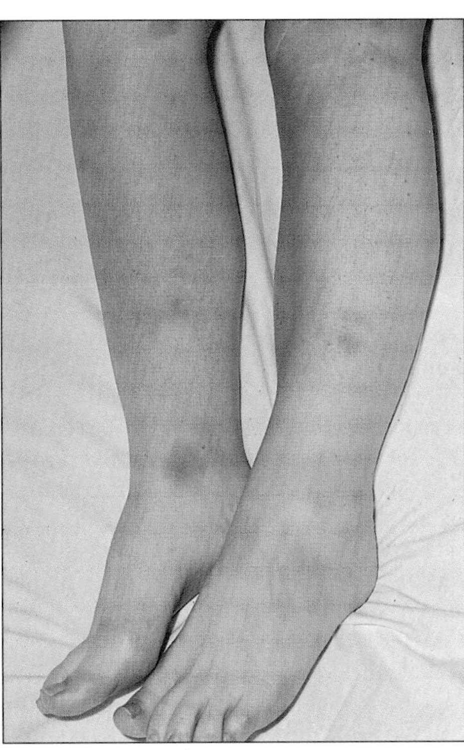

Fig. 3.19 Erythema nodosum - tender subcutaneous nodules on the lower legs. By permission of St Mary's Hospital Medical School, London.

patients with RA and a small fraction of lupus patients [47]. Nearly all of these patients are observed to be serologically positive for rheumatoid factor.

Rheumatoid nodules may be pathologically indistinguishable from necrobiosis lipoidica diabeticorum (NLD), or granuloma annulare (GA), but these disorders do not present a problem of clinical differential diagnosis since NLD is most commonly observed as a pretibial subcutaneous nodule in the diabetic patient and GA is usually intracutaneous rather than subcutaneous. However, generalized GA is more commonly seen in patients with RA and lupus [48].

Rheumatic-fever-associated nodules are also firm, nontender lesions in areas of pressure but tend to be smaller, usually less than 1cm [47], and shorter-lived (the average duration is 4–6 days, and the lesions rarely last longer than 1 month). These nodules tend to form in crops late in the course of the illness. Patients with rheumatic nodules usually manifest signs of carditis. Rheumatic nodules at the elbow tend to occur at the point of the olecranon, rather than several centimeters distal as with rheumatoid nodules.

Tophi secondary to uric acid deposits may produce subcutaneous nodules with a distribution similar to those of rheumatoid nodules. Helpful discriminating features include asymmetry, DIP joint involvement, involvement of the helix of the ear, origin at the joint margin rather than adjacent tissue, yellow appearance, overlying erythema, history of recurrent monoarthritis, asymmetric joint involvement, and absence of a positive rheumatoid factor. Such signs should prompt joint aspiration and possible nodule biopsy to define the histopathology. A portion of the pathologic specimen should be placed in ethanol rather than formaldehyde to prevent dissolution of monosodium urate crystals.

Periarticular deposits of calcium crystals (pyrophosphate dihydrate, hydroxyapatite and oxalate) may rarely produce subcutaneous nodules and inflammatory or mechanical joint symptoms [49–51]. In oxalosis, miliary intradermal papules of calcium are more characteristic than nodule formation.

Achilles tendonitis in association with subcutaneous nodules of cholesterol at the tendon may be observed in the homozygous and heterozygous forms of type II hyperlipoproteinemia. In the homozygous state patients may also develop subcutaneous nodules over extensor surfaces of the knees and elbows and a migratory polyarthritis of large joints [47].

Multicentric reticulohistiocytosis [52] is a rare disorder associated with a destructive polyarthritis and multiple nodules. These nodules are usually cutaneous rather than subcutaneous, light copper to red–brown and often involve the hands, forearm and face. Periungual lesions, 'coral beads', are also characteristic. Unlike RA, multicentric reticulohistiocytosis commonly involves the DIP joint. This entity is frequently associated with occult malignancy.

Farber disease is a rare autosomal recessive lysosomal storage disorder associated with subcutaneous periarticular swelling and mucopolysaccharide-containing nodules, peripheral joint arthropathy, and progressive neurologic deterioration which leads to death in early childhood [47]. Neurofibromatosis should be considered in the patient with soft nontender cutaneous or subcutaneous nodules, light brown macules (café au lait spots) and symptoms of nerve compression or signs of kyphoscoliosis [53]

Red and tender subcutaneous nodules may occur in panniculitis, arteritis, atypical infections and metastatic tumor. The location of nodules, their propensity to scar, and their histopathology assist differential diagnosis [3,54,55].

Erythema nodosum (EN) lesions are red or violet subcutaneous nodules, 1-5cm in diameter, without associated epidermal abnormalities (Fig. 3.19). The pathology shows a septal panniculitis without vasculitis. EN nodules usually develop in pretibial locations and resolve spontaneously over several weeks without ulceration or scarring. The lesions may develop less frequently on the thighs, arms, face, neck, and trunk [55]. Whether idiopathic or associated with a known precipitant, EN lesions are often accompanied by acute polyarthralgias or arthritis predominantly in large joints of the lower extremities. A diagnosis of EN should prompt consideration of primary immune processes, for example sarcoidosis (Lofgren's syndrome), or inflammatory bowel disease, Behçet's disease, the effects of drugs (sulfa, birth control pills), pregnancy and infections (post-β hemolytic streptococcus, *Mycobacterium tuberculosis* or *M. leprae,* fungus, *Yersinia, Chlamydia,* etc.)

Erythematous subcutaneous nodules that are unusually painful, develop in locations other than the pretibial region, ulcerate or scar, persist for more than several weeks, or are not in association with the above diseases, may be expressions of a different pathologic entity. Weber–Christian disease is an idiopathic lobular panniculitis with fever, polyarthralgias and painful subcutaneous nodules more widespread than in erythema nodosum and which often ulcerate or scar (secondary to fat necrosis). Panniculitis with pancreatitis or pancreatic carcinoma may manifest similar skin lesions and polyarthritis. Serum lipase levels are often elevated. Excisional biopsy will reveal a lobular panniculitis often with characteristic 'ghost-like' fat cells, presumed to be due to the enzyme effects upon the adipose cell.

Lupus profundus is a lobular panniculitis found on the face, upper arms or buttocks. Overlying cutaneous involvement with discoid lesions is common. The lupus band test in the overlying skin is positive in about 70% of cases [55]. This entity usually follows a chronic course associated with local scarring.

Diffuse granulomas in the subcutaneous tissue may also produce lobular panniculitis in sarcoidosis, although the septal panniculitis of EN is a much more common expression [56].

Erythema induratum (nodular panniculitis) is a lobular panniculitis with local vasculitis which may be idiopathic or associated with tuberculosis. Unlike EN nodules, the nodules of erythema induratum are commonly on the calf and tend to ulcerate [55]. Erythema nodosum leprosum lesions tend to be more widespread, and upper extremity joint involvement is seen more often than in primary EN [57].

Necrotizing arteritis such as polyarteritis nodosa may be associated with painful cutaneous and subcutaneous nodules. These lesions tend to be smaller than those of EN. They develop in crops and are found most commonly on the lower legs and feet, especially along the course of arteries, although they may have a widespread distribution. Other skin lesions, such as purpura and livedo reticularis, may also be present [3].

Polyarthralgias may accompany erythema elevatum diutinum, nodular skin lesions secondary to leukocytoclastic vasculitis. These vasculitic lesions have a predilection for extensor surfaces of joints as well as skin overlying the buttocks and Achilles tendons [58].

Nodules adjacent to an inflammatory joint or tendon sheath should prompt consideration of local infections, such as sporotrichosis (Fig. 3.20), atypical mycobacterial infection and treponemal infections [47]. Ulceration develops frequently.

Cutaneous and subcutaneous nodules may also result from infiltration of metastatic tumor cells. When there are multiple nodules, hematologic malignancies are most common [25].

VESICLES AND BULLAE

Vesicles and bullae result from a disturbance of intra-epidermal coherence or dermal–epidermal adherence [59]. A host of pathologic mechanisms may lead to blistering of the skin. Two blistering eruptions are seen in SLE. First, a generalized bullous eruption may develop in normal appearing or erythematous skin (bullous eruption of SLE). This eruption is bullous-pemphigoid-like and has histological similarities to dermatitis herpetiformis: it may be dapsone responsive. Unlike dermatitis herpetiformis, it is not pruritic and is more widespread. Immunofluorescence and electron microscopic studies may be helpful diagnostically [60,61]. Second, blistering may be seen in areas of photosensitive dermatitis. Such lesions must be distinguished from the rash of porphyria cutanea tarda, which is seen occasionally in the lupus patient [62].

Some primary immune skin disorders have been described at increased frequency in a number of rheumatic diseases [62]. Bullous pemphigoid is significantly more common in the rheumatoid patient and has been described in SLE, polymyositis, and primary biliary cirrhosis. Dermatitis herpetiformis is commonly associated with autoimmune thyroid disease and has been reported in RA, Sjögren's syndrome, dermatomyositis, and ulcerative colitis. Pemphigus has been described in patients with SLE, RA, Sjögren's syndrome and lymphomatoid granulomatosis. Pemphigus foliaceous may result from a D-penicillamine reaction.

Vesicles and bullae may accompany more characteristic lesions in patients with necrotizing vasculitis, ecthyma gangrenosum and disseminated intravascular coagulation (DIC). Blistering may also be a prominent feature in erythema multiforme major, and short-lived bullae may be seen in staphylococcal scalded skin syndrome. Musculoskeletal symptoms may accompany each of these entities.

Localized or generalized vesicles may also be seen in varicella or herpes viral infections. Tzanck test or culture may be helpful [63]. Lesions of ECM may vesiculate centrally.

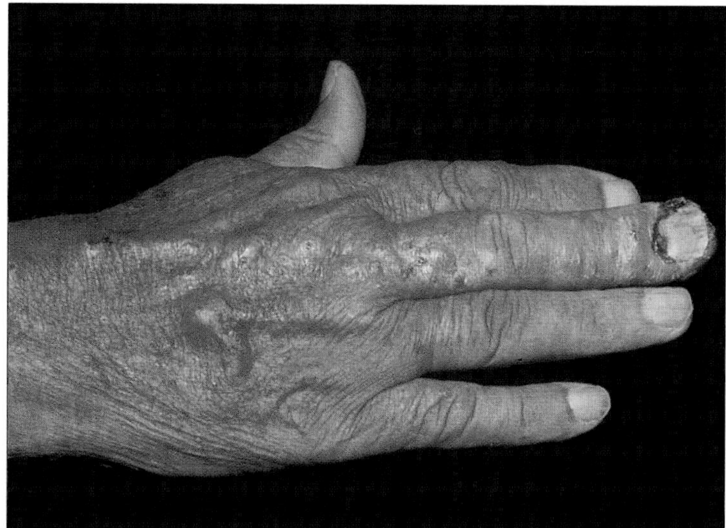

Fig.3.20 Sporotrichosis. Several secondary nodules are apparent along lymphatic channels. Courtesy of Dr TF Sellers Jr.

PUSTULAR LESIONS

Pustular skin lesions in patients with rheumatic disease include pustular vasculitis associated with several bowel-associated processes, Sweet's syndrome, Behçet's disease, disorders with palmar and plantar pustular skin lesions, and disorders associated with severe forms of acne. In addition, disseminated gonococcemia (Fig. 3.21), chronic meningococcemia, disseminated viral infections such as varicella and disseminated herpes simplex, and reactions to drugs (especially sulfa drugs, hydantoins and halogen compounds) may produce disseminated pustular lesions [63].

Patients who have undergone ileo-jejunal bypass surgery for obesity frequently manifest episodic painful cutaneous pustules on a purpuric base. The papules are seen primarily on the upper extremities and upper trunk and are associated with fever, polyarthralgias, and polyarthritis. A similar syndrome is seen in patients with inflammatory bowel disease and those having undergone Billroth II surgery, thus prompting the descriptive term bowel-associated dermatosis–arthritis syndrome [64].

Patients with Sweet's syndrome (acute febrile neutrophilic dermatosis) may also present with painful papulonodules or pustules [65] (Fig. 3.22). Although painful oral and genital ulcers are most characteristic of Behçet's syndrome, pustular skin lesions, especially at

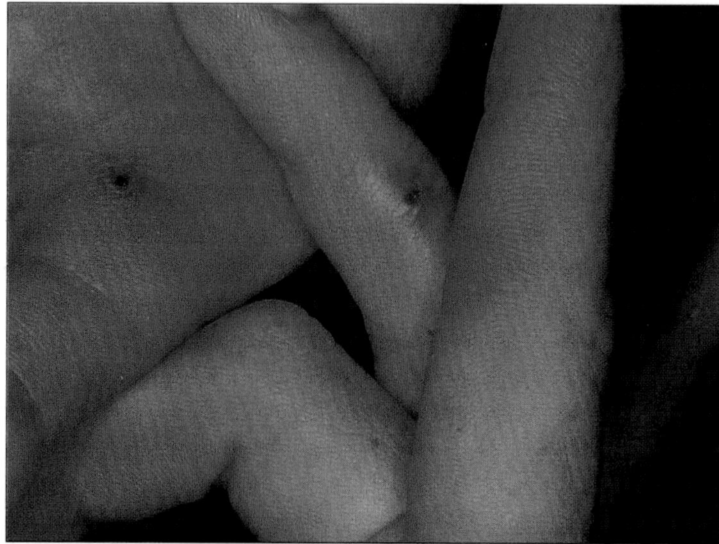

Fig. 3.21 Gonococcemia. Acral pustular lesions with central necrosis. Reproduced, with permission, from Clinical Atlas of Dermatology, 2E, Anthony du Vivier, London, Gower, 1992.

sites of minor trauma (e.g, needlestick pathergy), should also lead to its consideration. The arthritis is frequently pauciarticular in these disorders. Histology of pustular skin lesions may be similar in Behçet's syndrome, Sweet's syndrome and bowel-associated dermatitis–arthritis [64].

Isolated palmar and plantar pustulosis, pustular psoriasis, and keratodermia blennorrhagica are identical pathologically. Patients with psoriasis and keratodermia blennorrhagica may have symptoms of spondyloarthropathy. An association of palmar pustulosis with sternal clavicular hyperostosis and chronic recurrent multifocal osteomyelitis (CRMO) has been described [66].

Severe forms of acne have also been associated with rheumatic illnesses [67]. Acne fulminans has also been associated with sternal clavicular hyperostosis and CRMO. The patients described have usually been young, white males who become acutely ill with fever, weight loss, arthralgias, myalgias and multiple inflammatory skin lesions with ulceration on the back and chest. Acne conglobata and related illnesses exhibit extensive cystic and nodular acne on the buttocks, thighs and upper arms as well as the conventional locations of acne vulgaris. Some of these patients, most notably young black males, have a higher frequency of spondyloarthropathy and sternal clavicular hyperostosis. Isotretinoin, a vitamin A derivative used for severe acne, has been associated with mild myalgias and arthralgias which often resolve spontaneously without cessation of therapy, and with axial skeletal hyperostoses.

PURPURA

Purpura, nonblanching erythematous lesions, should be evaluated by size and palpability [68]. Petechiae are characteristic of platelet disorders. They result from leakage of erythrocytes from dermal capillaries where platelet plugs serve as the major source of coagulation. Larger collections of blood form ecchymoses that are due to leakage from arterioles or venules at sites of minor trauma; ecchymoses are also common in platelet and other bleeding disorders. These lesions are not usually palpable unless bleeding occurs into an unrelated inflammatory lesion.

Nonpalpable purpura result from extravasation of erythrocytes in the absence of inflammation. Causes of nonpalpable purpura in the patient with rheumatic complaints include: platelet deficiency states such as immune thrombocytopenia; vascular fragility as observed in primary amyloid, scurvy, and genetic disorders of collagen formation; reduced integrity of supportive connective tissue as observed in steroid therapy; and vessel thrombosis or nonseptic emboli such as thrombotic thrombocytopenic purpura, cholesterol emboli, and marantic endocarditis [28].

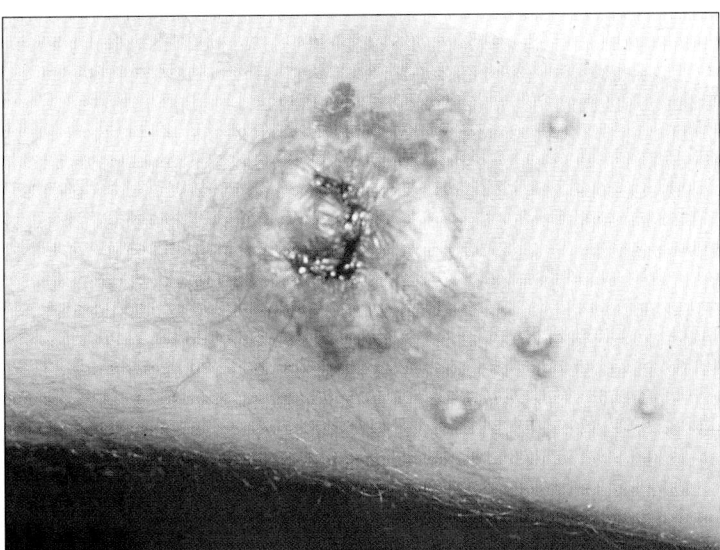

Fig. 3.22 Sweet's syndrome. Erythematous plaque with pustulation and ulceration. Courtesy of Dr Kenneth DeBenedictus.

In primary amyloid, vascular fragility results from infiltration of the vessel with amyloid light chain protein. Purpura is most common in the periorbital region, at skin folds and in areas of minor trauma (pinch purpura). Patients may manifest polyarthritis secondary to amyloid infiltration of synovium. In scurvy, altered collagen formation probably contributes to vascular fragility [69] and the lesions are rarely palpable. Perifollicular hemorrhage with central corkscrew hairs on the lower extremities is characteristic. Hemorrhage into muscle or joints may occur. Cholesterol emboli, a consequence of severe atherosclerotic vessel disease may mimic vasculitis and characteristically involves the lower extremity with purpura, livedo reticularis, nodules, and ischemic ulcers [28,70]. Rickettsial and certain viral illnesses (echovirus and coxsackie viral infections) may show petechial lesions in the course of the illness.

Palpable Purpura

Petechiae and flat purpuric lesions are rarely observed in necrotizing angiitis [71] because vascular inflammation leads to increased permeability. Palpable hemorrhage of lesions of the dermis should suggest vasculitis or embolus associated with an infectious agent.

Palpable purpura in dependent locations (areas with increased orthostatic pressure, such as the buttocks or lower extremities), is the most common presentation of necrotizing venulitis (Fig. 3.23). Lesions are round or oval secondary to radial diffusion of erythrocytes from the postcapillary venules of the upper vascular plexus of the dermis [71]. The differential diagnosis includes chronic bacterial infection, acute hepatitis B infection, drug reaction, associated lymphoproliferative disorder, associated rheumatic disease, and Henoch–Schönlein purpura (HSP). Biopsy within 24–48 hours helps define the inflammatory nature of the lesion. The presence of IgA immunofluorescent deposits at the dermal–epidermal junction supports the presence of HSP. In isolated leukocytoclastic vasculitis the prognosis is generally good; nevertheless, necrotizing venulitis may be associated with larger vessel vasculitis and should prompt a careful search for systemic necrotizing arteritis [72]. Signs of necrotizing arteritis include irregularly outlined purpura, since inflammation and thrombosis of deep dermal and subcutaneous vessels result

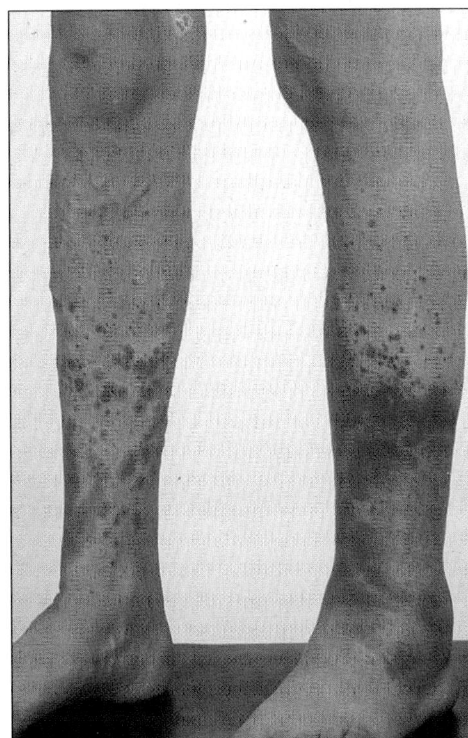

Fig. 3.23 Palpable purpura of necrotizing venulitis (Henoch-Shönlein purpura). Reproduced, with permission, from Dermatology in Practice, Anthony du Vivier, London, Gower, 1990.

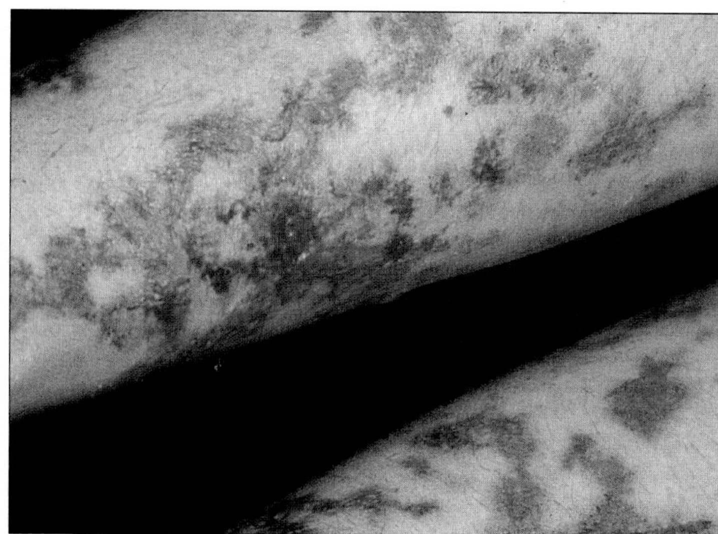

Fig. 3.24 Polyarteritis nodosa with irregular purpura, livedo reticularis, and necrosis. Courtesy of American Academy of Dermatology.

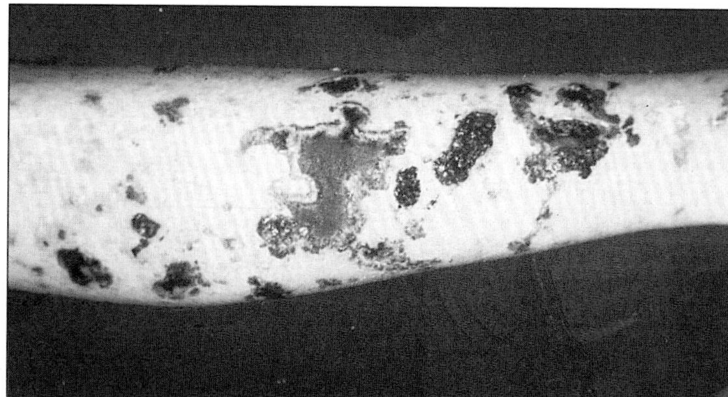

Fig. 3.25 Purpura fulminans with secondary skin necrosis. Reproduced, with permission, from Infectious Diseases, 2E, W Edmund Farrar et al., London, Gower, 1991.

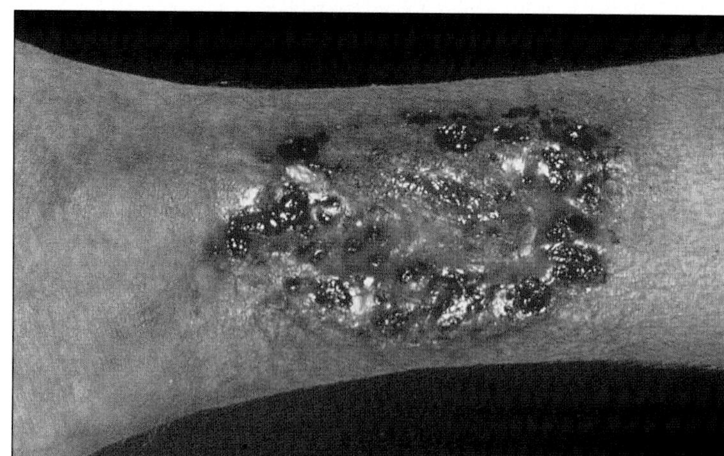

Fig. 3.26 Pyoderma gangrenosum. Reproduced, with permission, from Clinical Atlas of Dermatology, 2E, Anthony du Vivier, London, Gower, 1992.

in areas of hemorrhage and infarction [71]. Cutaneous nodules, livedo reticularis, digital infarcts and deep cutaneous ulcers (Fig. 3.24) are also seen.

Acute onset of purpuric lesions in the febrile patient is sepsis until otherwise proven [73]. Acute meningococcemia begins as small, irregular, often palpable purpura which are more widely distributed and less symmetrical than leukocyclastic vasculitis. The lesions may progress rapidly over hours to extensive bullous and irregular hemorrhagic lesions with central necrotic gunmetal gray patches (Fig. 3.25). The vascular lesions come from direct invasion of the organism as well as being secondary to DIC.

Gram-negative infection may embolize to the skin (ecthyma gangrenosum) and also seed the joint. The skin lesions are erythematous wheals or papules with irregular areas of purpura followed by necrosis and ulceration. The morphology of wheal or papule containing an irregular purpuric area is a specific sign of septicemia with gram-negative organisms including gonococcus, meningococcus, *Klebsiella* spp., *Pseudomonas* spp. and *Escherichia coli* [74].

ULCERS

Vascular, infectious and tumor-associated causes must be considered in the patient with cutaneous ulceration and musculoskeletal symptoms. Ulcerations secondary to ischemia may result from vasospasm in Raynaud's phenomenon, vascular thrombosis in antiphospholipid syndrome or paraproteinemia, and vascular necrosis in necrotizing venulitis or arteritis. Other skin findings and associated systemic signs and symptoms differentiate among these causes.

Lower extremity ulcers in the debilitated rheumatoid patient [75–78] present a common diagnostic dilemma. The differential diagnosis includes vasculitis, pyoderma gangrenosum, pressure sores, infection and vascular insufficiency. Pyoderma gangrenosum (Fig. 3.26) is observed more commonly in patients with RA, inflammatory bowel disease, Behçet's syndrome, Wegener's granulomatosis, paraproteinemias, or chronic active hepatitis [79].

Pyoderma gangrenosum is a rare ulcerating lesion of unknown cause which begins as a nodule or hemorrhagic pustule that breaks down to form a painful ulcer with an irregular, undermined, raised violacious border. The lesion is usually single and is most commonly observed in the lower extremities, buttock or abdomen. Such lesions often develop at sites of previous minor trauma. Pathologic specimens may be suggestive of this entity but are not diagnostic. Differential diagnosis of the lesion includes necrotizing arteritis and infectious causes, including atypical mycobacterial or fungal infection, amoebiasis, tropical ulcer and anaerobic bacterial synergistic gangrene (Meleney's ulcer) [28,79].

Rheumatoid vasculitic ulcers classically develop suddenly on the calves or dorsum of the foot [80] They are multiple, painful, have a 'punched out' appearance and an indurated base, and may enlarge rapidly (Fig. 3.27). They are most often seen in patients with long standing erosive nodular RA, especially those with Felty's syndrome or other signs of vasculitis. Chronic superficial leg or sacral ulcers are also observed in rheumatoid patients with other signs of vasculitis, but these lesions are less specific [80]. Venous stasis ulcers are most common in the ankle area, especially near the medial malleolus, and are painless unless there is secondary infection. These ulcers are shallow and wide and have an irregular outline. They are often surrounded by thick and hyperpigmented skin secondary to the chronic venous insufficiency.

Venous insufficiency ulcers are common in the rheumatoid patient because of reduced skin integrity, increased venous stasis due to inactivity, and possibly reduced venous muscle pump activity secondary to reduced ankle mobility [81].

Ulcers occur over bony prominences associated with undue pressure. They can become quite deep and are frequently infected in patients with severe peripheral neuropathies. Painful ulceration with pale edges on the toes and dorsum of the foot, or the heel, and poor granulation tissue in a leg with trophic changes and reduced peripheral arterial pulse pressures suggest arterial insufficiency ulcers on an atherosclerotic basis. Vasculitis may reduce the threshold of pressure or atherosclerotic disease that will produce ischemia and ulceration.

Other ulcerating lesions may be of assistance in differentiating various immune diseases. For example, perianal ulcers secondary to cutaneous granulomatous disease may be seen in Crohn's disease [82]. Genital ulcers are often a sign of Behçet's syndrome.

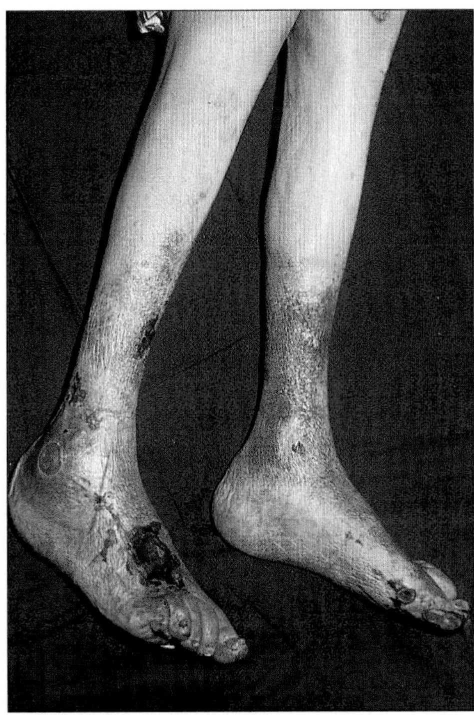

Fig. 3.27 Rheumatoid vasculitic ulceration in various stages of evolution.

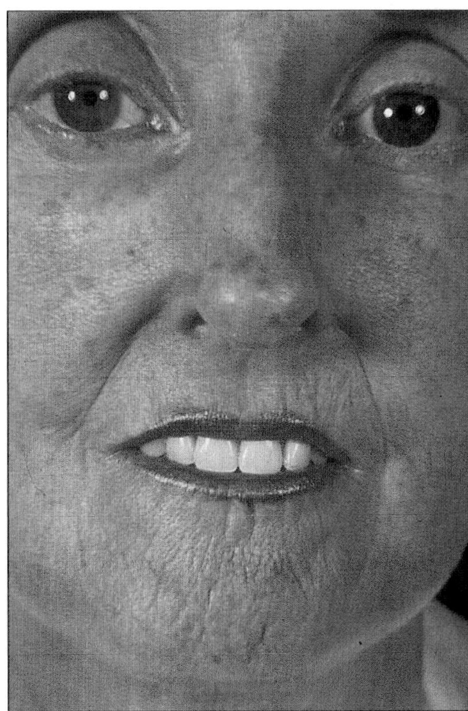

Fig. 3.28 Mat telangiectases in a patient with scleroderma. Reproduced, with permission, from Dermatology in Practice, Anthony du Vivier, London, Gower, 1990.

DERMAL SCLEROSIS

Fibrosis of the skin producing visible and palpable thickening is a characteristic feature of scleroderma. Attention to the appearance, distribution, and histopathology of the involved skin can be helpful in distinguishing between patients with scleroderma and those with scleroderma-like abnormalities [83]. The distribution of involvement helps to distinguish the limited form of scleroderma (formerly the CREST syndrome) variant from progressive systemic sclerosis. The CREST variant does not generally produce scleroderma of the proximal extremities or of the trunk and has a more benign prognosis.

Eosinophilic fasciitis [84] and eosinophilic myalgia syndrome associated with tryptophan ingestion might be suggested in a patient with cutaneous sclerosis of the extremities sparing the hands and feet. These patients usually lack Raynaud's phenomenon nailfold abnormalities and body telangiectases. Development of peau d'orange is common. Severe myalgias are common and polyarthritis has been described. The presence of fascial inflammation upon biopsy may be helpful in excluding scleroderma [85].

Sclerodactyly and bound down skin over the dorsum of the hands with joint contractures are common findings in the patient with long standing diabetes mellitus [86]. Obese, non-insulin-dependent diabetes mellitus patients may develop a benign skin tightening called scleredema that develops rapidly over the neck and upper back [86].

Patients with monoclonal gammopathies with scleroderma-like skin lesions have been described. POEMS syndrome (polyneuropathy, organomegaly, endocrinopathy, M protein and skin changes) is associated with hyperpigmentation and thickened, tight, but not bound down, skin [87,88].

Primary amyloid may rarely be associated with scleroderma-like lesions, but waxy cutaneous papules and purpura are more characteristic [83].

Scleromyxedema is a rare disorder associated with monoclonal gammopathy where dermal deposits of hyaluronic acid are observed. Patients develop induration of the hands, face, arms and, to a lesser degree, the trunk and lower extremities associated with multiple fine waxy papules. Patients may have myopathy and polyarthritis, but other features of scleroderma, like Raynaud's phenomenon, are rare [83,89].

Scleroderma-like lesions of the lower extremities have been described in carcinoid patients [87]. A paraneoplastic condition, palmar fasciitis, and polyarthritis syndrome may occasionally be confused with scleroderma [90]. Bound down palmar or plantar fascia may be helpful diagnostically. History of vasomotor instability in the early phase of illness and unilateral expression may be helpful in distinguishing the late phase of reflex sympathetic dystrophy from scleroderma.

Disorders of childhood associated with scleroderma-like skin include Werner's syndrome, progeria, and phenylketonuria [83].

TELANGIECTASES

Telangiectases result from dilated venules, capillaries and arterioles. Periungual telangiectases and broad lesions called mat telangiectases are important types to identify because of their specificity for scleroderma (Fig. 3.28). Mat telangiectases are broad, oval or polygonal macules 2–7mm in diameter and found on the face, mucous membranes and hands. These lesions are clinically distinguishable from the broad telangiectases of hereditary hemorrhagic telangiectasia. In this latter disease, telangiectases are actually arterio-venous malformations and are associated with epistaxis and gastrointestinal bleeding (Osler–Rendu–Weber Disease) [91].

Linear telangiectases are nonspecific and may be seen in sundamage, acne rosacea, venous hypertension (lower extremities), carcinoid, and hypercorticism. When linear telangiectases are present on the face, malar erythema may result which can be confused with a non-raised malar rash of lupus.

HYPERPIGMENTATION

Pigmentary changes of the skin may be a clue to diagnosis in patients with rheumatic complaints [28]. Joint pain and diffuse hyperpigmentation may be seen in primary biliary cirrhosis, hemochromatosis and Whipple's disease. Rarely, diffuse hyperpigmentation may antedate the more characteristic skin changes of scleroderma [31]. Generalized hyperpigmentation has also been reported rarely in SLE [31]. Hyperpigmentation may also be present without dermal sclerosis in patients with POEMS syndrome, but arthritis occurs infrequently.

Addison's disease and Cushing's syndrome with ectopic production of adrenocorticotrophic hormone are also important entities to consider in patients with generalized hyperpigmentation.

Brown to blue–gray discoloration of the skin secondary to drug deposition may occur in rheumatoid patients treated with gold (chrysiasis). Diffuse yellow discoloration is observed frequently with quinacrine therapy, and bluish–black pigmentation of the pretibial area, face and nailbeds is associated with the use of antimalarial drugs [93].

Hyperpigmentation over an inflamed finger joint may occasionally be seen. A diagnosis of ochronosis should be considered in the osteoarthritic patient with pigmentary changes overlying cartilage and tendons.

HAIR LOSS

Both diffuse nonscarring and localized hair loss are seen in SLE. Diffuse hair loss may result from telogen effluvium arising from a large fraction of hair follicles passing into the resting phase. This process may occur weeks to months after major emotional or physical stress or following pregnancy or surgery. Endocrinopathies including hyperthyroidism, hypothyroidism, hypopituitarism and hyperparathyroidism may also be associated with diffuse hair loss, as may deficiencies of protein, iron, biotin and zinc [94]. Diffuse alopecia may be associated with the use of drugs including corticosteroids, methotrexate, azathioprine, cyclophosphamide and colchicine. Discontinuation of corticosteroid has also been associated with diffuse alopecia [94].

Increased fragility of the hairshaft leading to broken hairs in the frontal hair line has been called lupus hair.

Scalp lesions of discoid lupus have alopecia, atrophy, erythema, scaling, telangiectases and follicular plugging occurring in well demarcated patches. The differential diagnosis includes alopecia areata, which usually presents with well demarcated patches of hair loss without erythema or scarring and with the presence of hair clubs within the follicles. Secondary syphilis may produce a moth-eaten pattern of hair loss with cutaneous scaling.

Tinea infection may mimic the localized alopecia of discoid lupus. The hair shaft may break at the level of the scalp, producing a black dot appearance. Diagnosis can be made by KOH examination and culture of scalp scraping and hair. A form of lichen planus, lichen planopilaris, may have features in common with discoid lesions, for example follicular plugging, mild atrophy and scarring alopecia. Characteristic lesions elsewhere on the body and lesional histopathology are distinctive[12]. Rarely, infiltrating sarcoid granulomas, metastatic carcinoma and granulomatous infections, such as tertiary syphilis, may produce localized scarring alopecia.

ORAL LESIONS

A careful evaluation of the mouth and pharynx is helpful in the evaluation of rheumatic disease. Findings of ulceration, xerostomia and gingivitis, and an assessment of tongue size and color, may all be of diagnostic importance.

Oral ulcers are common findings in Behçet's syndrome, Crohn's disease, Reiter's syndrome and SLE. Oral ulcerations of Behçet's syndrome and Crohn's disease may be indistinguishable from those of recurrent aphthous stomatitis. Patients with Behçets syndrome or Crohn's disease may experience painful, shallow, round to oval ulcers with discrete borders, which often occur in crops. These lesions tend to occur on mucosa not bound to periosteum as opposed to the lesions of recurrent intra-oral herpes which tend to be present upon the hard palate and gingiva [95]. Histopathology of the lesions of Behçet's syndrome or Crohn's disease is not helpful for differential diagnosis, and other clinical signs and symptoms are required to distinguish between these illnesses. In contrast, the lesions of Reiter's syndrome are painless, have an irregular border and are commonly located upon the palate or dorsum of the tongue [95].

Oral ulcers are common in patients with active lupus and may herald a disease flare. Lesions are usually painless, but may occasionally be painful, and are most common on the hard palate [33]. Discoid lesions may produce irregularly shaped white scars upon the mucosa that may be confused with lichen planus or leukoplakia. Histopathology and immunofluorescence studies are diagnostic of these discoid lesions. Nonspecific oral ulcers frequently develop in patients receiving nonsteroidal anti-inflammatory drugs or disease modifying drugs such as gold, D-penicillamine, methotrexate, and azathioprine.

Gingivitis secondary to immune disease has been described rarely in lupus [33] and may also be seen as an early manifestation of Wegener's granulomatosis [3].

Kawasaki disease and erythema multiforme major may both reveal signs of fever, conjunctivitis and oral mucosa lesions as well as a polymorphic skin eruption. In Kawasaki disease diffuse erythema of the oral cavity is seen, as well as erythema of the lips followed by dryness, fissuring and surface erosions which contrast to the bloody, crusting lips of a patient with erythema multiforme major. Erythema of the tongue with prominent ungual papillae leads to the strawberry tongue of Kawasaki disease which can be seen in scarlet fever but not in erythema multiforme major.

NAIL ABNORMALITIES

Nail abnormalities are common with psoriasis and psoriatic arthritis. The presence of many nail pits (more than 60) or a combination of nail pits with onycholysis (nailplate separation) and horizontal ridging strongly support a diagnosis of psoriatic arthritis in a patient with inflammatory polyarthritis [96]. Onycholysis and hyperkeratosis also occur in Reiter's syndrome, but pitting is absent in this case [97].

Hyperkeratotic nail changes of fungal disease may be indistinguishable from those of psoriasis, although psoriatic lesions tend to be more symmetric and are generally associated with skin lesions. Pitting is uncommon in onychomycoses. Hyperkeratosis confined to the distal or proximal portion of the nail supports a mycotic etiology. Microscopic examination and culture of the nailbed scrapings allow diagnosis of onychomycosis in some patients [98].

Onycholysis may result from a number of causes including fungal infection, psoriasis, hyperthyroidism and trauma. Splinter hemorrhages are also commonly the result of trauma but may occasionally be a sign of a systemic illness such as subacute bacterial endocarditis, RA or lupus. Simultaneous involvement of multiple nails and more proximal involvement of the nailbed increase the likelihood of a systemic process [99].

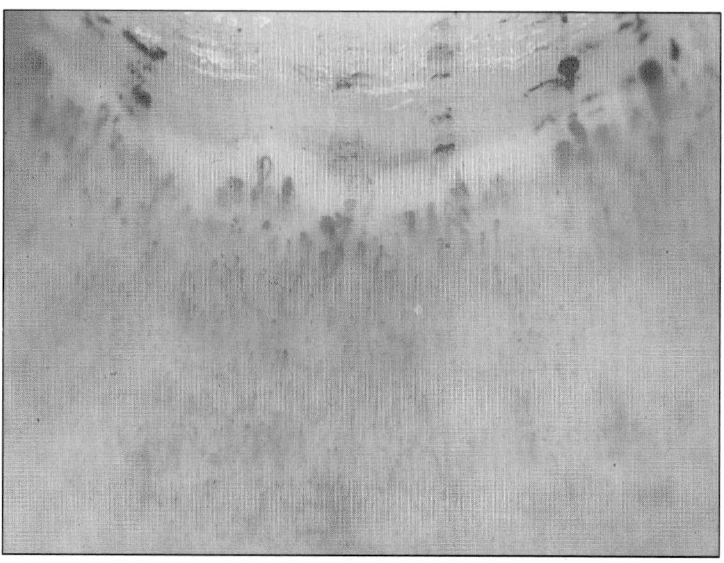

Fig. 3.29 Nailfold capillary pattern in a patient with scleroderma. Notice the avascular areas. Courtesy of Dr Hildegard Maricq.

Nailfold telangiectases observed by the naked eye, or, preferably, by capillary microscopy, are quite specific for the presence of systemic rheumatic disease, especially scleroderma (Fig. 3.29), dermatomyositis and occasionally lupus (Fig. 3.30), and may occur in as many as two-thirds of patients with such conditions. They may be helpful as early markers of these diseases [91,92]. The characteristic pattern of scleroderma and dermatomyositis is dilated capillaries frequently bordered by avascular areas. In SLE a tortuous pattern of capillaries without avascular areas is characteristic. In dermatomyositis and lupus, periungual erythema is commonly present as well.

Nail patella syndrome is an autosomal dominant disorder associated with abnormal development of nails and with absent or hypoplastic patellae.

Clubbing of the nail may be observed in association with hypertrophic pulmonary osteoarthropathy, thyroid acropachy and hereditary pachydermoperiostosis [100].

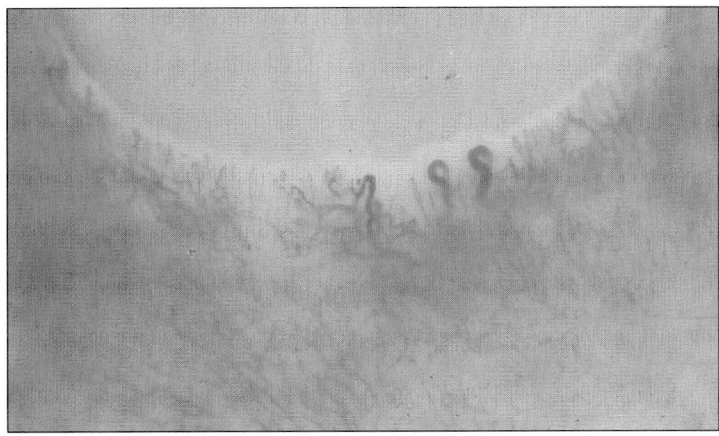

Fig. 3.30 Nailfold capillary pattern in a patient with discoid lupus erythematosus. Courtesy of Dr Hildegard Maricq.

REFERENCES

1. Braverman IM. Skin signs of systemic disease, 2E. Philadelphia: WB Saunders;1981.
2. Fitzpatrick TB, Eisen AZ, Wolff K, Freedberg IM, Austen KF, eds. Dermatology in general medicine, 3E. New York: McGraw-Hill;1987; 20–49.
3. Cupps TR, Fauci AS. The vasculitides. Philadelphia:WB Saunders; 1981.
4. Ansell BM. Rheumatic disorders in childhood. London: Butterworths;1980;50–51.
5. Case Records of the Massachusetts General Hospital. N Engl J Med. 1989; **321**:34–43.
6. Kidd BG, Hart HH, Gregor RR. Clinical features of meningococcal arthritis: a report of four cases. Ann Rheum Dis. 1985;**44**:790–2.
7. Weinberg AN, Schwartz MN. Gram-negative coccal and bacillary infections. In:Fitzpatrick TB, Eisen AZ, Wolff K, Freedberg IM, Austen KF, eds. Dermatology in general medicine, 3E. New York: McGraw-Hill;1987:2121–36.
8. Krober MS. Skeletal muscle involvement in Rocky Mountain spotted fever. South Med J. 1978;**71**:1575–6.
9. Case Records of the Massachusetts General Hospital. N Engl J Med.1971;**288**:1400–4.
10. Gerster JC, Weintraub A, Vischer TL, Fallet GH. Secondary syphilis revealed by rheumatic complaints. J Rheumatol. 1977;**4**:197–200.
11. Gertner E, Inman RD. Aseptic arthritis in a man with toxic shock syndrome. Arthritis Rheum. 1986;**29**:910–16.
12. Schwartz MN, Weinberg AN. Miscellaneous bacterial infections with cutaneous manifestations. In: Fitzpatrick TB, Eisen AZ, Wolff K, Freedberg IM, Austen KF, eds. Dermatology in general medicine, 3E. New York: McGraw-Hill;1987;2136–51.
13. Steere A. Viral arthritis. In: McCarty DJ, ed. Arthritis and allied conditions: a textbook of rheumatology. Philadelphia: Lea and Febiger; 1989:1938–51.
14. Tesh RB. Arthritis caused by mosquito-borne viruses. Ann Rev Med. 1982;**33**:31–40.
15. Woolf AD, Campion GV, Chishick A, et al. Clinical manifestations of human Parvovirus B19 in adults. Arch Intern Med. 1989; **149**:1153–6.
16. Hulsebosch HJ, Claesson FA, van Ginkel CJ, Kuiters GR, Goudsmit J, Lange JM. Human immunodeficiency exanthem. J Am Acad Dermatol. 1990;**23**:483–6.
17. Braverman IM. Skin signs of systemic disease, 2E. Philadelphia: WB Saunders;1981;825.
18. Huff JC, Weston WL, Tonneson MG. Erythema multiforme: a critical review of characteristics, diagnositic criteria and causes. J Am Acad Dermatol. 1983;**8**:763–75.
19. Braverman IM. Skin signs of systemic disease, 2E. Philadelphia: WB Saunders; 1981; 453–516.
20. Majeed HA, Quabazard Z, Hijazi Z, Farwana S, Harshani. The cutaneous manifestations in children with Familial Mediterranean Fever (Recurrent Hereditary Polyserositis). A six-year study. Q J Med. 1990;**278**:607–16.
21. Frizzera G, Moran EM, Rappaport H. Angioimmunoblastic lymphadenopathy. Am J Med. 1975;**59**:803–18.
22. Braverman IM. Skin signs of systemic disease, 2E. Philadelphia: WB Saunders;1981;740–60.

23. Sontheimer RD, Rothfield N, Gilliam JN, Lupus erythematosus. In: Fitzpatrick TB, Eisen AZ, Wolff K, Freedberg IM, Austen KF, eds. Dermatology in general medicine, 3E. New York: McGraw-Hill; 1987;1816–34.
24. Wintroub BU, Stern R. Cutaneous drug reactions: Pathogenesis and clinical classification. J Am Acad Dermatol. 1985;**13**:167–79.
25. Piette WW. An approach to cutaneous changes caused by hematologic malignancies. Dermatol Clin. 1987;**7(3)**:467–79.
26. Ansell BM. Rheumatic disorders in childhood. London: Butterworths;1980;155–6.
27. Malone MS, Grant-Kels JM, Feder HM, Luger SW. Diagnosis of Lyme disease based on dermatologic manifestations. Ann Intern Med. 1991;**114**:490–8.
28. Bolognia J, Braverman I. Skin manifestations of internal disease. In: Wilson JD, Brownwald E, Isselbacher KJ, et al., eds. Harrison's principles of internal medicine. New York: McGraw-Hill;1991;322–43.
29. Almeida L, Grossman M. Widespread dermatophyte infections that mimic collagen vascular disease. J Am Acad Dermatol. 1990;**23**:855–7.
30. Weigard DA. Cutaneous immunofluorescence. In: Callen JP, ed. Med Clin North Am. 1989;**73(5)**:1263–74.
31 Braverman IM. Skin signs of systemic disease, 2E. Philadelphia: WB Saunders; 1981;255–377.
32. Zax RH, Callen JP. Sarcoidosis. Dermatol Clin. 1989;**7(3)**:505–14.
33 Wallace DJ, Dubois EL. Dubois' lupus erythematosus, 3E. Philadelphia:Lea and Febiger;1987;362–71.
34. Plotz PH. Current concepts in the idiopathic inflammatory myopathies: polymyositis, dermatomyositis, and related disorders. Ann Intern Med. 1989;**111**:143–57.
35. Bligard CA, Storer JS. Photosensitivity in infants and children. Dermatol Clin. 1986;**4(2)**:311–19.
36. Bigby M, Stern R. Cutaneous reactions to non-steroidal anti-inflammatory drugs. J Am Acad Dermatol. 1985;**12**:866–76.
37. Bernhard JD, Pathak MA, Kochever IE, Parrish JA. Abnormal reactions to ultraviolet radiation. In: Fitzpatrick TB, Eisen AZ, Wolff K, Freedberg IM, Austen KF, eds. Dermatology in general medicine, 3E. New York: McGraw-Hill;1987;1481–507.
38. Epstein JH. Polymorphous light eruption. In: Beare JM, Ruiz Maldonaudo R, Parish LC, eds. Textbook of pediatric dermatology. Philadelphia: Grune and Stratton;1989; 706–10.
39. Bickers DR, Pathak MA. The Porphyrias. In: Fitzpatrick TB, Eisen AZ, Wolff K, Freedberg IM, Austen KF, eds. Dermatology in general medicine, 3E. New York: McGraw-Hill;1987;1666–715.
40. Barthelmy H, Chouvet B, Cambazard F. Skin and mucosal manifestations in vitamin deficiency. J Am Acad Dermatol. 1986;**15**:1263–74.
41. McElgunn PS. Dermatologic manifestations of hepatitis B virus infection. J Am Acad Dermatol. 1983;**8**:539–48.
42. Bielory L, Gascon P, Lawley TJ, Young NS, Frank MM. Human serum sicknes: A prospective analysis of 35 patients treated with equine anti-thymocyte globulin for bone marrow failure. Medicine. 1988;**67**:40–57.
43. Burrall BA, Halpern GM, Huntley AC. Chronic urticaria. West J Med. 1990;**152**:268–76.
44. Pasero G, Oliveri I, Gemignani G, Vitali C. Urticaria/ arthritis syndrome: report of four B51 positive patients. Ann Rheum Dis.1989;**48**:508–11.
45. Monroe EW. Urticarial vasculitis: An updated review. J Am Acad Dermatol. 1981;**5**:88–95.
46. Kaye B, Kaye D, Bobrove A. Rheumatoid nodules. Am J Med. 1984;**76**:279-292.
47. Moore CP, Willkens RF. The subcutaneous nodule: Its significance in the diagnosis of rheumatic disease. Semin Arthritis Rheum. 1977;**7**:63–79.
48. Dabski K, Winkelman RK. Generalized granuloma annulare: Clinical and laboratory findings in 100 patients. J Am Acad Dermatol. 1989;**20**:39–47.
49. Reginato AJ, Kurnik B. Calcium oxalate and other crystals associated with kidney diseases and arthritis. Semin Arthritis Rheum. 1989;**18**:198–224.
50. Resnick C. Tumorol calcinosis. Arthritis Rheum. 1989;**32**:1484–6.
51. Leisen JC, Austard ED, Bluhm GB, Sigler JW. The tophus in calcium pyrophosphate deposition disease. JAMA. 1980;**244**:1711–12.
52. Ginsburg WW, D'Duffy JD. Multicentric reticulohistiocytosis. In: Kelley WN, Harris ED, Ruddy S, Sledge CB, eds. Textbook of rheumatology. Philadelphia: WB Saunders;1989;1563–6.
53. NIH Consensus Conference. Neurofibromatosis. Arch Neurol. 1988; **45**:575–8.
54. Bondi EE, Lazarus GA. Panniculitis. In: Fitzpatrick TB, Eisen AZ, Wolff K, Freedberg IM, Austen KF eds. Dermatology in general medicine, 3E. New York: McGraw-Hill;1987;113–48.
55. Braverman IM. Skin signs of systemic disease, 2E. Philadelphia: WB Saunders;1981;710–40.
56. Kalb RE. Sarcoidosis with subcutaneous nodules. Am J Med.1988; **85**:731–6.
57. Albert DA, Weisman MH, Kaplan R. The rheumatic manifestations of leprosy. Medicine. 1980;**59**:442–8.
58. Katz SI. Erythema elevation diutinum. In: Fitzpatrick TB, Eisen AZ, Wolff K. Freedberg IM, Austen KF, eds Dermatology in general medicine, 3E. New York: McGraw-Hill;1987;1312–16.
59. Fritch PO, Elias PM. Mechanisms of vesicle formation and classification. In: Fitzpatrick TB, Eisen AZ, Wolff K, Freedberg IM, Austen KF, eds. Dermatology in General medicine, 3E. New York: McGraw-Hill;1987;546–54.
60. Hall RP, Lawley TJ, Katz SI. Bullous eruption of systemic lupus erythematosus (editorial). J Am Acad Dermatol. 1982;**7**:797–9.
61. Rappersberger K, Tschachler TM, Wolff K. Bullous disease in systemic lupus erythematosus. J Am Acad Dermatol. 1989;**21**:745–52.
62. Callen J. Internal disorders associated with bullous disease of the skin. J Am Acad Dermatol. 1980;**3**:107–19.
63. Fitzpatrick TB, Bernhard JD. The structure of skin lesions and fundamentals of diagnosis. In: Fitzpatrick TB, Eisen AZ, Wolff K, Freedberg IM, Austen KF, eds. Dermatology in general medicine, 3E. New York: McGraw-Hill;1987;20–49.
64. McNeely MC, Jorizzo JL, Solomon AR, Schmalstieg FC, Cavallo T. Primary idiopathic cutaneous pustular vasculitis. J Am Acad Dermatol. 1986;**14**:939–44.
65. Moreland LW, Brick JE, Kovach RE, O, Bartolomeo AG, Mullins MC. Acute febrile neutrophilic dermatosis (Sweet Syndrome): A review of the literature with emphasis on musculoskeletal manifestations. Semin Arthritis Rheum. 1988;**17**:143–55.
66. Laxer RM, Shore AD, King S, Silverman ED, Wilmot DM. Chronic recurrent multifocal osteomyelitis and psoriasis: A report of a new association and review of related disorders. Semin Arthritis Rheum. 1988;**17**:260–70.
67. Knitzer RH, Needleman BW. Musculoskeletal syndromes associated with acne. Semin Arthritis Rheum. 1991;**20**:247–55.
68. Schreiner DT. Purpura. Dermatol Clin. 1989;**7**:481–9.
69. Reuler JB, Broudy VC, Cooney TG. Adult scurvy. JAMA. 1985;**253**:803–7.
70. Cappiello RA, Espinoza LR, Adelman H, Aquilar J, Vassey FB, German BF. Cholesterol embolism: A pseudo-vasculitis syndrome. Semin Arthritis Rheumatol.1989;**18**:240–246.
71. Braverman IM. Skin signs of systemic disease. 2E. Philadelphia: WB Saunders;1981; 378–452.
72. Gibson LE, Daniel SU. Cutaneous vasculitis. Rheum Dis Clin North Am. 1990;**16**:309–24.
73. Spencer LV, Callen JP. Cutaneous manifestations of bacterial infections. Dermatol Clin. 1989;**7**:579–89.
74. Braverman IM. Skin signs of systemic disease. 2E. Philadelphia: WB Saunders;1981;809–922.
75. Cawley MI. Vasculitis and ulceration in rheumatic disease of the foot. Baillière's Clin Rheumatol. 1987;**1**:315–33.
76. Vollersten RS, Conn DL. Vasculitis with rheumatoid arthritis. Rheumatol Dis Clin North Am. 1990;**16**:445–61.
77. Jorizzo JL, Daniels JC. Dermatologic conditions reported in patients with rheumatoid arthritis. J Am Acad Dermatol;1983;**8**:439–57.
78. Levine JM. Leg ulcers: Differential diagnosis in the elderly. Geriatrics. 1990;**45**:32–42.
79. Wolff K, Stingl G. Pyoderma gangrenosum. In: Fitzpatrick TB, Eisen AZ, Wolff K, Freedberg IM, Austen KF, eds. Dermatology in general medicine, 3E. New York: McGraw-Hill;1987;1328–36.
80. Bacon DG, Tribe CR. Systemic rheumatoid vasculitis: A clinical and laboratory study of 50 cases. Medicine. 1981;**60**:288–97.
81. Gaylarde PM, Dodd HJ, Sarlcony I. Venous leg ulcers and arthropathy. Br J Rheumatol. 1990;**29**:142–4.
82. Burgdorf W. Cutaneous manifestations of Crohn's disease. J Am Acad Dermatol. 1981;**5**:689–95.
83. Rocco VK, Hurd ER. Scleroderma and scleroderma-like disorders. Semin Arthritis Rheum. 1986;**16**:22–69.
84. Lakhanapal S, Ginsburg WW, Michet CJ, Doyle JA, Moore SB. Eosinophilic fasciitis: Clinical spectrum and therapeutic response in 52 cases. Semin Arthritis Rheum. 1988;**17**:221–31.
85. Varga J, Peltonen J, Vitto J, Jimenez S. Development of diffuse fasciitis with eosinophilia during L-tryptophen: Demonstration of elevated type I collagen gene expression in affected tissues. Ann Intern Med. 1990;**112**:344–51.
86. Feingold KR, Elias P. Endocrine skin interactions. J Am Acad Dermatol. 1987;**17**:921–40.
87. Feingold KR, Elias P. Endocrine skin interactions. J Am Acad Dermatol.1988;**19**:1–20.
88. Viard J, Lasavre P, Boitard C, et al. POEMS syndrome presenting as systemic sclerosis. Am J Med. 1988;**84**;524–27.
89. Gabriel SE, Perry HO, Oleson GB, Bowles CA. Scleromyxedema: A scleroderma-like disorder with systemic manifestations. Medicine. 1988;**67**:58–65.
90. Pfinsgraff J, Buckingham RB, Killian PJ, Keister SR, et al. Palmar fasciitis and arthritis with malignant neoplasms: A paraneoplastic syndrome. Semin Arthritis Rheum. 1986;**16**:118–25
91. Braverman IM. Skin signs of systemic disease. 2E. Philadelphia: WB Saunders;1981; 532–65.
92. Minkin W, Rabhan NB. Office nail fold microscopy using ophthalmoscope. J Am Acad Dermatol. 1982;**7**:191–3.
93. Bailin PL, Matkaluk. Cutaneous reactions to rheumatologic drugs. Clin Rheumatol Dis. 1982;**8**:493–516.
94. Bertolino AP, Freedberg IM. Hair. In: Fitzpatrick TB, Eisen AZ, Wolff K, Freedberg IM, Austen KF, eds. Dermatology in general medicine, 3E. New York:McGraw-Hill;1987;627–51.
95 Archard HO. Biology and pathology of the oral mucosa. In: Fitzpatrick TB, Eisen AZ, Wolff K, Freedberg IM, Austen KF, eds. Dermatology in general medicine, 3E. New York: McGraw-Hill; 1987;1152-239.
96. Eastmond CJ, Wright V. The nail dystrophy of psoriatic arthritis. Ann Rheum Dis. 1979;**38**:226–8.
97. Arnett F. Reiter's syndrome. In: Fitzpatrick TB, Eisen AZ, Wolff K, Freedberg IM, Austen KF. Dermatology in general medicine, 3E. New York:McGraw-Hill;1987;1874–82.
98. Goslen JB, Kobayashi GS. Mycologic infections. In: Fitzpatrick TB, Eisen AZ, Wolff K, Freedberg IM, Austen KF, eds. Dermatology in general medicine, 3E. New York:McGraw-Hill; 1987;2193–248.
99. Daniel CR, Same WM, Scher RK. Nails in systemic disease. Dermatol Clin. 1985;**3(3)**:465–83.
100. Altman RD, Tenenbaum J. Hypertrophic osteoarthropathy. In: Kelley WN, Hanus ED, Ruddy S, Sledge CB, eds. Textbook of rheumatology. Philadelphia: WB Saunders;1989;1666–73.

4

ARTHRITIS AND ABDOMINAL SYMPTOMS

Herman Mielants & Eric M Veys

INTRODUCTION

For many years pathology of the gut has been related to clinical manifestations of inflammatory arthritis. In 1922 [1] colectomy was proposed as a treatment for rheumatoid arthritis (RA) and an association between a peripheral arthritis and chronic ulcerative colitis was suggested. An association between gut lesions and inflammatory joint disease has been established in intestinal bypass surgery, the inflammatory bowel diseases, coeliac disease and Whipple's disease. The gut likely plays a direct role in the pathogenesis of the arthritis in these diseases. In other inflammatory joint diseases, abdominal manifestations can be a symptom of a complication of the disease.

Major abdominal symptoms are diarrhea, abdominal pain and intestinal blood loss (Fig.4.1).

DIFFERENTIAL DIAGNOSIS

The differential diagnosis of inflammatory locomotor diseases associated with abdominal symptoms is aided by determining the location of the joint inflammation. Inflammatory symptoms of the locomotor system can be subdivided into peripheral joint involvement with or without tendinitis, and axial inflammation (of the spine and sacroiliac joints).

The peripheral arthritis can be subdivided into mono- or pauciarticular and polyarticular joint involvement.

THE GUT AND ARTHRITIS
Arthritis associated with diarrhea
Crohn's disease Ulcerative colitis Enterogenic (bacterial) reactive arthritis (Reiter's) Undifferentiated spondyloarthropathies Whipple's disease Blind loop syndrome Coeliac disease Behçet's disease Collagenous colitis
Arthritis associated with abdominal pain
Ulcerative colitis Crohn's disease Vasculitic syndromes Henoch–Schönlein (leukoclastic vasculitis) Rheumatoid arthritis Systemic lupus erythematosus Polyarteritis nodosa Scleroderma Amyloidosis Familial Meditteranean fever Behçet's disease Whipple's disease
Arthritis associated with intestinal blood loss
Ulcerative colitis Vasculitic syndromes Henoch–Schönlein Whipple's disease

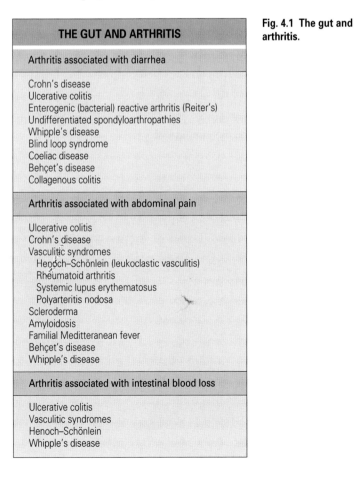

Fig. 4.1 The gut and arthritis.

PAUCIARTICULAR OR MONOARTICULAR INVOLVEMENT

This clinical picture is typical of the spondyloarthropathies (see Chapter 29). This concept consists of diseases in which the joint involvement is not only pauciarticular but also asymmetric, involving large and small joints, predominantly of the lower limbs, and frequently associated with tendinitis. Enthesitis, inflammation of the insertion of the tendon into the bone, is the hallmark of these diseases, and usually involves the feet (Achilles tendon, insertion of plantar fascia) or knee (insertion of patellar ligament). Sacroiliitis and spondylitis (which is also an enthesitis) can be associated. Other features include clinical overlap of the different diseases, familial aggregation among members of the group and the frequent association with HLA-B27 [2].

Diseases belonging to this group in which abdominal symptoms are present are Crohn's disease, ulcerative colitis, enterogenic reactive arthritis and undifferentiated spondyloarthropathies (see Fig. 4.2).

Crohn's Disease

The prevalence of Crohn's disease has increased during the last three decades to about 75 per 100,000 population.

Abdominal symptoms

Crohn's disease is characterized by the classic triad of diarrhea, abdominal pain and weight loss. Disease onset may be insidious and progression subclinical. Diarrhea consists mainly of frequent watery bowel actions and typically follows meals. The stool volume depends on the anatomic location of the disease. Intestinal bleeding is rather uncommon. Abdominal pain is present in the majority of patients and described as cramping, predominantly in the right lower quadrant of the abdomen. Pain is usually not reported as severe [3]. Weight loss is a common feature and is in the range of 10–20% of body weight. General debility is a common complaint together with low grade fever.

In the later stages of Crohn's disease perianal involvement appears, with fistulae and abscesses. A tender abdominal mass can be felt in the lower quadrant; intra-abdominal abcesses and fistulae can be present.

Peripheral arthritis

Peripheral arthritis, mainly pauciarticular and asymmetric, appears in about 17–20% of the patients, with an equal sex ratio. Peak age is between 25 years and 44 years. Large and small joints are involved, predominantly those of the lower limbs (most commonly the knees and ankles but also the metacarpophalangeal and the metatarsophalangeal joints). The arthritis is mainly migratory and transient and subsides within 6 weeks, but it may also become chronic and destructive. Recurrences are very common.

Enthesopathies, especially at the feet (Fig. 4.3) are frequent and can be considered as a peripheral location of the disease.

Relationship between arthritis and gut inflammation

In most cases gut symptoms antedate or coincide with the joint manifestations, but the articular symptoms may precede the intestinal

DISORDERS WITH MONOARTICULAR OR PAUCIARTICULAR JOINT INVOLVEMENT AND ABDOMINAL SYMPTOMS					
Diagnosis	Abdominal symptoms	General symptoms	Extra-articular features	Relationship between abdominal symptoms and arthritis	
				Onset	Course
Crohn's disease	Diarrhea Abdominal pain Fistulae	Weight loss Ill-being Fever	Erythema nodosum Clubbing Uveitis, conjunctivitis	Usually before arthritis, coincident or postdated	Flares rarely coincide
Ulcerative colitis	Diarrhea Blood loss	Rare	Erythema nodosum Uveitis	Before arthritis, frequently coincident	Flares directly related
Enterogenic reactive arthritis	Diarrhea Vomiting	Spiking fever Ill-being Dehydration	Uveitis Urethritis	1–4 weeks before arthritis	Longer arthritis duration
Undifferentiated spondyloarthropathies	Rare diarrhea	None	Uveitis Erythema nodosum Urethritis	Arthritis before abdominal symptoms 'subclinical' gut inflammation	Related

Fig. 4.2 Disorders with monoarticular or pauciarticular joint involvement and abdominal symptoms.

symptoms by years [4]. It is argued that in some cases of spondyloarthropathy, Crohn's disease can remain subclinical, joint or tendon inflammation being the only clinical manifestation [5]. Colonic involvement increases the susceptibility to peripheral arthritis. Attacks of arthritis can be related temporally to flares of the bowel disease although this is less pronounced than in ulcerative colitis.

Extra-articular features

Skin lesions, specifically erythema nodosum and pyoderma gangrenosum are frequently associated and occur in 10–21% of the patients. Erythema nodosum parallels the activity of the bowel disease and tends to occur in patients with active peripheral arthritis; it is probably a manifestation of Crohn's disease. Pyoderma gangrenosum is less common and more severe. It is not related to bowel and joint diseases and is probably an associated disorder [6]. Clubbing is also reported in this disease.

Acute anterior uveitis is the ocular manifestation most commonly associated with Crohn's disease, occurring in 3–11% of patients. It is acute in onset, unilateral and transient, but recurrences are common. It generally spares the choroid and retina, but a chronic evolution with lesions in the posterior part has been described. Mutton-fat keratic precipitates are a sign of granulomatous uveitis and can be present. Acute anterior uveitis is more related to those spondyloarthropathies showing axial involvement and associated with HLA-B27. Conjunctivitis and episcleritis are also described, in these cases a red eye without photophobia or pain is typically seen.

Secondary amyloidosis with involvement of major organs is not uncommon and is usually fatal.

Diagnosis

Histological evidence of Crohn's disease is essential and can be obtained at colonoscopy (in cases of colonic involvement) or ileo-colonoscopy. Macroscopically, the presence of patchy aphtoid ulcerations, and of cobblestones will raise suspicion and contribute to the diagnosis. Although the differential diagnosis with ulcerative colitis can be difficult, some histological features of Crohn's disease, such as the patchy distribution of the lesions, the involvement of different layers of the bowel wall, and the presence of aphtoid ulcerations, pseudopyloric metaplasia and sarcoid granulomas (Fig. 4.4) are pathognomonic.

Ulcerative Colitis

The prevalence of ulcerative colitis is 50–100 per 100,000 population; the disease seems to be more frequent in Whites than in non-Whites or Jews.

Abdominal symptoms

The most frequent abdominal manifestations of ulcerative colitis are diarrhea and blood loss. In distal locations, there can be passage of blood with each bowel movement. With more extensive colon involvement, the blood will be mixed with a soft, liquid and sometimes mucopurulent stool.

Diarrhea is practically always present. Defecation is frequent, sometimes every few minutes, and usually in small amounts. Abdominal pain, rectal cramps and fever are less frequent than in Crohn's disease, and considerable weight loss is distinctly uncommon.

Peripheral arthritis

The patterns of peripheral arthritis and enthesopathy associated with ulcerative colitis are identical to those seen in Crohn's disease, but their prevalence is much lower (5–10%).

Relationship between arthritis and gut inflammation

Disease onset usually precedes the joint symptoms but a coincidental onset of joint and abdominal symptoms is not uncommon. In the course of the disease the temporal relationship between attacks of arthritis and flares of the bowel disease is more marked than in Crohn's disease. Joint symptoms are more common in total than in partial colon involvement. Surgical removal of the inflamed colon has a therapeutic effect on the joint symptoms [7].

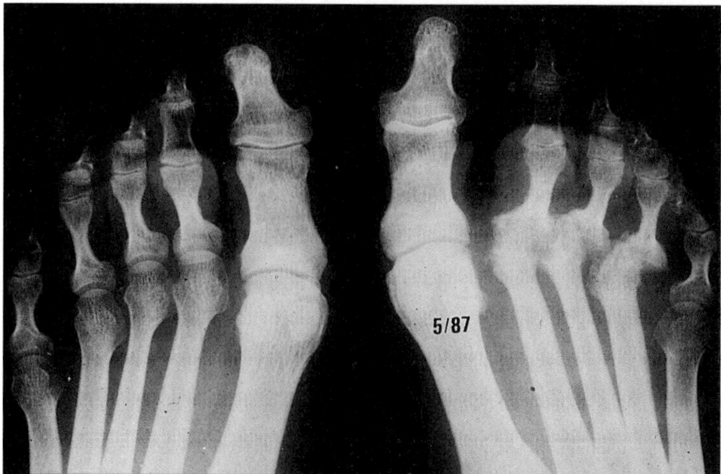

Fig. 4.3 Erosive metatarsophalangeal joint lesions in a patient with Crohn's disease (asymmetric joint involvement).

Extra-articular features

The dermatologic and ocular manifestations of ulcerative colitis are comparable to those seen in Crohn's disease, but they are less common. Clubbing and amyloidosis are absent.

The laboratory and radiographic findings are also identical to those of Crohn's disease.

Diagnosis

The endoscopic appearance is different from that seen in Crohn's disease: the mucosa is continuously involved, with edema, friability and bleeding on minor trauma. Subsequently, ulcerations and strictures may appear. The histological picture differs from Crohn's disease by the continuous involvement of only the mucosa, with no damage to the deeper layers (Fig. 4.5).

Enterogenic Reactive Arthritis

Different enterogenic bacteria are capable of initiating peripheral arthritis: *Shigella flexneri*, *Salmonella typhimurium*, *Yersinia enterocolitica* (especially serotype 3), *Y. pseudotuberculosis*, and *Campylobacter jejuni* are the most common species [8], although arthritis has frequently been reported in outbreaks of diarrhea in which no pathogens were identified.

The disease has been termed reactive arthritis, since the causative organisms cannot be isolated from the joint [9]. The sterile arthritis develops as a reaction to a distant infection.

Abdominal symptoms

The clinical picture mainly consists of very profuse diarrhea, accompanied by spiking fever, general ill-being, abdominal cramps, vomiting and progressive dehydration. In some cases blood loss in stools may be present. The delay between infection and intestinal symptoms is very short.

In salmonella epidemics the frequency of persons reporting gastrointestinal distress is between 1% and 10% depending on the antimicrobial resistance pattern. Most patients recover within 1 month although a fatal outcome is not uncommon.

Peripheral arthritis

The peripheral arthritis related to intestinal bacterial infections resembles the clinical picture of the spondyloarthropathies: an asymmetrical oligoarticular pattern of joint involvement, predominantly of the lower limbs, accompanied by tendinitis (10%). Monoarthritis is a common finding, as well as dactylitis (sausage-like toes and fingers). Men are more frequently affected than women (1.5:1).

The duration of the joint symptoms is usually restricted and in more than 70% of the cases the patient is symptom-free after approximately 19 weeks. Nevertheless, about 20% of the patients experience multiple episodes of flare-up of the joint disease and in about 10–30% of the cases (depending on the causative organism) the joint inflammation becomes chronic. In the majority of cases antibiotic treatment has no effect on the joint manifestations.

Relationship between arthritis and gut inflammation

The arthritis develops generally 6–14 days after the diarrhea. The interval is less than 30 days in 80% of the patients, although it may amount to 3 months. The joint symptoms usually take longer to subside than the abdominal symptoms. In some cases, mainly of *Yersinia* arthritis, diarrhea can be absent.

There is no relationship between the severity of the gut symptoms and the severity of the joint symptoms.

Extra-articular features

The most common extra-articular lesions are ocular manifestations. Acute anterior uveitis and conjunctivitis occur in about 5–30% of the cases and are usually self-remitting. The uveitis is frequently associated with attacks of arthritis, but can subsequently follow an independent course.

Urogenital inflammation (urethritis, balanitis, vaginitis) occurs in about 12–20% of cases, although the infectious organism is usually absent from the urogenital tract: the urogenital inflammation is probably reactive in nature.

Oral ulcers and erythema nodosum (especially in *Yersinia* enteritides) are not uncommon, while keratodermia blenorrhagica is never seen in enterogenic reactive arthritis. Neurological, cardiac and renal complications are rare.

Laboratory and radiographic features

During the initial stage of reactive arthritis the patients develop the specific laboratory features of an acute bacterial infection. The causative organisms can be cultured from the stools during the active stage of intestinal manifestations. Increased levels of immunoglobulins can be detected in the serum: the IgM increase is very short-lived, but the increase in IgG and IgA levels may be persistent. It appears, however, that these immunoglobulins are not very organism-specific.

The joint fluid is inflammatory and contains 4000–120,000 cells/mm^3, mainly polymorphonuclear cells. A characteristic of reactive arthritis is that the causative organism cannot be detected in the joint fluid or synovium. In recent papers, however, specific bacterial antigenic material (lipopolysaccharide) has been demonstrated in the synovial fluid cells [10] and the synovium of patients with reactive arthritis. Other work suggests the persistence of the causative

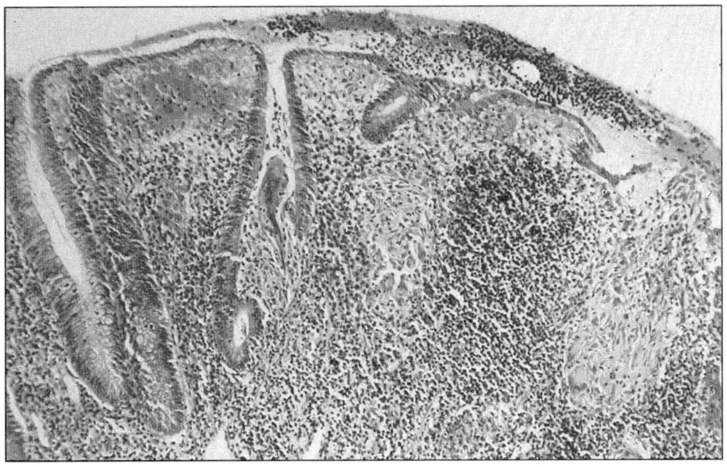

Fig. 4.4 Crohn's disease of colon. Microscopic aspect of colon biopsy showing irregular distorted crypts which are interrupted by infiltrations of inflammatory cells. The lamina propria contains sarcoid granulomas and a mononuclear infiltrate. (H&E stain, × 120.)

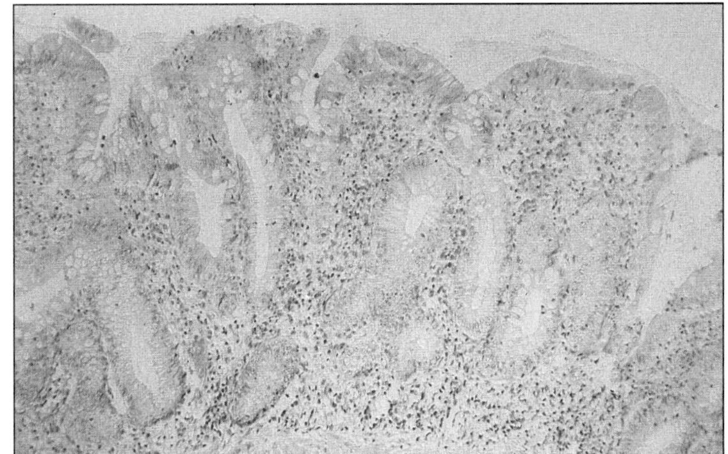

Fig. 4.5 Ulcerative colitis. Microscopic aspect of colon biopsy showing irregular villous surface with distorted and branching crypts. There is mucin depletion. The lamina propria contains infiltrates with mononuclear cells and granulocytes. The bottom of the crypts does not reach the muscularis mucosa. (H&E stain, × 120.)

organism in the gut submucosa of patients with chronic joint disease due to defective local defense mechanisms [11].

Erosive lesions of the involved joint are uncommon but may be present. Typical aspects are the combined presence of bone proliferation and bone erosions, and the asymmetric pattern of involvement.

Diagnosis

The diagnosis is made by stool cultures obtained during the active episode of intestinal symptoms, or by determining specific immunoglobulins in the serum (although the specificity of these tests is questionable).

Endoscopic confirmation can be obtained: the histology mainly demonstrates an infiltrate with polymorphonuclear cells, mucosal ulceration and crypt abscesses. The architecture of crypts and villi is usually preserved.

Undifferentiated Spondyloarthropathies

A large number of patients presenting with clinical, biologic, radiographic and genetic features of the spondyloarthropathies cannot be classified into one of the known clinical entities. These patients are classified under 'undifferentiated spondyloarthropathies'.

Abdominal symptoms

The majority of these patients do not present pronounced abdominal symptoms. However, about 20–30% regularly experience short episodes of diarrhea or regularly have more than two stools per day [12].

Peripheral arthritis

The clinical picture is identical to that seen in other forms of spondyloarthropathy. There is asymmetric involvement of the small and large joints, predominantly of the lower limbs. Enthesopathies, mainly of the feet, and dactylitis are frequently associated.

Relationship between arthritis and gut inflammation

The gut inflammation in undifferentiated spondyloarthropathies is mainly subclinical and can only be demonstrated by ileocolonoscopy [5]. In about 60% of the patients inflammatory gut lesions can be detected on biopsy. These lesions either resemble acute bacterial enteritis and are then classified as 'acute', or resemble idiopathic inflammatory bowel disease and are then classified as 'chronic' [13].

Repeat ileocolonoscopy has demonstrated a strong relationship between the persistence of intestinal inflammation and that of joint inflammation [14], which supports the hypothesis that the gut triggers the joint disease in the majority of the spondyloarthritic patients.

Extra-articular features

Acute anterior uveitis, erythema nodosum and urogenital symptoms are the most frequent extra-articular features.

Laboratory and radiographic features

Most patients present elevated inflammatory serum parameters; the parameters are significantly more raised in patients with 'chronic' inflammatory gut lesions than in those presenting acute lesions or a normal histology. Erosive joint lesions, particularly of the small joints of hands and feet, are not uncommon. They resemble the lesions seen in RA, but differ by their asymmetric and pauciarticular pattern. Destructive lesions of the hip joint, mimicking RA hip involvement and different from the concentric hip involvement in ankylosing spondylitis (AS), have been described [15] (Fig. 4.6). Like the erosive joint lesions they are related to the presence of subclinical gut inflammation.

Diagnosis

The diagnosis is made by the clinical picture and by excluding proven enteric infections. Ileocolonoscopy can confirm the presence of subclinical gut inflammation.

POLYARTICULAR INVOLVEMENT

As a rule, abdominal symptoms are not prominent in those forms of joint disease characterized by polyarticular involvement (Fig. 4.7), and they frequently appear as a complication. There is no specific relationship between these different diseases.

Whipple's Disease

Whipple's disease is probably a form of enterogenic reactive arthritis, caused by an infection of the gut, although no classic organisms have been described. Characteristic periodic acid Schifff (PAS) staining deposits are found in macrophages of the small intestine and in the mesenteric nodes; these cells contain rod-shaped free bacilli [16]. These bacilliform bodies are considered to be the etiologic agent since they disappear when a patient is successfully treated with antibiotics [17]. The ratio of affected males to affected females is 9:1.

The clinical picture is characterized by weight loss, pyrexia, lymphadenopathy, abdominal pain and migratory polyarthritis. Diarrhea with steatorrhea usually is the chief complaint and is observed in 75% of the cases.

The peripheral arthritis may be transient or chronic, it involves larger joints more often than small ones, and is predominantly polyarticular and symmetric. The arthritis may antedate the intestinal complaints. Flares of arthritis are not related to exacerbations of intestinal symptoms. The synovial fluid usually contains a high number of cells (4000–100,000/mm^3), predominantly polymorphonuclear cells (up to 100%).

Erosive lesions on radiographs are absent, although destructive lesions have been reported. The incidence of sacroiliitis and spondylitis is controversial and ranges between 8% and 20%. The relationship with HLA-B27 has also been described.

The disease responds very well to antibiotic treatment, usually with tetracyclines, which have to be continued for more than one year.

Blind Loop Syndrome

Intestinal bypass surgery can cause a syndrome associated with arthritis and dermatitis. The pathogenesis involves bacterial overgrowth and mucosal alterations in the blind loop and is probably immune-mediated [18].

Polyarthritis develops in 20–50 % of patients with the blind loop syndrome, 2–30 months following surgery. The arthritis is polyarticular, symmetric, and migratory and may become chronic. The most frequently affected joints are the knees, wrists, metacarpophalangeal and metatarsophalangeal joints. The duration of the arthritis is unpredictable. Radiographic deformities or erosions are not seen. There is no relationship between joint symptoms and gut symptoms. Erythema nodosum, vesicopustular eruptions and urticaria may be associated. Surgical reanastomosis gives complete resolution of all symptoms.

Coeliac Disease

Coeliac disease (gluten-sensitivity enteropathy) is known to be associated with abnormal intestinal permeability. Bowel symptoms are absent in 50% of patients. Many disorders, such as dermatitis herpetiformis, hyposplenism and autoimmune disorders, have been associated with the disease.

Coeliac disease can be divided into 3 types:

- one in which diarrhea (usually steatorrhea) is the main feature;
- one with constitutional disturbances such as lassitude, weight loss and malaise;
- one with varied symptoms such as neuropathy and osteomalacia.

The distribution of the arthritis varies widely but is mainly polyarticular and symmetric, involving predominantly the large joints, hips, knees, and shoulders. Radiographic changes are rare. A higher frequency of HLA-B8, DR3 has been described. There is a striking

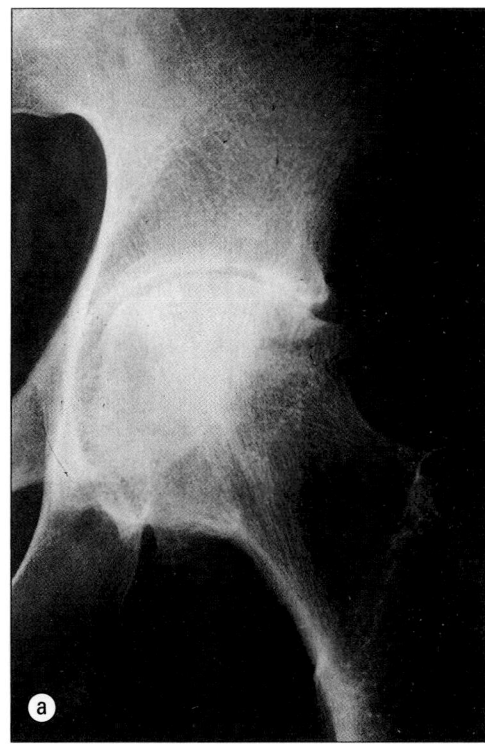

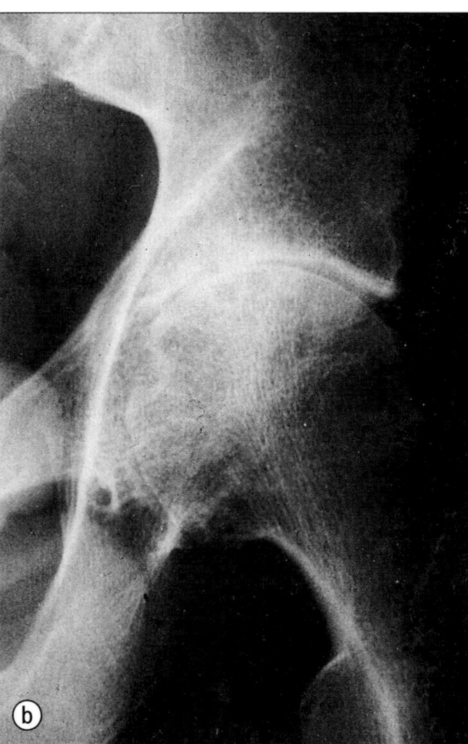

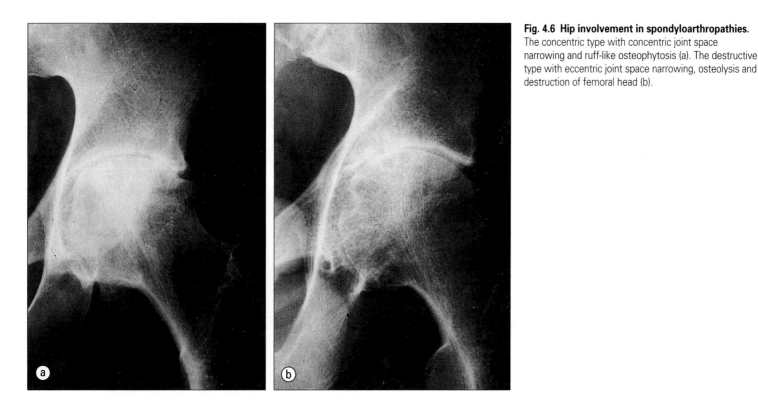

Fig. 4.6 Hip involvement in spondyloarthropathies. The concentric type with concentric joint space narrowing and ruff-like osteophytosis (a). The destructive type with eccentric joint space narrowing, osteolysis and destruction of femoral head (b).

response of the joint manifestations to a gluten-free diet [19], although rechallenge does not provoke arthritis.

Other Systemic Diseases

Other systemic diseases that have an element of arthritis and can be associated with gastrointestinal disorders include vasculitic syndromes and Henoch–Schönlein purpura, RA, systemic lupus erythematosus, scleroderma, Behçet's syndrome, amyloidosis and familial Mediterranean fever.

AXIAL INVOLVEMENT

The axial involvement related to intestinal inflammation consists of sacroiliitis and syndesmophytes. Both lesions can be regarded as forms of enthesopathy. Sacroiliitis can be present without vertebral lesions; in cases of spondylitis, sacroiliitis is practically always associated.

Inflammatory Bowel Disease (Crohn's Disease and Ulcerative Colitis)

There is no significant difference between the axial involvement in these diseases. The true prevalence of sacroiliitis is difficult to estimate since the onset frequently is insidious. Prevalence rates of 10–15% for sacroiliitis and of 7–12% for spondylitis have been described, although the real figures are probably higher. The male to female ratio is 3:1, which is comparable to uncomplicated ankylosing spondylitis (AS) [20].

The clinical picture is indistinguishable from uncomplicated AS. The patient complains of inflammatory low back pain, thoracic or cervical pain, alternate buttock pain or chest pain. Limitation of motion in the lumbar or cervical region and reduced chest expansion are classical clinical signs.

The onset of axial involvement does not parallel that of bowel disease and frequently precedes it. Its course is also totally independent of the course of the gut disease; neither colectomy in ulcerative colitis nor surgery in Crohn's disease alter the course of any associated sacroiliitis or spondylitis.

DISORDERS WITH POLYARTICULAR JOINT INVOLVEMENT AND ABDOMINAL SYMPTOMS				
Diagnosis	Abdominal symptoms	General symptoms	Extra-articular features	Relationship between abdominal symptoms to arthritis
Whipple's disease	Diarrhea (steatorrhea) Abdominal pain	Fever Weight loss Lymphadenopathy	Neurologic Dermatologic	Onset Different Course No relationship
Blind loop syndrome	Abdominal pain Diarrhea	Fever Weight loss	Erythema nodosum Vesicopustulae Urticaria	Onset 2–30 months after surgery Course No relation
Coeliac disease	Absent in 50% Abdominal pain Steatorrhea	Malaise Weight loss	Osteomalacia	Relationship unknown
Vasculitic syndromes Henoch–Schönlein Rheumatoid arthritis Systemic lupus erythematosus Polyarteritis nodosa	Abdominal pain Intestinal bleeding Perforation	Disease-related	Purpura Disease-related	No direct relationship
Scleroderma	Obstipation Abdominal cramps	Disease-related	Disease-related	No direct relationship

Fig. 4.7 Disorders with polyarticular joint involvement and abdominal symptoms.

Radiographically, the axial involvement is indistinguishable from uncomplicated AS. The frequency of asymmetric sacroiliitis could be higher (Fig. 4.8).

Sacroiliitis and spondylitis are opposed to the peripheral arthritis associated with HLA-B27, but to a lesser degree than in uncomplicated AS.

HLA-B27 positivity is found in 66% of ulcerative colitis patients and in 53% of the Crohn's disease patients with spondylitis. The prevalence of HLA-B27 is lower in patients with inflammatory bowel disease (IBD) and sacroiliitis alone. AS patients not carrying the HLA-B27 antigen are at a higher risk of developing IBD than HLA-B27$^+$ AS patients. In first degree relatives of patients with IBD, there is an increased prevalence of IBD and of AS. The HLA-B27-B44 phenotype has been found to place patients at a higher risk of developing the common manifestations of Crohn's disease and AS [21].

It has been postulated that the axial involvement in inflammatory bowel disease is not a manifestation of this disease but an associated disorder [6].

Enterogenic Reactive Arthritis

Axial involvement in patients with reactive arthritis caused by enterogenic bacteria is relatively rare. Radiographic evidence of sacroiliitis has been found in 6–9% of patients and is more likely in chronic and recurrent disease. Ankylosing spondylitis is relatively rare.

The presence of sacroiliitis and spondylitis may be accounted for by a common genetic basis rather than by a predisposition to one as a result of the other.

Other Spondyloarthropathies

In AS subclinical gut inflammation was found in about 52% of the patients [12]. Most of these patients, however, did not present abdominal symptoms, although 15–20% often passed more than two stools per day.

Sacroiliitis and spondylitis have also been described in Whipple's disease and in Behçet's syndrome but the relation of these diseases to the spondyloarthropathies remains speculative. Axial involvement in these diseases is rare and the association with HLA-B27 is questionable.

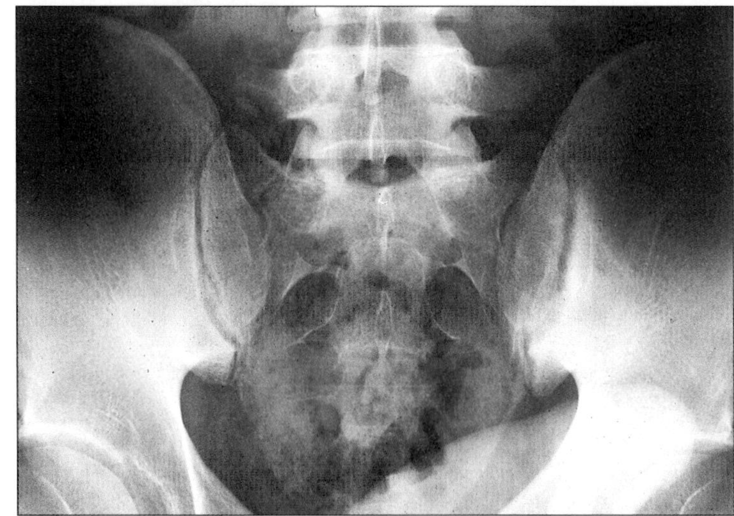

Fig. 4.8 Asymmetric sacroiliitis in a patient with inflammatory bowel disease.

REFERENCES

1. Smith R. Treatment of rheumatoid arthritis by colectomy. Ann Surg. 1922;**76**:515–78.
2. Wright V, Moll JHD. Seronegative polyarthritis. Amsterdam: North-Holland;1976.
3. Kirsner JB, Shorter RG. Inflammatory bowel disease. Philadelphia: Lea & Febiger;1988.
4. Haslock I. Arthritis and Crohn's disease. Ann Rheum Dis. 1973;**32**:479–86.
5. Mielants H, Veys EM. The gut in the spondyloarthropathies. J Rheumatol. 1990;**17**:7–10.
6. Schorr-Lesnick B, Brandt LJ. Selected rheumatologic and dermatologic manifestations of inflammatory bowel disease. Am J Gastroenterol. 1988;**83**:216–23.
7. Wright V, Watkinson G. The arthritis of ulcerative colitis. Br Med J. 1965;**2**:670–75.
8. Keat AE. Reiter's syndrome and reactive arthritis in perspective. N Engl J Med. 1983;**309**:1606–15.
9. Ahvonen P, Sievers K, Aho K. Arthritis associated with *Yersinia enterocolitica* infection. Acta Rheum Scand. 1969;**15**:323–32.
10. Granfors K, Jalkanen S, Von Essen R, et al. Yersinia antigens in synovial fluid cells from patients with reactive arthritis. N Engl J Med. 1989;**320**:216–21.
11. De Koning J, Heeseman J, Hoogkamp-Korstanje JAA, et al. Yersinia in intestinal biopsy specimens from patients with seronegative spondylarthropathies: correlation with specific serum IgA antibodies. J Infect Dis. 1989;**159**:109–12.
12. Mielants H, Veys EM, Goemaere S, Goethals K, Cuvelier C, De Vos M. Gut inflammation in the spondylarthropathies: clinical, radiological, biological and genetic features in relation to the type of histology. A prospective study. J Rheumatol. 1991;**18**:1542–51.
13. Cuvelier C, Barbatis C, Mielants H, De Vos M, Roels H, Veys EM. The histopathology of intestinal inflammation related to reactive arthritis. Gut. 1987;**2**:394–401.
14. Mielants H, Veys EM, Joos R, Cuvelier C, De Vos M. Repeat ileocolonoscopy in reactive arthritis. J Rheumatol. 1987;**14**:456–8.
15. Mielants H, Veys EM, Goethals K, Van Der Straeten C, Ackerman C, Goemaere S. Destructive hip lesions in seronegative spondylarthropathies. Relation to gut inflammation. J Rheumatol. 1990;**17**:315–40.
16. Fleminc JL, Wiesner RH, Shorter RG. Whipple's disease: clinical, biochemical and histopathologic features and assessment of treatment in 29 patients. Mayo Clin Proc. 1988;**63**:539–52.
17. Dobbins WO. Whipple's disease: an historical perspective. Q J Med. 1985;**56**:523–31.
18. Wands JA, Le Mont JT, Mann E, Isselbachter K. Arthritis associated with intestinal bypass procedure for morbid obesity. Complement activities and characterization of circulatory cryoproteins. N Engl J Med. 1976;**294**:121–4.
19. Bourne JT, Kumar P, Huskisson E. Arthritis and coeliac disease. Ann Rheum Dis. 1985;**44**:592–8.
20. Isdale A, Wright V. Seronegative arthritis and the bowel. In: Baillières Clinical Rheumatology: The gut and rheumatic diseases 1989;**3**:285–301.
21. Purmann J, Zeidler H, Bertram S, et al. HLA-antigens in ankylosing spondylitis associated with Crohn's disease. Increased frequency of the HLA phenotype B27–B44. J Rheumatol. 1988;**15**:1659–61.

NECK PAIN

John A Mathews

INTRODUCTION

The neck is often admired for its aesthetic properties, but its main function is to connect the head with the trunk. Its stability depends mainly upon the spine, which in the cervical region has seven vertebrae. These articulate with each other through a system of joints of unusual complexity. Not only is each pair of vertebrae separated by the usual intervertebral disc and pair of apophyseal joints, but in the cervical spine the bodies articulate by an additional pair of synovial joints at their postero-lateral aspects. These develop during adolescence. The need to move the head to communicate, breathe and eat places an almost continuous demand on this system, and the wonder is that this does not lead to even more frequent problems.

The cervical spine provides a protective passageway for structures vital to life. The blood supply of the brain depends partly on the vertebral arteries which pass through the cervical vertebrae, and the spinal cord is enclosed in the spinal canal. These features indicate the crucial importance of the cervical spine. It thus occupies a uniquely important place in the system of joints of the body.

Most cervical problems are mechanical and mainly affect the joints and associated ligaments and muscles [1]. The term cervical spondylosis is used to describe this pathology and the accompanying radiologic changes. Less common, but more serious, is an extension of this process, with osteophytes involving nerve roots, the vertebrobasilar circulation, and the spinal cord itself. Occasionally the cervical spine is affected by inflammatory or neoplastic diseases.

EPIDEMIOLOGY

The commonly held idea that human spinal problems result largely from adopting the upright posture is shaken by Lewin's claim that hominids were walking upright 3,750,000 years ago [2], surely sufficient time for adaptation. Davis [3] has suggested that the huge modification in the use of the trunk that occurred between the hunter-gatherer stage of evolution and modern times might explain the current high rate of complaints related to the neck.

Since the vast majority of patients with neck pain are suffering from mechanical problems, their symptoms are likely to be induced by trauma, posture or faulty use. They often settle with rest. The problem of how best to help these patients often lies in the field of rheumatology. Sometimes there is an important neurologic component needing specialist help.

Treatment is rarely surgical, but when there is major instability or progressive neurologic pressure the help of an orthopedic surgeon or neurosurgeon should be sought. As mechanical neck problems are rarely progressive and crippling, spondylosis could be called 'minor', but this would underestimate the effects on patients' lives.

Neck pain is less common than low back pain and the figures for its prevalence are harder to obtain. Lawrence of the Arthritis and Rheumatism Council Epidemiology Unit [4] showed in a study population that 28% of males and 34% of females give a history of neck–shoulder–brachial pain and that 9% of males and 12% of females over the age of 15 years actually had neck–shoulder–brachial pain at the time of the survey (Fig. 5.1). In a general practice 1000 new patients were screened for rheumatologic presenting symptoms [5]. Spinal problems formed 46% of all cases, the majority, however, being lumbosacral. Wood and McLeish [6], recording 'certified incapacity' for 1 year, showed that back troubles per 1000 insured population accounted for 21.09 spells and 627 days of incapacity in males – 42.9% of all rheumatic complaints. The corresponding figures for females were 10.53 spells and 347 days – 36.7% of all rheumatic complaints. Anderson [7], surveying rheumatic complaints in 2684 male employees, showed that cervical problems occur at a rate of one half to one quarter of lumbar disorders. Formal, detailed studies of the relationship of neck pain to age, weight, climate etc, are not available. The clinical impression is that neck pain and stiffness is a common problem. Westerling and Jonsson [8] found an 18% prevalence among 2500 randomly selected men and women, 20% of the women and 16% of the men. Holt [9] looked at 1137 working men aged 25–54 years, of whom half were engaged in light work and the others in heavy jobs. Attacks of stiff neck recurred in 27% of those aged under 30 years and in 50% of those over 45 years. Brachial pain occurred later, affecting 8% of those below 30 years of age and 38% of those aged over 45 years. No definite difference between light and heavy workers was seen in this study. However spontaneous recovery occurs in 1–4 days but shoulder and arm pain follows in a proportion of subjects; 5–10% in the group aged 25–29 years and 25–40% of those aged over 45 years.

There is a clear relationship between musculoskeletal complaints and occupation [10]. The lowest incidences are found in sedentary office workers and the higher figures are found in heavy jobs. Particularly 'at risk' seem to be workers in assembly lines whose posture, attitude at work, and prolonged stationary position seem to be aggravating factors. An individual gross example is 'Porters' neck' [11]: when bags of meal weighing 90.7kg are loaded onto a porter's head, radiologic straightening of the cervical spine can be shown, as well as disc compression and occasionally forward angulation. This results in episodes of pain or even dislocation with spinal cord compression.

DISTRIBUTION OF NECK–SHOULDER–BRACHIAL PAIN, BY SEX

	Males (n=1803)		Females (n=1572)	
Site of pain	Past	Present	Past	Present
Neck only	152	13	179	22
Shoulder only	174	48	112	23
Brachial only	22	6	35	8
Neck and shoulder	83	35	110	38
Neck and brachial	18	13	24	14
Shoulder and brachial	34	20	31	30
Neck–shoulder–brachial	18	20	38	46
Total	501	155 (9%)	529	181 (12%)

Fig. 5.1 The prevalence of neck pain. Data from Lawrence [4].

RADIOLOGIC FEATURES

It might be supposed that disc degeneration and osteoarthritis of facet joints would proceed hand in glove. This does not seem to be the case, since Hirsch *et al.* [12] found no evidence of a relationship between the two processes in an autopsy examination of 111 cervical spines. Lawrence [4] also studied the distribution of cervical disc degeneration on radiography in a population sample (Fig. 5.2) composed of 1803 males and 1572 females aged from 15 years to over 65 years. In the 15–24 age group only 5% of males and 4% of females were found to have mild spondylotic changes, but by the age of 65 years and over the figure had risen to 96% of males and 84% of females and the changes were more severe. The figure was 63% in those aged 45–55 years. Although 15% of men and 19% of women reported symptoms at the time of the survey, there was a dramatic rise in the history of painful episodes in those who were older and had moderate or severe disc degenerative changes. Painful episodes were reported as occurring in nearly 60% of those with severe degenerative changes and age over 65 years. There was also a very strong relationship between cervical and lumbar spondylotic changes. The greatest prevalence of disc degeneration was found in male manual workers, especially coal miners, but no association with the specific types of work being performed by females. Dampness in the environment could not be related to radiologic changes. The epidemiology of disc disorders is reviewed by Lawrence [13].

ANATOMY

The neck is the most mobile section of the spine and is capable of movement in all directions. It supports the head, which weighs a little over 3kg and is supported on seven vertebrae.

The atlas and axis are particularly specialized variants of standard cervical vertebrae. The atlas is designed to support the skull, which is perched on a pair of convex/concave lateral joints between the occipital condyles and lateral masses of the atlas (Fig. 5.3). These permit a nodding movement of about 35°. The atlas has no body, the equivalent being the odontoid process, which is fused with the body of the axis forming a vertical rod. This rod permits rotation with a gliding movement of the synovial joints between the lower articular facets of the atlas and the upper articular surfaces of the axis. Those nerve roots emerging either between the base of the skull and the atlas, or between the atlas and axis, may be compressed, leading to severe neuralgia .

The remaining cervical vertebrae conform to a more standard pattern (Fig. 5.4). Each has anteriorly a bony body separated from its neighbor by an intervertebral disc. In childhood the opposing surfaces of the vertebral bodies are covered by thin plates of cartilage which form epiphyses. These fuse soon after the age of 21 years. The peripheral parts of the cartilaginous plates ossify, thus forming a bony ring. Only in later life does the central part become ossified. The disc consists of a semi-fluid central core, the nucleus pulposus, encircled by and enclosed within the tough, fibrous annulus. This is largely composed of concentric layers of fibrous tissue arranged as parallel fibers running at 45° to the vertebral bodies, alternate layers lying at right angles to each other. This format results in great strength of union of the vertebral bodies and resistance to torsional and flexion deformities. In addition there is a great resistance to rupture. The nucleus pulposus is semi-gelatinous, consisisting of a ground substance of collagen and protein-polysaccharide, and composed overall of about 80% water. The whole is incompressible and under normal circumstances the end plates of the vertebrae and the encircling annulus will resist the high pressures generated. There is a decrease in the water content of the disc with aging.

The spinal canal is surrounded by bony and ligamentous structures. Laterally, the transverse processes contain the vertebral arteries and sweep posteriorly to form laminae and a spinous process. Blood ascends in the vertebral arteries (Fig. 5.4) to feed the circle of Willis. Occlusion of the vertebral circulation may lead to ischemic episodes and drop attacks. The articular facets face postero-laterally and are oblique to allow flexion, extension, and rotations at the synovial zygapophyseal (synovial facet) joints. The atlantoaxial joint is

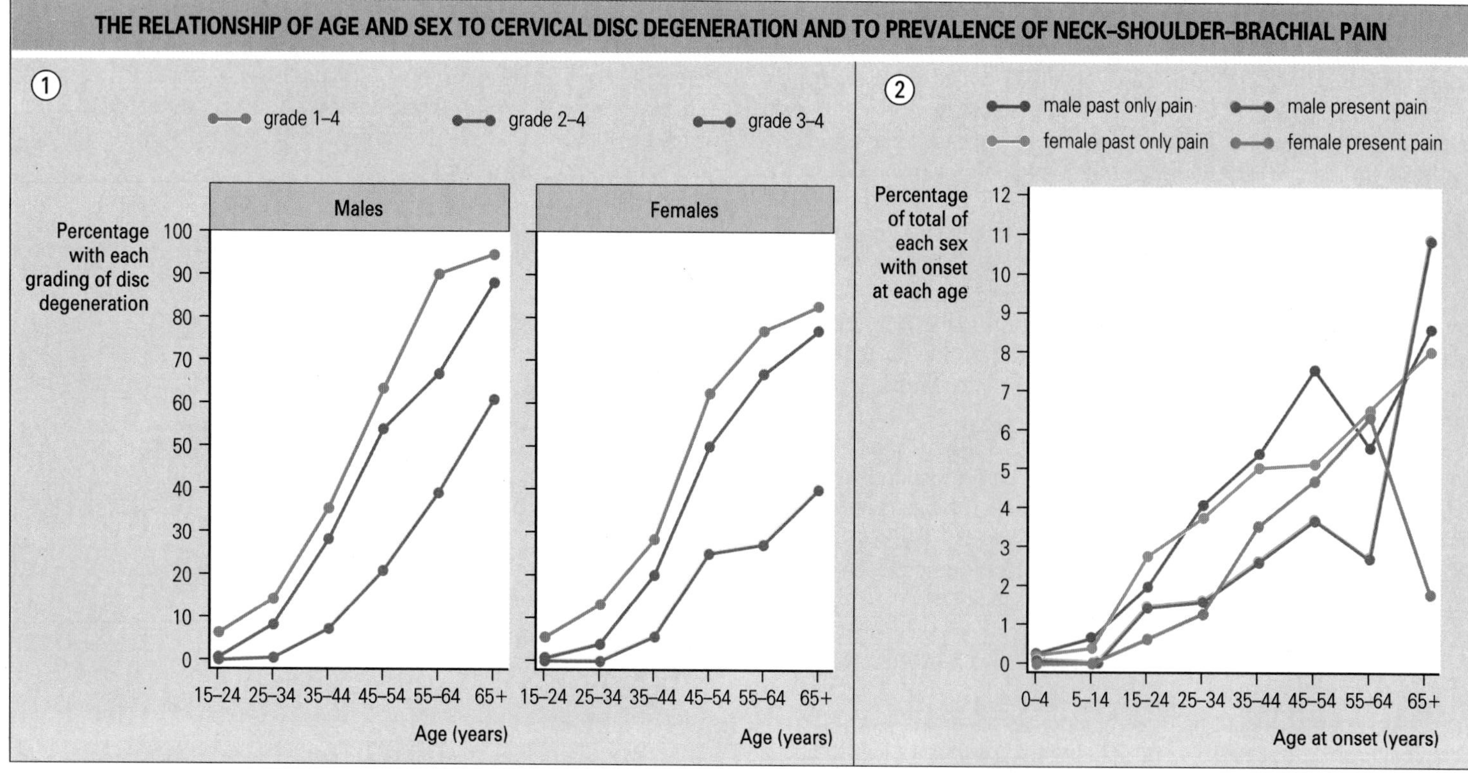

Fig. 5.2 Radiological evidence of cervical disc degeneration by age and sex (1). The prevalence of neck–shoulder–brachial pain by age and sex (2). Both increase with age, but not with sex. Data from Lawrence [4].

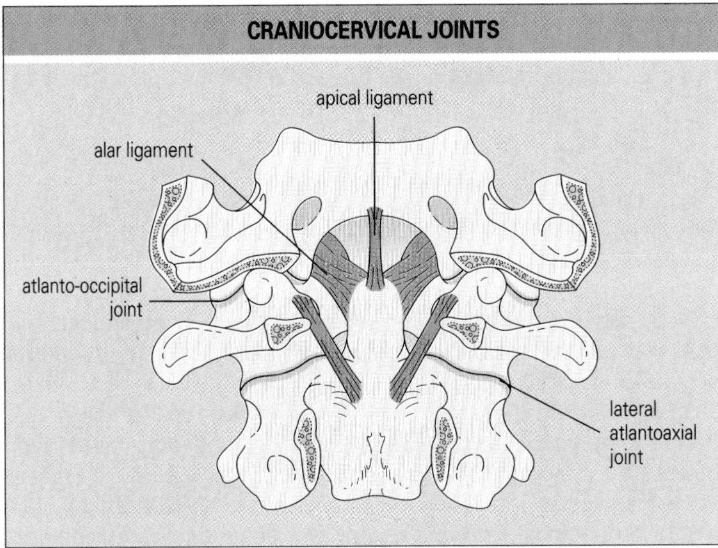

Fig. 5.3 The occipital condyles of the skull are supported by the lateral masses of the atlas and these in turn by the upper articular surfaces of the axis.

prevented from subluxing antero-posteriorly primarily by the transverse ligament of the atlas but is also restrained by the suspensory and oblique ligaments of the odontoid process.

The spinal cord is protected inside the spinal canal. Nerve roots emerge at every level, being numbered according to the vertebra above which they pass. Thus, C1 passes between skull and atlas, C7 between C6 and C7, and C8 between C7 and T1; but T1 passes between T1 and T2 and is thus partly protected from mechanical and degenerative changes.

The spinal cord is nourished largely by the anterior spinal artery, which is formed from branches of the right and left vertebral arteries. Blood flow is caudal and supplies the spinal cord with segmental sulcal and coronal branches. There is also a posterior longitudinal artery of slightly lesser importance. Embryologically, feeders enter at each level, but in adult life only a few remain, generally at C4 or C5, and T1 or T2. Thus, occlusion of the vertebral artery can lead to a watershed area of ischemia.

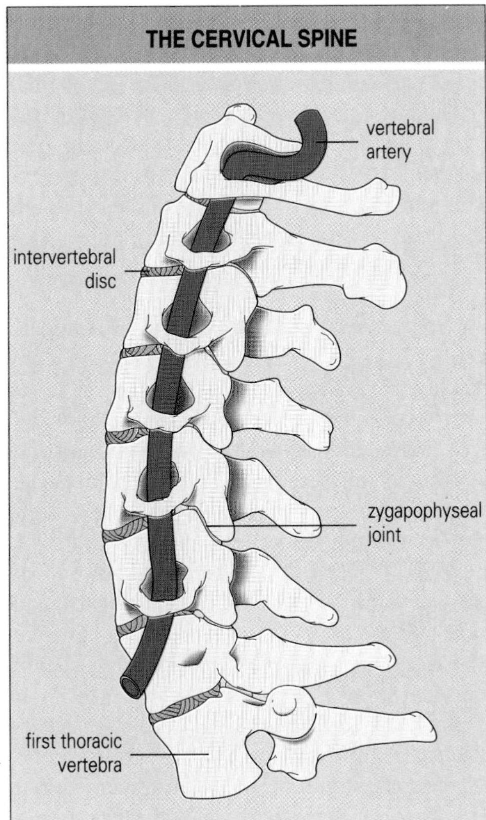

Fig. 5.4 The vertebrae from C3–C7 form a gentle lordotic curve and conform to a standard pattern. The vertebral arteries pass through the transverse processes of the cervical vertebrae to feed the circle of Willis.

CLINICAL APPROACH

Introduction

Pain is by far the most common feature leading a patient with a cervical spine disorder to seek advice. Alternative presentations include deformity (torticollis) or neurologic features, for example paresthesia, arm weakness, or spasticity. An important feature of mechanically induced pain is its intermittent nature. It is frequently produced by alteration in position or a prolonged awkward posture. It is often relieved by a change in position or by rest – i.e. recumbency, when the weight of the head is taken through a pillow. By contrast, inflammatory and neoplastic disorders often produce prolonged and unremitting pain.

Mechanical lesions occur most commonly in the mid and lower cervical region, in particular at the C5–C6 and C6–C7 levels. The origin of the pain may be bone, joint, ligament or muscle. The classic provocation experiments performed by Cloward provide information about pain referral [14,15]. He showed that needling the anterior surface of a disc in a conscious patient would provoke pain in the shoulder blade area. By contrast, touching the vertebral bodies above and below the disc caused no pain. Upper cervical discs referred pain more cephalad on the scapula, and lower discs more caudad. Other experiments performed by discographic stimulation provided further documentation of pain referral from discs. Pain could also be produced by injections under pressure into an intact disc and this was termed 'discogenic'. Commonly the bulging annulus would cause a deep dull aching sensation, referred to the medial scapular border. This could be made to spread over the back or top of the shoulder in a broad area and then down the posterior surface of the upper arm to the elbow. When the annulus fibers were leaking, allowing discographic fluid to pass through the defect, a different type of pain termed 'neurogenic' was produced. This was sharper, more intense in quality and often described as an electric shock, or a hot burning sensation. It would shoot into the arm and be felt in a strictly dermatomal distribution. In midline protrusions with spinal cord compression a further type of pain was produced and termed 'myelogenic'. This was a shock-like sensation spreading down the spine, at times into all four extremities.

An interesting concept is that pain is produced locally. Thus Weddell *et al.*[16] demonstrated by electromyography that the sites of muscular pain were producing abnormal action potentials. Thus, they argue, the nerve impulse must be propagated by way of the anterior nerve root.

These hypotheses for pathways of pain referral propose the passage of impulses along the sinuvertebral nerve (of Luschka). This nerve supplies the vertebral column, the intervertebral discs, the intravertebral ligaments, the epidural tissue of the vertebral canal, and the dura mater. It is largely sensory and emerges through the intervertebral foramen and curls back to join the spinal nerve just within the spinal canal. Typically, an impulse will travel along the sinuvertebral nerve to join the posterior primary ramus, pass through the dorsal root ganglion and emerge through the anterior ramus to be transmitted to the muscle concerned.

The posterior primary ramus serves the posterior ligaments, the apophyseal joints and the posterior musculature of the cervical spine. It probably also can be a pathway for myalgic and referred pain. Experimental work in the lumbar spine [17] has shown that injections of hypertonic saline into deep ligaments can produce considerable local and distal referral of pain. The situation is presumably analogous in the neck, but the work has not been done at cervical levels.

Thus, pain originating in the cervical spine may be referred to a wide range of sites. Headache and occipital pain may clearly result from direct C1 or C2 root irritation. This pain can be so severe as to make the patient 'cradle' the head in the hands in order to prevent jarring. However, a destructive pathology rather than spondylosis is usually required to cause this. At this level destructive rheumatoid changes, trauma and infections occur. More common is dull, diffuse headache and this may be referred through the deeper longitudinal anastomoses already mentioned, for example those of the sinuvertebral nerve .

True and severe C3 or C4 root pain is felt over the shoulder. This may occur after trauma or may be confused with neuropathy due to diabetes, virus or allergy. Again, a dull ache may be referred from deep spinal structures with a degenerative process. Lesions at levels C5, C6, C7 or C8 are the most common and often arise with spondylosis. The pain may originate from discs, apophyseal joints or other deep structures and may have the referral patterns discussed. However, true root pain also occurs most frequently involving the C7 level. Root compression pain is classically severe, well delineated and exacerbated by spinal movement or changes in cerebrospinal fluid pressure, for example with coughing or sneezing. Unusually large anterior osteophytes may compromise swallowing, leading to dysphagia. Occasionally, referred anterior chest pain is produced and can be confused with myocardial ischemia.

Whiplash Injuries

Crowe [18] coined the term whiplash to 'describe only the manner in which a head was moved suddenly to produce a sprain in the neck'. The injury is said to occur in 18–60% of motor accidents. The causative injury is usually a sudden flexion and hyperextension of the cervical spine, perhaps preceded by forced extension. The phrase 'acceleration–deceleration' is sometimes used, especially when the injury is sustained in the most common circumstances, a rear-end motor collision. However, the term whiplash syndrome is used to describe a cluster of symptoms which can follow an injury sustained in this manner, and is reserved for the situation in which there is no demonstrable radiologic lesion. Seat belts prevent serious bodily or head injury but make neck sprains more likely: head restraints are protective if correctly adjusted. Typically, symptoms and signs are like those of other mechanical neck disorders, but there is sometimes an impression that anxiety about a compensation claim may aggravate the features.

This subject has recently been reviewed by Barry [19]. Radiographic changes are variable and of debatable relevance. Soft tissue swelling and angular deformity have been described, and magnetic resonance imaging (MRI) is indicated with neurological symptoms or signs. Management generally consists of rest, sometimes using a collar in slight flexion, and analgesics for 1–2 weeks. The role of mobilizing physiotherapy is difficult to understand and has been reviewed by Newman [20]. Over 70% of patients settle in 2–3 months. However, in a proportion as high as 26% symptoms persist for more than 6 months, the 'late whiplash syndrome'. In these patients, MRI and neurophysiologic studies have produced abnormal findings whose implications are not clear. Long-term psychological and litigation problems are common and the treatment empirical.

Hyperextension in the Elderly

Central cervical cord syndromes may be overlooked, particularly in the elderly. Features including the combination of weakness in the arms and pyramidal signs in the legs are often misinterpreted. Exacerbation of pre-existing cervical spondylosis should be considered [21,22].

Sporting Injuries

Attention has been given recently to the incidence of injuries to the cervical cord in sports such as rugby football [23,24].

The Welsh Rugby Union recorded two fractures of the cervical spine with serious neurologic sequelae between 1945 and 1964 in a population of 18,000–20,000 players. In South Africa 20 cervical cord injuries were described in nearly 45,000 schoolboys over a 12-year period [25]. Of these, 60% occurred while tackling and 40% while scrummaging. A range of fractures is reported, including fracture-dislocations and compression fractures. Scrummaging lesions were generally a fracture-dislocation of the cervical spine with bilateral 'locking' of facet joints. The lesion is caused by a combination of flexion and rotation of the cervical spine and may be lethal.

Musicians

The particular stresses of those involved in performing arts lead to their own idiosyncratic problems [26]. Instrumental players are understandably sensitive to painful problems. In students this is perhaps due to their career anxieties and in mature artistes may follow excessive physical demands. Those performers whose instruments are held between the jaw and chest, for example violinists and violists, need to take particular care. Electromyographic studies of the muscles used are providing a valuable insight into the problems [27]. Rather than resort to aggressive physical methods of treatment, or potent drugs, the approach should be to exclude significant organic disease and then proffer advice. Sound advice should usually start with a professional teacher's assessment of posture and technique, sometimes followed by a therapist's advice on posture and position. Seldom is prolonged abstinence from playing essential but rather a gradual return in modified circumstances.

PHYSICAL EXAMINATION

General

The clinical examination should start with a general assessment. Although most neck pain is due to local mechanical problems, the cumulative prevalence of less common causes with sytemic features makes general examination mandatory on the least pretext. The examiner should look for evidence of weight loss, anemia or adenopathy as well as abnormalities of the heart, chest and abdomen. Abnormalities of posture, movement, expression and gestures should also be recorded. Finally, cervical problems often require examination of the shoulders, arms and peripheral nervous system.

Local

Local examination should include a careful inspection of the skin, noting blemishes such as scars, pigmentation and swellings. The attitude of the head and neck will be noted.

Palpation of both anterior and posterior structures of the neck should follow, including in particular the spinous processes, spinal joints, paraspinal muscles and soft tissues. Deep palpation for spinal joint tenderness may be of value and often reassures the patient. The carotid, temporal and occipital arteries should be felt for tenderness and pulsation and auscultated for bruits in relevant cases. Lymph and salivary gland swelling may also be relevant.

Movement

The normal neck moves freely through a large range. Movements should be recorded in three planes; flexion/extension, left and right rotation, and left and right lateral flexion (Fig. 5.5).

Flexion and extension have a combined excursion of approximately 70°. About half of this occurs between the occiput and C1, the remainder being distributed fairly evenly through the cervical spine. Thus, if the cervical spine is fused, for example by spondylitis, a substantial nodding movement only remains. Left and right rotations are appoximately 90° in each direction, and about half of this occurs at the atlantoaxial joint, the remainder being distributed evenly through the cervical spine. Lateral flexions are approximately 45° to the left and to the right, the whole excursion being shared along the length of the cervical spine.

Movement can be tested actively or passively. Active movements require cooperation, volition and an intact neuromuscular system. They also serve to demonstrate the range of movement but can be restricted by pain. Passive movements in which the power

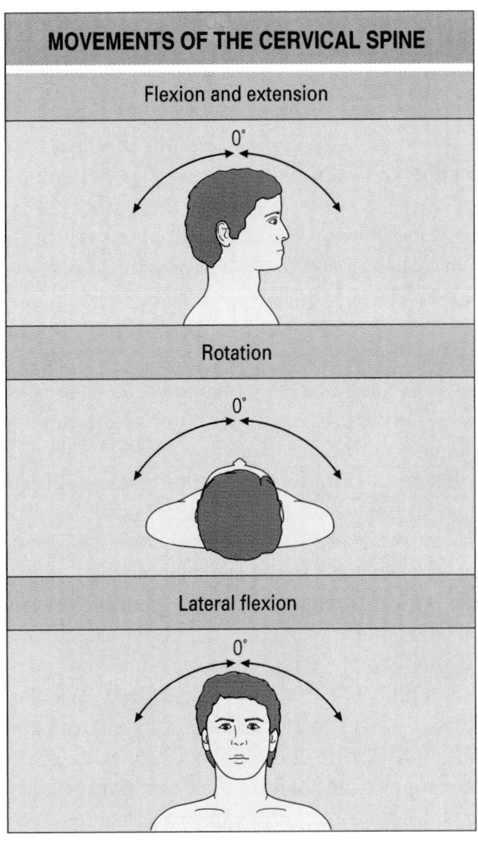

Fig. 5.5 Movements of the cervical spine are recorded in three planes; flexion/extension, rotation, and lateral flexion.

and volition are supplied by the examiner give an indication of the range of motion in isolation. Most mechanical disorders are caused by a local mechanical problem, due to injury or the process of wear and tear. The lesion is usually asymmetrical and the range of movement will be asymmetrically painful and/or limited. By contrast, inflammatory or neoplastic disorders cause a widespread and more or less symmetrical pathology so that pain and restriction are also symmetrical. Often the lateral flexions are restricted earliest and most obviously. Perhaps this is because so much flexion/extension and rotation is spared, occurring as it does largely at the occipito-atlanto-axial levels. Restricted movements are a test of neuromuscular power or a local musculotendinous pathology. Thus, weakness is a sign of a proximal neuropathy or myopathy, and pain a feature of a muscle or tendon lesion.

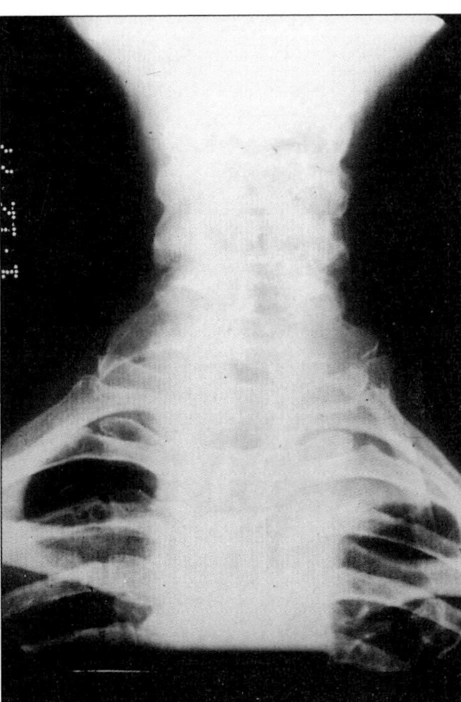

Fig. 5.6 A 'cervical rib' or an analogous fibrous band may encroach on the space between the clavicle and the first rib.

The standard procedure begins by asking the patient to sit facing the examiner. Extension followed by flexion should be requested, followed by left then right rotation, then left and right lateral flexions. A measurement can be made by fixing a reflex hammer onto the occiput (for flexion/extension and lateral flexions) or forehead for rotations. Alternatively a spirit level goniometer can be used.

In the normal person, the active and passive ranges of movement will be full and equal. There will be no pain or discomfort at any time. Resisted movements are not a test of joint range, but of neuromuscular power or painful intramuscular pathology. Increasing severity of pathology will provide increasing and more definitely abnormal signs. Minimal pathologic processes will produce mere discomfort at the extreme of range, with no actual restriction of movement. A more distinct process will produce actual restriction of range.

Thoracic Outlet

So frequently are the symptoms of cervical problems felt in the arms that examination of the thoracic outlet should be routine in such patients. For practical purposes, this space is bounded superiorly by the clavicle and inferiorly by the first rib. The two main structures whose function may be compromised in this space are the brachial plexus and the subclavian artery. Classically, the space is intruded upon by an extra or 'cervical' rib (Fig. 5.6). This can be either a large transverse process to C7 or a radiologically invisible fibrous band in the same position and can cause problems due to compression of nerve root or blood vessel.

The positive physical signs used to support the diagnosis suspected on the history are those which provoke symptoms.

NEUROLOGIC EXAMINATION

Examination of the nervous system is often important in considering patients with neck pain. Vertebral disease may affect the spinal cord and/or nerve roots. For example if the cervical canal is shallow or narrow the cord will have a tight fit and be more readily prone to pressure. If the sagittal measurement of the canal is under 13mm then the cord is particularly liable to compression. Abnormal nerve root signs are unusual at upper and midcervical levels, but more frequently found related to the more common lower cervical lesions. Cord pressure features may occur with lesions at any level.

Segmental Examination

Involvement of C1 or C2 nerve roots causes severe occipital pain. Rather more diffuse pain in the upper neck and occiput may be referred from other levels, and this may be difficult to differentate from the mechanical pain which is believed, on circumstantial evidence, to arise from more mundane midcervical lesions. True pain in the C1 or C2 distribution has no detectable motor or reflex abnormalities but may be suspected because of its severe, well circumscribed nature and accompanying sensory loss. The pathology is more likely to be traumatic or inflammatory.

Pain originating at C3 may occur in the neck in association with numbness in the pinna, posterior cheek, temporal area, and chin. Paresthesia may occur but detectable weakness is rare .

Pain originating at C4 may spread from the mid cervical spine to the shoulder with a band of impaired sensation along the spine of the scapula, the mid-deltoid area, and the clavicle. Detectable muscle weakness is rare. It may occur after trauma.

The most common levels for mechanical/degenerative lesions are in the low cervical spine. Exact allocation to a root level is not possible on clinical grounds alone and some overlap and variation is found in motor, reflex and sensory findings. However, C6 and C7 each accounts for about 35% of lesions, C8 for 25% and C5 for about 5%. Lesions which are outside these levels, or those which

COMMONLY AFFECTED NERVE ROOTS IN THE CERVICAL SPINE			
Root	Motor weakness	Reflex diminution	Sensory impairment
C6	Biceps Brachioradialis	Biceps Supinator (may be inverted)	Lateral forearm Thumb and index finger
C7	Triceps Forearm extensors	Triceps	Strip posteriorly along forearm, dorsum of middle and one other finger
C8	Thumb and finger extensor	None	Ulnar border of forearm Ring and small finger flexors

Fig. 5.7 Commonly affected nerve roots in the cervical spine.

involve more than one level or which are bilateral usually imply gross or sinister pathology. Motor findings consist of weakness, flaccidity, wasting and electromyographic (EMG) evidence of denervation. Reflex changes are indicated by diminution of the tendon reflex. Sensory loss can be to all modalities, but especially light touch and pinprick. Figure 5.7 summarizes the most common findings associated with cervical nerve root compression .

Lesions of the lower root of T1 are very rare in uncomplicated cervical spondylosis, presumably because the root emerges between the relatively well supported and rather immobile first and second thoracic vertebrae. Their presence should prompt a search for an alternative pathology. It leads to wasting of the small muscles of the hand of both median and ulnar supply. There is no reflex change or reliable sensory impairment, although there may be a patch of numbness medial to the elbow.

Spinal Cord Pressure

Symptoms usually start with pain in the neck and are followed by weakness and sensory symptoms in the arms or in all four limbs. There may be paresthesias in the arms or all four limbs provoked by neck movement, especially cervical flexion (Lermitte sign). The weakness may be multisegmental, affecting one or both arms. Difficulty in walking may be observed in the presence of pyramidal tract involvement. On examination there is a flaccid weakness in the arms involving segments from C5–T1 inclusive, with muscle wasting more apparent distally. Some of these changes have been shown in an analogous situation to be due to anterior spinal artery compression [28] and cord ischemia in a watershed area [29]. Reflexes are patchily reduced and the sensory impairment is diffusely diminished distally. The legs show spastic weakness with hyper-reflexia and extensor plantar responses. Vibration and position sensation are often reduced.

SYSTEMATIC APPROACH TO NECK DISORDERS

Etiology of Spondylosis

The most common cause of pain in the neck is the combined mechanical/traumatic/over-use syndrome generally described under the heading cervical spondylosis. The question as to why it occurs and why especially in two areas of the spine – the low cervical and the low lumbar – is not completely answered. In both instances the site is related to the secondary lordosis. At the cervical level it is acknowledged that exceptional demands are made in terms of the frequent movements required by visual, auditory, balance and eating processes as well as the frequent movements needed to stabilize the head when any other part of the trunk is moved. Certain specific etiological factors have already been mentioned: the flexion/extension injury (whiplash); sports (rugby, football, diving); and other specific injuries often occurring during falls. These may be injuries related to a single traumatic event or caused by repeated minor trauma. Curiously, a case of multiple subaxial subluxation has been attributed to corticosteroids [30].

Pathology of Spondylosis

The pathology of cervical spondylosis centers around the disc and the apophyseal synovial joints [31]. There is a difference in the pathogenesis of the two parts of the process, although radiographically they generally occur together. Autopsy studies show a very high pathological prevalence of spondylosis, even higher than radiological surveys. For example, Schmorl [32] found evidence of the condition by the age of 49 years in 60% of women and 80% of men and in 95% of both sexes by the age of 90 years. The shortfall in prevalence on standard radiographic techniques is presumed to be due to technical shortcomings, and may lessen with computerized tomography (CT) scanning or magnetic resonance imaging (MRI). There is also a discrepancy between radiographic and pathological findings and recorded neck pain. It might be assumed that all pathology is painful, but this clearly is not the case. Severe spondylosis and other pathological problems may be detected in the absence of pain.

After middle age, clefts appear in the cervical discs parallel to the end plates; the central part of the disc may even become isolated and loose. This is believed to happen by a tearing process. Clefts pass through the annulus to the epidural space. The associated vascular response observed suggests a repair reaction. Clefts may also appear in the annulus at 90° to the bundles of collagen, and again the presence of vascular ingrowth suggests an attempt at repair. Rim lesions have been found pathologically in the majority of subjects aged over 50 years, most often in the upper anterior portion of a vertebra; their significance is not clear. In the lumbar region, postmortem studies have shown vertical disc prolapse in the form of Schmorl's nodes in 50% and posterior prolapse in 10% of spines [33]. Vascular invasion of a disc may occur where there has been a breach in the cartilage end plate, and this may be followed by calcification or ossification. Disc height lessens with dehydration and is accelerated by protrusion.

Herniation of the nucleus pulposus is prevented by a normal end plate and an intact annulus. However, herniation can occur at either of the two weak places; the cartilage end plate, or the posterior segment of the annulus, usually to either side of the tough posterior longitudinal ligament. Anterior and lateral protrusions are rare. The usual cause of herniation is trauma, but congenital defects of end plate and annulus are possible. Cadaveric experiments and observations during surgery show that protrusions may project and retreat alternately with position, pressure and relaxation. Stabilization of a prolapse usually occurs due to periosteal elevation and osteophyte formation [34]. These protective bony processes encase the prolapsed tissue. When this does not occur the protruding disc may compress nerve root tissue.

Osteoarthritis of the Apophyseal Joints

Anatomical abnormalities in the disc are always accompanied by apophyseal joint changes, and the converse applies; when the apophyseal joints are normal, so are the discs. This is relevant to degenerative changes, fractures, block vertebrae and deformities. Osteoarthritis in apophyseal joints may differ slightly from that found in major weight-bearing joints. Often, hyaline cartilage is preserved even when large osteophytes have formed. However, when osteoarthritis is severe there may be eburnation and subarticular cyst formation. The osteophytic outgrowths from apophyseal joints often project into intervertebral foramina and may compress nerve roots. Capsule and soft tissue, including ligamentum flavum, may hypertrophy. It can be surmised that pain arises from:

- abnormal (vascularized) disc;
- trabecular fractures in vertebral bone;
- osteoarthritis of apophyseal joints;
- pressure on ligaments;
- pressure on nerve roots.

Nerve Roots

Although the 'pathology' of spondylosis is so common as to make it almost the rule rather than an exception, true nerve root features, as opposed to deep joint or ligamentous pain and stiffness, are less common. The process by which a nerve root is compromised may be associated with either disc prolapse or osteophyte formation. It is relatively uncommon for annulus defects to occur so laterally and cause root compression. However, osteophytes may arise from the annulus attachment to the vertebra, from the apophyseal joints or from the uncovertebral joints (of Luschka). All of these can cause foraminal encroachment with the consequent neurologic sequelae.

Spinal Cord

Myelopathy is probably a less common complication of cervical spondylosis. In his neurological practice, Brain [35] reviewed 100 consecutive patients and found that brachial radiculitis was a presenting feature in 32, headache in 28, vertigo in 17, myelopathy in 13, neck pain in 13, vertebro-basilar ischemia in five, attacks of unconsciousness in four, drop attacks in three, and acute lesions of the spinal cord in three. Features were sometimes multiple and probably represent a rather different selection from patients coming to rheumatologists. Degeneration of discs with protrusions, osteophytic outgrowths, osteoarthrosis of apophyseal joints and thickening of the ligamentum flavum can cause narrowness and shallowness of the cervical spinal canal. This may physically compress the spinal cord either by direct pressure or by compression of the anterior and posterior spinal arteries [36]. This may lead to lower motor neuron weakness at the level of the lesion, commonly the fifth cervical level, with weakness of shoulder abduction (deltoid) and external rotation (infraspinatus) associated with a diminution of the supinator reflex (C6) and a brisk finger jerk (inverted supinator reflex) due to a combination of lower and upper motor neuron features. The legs usually show weakness of a spastic type with hyper-reflexia and extensor plantar responses. Compression of the circulation of the spinal cord may lead to cord damage suspended to a distal level.

The supply of blood to the cervical cord is dependent on two main longitudinal vessels; the anterior median longitudinal artery and a lesser posterior vessel. The anterior is by far the more important. Disturbance of flow has been shown to lead to ischemia in the several 'watershed areas' [37]. The great variability is of interest and importance in explaining neurological sequelae of spinal column lesions. Dommisse [38] showed that the thoracic cord is least generously supplied from T4–T9, but at the cervical levels reliance is often placed on a unilateral segmental radicular feeding vessel at C5, often the next not occurring until C8 or T1. Thus, otherwise inexplicable lower cervical cord lesions with T1 wasting can be seen to occur with upper and mid-cervical compression. This clinical phenomenon has been illustrated with clinical examples, radiography, electrophysiology and postmortem studies [28].

Vertebro-basilar Ischemia

Vertebro-basilar ischemia may be produced by osteophytes projecting from the tips of the intervertebral joints that displace the vertebral arteries anteriorly and laterally [39]. Osteophytes are especially likely to distort the vertebral artery between the second and third vertebrae because the vessel at this level is placed laterally so as to reach the transverse process of the atlas. These effects tend to accentuate the consequences of pre-existing atheroma. It is also possible for a plaque of atheroma to become detached and embolize in the cerebral circulation.

Drop Attacks

Drop attacks are defined as sudden falls due to involuntary loss of power in the legs and may be due to temporary and reversible loss of the brainstem circulation. Vertigo may occur simultaneously in some patients by the same mechanism.

Torticollis

The term torticollis describes an abnormal position of the cervical spine. This often results from minor mechanical disorders and derangements in the cervical spine. In this case the mechanism is presumed to be an acute joint derangement. Other forms of torticollis need to be considered.

Congenital torticollis is painless, and results from contracture of one sternomastoid, pulling the head and neck into flexion and rotation away from the contracted side.

Acute torticollis has many known causes. In children it may follow a sore throat and stiff neck. It is due to a painful adenitis causing muscular spasm. It also occurs with inflammatory disorders of the cervical spinal joints such as may occur in juvenile chronic arthritis. In adolescents and adults it may also be caused by inflammation, but mechanical causes such as injury become more common.

Spasmodic torticollis is produced by sudden contraction of neck muscles rotating and tilting the head to the most extreme position. Relaxation may be quite sudden and unheralded. The cause of spasmodic torticollis may be psychogenic or post-encephalitic, or it may be part of an extrapyramidal or tonic muscle disorder. Explanation and instruction may be helpful at first, but physiotherapy is useless. Heroic neurosurgery is of unproven value.

Spastic torticollis describes the situation where the altered position has become almost fixed into rotation and lateral flexion. A powerful traction pull may temporarily restore the normal posture, as may recumbency. These observations suggest a postural tone disorder.

DIFFERENTIAL DIAGNOSIS OF NECK PAIN

Although spondylosis is the most common cause of pain in the neck and results from a blend of trauma, wear and tear and degeneration, there is often no clear history of injury. Frequently there is no more than a conjecture of poor posture, unaccustomed activity, or an inconspicuous injury.

Rheumatoid Arthritis

Rheumatoid arthritis commonly affects the upper cervical spine, this being a site rich in synovial tissue (see Chapters 15 and 18). Studies have shown antero-posterior subluxation in 25% and vertical subluxation in 5% of rheumatoid patients [40]. Antero-posterior subluxation can result from ligamentous laxity. However this needs to involve not merely the transverse ligament of the atlas, section of which in the cadaver leads only to a few millimeters of subluxation, but also the alar, oblique and suspensory ligaments. Follow-up studies show that this can be progressive, and in patients with severe rheumatoid disease deterioration is common [41]. Antero-posterior subluxation may be sudden, following minor trauma, and accompanied by a click and followed by a dull pain in the neck or occiput. Alternatively the pain may be extremely severe, occipital, and clearly due to occipital nerve root compression. Such patients cradle their heads in their hands to relieve pain, and move in terror of any jarring activity. However, such severe pain is more frequent in patients with vertical subluxation. This follows destructive rheumatoid changes which cause erosion of the lateral mass of the atlas [42]. The ensuing vertical descent of the skull 'wedges' the foramen magnum over the odontoid process. This may cause dangerous medullary compression in the foramen magnum in addition to the severely painful occipital neuralgia. Subaxial subluxations may also cause neck pain and quadraplegia [43] by direct cord compression [44,45] or pressure on the anterior spinal artery [28].

Spondylitis

The term spondylitis indicates a fundamentally inflammatory disease process. The classical disorder is ankylosing spondylitis, but atypical forms may occur with Reiter's syndrome, psoriatic arthritis and chronic intestinal disorders (see Chapters 22 and 29). In ankylosing spondylitis the spinal disease always appears to start in the sacroiliac joints, and frequently spreads up the spine. In the atypical spondyloarthropathies this is much less often the case and the cervical spine may even be affected first. The inflammatory process affects the apophyseal joints with a synovitis and causes calcification of the annulus of the discs forming syndesmophytes. Calcification also occurs at muscle and tendon attachments; this is termed 'enthesopathy'. The pathology generally becomes bilateral and symmetrical, so that pain can affect either or both sides of the neck. Symptoms are often prolonged and characteristically there is stiffness after immobility. Restriction of movement is also generally symmetrical, lateral flexions usually being affected first, followed by the rotation movements. Flexion and extension are affected last and, even in severe cases, to a lesser extent. This is due to the sparing of the atlanto-occipital joint which allows preservation of the nodding movement.

Infection

In developed Western countries, infections of the spine always seem to take the physician by surprise. Perhaps this is partly because of their relative rarity, and partly because the more acute infections often seem less aggressive than in classical descriptions. A source of infection is often only discovered retrospectively. A history of trauma should never put the clinician off the diagnosis of infection.

Acute infection

Bacterial infection generally spreads to the spine via the blood stream, but local spread is possible from the throat and retropharyngeal space, or glands . The organisms are generally *Staphylococcus*, *Streptococcus*, or *Escherichia coli*. Systemic features may be present, such as fever, tachycardia and weight loss. Local pain is usually very prominent and characteristically is constant, progressive and becomes very severe. The neck may be tender to pressure, and movements soon become symmetrically and severely restricted. Sometimes infection can spread into the epidural space with abscess formation and neurologic compromise.

Diagnosis of bacterial infection should be suspected on the history and physical examination. The ESR will usually be elevated. An increase in the total white blood cell count is less constant. Early changes may be spotted clinically or radiologically, as with a retropharyngeal soft tissue mass. In effect this is an abscess arising from the underlying, but radiologically still normal, infected bone. Bony radiographic changes themselves are relatively late, taking 2–3 weeks to appear. They generally show as erosion of a vertebral end plate, osteoporosis, or collapse (Fig. 5.8). Generally two vertebrae and the enclosed disc space are affected. An isotope bone scan will often show the abnormality at an earlier stage and is an important additional investigation [46] but diagnosis should be confirmed by needle aspiration or blood culture. Untreated abscess formation, septicemia, and death may ensue.

Chronic Infection

Cervical spine tuberculosis is rare, and less common than at other levels, but by no means extinct. The organism is usually *Mycobacterium tuberculosis*. The portal artery may be pulmonary or intestinal. The infection is blood-borne to a single vertebra, which collapses, infecting the adjacent disc and the next vertebra. Caseous material is discharged and may press on the cervical cord or into paraspinal tissues forming a 'cold abscess'. Bony destruction and wedging of vertebrae may occur.

There is often a long and insidious period of ill health and pain is often slight, only being apparent on jolting or movement. Sometimes pain is not reported at all and the patient presents with a swelling or paraplegia. Clinically, the general features of ill health should be spotted and a blood count and ESR may reveal evidence of an inflammatory process. Mantoux testing is of dwindling value but a chest radiograph may show the source of infection. As with acute infections, a bone scan may show the abnormality early. Retropharyngeal abscess will soon show on a lateral radiograph (Fig. 5.9) but definitive bony changes will occur later. CT or MRI may be useful in showing the extent of abscess formation, and radiculography with or without CT may give further information about intraspinal extension.

Giant Cell Arteritis

The distribution of lesions in giant cell arteritis has been shown to be widespread, involving the elastic coating of extradural arteries [47] (see Chapter 39). Although the most prominent rheumatologic feature is polymyalgia, the arterial inflammation in itself may cause pain in the form of headache. Involvement of the occipital arteries is an occasional and very important cause of neck pain and tenderness, especially in the elderly.

Tumors

Malignant tumors in the cervical spine are usually metastases. The primary source may be bronchus, kidney, thyroid, prostate or breast. Multiple myeloma is much rarer in this location. Pain is the most common feature. Although it may be intermittent at the onset, it characteristically becomes severe and constant. Restriction of movement of the cervical spine may be mild and intermittent at the onset, but eventually the spine becomes rigid. Swelling is seldom detected, but a misleading history of trauma can be obtained. Tumors may cause nerve root pain and damage. Whereas in spondylotic problems one root only is generally affected, with neoplasms the lesion may involve two or more roots or be bilateral with pain, weakness, reflex changes and sensory loss. Infiltration intraspinally may also lead to spasticity with long tract signs.

Primary tumors are much less common. Benign soft tissue tumors, such as meningiomas, neurofibromas (Fig. 5.10) and schwannomas, will usually present with mixtures of skeletal and neurologic features. Not uncommonly there will be a history of recurrent neck pain with restriction of movement, indistinguishable from a spondylotic problem and arousing no suspicion. Subsequently, neurologic features

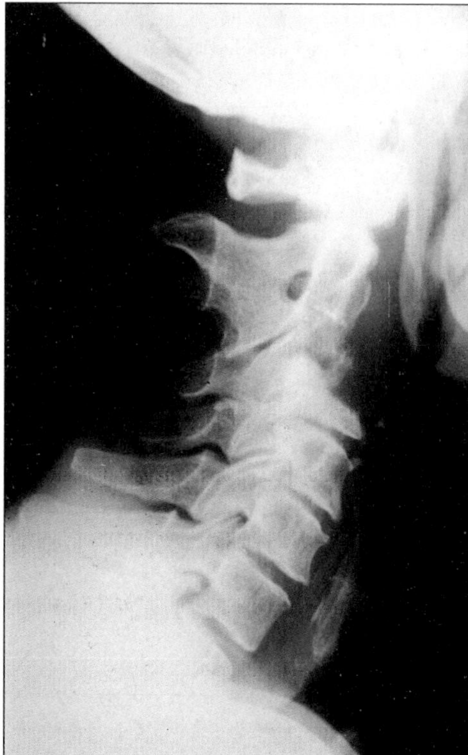

Fig. 5.8 This patient presented with severe neck pain, and also had shoulder and lumbar pain. Destruction is shown of the bodies of C2, C3, C4, and a staphylococcus was grown from the shoulder biopsy.

appear, with weakness in the arms, a sensory level in the trunk, and spasticity of the legs. Neurofibromas occur at a younger age than spondylotic problems and symptoms may be very persistent .

Involvement of more than one nerve root is a suggestive feature, as are bilateral features and long tract involvement. Hemangioma, osteoid osteoma, and osteoblastoma very rarely occur in the spine and usually do not cause neurologic impairment.

Trauma

Spondylosis, whiplash and occupational problems have already been discussed. One other relatively minor problem deserves mention; Clay-shoveller's fracture, in which the seventh cervical spinous process is avulsed by an injury following unaccustomed exertion. There is local tenderness.

NEUROLOGIC FEATURES

Osteophyte Root Palsy

Just occasionally an osteophyte will impinge gradually and steadily onto an intervertebral foramen. Neck ache is not a prominent feature, but insidious scapular or arm aching can be followed by weakness, wasting and reflex change and also by sensory loss. Sometimes the root pain is more severe. The patient is usually elderly, the neck movement is restricted from spondylosis, and a radiograph shows the foraminal encroachment (Fig. 5.11). Surgical decompression is indicated if pain is severe and often provides relief.

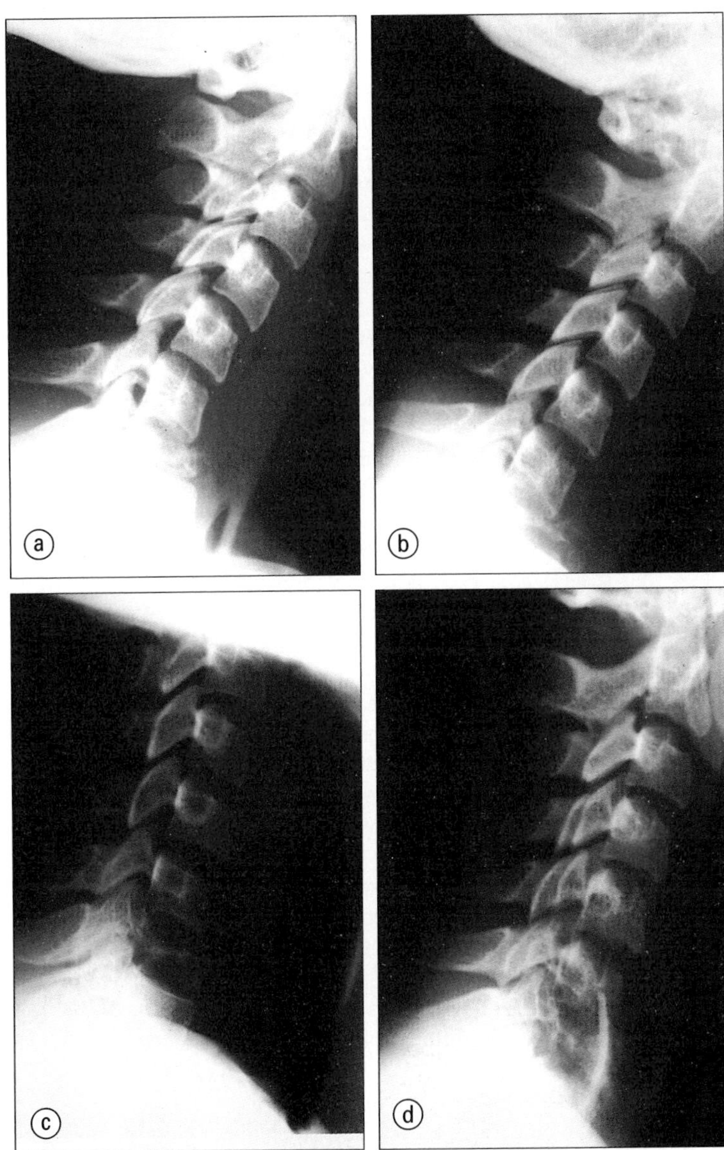

Fig. 5.9 Despite a recent road traffic accident, whiplash injury and the appearance of a burst fracture of C7 (a) this patient continued to absorb the vertebral body and developed a retropharyngeal abscess (b). Healing followed antituberculous chemotherapy and surgical fusion (c&d).

Neuralgic Amyotrophy

As the term neuralgic amyotrophy describes, this condition starts with very intense pain in the distribution of one or more nerves, which is followed by muscle wasting. Recognized causes include viral infections, foreign protein injections and blood transfusions. Thus, it is sometimes seen postoperatively and can be difficult to differentiate from a shoulder lesion such as subacromial bursitis. The distribution may involve more than one branch of a nerve and only rarely is it bilateral. The condition is said to always recover completely, although the pain often takes 12–18 months to subside. Weakness settles in the regeneration time of the nerve involved. It is claimed that steroids given within a few days of onset can cut short the duration of the syndrome.

Multiradicular Cervical Lesions

When more than one nerve root is involved, alternatives to simple disc prolapse/spondylosis must be considered. The prolapse may be of extraordinary size or may have caused a vascular myelopathy. However, infection and secondary neoplasms must be considered.

Thoracic Outlet Syndrome

The most common problem is caused by pressure on the lower trunk of the brachial plexus. This is formed from the C8 and T1 nerve roots. The first symptom is usually paresthesia felt rather diffusely in the hand and not confined to median or ulnar distribution. Symptoms are of gradual onset, may be bilateral and are sometimes noticed with activities that depress the shoulders. Thus, wearing a heavy overcoat or carrying shopping bags may be troublesome. Alternatively, paresthesia may come on at night disturbing sleep, presumably due to a 'release' phenomenon, the nerve 'recovering' when not compressed. Features may progress so that the forearm and upper arm ache. There is no associated color change in the arm

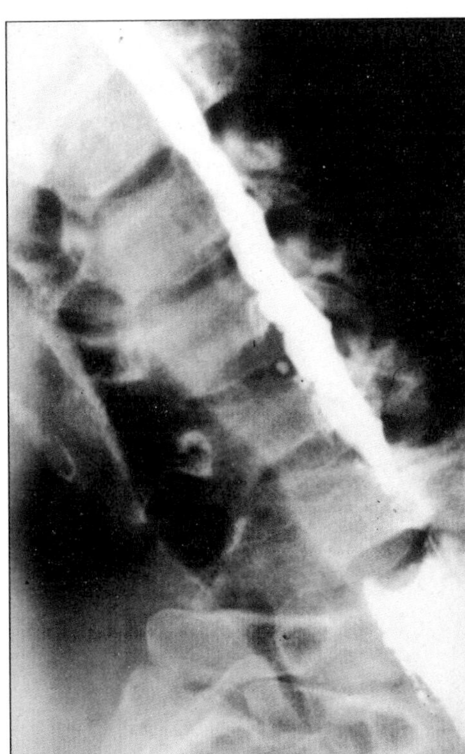

Fig. 5.10 During a round-the-world trip this patient reported neck pain and stiffness at many ports of call. By the time he arrived back in the UK the problem was constant, with neurologic features. The filling defect was a neurofibroma, which was successfully removed.

or hand. With more severe pressure, denervation and subsequent weakness and wasting can occur in those hand muscles innervated by T1. Electromyography and nerve conduction tests may be required in order to differentiate this from peripheral median or ulnar nerve lesions.

Vascular features are due to compression of the subclavian artery [48], or less often the vein. The hand may be cold and ache when hanging by the side, or Raynaud's phenomenon may occur.

Physical examination reveals a normal cervical spine, in particular sustained over-pressure should not provoke neurologic symptoms. By contrast, depressing the shoulder either by direct pressure or by downward traction on the arm may produce paresthesia. This acts by further compressing the tight fitting thoracic outlet. Bracing backwards of the shoulder girdle may have a similar effect.

Treatment may be prophylactic – avoidance of the provoking factors; elevating the arms before retiring at night. Physiotherapeutic posture instruction and exercises to elevate the shoulder girdle may help. On rare occasions, surgical release may be indicated, but only after confirming the site of nerve and/or vascular compression.

MANAGEMENT OF MECHANICAL NECK PAIN

Reassurance

Many patients with neck pain have suffered repeated episodes of disability and are anxious that the problem might be progressive and more crippling. Although no relevant statistics are available the impression is that serious sequelae are uncommon. Thus reassurance can be given along these lines. Equally, it is not possible to give guarantees against recurrence and the possibility should be discussed openly so as to avoid loss of confidence.

Symptomatic

A wide range of treatments is available and in widespread use – a situation that results from lack of clinical trials and poorly studied efficacy. There is no good reason to suppose that any of them favorably influences the underlying process, except to say that rest and support generally favor tissue repair.

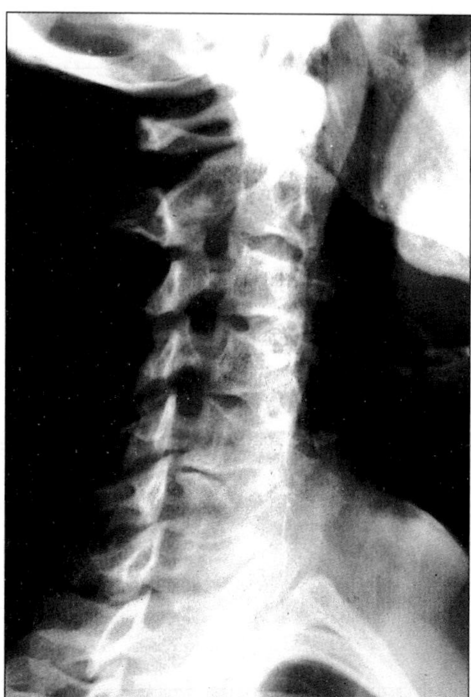

Fig. 5.11 Osteophytic encroachment into an intervertebral foramen. This may be harmless or there may be insidious nerve root interruption or severe root pain.

Analgesics

A mild analgesic, such as paracetamol, will often have been tried by the patient. Co-proxamol or dihydrocodeine may be needed for pain of moderate severity and opiates reserved for severe short-lived episodes.

Nonsteroidal Anti-inflammatory Drugs and Muscle Relaxants

These undoubtedly give short term symptomatic relief. The same principles apply as in their use for other rheumatic disorders, and the same benefits and side effects can be expected.

Heat

A wide range of physiotherapeutic techniques for giving superficial or deep heat is in use. No controlled clinical trials of their efficacy have been published. Their main role is to provide analgesia and relaxation prior to some mechanical form of treatment.

Rest

The fundamental treatment for most mechanical disorders of the cervical spine would seem to be rest. This provides a basis for spontaneous relief of pain, minimizes the need for analgesics and provides a basis for the natural resolution of the pathologic process.

Rest may be complete, with bed rest and recumbency, and even enhanced by continuous traction. More often it is partial and provided by a restricting collar, often termed tortologically a 'cervical collar'. It is presumed that the more restricting a collar is the more effective it will be. When pain relief is the main objective, the collar can be soft or firm, only partly limiting movement (Fig. 5.12). However, demands of tolerance need to be taken into account. In patients with dangerous instability and important neurologic features complete immobilization is the objective and the collar needs a contact on chin and occiput, chest and posterior thorax (Fig. 5.13). Many intermediate versions are available. Atlanto-axial subluxation, fracture dislocations and infections come into the dangerous category and require immobilization; spondylosis generally causes pain only and pain relief will suffice. A comparative study of collars has been performed [49]. Collars were classified into three main types by their construction. They were made either from soft flexible foam, plastic or leather, or they could have rigid supports from chin to anterior chest and occiput to posterior chest. The amount of restriction depends upon the overall rigidity and the closeness of fit. The restriction achieved could limit movement to 75% of the normal range with a soft collar, and to 15% with a rigid 'brace'. This suggests that the flexible type is acceptable for analgesia but a rigid type is needed if there are neurological warnings of destructive pathologic processes.

There is scarcity of controlled clinical trials of rest treatments. However, a study has been published [50] of a multicenter trial comparing traction, 'positioning', collar, placebo tablets and placebo shockwave diathermy. Patients were selected with pain and restriction of neck movement, and/or neurologic symptoms in the arms. A total of 493 patients entered the trial, of whom 57% were having their first attack. Temporary relief of pain was recorded in 92% of patients receiving traction and 86% of those with its control, 'positioning'. At 2 and 4 weeks all groups showed a similar rate of recovery. This recovery rate was related to age, initial severity of symptoms and the number and duration of previous attacks. The clear message is that rest treatments are being given with incomplete knowledge of the natural history of the condition or the effects of the treatments on it.

Mechanical Techniques

There is a wide range of manipulation techniques (literally treatment with hands) in use. These range from gentle repetitive oscillations with the patient fully conscious, to more forceful manipulations under general anesthesia. Generally the term manipulation is used for a definitive forceful movement applied to the cervical spine, while mobilization is used for the repeated movements. In either case the objective is to restore a fuller range of movement and thus relieve pain. Conceptually it may be that manipulation 'reduces a displaced fragment' and mobilization 'stretches contracted joints' – presumably the capsules of degenerative joints in the cervical spine. Despite the continuing proliferation and popularization of rival methods of manipulation there seem to be no reliable controlled clinical trials of their effects. For more detailed descriptions of the principles and indications seen from a physiotherapists viewpoint one is referred to a physiotherapy textbook [51]. Here the standard physiotherapy techniques together with osteopathy and chiropractic, are described and discussed. Complications of manipulation are reported sporadically. Although alarming, these occasional reports should not be used to deny a treatment form that has a generally accepted, albeit unproved, value. Provided the patient is generally fit and free of neurologic or vascular symptoms or signs these techniques are 'acceptable'. The practitioner should choose patients who have mainly articular features, i.e. painful restriction of neck movement. He should be experienced in the principles of diagnosis of more sinister disorders, and should not continue with treatments unless progress is clearly being made.

Traction

Cervical traction literally means pulling longitudinally on the cervical spine. This can be achieved manually or with machinery. Manual treatment involves pulling with one hand under the chin and another beneath the occiput. A mechanical device, powered either by a weight or motor can be applied with a halter applied to a similar area and the cervical vertebrae can be distracted. This will have a mechanical effect on both disc and apophyseal joint. Outpatient traction can be brief or sustained for half an hour. In hospital the traction can be sustained for days on end, but at lower intensity. When low, the force applied merely achieves rest and a degree of immobilization. Greater forces undoubtedly distract vertebrae and can relieve the pain associated with nerve root pressure. Some patients have obtained relief with domestic traction apparatus, partially suspending themselves from a frame with a halter.

The main accepted indication for traction is an articular problem in the cervical spine associated with signs of nerve root compression. Again the practitioner must be fully aware of the features of severe or sinister disorders, and should withdraw from treatment if progress is not being made .

Injections

Epidural injections can be given at the cervical level and some pain clinic practitioners are familiar with the technique. The usual indication would be persistent cervical root pain, unresponsive to rest and analgesics.

Facet joint injections have been tried under radiologic control and may give short-term relief.

Surgery

This is only occasionally necessary in cervical disorders. There are three main indications for surgery. Firstly there is the presence of severe, unremitting root pain. If this is confirmed clinically and electrophysiologically with root damage, root decompression is usually successful. The actual root involved and the level of the lesion need to be confirmed radiologically. Often, decompression of a foramen will give good results. Secondly, cord compression with long tract signs is an important indication for cervical decompression. Again, clear radiologic confirmation is needed, and CT radiculography remains the 'gold standard'. Unfortunately chronic lesions may be accompanied by ischemia and gliosis, so that some changes are irreversible. Thirdly, the presence of instability, with either pain or neurologic disturbance, may be an indication for combined decompression and fusion. This will necessitate wiring and/or bone grafts and can be very successful.

Prophylaxis

It is quite difficult to do better than heed the natural warnings. If pain is being caused by any activity or posture, then harm is being done. So the first instruction is to avoid activities which cause the neck to protest. In general the patient should avoid awkward posture, and sustained extremes of range of movement. The head may need support in a neutral and pain-free position, with attention paid to pillows and mattresses when at rest. In particular, careful attention should be paid to posture at work and during leisure pursuits.

CONCLUSION

Pain in the neck is common and usually self-limiting. It is usually due to a degenerative or traumatic pathology. However, exclusion of more serious causes of neck pain and differentiation of neurologic sequelae from other disorders is crucial for the correct management of patients.

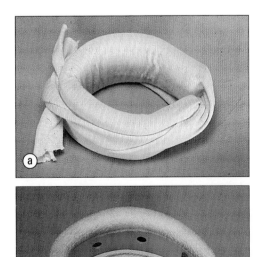

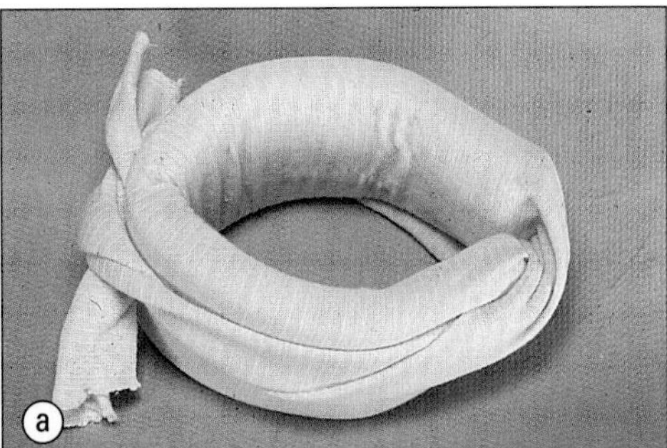

Fig. 5.12 Collars may be soft (a) or firm (b).

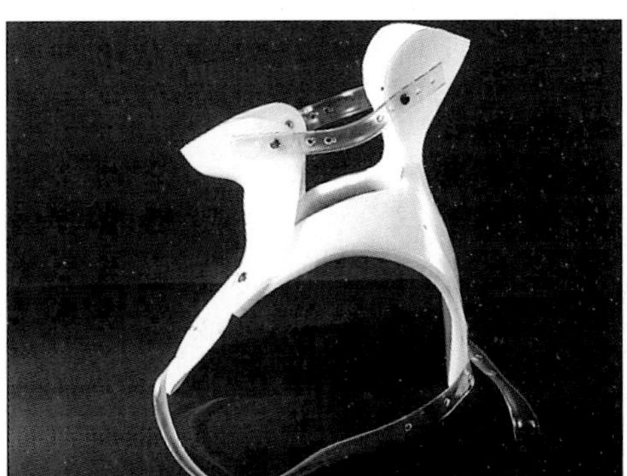

Fig. 5.13 If there is dangerous instability a rigid cervical brace with purchase on chin and occiput is needed.

REFERENCES

1. Mathews JA . Acute neck pain. Differential diagnosis and management. Reports on rheumatic diseases (series 2). 1989; no 13.
2. Lewin R. Ancient footprints mark time. New Scientist.1979; **82**:931.
3. Davis PR. The physical causation of disease. R Soc Health J. 1972;**92**:63–4.
4. Lawrence JS. Disc degeneration, its frequency and relationship to symptoms. Ann Rheum Dis. 1969;**28**:121–38.
5. Billings RA, Mole KF. Rheumatology in a general practice: a survey in World Rheumatism Year . J R Coll Gen Pract. 1977;**27**:721
6. Wood PHN, McLeish CL. Statistical appendix. Ann Rheum Dis. 1974;**33**:93–105.
7. Anderson JAD. Rheumatism in industry: a review. Indust Med. 1971;**28**:103–21.
8. Westerling D, Jonsson BG. Pain from the neck shoulder region and sick leave. Scand J Soc Med. 1980;**8**:131.
9. Holt L. The Munkfors investigation. Acta Orthop Scand. 1954;Suppl 17.
10. Holt L. Frequency of symptoms for different age groups and professions. In: Hirsch C, Zotterman Y, eds. Cervical pain. New York: Pergamon Press;1971:17–20.
11. Levy LL. Porter's neck. Br Med J. 1968;**2**:16–9.
12. Hirsch C, Schajowicz F, Galante T. Structural changes in the cervical spine. Acta Orthop Scand. 1967;**109**(Suppl):9
13. Lawrence JS. Disc disorders. In: Rheumatism in populations. Heinemann: London; 1977.
14. Cloward R B. The clinical significance of the sinuvertebral nerve or the cervical spine in relation to the cervical disk syndrome. J Neurol Neurosurg Psychiatry. 1960;**23**:321–6.
15. Cloward R B. Cervical diskography. A Contribution to the etiology and mechanism of neck, shoulder and arm pain. Ann Surg. 1959;**150**:1052–64.
16. Weddell G, Feinstein B, Pattee RE. The clinical application of electromyography. Lancet. 1943;**1**:236–9 .
17. Kellgren JH. On the distribution of pain arising from deep somatic structures with charts of segmental pain areas. Clin Sci. 1939;**4**:35–46.
18. Crowe H, cited in Breck LW, Van Norman RW. Medico-legal aspects of cervical spine sprains. Clin Orthop. 1971;**74**:124–8.
19. Barry M. Whiplash injuries. Editorial. Br J Rheumatol. 1992;**301**:579–81.
20. Newman PK. Whiplash injury. Leading article. Br Med J. 1990;**301**:395–6.
21. Crawford PM, Shepherd DI. Hyperextension in the elderly. Br Med J. 1989;**229**:669–70.
22. Young S, Tamas L, O'Lavire SA. Prolapse of a cervical disc in elderly patients with cervical spondylosis. Br Med J. 1986;**293**:749–50.
23. Leading article. Rugby injuries to the cervical cord. Br Med J. 1977;**6076**:155–6.
24. Schneider RC. Head and neck injuries in football. Baltimore: Williams and Wilkins; 1973:126.
25. Scher AT. Rugby injuries to the cervical cord. S Afr Med J. 1977;**51**, 473–5.
26. Bird H. Overuse injuries in musicians. Br Med J. 1989;**298**:1128–30.
27. Levy CE. Electromyographic analysis of muscular activity in the upper extremity generated by supporting a violin with and without a shoulder rest. Paper at 10th Annual Symposium on Medical Problems of Musicians and Dancers. 1992.
28. Mathews JA. Rheumatoid cervical myelopathy; a clinical, radiological and pathological study of flaccid arm weakness. Arthritis Rheum. 1988;**31**(Suppl. 4):480.
29. Symonds CP, Meadows SP. Compression of the spinal cord in the neighbourhood of the foramen magnum. Brain. 1937;**60**:52–84.
30. Dunn NA, Lewis-Barned NJ, Lloyd Jones JK. Multiple subaxial subluxation of cervical spine: a side effect of corticosteroids? Br Med J. 1985;**290**:299–303.
31. Vernon-Roberts B. Pathology of intervertebral discs and apophyseal joints. In: Malcolm I V Jayson, eds. The lumbar spine and back pain, 3E. Edinburgh: Churchill Livingstone; 1985.
32. Schmorl G, Junghanns H. The human spine in health and disease (translated by EF Besemann). New York: Grune & Stratton; 1971.
33. Hilton RC, Ball J. Vertebral rim lesions in the dorsolumbar spine. Ann Rheum Dis. 1984;**43**:302.
34. Vernon Roberts B, Pirie CJ. Degenerative changes in the vertebral discs and their sequelae. Rheumatol Rehab. 1977;**16**:13–21.
35. Brain, Lord. Some unsolved problems of cervical spondylosis. Br Med J. 1963;**1**:771–7.
36. Wilkinson M. Cervical spondylosis. London: Heinemann; 1971.
37. Henson RA, Parsons, M. Ischaemic lesions of the spinal cord: an illustrated review. Q J Med. 1967;**new series XXXVI, no 142**:205–22.
38. Dommisse GF. The blood supply of the spinal cord. A critical vascular zone in spinal surgery. J Bone Joint Surg. 1974;**56B, 2**:225–35.
39. Hutchinson EC, Yates PO. The cervical portion of the vertebral artery. A clinico-pathological study. Brain. 1956;**79**:319–31.
40. Mathews JA. Atlanto-axial subluxation in rheumatoid arthritis. Ann Rheum Dis. 1969;**28**:260–5.
41. Mathews JA. Atlanto-axial subluxation in rheumatoid arthritis: a 5 year follow up study. Ann Rheum Dis. 1974;**33**:526–31.
42. Swinson DR, Hamilton EBD, Mathews JA, Yates DAH. Ann Rheum Dis. 1972;**31**:359–63.
43. Hopkins JA. Lower cervical rheumatoid subluxation with tetraplegia. J Bone Joint Surg. 1967;**49B**:46–51.
44. Meijers KAE, Van Beusekom GTH, Luyendijk W, Duijfjes F. Dislocation of the cervical spine with cord compression in rheumatoid arthritis. J Bone Joint Surg. 1974;**1**:668–80.
45. Mark JS, Sharp J. Rheumatoid cervical myelopathy. Q J Med. 1981;**199**:307–19.
46. Choong K, Monaghan P, McGuigan L, McLean R. Role of bone scintigraphy in the early diagnosis of discitis. Ann Rheum Dis. 1990;**49**:932–4.
47. Wilkinson MS, Russell RWR. Arteries of the head and neck in giant cell arteritis. Arch Neurol. 1972;**27**:378–91.
48. Lewis T, Pickering GW. Observations upon maladies in which the blood supply to the digits ceases intermittently or permanently, and upon bilateral gangrene of the digits, observations relevant to so-called 'Raynaud's disease'. Clin Sci. 1934;**1**:327–66.
49. Johnson RM, Hart DL, Simmons EF, Ramsby GR, Southwick WO. Cervical orthoses. A study comparing their effectiveness in restricting cervical motion in normal subjects. J Bone Joint Surg. 1977;**59a**:332–9.
50. British Association of Physical Medicine. Pain in the neck and arm: a multicentre trial of the effects of physiotherapy. Br Med J. 1966;**1**:253–8.
51. Grieve GP. Common Vertebral joint problems. 2E. Edinburgh: Churchill Livingstone; 1988.

REGIONAL PAIN PROBLEMS

6

LOW BACK PAIN

David G Borenstein

INTRODUCTION

Low back pain is a ubiquitous health problem. It represents the most frequent illness of mankind after the common cold [1–2]. Between 65% and 80% of the world's population will develop back pain at some point during their lives. Back pain accounts for 30–50% of the rheumatic complaints in a general medical practice [3]. Data from the US Health Interview Survey indicate that impairments of the back and spine are the chronic conditions that most frequently cause activity limitation among people aged 45 years or under and is the third most common reason for impairment in people aged 45–64 years [4].

The surgical subspecialties of orthopaedics and neurosurgery are most frequently associated with low back pain evaluation and treatment, despite the fact that the vast majority of patients do not require surgical intervention. Surgeons evaluate a large number of patients with non-surgical lesions in order to identify the relative few who require back surgery. In regard to back pain, rheumatologists have concentrated their efforts on the spondyloarthropathies and have shied away from patients with mechanical low back pain. Since they are experts in the conservative management of musculoskeletal disorders, rheumatologists are in many ways the most appropriate physicians to complete the initial and subsequent evaluation of patients with low back pain of any etiology and to plan a treatment program. They constantly use patient education, physical modalities, and drug therapy, which are the cornerstones for treatment of back patients.

EPIDEMIOLOGY

Most episodes of back pain are not incapacitating. Over 50% of all patients with back pain improve after 1 week, while more than 90% are better at 8 weeks [5]. The remaining 7–10% continue to experience symptoms for longer than 6 months. The high costs associated with low back pain are related to these individuals with chronic pain. For example, in the state of Tennessee in 1986, 10% of cases with chronic low back pain accounted for 57% of the total expenditures (US$31.8 million) spent on work-related sickness payments [6]. Frymoyer has estimated that the direct cost of back pain in the United States in 1990 was over US$24 billion [7]. This excludes the US$3.6 billion of indirect costs of work-related sickness payments, litigation, and lost days from work.

Many risk factors described for back pain involve occupational or psychologic characteristics. Occupational factors include jobs that require lifting beyond the worker's physical capabilities, or in an awkward position. Workers involved in heavy duty labor who are aged over 45 years have a 2.5 times greater risk of absence from work secondary to back pain compared to workers aged 24 years or younger [8].

A number of psychologic conditions are associated with back pain. Neurosis, hysteria and conversion reaction are more frequent than depression as primary causes of acute back pain [9]. Depression is a frequent complication of patients who develop chronic low back pain. Obesity and cigarette smoking are also associated with an increased risk of back pain [10].

As many as 90% of patients with back pain have a mechanical reason for their pain [11]. Mechanical low back pain may be defined as pain secondary to overuse of a normal anatomic structure (muscle strain) or pain secondary to trauma or deformity of an anatomic structure (herniated nucleus pulposus). The remaining 10% of adults with back pain have the symptom as a manifestation of a systemic illness [12]. Over seventy nonmechanical illnesses may be associated with back pain [13]. Careful clinical evaluation helps separate patients with mechanical back pain from those with nonmechanical back pain.

CLINICAL EVALUATION

The evaluation of a patient with low back pain requires an organized and thoughtful approach that should be tailored to the specific complaints of the patient. In rare circumstances, a patient's symptoms and signs can be related to an identifiable pathologic process involving a specific anatomic structure. In these cases, specific therapy can be given. However, in most cases, the offending anatomic structure, be it bone, muscle, ligament, fascia, or nerve, cannot be identified as the specific source of back pain. Fortunately, the natural history of the symptom is resolution frequently over a short period of time, so all interventions seem to work whether it is limitation of activity, over-the-counter medications, temperature modalities or chiropractors. Although the diagnostic process is inexact for many patients, it nevertheless remains essential to identify a specific abnormality.

The physician plays an essential role in the evaluation and treatment of low back pain patients and their recovery. The very nature of the interaction of a person and a physician makes that individual view themselves as being sick. The physician may encourage this behavior by evaluating or treating an individual in too aggressive a manner. This may be a particular problem for individuals who have been injured at work. It is essential for the physician to downplay 'illness behavior' in these patients. Patients with low back pain need to be encouraged to resume normal activities as soon as possible and be constantly reminded that the vast majority of individuals improve over a 2–3 week period.

History

The clinical history is an essential step in evaluating patients with low back pain. The astute clinician allows the patient to tell his story in his own words, but also steers him in directions that elicit the essential information needed for the diagnostic process. The age of the patient is helpful in determining the potential cause of their back pain. Certain disorders occur more commonly in younger individuals while others are associated with older patients (see Fig. 6.1). The sex of the patient may also help select potential causes of low back pain. Certain disorders occur more frequently in men while others are associated more commonly with women. Others occur equally in both sexes (see Fig. 6.2).

The duration and location of pain help decide the subsequent kinds of questions that the evaluating physician will ask. Mechanical low back pain tends to have an onset associated with a physical task and is usually of short duration (days to weeks). Medical causes of low back pain tend to have a more gradual onset with no identifiable precipitating factor. These causes of low back pain are frequently present from weeks to months. Most back pain is limited to the lumbosacral area of the low back. Radiation of pain in the thighs, or to

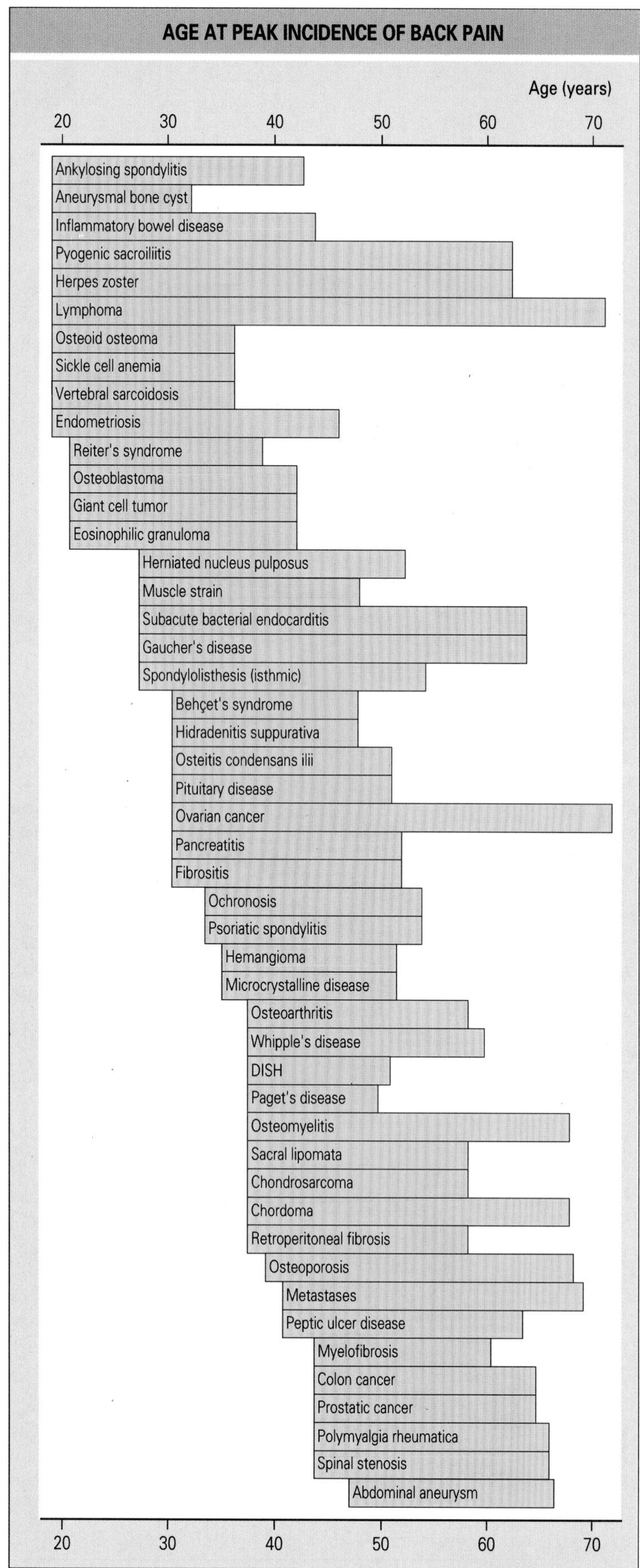

Fig. 6.1 Age of peak incidence of back pain. (Adapted with permission from Borenstein DG, Wiesel SW. Low Back Pain: medical diagnosis and comprehensive management. Philadelphia: WB Saunders; 1989).

the knees may be related to referred pain from elements of the spine (muscle, ligaments or apophyseal joints). Pain that radiates from the low back to below the knees is usually neurogenic in origin and suggests a pathologic process affecting spinal nerve roots.

SEX PREVALENCE OF LOW BACK PAIN CONDITIONS
Male predominant
Spondyloarthropathies Vertebral osteomyelitis Benign and malignant neoplasms Paget's disease Retroperitoneal fibrosis Peptic ulcer disease Work-related mechanical disorders
Female predominant
Polymyalgia rheumatica Fibromyalgia Osteoporosis Parathyroid disease
Equal frequency
Inflammatory bowel disease Pituitary disease Subacute bacterial endocarditis

Fig. 6.2 Sex prevalence of low back pain conditions.

CATEGORIES OF LOW BACK PAIN		
Category	Source/Pathologic Entity	Quality
Superficial somatic	Skin, subcutaneous tissues (cellulitis)	Sharp, burning
Deep somatic	Muscles, fascia, periosteum, ligaments, joints, vessels, dura (arthritis)	Sharp, dull ache, boring
Radicular	Spinal nerves (herniated disc, spinal stenosis)	Radiating, shooting, tingling
Neurogenic	Mixed motor sensory nerves (femoral neuropathy)	Burning
Visceral-referred	Abdominal viscera, pelvic viscera, aorta (autonomic sensory nerves)	Boring, colicky, tearing
Psychogenic	Cerebral cortex (conversion reaction, malingering)	Variable

Fig. 6.3 Categories of back pain.

Present illness

Most of the time spent in obtaining the clinical history is used to elucidate the factors that affect the pain. The history is directed toward understanding the chronological development of low back pain, its character, and its response to therapy. The anatomic structures of the lumbosacral spine receive specific types of sensory innervation that are associated with distinct qualities of pain. The major categories of pain include superficial somatic, deep somatic (spondylogenic), radicular, neurogenic, visceral-referred and psychogenic (Fig. 6.3).

Superficial somatic pain

Superficial somatic pain is associated with disorders that affect the skin and subcutaneous tissues. These tissues are well innervated by cutaneous A fibers that cover very small fields. Pathogenic processes in these tissues cause sharp or burning pain. Areas of cellulitis are rapidly recognized because of their superficial location and are not diagnostically difficult. The exception may be in patients who present with the burning pain of herpes zoster prior to the appearance of vesicles. The acute onset and distribution in a dermatomal pattern should alert the clinician to this possibility.

Deep somatic pain

Deep somatic pain has its source in the vertebral column, the surrounding muscles, and the attaching tendons, ligaments, and fascia. These structures are supplied by the sinuvertebral nerves and the unmyelinated pain fibers of the posterior primary rami of the spinal nerves. Deep somatic pain is characterized by a deep, dull ache that is maximal over the involved site and often radiates into the thighs but rarely below the knees. Acute injury to these tissues is associated with a sharp stab of pain at the moment of injury followed by a dull ache that may persist for weeks and may be associated with tenderness on palpation and reflex muscle spasm.

Radicular pain

Radicular pain is related to involvement of the proximal spinal nerves with inflammation, or any processes that decrease blood flow to the nerve. This type of pain is lancinating, shooting, burning, sharp and tender in quality and radiates from the low back to the lower extremity in the distribution of the compromised spinal nerve. In addition to the shooting pain, achiness and spasm may be experienced in the thigh and calf muscles. Herniated intervertebral discs are the most common cause of radicular pain. Other causes include overgrowth of bone from apophyseal joints intruding into the spinal canal, spinal stenosis, fracture-dislocation of the spine, infections and neoplasms.

Neurogenic pain

Neurogenic pain results from involvement of the sensory portion of a peripheral nerve. Diabetic neuropathy is a good example. This type of pain is described as burning, tingling, crushing, gnawing or skin crawling and tends to be sustained in most circumstances.

Visceral-referred pain

Visceral-referred pain arises from abnormalities in organs that share segmental innervation with the lumbosacral spine. The back pain may be gripping, cramping, aching, squeezing, crushing, tearing, stabbing or burning, depending on the affected organ. The wider distribution of viscerogenic pain differs from the more precise localization of somatic pain.

Psychogenic pain

Psychogenic pain is perceived at the level of the cerebral cortex. It does not follow any dermatomal pattern and may be of any quality. The patient may describe the pain in terms of suffering or punishment. Some terms used in this circumstance might include 'being hit', or 'being burned with a red hot poker' [14]. Duration may be extremely short or prolonged. In most circumstances psychogenic pain is resistant to all therapies. Patients who suffer from depression, hysteria or conversion reaction tend to exhibit psychogenic pain.

In addition to the quality of pain, elucidating factors that aggravate and alleviate pain are helpful in defining potential sources for the symptom. Typically, mechanical disorders worsen with activity, including prolonged sitting and standing and improve with recumbency. The pain tends to occur on a recurring basis with the same degree of physical activity.

While some patients with medical disorders that affect the spine, such as compression, pathologic fractures or acute infection, may also find relief of their pain with recumbency and even complete immobility, most find no association with body position. Exceptions include patients with a spondyloarthropathy who classically report increased pain and stiffness when they remain in bed for a few hours; patients with tumors that involve the structures of the lumbar spine who are worse with recumbency; and patients with viscerogenic pain, in whom moving around trying to achieve a comfortable postion is characteristic.

Increases in cerebrospinal fluid pressure brought about by coughing or sneezing exacerbate radicular pain in patients with intervertebral disc herniation. Sudden motion may also cause reflex contraction of paraspinous muscles but no radiation of pain into the lower extremities.

The severity of pain may be measured by a number of means. The patient may describe how the pain has interfered with activities of daily living. The more severe the pain, the greater the intrusion on leisure time pursuits. Patients may fill in a diagram with the location, quality and severity of pain (Fig. 6.4). These pain diagrams are a helpful way of documenting the extent of pain involvement and subsequent response to therapy.

Family and Social History

In addition to the present illness, other components of the history may help to identify any underlying abnormality which is a cause of back pain. Familial predisposition does occur in certain medical illnesses associated with back pain. Of particular importance is the group of illnesses that cause spondyloarthropathy. The ethnic background of the family may predispose individuals to specific illnesses. For example, Caucasian women of Northern European origins are at greater risk of developing osteoporosis. Mechanical disorders such as intervertebral disc herniation and spinal stenosis may have a familial predilection.

Occupational and social history are important for identifying those patients at risk of developing mechanical low back pain. The association of work and the onset of pain is important in regard to compensation. The patient's opinion about the association of the pain and their work must be determined as well as their expectation of work-related sickness payments for injury and return to work. Some workers may be afraid to return to their job because of fear of reinjury. They may amplify their symptoms and may be slow to respond to therapy.

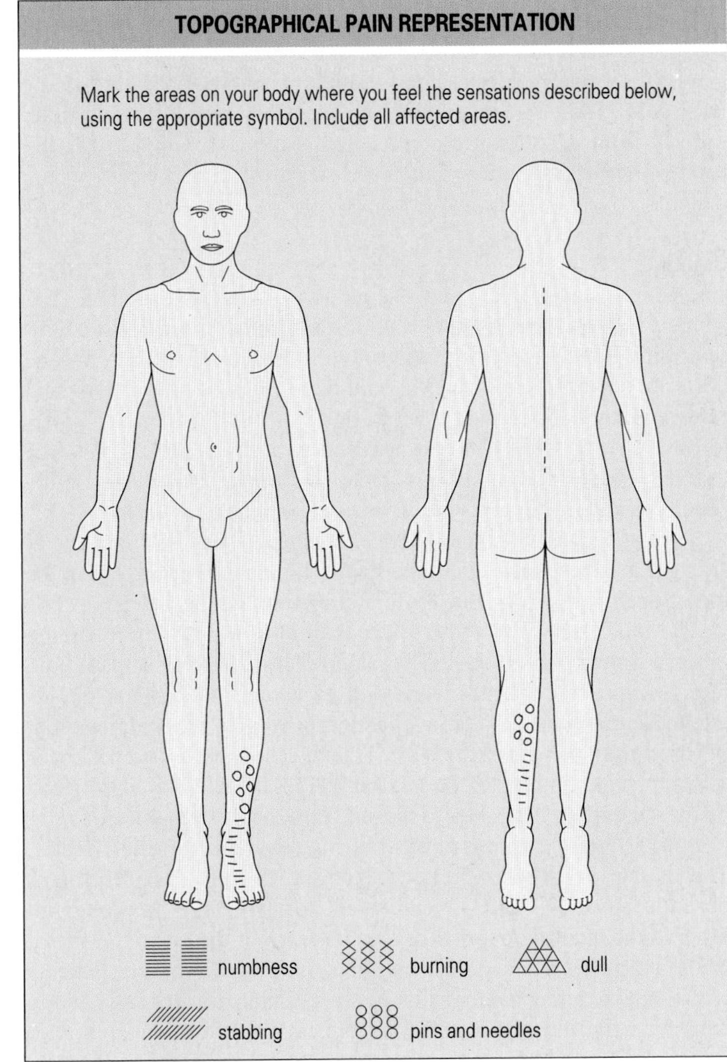

Fig. 6.4 Pain diagram. Pain distribution of a patient with radiculopathy secondary to a lumbar intervertebral disc herniation

Social habits also need to be determined, particularly in regard to smoking, consumption of alcohol, and the use of recreational drugs. Smoking is an independent risk factor for low back pain [10]. Increased use of alcohol is associated with osteoporosis, while illicit drug use causes immunosuppression and predisposition to infection.

Past Medical History

Past medical history and a review of systems should be discussed briefly. In most circumstances, these components of the history add little additional information. However, for the patient with medical low back pain, these components of the medical history are particularly pertinent. Previous history of malignancy, arthritis, or metabolic bone disease may be significant. The review of systems may identify the patient who had a systemic disorder causing back pain but does not realize the association between the two (skin rash and spondyloarthropathy).

Physical Examination

In patients with a history suggestive of mechanical low back pain, the physical examination will concentrate on the evaluation of musculoskeletal and neural tissues of the lumbosacral spine. However, a full examination should be completed at a subsequent visit if the patient does not improve in a short period of time.

When a medical cause of low back pain is suspected, a general medical physical examination should be completed before evaluation of the back. Clues to the specific cause of back pain may be discovered during the general examination. Changes in various organ systems (skin, ocular, gastrointestinal, for example) may be noted in patients with medical low back pain.

The objective of the physical examination of the lumbosacral spine is to demonstrate those static and dynamic abnormalities that can help sort out the disease entities that may be responsible for low back pain. The tests for motion and function should be done in an orderly fashion following a consistent pattern that minimizes the time of the examination and the discomfort experienced by the patient.

Standing

The patient stands undressed, facing away from the examiner. The spine is viewed for curvatures and postural deformities. A list is present if the first thoracic vertebra is not centered over the sacrum. The posterior superior iliac spines should be of equal height. The gluteal folds and knee joints should be at identical levels. Laterally, hyperlordosis or a flattened lumbosacral curve may be identified while marked kyphosis is noted best from this position. Anteriorly, the shoulders and iliac wings should be of equal height.

The patient should squat in place. This maneuver tests the general strength and integrity of the function of the joints from the hip to the toes. Specific areas of decreased function must be identified.

The muscle power of the lower extremity can be tested by toe raises standing on both feet. The patient is asked to raise up on both feet 10 times and 10 more times on each foot independently. This test measures first sacral root function primarily. Fifth lumbar root function may be assessed by the Trendelenburg test. The patient is asked to stand on one leg. Weakness of hip abduction is highlighted by the sagging of the pelvis to the side opposite to the affected leg.

Spinal motion is important in terms of symmetry and rhythm. The patient is asked to flex, extend, and laterally bend the lumbosacral spine. As the patient bends forward, it is important to observe the quality of spinal flexion in terms of the smooth reversal of the normal lumbar lordosis as the spine flexes forward. Patients with localized mechanical disorders maintain the lordosis while bending from the hips when asked to forward flex. Patients with injuries in musculoskeletal structures at the L4–L5 and L5–S1 interspaces will experience abnormal motion secondary to protective muscle contraction.

After full flexion, it is helpful to observe how the patient regains the erect posture. Patients with back lesions return to the erect position utilizing a fixed lordosis and rotating the pelvis with the help of knee and hip flexion. Pain that increases with forward flexion suggests an abnormality in the anterior elements of the spine, including discogenic disease.

The patient should then be asked to extend the spine while limiting movement of the hip or knee. Pain that is increased by extension suggests disease in the posterior elements of the spinal column, including the apophyseal joints.

The exact source of pain with lateral bending is difficult to determine. Pain that is elicited on the same side as the bending motion suggests an apophyseal joint origin for the discomfort. Pain that is produced in a paraspinous location on the side opposite to the lateral bending motion may be of muscular, ligamentous, or fascial origin. Spinal rotation is best examined when the patient is seated.

Bending forward over a table

Palpation of the spine and surrounding tissues with the back supported by the arms, is possible with the patient bent forward over a table. Palpation detects local tenderness, increased muscle tone, or bony defects over the spinous processes. Sacroiliac tenderness may be elicited with direct percussion over these joints.

Kneeling

The ankle reflex is best determined in the kneeling position. It may also be elicited with the patient seated on the examining table.

Seated on a chair

Dorsiflexion power of the foot, a fifth lumbar nerve root function, is best tested by seating the patient on a chair and by pushing down on the patient's foot with the heel on the floor. The maneuver should be continued for a minute to allow for detection of weakness in the muscle. Patients who feign weakness may either resist pressure for a few seconds and then release the muscle suddenly, or in a manner resulting in a 'cogwheel' effect. Function of the L5 nerve root may also be tested by asking the patient to dorsiflex the large toe of the foot.

Seated on the examining table

Reflexes may be elicited when the patient is seated on the examining table. The knee reflex reflects the integrity of the L4 nerve root. Asymmetry of the reflexes should only be accepted if the abnormality persists on repeated testing.

In the seated position, the plantar response may be tested by lifting the straight leg and stroking the lateral aspect of the foot. Patients with radicular abnormalities will experience pain down the leg below the knee to the ankle or foot. Patients will also lean backwards to minimize the traction on neural elements (tripod sign). Patients with hamstring tightness will experience thigh pain but no pain radiation below the knee. A Babinski reflex (extension of the large toe and spreading of the other toes) should be plantar, since the spinal cord conus is situated at L1–L2 level.

Hip flexor strength is tested by asking the patient to lift their thigh off the examining table. Downward pressure by the examiner helps distinguish differences in strength from side to side.

Lying supine

The supine position is excellent for testing the status of the nerve roots, peripheral nerves, and hip joints. Assessment of the neurologic status of the patient is very important in the overall back evaluation. A neurologic abnormality will give objectivity to a patient's subjective complaints. Any compression or traction on the dura surrounding a nerve will compress its contents and encroach upon the nerve and its blood supply. With inflammation of the nerve, pain is produced along the course of the peripheral nerve causing dysesthesias, motor weakness, and decreased reflex function associated with the affected nerve

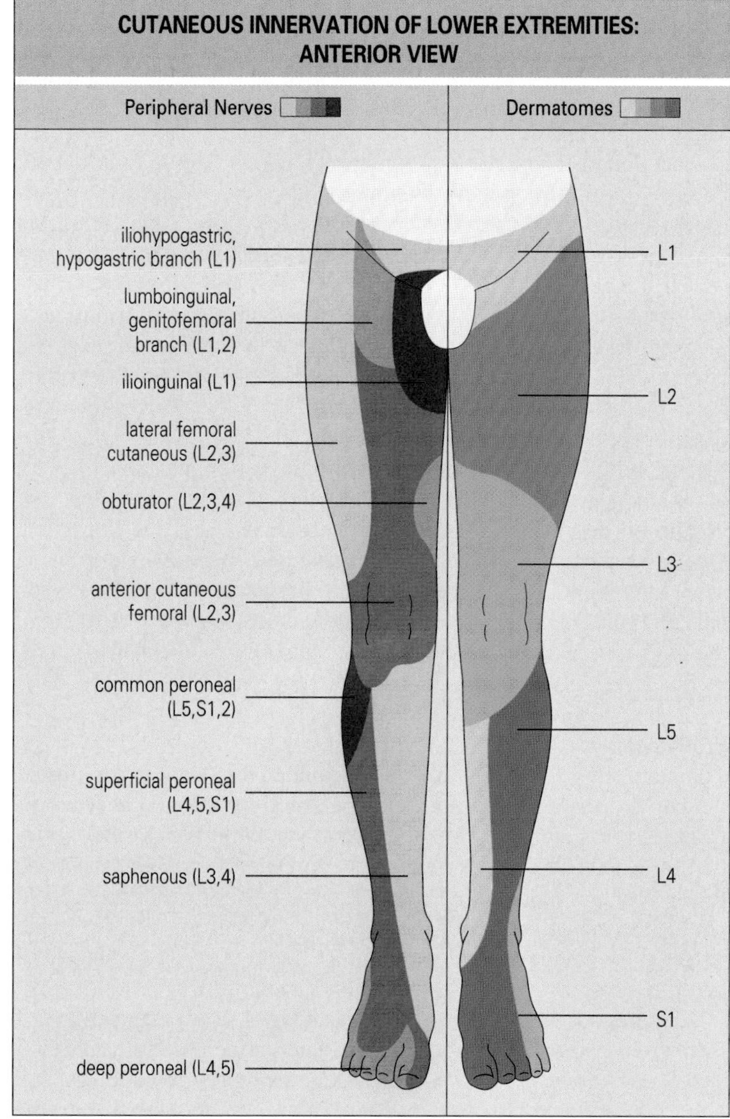

Fig. 6.5 Cutaneous sensory innervation. Anterior view of lower extremities illustrating skin areas supplied by nerve roots (right) and peripheral nerves (left).

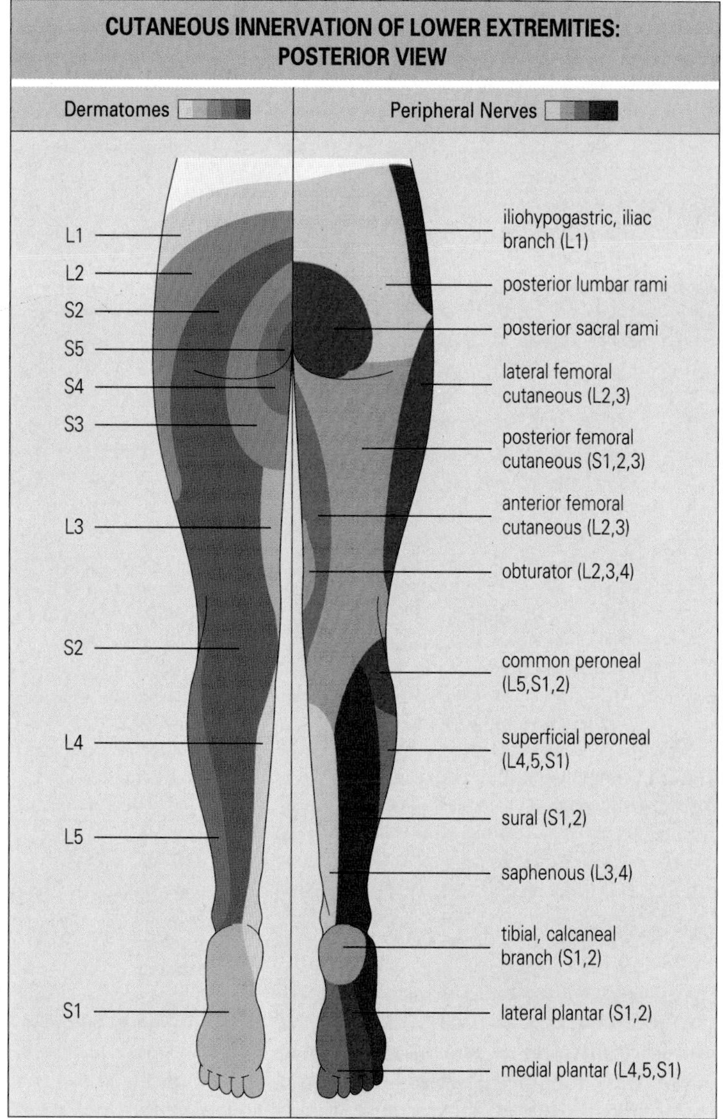

Fig. 6.6 Cutaneous sensory innervation. Posterior view of lower extremities illustrating skin areas supplied by nerve roots (left) and peripheral nerves (right).

root. Tests that increase nerve compression result in increased nerve pain or dysfunction. Of the possible neurologic abnormalities, persistent muscle weakness is the most reliable indicator of persistent nerve compression with loss of nerve conduction [15]. Sensory findings are less reliable since they are affected by the state of fatigue and emotional state of the patient. Reflex changes are also not as reliable as motor function. Previous episodes of nerve compression may cause a loss of reflexes, which may not return even with recovery of motor and sensory function [16]. Older individuals may lose reflex function particularly in the ankles. The loss of reflexes is then symmetrical. Patients who lose reflex function in both lower extremities acutely on the basis of compression have impingement of the cauda equina.

Upper motor neuron and peripheral nerve abnormalities may also cause neurologic dysfunction. Patients with upper motor neuron dysfunction develop muscle spasticity, hyperreflexia, and a Babinski reflex. Sensory and motor abnormalities associated with peripheral nerve injuries depend on the location of the damaged nerve. Peripheral nerves receive innervation from a number of nerve roots. An injury to a single nerve root may have little effect on motor or cutaneous function if the area is supplied by nerves from multiple levels. However, if a peripheral nerve is injured, a specific muscle may become paralyzed or specific skin areas become anaesthetic (Figs 6.5 & 6.6) The distinction between upper motor, nerve root, and peripheral nerve lesions is essential for the differential diagnosis of back pain. Different disease processes preferentially effect upper motor (multiple sclerosis), nerve root (disc herniation) or peripheral nerve (diabetes).

The straight leg raising test detects irritation of the sciatic nerve (L4, 5, S1). The passive raising of the leg by the foot with the knee extended stretches the sciatic nerve, its nerve roots, and dural attachments (see Fig. 6.7). When the dura is inflamed and stretched, the patient will experience pain along its anatomic course to the lower leg, ankle, and foot. Dural movement starts at 30° of elevation. Pain of dural origin should not be felt below that degree of elevation. Pain is maximum between 30° to 70° of elevation. Symptoms at greater degrees of elevation may be of nerve root origin, but may also be related to mechanical low back pain secondary to muscle strain or joint disease [17]. Dorsiflexion of the foot will exacerbate the radicular pain. Pain may also be experienced in the leg below the knee when the contralateral normal leg is raised. The presence of contralateral pain suggests a large central lesion in the spinal canal causing traction on the opposite nerve root when the normal leg is raised.

A bilateral straight leg raising test may also detect sciatic nerve irritation. The test is performed by lifting the legs by both ankles with the knees extended. This motion causes the pelvis to tilt upwards diminishing the stretch on the neural elements. Pain that occurs in an arc of elevation of 70° is related to stress on the sacroiliac joints. Above 70°, pain is related to lesions in the lumbar spine. The bilateral straight leg raising test is useful to identify patients with psychogenic pain who frequently complain of pain at a lower elevation than noted during the unilateral straight leg raising test.

In the supine position, leg lengths should be measured to document discrepancies. The hip joints should be moved through their

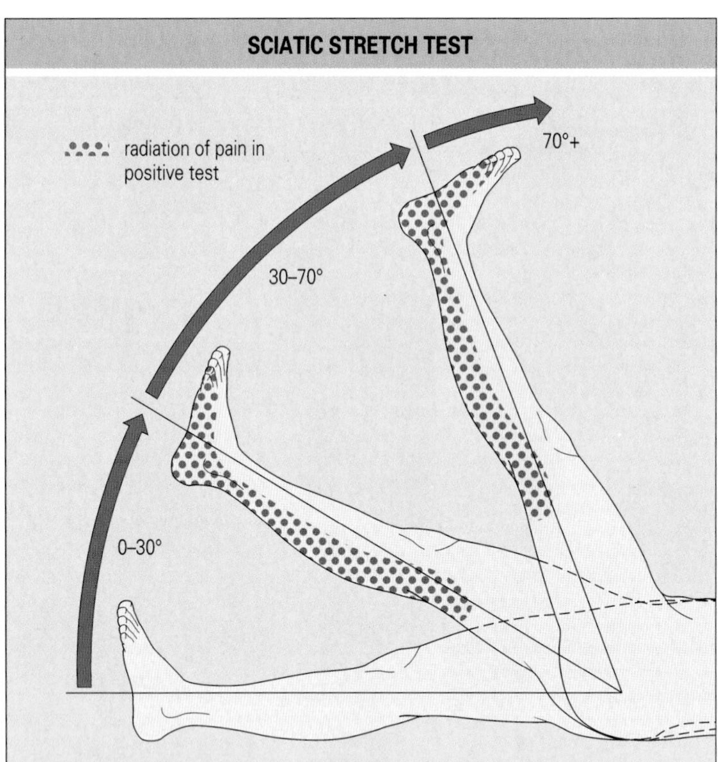

Fig. 6.7 Straight leg raising test. The leg is lifted with the knee extended. Sciatic roots are tightened over a herniated disc between 30 degrees and 70 degrees. Dorsiflexion of the foot increases pain with nerve impingement.

range of motion. Differentiation of hip pain versus sacroiliac joint pain may be determined by the Patrick or 'faber' (flexion, abduction, external rotation) test.

Neurologic function may be tested with the patient in the supine position. The sensory, motor and reflex functions of the lumbar spine and lower extremities should be assessed. Sensory function may be assessed by running the hands down the lower extremities, to elicit differences in the legs. Any abnormality should result in a more detailed examination of pain, light touch, and vibratory function.

Useful in screening is muscle testing of the legs, which measures strength on a five-point scale for: extension and flexion (knee); abduction and adduction (hip); and eversion and inversion and dorsiflexion and plantar flexion (foot) (Fig. 6.8).When testing muscle power, the intervening joints should be in a neutral position. Pressure is applied by the examiner to a nonarticular structure for a minimum of 5 seconds. When feasible, both sides should be tested simultaneously. The innervation of the muscles to the legs follows a sequential pattern. L2 and L3 supply hip flexion and L4 and L5 hip extension; L3 and L4 supply knee extension and L5 and S1 knee flexion; L4 and L5 supply ankle dorsiflexion and S1 and S2 ankle plantar flexion; ankle inversion is a function of L4 and ankle eversion is a function of L5 and S1.

Tender motor points are important diagnostically and prognostically. Motor points represent the main neuromuscular junctions for the involved muscle groups and are constant for an individual patient. Patients with radiculopathy and tender motor points have a nerve root lesion at the corresponding level for the affected myotome. Patients with tender motor points remain symptomatic for longer than do those without [18].

Function of the three most commonly affected nerve roots should be tested while the patient is supine and prone. When S1 is compressed, the gastrocnemius becomes weak. The Achilles reflex (ankle jerk) is diminished or absent, and atrophy of the calf is present if the nerve compression is chronic. The posterior calf and lateral side of the foot may have decreased sensation (S1 distribution).

Compression of L5 leads to weakness in the extension of the large toe and, less completely, in the everters and dorsiflexors of the foot. The sensory deficit associated with L5 is noted over the anterior tibia and the dorsomedial aspect of the foot down to the great toe. No reflex other than the posterior tibial reflex, which is difficult to obtain, is associated with the L5 nerve root.

The L4 nerve supplies the quadriceps muscles of the upper leg. Quadriceps muscle weakness, demonstrated in knee extension, is associated with L4 nerve compression. The patient complaint associated with this lesion is frequently one of an unstable knee. Atrophy of the thigh musculature may be marked. Sensory loss affects the anteromedial aspect of the thigh. The patellar tendon reflex is lost (Fig. 6.9).

Prone position

The neurologic examination is completed by testing for higher lumbar and sacral nerve root function. Dural irritation of nerve roots from L2 to L4 are tested by the femoral stretch test (Fig. 6.10). With the knee bent, the thigh is elevated from the examining table. The test is positive if pain is reproduced in the front of the thigh (L2 and L3) or the medial aspect of the leg (L4). Gluteus maximus strength is tested by having the patient contract the buttocks. Asymmetry of contraction or atrophy suggests an abnormality of S1.

Upper and lower sacral roots are tested by sensory examination of the skin over the lower legs, buttocks, and perineum. If a patient has saddle anesthesia, a positive straight leg raising test in both legs, and abnormal sphincter tone, a cauda equina compression syndrome should be suspected.

The final part of the evaluation are the genital and rectal examinations. This part of the examination is completed in patients who have symptoms and signs suggestive of medical low back pain. These examinations are helpful in detecting patients with prostatic abnormalities, rectal cancer, or endometriosis.

A number of ancillary physical examination tests may be used to confirm abnormalities discovered during the routine examination. These tests are listed in Fig. 6.11.

MOTOR INNERVATION OF LOWER EXTREMITIES

Region	Backward	Forward
Hip	L4,5 extension	Flexion L2,3
Knee	L5,S1 flexion	Extension L3,4
Ankle	S1,2 plantar flexion	Inversion L4 Dorsiflexion L4,5 Eversion L5,S1

Fig. 6.8 Motor innervation of the lower extremities.

LUMBAR ROOT LESIONS

Root	Muscle weakness/movement affected	Tendon reflex decreased
L2	Hip flexion/adduction	
L3	Hip adduction Knee extension	Knee jerk
L4	Knee extension Foot inversion/dorsiflexion	Knee jerk
L5	Hip extension/abduction Knee flexion Foot/toe dorsifexion	
S1	Knee flexion Foot/toe plantar flexion Foot eversion	Ankle jerk

Fig. 6.9 Lumbar root lesions. Cutaneous, motor, and reflex functions of the lower extremity.

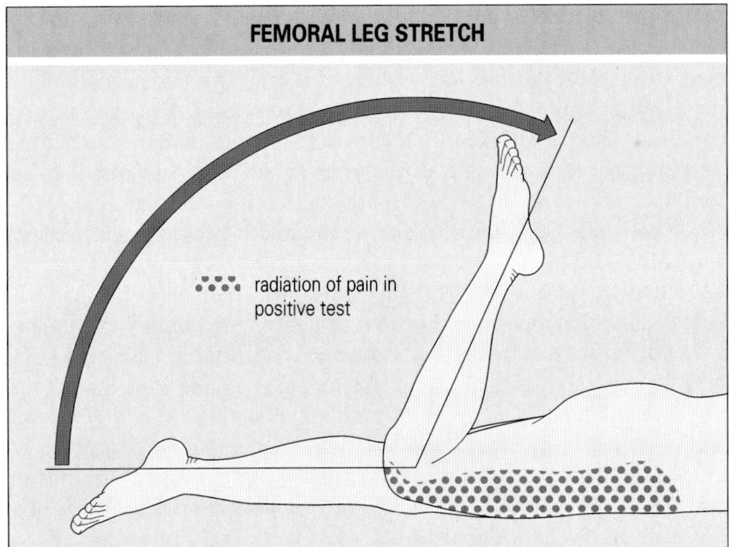

Fig. 6.10 Femoral stretch test. The knee is flexed and lifted superiorly. Sharp pain that is generated in the anterior thigh is considered a positive test.

Non-organic physical signs

Patients who are involved with litigation or claims for work-related sickness payment occasionally exaggerate their symptoms. In these patients, the objective findings do not match the subjective complaints [19]. Close observation of the patient helps identify the inconsistencies. Waddell has described five tests that identify individuals with 'functional' or 'exaggerated' symptoms (Fig. 6.12) [20]. A finding of three or more of the five signs is clinically significant. Isolated positive signs are ignored. These tests can be incorporated unobtrusively into the physical examination. Using the tests on a consistent basis allows the examiner to become familiar with the spectrum of normal and abnormal findings. Once familiar with the tests, the physician will have less difficulty in identifying the patient who exaggerates symptoms for ulterior motives.

Value of results

Although the physical examination adds essential information for the evaluation of patients with low back pain, problems exist in the reproducibility and significance of abnormal findings. Part of the difficulty in the evaluation of low back pain is the lack of definition for physical signs. McCombe evaluated the reproducibility between three observers of 54 physical signs used for back pain evaluation [21]. Reproducible signs included measurements of lordosis (by tape measure from the maximum kyphosis of the thoracic spine to that of the sacrum), and flexion range (Schober test); determination of pain location on flexion and lateral bend; straight leg raising test (pendulum goniometer measurement of the angle at which pain was first experienced and angle of maximum tolerance); determination of pain location in the thigh and legs, and sensory changes in the legs. Nerve root tension signs were reliable if the location of pain was described. Reproducibility of bone tenderness over the sacroiliac joints, spinous processes, and iliac crests was greater than that associated with soft tissue structures. Although the better description of test results will allow greater agreement between physicians in regard to the presence or absence of physical signs, these descriptions do not have diagnostic validity.

The question of diagnostic validity was tested prospectively by Jensen in 52 patients with lumbar disc herniations confirmed at surgery for correlation of disturbed sensory and motor function and anatomic abnormalities [22]. The positive predictive value of disturbed sensation in the L5 dermatome and weakness of foot dorsiflexion was 76% for herniation from the fourth lumbar disc. The positive predictive value of altered sensation in the S1 dermatome was only 50%. Therefore, although the history and physical examination are important and may identify levels of nerve impingement, they are not sufficient to make a correct diagnosis in all circumstances of spinal nerve compression [23].

With information obtained from the history and physical examination the physician should formulate a working diagnosis for the low back pain patient. The diagnosis of low back pain of undetermined etiology is inadequate. Patients may have mechanical low back pain, apophyseal joint disease, intervertebral disc herniation with or without nerve root impingement, or a systemic inflammatory disease. Patients with mechanical disorders may be treated without an additional laboratory test during the initial visit. Patients who are aged 50 years or over, or those with systemic symptoms, may benefit from further diagnostic tests.

ANCILLARY TESTS FOR EVALUATION OF LOW BACK PAIN	
Schober test	Lumbosacral motion
Contralateral straight leg raising test	Nerve root compression
Bow string sign	Nerve root compression
Hoover test	Patient effort

Fig. 6.11 Ancillary tests for evaluation of low back pain.

DIFFERENTIAL DIAGNOSIS

Each patient with back pain presents to the physician a different set of complaints. These complaints may be associated with a broad range of disorders, from mechanical muscle strain, to spondyloarthropathy, to metastatic disease. The problem confronting the examining physician is to integrate the patient's symptoms and physical signs into a logical diagnosis and initial treatment plan and to identify those individuals with more serious ailments from the vast majority with mechanical disorders. With the myriad of symptoms, signs, laboratory tests, radiographic methods and possible diagnoses, the physician must be organized in his approach to the patient with low back pain. Most patients with low back pain will improve and will not require additional diagnostic testing. In times of increasing medical financial costs, diagnostic tests must be obtained in a thoughtful and time-efficient manner. A standardized approach to the diagnosis and treatment of low back pain is possible

WADDELL TESTS FOR FUNCTIONAL LOW BACK PAIN
Tenderness to superficial touch
Simulation tests Axial loading Spinal rotation in one plane
Distraction tests Inconsistent results on confirmatory testing
Regional disturbances Abnormalities not following neuroanatomic structures
Overreaction Disproportionate verbalization

Fig. 6.12 Waddell tests for functional low back pain.

MECHANICAL LOW BACK PAIN					
	Muscle strain	Spondylothesis	Herniated disc	Osteoarthritis	Spinal stenosis
Age (years)	20–40	20–30	30–50	over 50	over 60
Pain pattern					
Initial location	Back	Back	Back	Back	Leg
Onset	Acute	Insidious	Acute	Insidious	Insidious
Standing	+	+	–	+	+
Sitting	–	–	+	–	–
Flexion	+		+	–	–
Extension	–	+	–	+	+
Straight leg raising	–	–	+	–	+ (stress)
Plain radiograph	–	+	–	+	+

Fig. 6.13 Mechanical low back pain.

if basic rules are followed. This approach has been utilized in the evaluation of thousands of patients and has been useful in the vast majority of those individuals [24].

The primary objective for the physician is to return the patient with acute low back pain to regular activity as quickly as possible. Patients who continue with low back pain for six months or longer are unlikely to have resolution of pain and rarely return to their usual employment. The effort required to evaluate and treat patients effectively to prevent the evolution into a chronic pain syndrome is worthwhile. In achieving this goal, the physician must be concerned with making efficient and precise use of diagnostic studies, avoiding ineffectual surgery, and making therapy available at a reasonable cost.

Systemic Approach to Low Back pain

Most patients with low back pain have a mechanical cause for their symptoms and do not require any diagnostic tests (Fig. 6.13). Individuals who must be evaluated more intensively are those with life-threatening disorders, such as cauda equina compression or expanding abdominal aneurysms (Fig. 6.14).

Patients with cauda equina compression have a symptom complex that may include low back pain, bilateral sciatica, saddle anesthesia, or bladder and bowel incontinence. The most common mechanical causes of cauda equina compression are central herniations of intervertebral discs while epidural abscesses and tumor masses constitute the most frequent nonmechanical causes. Once the diagnosis is suspected, the patient should undergo a radiographic procedure to visualize the affected anatomic area of the lumbosacral spine. MRI is the most sensitive radiographic technique for detecting these lesions. Patients are treated appropriately for their underlying abnormalities.

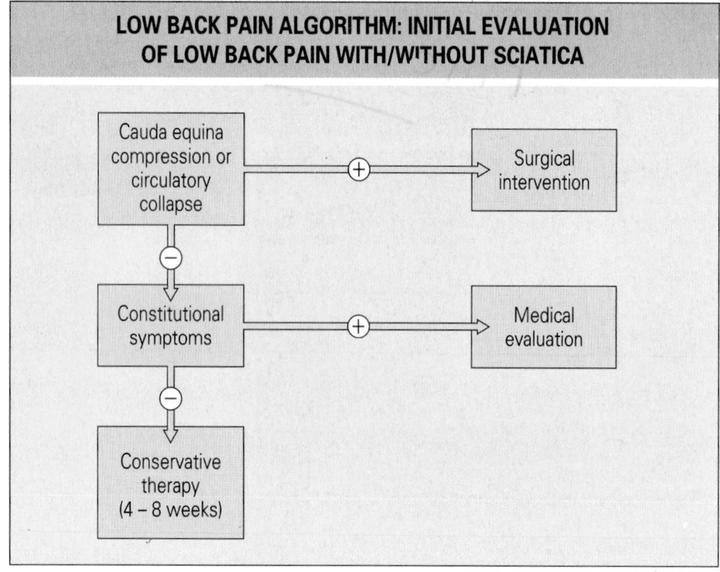

Fig. 6.14 Low back pain algorithm. Initial evaluation.

A patient with tearing or throbbing back pain who has experienced acute dizziness may have an expanding abdominal aneurysm. Any change in the frequency, intensity or location of the pain suggests expansion in the size of the aneurysm. Patients with an abdominal aneurysm are usually older individuals who have had a history of lower extremity claudication. If patients complain of syncope or are hypotensive, they must be evaluated for an aneurysm on an emergency basis. Physical examination of the abdomen may reveal a pulsatile mass, abdominal bruits, and decreased pulsations in the lower extremities. Patients with expanding aneurysms may be evaluated with CT or ultrasonography, depending on the patient's hemodynamic status. Patients with an expanding aneurysm require surgical correction of the aneurysmal defect.

Other patients with low back pain who need to be identified before therapy is initiated are those with medical low back pain. Most of these patients can be identified during the history portion of the evaluation since they usually present with one of the following:

- fever and/or weight loss;
- increased pain on recumbency (sleeping in a chair);
- morning stiffness lasting hours;
- acute, localized lumbosacral bone pain;
- visceral pain associated with alterations in gastrointestinal or genitourinary function.

Patients with any of these symptoms, should be evaluated thoroughly.

The remaining patients without cauda equina syndrome or a medical illness may be started on conservative therapy without a laboratory or radiographic evaluation. One exception to this guideline is older individuals (aged over 50 years) with new onset back pain. These patients may benefit from a plain radiograph of the lumbar spine and ESR measurement to detect neoplastic, or infectious disorders [25].

Conservative management for acute low back pain includes patient education, controlled physical activity, nonsteroidal anti-inflammatory drugs, muscle relaxants, or physical therapy. Any or all of these components of conservative management may be used in an individual patient.

The physician should decide on a course of therapy and continue it for a 4–6 week trial. The determination of a specific diagnosis, whether it be a muscular strain of the paraspinous muscles of the lumbar spine or a herniated intervertebral disc, is not important at this stage of the evaluation. The entire population of individuals with low back pain are treated in a similar manner. Some of these may require more elaborate diagnostic tests or more invasive therapy. However, conservative therapy and time is so effective (90% or more at 2 months) that most patients do not require expensive tests or therapies. The opportunity to treat patients in this manner results from the fact that the vast majority of patients have nonradiating low back pain or back strain. The etiology of the pain associated with back strain is unclear. Possibilities include injury to muscle bundles, ligamentous or fascial attachments, mechanical stress associated with poor posture, or tears of the annulus fibrosus, among others. Patients complain of pain with an acute onset, frequently related to some traumatic event that involved excess effort in an awkward position or a contusion. The pain is localized to areas lateral to the midline near the lumbosacral junction. On occasion the pain may radiate across the midline or into the buttocks. On physical examination, they demonstrate a decreased range of lumbar spine motion, tenderness to palpation over the involved muscle and increased muscle contraction. Laboratory and radiographic evaluation of these patients are normal. Any variation from normal should result in an evaluation for alternative diagnoses.

After 4–6 weeks have passed, patients in whom the initial treatment regimen fails are sorted into four groups, based upon the location and radiation of the residual pain. These groups include those with localized low back pain, leg pain below the knee (sciatica), anterior thigh pain, and posterior thigh pain.

Localized Low Back Pain

Patients with localized low back pain make up the largest group with residual pain (Fig. 6.15). Evaluation with plain radiographs of the lumbar spine is indicated, with flexion and extension views if spinal instability is suspected. Spondylolysis, with or without spondylolisthesis, is the most common structural abnormality to cause significant low back pain. Spondylolysis is a break in the pars interarticularis. If the defect permits displacement of one vertebra on another, it is termed a spondylolisthesis (Fig. 6.16). Individuals may have this abnormality without symptoms. Most patients with symptomatic spondylolisthesis complain of pain when their spine is placed in extension (increased displacement) as opposed to flexion (that tends to normalize vertebral body position). Most patients have a good response to nonoperative measures, including patient education, flexion exercises, and a flexion back support. A small group will fail conservative management and require a fusion of the unstable segment.

Localized low back pain may also be associated with disorders of the intervertebral discs and related apophyseal joints. Abnormalities may be noted on plain radiographic evaluation of the lumbar spine. Decreased disc height and apophyseal joint sclerosis may not cause low back pain. However, articular degeneration with apophyseal joint sclerosis may be associated with decreased back motion and back pain. Patients may have mild stiffness in the morning. During the day, these patients experience an improvement in their symptoms only to have a return of pain at the end of the day, after they have been physically active. Patients with osteoarthritis of the lumbar spine should be treated as other patients with this disorder affecting other joints in the skeleton. Therapy includes analgesics, nonsteroidal anti-inflammatory drugs (NSAIDs) and appropriate exercises. A point to remember is that older individuals who develop osteoarthritis are also more likely to develop more ominous causes of low back pain. These disorders (malignancy, infection, osteoporosis, for example) should be considered before the physician ascribes the patient's pain to osteoarthritis.

Another abnormality occasionally seen is disc calcification. This is associated with ochronosis, calcium pyrophosphate dihydrate disease, hemochromatosis, hyperparathyroidism, and acromegaly. Patients with disc calcification should be evaluated for the associated endocrinologic or metabolic disorder.

Patients who fail to respond to conservative management and who have no specific radiographic abnormalities may improve with a local injection of a combination of an anesthetic and a semi-soluble corticosteroid preparation into the area of maximal tenderness. Many patients with local muscle strain experience complete relief of symptoms with the injection. This therapy should be given to individuals who will be compliant with the instructions regarding limitation of activity. Patients who have undergone an anesthetic injection will not experience pain if they engage in physical activity that causes additional damage to musculoskeletal structures. These individuals should be cautioned to limit their activities for 24–48 hours to be sure that additional healing has occurred so that usual activities can be resumed.

Patients who persist with low back pain who do not have spondylolysis, disc calcification, or osteoarthritis must be re-evaluated for the possibility of a systemic disorder causing their symptom. This re-evaluation should commence with a review of the patient's history and physical examination. The patient may have forgotten to mention an important symptom during the initial evaluation or may have developed a new one during the course of therapy. The histories of patients with medical low back pain may be divided into five groups according to symptoms. These groups include individuals with fever or weight loss, pain with recumbency, morning stiffness, acute localized lumbosacral bone pain or visceral pain.

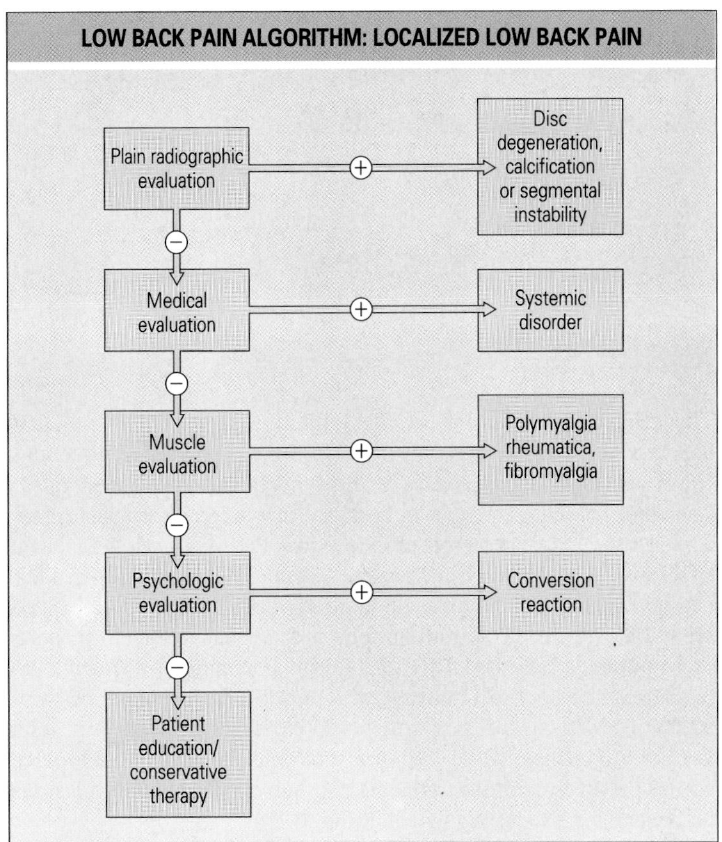

Fig. 6.15 Low back pain algorithm. Localized low back pain.

Fever and/or Weight Loss

Patients with fever and/or weight loss frequently have an infection or tumor as a cause of their pain. Neoplastic lesions also cause pain with recumbency.

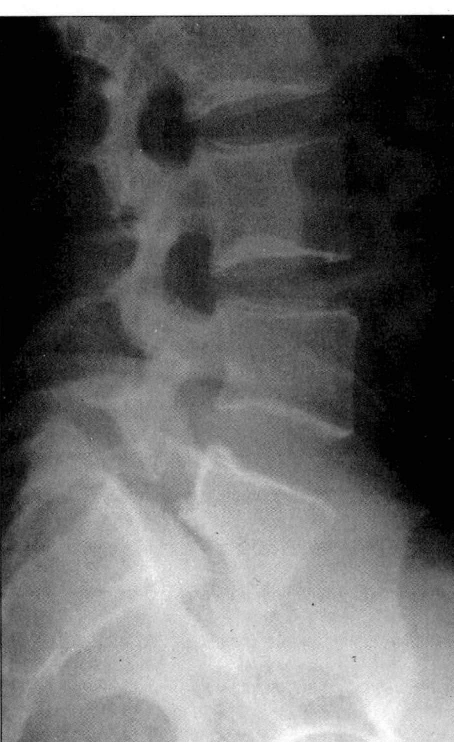

Fig. 6.16 Grade II developmental spondylolisthesis. At the L5–S1 level.

INFECTIOUS DISORDERS AFFECTING THE LUMBOSACRAL SPINE
Vertebral osteomyelitis Bacterial Tuberculous Fungal Spirochetal Parasitic
Discitis
Pyogenic sacroiliitis

Fig. 6.17 Localized low back pain. Infectious disorders affecting the lumbosacral spine.

The clinical presentation of the patient with a spinal infection depends on the infecting organism (Fig. 6.17). Bacterial infections cause acute, toxic symptoms, while tuberculous and fungal infections are indolent. The pain in bacterial infections is persistent, present at rest, and is exacerbated by motion. Physical findings include decreased range of motion, muscle spasm, and percussion tenderness over the involved bone. Plain radiographs may reveal localized areas of osteopenia. If radiographs are normal, technetium bone scintigraphy is indicated. MRI is a sensitive technique with which to investigate the entire lumbosacral spine for the presence of local infection. MRI also detects soft tissue extension of lesions beyond the bony confines of the vertebral column. CT should take place after MRI evaluation to delineate the bony architecture of lesions not visualized adequately by MRI (Fig. 6.18).

Vertebral osteomyelitis follows hematogenous spread from an extraosseous source and can be identified in 40% of patients [26]. Organisms may enter bone from nutrient arteries, or from the venous plexus of Batson, a valveless system of veins that supplies the spinal column. Organisms that cause osteomyelitis include bacteria, mycobacteria, fungi, spirochetes, and parasites. The primary sources for spinal infections include the genitourinary tract, respiratory tract, and skin. The most frequently encountered organism causing infection in 60% of cases is *Staphylococcus aureus* [27]. Gram-negative organisms are often grown from the elderly and from parenteral drug abusers (*Escherichia coli* and *Pseudomonas aeruginosa* [28] respectively). In patients who have undergone surgery or trauma to the spine, nonpathogenic organisms (diphtheroids, *Staphylococcus epidermidis*) may be associated with an indolent infection of the vertebral column [29]. Workers in the meat-processing industry may acquire a brucellosis infection [30]. Tuberculous and fungal infections of the vertebral column occur most often in the elderly and other immunocompromised individuals. Fifty to sixty percent of individuals with skeletal tuberculosis have axial skeletal disease. The clinical presentation of a patient with tuberculous spondylitis is pain over the involved vertebrae, low-grade fever, and weight loss. The process is indolent and may be present for years before diagnosis (Fig. 6.19) [31].

The definitive diagnosis of infection is based on the recovery and identification of the causative organism from blood cultures, or from aspirated material or biopsy of the lesion. Antibiotic therapy is adequate to cure most spinal infections. Surgical intervention for drainage is needed if neurologic dysfunction has occurred secondary to the infection.

Other infections that affect the lumbosacral spine include discitis and pyogenic sacroiliitis. Infection of the intervertebral disc space in adults is most frequently associated with lumbar disc surgery. Approximately 3% of lumbar disc surgery patients develop disc space infections [32]. Diagnosis is confirmed by identifying the causative organism from blood cultures of aspirated disc material. Pyogenic sacroiliitis is an unusual form of septic arthritis [33]. The disease is associated with acute symptoms, severe sacroiliac joint pain, and fever. Bone scinitigraphy with early perfusion views will identify the affected joint. Diagnosis of the causative organism may be obtained by blood cultures, fluoroscopic fine needle aspiration, or open biopsy. Antibiotic therapy for 6 weeks is usually adequate to heal the infection without the need for surgical drainage.

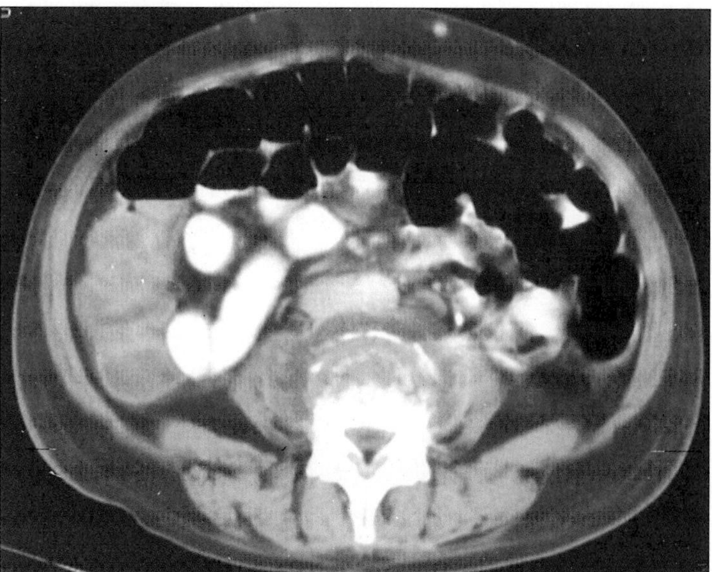

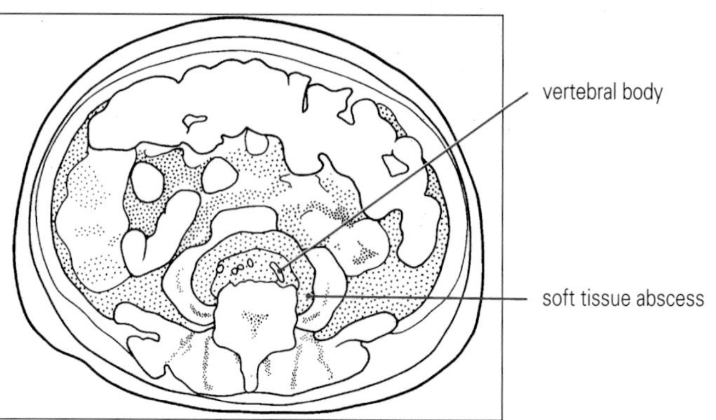

Fig. 6.18 Vertebral osteomyelitis. CT scan, axial view, demonstrating destruction of vertebral body with soft tissue extension into the paravertebral space.

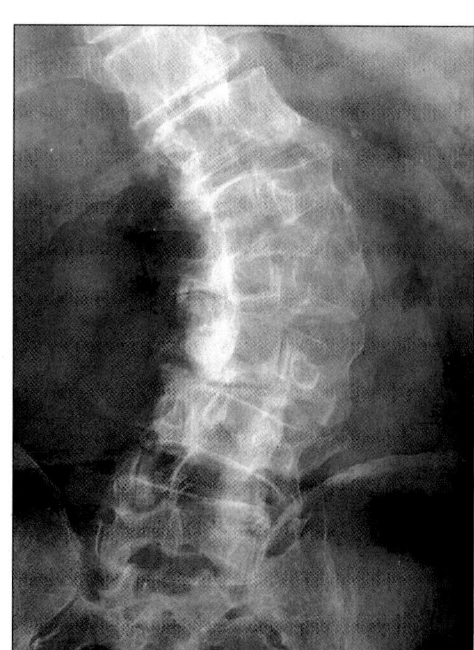

Fig. 6.19 Lumbosacral spine involvement. Pott's disease affecting the lumbosacral spine at L3, resulting in rotatory scoliosis and lateral calcification.

NEOPLASTIC LESIONS OF THE LUMBROSACRAL SPINE		
Benign	**Malignant**	**Spinal cord tumors**
Osteoid osteoma	Multiple myeloma	Extradural
Osteoblastoma	Chondrosarcoma	Metastases
Osteochondroma	Chordoma	
Giant cell tumor	Lymphoma	Intradural-Extramedullary
Aneurysmal bone cyst	Skeletal metastases	Neurofibroma
Hemangioma		Meningioma
Eosinophilic granuloma		
Sacoiliac lipoma		Intramedullary
		Ependymoma
		Astrocytoma

Fig. 6.20 Localized low back pain. Neoplastic disorders affecting the lumbosacral spine.

Nocturnal Pain/Pain with Recumbency

Tumors of the spinal column or spinal cord cause pain at night or with recumbency. Both benign and malignant neoplasms cause these symptoms. Nocturnal pain may be caused by swelling of neoplastic tissues associated with inactivity in the supine position or by stretching the neural tissues over the neoplastic mass.

A number of benign and malignant tumors are associated with involvement of the lumbosacral spine (Fig. 6.20). Benign lesions tend to cause local pain and involve the posterior elements of vertebrae. Malignant lesions cause more diffuse pain, systemic symptoms, and involve the anterior elements of vertebrae.

Patients with malignancies have pain that is gradual in onset but persistent in character and increasing in intensity. Physical examination shows localized tenderness over the lesion along with neurologic dysfunction if neural elements are compressed. Radiographic evaluation is very useful in detecting the location and characteristics of the neoplastic lesion.

An example of a benign tumor of bone that affects the lumbar spine is an osteoid osteoma. The tumor is most frequently found in young adults aged 20–30 years. Approximately 7% of osteoid osteomas occur in the spine, most frequently in the lumbar area [34]. The pain associated with this lesion is intermittent and vague initially, but with time becomes constant and aching, with a boring quality. The pain is not relieved with rest or application of heat. The pain is frequently exacerbated at night and disturbs sleep. In the spine, osteoid osteomas are associated with nonstructural scoliosis. The appearance of marked paravertebral muscle spasm and the sudden onset of scoliosis in a young adult requires an evaluation for the presence of this lesion. The lesion is on the concave side of the scoliosis. The symptoms of osteoid osteoma may be present for considerable time before plain radiographic findings become evident. The pain is relieved with low doses of NSAIDs.

Physical examination reveals local tenderness. Scoliosis is reversible early in the course of the lesion. With prolonged spasm, muscle atrophy may occur. Vertebral deformity may occur in young individuals who are growing. Hyperemia of the tumor may cause swelling and erythema of the skin if the lesion is superficial in location.

The radiographic finding of a lucent nidus with a diameter of 1.5cm and a surrounding well-defined area of dense sclerotic bone is virtually pathognomonic of osteoid osteoma. The lesions are in the neural arch in 75% of vertebrae, articular facets in 18%, and 7% in vertebral bodies (Fig. 6.21). Bone scans or CT scans should be utilized if an osteoma is suspected and not found on plain radiographs (Fig. 6.22) [35,36].

The treatment for an osteoid osteoma is simple excision of the nidus and surrounding sclerotic bone. If the nidus is not entirely removed, recurrence of the lesion is possible and symptoms may persist. On occasion, osteoid osteomas may undergo spontaneous healing.

Multiple myeloma is the most common primary malignancy of bone in adults (27% of biopsied bone tumors) [37]. Patients range in age from 50 to 70 years, with only a rare patient below the age of 40. Low back pain is the initial complaint in 35% of patients. The pain is aching and intermittent at onset, is aggravated by weight-bearing and improved with bed rest. Some patients may have radicular symptoms that mimic those of sciatica and arthritis [38]. Significant neurologic dysfunction, including paraplegia, occurs more commonly with solitary plasmacytoma than with multiple myeloma [39].

Physical examination may demonstrate diffuse bone tenderness, fever, pallor, and purpura in the later stages of the illness. Signs of spinal cord compression are present if vertebral body collapse has progressed to a significant degree.

Laboratory testing reflects the systemic nature of this malignancy. Included in the abnormal findings may be anemia, leukocytosis, thrombocytopenia, elevated ESR, hypercalcemia, hyperuricemia, elevated creatinine, and positive Coomb's test. An increase in serum proteins is secondary to the presence of abnormal immunoglobulins of any of the five classes. Urinalysis may detect Bence Jones protein formed by the production of excess immunoglobulin light chains. Bone marrow aspirate or biopsy reveals an excess number of plasma cells of varied histologic grades.

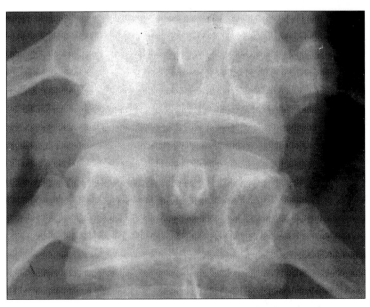

Fig. 6.21 Osteoid osteoma. Plain radiograph of thoracic spine demonstrating sclerosis affecting the right pedicle of T11.

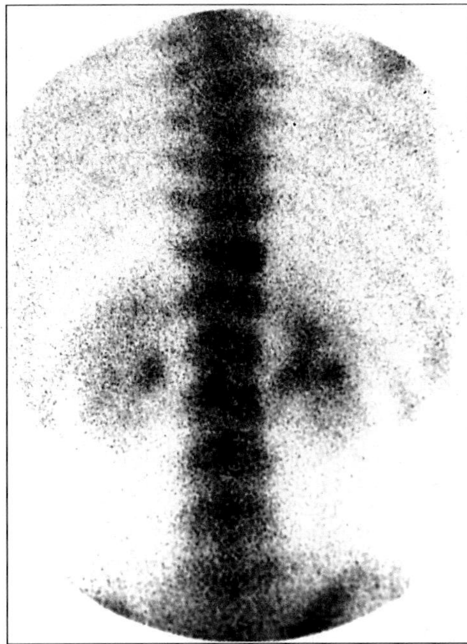

Fig. 6.22 Osteoid osteoma. Bone scintigraphy demonstrating increased uptake in T11. There is no other area of increased uptake in the skeleton.

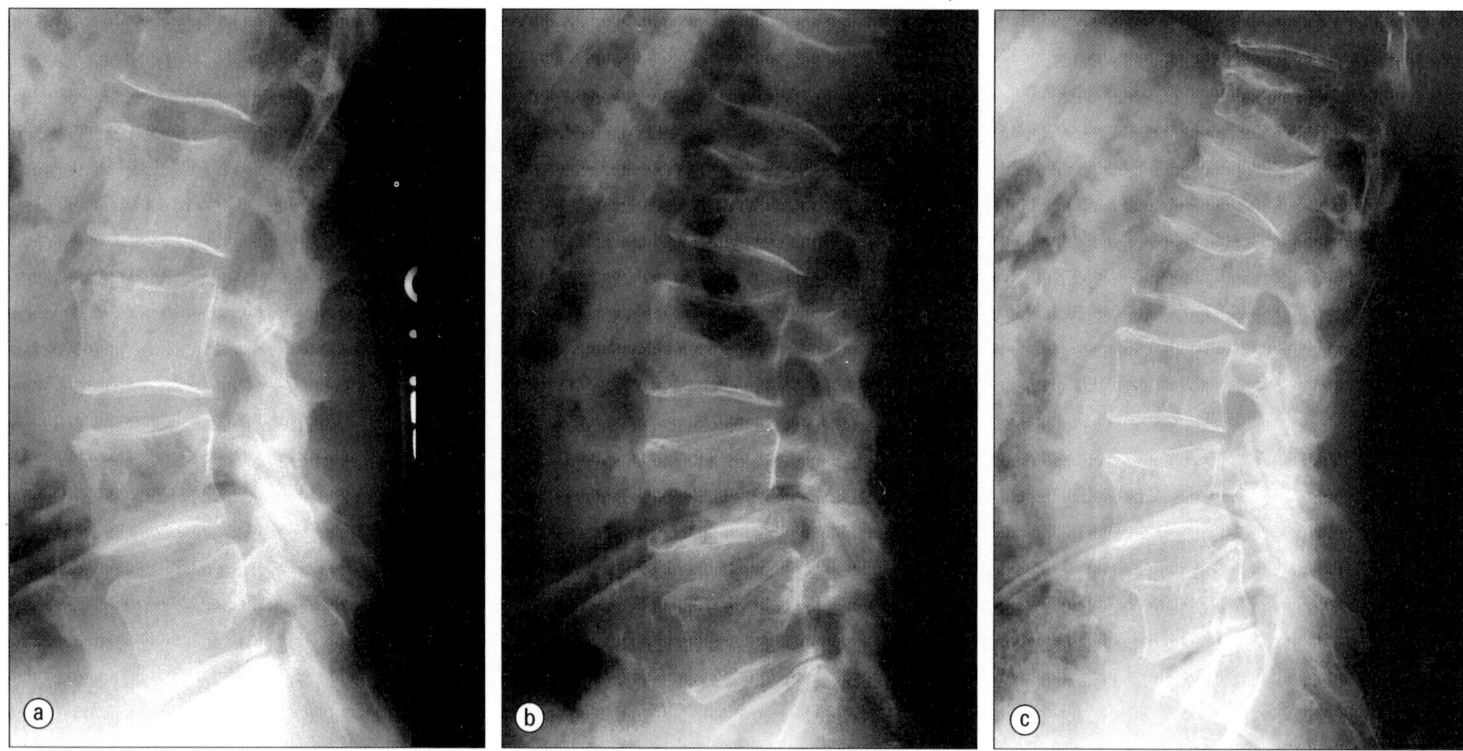

Fig. 6.23 Multiple myeloma. A series of plain radiographs taken over a 3-month period. Progressive osteopenia and pathologic compression fractures are noted. (a) Initial evaluation; (b) at 12 weeks; (c) at 14 weeks. Diagnosis was made at 12 weeks after initial presentation.

Plain radiographs demonstrate osteolysis without reactive sclerosis and sparing of the posterior elements of the spine (Fig. 6.23) [40]. Solitary plasmacytomas in the spine have variable radiographic appearances. They may be expansile, with or without reactive bone. They may invade an intervertebral disc space and mimic discitis. Bone scintigraphy does not detect myeloma since there is no reactive component of osteoblasts to the myeloma cells. MRI and CT are better techniques for identifying the presence and extent of myeloma lesions in the bone and soft tissues.

The diagnosis of multiple myeloma is based upon clinical data, along with the detection of abnormal plasma cells on biopsy. Myeloma is treated with the use of chemotherapeutic agents to control the growth of the malignant plasma cells. In patients with cord compression, decompression laminectomy with or without local radiotherapy is indicated.

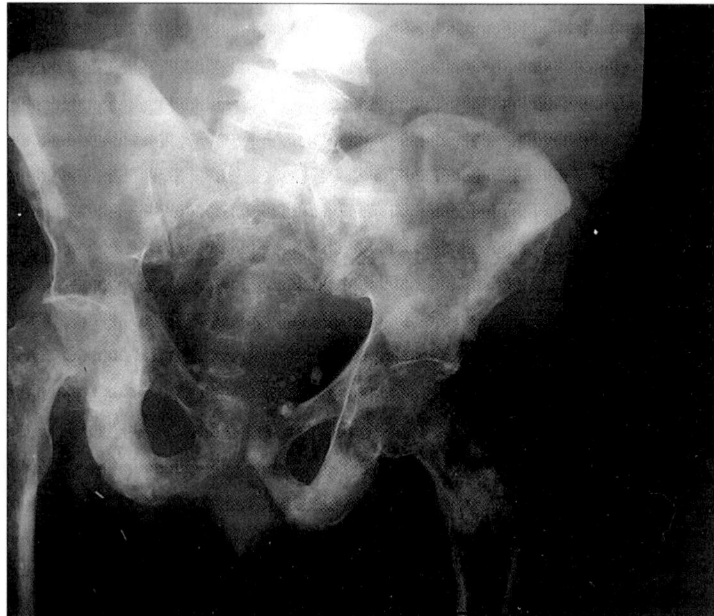

Fig. 6.24 Metastatic prostate cancer. Plain radiograph demonstrating osteoblastic lesions replacing lower lumbar vertebral bodies and most of the bony pelvis.

Skeletal metastases are 25 times more common than primary tumors as the cause of neoplastic lesions in the spine. Patients who are aged over 50 years are at greatest risk of developing metastatic disease. Autopsy results demonstrate that 70% of patients with primary tumors develop metastases to the thoracolumbar spine [41]. The common sources for skeletal metastases include tumors of the breast, prostate, lung, kidney, thyroid, colon, uterine cervix, and bladder.

Lumbar pain is of gradual onset and increasing intensity. The symptoms are increased with motion, sneezing, or coughing. The pain is local at the onset but may become radicular in character. Neurologic abnormalities may occur abruptly over a 4–6 month period.

Physical examination may demonstrate pain on palpation over the affected bone. Muscle spasm and limitation of motion are associated findings. Neurologic abnormalities are indicative of nerve root or spinal cord impingement.

Laboratory findings may include anemia, elevated ESR, abnormal urinalysis, increased alkaline phosphatase, and in metastatic prostate cancer, increased prostatic acid phosphatase. Histologic features of biopsy specimens may suggest the identity of the primary tumor, but some lesions are too undifferentiated for identification.

Radiographic abnormalities depend on the character of the underlying malignancy. Kidney and thyroid metastases are typically osteolytic while colon lesions are osteoblastic. Mixed lytic and blastic lesions are noted with breast, lung, prostate, or bladder tumors (Fig. 6.24). Plain radiographs may not show any abnormalities until 30–50% of bone calcium is lost [42]. Bone scans are positive in over 85% of patients with metastases. MRI is able to show tumor in the spinal cord, extraosseous extension, and bone marrow replacement, while CT is more helpful for detecting cortical bone involvement and bone mineralization [43].

Neoplastic lesions may also occur inside the spinal canal. These intraspinal neoplasms may be extradural, between bone and the outermost covering of the spinal cord (the dura); intradural extramedullary, between the dura and the spinal cord; and intramedullary, in the spinal cord proper. Extradural tumors are most commonly metastatic in origin. Intradural–extramedullary tumors are primarily meningiomas, neurofibromas, or lipomas. Intramedullary tumors are

RHEUMATOLOGIC DISORDERS AFFECTING THE LUMBOSACRAL SPINE
Spondyloarthropathies Ankylosing spondylitis Reiter's syndrome Psoriatic arthritis Enteropathic arthritis
Behçet's syndrome Familial Mediterranean fever Whipple's disease Diffuse idiopathic skeletal hyperostosis

Fig. 6.25 Rheumatic disease causing pain in the lumbosacral spine.

ependymomas or gliomas. The neurologic abnormalities associated with these unusual neoplasms are dependent on their location in the spinal cord and cauda equina. MRI, by its ability to define the exact location, size, and character of the lesions, has revolutionized the visualization of intraspinal lesions [44].

Treatment of metastatic disease of the spine is directed toward pain palliation. A cure is rarely possible since most metastatic lesions are rarely solitary. Radiotherapy is useful to control spinal pain. Decompressive laminectomy is recommended for patients who have recently developed neurologic dysfunction.

Morning Stiffness

Morning stiffness of the lumbosacral spine is a frequent symptom in patients with inflammatory arthropathies that affect the axial skeleton (Fig. 6.25). While morning stiffness of mechanical origin may last an hour or less, stiffness associated with the spondyloarthropathies typically lasts for hours. The spondyloarthropathies include a group of arthritides that inflame the sacroiliac joints and the axial skeleton. Patients with a spondyloarthropathy may have unilateral or bilateral sacroiliac pain. Patients with ankylosing spondylitis or enteropathic spondylitis have sacroiliitis initially and subsequently develop spondylitis. On rare occasions, patients have pain that is primarily in the lumbar spine and spares the sacroiliac joints (Reiter's syndrome, psoriatic spondylitis). The spondyloarthropathy group of patients have great difficulty getting out of bed in the morning because of stiffness. They may also awaken during the night after they have been sleeping because of back pain.

Spondyloarthropathies are systemic illnesses that affect nonosseous organs. In these conditions, the extra-articular manifestations of the disease help characterize the specific form of arthritis causing the patient's low back pain. Iritis is associated with ankylosing spondylitis. Conjunctivitis, urethritis, keratoderma blennorrhagicum, and circinate balanitis are seen in patients with Reiter's syndrome. Psoriatic skin and nail changes are noted in patients with psoriatic spondylitis. Patients with inflammatory bowel disease are also at risk of developing arthritis that affects the appendicular and axial skeleton joints.

Physical examination of the musculoskeletal system may demonstrate decreased mobility in the axial skeleton (i.e. Schober test, chest expansion). The general physical examination may discover physical findings unsuspected by the patient that helps diagnose the specific spondyloarthropathy (oral ulcers, psoriatic skin lesions).

Laboratory tests may show a mild anemia and elevated ESR. Histocompatibility testing for the HLA-B27 haplotype is confirmatory but not diagnostic. Approximately 8% of the Caucasian population is HLA-B27$^+$ but is unaffected by a spondyloarthropathy.

Plain radiographs of the sacroiliac joints represent the initial investigation of choice in patients suspected of having an inflammatory arthropathy of the axial skeleton (Fig. 6.26). Thoracolumbar radiographs are less helpful initially since squaring of the vertebral bodies and syndesmophytes rarely occur in the absence of sacroiliitis. Sacroiliac radiographs may show joint erosions in the lower third of the joints. Lumbar radiographs may show loss of lumbar lordosis and squaring of the vertebral bodies (Fig. 6.27). If plain radiographs are normal, tilting the radiography tube by 30° results in an image taken with the sacroiliac joint in one plane (Ferguson view). This view is helpful in detecting early changes of sacroiliitis. Bone scintigraphy can detect increased uptake in the sacroiliac joints but false positive results frequently occur. CT scan is the most sensitive test and may show early involvement of the sacroiliac joint when plain radiographs are normal or equivocal [45].

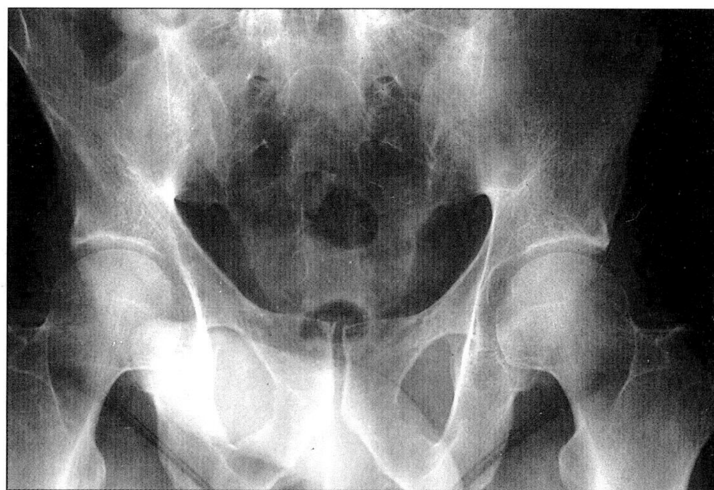

Fig. 6.26 Ankylosing spondylitis. Plain radiograph of the pelvis demonstrating bilateral sacroiliitis with fusion of the sacroiliac joints.

Patients with spondyloarthropathy are treated with a combination of NSAIDs and physical therapy. Additional therapies may be used to control the underlying illness that has caused the arthritis (topical preparations – psoriasis; corticosteroids – bowel disease).

Acute Localized Bone Pain

Another group of patients with medical low back pain may present with acute onset of pain in the midline of the back. Pain localized to the midline is frequently associated with disorders that affect osseous structures of the lumbar spine. Acute localized bone pain is usually caused by a fracture or expansion of bone. Any systemic process that increases mineral loss from bone, causes bone necrosis, or replaces bone cells with inflammatory or neoplastic cells will weaken vertebral bone to the point where fracture may occur spontaneously or

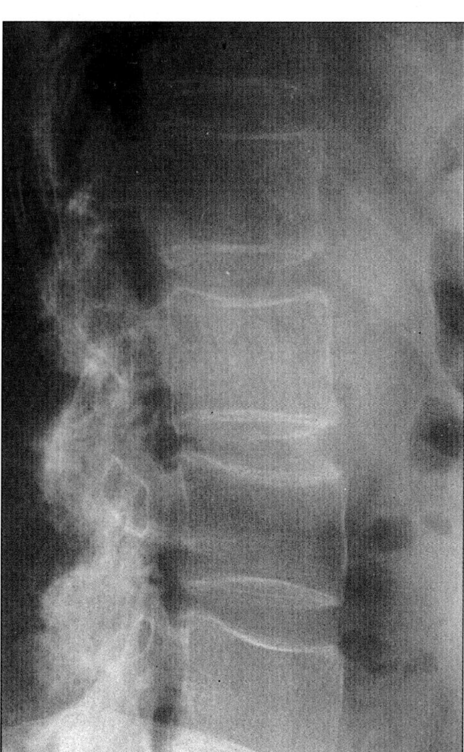

Fig. 6.27 Ankylosing spondylitis. Lateral view of lumbar spine demonstrates squaring of vertebral bodies, thin syndesmophytes, disc calcification, and diffuse osteopenia.

ENDOCRINOLOGIC, HEMATOLOGIC, AND MISCELLANEOUS DISORDERS AFFECTING THE LUMBOSACRAL SPINE

Endocrinologic/Metabolic
- Osteoporosis
- Osteomalacia
- Hyperparathyroidism

Hematologic
- Hemoglobinopathy
- Myelofibrosis
- Mastocytosis

Miscellaneous
- Paget's disease
- Subacute endocarditis
- Sarcoidosis
- Retroperitoneal fibrosis

Fig. 6.28 Endocrinologic, hematologic, and neoplastic disorders that cause acute localized bone pain.

with minimal trauma (Fig. 6.28). Patients with acute fractures experience sudden onset of pain localized to the affected bone. Bone pain may be the initial manifestation of disease or may occur in the setting of associated symptoms. A medical history, including the review of systems, may elicit responses that suggest the underlying cause of the patient's back pain (kidney stones – hyperparathyroidism; chronic cough – sarcoidosis).

Physical examination shows localized tenderness with palpation of the affected areas of the spine. Muscle spasm may surround the area of bony tenderness.

Laboratory evaluation of patients with acute localized bone pain may be quite extensive. Therefore, screening tests should suit the most likely causes of the patient's symptoms. Anemia or an increased ESR should raise the suspicion of an inflammatory process. Serum chemistries may detect abnormalities of calcium metabolism associated with vitamin D deficiency (osteomalacia) or elevated parathormone level (hyperparathyroidism). Elevations in alkaline phosphatase may suggest increased bone activity associated with neoplasms or Paget's disease.

Radiographic evaluation concentrates on the tender area noted with physical examination. Plain radiographs may show osteopenia if greater than 30–50% of the bone calcium has been lost (Fig. 6.29). Areas of sclerosis related to healed fractures or Paget's disease may be identified (Fig. 6.30). Microfractures cause significant pain and may not be detected with plain films. Bone scintigraphy is useful in this context for detection of increased bone activity associated with fractures. CT scans may identify the location of a fracture or an area of bone that has been replaced by inflammatory tissue.

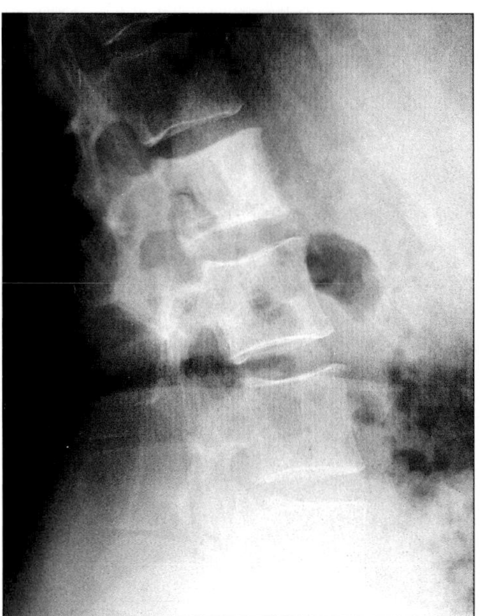

Fig. 6.30 Paget's disease. Plain radiographs demonstrating osteosclerotic alterations of bony trabeculae in L2 vertebral body. The body is slightly increased in size. This patient had elevation of serum alkaline phosphatase.

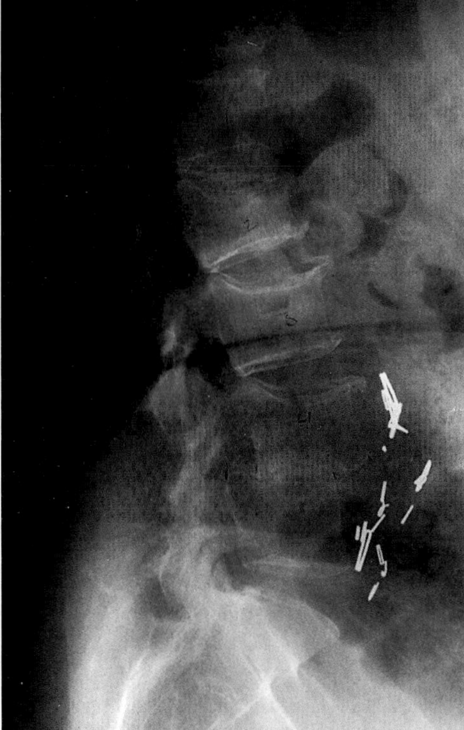

Fig. 6.29 Osteoporosis. Plain radiograph, lateral view, demonsting diffuse osteopenia and multiple compression fractures.

Therapy for patients with acute localized bone pain must be tailored to the specific disease process causing their illness.

Visceral Pain

Disorders of the vascular, genitourinary, and gastrointestinal systems can cause stimulation of sensory nerves that results in the perception of pain both in the damaged area and in superficial tissues supplied by the same segments of the spinal cord (Fig. 6.31). Visceral sensory input travels to the brain in the same pathways as somatic sensory input. Sensory stimulation may result in pain felt only in somatic locations, or may stimulate anterior horn cells to produce muscular contractions. True visceral pain is felt at the site of primary stimulation and is dull, aching, diffuse, and deep. Referred pain to the lumbosacral spine is sharp, well localized and may be associated with hyperalgesia.

The duration and sequence of visceral pain follows the periodicity of the involved organ. Colicky pain occurs in peristaltic waves and is associated with a hollow viscus, such as a ureter, uterus, gall bladder, or colon. Throbbing pain is associated with vascular structures.

Back pain is rarely the only symptom of visceral disease. Changes in genitourinary or gastrointestinal function may be clues to the potential source of the patient's low back pain. Patients with viscerogenic pain get little relief from bed rest. Many patients prefer to move in order to find a comfortable position.

Vascular lesions cause dull, steady abdominal pain that is unrelated to activity. Back pain is usually associated with epigastric

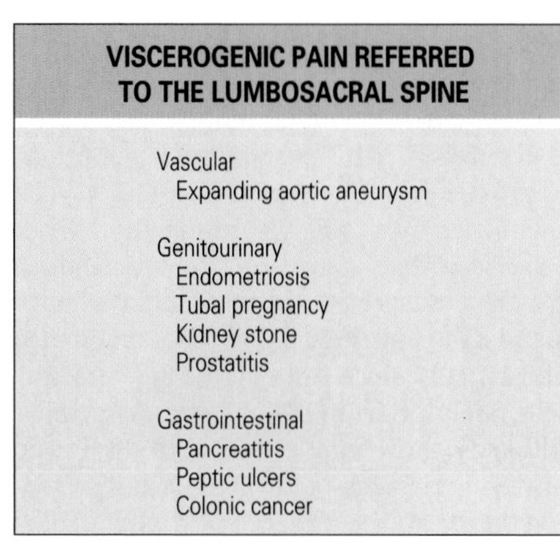

VISCEROGENIC PAIN REFERRED TO THE LUMBOSACRAL SPINE

Vascular
- Expanding aortic aneurysm

Genitourinary
- Endometriosis
- Tubal pregnancy
- Kidney stone
- Prostatitis

Gastrointestinal
- Pancreatitis
- Peptic ulcers
- Colonic cancer

Fig. 6.31 Viscerogenic disorders that cause referred pain to low back.

discomfort and may radiate to the hips or thighs if retroperitoneal structures are irritated. Rupture or acute expansion of an aneurysm is associated with tearing pain and circulatory collapse.

Back pain from genitourinary disorders may arise from the kidney, ureter, bladder, or genital organs. Kidney pain is felt in the costovertebral angle. The pain is due to acute distension of the capsule of the kidney and is constant. Ureteral pain from nephrolithiasis may cause dull flank pain with chronic distension or colic if obstruction occurs at the ureteropelvic junction. Stones in the ureter or bladder may cause pain in the testicle or vulva. Patients with bladder infections may develop diffuse low back pain centered near the sacrum. Pain from genital organs may occur locally or in a referred pattern.

Back pain that recurs on a regular basis associated with eating or with alcohol intake is suggestive of a gastrointestinal source. Pain may be related to pancreatitis, peptic ulcer disease, or colon or rectal disorders. Examination of the abdomen may be able to identify the maximum source of pain. Laboratory tests may be able to document the presence of pancreatic inflammation (elevated amylase). Endoscopic evaluation of the upper tract or colon may identify the presence of an ulcer or mass respectively.

Patients who do not have constitutional symptoms should be asked specifically about muscle pain and stiffness. Patients aged over 50 years may have proximal stiffness around the hips and shoulders. These patients may present with low back pain as well. Polymyalgia rheumatica must be considered in these older individuals. In younger individuals with more localized areas of pain, fibromyalgia may be the cause of low back pain. Tender points are found in characteristic locations throughout the musculoskeletal system. Some patients may not even be aware of the tender points until they are pressed by the examiner.

The diagnosis of these disorders is a clinical one. Polymyalgia rheumatica is associated with an elevated ESR. Fibromyalgia has a normal ESR. The therapy for these illnesses is very different. Polymyalgia is treated with low-dose corticosteroids (prednisone, 10–15 mg/day). Fibromyalgia is treated with mild aerobic exercise, and moderate doses of tricyclic antidepressants.

Some patients will remain undiagnosed. A surreptitious illness may be present but has not progressed to the point of detectability. These patients need to be watched carefully for the development of additional symptoms and signs while they continue to receive therapy for their low back pain. A repeat ESR is a cost-effective method to identify those patients who develop an inflammatory process.

If the medical evaluation remains unrevealing, the patient should be evaluated for any psychosocial difficulties. Drug habituation, depression, alcoholism, and hysteria may be associated with low back pain. These patients will benefit from therapy directed at controlling their addiction or psychiatric difficulties.

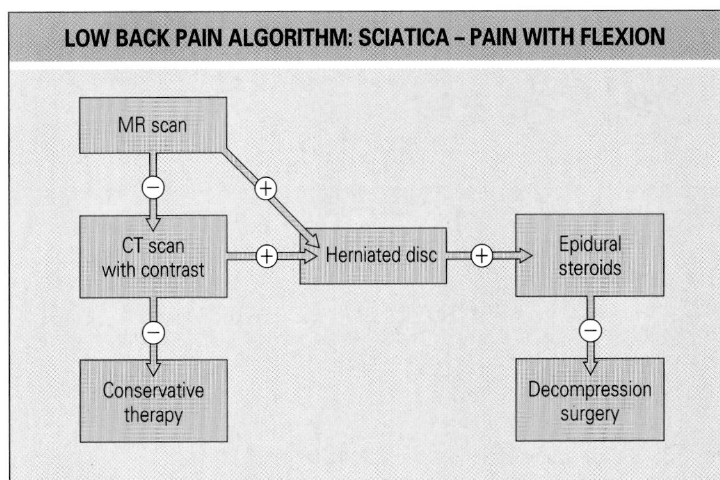

Fig. 6.32 Low back pain algorithm. Sciatica – herniated disc.

Those patients who do not show any evidence of systemic medical illness or psychiatric difficulties should be educated about their back problem individually by the physician or in a back school. Back school reviews proper and efficient use of the body in work and recreation. Patients are given methods for dealing with the stresses of chronic pain. Many individuals are able to be more functional once they realize that their pain is not related to an acute illness. These individuals concentrate on maximizing their physical function in their daily activities as opposed to concentrating on the presence of pain.

Leg Pain Below the Knee (sciatica)

Other patients who may continue to experience musculoskeletal pain despite a 4–6 week course of conservative management are those with sciatica. Further diagnostic tests are indicated to document the anatomic abnormalities associated with the patient's symptoms (Figs 6.32 & 6.33). Depending on the circumstances, the patient should undergo MRI or CT evaluation. Once the abnormality is identified (herniated disc, spinal stenosis) and medical disorders have been ruled out as possible causes of the patient's pain, additional therapy in the form of epidural steroid injections may be given [46]. An injection of long-acting corticosteroid is injected into the epidural space close to the location of nerve root compression. The procedure can be done in the outpatient setting. Although well-designed controlled studies are needed to prove the efficacy of this therapy, over 90% of patients with sciatica have described improvement in rest and walking pain over a 1-month period [47]. The maximum benefit is noted after 2 weeks. The injection may be given as a series of three over a 3 to 6 week period.

If epidural steroids are effective in alleviating the patient's leg pain, the patient should be encouraged to increase physical activity, although limiting activities that increase intradiscal pressure, such as heavy lifting or sitting for long periods of time. Patients with a disc herniation should be on restricted work for a 3-month period before resuming more typical physical activities.

If the epidural steroid therapy has not been effective and the patient is considering surgical intervention, the individual must be re-evaluated for the persistence of a neurologic deficit, and a positive tension sign. Electrodiagnostic tests may be obtained to confirm the presence of a radiculopathy and its level in the spinal cord. Some surgeons obtain a metrizamide myelogram before contemplating surgery, while others rely on the anatomic changes demonstrated by MRI (see Figs 6.34 & 6.35).

The choice of surgical procedure (laminectomy with discectomy, versus chymopapain injection, versus percutaneous discectomy) is

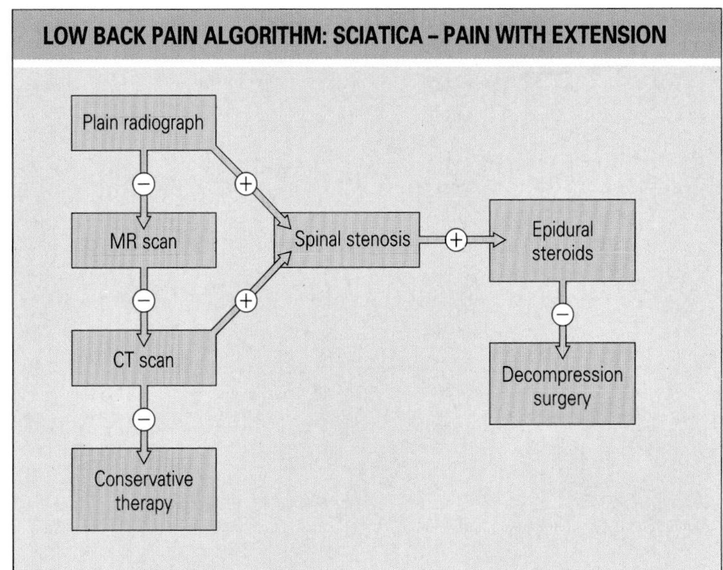

Fig. 6.33 Low back pain algorithm. Sciatica - spinal stenosis.

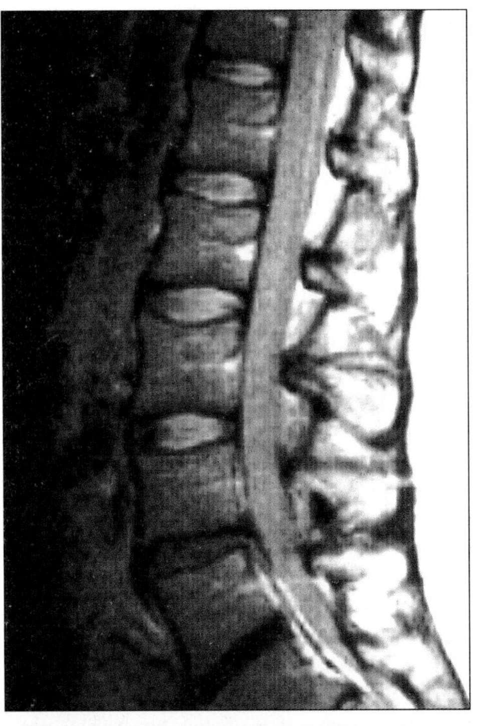

Fig. 6.34 Herniated intervertebral lumbar disc. Sagittal view of an MR scan demonstrated a herniated disc with caudal migration of the disc at the L4-L5 interspace.

beyond the scope of this chapter. Needless to say, the success of any of these surgical procedures is dependent on choosing the patient who requires surgery. Surgery for sciatica is helpful in relieving leg pain. It should not be done to improve back pain.

The second group of patients whose symptoms are based upon mechanical pressure on the neural elements are those with spinal stenosis. Spinal stenosis is narrowing of the spinal canal secondary to degenerative changes that occur in the spinal canal with time. The most commonly affected group with spinal stenosis are those who are aged over 60 years (Fig. 6.36).

Anterior Thigh Pain

A small group of individuals develop anterior thigh pain in conjunction with back pain. Such pain has a number of possible sources (Fig. 6.37). Pain in the anterior thigh is related either to hip disease, a hernia, kidney disorders, femoral neuropathy, or retroperitoneal process (anterior). Hip arthritis causes pain that is primarily in the groin. However, the peripheral nerves that supply the hip joint also innervate muscles in the low back and anterior thigh. Hip disease may present as lateral low back and anterior thigh pain. A careful physical examination, including range of motion of the hips, will identify those individuals with decreased hip motion. The patient's pain

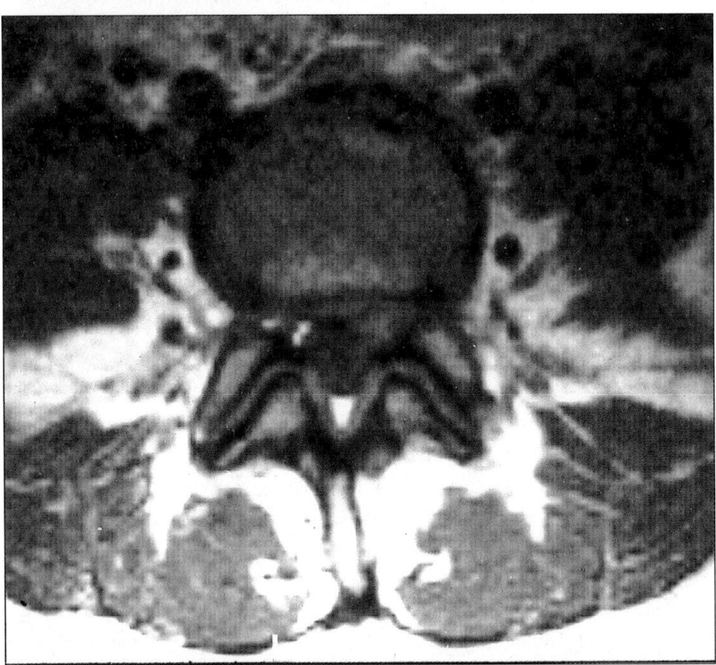

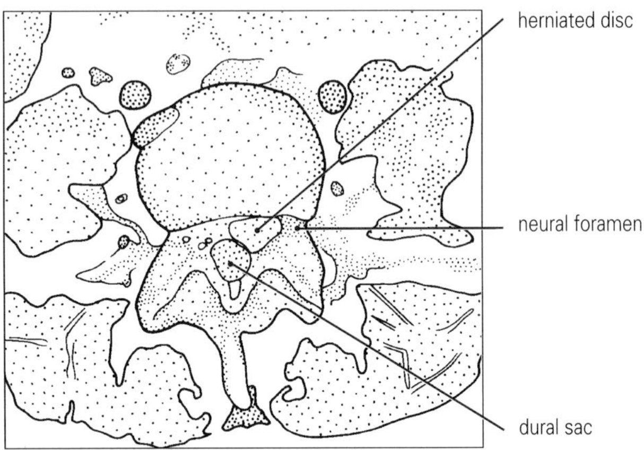

Fig. 6.35 Herniated intervertebral lumbar disc. Axial view of an MR scan demonstrates a herniated disc blocking the left neural foramen.

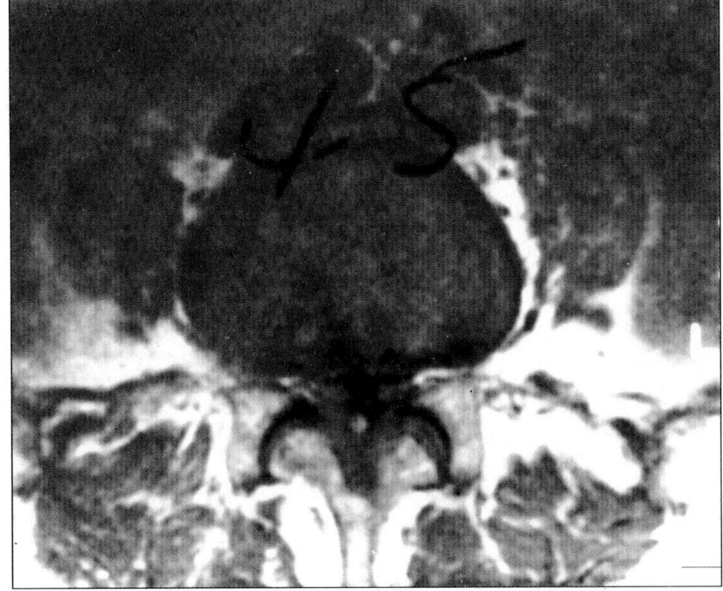

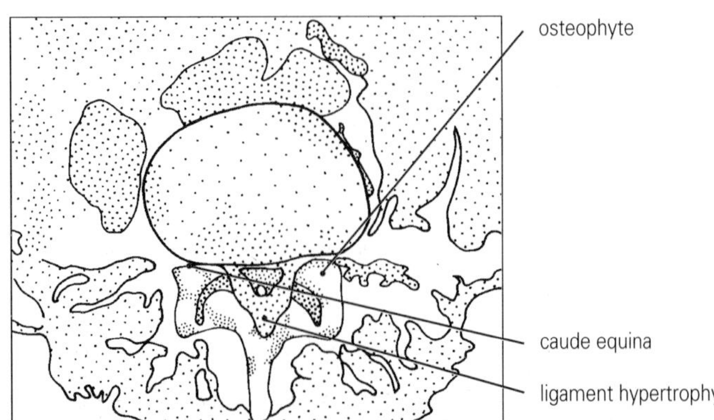

Fig. 6.36 Spinal stenosis. MR scan, axial view, of the L4–L5 disc level demonstrating osteophytic overgrowth, disc degeneration, and ligamentous hypertrophy. The cauda equina is compressed in the central area of the cord.

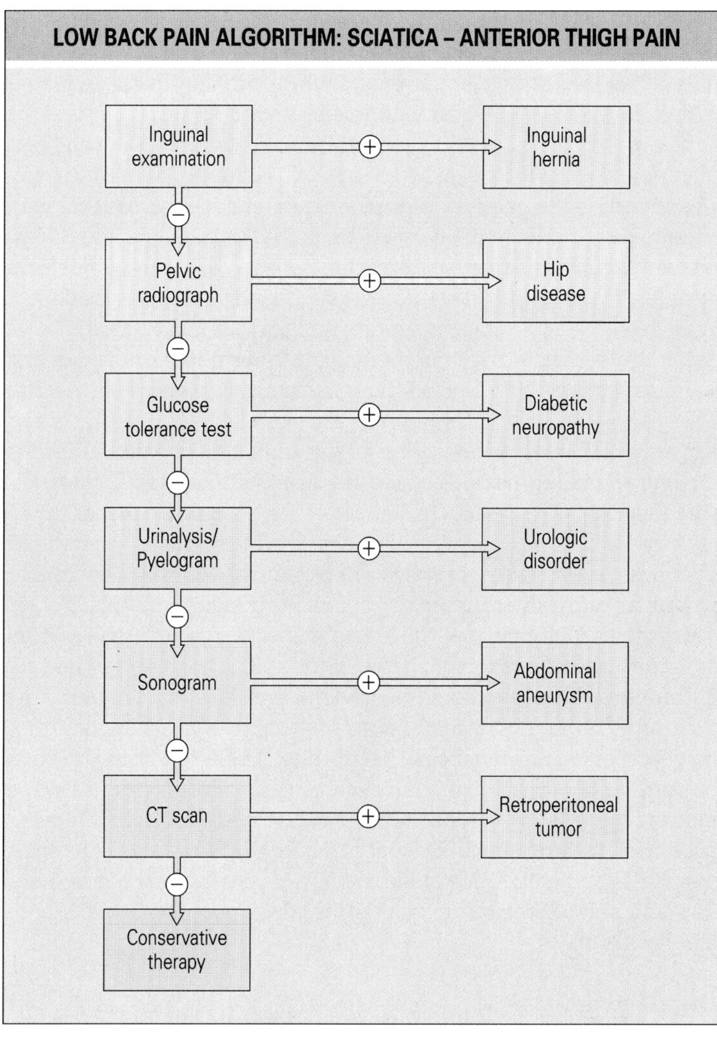

Fig. 6.37 Low back pain algorithm. Anterior thigh pain.

should be recreated by putting tension on the hip joint. Plain films of the hips should document the presence of joint disease (Fig. 6.38).

An inguinal hernia can cause anterior thigh pain. Occasionally, the pain radiates into the lateral low back. Physical examination will identify patients with direct and indirect hernias.

Patients with kidney disease may present with anterior thigh pain. Nephrolithiasis will cause pain that radiates from the back into the genitalia or anterior thigh. A simple urinalysis may identify hematuria or pyuria suggesting a renal source for the pain. An intravenous pyelogram may be obtained to evaluate more fully the urinary system.

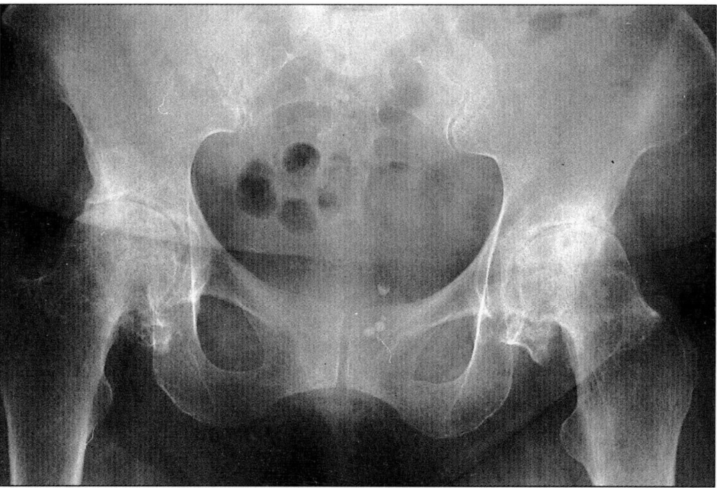

Fig. 6.38 Hip arthritis. Plain radiograph of pelvis demonstrating severe osteoarthritis of both hips. The patient had presented with back and knee pain. Hip examination revealed no motion of the joint. Back pain reduced with joint replacement.

Disorders of the femoral nerve may be associated with anterior thigh pain. The anterior femoral cutaneous nerve (L2, L3) supplies the anterior thigh. Peripheral neuropathies may affect the femoral nerve. Diabetes is the most frequent cause of peripheral neuropathy. Evaluation for diabetes is appropriate for evaluating a patient with femoral neuropathy.

Any retroperitoneal process may refer pain to the anterior thigh. Retroperitoneal structures that may cause pain include the aorta and kidneys. Tumor or infiltrative processes that involve the retroperitoneum may also cause back and anterior thigh pain. If a retroperitoneal process is suspected, CT evaluation is appropriate to determine the status of the aorta, kidney, and lymph nodes.

Posterior Thigh Pain

The fourth group of patients will complain of pain that radiates from the low back into the posterior thigh. These patients may have referred or radicular pain (Fig. 6.39). Patients with referred pain have it on the basis of injury to the bony, ligamentous, and muscular components of the lumbar spine. The muscles of the posterior thigh and buttocks have the same embryologic origin as those of the lumbar spine. An injury to these structures in the lumbar spine may be referred to the posterior thigh. These patients may respond to a local injection of corticosteroid and anesthetic into the maximum point of tenderness in the lumbar spine. Patients with referred pain do not improve with surgical intervention.

Patients with lesions compressing the L2 and L3 nerve roots may experience pain on the medial and lateral portions of the posterior thigh. These areas are supplied with cutaneous nerves that have their origin at the L2 and L3 spinal cord levels. MRI evaluation can identify causes of nerve impingement at higher levels of the spinal cord. Electrophysiologic studies can corroborate the presence of a radiculopathy. Surgical intervention should only be contemplated when the clinical and laboratory data document a radiculopathy.

MANAGEMENT

No single form of therapy is effective for all forms of back pain. Patients with medical causes for back pain must be treated with specific therapies effective for their underlying disease. Antibiotics are effective for osteomyelitis while chemotherapeutic agents are effective in slowing the growth of malignant plasma cells in multiple myeloma.

The vast majority of patients have low back pain on a mechanical basis. In most circumstances, the mechanical disorder causing the symptoms cannot be identified. Despite the inability to identify the specific source of the patient's pain, the physician is faced with

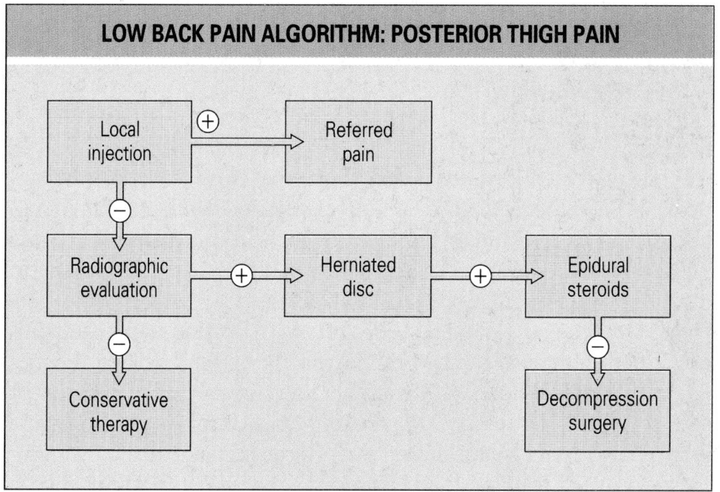

Fig. 6.39 Low back pain algorithm. Posterior thigh pain.

treating the patient to decrease their symptoms. Ideally, therapy would decrease symptoms without any toxicities. This circumstance does not exist, and even conservative therapy has its potential risks. The risks associated with NSAIDs, muscle relaxants, and injection therapy must be compared to the possibilities of infection, paralysis, and death associated with surgical intervention. It is the role of the physician to maximize medical therapy so that surgical intervention is considered in the appropriate clinical setting. Only 1-2% of patients with low back pain will undergo lumbar spine surgery [48].

Controlled Physical Activity

Components of a conservative management program for low back pain patients include patient education, 'controlled physical' activity, bed rest, exercise, and drug therapy in the form of NSAIDs and muscle relaxants. Of all the therapies, controlled physical activity is utilized most frequently. Many patients spontaneously take to bed to assume a supine position when they develop mechanical back pain. The amount of scientific data to support this form of therapy is small [49,50]. Despite the lack of data, bed rest remains a mainstay of therapy.

The biomechanical rationale for bed rest is that intradiscal pressures are lower in the supine position. However, rolling over in bed may result in increased intradiscal pressure. In addition, the number of patients with herniated discs compared to muscle strain is small. The exact mechanism that causes improvement in pain associated with muscle and ligament injury is unknown.

Bed rest is not benign if it is continued for too long a duration. Muscles become deconditioned. Cardiovascular function diminishes. Individuals lose time from work and, with continuing bed rest, start to view themselves as ill.

Busy patients rarely stay in bed unless their back pain is severe. Most patients strictly limit their recreational activities and minimize the time lost at their job. Explaining the importance of bed rest as the cornerstone of conservative therapy cannot be overemphasized.

Physical Modalities

Physical modalities may be used to diminish symptoms for short periods of time. These counter-irritant forms of therapy include ice massage, hot packs, diathermy, ultrasound, and transcutaneous electrical stimulation (TENS). These therapies may be applied by the patient themselves or by a therapist.

Patients with acute low back pain may experience analgesia with ice massage or cold packs. Cold temperatures decrease swelling, pain, and muscle spasm during the acute phase of an injury. Cold reduces metabolic activity locally, decreases muscle spindle activity, and slows nerve conduction. A cold pack may be placed in a towel and applied to the painful area of the back if the patient cannot tolerate the stroking of the skin with ice massage. Cold relieves pain and spasm longer than superficial heat. Patients who experience increased alpha motor neuron discharges with cold application will experience increased muscle spasm and cannot tolerate this form of therapy. Patients may experience at least 33% reduction in pain following ice massage [51].

Heat is another form of counter-irritant therapy that has utility in the treatment of low back pain patients. Heat should not be used in patients with back pain secondary to trauma. Heat causes vasodilatation and increased blood flow. This can cause increased damage to an area recently traumatized. However, heat increases the elastic properties of connective tissues and may be of particular utility in patients who complain of stiffness associated with their back pain. Heat also decreases gamma fiber activity, muscle spindle excitability, and resting muscle tension. Heat may be applied to superficial or deep structures. Superficial heat penetrates to the subcutaneous tissues. Hydrocollator packs, heating pads, infrared heat, and whirlpools generate superficial heat. The maximal safe exposure for these forms of therapy is 30 minutes applied directly to the skin at 45°C. Deep heat generated by diathermy or ultrasound penetrates to structures below the subcutaneous tissues. Deep heat is given in 20 minute sessions. Heat has been shown to be helpful for reducing pain in hospitalized patients with low back discomfort [52].

The practical application of temperature modalities depends on the response of the patient. Although physiologically, cold therapy should be used in patients with acute pain, and heat in patients with chronic pain, these modalities may have the opposite effect. The recommendation should be cold for acute pain and heat for chronic pain initially. If the patient does not respond, or has an exacerbation of symptoms, the opposite temperature modality should be tried.

TENS therapy is based upon the gate control theory of pain that suggests that counterstimulation of the sensory system will modify pain perception in the cerebral cortex. TENS preferentially stimulates low-threshold alpha-A fibers. The stimulation of these fibers is thought to inhibit the nociceptive impulses of the small C unmyelinated and alpha-D fibers. The effect of TENS on pain is not mediated through opiate receptors. The electrical stimulation is produced by an electrical pulse generator which delivers current that can be varied in form, intensity, and frequency to superficial electrodes. The optimal placement of the electrodes is proximal to the painful area. The average time for the onset of analgesia is approximately 20 minutes. Therapy should be given for at least 30 minutes. The pain relief from TENS may be present only during stimulation or may last for a considerable period of time. TENS has been shown to be superior to massage or equivalent to cold therapy [53]. However, a more recent, large, randomized, placebo-controlled study for low back pain patients found no benefit of TENS for chronic low back pain [54]. The role of TENS in the therapy of low back pain is in question and should not be considered usual therapy for patients with low back pain.

Drug Therapy

A variety of drugs is widely used in the therapy of patients with acute and chronic low back pain. The types of medications that have been utilized have included analgesics, NSAIDs, muscle relaxants, and antidepressants. Medications should be used for a limited period and monitored constantly. The potential toxicities of the agents must also be considered when choosing an agent for a patient.

Analgesics

Non-narcotic (acetaminophen) and narcotic (codeine, oxycodone, meperidine) analgesics have been utilized for low back pain. Patients who are intolerant of NSAIDs may benefit from acetaminophen, in doses of 500–650mg every 4 hours. Acetaminophen is less effective than aspirin as an analgesic, but does not cause gastrointestinal bleeding, a frequently encountered toxicity of aspirin. The drug has a synergistic effect with the NSAIDs and may be used in combination to increase analgesia without increasing toxicity.

Narcotic analgesia should be reserved for patients with severe pain associated with a herniated disc. Codeine in doses of 30–60mg every 4–6 hours, in combination with an NSAID or acetaminophen, is an effective analgesic. This form of therapy may be used in an outpatient setting along with controlled physical activity and temperature modalities. However, codeine does have the potential to cause constipation that may exacerbate low back pain. Patients should be told to increase fiber in their diets and consume increased amounts of liquids to decrease the potentia! for this side effect. Stronger narcotic analgesia should be reserved for hospitalized patients. The continuation of narcotic analgesics in the outpatient setting should be discouraged. Addiction and tolerance frequently result from the continued use of narcotics. In addition, the efficacy of the narcotic analgesics diminishes over time. Narcotic analgesics have no role in chronic low back pain therapy.

NSAIDs

NSAIDs have analgesic properties in low doses and anti-inflammatory properties at higher doses. Different NSAIDs have greater potentials as analgesics or as anti-inflammatory agents. Some NSAIDs combine both characteristics. The onset of action of the agents is also an important characteristic. In acute back pain, a rapid onset of action is important to control symptoms quickly. In chronic pain, the onset of action is not as important as efficacy and safety over extended periods of time.

NSAIDs have been studied in patients with acute and chronic back pain. Naproxen, piroxicam, and diflunisal have been reported to be more effective than placebo in relieving low back pain [55,56]. From a practical viewpoint, NSAIDs as a class of agents are effective in low back pain therapy. The problem that remains is that there is no specific selection criteria for the choice of a single agent for a specific patient with pain. The patient is given an NSAID with characteristics that fit the patient's symptoms and complicating medical problems (renal failure, gastric ulcer). The drug is given for a period of 2–4 weeks as a therapeutic trial, and is continued if efficacious and well tolerated. The drug is changed if the initial agent is ineffective or associated with serious toxicity. In that circumstance, an NSAID from a different chemical group is selected with the hope that it will be efficacious. The process is continued until an effective NSAID is identified.

The NSAID is continued while the patient increases physical activity and regains confidence. It is discontinued once the individual resumes their normal daily activities in work and recreation. Patients with chronic low back pain may require NSAIDs for extended periods of time. NSAIDs are not used so much to relieve pain as to support the patient's efforts to be physically active. Patients with chronic pain may not achieve a total resolution of pain, but should be encouraged to engage in as much physical activity as can be tolerated. NSAIDs help support the patient in this endeavor.

Muscle relaxants

Muscle relaxants are a group of drugs used to decrease muscle contraction present in patients with low back pain. The use of muscle relaxants in low back pain remains controversial [57]. The muscle relaxants used for low back pain patients work centrally to affect the activity of muscle stretch reflexes. Despite the skepticism concerning the pathophysiology of muscle spasm and the mechanism of action of these drugs, the muscle relaxants have been found to be effective for muscle contraction in the lumbar spine in scientific studies. Drugs including cyclobenzaprine, carisoprodol, and chlorzoxazone, have been shown to be more effective than placebo in treating patients with muscle spasm [58]. Of interest is the lack of efficacy of diazepam as a muscle relaxant for low back pain. In appropriately selected patients with acute muscle spasm, the combination of an NSAID and a muscle relaxant alone is more effective than the same NSAID alone [59]. The major toxicity of muscle relaxants is drowsiness. Also noted are headache, dizziness and dry mouth. Muscle relaxants should be used only during the time the spasm is palpable. Once the spasm has subsided, the drug should be discontinued.

Antidepressants

Tricyclic antidepressants have been used for the treatment of chronic pain for patients with or without depression. A number of mechanisms have been suggested to explain the pain relief associated with the tricyclics. One theory suggests that tricyclic antidepressants increase serotonin levels in the pain inhibitory pathway in the central nervous system. Double blind studies have documented the role of tricyclics for relieving chronic pain. Low doses in the range of 10mg to 25mg may be needed to control symptoms [60]. Rare patients may require up to 150mg per day. The drug does not work immediately and may need to be continued for a number of weeks before decreased symptoms are noted.

Injection therapy

Local or regional anesthesia given by injection is part of the therapeutic regimen for some patients with low back pain. By blocking peripheral pain input, the local area of pain can be eased as well as areas of referred pain and increased muscle tension. Patients who describe localized areas of muscle or ligamentous tenderness are candidates for local anesthetic therapy. The area injected may be an area of local trauma or a myofascial trigger point [61]. Trigger points are areas of the muscle that are painful at rest, prevent full lengthening of the muscle, weaken the muscle, refer pain in the muscle group on direct palpation and cause a local contraction when palpated. Trigger points may be found in the paraspinous muscles, the quadratus lumborum and the gluteal muscles. The point of maximum tenderness is injected with a combination of 1% xylocaine and a depository form of corticosteroid [62]. A study by Garvey suggests that needling the area with or without medication may have a beneficial effect [63]. Injections may be given on a weekly basis for 3–4 additional weeks. Controlled studies designed to evaluate the efficacy of this treatment modality have yet to be done.

Epidural corticosteroid injections are used for patients with nerve root compression that do not respond to conservative management. Corticosteroids are injected directly into the epidural space with the intention of increasing the anti-inflammtory effect in comparison to oral corticosteroids. The injections may be given on an outpatient basis. The course of therapy includes three injections given at variable intervals (days to weeks). The efficacy of these injections for the therapy of herniated discs and spinal stenosis with radiculopathy has been questioned. Epidural injections have been found to be effective in some patients [64]. Other studies have documented no improvement compared to a placebo group. Until larger studies are done, the utility of epidural corticosteroids is undetermined. In patients who have radiculopathy secondary to compression and are poor candidates for surgical intervention, epidural steroids may be considered.

Patients who have apophyseal joint disease may develop pain on a referred basis that simulates radicular pain. In this circumstance, patients have received injections of anesthetic and corticosteroid to decrease pain [65]. The injections are done under fluoroscopic control to document the appropriate placement of the needle into the facet joint. Facets both at and above the level of the involved joint must be blocked in order to obtain adequate analgesia since each facet joint receives sensory innervation from two spinal levels. Injections are given every 2–4 weeks for three sessions. The efficacy of these injections has been questioned [66]. Even in studies reporting a good response, the mean pain relief is only 30%. With the results of these studies, the use of facet joint blocks must be limited.

Exercise

Physical therapy, particularly in the form of therapeutic exercises, may be particularly helpful in controlling mechanical low back pain [67]. A number of different exercise programs are available for patients with low back pain. These include flexion exercises, extension exercises, stretching regimens, and aerobic conditioning. As a generalization, patients with mechanical disorders of the discs prefer extension exercises, while those with posterior component disease prefer flexion exercises. In most circumstances patients eventually receive a combination of both forms of exercises.

A recent study suggests that with an exercise program, patients may feel worse before they feel better [68]. In this study, 2 months were required in patients with chronic low back pain before benefit was noted. The treating physician should find a physical therapist who is interested in taking care of back patients and communicate their concerns about patients to the therapist. The therapist can then try various exercise programs and modify them according to the response of the patient. The time spent in encouraging the patient to participate in exercises and becoming physically fit is well worth the effort.

Doctor–Patient Relationship

The importance of the interaction of the physician and patient education in the therapy of low back pain patients cannot be overlooked. Educational programs such as back school where a number of individuals with back pain gather together to discuss ways of improving their situation has been shown to be an effective way of controlling patients' symptoms. Some schools are directed at groups. Some are organized for individuals with acute or chronic back pain [69]. Back school has been shown to decrease pain and time missed from work compared to placebo interventions [70].

The significance of the doctor-patient relationship has been shown by the studies that have documented the benefit of chiropractic therapy for low back pain [71]. In this study of 215 patients who visited a physician and 242 who visited a chiropractor, overall satisfaction with care was 3 times greater with the chiropractors than with the physicians. Patients had greater satisfaction with the information imparted by the chiropractors, which included graphic descriptions of the causes of pain and instructions on physical measures to improve back pain. Physicians were perceived as being less concerned about the patient's condition and pain and were less confident about the underlying cause of the patient's discomfort.

Many factors play a role in the therapy and outcome of patients with low back pain. A positive attitude about diagnosis and treatment play an important role in alleviation of pain. Physicians should not rely on machines alone to diagnose and treat patients with back pain. Communication between physican and patient that includes education about the patient's illness is an important component of back pain therapy.

REFERENCES

1. Kelsey JL, White AA III. Epidemiology and impact of low back pain. Spine. 1980;**5**:133–42.
2. Frymoyer JW, Pope MH, Costanza MC, Goggin JE, Wilder DG. Epidemiology studies of low back pain. Spine. 1980;**5**:419–23.
3. Wood PHN, MacLeish CL. Digest of data on the rheumatic diseases 5. Morbidity in industry and rheumatism in general practice. Ann Rheum Dis. 1974;**33**:93–105.
4. National Center for Health Statistics: Limitation of activity due to chronic conditions, United States 1969-1970. Vital and Health Statistics Series. 10, No. 80, 1973.
5. Dixon A StJ. Progress and problems in back pain research. Rheumatol Rehabil. 1973;**12**:165–75.
6. Federspiel CF, Guy D, Kane D, Spengler D. Expenditures for nonspecific back injuries in the workplace. J Occup Med. 1989;**31**:919–24.
7. Frymoyer JW, Cats-Baril WL. An overview of the incidences and costs of low back pain. Orthop Clin North Am.1991;**22**:263–71.
8. Rossignol M, Suissa S, Abenhaim L. Working disability due to occupational back pain: three year follow-up of 2,300 compensated workers in Quebec. J Occup Med. 1988;**30**:502-5.
9. Merskey H. The characteristics of persistent pain in psychological illness. J Psychosom Res. 1965;**9**:291–98.
10. Deyo RA, Bass JE. Lifestyle and low back pain: the influence of smoking and obesity. Spine. 1989;**14**:501–6.
11. Nachemson A. The lumbar spine: an orthopaedic challenge. Spine. 1976;**1**:59–71.
12. Hadler NM. Regional back pain. N Engl J Med. 1986;**315**:1090–2.
13. Borenstein DG, Wiesel SW. Low back pain: medical diagnosis and comprehensive management. Philadelphia: Saunders; 1989:145–450.
14. Klein RF, Brown W. Pain descriptions in medical patients. J Psychosom Res. 1967;**10**:367–72.
15. Spengler DM, Freeman CW. Patient selection for lumbar discectomy. Spine. 1979;**4**:129–34.
16. Blower PW. Neurologic patterns in unilateral sciatica. A prospective study of 100 new cases. Spine. 1981;**6**:175–9.
17. Fahrni WH. Observation on straight leg raising with special reference to nerve root adhesions. Can J Surg. 1966;**9**:44–8.
18. Gunn CC, Chir B, Milbrandt WE. Tenderness at motor points: A diagnostic and prognostic aid to low back pain injury. J Bone Joint Surg. 1976;**58A**:815–25.
19. Vallfors B. Acute, subacute, and chronic low back pain: clinical symptoms, absenteeism, and working environment. Scand J Rehabil Med. 1985;**11**(suppl):1-98.
20. Waddell G, McCullogh JA, Kummel E, Venner RM. Non-organic physical signs in low back pain. Spine. 1980;**5**:117–25.
21. McCombe PF, Fairbank JCT, Cockersole BC, Pynsent PB. Reproducibility of physical signs in low back pain. Spine. 1989;**14**:908–18.
22. Jensen OH. The level-diagnosis of a lower lumbar disc herniation: The value of sensitivity and motor testing. Clin Rheumatol. 1987;**6**:564–69.
23. Hudgins WR. Computer-aided diagnosis of lumbar disc herniation. Spine. 1983;**8**:604–15.
24. Wiesel SW, Feffer HL, Rothman RH. Industrial low back pain: a prospective evaluation of a standardized diagnostic and treatment protocol. 1984;**9**:199–203.
25. Tumeh SS, Tohmeh AG. Nuclear medicine techniques in septic arthritis and osteomyelitis. Rheum Dis Clin North Am. 1991;**17**:559–84.
26. Ross PM, Flemming JL. Vertebral body osteomyelitis: Spectrum and natural history: A retrospective analysis of 37 cases. Clin Orthop. 1976;**118**:190–8.
27. Digby JM, Kersley JB. Pyogenic non-tuberculous spinal infection: an analysis of thirty cases. J Bone Joint Surg.1979;**61B**:47–55.
28. Kido D, Bryan D, Halpern M. Hematogenous osteomyelitis in drug addicts. AJR. 1973;**118**:356–63.
29. Schofferman L, Schofferman J, Zuckerman J, et al. Occult infection causing persistent low back pain. Spine. 1989;**14**:417–9.
30. Young EJ. Human brucellosis. Rev Infect Dis. 1983;**5**:821–42.
31. Gorse GJ, Pais MJ, Kusske JA, Cesario TC. Tuberculous spondylitis: a report of six cases and a review of the literature. Medicine. 1983;**62**:178–93.
32. Pilgaard S. Discitis following removal of lumbar intervertebral disc. J Bone Joint Surg. 1969;**51A**:713–6.
33. Vyskocil JJ, McIlroy MA, Brennan TA, Wilson FM. Pyogenic infection of the sacroiliac joint: Case reports and review of the literature. Medicine. 1991;**70**:188–97.
34. Cohen MD, Hanington DM, Ginsburg WW. Osteoid osteoma: 95 cases and a review of the literature. Semin Arthritis Rheum. 1983;**12**:265–81.
35. Winter PF, Johnson PM, Hilal SK, Feldman F. Scintigraphic detection of osteoid osteoma. Radiology. 1977;**122**:177–8.
36. Wedge HJ, Tchang S, MacFadyen DJ. Computed tomography in localization of spinal osteoid osteomas. Spine. 1981;**6**:423–7.
37. Dahlin DC, Unni KK. Bone Tumors: General Aspects and Data on 8,542 Cases. 4th ed. Springfield: Charles Thomas; 1986:193–207.
38. Bayrd ED, Heck FJ. Multiple myeloma: a review of 83 proved cases. JAMA. 1947;**133**:147–57.
39. Valderrama JAF, Bullough PG. Solitary myeloma of the spine. J Bone Joint Surg. 1968;**50B**:82–90.
40. Jacobson HG, Poppel MH, Shapiro JH, Grossberger S. The vertebral pedicle sign: a roentgenographic finding to differentiate metastatic carcinoma from multiple myeloma. AJR. 1958;**80**:817–21.
41. Fornasier VL, Horne JG. Metastases to the vertebral column. Cancer. 1975;**36**:590–4.
42. Edelstyn GA, Gillespie PG, Grebbel FS. The radiological demonstration of skeletal metastases: Experimental observations. Clin Radiol. 1967;**18**:158–62.
43. Zimmer WD, Berquist TH, McLeod RA, et al. Magnetic resonance imaging versus computed tomography. Radiology. 1985;**155**:709–18.
44. Sze G, Stimac GK, Bartlett C, et al. Multicenter study of gadopentetate dimeglumine as an MR contrast agent: evaluation in patients with spinal tumors. AJNR. 1990;**11**:967–74.
45. Kozin F, Camera GF, Ryan LM, Foley D, Lawson T. Computed tomography in diagnosis of sacroiliitis. Arthritis Rheum. 1981;**24**:1479–85.
46. White AH, Derley R, Wynne G. Epidural injection for the diagnosis and treatment of low back pain. Spine. 1980;**5**:78–86.

47. Ridley MG, Kingsley GH, Gibson T, Grahame R. Outpatient lumbar epidural corticosteroid injection in the management of sciatica. Br J Rheumatol. 1988;**27**:295–99.
48. Deyo RA, Tsui-Wu YJ. Descriptive epidemiology of low back pain and its related medical care in the United States. Spine. 1987;**12**:264–8.
49. Deyo RA, Diehl AK, Rosenthal M. How many days of bed rest for acute low back pain? A randomized clinical trial. N Engl J Med. 1986;**315**:1064–70.
50. Gilbert JR, Taylor DW, Hildebrand A, Evans C. Clinical trial of common treatment for low back pain in family practice. Br Med J. 1985;**291**:791–4.
51. Melzack R, Jeans ME, Stratford JG, Monks RC. Ice massage and transcutaneous electrical stimulation: Comparison of treatment of low back pain. Pain. 1980;**9**:209–17.
52. Landon BR. Heat or cold for the relief of low back pain? Phys Ther. 1967;**47**:126–30.
53. Melzack R, Vetere P, Finch L. Transcutaneous electrical nerve stimulation for low back pain. A comparison of TENS and massage for pain and range of motion. Phys Ther. 1983;**63**:489–93.
54. Deyo RA, Walsh N, Martin D, Schoenfeld L, Ramamurthy S. A controlled trial of transcutaneous electrical nerve stimulation (TENS) and exercise for chronic low back pain. N Engl J Med. 1990;**322**:1627–34.
55. Berry H, Bloom B, Hamilton EBD, Swinson DR. Naproxen sodium, diflunisal, and placebo in the treatment of chronic back pain. Ann Rheum Dis. 1982;**41**:129–32.
56. Videman T, Osterman K. Double-blind parallel study of piroxicam versus indomethacin in the treatment of low back pain. Ann Clin Res. 1984;**16**:156–60.
57. Johnson EW. The myth of skeletal muscle spasm. Am J Phys Med Rehabil. 1989;**68**:1.
58. Elenbaas JK. Centrally acting oral skeletal muscle relaxants. Am J Hosp Pharm. 1980;**37**:1313–22.
59. Borenstein DG, Lacks S, Wiesel SW. Cyclobenzaprine and naproxen versus naproxen alone in the treatment of acute low back pain. Clin Therapeutics. 1990;**12**:125–131.
60. Hameroff SR, Crago BR, Cork RC, Schein K, Leeman E. Doxepin effects on chronic pain, depression and serum opiods. Anesth Analg. 1982;**61**:187.
61. Travell JG, Simons DG. Myofascial pain and dysfunction: the trigger point manual. Baltimore: Williams & Wilkins; 1983.
62. Swezey RL, Clements PJ. Conservative treatment of back pain. In: Jayson MIV, ed. The lumbar spine and back pain. 3rd ed. Edinburgh: Churchill Livingstone; 1987:299–314.
63. Garvey TA, Marks MR, Wiesel SW. A prospective, randomized, double-blind evaluation of trigger point injection. Spine. 1989;**14**:962–4.
64. Dilke TFW, Burry HC, Grahame R. Extradural corticosteroid injection managment of lumbar nerve root compression. Br Med J. 1973; **2**:635–7.
65. Jackson RP, Jacobs RR, Montesano PX. Facet joint injection in-low back pain: a prospective statistical study. Spine. 1988;**13**:966–71.
66. Carette S, Marcoux S, Truchon R, et al. A controlled trial of corticosteroid injections into facet joints for chronic low back pain. N Eng J Med. 1991;**325**:1002–7.
67. Jackson CP, Brown MD. Is there a role for exercise in the treatment of patients with low back pain? Clin Orthop. 1983;**179**:39–45.
68. Manniche C, Hesselsoe G, Bentzen L, Christensen I, Lundberg E. Clinical trial of intense muscle training for chronic low back pain. Lancet. 1988;**ii**:1473–6.
69. White AH Back school and other conservative approaches to low back pain. St Louis: Mosby; 1983.
70. Mooney V. Alternative approaches for the patient beyond the help of surgery. Orthop Clin North Am. 1975;**6**:331–4.
71. Cherkin DC, MacCornack FA. Patient evaluations of low back pain care from family physicians and chiropractors. West J Med. 1989;**150**:351–5.

7

THE SHOULDER

Seamus E Dalton

FUNCTIONAL ANATOMY

Introduction

The clavicle, scapula and humerus make up the bony skeleton of the shoulder girdle, the relationship of which with the axial skeleton is maintained largely through muscular attachments and also the articulation of the clavicle with the thoracic cage at the sternoclavicular joint. Shoulder movement occurs through many planes and is achieved through motion at four articulations: the glenohumeral, acromioclavicular, sternoclavicular and scapulothoracic. Some constraint is also afforded to the head of the humerus through the subacromial joint by the overlying acromion and coracoacromial ligament. The glenohumeral joint is a multiaxial joint that allows the greatest freedom of movement of any joint of the body, although this is at the expense of stability. The bones of the shoulder girdle combine to provide a mobile framework upon which glenohumeral motion can take place.

Ligamentous support is important in maintaining the stability of the joints of the shoulder and allowing synchronous movements to take place. Muscles act as prime movers at the shoulder as well as providing some dynamic stability to the glenohumeral joint.

THE GLENOID FOSSA: ITS ATTACHMENTS AND RELATIONSHIP TO SCAPULAR STRUCTURES

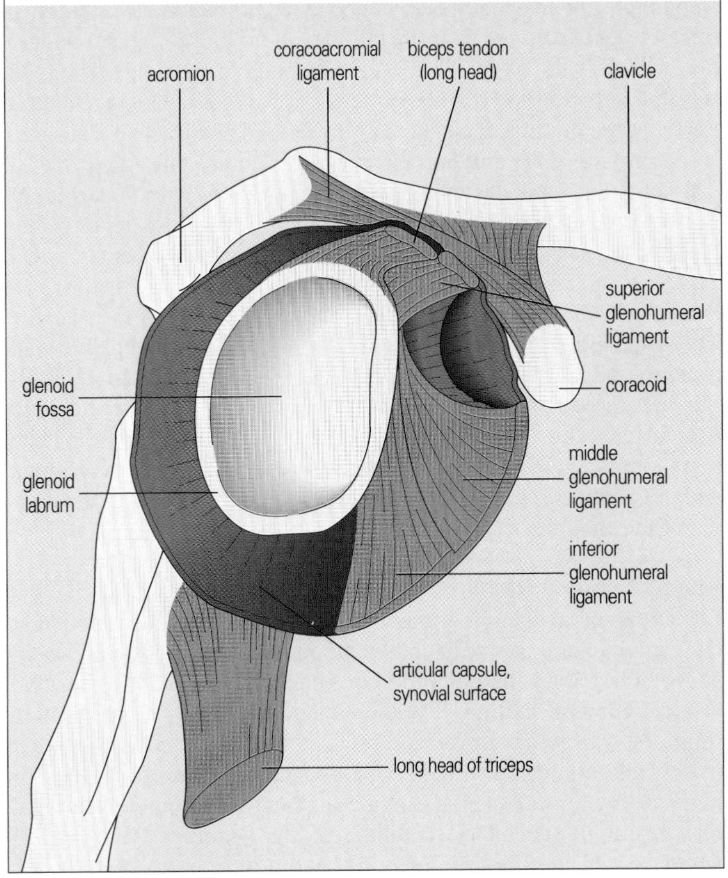

Fig. 7.1 The glenoid fossa. Its attachments and relationship to scapular structures.

Glenohumeral Joint

This is not a true ball and socket joint and allows a certain amount of gliding movement, which is increased when there is laxity of the musculoligamentous support to the joint. Inherent bony stability is poor due to the shallow glenoid fossa and larger humeral head. The glenoid labrum is a rim of fibrocartilage at the periphery of the glenoid which effectively deepens the glenoid fossa and increases its diameter and contact with the humeral head, thereby affording some increased stability (Fig. 7.1). The joint capsule is lax, especially inferiorly, which allows rotation and elevation. In conditions where this capsule contracts there is restriction of glenohumeral motion. Restriction in this capsule posteriorly can aggravate or even give rise to secondary impingement.

The joint capsule is thickened anteriorly to form separate components known as the glenohumeral ligaments, which act to strengthen the anterior and inferior capsule. The superior glenohumeral ligament runs from the anterosuperior aspect of the glenoid to the proximal edge of the lesser tuberosity of the humerus, with the middle glenohumeral ligament running just below this.

The inferior glenohumeral ligament runs from the anteromedial aspect of the glenoid to the distal edge of the lesser tuberosity and proximal shaft of the humerus and has three components [1]. It is important in the provision of anteroinferior stability to the joint, particularly with the arm in abduction and external rotation, and has also been shown to provide some posterior stability [2]. Deficiencies in this ligament complex are important in the etiology of instability. The coracohumeral ligament runs from the coracoid process to the greater tuberosity and capsule and has a minor role to play in stabilizing the humeral head. The coracoacromial ligament extends from the undersurface of the medial acromion to the superolateral border of the coracoid process. Therefore, along with the acromion, it acts as a roof over the subacromial space under which the rotator cuff tendons slide, with the subacromial bursa lying between. This structure has been implicated in the pathology of impingement of the shoulder [3]. The transverse humeral ligament runs between the greater and lesser tuberosities, covering the long head of the biceps tendon (see Fig. 7.2).

The stabilizers of the shoulder can be divided into two groups; static and dynamic. The capsule, labrum, glenohumeral and, to a lesser extent, coracohumeral ligaments can be thought of as static stabilizers of the glenohumeral joint. There are two sleeves of muscles about the shoulder; superficial and deep. The deep group comprises the rotator cuff muscles (supraspinatus, subscapularis, infraspinatus and teres minor) and the tendon of the long head of biceps. This layer acts dynamically to stabilize the humeral head in the glenoid fossa during shoulder movement, while simultaneously providing rotation (through subscapularis, teres minor and infraspinatus) and abduction (through supraspinatus). During the initiation of shoulder abduction or elevation, the larger more powerful deltoid muscle, if unopposed, would pull the humeral head superiorly towards the acromion. The rotator cuff muscles and the biceps tendon act as humeral head depressors to prevent this translational movement superiorly. This is known as the 'force-couple'. The subscapularis also acts to resist the tendency of the humeral head to sublux anteriorly in the upper ranges of abduction. Dysfunction of the rotator cuff muscles, either through weakness or a tear, results in

LIGAMENTOUS AND MUSCULOTENDINOUS ATTACHMENTS ABOUT THE SHOULDER JOINT

acromioclavicular ligament
coracoid
coracoclavicular ligament (trapezoid and conoid)
coracoacromial ligament
biceps tendon (intra-articular)
rotator cuff
greater tuberosity
transverse humeral ligament
lesser tuberosity
long head of biceps tendon
short head of biceps
pectoralis minor

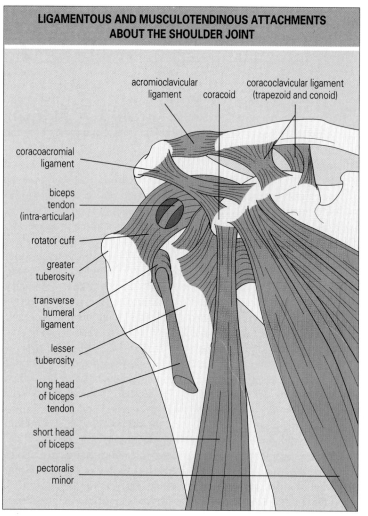

Fig. 7.2 Ligamentous and musculotendinous attachments about the shoulder joint.

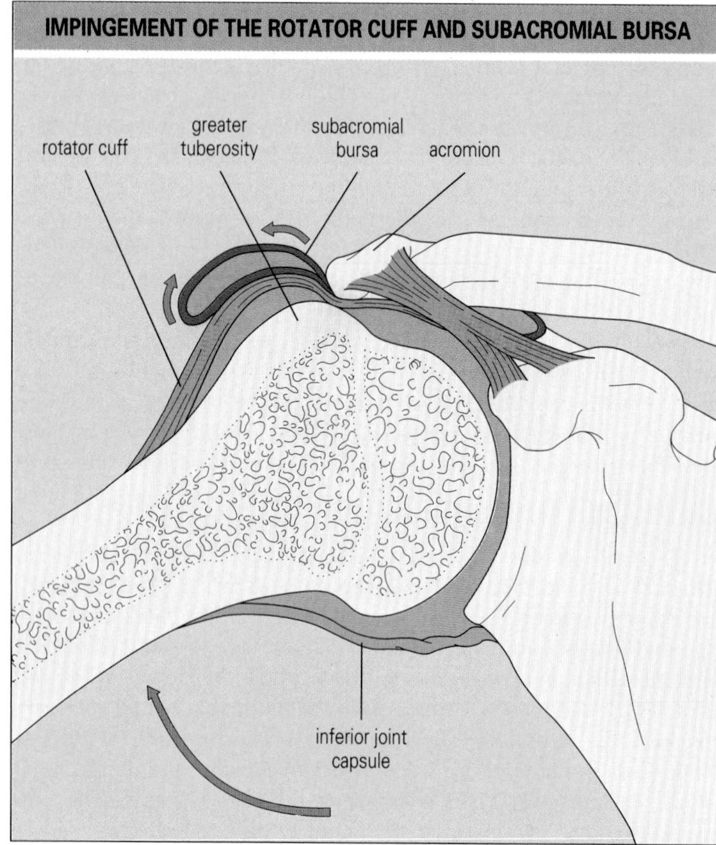

Fig. 7.3 Mechanism of impingement of the rotator cuff and subacromial bursa between the humeral head and overlying coracoacromial arch.

diminished stabilization of the humeral head. This leads to weakness of the arm in elevation as well as superior migration of the humeral head, increasing the likelihood of subacromial compression or impingement (Fig. 7.3). Therefore, the four tendons of the rotator cuff grip the humeral head and act as guy-ropes to stabilize it during shoulder movement, resisting this sliding tendency within the joint. The biceps tendon inserts into and reinforces the superior labrum and also acts as a humeral head depressor in full abduction.

The outer sleeve of muscles comprises the deltoid, teres major, pectoralis major, latissimus dorsi, and trapezius muscles. They act as prime movers of the humerus, although the trapezius acts through movement of the scapula and clavicle. The combination of these large muscles (which provide abduction, flexion, extension, adduction and a degree of rotation) with the deep layer of rotator cuff muscles (which provide more rotation of the humeral head) allows the expansive movement of the arm in actions such as reaching behind one's back or behind the head.

The deltoid muscle has three bellies: anterior, middle and posterior, producing respectively flexion, abduction and extension of the shoulder. All three muscles converge to an insertion on the deltoid tubercle on the lateral aspect of the humeral shaft. The rotator cuff muscles originate from the scapula and attach to the greater (supraspinatus, infraspinatus and teres minor) and lesser (subscapularis) tuberosities of the humerus.

Nerve supply to the glenohumeral joint is provided by those peripheral nerves supplying muscles acting upon the joint, namely the axillary, suprascapular, subscapular and musculocutaneous nerves. Innervation is via the fifth, sixth and seventh cervical roots, and the brachial plexus passes anterior and inferior to the glenohumeral joint.

Acromioclavicular Joint

A fibrous disc separates the non-congruous surfaces of the distal end of the clavicle and the acromion and allows movement at this joint. During abduction and elevation the clavicle rotates through 30–40° and this largely occurs at the sternoclavicular joint [4]. There is a small amount of movement at the acromioclavicular joint and compressive force is applied to the joint in full elevation and horizontal adduction, which is the basis of stress tests applied to this joint. The joint is stabilized posteriorly by the posterior transverse ligament and inferiorly by the inferior ligament, and the deltoid and trapezius muscles act to provide some anterior and superior stability through their fascial layer. Of particular importance are the conoid and trapezoid, or coracoclavicular, ligaments which maintain the close relationship between the scapula and clavicle during shoulder movement.

Scapulothoracic Joint

The scapula lies against the posterolateral aspect of the thoracic wall rotating and sliding laterally in abduction, elevation and flexion. It provides the origin for the rotator cuff muscles as well as the deltoid muscle and the trapezius inserts along its superior aspect. The scapulothoracic joint represents that articulation between the scapula and thoracic cage, and motion here is important for normal functioning of the shoulder.

Scapulohumeral Rhythm

Elevation and abduction of the arm involves synchronous motion at the glenohumeral and scapulothoracic joints. As elevation increases above 90° so does the proportion of scapulothoracic motion relative to glenohumeral motion. Scapulohumeral rhythm is representative of the ratio between movement at these two joints and is important in several shoulder disorders. Disturbance of the normal scapulohumeral rhythm affects the biomechanics of the shoulder joint and may result in secondary tendinitis of the shoulder. This is well demonstrated in elite swimmers, in whom muscle imbalances can give rise to tendinitis or impingement in this manner.

Several muscles (levator scapulae, serratus anterior, trapezius, rhomboids) act to stabilize and control movement of the scapula, and the balance between scapula elevators, rotators, depressors, retractors and protractors provides scapular control and determines scapulothoracic movement. Scapular control by these muscles is becoming better understood as an important factor in glenohumeral instability and rotator cuff dysfunction.

Sternoclavicular Joint

Like the acromioclavicular joint the sternoclavicular joint contains an intra-articular fibrous disc which allows rotation of the clavicle during abduction and elevation. Strong ligaments stabilize this joint anteriorly and posteriorly.

Bursae

Significant variation exists in regard to the number and extent of bursae around the shoulder. The subacromial bursa lies between the rotator cuff (mainly supraspinatus tendon) and overlying acromion. This bursa does not consist of a distinct sac and its synovial layers blend in with and are firmly attached to the acromion and rotator cuff. In subacromial impingement and rotator cuff tendinitis there is reactive inflammation of this bursa. The subscapularis bursa communicates with the synovial joint cavity between the superior and middle glenohumeral ligaments, and the synovial membrane of the joint invests the tendon of the long head of biceps. Other bursae include the subdeltoid, coracoid, infraserratus, and bursae at the insertion of the tendon of trapezius and the tendon insertions on the humerus.

PHYSICAL EXAMINATION

History

Shoulder pain may be seen in association with several medical conditions and may be referred from cervical, thoracic, or abdominal sources. Any history of diabetes, Raynaud's, cervical spondylitis, cerebrovascular or cardiac disease needs to be established. The mechanism of any injury will assist in making a diagnosis. A fall onto an outstretched arm can give rise to instability in the younger patient or a rotator cuff tear in the elderly. A fall onto the point of the shoulder may result in injury to the rotator cuff or acromioclavicular joint. Throwing injuries tend to stress the capsule and ligaments of the glenohumeral joint and can also give rise to rotator cuff or bicipital tendinitis. A good pain history is essential, since the location and type of pain varies between conditions. Pain referred from the cervical spine is often maximal over the suprascapular region with associated paresthesia or pain referred into the upper limb. Acromioclavicular and sternoclavicular pain is usually well localized to the involved joint. Pain from rotator cuff pathology is usually felt at the outer aspect of the upper arm or deltoid region. Adhesive capsulitis tends to give rise to an intense aching deep in the shoulder although features similar to rotator cuff pathology are common in the early stages. Radiating pain into the arm may indicate cervical pathology, thoracic outlet syndrome, compressive neuropathy, brachial neuritis, or reflex sympathetic dystrophy. Night pain tends to be of two main types: either sharp pain associated with movement of the individual, indicative of a rotator cuff tendinitis or acromioclavicular pathology; or pain of a deep, constant aching nature more suggestive of capsulitis or a chronic tear of the rotator cuff.

Inspection

This should be carried out from anterior, posterior and lateral aspects and the patient's ability to undress may indicate functional limitations. Areas of erythema and bruising should be noted. Although uncommon, swelling of the shoulder joint will be seen anteriorly in the projection of the subscapularis bursa. Deformity of the shoulder girdle exists with acromioclavicular joint separation or fractures of the clavicle or humerus. It is important to look for positioning of the shoulder such as asymmetrical elevation or overprotraction. Neck positioning should also be recorded. Rupture of the long head of biceps tendon is readily seen. Muscle wasting may be present in cases of cervical or brachial neuropathy but is also seen with chronic rotator cuff pathology in the supraspinatus and infraspinatus muscle bellies. Scapulohumeral and scapulothoracic rhythm during elevation should be assessed and any asymmetry noted. Winging of the scapula can be demonstrated by asking the patient to do a push-up against the wall. It is indicative of serratus anterior weakness (as in long thoracic nerve palsy) but can also occur with muscular dysfunction.

Palpation

This should assess the presence of tenderness, swelling and instability of the acromioclavicular, sternoclavicular and glenohumeral joints. Tenderness over the tendon of the long head of biceps and the bicipital groove is common in bicipital tendinitis but comparison with the normal shoulder is necessary as this tendon is normally sensitive to touch. There may be tenderness over the rotator cuff insertions to the greater and lesser tuberosities but this is not always present in rotator cuff tendinitis. Acute calcific tendinitis is exquisitely tender over the involved tendon. The lateral margin of the subacromial joint can be palpated for swelling and tenderness and the glenohumeral joint itself may be tender in chronic or acute instability or capsulitis. An effusion of the glenohumeral joint should be differentiated from subacromial swelling, although communication between the two may exist in degenerative conditions where there is a full-thickness tear of the rotator cuff. Osteophytes can also be palpated at the margins of these joints, as can any crepitus present. Instability of the acromioclavicular and sternoclavicular joints is readily demonstrable but glenohumeral instability requires a more detailed examination combining assessment of laxity in anterior, posterior and inferior directions with stress and apprehension tests to determine the presence of symptomatic instability. This assessment needs to be carried out in the young adult presenting with shoulder pain since underlying instability is a frequent cause of tendinitis around the shoulder. Muscles of the shoulder girdle and neck region should be palpated for trigger points and tender points, typically present with myofascial syndromes and fibromyalgia respectively.

Mobilization

Active and passive ranges of motion of both shoulders should be assessed in the planes of abduction, forward flexion, and external rotation both with the arm by the side and at 90° abduction. Internal rotation is frequently assessed as a combined maneuver with extension in bringing the arm up behind the back. This is limited in many periarticular conditions and a better assessment of true glenohumeral joint restriction is done by measuring true internal rotation with the arm by the side and the elbow extended, using the epicondyles as markers for comparison with the other shoulder. Any limitation of movement should be noted as well as any discrepancy between active and passive motion. Glenohumeral joint pathology is unlikely in the presence of a normal range of passive motion.

Further assessment should include passive adduction of the flexed and internally rotated shoulder to look for tightness of the posterior structures, namely the posterior capsule and external rotator cuff muscles, as this is often seen in chronic cuff pathology. Resisted shoulder movements are performed to assess involvement of muscles and tendons. The patient is asked to resist a specific movement in order to elicit an isolated, isometric contraction in the particular muscle group. The supraspinatus is tested with the arm abducted to 90°, flexed to 30° and internally rotated (i.e. thumb downwards). The examiner then resists abduction from this position. Resisted internal rotation tests subscapularis and resisted external rotation tests infraspinatus and teres minor. Resisted abduction should also

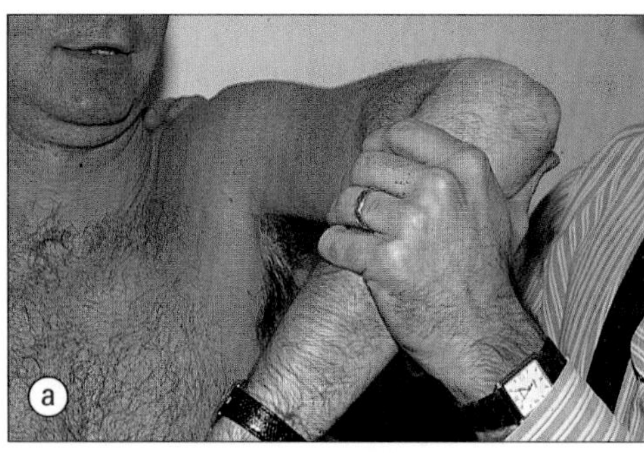

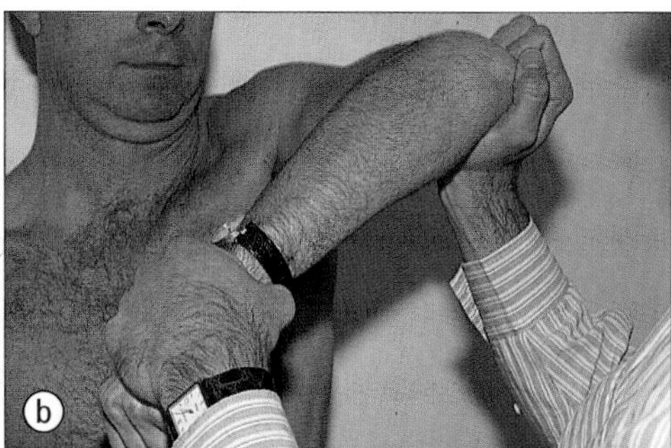

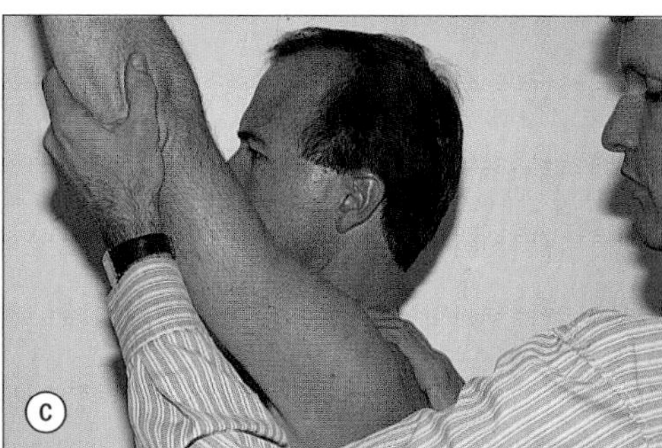

Fig. 7.4 Impingement tests: forced passive internal rotation (a); resisted external rotation (b); forced passive full forward flexion (c).

be carried out with the arm by the side. Biceps function can also be tested by resisting shoulder flexion with the elbow extended (Speed's test) or resisting supination with the elbow flexed to 90° (Yergason's test). Any assessment must include an examination of the cervical spine to assess range of motion and the presence of any referred upper limb pain (see Chapter 5).

Special Movements

Specific examination techniques can be employed to further localize the source of pain in the shoulder region. Various tests for impingement have been described. In one of these the arm is flexed to 90°, adducted and then forcefully internally rotated and slightly elevated by the examiner, with the scapula stabilized by the examiner's other hand (Fig. 7.4a). In another variation the arm is placed in the adducted, flexed, internally rotated position and the patient is asked to externally rotate the arm against resistance (Fig. 7.4b). A further impingement test is carried out by passively forcing the arm into full forward flexion while the examiner stabilizes the top of the scapula with the other hand (Fig. 7.4c). In all situations a positive test is recorded if pain is felt as the subacromial bursa and the rotator cuff is forced against the undersurface of the acromion.

Apart from Speed's and Yergason's tests a further bicipital provocation test can be performed by asking the patient to abduct the arm to 90° with the palm upwards. The arm is then slowly adducted (with the elbow extended) across the midline and the chest against resistance [5]. In cases of bicipital tendon involvement a catching pain is felt in the region of the bicipital groove as the arm crosses in front of the shoulder joint (Fig. 7.5).

Pain at the acromioclavicular joint can be localized by performing various stress tests. In one the arm is held with the elbow and shoulder extended and then passively adducted across behind the back (Fig. 7.6). In another less specific maneuver the arm is abducted to 90° and then adducted across the patient's chest under the chin. In both tests pain is felt over an inflamed acromioclavicular joint at the limits of these movements. Assessment for a thoracic outlet syndrome is always difficult and several maneuvers are described which may provoke the symptoms of neurovascular compression.

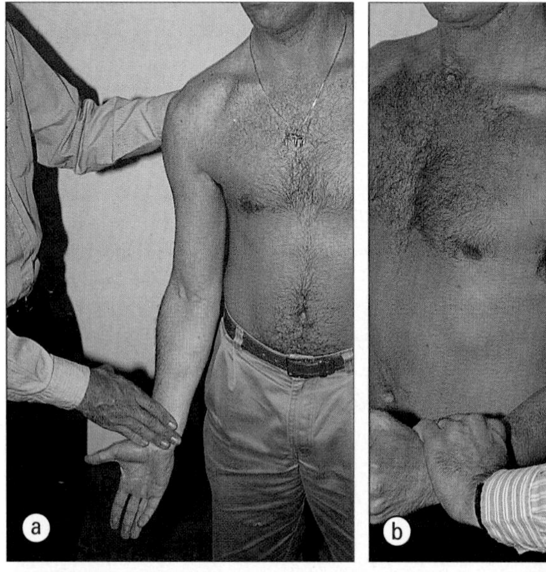

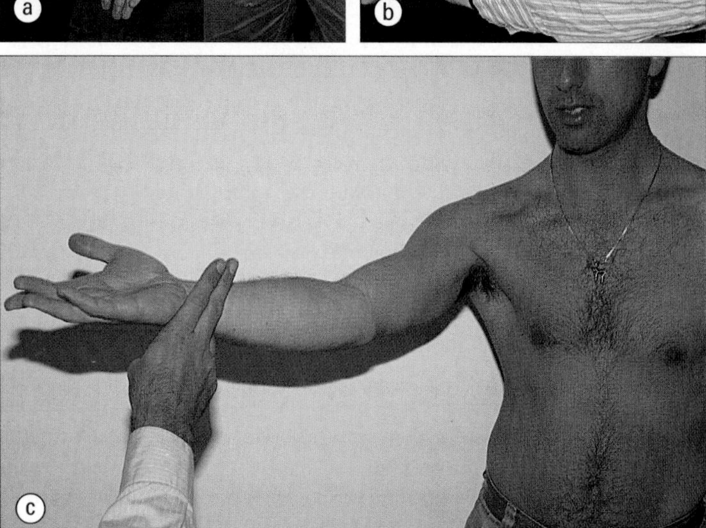

Fig. 7.5 Clinical tests for bicipital tendinitis: Speed's test (a); Yergason's test (b); bicipital provocation test (c).

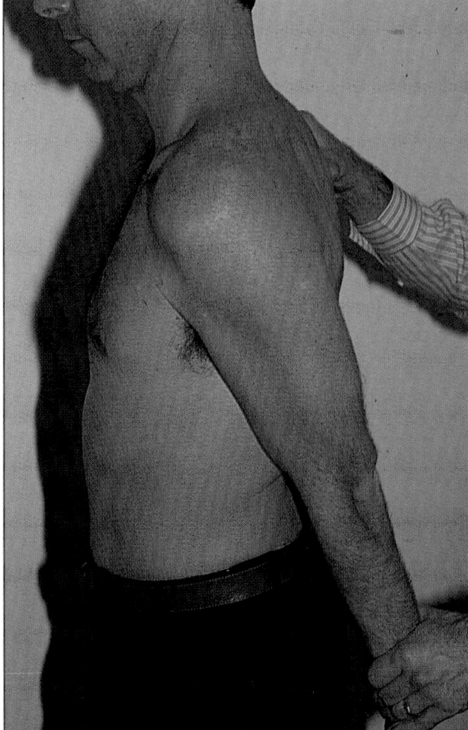

Fig. 7.6 An adduction stress test of the acromioclavicular joint.

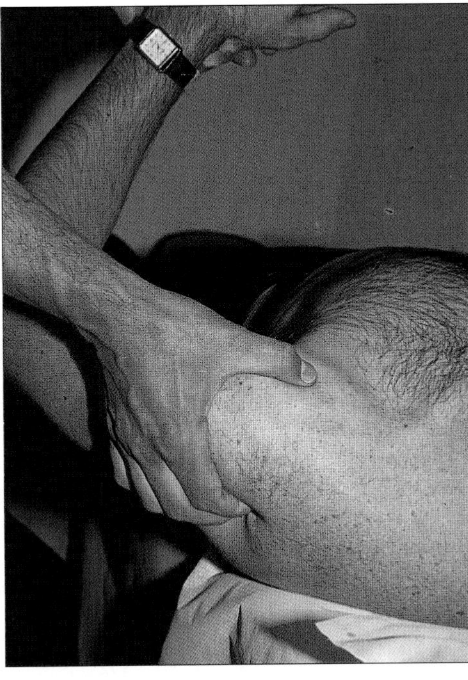

Fig. 7.7 The anterior drawer test.

The patient should be assessed for the presence of joint hypermobility. Laxity of the glenohumeral joint in anterior and posterior directions is determined by carrying out drawer tests in which the humeral head is gripped firmly and translated backwards and forwards in the glenoid fossa. This is best carried out with the patient lying supine and the abducted arm supported by the examiner's hand (Fig. 7.7). Inferior laxity is assessed by applying distal retraction to the arm while palpating the gap between the humeral head and acromion. Presence of a distinct gap can be felt and even seen, and is referred to as a positive sulcus sign. If present this is indicative of multidirectional laxity of the joint. Anterior apprehension and stress tests are carried out with the examiner slowly extending and externally rotating the abducted arm with the patient supine. A positive test occurs when the patient experiences pain or apprehension during this maneuver and is confirmed when these symptoms disappear as the examiner's free hand applies a downward, i.e. stabilizing, force to the anterior aspect of the upper humerus. This often allows further external rotation of the arm (Fig. 7.8). Symptoms return as this stabilizing force is slowly withdrawn. The posterior stress test is carried out by applying gentle axial pressure to the humerus with the arm in the forward flexed, internally rotated and slightly adducted position, again in an attempt to reproduce pain and apprehension.

DIFFERENTIAL DIAGNOSIS OF SHOULDER PAIN

The glenohumeral joint may be affected as part of widespread joint disease, i.e., a polyarthropathy such as rheumatoid arthritis, crystal arthropathy, other inflammatory arthropathies or generalized osteoarthritis. Septic arthritis, neuropathic (Charcot's) arthritis, osteonecrosis and idiopathic destructive arthritis are all conditions which can affect the shoulder joint in isolation. In articular disorders of the shoulder there may be swelling or synovitis, and invariably there is an effect on passive and active motion of the glenohumeral joint with pain, restriction of motion and often crepitus.

Periarticular conditions affecting the shoulder can be loosely grouped into those with and those without capsulitis. If there is no capsular involvement then passive joint motion is largely unaffected, whereas active movement may be limited by pain and/or weakness (e.g., rotator cuff disorders). With capsulitis there is multidirectional restriction of passive motion, and differentiation from articular conditions of the shoulder is made on clinical and radiological grounds.

Referred pain to the shoulder can occur with cervical disorders, Pancoast tumor of the lung, subphrenic pathology, entrapment neuropathies and brachial neuritis. In these conditions passive and often active movement of the shoulder are largely unaffected and there is usually little or no pain when testing rotator cuff function. Again, differentiation from disorders of the shoulder is possible with an adequate history and examination (see Fig. 7.9).

ROTATOR CUFF DISORDERS

The spectrum of disorders affecting the rotator cuff ranges from the mild transient tendinitis following an episode of glenohumeral instability in the young patient, to the complete tear in the degenerative rotator cuff of the older patient. The anatomical configuration of the shoulder joint is such that the cuff is subjected to stresses when the arm is in the elevated position. Impingement can occur as the supraspinatus tendon is compressed between the humeral head and the overlying anterior acromion, coracoacromial ligament and even the inferior border of the acromioclavicular joint [3]. Impingement may be structural due to the presence of an acromial spur or degenerative acromioclavicular joint, but it may also be functional, due to superior migration of the humeral head during abduction and elevation. Underlying glenohumeral instability is a frequent cause of rotator cuff tendinitis, particularly in the younger patient, as is eccentric overload in the throwing athlete, where the rotator cuff muscles act as decelerators of the throwing arm. As the rotator cuff becomes inflamed, thinned or torn, so its function as a humeral head depressor

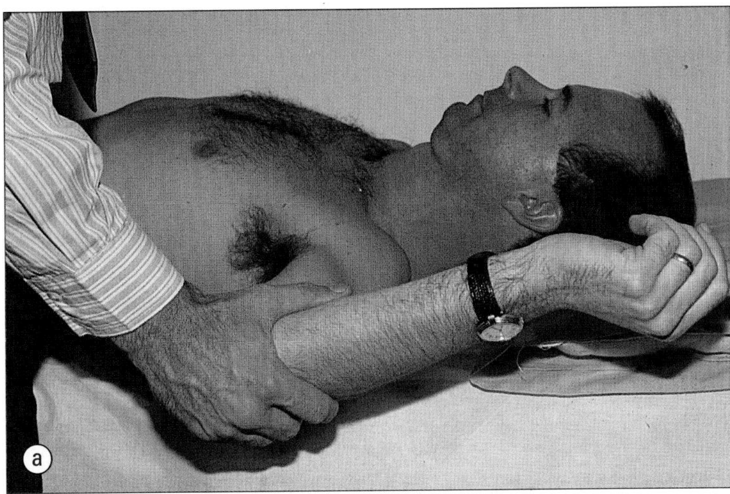

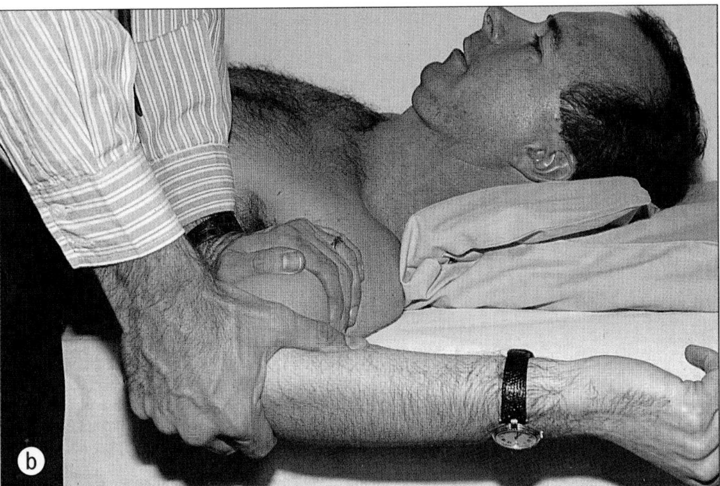

Fig. 7.8 A stress test for anterior glenohumeral instability (a). Containment sign: applying pressure anteriorly relieves the symptoms and allows further external rotation (b).

DIFFERENTIAL DIAGNOSIS OF SHOULDER PAIN													
Diagnosis	Age	Type of onset	Location of pain	Night pain	Active range of motion	Passive range of motion	Impinge-ment signs	Radiation of pain	Paras-thesia	Weakness	Instability	Radio-graphic changes	Special features
Rotator cuff tendinitis	Any	Acute or chronic	Deltoid region	+	↓↓ guarding	Normal	+++	–	–	Only due to pain	Look for	In chronic cases	Painful arc of abduction
Rotator cuff tears (chronic)	Over 40 years	Often chronic	Deltoid region	++	↓↓↓	Normal (may ↓ later)	++	–	–	++	–	+	Wasting of cuff muscles
Bicipital tendinitis	Any	Overuse	Anterior	–	↓ guarding	Normal	+	Occasionally into biceps	–	Only due to pain	Look for	None	Special exam-ination tests
Calcific tendinitis	30–60 years	Acute	Point of shoulder	++	↓↓↓ guarding	Normal except for pain	+++	–	–	Only due to pain	–	++	Tenderness ++
Capsulitis 'frozen shoulder'	Over 40 years	Insidious	Deep in shoulder	++	↓↓	↓↓	+	–	–	–	–	–	Global range of motion ↓
Acromioclavicular joint	Any	Acute or chronic	Over joint	Lying on side	↓ full elevation	Normal	–	–	–	–	–	In chronic cases	Local tenderness
Osteoarthrosis of glenohumeral joint	Over 40 years	Insiduous	Deep in shoulder	++	↓↓	↓↓	–	–	–	May have mild	–	+++	Crepitus
Glenohumeral instability	Usually <25 years	Episodic	Anterior or posterior	–	Only appre-hension	Only appre-hension	Possible	–	+ with acute episodes	+ with acute episodes	+++	Often	Stress tests
Cervical spondylitis	Over 40 years	Insiduous	Supra-scapular	Often	Normal	Normal	–	++	+++	+	–	In cervical spine	Pain with neck movement
Thoracic outlet syndrome	Any	Usually with activity	Neck shoulder. arm	–	Normal	Normal	–	++	++	++	–	–	Special exam-ination tests

Fig. 7.9 Differential diagnosis of shoulder pain: clinical and radiographic features of common causes of shoulder pain.

is compromised and superior migration of the humeral head can occur due to the unopposed action of the deltoid, giving rise to further impingement. In the degenerative cuff with a complete tear this can eventually result in a cuff arthropathy with degenerative changes taking place at the subacromial and glenohumeral joints. The subacromial bursa lies between the rotator cuff tendons and the overlying acromial arch and becomes inflamed with this impingement. This is a reactive process and is usually a secondary phenomenon, although primary subacromial bursitis can result from trauma.

Rotator Cuff Tendinitis

Clinical presentation and features

Presentation depends to a degree on the age of the patient and the likely etiology. Tendinitis resulting from eccentric overload or glenohumeral instability in the young adult usually presents acutely following an activity such as throwing. In the middle-aged individual, onset may be more gradual, reflecting the underlying chronic changes seen in the involved tendon. The patient may present with aching and discomfort in the shoulder, pain on movement and a history of repetitive or strenuous upper limb activity. The elderly patient may present with no history of antecedent trauma or repetitive activity and there is usually a gradual history of increasing shoulder discomfort, night pain, pain with movement, and weakness if a degenerative tear is present. Except in the young patient with a history of explosive arm activity or trauma, onset tends to be gradual and aggravated by movements into abduction and elevation or sustained overhead activity, which are commonly sports- or occupation-related. Patients frequently complain that they have difficulty reaching up behind their back when dressing. The pain at night usually occurs when rolling onto the affected side and is typically felt in the deltoid region rather than the point of the shoulder, although this can occur. Active movements may be restricted by pain and in the more severe or chronic cases a secondary capsulitis can develop, further restricting movement at the shoulder.

Findings on examination include a painful arc of abduction usually occurring between 70–120° abduction. When lowering from full abduction there is often a 'catch' of pain usually at midrange as impingement occurs. Passive motion tends to be full and pain-free if adequate muscle relaxation can be achieved. Point tenderness over the greater tuberosity can occur but is not always present and the diagnosis is confirmed by reproducing pain when resisting movement of the affected tendon and on impingement testing. In the older patient acromioclavicular joint involvement is often present and there may be early joint stiffness.

Pathology

Impingement has been shown to occur in forward flexion when the anterior margin of the acromion impinges on the supraspinatus tendon [3]. Vascular studies have demonstrated that there is a constant area of avascularity or 'critical zone' extending from a point approximately 1cm proximal to the point of insertion of the tendon into the greater tuberosity, and this compromise in microvascularity is seen with the arm in the adducted (neutral) position [6]. However, studies by Iannotti *et al.* have detected substantial blood flow in this critical zone using a laser Doppler [7]. It has long been supposed that this region of relative hypovascularity is compromised in elevation and abduction, thereby producing an inflammatory response and subsequent tendinitis. Sigholm *et al.* found that in flexion of the shoulder there is a significant increase in subacromial pressure [8]. The high incidence of complete rotator cuff tears seen in cadaver studies

(7–27%)[9–12] would indicate that with time attrition of the cuff leads to degenerative change and eventual tears. The pathology of this impingement syndrome has been classified by Neer into three stages:

- stage I, edema and hemorrhage of the tendon;
- stage II, fibrosis of the subacromial bursa and tendinitis of the rotator cuff;
- stage III, tendon degeneration, bony changes at the acromion and humeral head and eventual tendon rupture.

The bicipital tendon is frequently involved as part of this condition but is not usually the primary pathology. Generally, stage II occurs in patients aged 25–40 years, stage III in those aged over 40 years and stage I is the pathology found in those under 25 years of age.

Investigations

Plain radiographs may show evidence of calcification in the rotator cuff tendons in chronic cases, and in longstanding cases there are changes suggestive of rotator cuff degeneration, i.e. cystic and sclerotic changes of the greater tuberosity insertion. Diagnostic ultrasound and magnetic resonance imaging (MRI) can be used to demonstrate partial tears of the rotator cuff, although observer-dependence may present a problem with interpretation. Dynamic ultrasound scans can also demonstrate thickening of the subacromial bursa and impingement.

Diagnostic pitfalls

Pain felt in the deltoid may suggest referred cervical pain, although this is more likely to present with upper trapezius or suprascapular pain referring down into the arm. Pain on active arm movement and impingement testing will assist in differentiation, and preservation of passive range of movement will differentiate a capsulitis from rotator cuff tendinitis. In cases of tendinitis due to underlying instability, and this must be suspected in patients under 25 years of age, examination should confirm symptomatic instability.

Management

The treatment of rotator cuff tendinitis is often difficult and usually made impossible by continued participation in aggravating activities. Rest and activity modification are necessary to prevent the problem becoming chronic. Initial treatment should be directed at reducing inflammation by means of physical modalities and a nonsteroidal anti-inflammatory drug (NSAID) if required. When there is failure to settle symptoms by these means, a subacromial injection of corticosteroid can be used. As well as reducing pain, treatment should be directed at restoring range of motion and the normal biomechanics of shoulder movement, paying particular attention to scapular control and scapulohumeral rhythm. This is especially important in cases where such disturbance in biomechanics has aggravated or even precipitated the problem. Once the pain has reduced and normal shoulder movement patterns have been restored, a strengthening program should be instituted concentrating on rotator cuff exercises in order to restore their function as humeral head stabilizers and depressors, thereby reducing the likelihood of further injury.

The younger patient with instability needs a full stabilization rehabilitation program and rarely requires injection to the shoulder. The older patient with a degenerative rotator cuff and associated acromioclavicular joint pathology may be resistant to conservative treatment.

Indications for surgery vary according to the age of the patient, stage of impingement or tendinitis, and the symptoms. The major indication for surgical intervention is pain, and in the presence of an intact rotator cuff, failure to respond to a conservative program within 1 year is a reasonable indication for surgery. This involves subacromial decompression and encompasses an anterior acromioplasty and resection of the coracoacromial ligament, both of which can be carried out arthroscopically. Any impingement due to acromioclavicular joint pathology must also be addressed at operation.

Prevention

In the young patient or athlete attention to proper preparation for exercise and correct technique are important. Many athletes develop muscular imbalances about the shoulder, either through tightness or weakness, and if these are not corrected secondary impingement and tendinitis can result. In the older patient avoidance of sustained above-shoulder activities or explosive lifting will help prevent this condition from deteriorating or perhaps even developing.

Rotator Cuff Tears

Clinical presentation and features

Rotator cuff tears may be acute or chronic, partial or full thickness. Partial tears may occur in any age group following trauma, but the full thickness (or complete) tear is rarely seen in the patient under 40 years of age. In the young adult a partial tear can result from a fall or explosive shoulder movement and presents very much as a rotator cuff tendinitis, although onset is acute. Also, full active range of motion may be preserved. The acute complete rupture after trauma should be readily diagnosed. The mechanism of injury is usually a fall onto the outstretched arm, a hyperabduction injury or a fall onto the side of the shoulder. Bruising is often delayed and occurs in the upper arm, and there is an immediate loss of active abduction with weakness of abduction and external rotation. There is a close association between dislocation of the shoulder in the patient over 40 years of age and partial or complete tears of the rotator cuff. In one review of 40 patients the incidence of full-thickness tears was 90%[13].

Chronic full thickness tears are found in 7–27%[9–12] of patients at autopsy, and many patients with a documented complete tear of the supraspinatus tendon have full active abduction, occasionally in the absence of pain. There may be no history of trauma and symptoms frequently become apparent with increased activity. The usual picture is one of pain on abduction and flexion with varying degrees of loss of active movement depending on the size of the tear. The patient may complain of weakness of abduction, flexion or external rotation depending on the tendon involved.

Night pain is common and often severe. Examination reveals many of the features of rotator cuff tendinitis but there is often an inability to maintain the arm in abduction when lowering from the elevated position, i.e. a positive 'drop-off' sign. Subacromial crepitus and pain on impingement testing are present. A common clinical finding is wasting of the infraspinatus, and to a lesser extent supraspinatus, muscle bellies, together with weakness of abduction, but more often weakness of external rotation reflects the size of the tear. Rupture of the long head of biceps tendon is frequently associated with chronic rotator cuff pathology.

Pathology

Cuff arthropathy occurs when there is superior migration of the humeral head against the undersurface of the acromion. This occurs as the incompetent rotator cuff fails to stabilize and depress the humeral head and therefore counteract the pull of the deltoid. This leads to degenerative change both at the subacromial joint and secondarily at the glenohumeral joint. Management is difficult due to the combination of cuff deficiency and arthritic change. Neer estimates that 4% of cuff tears ultimately progress to a cuff arthropathy[14].

Investigation

Features of chronic rotator cuff degeneration can be seen on plain radiography with sclerosis and cystic changes at the greater tuberosity. Osteophyte formation may be present along the anterior inferior acromion, with possible acromioclavicular joint osteoarthrosis. With a complete tear there may be superior migration of the humeral head and narrowing of the subacromial space (less than 6mm indicates a tear). This finding is seen in cuff arthropathy where there is degenerative change in the subacromial compartment and glenohumeral joint.

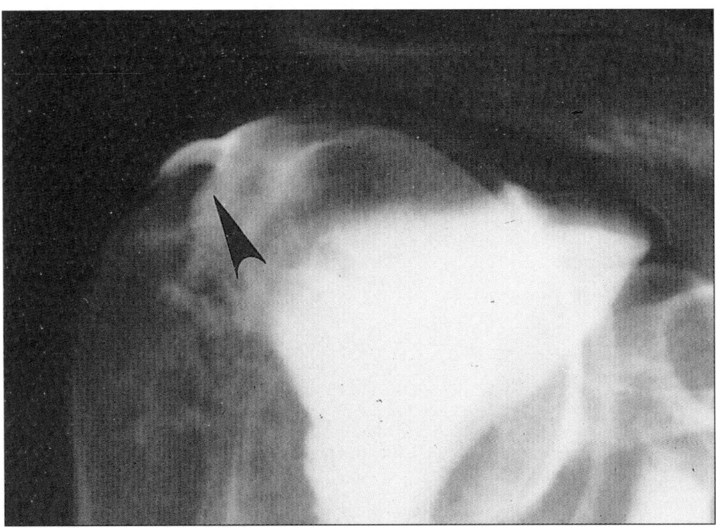

Fig. 7.10 Arthrogram of the shoulder showing leakage of dye into the supraspinatus tendon confirming a partial tear (arrow). This investigation is more accurate in the assessment of full thickness tears of the rotator cuff.

Full thickness tears are readily demonstrated with single or double contrast arthrography, and although false negatives can occur, sensitivity approaches 90%. Partial tears can occasionally be seen (Fig. 7.10). Estimation of the size of the defect using this technique is unreliable. Ultrasound techniques allow diagnosis of tears, both full and partial thickness, although the performance and interpretation of these scans are fairly observer-dependent. Magnetic resonance imaging compares favorably with arthrography in the diagnosis of complete tears (Fig. 7.11) but is less consistent in the assessment of partial tears, and interpretation is difficult (Fig. 7.12). Arthroscopy is now readily available as a means of establishing the diagnosis in the patient with shoulder pain who requires further assessment. It is particularly useful in the assessment of instability while at the same time allowing visualization of the rotator cuff, subacromial bursa, intra-articular bicipital tendon and glenoid labrum. It also has a role in the estimation of the size of a cuff tear prior to more definitive surgery.

Management

Initially, partial rotator cuff tears should all be managed conservatively, as for rotator cuff tendinitis, although corticosteroid injection is probably not advisable within 4–6 weeks of an acute injury. The management of complete tears is somewhat controversial in terms of if and when to operate. Acute ruptures in the young or active patient should be managed surgically earlier rather than later. In the older or less active patient it is reasonable to have a trial of conservative management, but if there is no substantial improvement within 3 months then subacromial decompression and repair is advisable [15].

Chronic complete tears should all be treated with an adequate conservative program in the first instance. Failure to achieve pain relief is a major indication for surgical intervention. Any operative procedure should be directed primarily at relief of impingement, debridement of the cuff tear and usually, but not always, repair of the defect. Surgery should also be considered where there is an associated rupture of the biceps tendon as these cases appear more likely to develop a cuff arthropathy.

BICIPITAL TENDINITIS

Clinical Presentation and Features

Although frequently diagnosed, bicipital tendinitis is not often seen in isolation and usually occurs in association with rotator cuff tendinitis or impingement, or with glenohumeral instability. Primary involvement of the tendon is seen as an overuse injury in sports such as weight-lifting where there is a repetitive stress placed upon the tendon, or after prolonged and repetitive carrying, e.g. of small children. The bicipital tendon acts as a secondary stabilizer of the humeral head and the translational movement seen with glenohumeral laxity can place increased stress upon the tendon leading to tendinitis. As with rotator cuff tendinitis the young patient with bicipital tendinitis should be assessed for instability. With chronic impingement or rotator cuff degeneration the biceps tendon may become fibrotic and attentuated and eventually rupture. Acute ruptures are also seen in young power-lifters and the diagnosis is made easy by the acute presentation.

Pain is usually felt over the anterior aspect of the shoulder, often radiating into the biceps muscle with well localized tenderness over the tendon as it runs in the bicipital groove. Pain is felt with overhead activities and often with shoulder extension and elbow flexion. Examination may reveal features of impingement, rotator cuff tendinitis and instability, all of which are important in determining the etiology of bicipital tendinitis. Pain may be reproduced with resisted elbow flexion, supination and shoulder flexion and various provocation tests are described, although none appears to be consistently positive. Passive shoulder extension stretches the biceps and may be painful. Rupture of the tendon is evident when there is the characteristic deformity of the upper arm with bunching up of the lateral muscle belly of the biceps best seen with resisted elbow flexion and supination.

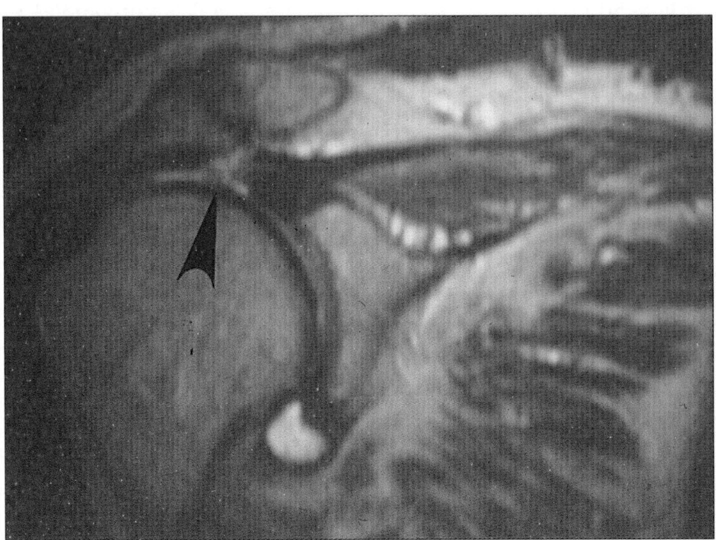

Fig. 7.11 MRI of the shoulder (T2-weighted image). There is a complete tear in the supraspinatus tendon (arrow).

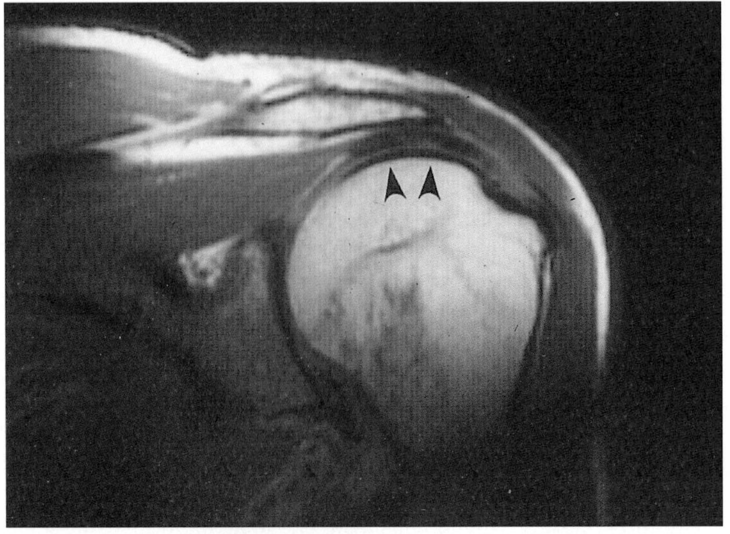

Fig. 7.12 MRI of the shoulder. A partial tear (right-hand arrow) and thinning and degeneration (left-hand arrow) are seen in the supraspinatus tendon.

Acute rupture of the transverse humeral ligament can result in subluxation or dislocation of the tendon. This can present with symptoms similar to bicipital tendinitis but often a more specific complaint is made of catching and a clicking sensation at the shoulder. Clinical examination may demonstrate subluxation of the tendon, which is felt as the arm is passively moved through internal and external rotation while in the 90° abducted position.

Pathology

The tendon of the long head of biceps may be involved at several sites: its attachment to the superior glenoid labrum, which may be injured in a fall or throwing action; as it runs across the glenohumeral joint (intra-articular); or as it runs in the bicipital groove (extra-articular). The transverse humeral ligament stabilizes the tendon in the bicipital groove and if this mechanism is disrupted subluxation or dislocation of the tendon can result. This tends to occur as the arm is rotated in the abducted position. The tendon can become inflamed and thickened and fibrotic in chronic cases. In the older patient there may be attenuation and thinning of the tendon and eventual rupture. This latter presentation is almost always indicative of underlying rotator cuff degeneration as the bicipital tendon appears to become stressed in its attempt to act as a humeral head depressor in cases of rotator cuff incompetence. Also, the presence of a complete rotator cuff tear exposes the intra-articular portion of the bicipital tendon to the overlying acromion and further impingement.

Investigation

Special radiographic views demonstrate the bicipital groove, allowing assessment of its depth and the presence of any degenerative spurring. Filling of the synovial extension around the tendon is seen on arthrography and may be reduced in cases of chronic fibrosis. Computed tomographic arthrography can be used to demonstrate subluxation and dislocation of the tendon. The tendon and any surrounding fluid can be seen well with diagnostic ultrasound, and this assists in the diagnosis of tears, both partial and complete, as well as tendinitis. Arthroscopy allows visualization of the intra-articular portion of the tendon and its labral attachment.

Management

It is necessary to establish whether the tendinitis is primary or secondary, since a failure to address any underlying rotator cuff pathology or instability will lead to a recurrence of symptoms. The principles of management are rest, and physical modalities, such as laser, coupled with NSAIDs as required. Corticosteroid injection is helpful in chronic cases but care should be taken not to inject the tendon itself. Since most cases of bicipital tendinitis are secondary, they usually settle as the primary condition is treated. The primary cases due to lifting or other activities respond to rest and simple anti-inflammatory measures. In chronic resistant cases surgery can be considered and this may involve subacromial decompression in cases of impingement, or tenodesis when there is chronic thickening of the tendon in the groove. Rupture of the tendon is normally treated conservatively except in the occasional young patient where upper arm strength is critical to their sport or profession. Usually, weakness following this injury is not significant. Subluxation of the tendon is usually treated conservatively, although occasionally surgery is necessary. Any conservative program must include range of motion exercises, stretches and, once symptoms have settled, a graduated eccentric and concentric biceps and rotator cuff strengthening program.

SUBACROMIAL BURSITIS

The close relationship between the subacromial bursa and the rotator cuff, specifically the supraspinatus tendon, is such that the term subacromial bursitis is frequently used when describing the pathology of impingement. In most cases inflammation of the bursa arises as part of the impingement process and co-exists with an underlying rotator cuff tendinitis. This bursitis is therefore a reactive phenomenon. In chronic cases the bursa becomes thickened and fibrotic and surgical excision or debridement may be necessary. Treatment of rotator cuff tendinitis is directed at reducing the inflammation in the subacromial space or bursa as well as reducing the impingement.

Acute traumatic bursitis in the form of hemorrhage and edema can occur as a result of a fall or a direct blow to the point of the shoulder. Pain on abduction is present but differentiation from rotator cuff tendinitis is possible by the presence of increased tenderness and fluid at the subacromial space. A period of rest combined with simple measures, such as ice, usually allows resumption of normal activities, but occasionally persistent impingement develops, requiring further treatment.

CAPSULITIS

Introduction

Capsulitis of the shoulder remains a condition both difficult to define and universally awkward to manage. Many labels have been given to the situation where there is a painful restriction of shoulder movement apparently of soft tissue origin. These include frozen shoulder, periarthritis or pericapsulitis of the shoulder, adhesive capsulitis and adherent or obliterative bursitis. More recently there has been an attempt to classify patients with a painful stiff shoulder according to the presence or absence of capsular joint restriction as seen at arthrography [16]. Perhaps incorrectly, the term 'frozen shoulder' is applied to many conditions where restriction of movement is largely due to pain from an underlying condition, such as rotator cuff tendinitis, rather than to the classical global restriction of glenohumeral joint motion seen with a true adhesive capsulitis. Primary capsulitis of the shoulder can be defined as a condition of unknown etiology in which there is a painful global restriction of glenohumeral movement in all planes, both active and passive, in the absence of joint degeneration sufficient to explain this restriction. A condition known as secondary capsulitis exists in which is seen a similar clinical condition but in association with a clearly defined clinical disorder or precipitating event. Underlying diseases associated with this condition are diabetes mellitus, thyroid disease, pulmonary disorders such as tuberculosis or carcinoma, and cardiac disease or surgery. Myocardial infarct, cerebrovascular accident or shoulder trauma may precipitate the development of a shoulder capsulitis.

Clinical Presentation and Features

Estimation of the prevalence of adhesive capsulitis is difficult due to variation in populations studied and diagnostic criteria used, but it appears to be in the order of 2–3% in non-diabetics [17-19]. Onset under the age of 40 years is rare, with the mean age of onset being in the sixth decade. Women are slightly more affected than men. Involvement of the contralateral shoulder occurs in 6–17% of patients over the subsequent 5 years [20]. It is commonly stated that recurrence in the same shoulder does not occur. There is a frequent history of minor shoulder strain or injury prior to the onset of symptoms but whether this represents a true strain of the shoulder or simply the earliest awareness of pain is unclear. The natural history of this condition has been assessed by various authors and it appears that there are three phases in its development and progression. The shoulder moves from being simply painful, to being painful and stiff and eventually to being less painful but profoundly stiff. This last stage appears to be self-limiting and recovery is gradual and spontaneous. These stages have been termed painful, adhesive and resolution [21]. The duration of each stage in the overall condition varies considerably, but approximate durations are 3–8 months for the painful phase, 4–6 months for the adhesive phase and 1–3 years for the resolution phase. The extent of recovery is variable, with quoted figures of 33–61% of patients having a clinically detectable limitation of shoulder movement, and although many remain asymptomatic 7–15% of patients may have a persisting functional disability [22–25]. The extent to which the duration of the painful and adhesive phases determine the degree of residual disability remains controversial.

Painful phase

This is characterized by the insidious onset of symptoms, usually in the form of pain on shoulder movement and background ache in the shoulder region, often in the upper trapezius muscle. As the condition becomes established there is the development of increasing pain at rest and at night, the latter becoming quite disturbing and frequently waking the patient in the absence of a history of precipitative movement. Muscle spasm may develop, further limiting shoulder movement, which becomes restricted, with the increase in pain and stiffness at the shoulder. Towards the end of this phase stiffness becomes a major complaint.

Adhesive phase

Usually after several months the character of pain alters and becomes less severe. There is a reduction in pain at rest and at night but discomfort and a more severe pain at the limits of movement persist. Shoulder movement becomes more restricted during this phase.

Resolution phase

The pain is less evident and the dominant symptom is restriction of shoulder movement, which often appears less distressing for the patient now that the pain has eased. There is a slow and gradual improvement in range of motion, although this is frequently incomplete. The onset and rate of recovery are variable and unpredictable.

Clinical Examination

The physical signs alter to a degree as the condition progresses, with pain, often severe, present in the earlier stages. Differentiation from rotator cuff tendinitis is possible on the basis of there being a global restriction of passive movement rather than simply the loss of abduction and flexion which is often seen with chronic rotator cuff conditions. In the painful phase there is painful restriction of active and passive motion (often mild in the earlier stages). There may be pain on impingement testing and resisted movement, although this is less evident than in rotator cuff tendinitis. Associated findings are tenderness in the upper trapezius muscle and early scapula hitching in elevation. In the latter phases the important finding is significant restriction of glenohumeral movement with a compensatory increase in scapulothoracic motion during flexion and abduction. Pain may be present but there is less discrepancy between active and passive range. Disuse atrophy of the rotator cuff and deltoid muscles may exist. Joint line tenderness is not a universal finding but is common in the painful phase.

Pathophysiology

Although the etiology of adhesive capsulitis is not known, there are associations with the aforementioned conditions. Capsulitis is more prevalent in diabetics (prevalence 10–20%), usually occuring at a younger age and often associated with prolonged duration of the diabetes, insulin dependence, the development of limited joint mobility syndrome and widespread microvascular disease. Also bilateral involvement is more common in diabetes [18,19]. The links between diabetes and capsulitis may revolve around microvascular disease, abnormalities of collagen repair or predisposition to infection [21]. An association between capsulitis and thyroid disease and pulmonary conditions has been noted but provides little information regarding its pathogenesis [26-29]. Laboratory investigation has revealed little to support the notion that an autoimmune process is involved and there has been no convincing response to immunosuppressive therapy. Histologic studies have failed to demonstrate the presence of inflammatory cell infiltrates, granulomas or vasculitis in the joint capsule or synovium. Also, there is nothing to implicate infection, crystal arthropathy or trauma. Histologic studies of the joint capsule early in the disease are difficult to perform and the heterogenicity of patients loosely labelled as having capsulitis makes study of this condition difficult. However, Lundberg [17] noted an increase in fibrous tissue, fibroblast numbers and vascularity with no change in the synovial lining and no inflammatory cell infiltrate. To date there has been no association noted between capsulitis and histocompatability antigen carriage in the population and no immunologic disturbance has been demonstrated. Several studies have looked at a variety of immunologic factors [30,31].

Investigation

Diagnosis is made largely on clinical grounds since there are few abnormalities found on investigation. Elevations of erythrocyte sedimentation rate (ESR), acute phase reactants and globulin levels are not usually seen, and calcium metabolism appears normal on testing. Plain radiographs are not helpful in making the diagnosis except to exclude widespread degenerative changes, calcific tendinitis or neoplasm. Classical features at arthrography are limitation of joint volume with a loss of the normal dependant axillary fold or pouch and irregularity of the capsular insertion to the anatomical neck of the humerus. Some authors insist that these changes need to be present in order to make a diagnosis of adhesive capsulitis. Ten to thirty percent of patients having arthrography have a demonstrable complete tear of the rotator cuff [17,24]. Other studies have suggested that a significant number of patients with a clinical diagnosis of adhesive capsulitis have normal findings at arthrography [24]. Arthroscopy allows further evaluation of these patients and different stages of synovitis and contracture have been described although variation in the patient population studied exists [16]. Bone scintigraphy may demonstrate increased isotope uptake in the affected shoulder region but this appears to have no predictive value in terms of outcome or response to treatment and is therefore of limited diagnostic value [32]. An average 50% reduction in bone mineral content in the affected humeral head has been demonstrated in bone densitometric studies, although again this is of little diagnostic or therapeutic value [17].

Management

Many therapies have been tried in an attempt to modify the natural history of capsulitis, and clinical studies of the efficacy of various treatment methods have been compromised by the difficulties with patient selection, diagnostic criteria and the variability in the natural resolution of the condition. The emphasis of treatment in the early stages should be on pain reduction and minimization of joint restriction. Analgesics and anti-inflammatory drugs provide limited relief of pain but do little to alter the course of the disorder. Physiotherapy utilizes physical modalities to modify pain and reduce protective muscle spasm while attempting to encourage range of motion exercises early on in order to maintain joint mobility. Shoulder immobilization should be discouraged if at all possible, although in the painful phase the patient tends to minimize shoulder movement.

Intra-articular corticosteroid injections have been shown to improve pain and range of movement to a degree, although no long-term benefit has been demonstrated [33–35]. Oral corticosteroids have also been shown to improve pain but not affect the rate of recovery [36]. Few treatments have been shown to consistently affect rate of recovery or limit restriction of movement. Careful utilization of analgesic or anti-inflammatory drugs with physiotherapy may assist, although this may be due to a reduction in the protective spasm which is seen in the untreated patient. Judicious and occasional injection of corticosteroid to the affected joint may help but is of little benefit in the adhesive phase. Manipulation under anesthetic has been advocated as a means of restoring joint motion by way of rupturing the inferior capsule and possibly the subscapularis tendon at its insertion. Care should be taken when carrying out this procedure, especially in the elderly patient, in order to avoid humeral fracture, shoulder dislocation or a significant rotator cuff rupture. Aggressive early rehabilitation in the immediate post-manipulation period is needed in order to maintain joint mobility, and patient co-operation with and tolerance of this treatment is essential. Manipulation during the painful phase is not recommended since possible recontraction of the capsule may occur, and this treatment method is usually reserved for the adhesive phase once the pain has settled [22]. For many patients, however, once the painful phase of their condition has subsided the prospect of this painful procedure is not appealing. Improvement in range of movement following this procedure is variable and is perhaps dependent upon patient selection. Long-term recovery appears unchanged although resolution may be accelerated immediately following manipulation [17,23,25].

Summary

Essentially, true adhesive capsulitis remains a condition largely unaffected by medical management. Symptomatic relief and preservation of movement are the aims of treatment, and an individual's response seems to depend on factors not well understood at this time. What is important is for the patient to understand the condition and for their expectations to be appropriate and proportional to our knowledge of the natural history of the untreated disorder.

ACROMIOCLAVICULAR SYNDROMES

Introduction

Pain localized to the acromioclavicular joint is commonly seen either as an acute or a chronic condition. In the younger patient this joint is frequently subjected to trauma as a result of falls or contact sport. This may result in an acute injury and may also predispose the joint to further problems, such as instability or secondary osteoarthritis. Infection of this joint is rare but septic arthritis has been described [37].

Trauma

Disruption of the acromioclavicular joint may be seen in association with fractures of the outer end of the clavicle and often leads to the development of secondary osteoarthritis. More common are injuries to the joint itself, which are graded according to the degree of disruption of the joint capsule and supporting ligaments. Grade I injury involves minor sprain to the joint capsule without ligament disruption. Grade II injury involves subluxation of the joint with downward displacement of the acromion relative to the distal end of the clavicle. There is stretching of the inferior acromioclavicular ligaments, and stretching and possibly a partial tear, but not complete rupture, of the coracoclavicular ligaments. In a Grade III injury complete dislocation of the joint occurs due to rupture of the coracoclavicular ligaments. Grade III injuries can be further classified according to the extent of disruption or perforation of the overlying deltotrapezius fascial or muscle layer by the displaced outer end of the clavicle.

Clinical presentation and features on physical examination

The mechanism of injury usually involves a fall directly onto the point of the shoulder. Pain is well localized to the top of the shoulder in the region of the involved joint, which is tender and often swollen to palpation. Abduction is often limited, both actively and passively, according to the degree of joint disruption. With a minor injury where there is good preservation of movement, acromioclavicular joint stress tests can be carried out to localize symptoms. In complete dislocation of the joint a visible step deformity is seen and examination will determine whether or not this dislocation can be reduced. This is important in the determination of the extent of any Grade III injury. The patient often describes a feeling of their shoulder having dropped due to the downward displacement of the acromion.

Management

For the Grade I or Grade II injury, treatment is largely symptomatic, with analgesics and provision of a sling for days to weeks depending on the symptoms. Shoulder movements should be encouraged as pain settles, and functional recovery is excellent. Controversy exists over the management of Grade III injuries. Provided perforation of the overlying muscle or fascial layer has not occurred, most patients settle with conservative treatment over a period of 6–10 weeks. Strapping of the joint has no effect on long-term stability and is not indicated in these patients [38]. Although effective, surgical stabilization by means of internal fixation is usually unnecessary and associated with a significantly high complication and failure rate. Surgery should therefore be reserved for severe Grade III disruptions or where an individual's occupation may be compromised by persistent deformity or instability at that joint.

Late sequelae

Patients may present with persistent pain at the acromioclavicular joint. This represents low-grade joint inflammation and may be associated with an underlying instability, early development of secondary osteoarthritis, or osteolysis of the distal end of the clavicle. Persistent pain following joint injury may also result from damage to the intra-articular fibrocartilage sustained at the time of injury. Treatment is symptomatic, with anti-inflammatory medication or injection of intra-articular corticosteroid for resistant cases. Delayed surgical stabilization may be carried out in cases of gross instability. Long-term treatment is as for osteoarthritis of the joint.

Osteolysis of the Clavicle

Osteolysis of the distal clavicle is a condition which may follow an acute injury or repetitive stress to the shoulder [39,40].

Symptoms are usually similar to those of acromioclavicular inflammation, with aching and pain at the limits of flexion and abduction. Radiographic changes typically show resorption of the distal clavicle, often with osteophyte formation, osteoporosis or tapering (Fig. 7.13). Response to activity modification and conservative treatment is usually satisfactory, but excision of the distal clavicle may be necessary. There may even be reconstitution of the distal clavicle with rest [41].

Osteoarthritis

Acromioclavicular joint morphology appears to be associated with the development of osteoarthritis with the Type I vertical joint more prone to degenerative change [42]. A previous history of joint injury is common when osteoarthritis of this joint occurs in isolation, but the joint may also be involved as part of widespread osteoarthritic joint disease.

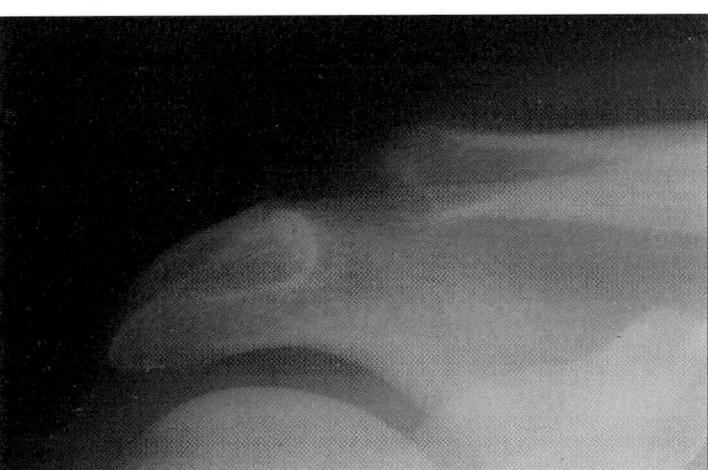

Fig. 7.13 Radiographic changes of osteolysis of the clavicle.

Clinical features

Pain and tenderness is well localized to the joint, which is often prominent due to osteophyte formation. Pain exists on full abduction or horizontal adduction and can also be reproduced with adduction of the extended arm. Crepitus is frequently localized to the joint. It is important to note that osteoarthritis of the joint is often seen in association with rotator cuff degeneration, and inferior osteophytes at the acromioclavicular joint may contribute to the development of a rotator cuff tear. Clinical features of both conditions frequently coexist, especially in the older patient.

Investigation

Degenerative change can be clearly seen on plain radiography and an arthrogram may reveal the presence of a complete tear of the rotator cuff. Traction or weight-bearing views can be taken in order to demonstrate joint instability.

Management

Initial management consists of local modalities and the use of analgesic or anti-inflammatory drugs. A suitable exercise program should be provided in order to restore normal scapulohumeral rhythm, glenohumeral range of motion and deltoid and rotator cuff strength once symptoms have settled. Cases resistant to conservative treatment may require surgery, which usually consists of excision arthroplasty of the joint while ensuring that instability is minimized. Careful assessment of rotator cuff function is important and in the presence of a significant tear rotator cuff repair or an acromioplasty may be indicated. Excision arthroplasty may also be indicated in the younger patient with chronic symptoms whether due to degenerative change, osteolysis or instability.

CALCIFIC TENDINITIS

Radiologically detectable calcification in the rotator cuff tendons has a reported prevalence of 2.7–7.5%, occuring in symptomatic and asymptomatic shoulders [43,44]. It is most common in the supraspinatus tendon and has been reported as being more common in women, housewives and sedentary individuals. Bosworth [45] estimated that 35–45% of individuals with calcification seen on radiography developed symptoms. Frequently bilateral, it usually occurs between the ages of 40 years and 60 years but can present as an acute condition in the younger patient. Patients may present with chronic symptoms of pain on movement with a catching sensation probably due to impingement. Acute calcific tendinitis has a quite different presentation with acute severe pain limiting passive or active shoulder movement almost completely, with exquisite point tenderness and occasionally erythema over the involved tendon. The onset of symptoms can be rapid with no history of injury or overuse and this occurs during the resorptive phase of calcification. Patients can therefore be divided into two groups. Firstly, those patients with an acute onset of severe pain and limitation of movement often in the absence of any previous shoulder symptoms. Secondly, patients who have a more chronic catching pain associated with movement presenting as an impingement problem.

Pathophysiology

It has been argued by various authors that calcification occurs as part of a degenerative process involving the rotator cuff tendons, largely because it is rarely seen in people before the fourth decade [9,46]. Histologic studies have confirmed that calcification follows on from tendon fibrosis and subsequent necrosis [46,47]. However Uhthoff and colleagues [48,49] have proposed a model for the pathogenesis of calcific tendinitis based on its clinical presentation as a self-healing condition in which the calcific process is actively mediated by cells in a viable environment. They classify the disease in three stages: precalcific, calcific and postcalcific. In the precalcific stage it is thought that there is fibrocartilaginous transformation in the avascular or 'critical' zone of the supraspinatus tendon. In the calcific stage calcium crystals are deposited in matrix vehicles to form large deposits (known as the formative phase). After a variable period of inactivity (resting period) there is spontaneous resorption of the calcium by means of peripheral vascularization and phagocytosis of the deposit (resorptive phase). Following removal of the calcium the space is filled with granulation tissue (postcalcific stage). Occasionally a deposit can rupture into the overlying subacromial bursa. There has been a reported association between this condition and HLA-Al [50].

Investigation

A plain radiograph will identify and localize the calcific deposit to a particular tendon, usually the supraspinatus. In the formative phase of calcification the deposit is well defined and homogenously dense. In the resorptive phase, usually presenting as the acute condition, the deposit is less well defined, irregular and has a fluffy, less dense appearance (Fig. 7.14). Degenerative rotator cuff disease and arthropathy may have radiologically detectable calcification but this is usually associated with other features of these conditions and the areas of calcification are usually small, stippled and close to the tendon insertion at the greater tuberosity.

Laboratory investigation usually does not reveal any abnormality of calcium or phosphate metabolism. There is no associated leukocytosis, raised ESR or change in serum alkaline phosphatase activity.

Management

Asymptomatic patients require no specific treatment. In patients with chronic symptoms conservative management should consist of mobility and strengthening exercises about the glenohumeral joint, physical modalities and NSAIDs for symptom relief if required. An injection of corticosteroid should only be given if there are clear-cut features of impingement and subacromial inflammation and should only be repeated with caution. In the acute stages treatment should include resting the arm in a sling, analgesics, anti-inflammatory medication and local application of ice. Injection of corticosteroid should be avoided as this may inhibit the resorption of calcium, but occasionally needling and aspiration of the deposit is possible with a subsequent reduction in pain. Injection of subacromial lidocaine should also be given for temporary relief of pain. Some authors advocate corticosteroid injection in the acute phase [49].

Surgical intervention is indicated when conservative management of the chronic condition has failed and there are persistent features of impingement. The deposit can be removed arthroscopically or at an open procedure and may be followed up by resection of the coracoacromial ligament and anterior acromioplasty.

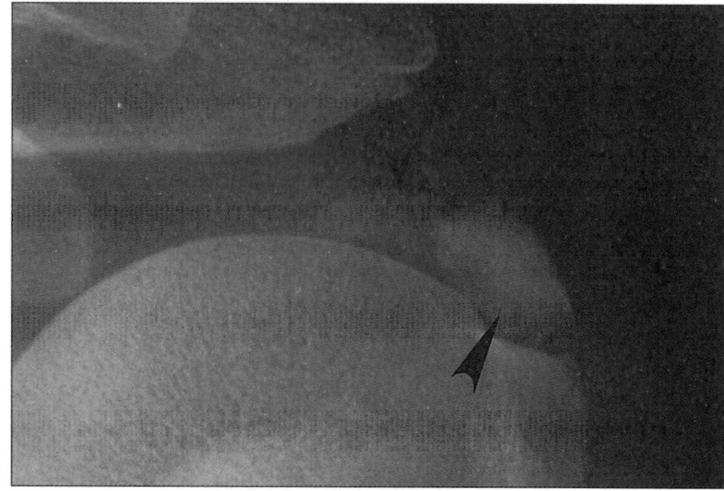

Fig. 7.14 Calcific tendinitis: formative phase (large arrow) and resorptive phase (small arrow).

SCAPULOTHORACIC BURSITIS

Scapulothoracic crepitus should by no means always be considered a pathological symptom since it is found in 8–70% of the normal population [51]. Rarely, it may represent changes in the bony structure of the deep surface of the scapula or underlying ribs, such as an osteochondroma of the scapula or a rib exostosis. These lesions tend to give rise to a more pronounced snapping sound and may result in deviation of the scapula away from the chest wall. Soft tissue causes are more common, and frequently a diagnosis of scapulothoracic bursitis is made, although the exact pathology if present is difficult to define. Crepitus is frequently found in association with muscular complaints, such as fibrositis, and probably represents a frictional sound as the scapula glides across the underlying muscle layers. Treatment is probably best directed at relief of symptoms and postural exercises, although subscapular injections have been given with variable results and at considerable risk of pneumothorax.

GLENOHUMERAL INSTABILITY

Glenohumeral instability is becoming better understood as a major cause of symptoms and pathology of the shoulder joint. The more traditional orthopedic model of shoulder dislocation, whether acute or recurrent, has been expanded to encompass the more subtle but equally important subluxations and minor instabilities which can play an important role in the development of shoulder pain, especially in a young active population. Glenohumeral instability can be classified according to the etiology, direction, type and circumstance of the instability, although in reality this represents a spectrum of disorders ranging from the traumatic unidirectional dislocation with a Bankart lesion to the atraumatic multidirectional instability with bilateral glenohumeral laxity [52]. Symptomatic subluxation or instability often presents as a painful shoulder with all the signs and features of a rotator cuff or bicipital tendinitis, but a careful history and examination coupled with a high index of suspicion in the young adult should confirm the presence of instability.

Management of tendinitis in the young patient with instability should be directed at the resolution of symptoms, restoration of normal flexibillty and scapular control, correction of faulty technique in athletes and then a suitable strengthening program for the dynamic stabilizers of the shoulder joint, notably the rotator cuff muscles. Also, correction of any muscle imbalance about the shoulder girdle is important. Arthroscopy allows closer evaluation of shoulder pathology and has an important role in the treatment of symptomatic instability, even to the extent of carrying out stabilization procedures.

REFERENCES

1. Turkel SJ, Panio MW, Marshall JL, Girgis FG. Stabilizing mechanisms preventing anterior dislocation of the glenohumeral joint. J Bone Joint Surg. 1981;**63A**(8):1208–17.
2. O'Brien SJ, Neves MC, Arnoczky SP, et al. The anatomy and histology of the inferior glenohumeral ligament complex of the shoulder. Am J Sports Med. 1990;**18**(5):449–56.
3. Neer CS. Anterior acromioplasty for the chronic impingement syndrome in the shoulder: a preliminary report. J Bone Joint Surg. 1972;**54A**:41-50.
4. Inman VT, Saunders JB de CM, Abbott LC. Observations on the function of the shoulder joint. J Bone Joint Surg. 1944;**26**:1–30.
5. Dalton SE. Clinical examination of the painful shoulder. In: Hazleman BL, Dieppe PA, eds. The shoulder joint. Bailliere's Clinical Rheumatology. London: Bailliere Tindall; 1989:453–74.
6. Rathbun JB, MacNab I. The microvascular pattern of the rotator cuff. J Bone Joint Surg. 1970;**52B**:540–53.
7. Iannotti JP, Swiontkowski M, Esterhafi J, Boulas HJ. Intraoperative assessment of rotator cuff vascularity using laser Doppler flowmetry. Abstract presented to AAOS Meeting, Las Vegas, 1989.
8. Sigholm G, Styf J, Korner L, Herberts P. Pressure recording in the subacromial bursa. J Orthop Res. 1988;**6**(1):123–8.
9. Codman EA. Rupture of the supraspinatus and other lesions in or about the subacromial bursa. In: The Shoulder, 2E. Boston: Todd; 1934:155.
10. Grant JCB, Smith CG. Age incidence of rupture of the supraspinatus tendon. Anat Rec. 1948;**100**:666.
11. Hazlett JW. Tears of the rotator cuff. J Bone Joint Surg. 1971;**53**B:772.
12. Nixon JE, DiStefano V. Ruptures of the rotator cuff. Orth Clin North Am. 1975;**6**:423-47.
13. Hawkins RJ, Bell RH, Hawkins RH, Koppert GJ. Anterior dislocation of the shoulder in the older patient. Clin Orthop. 1986;**206**:192–8.
14. Neer CS. Rotator cuff arthropathy. J Bone Joint Surg. 1983, **65A**:1232–44
15. Hawkins RJ, Misamore GW, Hobeika PE. Surgery for full-thickness rotator cuff tears. J Bone Joint Surg. 1985;**67A**:1349–55.
16. Neviaser RJ, Neviaser TJ. The frozen shoulder. Diagnosis and management. Clin Orthop, 1987;**223**:59–64.
17. Lundberg BJ. The frozen shoulder. Acta Orthop Scand. 1969;**119** (suppl.):1–59.
18. Bridgman JF. Periarthritis of the shoulder and diabetes mellitus. Ann Rheum Dis. 1972;**31**:69–71.
19. Satter MA, Luqman WA. Periarthritis: another duration-related complication of diabetes mellitus. Diabetes Care. 1985;8:507–10
20. Risk TE, Pinals RS. Frozen shoulder. Semin Arthritis Rheum.1982;**11**(4):440–452.
21. Nash P, Hazleman BL. Frozen shoulder. In: Hazleman BL, Dieppe PA, eds. The shoulder joint. Bailliere's Clinical Rheumatology. London: Bailliere Tindall; 1989:551–66.
22. Lloyd-Roberts GC, French PR. Periarthritis of the shoulder. A study of the disease and its treatment. Br Med J. 1959;**1**:1569–71
23. Reeves B. The natural history of the frozen shoulder syndrome. Scand J Rheumatol. 1976;**4**:193–6.
24. Binder A, Bulgen DY, Hazleman BL, Roberts S. Frozen shoulder: a long-term prospective study. Ann Rheum Dis. 1984;**43**:361–4.
25. Hazleman BL. The painful stiff shoulder. Rheumatol Rehabil. 1972;**11**:413–21.
26. Wohlgethan JR. Frozen shoulder in hyperthyroidism. Arthritis Rheum. 1987;**30**:936–9.

27. Bowman C, Jeffcoate W, Patrick M, Doherty M. Bilateral adhesive capsulitis, oligoarthritis and proximal myopathy as a presentation of hypothyroidism. Br J Rheum. 1988;**27**:62–4.
28. Johnson JTH. Frozen shoulder syndrome in patients with pulmonary tuberculosis. J Bone Joint Surg. 1959,**41A**:877–82.
29. Saha ND. Painful shoulder in patients with chronic bronchitis and emphysema. Am Rev Respir Dis. 1966;**94**:455–6.
30. Kessel L, Bayley I, Young A. The frozen shoulder. Br J Hosp Med. 1981;**25**:334–8.
31. Bulgen DY, Binder A, Hazleman BL, Park JP. Immunological studies in frozen shoulder. J Rheumatol. 1982;**9**(6):893–8.
32. Binder A, Bulgen DY, Hazleman BL. Frozen shoulder: an arthrographic and radionuclear scan assessment. Ann Rheum Dis. 1984;**43**:365–9.
33. Bulgen DY, Binder A, Hazleman BL. Frozen shoulder: prospective clinical study with an evaluation of three treatment regimens. Ann Rheum Dis. 1984;**43**:353–60.
34. Lee PN, Lee M, Haq AM, et al. Periarthritis of the shoulder: trial of treatments investigated by multivariate analysis. Ann Rheum Dis. 1974;**33**:116–9.
35. Richardson AT. The painful shoulder. Proc R Soc Med. 1975;**8**:731–6.
36. Binder A, Hazleman BL, Parr G, Roberts S. A controlled study of oral prednisolone in frozen shoulder. Br J Rheum. 1986,**25**:288–92.
37. Griffith PH III, Boyadjis TA. Acute pyoarthrosis of the acromioclavicular joint: a case report. Orthopedics. 1984;**7**(11):1727–8.
38. Rockwood CA, Young DC, Disorders of the acromioclavicular joint. In: Rockwood CA, Matsen FA, eds. The shoulder, Vol 2. Philadelphia:WB Saunders;1990:413–76.
39. Cahill BR. Osteolysis of the distal part of the clavicle in male athletes. J Bone Joint Surg. 1982;**64A**(7):1053–8.
40. Madsen B. Osteolysis of the acromial end of the clavicle following trauma. Br J Radiol. 1963;**36**(431):822.
41. Levine AH, Pais MJ, Schwartz EE. Post traumatic osteolysis of the distal clavicle with emphasis on early radiologic changes. AJR. 1976;**127**:781-4.
42. De Palma AF. Surgery of the shoulder, 2E. Philadelphia:JB Lippincott; 1973.
43. Bosworth BM. Calcium deposits in the shoulder and subacromial bursitis: A survey of 12 122 shoulders. JAMA.1941;**116**:2477–82.
44. Welfling J, Kahn MF, Desroy M, Paolaggi JB, De Seze S. Les calcifications de l'epaule.II. La maladie des calcifications tendineuses multiples. Revue de Rhumatisme.1965;**32**:325–34.
45. Bosworth BM. Examination of the shoulder for calcium deposits. J Bone Joint Surg. 1941;**23:**567–77.
46. McLaughlin HL. Lesions of the musculotendinous cuff of the shoulder. III: Observations on the pathology, course and treatment of calcific deposits. Ann Surg.1946;**124**:354-62.
47. MacNab I. Rotator cuff tendinitis. Ann R Coll Surg Engl. 1973;**53**:271–87.
48. Uthoff HK. Calcifying tendinitis: An active cell-mediated calcification. Virchows Arch [A]. 1975;**366**:51–8
49. Uthoff HK, Sarkar K. Calcifying tendinitis. In: Hazleman BL, Dieppe PA, eds. The Shoulder joint. Bailliere's Clinical Rheumatology. London: Bailliere Tindall; 1989: 567–81.
50. Sengar DPS, McKendry RJ, Uthoff HK. Increased frequency of HLA-AI in calcifying tendinitis. Tissue Antigens.1987;**29**:173–4.
51. Milch H. Snapping scapula. Clin Orthop.1961; **20**:139-50.
52. Dalton SE, Snyder SJ. Glenohumeral instablity. In:Hazleman BL, Dieppe PA, eds. The Shoulder joint. Bailliere's Clinical Rheumatology. London: Bailliere Tindall; 1989: 511–34.

WRIST AND HAND

Adel G Fam

INTRODUCTION

The hand is the chief sensory organ of touch and is uniquely adapted for grasping. The radial side of the hand performs pinch grip between the fingers and thumb, while the ulnar side performs power grip between the fingers and palm.

FUNCTIONAL ANATOMY

The bones of the hand are divided into a central fixed unit for stability, and three mobile units for dexterity and power[1]. The fixed unit comprises the eight carpal bones tightly bound to the second and third metacarpals (Fig. 8.1). The three mobile units projecting from the fixed unit are:

- the thumb, the first carpometacarpal (CMC) joint which permits extension, flexion, abduction and adduction for powerful pinch and grasp, and fine manipulations;
- the index finger, endowed with independent extrinsic extensors and flexors and powerful intrinsic muscles for precise movements alone or with the thumb;
- the middle, ring and little fingers for power grip, a function enhanced by slight movements of the fourth and fifth metacarpals at their CMC articulations.

The axis of the wrist and hand is an extension of the longitudinal axis of the radius and the third metacarpal, with the wrist in the neutral position and the dorsal surface of the hand in the same plane as that of the distal radius [2].

Wrist (Radiocarpal) joint

This is an ellipsoid joint between the distal radius and articular disc proximally, and the scaphoid, lunate and triquetrum distally [1–3] (Fig. 8.1). The articular capsule is strengthened by the radiocarpal (dorsal and palmar), and collateral (radial and ulnar) ligaments. The articular disc, or triangular fibrocartilage of the wrist, joins the radius to the ulna. Its base is attached to the ulnar border of the distal radius and its apex to the root of the ulnar styloid process The synovial cavity of the distal radioulnar joint is L shaped and extends distally beneath the triangular fibrocartilage but is usually separated from the radiocarpal joint.

The radiocarpal, intercarpal, midcarpal (located between the proximal and distal rows of the carpal bones), CMC and intermetacarpal joints often intercommunicate through a common synovial cavity (Fig. 8.1).

The carpal bones form a volar concave arch or carpal tunnel, with the pisiform and hook of the hamate on the ulnar side and the scaphoid tubercle and crest of the trapezium on the radial side [1–3]. The four bony prominences are joined by the flexor retinaculum (transverse carpal ligament), which forms the roof of the carpal tunnel. The palmaris longus (absent in 10–15% of the population) partly inserts into the flexor retinaculum and partly fans out into the palm forming the palmar aponeurosis (fascia). The aponeurosis broadens distally and divides into four digital slips which attach to the finger flexor tendon sheath, metacarpophalangeal joint capsules and proximal phalanges. There is usually no digital slip to the thumb.

Tendons crossing the wrist are enclosed for part of their course in tenosynovial sheaths. The common flexor tendon sheath encloses the long flexor tendons of the fingers (flexor digitorum superficialis and flexor digitorum profundus) and extends from approximately 2.5cm proximal to the wrist crease to the mid-palm. It runs with the flexor pollicis longus tendon sheath and the median nerve through the carpal tunnel (see Fig. 8.2). The tendon sheath of the little finger is usually continuous with the common flexor sheath. The flexor pollicis longus tendon to the thumb runs through a separate tenosynovial sheath, but may join the common flexor sheath. The flexor carpi radialis is invested in a short tendon sheath as it crosses the volar aspect of the wrist between the split radial attachment of the flexor retinaculum. The flexor retinaculum straps down the flexor tendons as they cross at the wrist. The ulnar nerve, artery and vein cross over the retinaculum but are sometimes covered by a fibrous band – the superficial part of the transverse carpal ligament – to form the ulnar tunnel, or Guyon's canal.

On the dorsum of the wrist, the extensor tendons pass through six tenosynovial, fibro-osseous tunnels beneath the extensor retinaculum

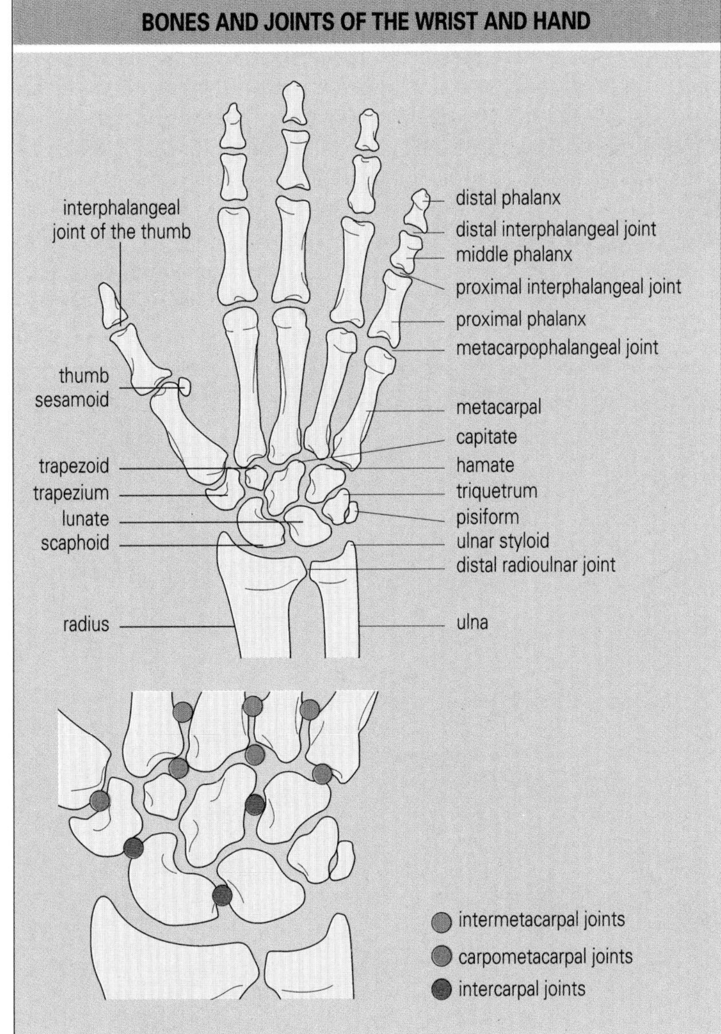

Fig. 8.1 The bones and joints of the wrist and hand.

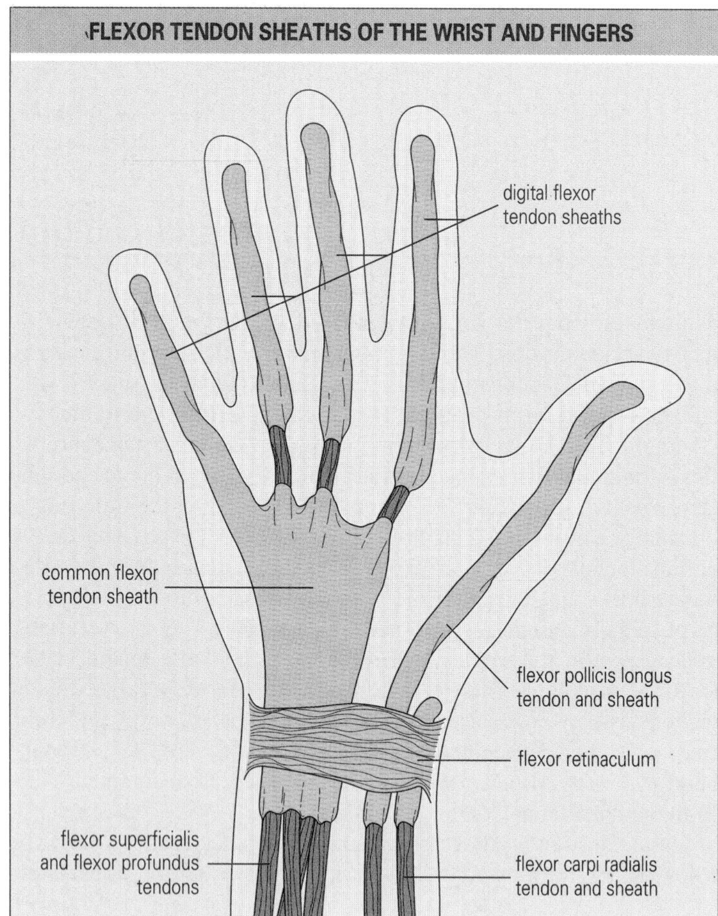

Fig. 8.2 The flexor tendon sheaths of the wrist and fingers.

(dorsal carpal ligament): abductor pollicis longus and extensor pollicis brevis are usually in a single sheath (first extensor compartment, most radial) (Fig. 8.3). Each tenosynovial sheath extends about 2.5cm proximally and distally from the retinaculum. The extensor retinaculum, by its deep attachments to the distal radius and ulna, binds down and prevents bowstringing of the extensor tendons as they cross the wrist. The anatomic snuffbox corresponds to the depression between the extensor pollicis longus tendon and the tendons of the abductor pollicis longus and extensor pollicis brevis.

Movements of the wrist include palmar flexion, dorsiflexion (extension), ulnar deviation, radial deviation and circumduction. The intercarpal joints contribute to wrist movements, particularly palmar flexion. Prime wrist palmar flexors are the flexor carpi radialis, flexor carpi ulnaris and palmaris longus. The prime dorsiflexors are the extensor carpi radialis longus and brevis and the extensor carpi ulnaris.

Pronation (palm of the hand turned backwards) to 90°, and supination (palm turned forward) to 90° of the hand and forearm occur at the proximal and distal radioulnar joints.

The Carpometacarpal Joints

The first CMC joint is a saddle-shaped, very mobile joint between the trapezium and the base of the first metacarpal [1,3,4]. It allows 40–50° of thumb flexion-extension (parallel to the plane of the palm) and 40–70° of adduction-abduction (perpendicular to the plane of the palm). These movements are important in bringing the thumb in opposition with the fingers. The second and third CMC joints are relatively fixed, but the fourth and fifth are mobile, allowing the fourth and fifth metacarpals to flex forward (15–30°) toward the thumb during power grip.

The Metacarpophalangeal Joints

The metacarpophalangeal (MCP) joints are modified hinge joints which lie about 1cm distal to the knuckles (metacarpal heads) [1,4,5] (see Fig. 8.1). Their capsule is strengthened by the radial and ulnar collateral ligaments on the sides and by the palmar (volar) plate on the volar surface. The collateral ligaments are loose in the neutral position, allowing radial and ulnar deviations, but become tight in the flexed position, preventing side-to-side motion (referred to as sagittal cam effect). The deep transverse metacarpal ligament joins the volar plates of the second to fifth MCP joints. The MCP joint of the thumb is large and has two sesamoid bones overlying its volar surface.

When the long extensor tendon of the digit reaches the metacarpal head, it is joined by the tendons of the interossei and lumbrical and expands over the dorsum of the MCP joint and digit forming the extensor hood or expansion (Fig. 8.4). The expansion divides over the dorsum of the proximal phalanx into an intermediate slip, which is inserted principally into the base of the middle phalanx, and two collateral slips which are inserted into the base of the distal phalanx.

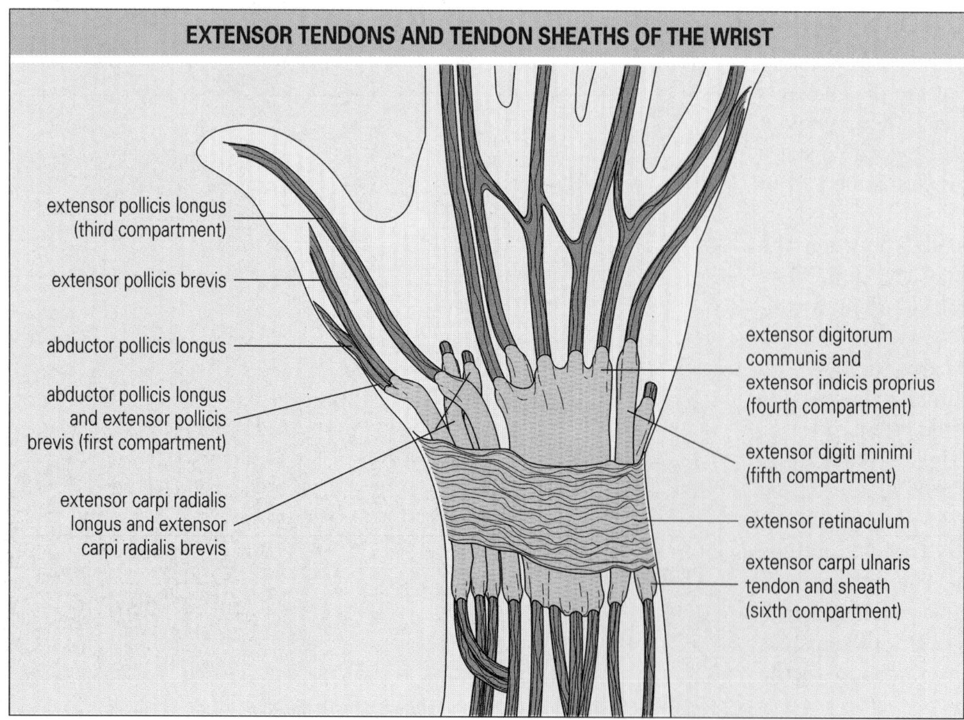

Fig. 8.3 The extensor tendons and tendon sheaths of the wrist.

The first MCP joint permits 50–70° palmar flexion and 10–30° dorsiflexion. Radial and ulnar deviations are limited to <10–20°. The other MCP joints allow 90° palmar flexion, 30° dorsiflexion, and 35° of radial and ulnar movements. The extensor pollicis brevis, extensor indicis proprius, extensor digitorum communis and extensor digiti minimi dorsiflex the MCP joints. The palmar flexors are the flexor pollicis brevis, lumbricals, interossei and flexor digiti minimi brevis assisted by the long flexors. Radial and ulnar movements at the second to fifth MCP joints are a function of the intrinsic muscles.

The Interphalangeal Joints

The proximal and distal interphalangeal (PIP and DIP) joints of the fingers and the IP joint of the thumb are hinge joints [1,4,5]. Their capsules are strengthened by the collateral ligaments on the sides and by the volar plates on the palmar surface, which serve to limit hyperextension, particularly at the PIP joints. Unlike the MCP joints, the radial and ulnar collateral ligaments remain taut in all positions, providing side-to-side stability throughout the range of movement.

The flexor tendon sheaths for the fingers enclose the tendons of flexor digitorum superficialis and profundus to their insertions on the middle and distal phalanges respectively. The sheaths extend from just proximal to the MCP joints to the bases of the distal phalanges (Fig. 8.2). The thumb flexor pollicis longus tendon sheath extends proximally to the carpal tunnel.

The flexor sheath of the little finger is often continuous with the wrist common flexor tendon sheath. Segmental condensations, or annular pulleys, in the digital flexor sheaths prevent bowstringing of the tendons and are mechanically critical for full digital flexion [1,4,6].

The PIP joints do not normally hyperextend. They allow 100–120° palmar flexion. The DIP joints permit 50-80° palmar flexion and 5–10° dorsiflexion. The IP joint of the thumb allows 80–90° palmar flexion and 20–35° dorsiflexion. The flexor digitorum superficialis flexes the PIP joints, and the flexor digitorum profundus flexes the DIP joints of the fingers. The prime dorsiflexors are the interossei and lumbrical muscles. The flexor pollicis longus flexes the IP joint of the thumb and the extensor pollicis longus dorsiflexes the joint.

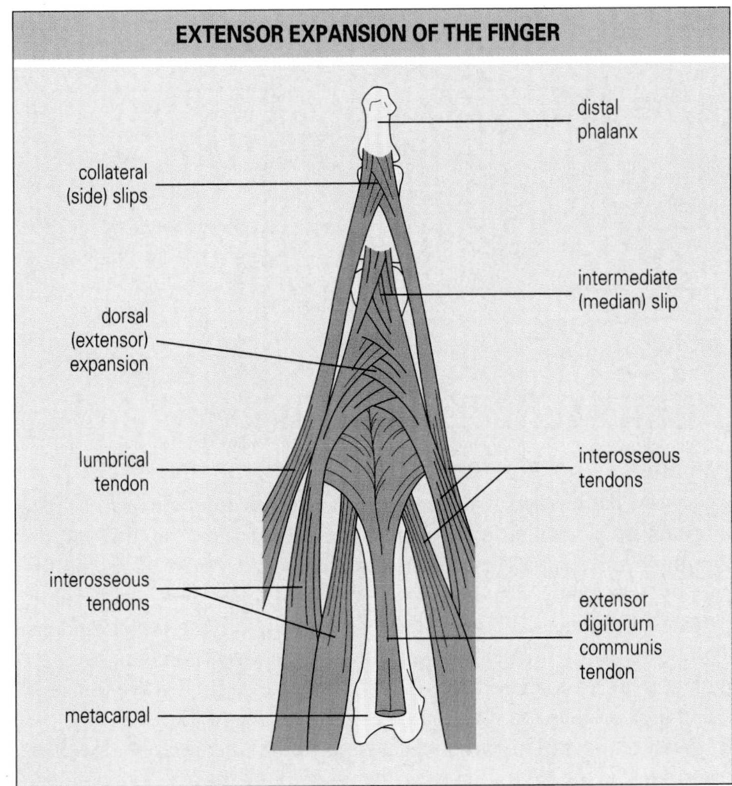

Fig. 8.4 The extensor expansion of the finger.

PHYSICAL EXAMINATION

Inspection

The wrist and hand are inspected for any swelling or deformity [2–5]. Arthritis of the radiocarpal joint produces a diffuse swelling distal to the radius and ulna. Extensor wrist tenosynovitis, by contrast, presents as a linear or oval-shaped dorsal swelling localized to the distribution of the tendon sheath. When the fingers are actively extended, the distal margin of the swelling moves proximally and folds in, like a sheet being tucked under a mattress (tuck sign) [2]. Tenosynovitis of the common flexor tendon sheath presents as a swelling over the volar aspect of the wrist just proximal to the carpal tunnel. The wrist is a common site for ganglia (Fig. 8.5). A ganglion is a cystic swelling arising from a joint capsule or from a tendon sheath. It is synovial lined and contains a clear, thick, jelly-like fluid.

Wrist deformities are common in rheumatoid arthritis (RA) and other chronic inflammatory arthritides. They include volar subluxation of the carpus with a visible step opposite the radiocarpal joint, carpal collapse (loss of carpal height to less than half the length of the third metacarpal, with inability to admit the tips of the patient's index and middle fingers), and radial posturing of the carpus (radial deviation of the carpus from the axis of the wrist and hand). Chronic arthritis of the distal radioulnar joint results in instability and dorsal subluxation of the ulnar head with a piano key movement on downward pressure.

Entrapment of the median nerve in the carpal tunnel (carpal tunnel syndrome) can lead to atrophy of the thenar muscles. In RA, rupture at the wrist of an extensor tendon to the little or ring finger is associated with inability to actively dorsiflex the digit at the MCP joint.

Deformities of the fingers and thumb are common in RA. The fingers are inspected for swelling of the MCP, PIP or DIP joints, deformities, clubbing, subcutaneous RA nodules, gouty tophi, osteoarthritic Heberden's or Bouchard's nodes, sclerodactyly, telangiectasia, ischemic digital ulcers, pitted scars, nailfold infarcts, periungual erythema or psoriatic skin/nail lesions [5]. MCP synovitis produces a diffuse swelling of the joint that may obscure the valleys between the knuckles. Swelling of a PIP joint produces a fusiform or spindle-shaped finger. Digital flexor tenosynovitis produces a diffuse tender swelling over the volar aspect of the finger (sausage finger). MCP joint deformities include ulnar drift, volar subluxation (often visible as a step) and flexion deformities. Boutonniere deformity describes a finger with flexion of the PIP joint and hyperextension of the DIP joint (Fig. 8.6). A swan-neck deformity describes the appearance of a finger in which there is hyperextension of the

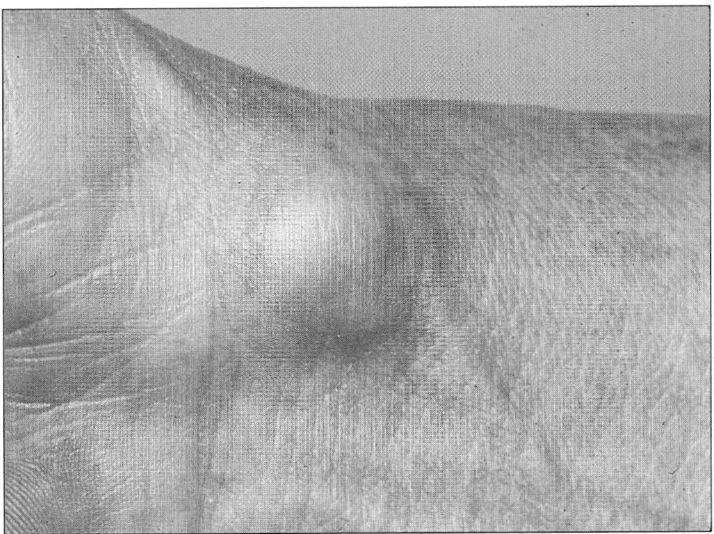

Fig. 8.5 A ganglion on the volar aspect of the wrist.

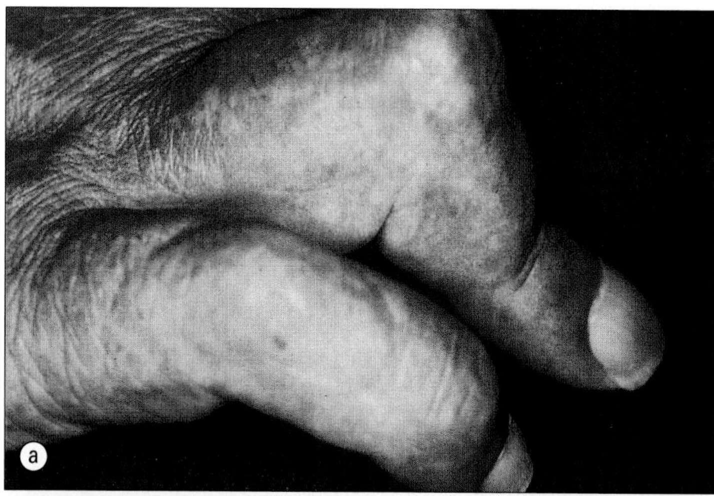

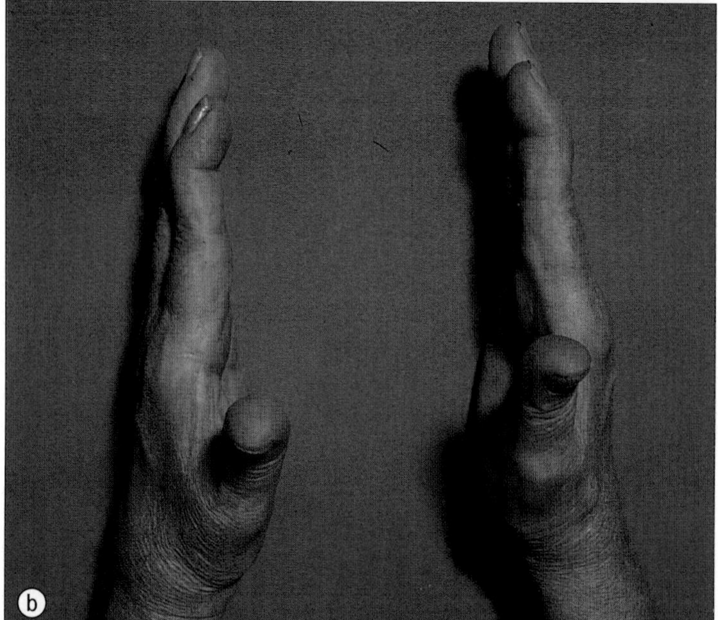

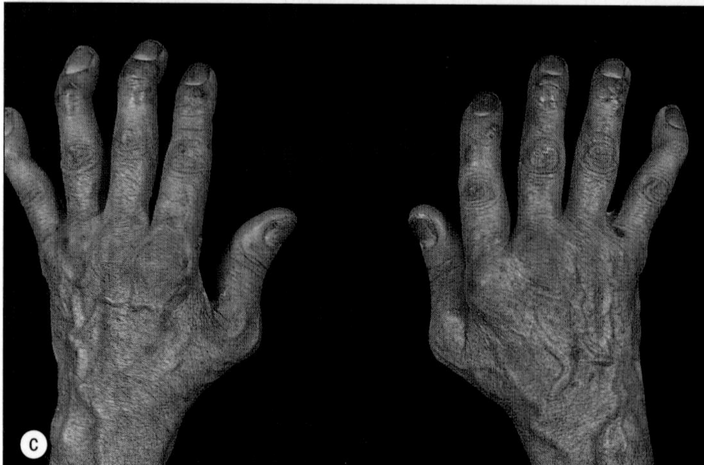

Fig. 8.6 Boutonniere (a) and swan-neck (b) deformities of the fingers, and 'Z' shaped deformity of the thumb (c).

PIP joint and flexion of the DIP joint (Fig. 8.6). A Z- deformity of the thumb is flexion of the MCP joint and hyperextension of the IP joint (Fig. 8.6). Telescoped shortening of the digits, produced by partial resorption of the phalanges secondary to psoriatic arthritis, RA or other destructive arthritis, is often associated with concentric wrinkling of the skin (opera-glass hand).

Thickening and contracture of the palmar aponeurosis (Dupuytren's contracture) often produces flexion deformities of the ring, and less commonly, the little and middle fingers.

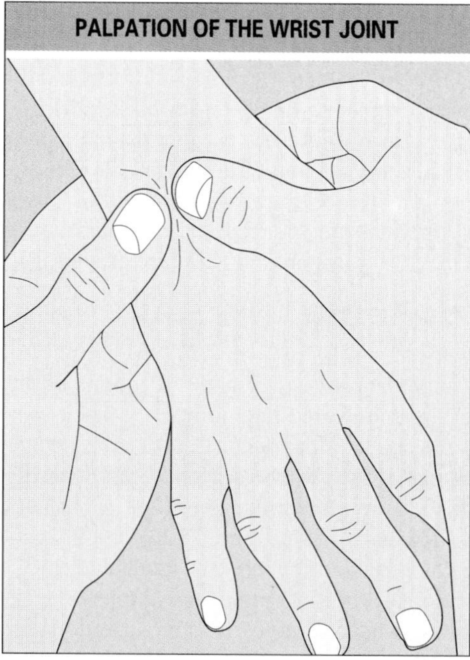

Fig. 8.7 Palpation of the wrist joint.

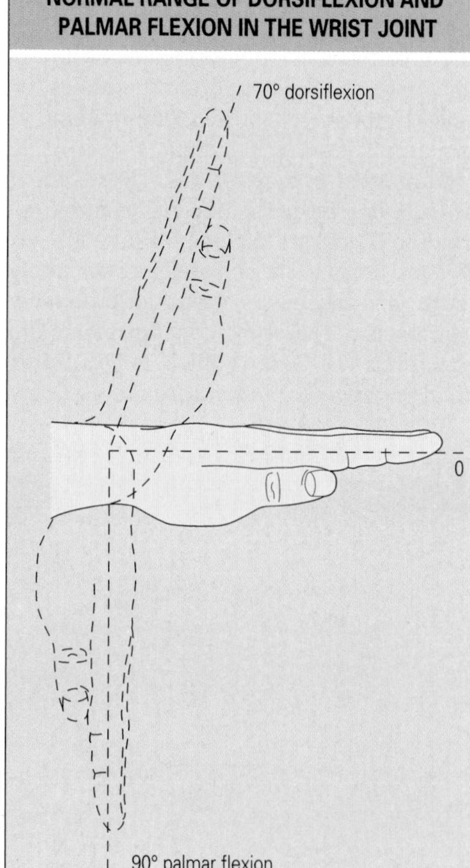

Fig. 8.8 Wrist joint: normal range of dorsiflexion and palmar flexion.

Palpation

The wrist is palpated with the joint in slight palmar flexion [2,3]. The margins of a swollen synovium are detected most reliably by the thumbs firmly palpating the dorsal surface of the wrist while the fingers of both hands support the joint (Fig. 8.7). The joint is difficult to palpate from the volar surface because of the overlying flexor tendons. The presence of fluctuation indicates a large wrist effusion; pressure with one hand on one side of the joint produces a fluid wave transmitted to the second hand placed on the opposite side of the wrist.

Wrist tenosynovitis produces a superficial, linear, tender swelling extending beyond the joint margins. A crepitus may be palpable and movements of the involved tendon often produce pain.

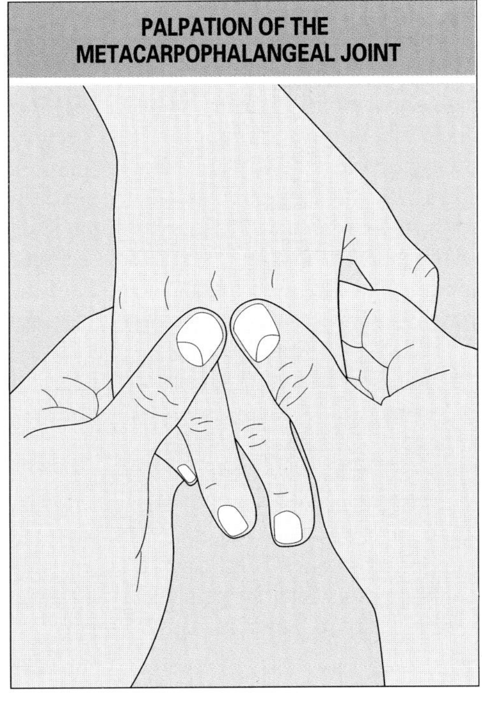

Fig. 8.9 Palpation of the MCP joint.

The normal range of movement at the wrist comprises 80–90° palmar flexion, 70–80° dorsiflexion, 40–50° ulnar deviation, and 15–20° radial deviation (Fig. 8.8).

The first CMC is palpated for tenderness, swelling or crepitus. Osteoarthritis is associated with crepitus and squaring of the joint.

Synovitis of the MCP joint is detected most reliably by palpating firmly with the thumbs over the dorsal surface of the joint on each side of the extensor tendon, while the forefingers support the joint over the volar aspect (Fig. 8.9).

The joint is difficult to palpate from the volar aspect because of the thickened skin of the palm, overlaying fat pad and intervening flexor tendon sheath.

The PIP and DIP joints are palpated for tenderness, synovial thickening, or effusion using the thumbs and forefingers of both hands placed on opposite sides of the joint [5] (Fig. 8.10). To detect an effusion, compression of the joint by one hand produces ballooning or a hydraulic lift sensed by the other hand (balloon sign). Unlike PIP synovitis, dorsal knuckle pads produce a non-tender thickening of the skin localized to the dorsal surface of the PIP joints.

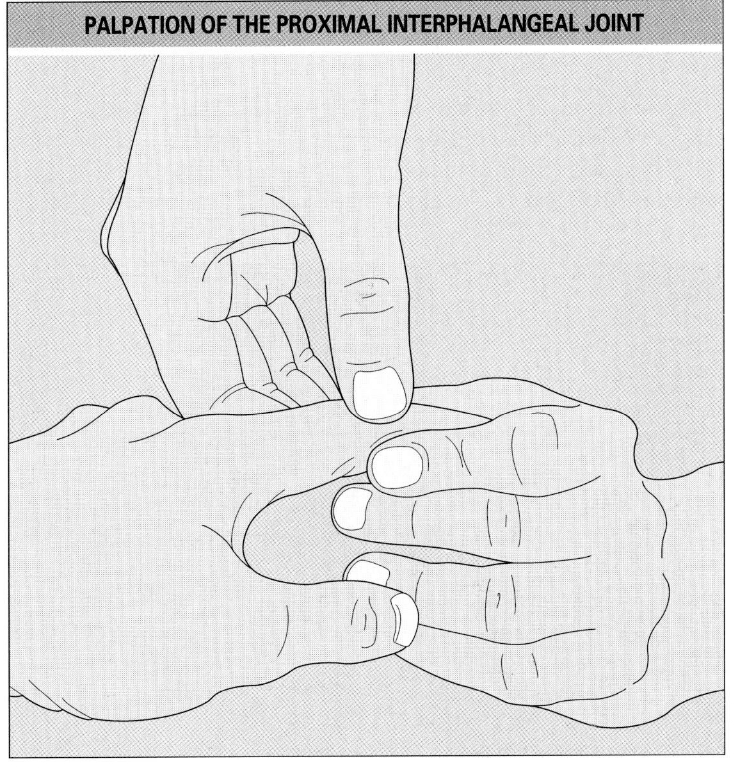

Fig. 8.10 Palpation of the proximal interphalangeal joint.

Finger tenosynovitis produces linear tenderness, volar swelling, thickening, nodules and/or crepitus of the flexor tendon sheath. Tendon nodules usually occur at the level of the metacarpal heads opposite the proximal annular pulley of the sheath. They can be palpated in the palm while the patient slowly flexes and extends the affected finger.

The range of movements at the MCP, PIP, and DIP joints is assessed by asking the patient to extend the fingers, make a fist, then flex the fingers so that the fingertips touch the palm opposite the MCP joints. To test for stability of the MCP joint, the joint is palmar flexed to 90° to tighten the radial and ulnar collateral ligaments, and the corresponding metacarpal is then held in one hand while the other hand moves the finger from side-to-side to test the integrity of the collateral ligaments. The stability of the radial and ulnar collateral ligaments of the PIP and DIP joints can be assessed by applying side strain with the joint in the neutral position.

Special Maneuvers

In carpal tunnel syndrome, percussion of the median nerve at the flexor retinaculum (just radial to the palmaris longus tendon at the distal wrist crease) produces paresthesia in the median nerve distribution: thumb, index and middle fingers and the radial half of the ring finger (Tinel's sign) [2,3]. Sustained palmar flexion of the wrist for 30–60 seconds may induce finger paresthesia (Phalen's wrist flexion sign). If the wrist cannot be flexed because of arthritis, pressure over the median nerve for 30 seconds often produces the same effect.

In de Quervain's stenosing tenosynovitis of the abductor pollicis longus and extensor pollicis brevis (*vide infra*), Finkelstein's test is a useful diagnostic maneuver. Passive ulnar deviation of the wrist with the fingers flexed over the thumb placed in the palm, stretches the tendons and reproduces the pain over the distal radius and the radial side of the wrist [2].

In vascular disorders of the hand, the patency of the radial and ulnar arteries can be assessed by Allen test [1]. The patient elevates the hand and makes a fist while the examiner occludes both the radial and the ulnar arteries at the wrist. The patient then extends the fingers and repeats the maneuver until blanching of the hand is seen. Each artery is then released and the color of the hand returns to normal. If either artery is occluded, the hand remains blanched when this artery alone is released.

In swan-neck finger deformity, tightness and shortening of the intrinsic muscles (interossei and lumbricals) results in restriction of PIP flexion when the MCP joint is dorsiflexed. Thus, with the MCP joint dorsiflexed, the range of PIP flexion is less than that when the MCP joint is palmar flexed (positive Bunnell's test) [4].

DIFFERENTIAL DIAGNOSIS OF WRIST AND HAND PAIN

Pain in the wrist is of diverse causes [7]. It may have its origin in the bones and joints of the wrist and hand, periarticular soft tissues (cutaneous and subcutaneous tissues, palmar fascia, tendon sheaths), nerve roots and peripheral nerves, or vascular structures, or be referred from the musculoskeletal structures of the cervical spine, thoracic outlet, shoulder, or elbow. Figure 8.11 provides a classification of painful disorders of the wrist and hand based upon the site of origin of pain and its predominant location. Precise diagnosis rests upon a meticulous history, a thorough examination of the joints, periarticular structures, cervical spine, nerve and blood supplies to the hand, and a few rationally selected diagnostic studies. As with any other clinical problem, assessment begins with a complete history, which should take account of the onset, location, character, duration and modulating factors of pain. A history of unaccustomed, repetitive or excessive hand activity is particularly important in the diagnosis of wrist and/or finger tenosynovitis due to an overuse syndrome. Initial diagnostic studies include hematologic, biochemical and immunological screening tests, and hand radiographs. Additional studies are sometimes required, including synovial fluid analysis, skeletal scintigraphy, nerve conduction studies, noninvasive vascular (Doppler) studies, arteriography, computed tomography, arthrography and synovial biopsy.

DIFFERENTIAL DIAGNOSIS OF WRIST AND HAND PAIN
Articular
Arthritis of wrist, MCP, PIP, and/or DIP due to Trauma, hypermobility, sprain RA (wrist, MCP, PIP joints) Osteoarthritis (first carpometacarpal, PIP and DIP joints) Other forms of arthritis: gout, psoriatic arthritis, infection Joint neoplasms
Periarticular
Subcutaneous RA nodules, gouty tophi, painful subcutaneous calcific nodules in scleroderma, glomus tumor of nail bed Palmar fascia Dupuytren's contracture Tendon sheath Wrist extensor tenosynovitis including de Quervain's tenosynovitis and extensor carpi radialis tenosynovitis Wrist volar flexor tenosynovitis (including carpal tunnel syndrome) Thumb flexor tenosynovitis (trigger or snapping thumb) Finger flexor tenosynovitis (trigger finger) Pigmented villonodular tenosynovitis (giant cell tumor of the tendon sheath) Acute calcific periarthritis: Wrist, MCP, and rarely PIP and DIP Ganglion
Osseous
Bone lesions Fractures, neoplasms, infection, osteonecrosis including Kienbock's disease (lunate) and Preiser's disease (scaphoid)
Neurologic
Nerve entrapment syndromes Median nerve Carpal tunnel syndrome (at wrist) Pronator teres syndrome (at pronator teres) Anterior interosseous nerve syndrome Ulnar nerve Cubital tunnel syndrome (at elbow) Guyon's canal (at wrist) Posterior interosseous nerve syndrome Radial nerve palsy (spiral groove syndrome) Lower brachial plexus Thoracic outlet syndrome, Pancoast's tumor Cervical nerve roots Herniated cervical disc, tumors Spinal cord lesions: spinal tumors, syringomyelia
Vascular
Vasospastic disorders with Raynaud's phenomenon Scleroderma, occupational vibration syndrome, etc Small- or large-vessel vasculitis With digital ischemia, ischemic ulcers, e.g., SLE, RA, and Takayasu's arteritis
Referred pain
Cervical spine disorders Reflex sympathetic dystrophy syndrome (RSDS) e.g., shoulder-hand syndrome and causalgia Cardiac Angina pectoris

Fig. 8 11 Differential diagnosis of wrist and hand pain.

SPECIFIC DISORDERS OF THE WRIST AND HAND

De Quervain's Tenosynovitis

De Quervain's stenosing tenosynovitis of the abductor pollicis longus and extensor pollicis brevis typically represents an occupation- or vocation-related repetitive strain injury due to chronic overuse of the wrist and hand. It is most common in women between 30 and 50 years of age [8,9]. Repetitive activity, involving pinching with the thumb while moving the wrist in radial and ulnar directions, results in frictional inflammation with thickening and stenosis of the fibrous tendon sheath as it passes over the distal radius beneath the flexor retinaculum.

De Quervain's tenosynovitis may also occur in association with RA [10], psoriatic arthritis, other inflammatory synovitides, direct trauma, pregnancy and during the postpartum period [11].

Most patients report several weeks or months of pain on the radial aspect of the wrist and at the thumb base during pinch grip, grasping, and other thumb and wrist movements. The affected tendon sheath is tender and often swollen (Fig. 8.12). Finkelstein's test is positive and a tendon crepitus may be palpable [8,9]. Patients may have other forms of tenosynovitis such as carpal tunnel syndrome, or trigger finger or thumb.

The diagnosis of de Quervain's tenosynovitis is often confused with osteoarthitis of the first CMC joint and with the intersection syndrome due to tenosynovitis of the second extensor compartment (extensor carpi radialis longus and brevis) at its intersection with the tendons of the first extensor compartment (abductor pollicis longus and extensor pollicis brevis) [9].

Treatment of de Quervain's tenosynovitis consists of heat therapy, nonsteroidal anti-inflammatory drugs (NSAIDs), and wrist and thumb immobilization by thermoplastic splinting [8–11]. A radial gutter light support splint immobilizes the wrist in slight extension and radial deviation and the first MCP joint in slight extension. The IP joint of the thumb is left unrestricted. Alteration of hand activities, avoiding tasks that require repetitive thumb movements or pinch grasping, is important. These measures are usually effective in alleviating symptoms. In patients with more severe or persistent pain, one or more local corticosteroid injections can be helpful, giving complete and lasting relief in about 70% of patients [12,13]. Surgical decompression of the first extensor compartment, with or without tenosynovectomy, is indicated in those with persistent or recurrent symptoms for more than 6 months [8–10,12,13].

Trigger Finger or Thumb (Stenosing Digital Tenosynovitis)

Trigger finger or thumb, also known as stenosing digital tenosynovitis or snapping finger or thumb, is the most common repetitive strain injury of the hand [9]. The anatomic lesion is a tenosynovitis of the

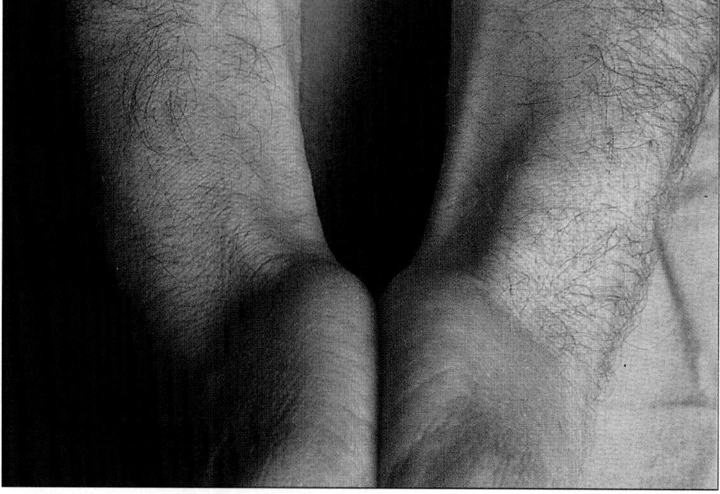

Fig. 8.12 De Quervain's tenosynovitis of the wrist.

flexor tendons of the finger or thumb, which results in fibrosis and constriction localized to the first annular pulley that overlies the MCP joint [9,12,14-17]. A tendon nodule often develops at the site of stenosis.

The nodule and/or tendon sheath constriction interfere mechanically with normal tendon gliding, resulting in pain over the area of the pulley and snapping or triggering movement of the finger or thumb. Pain along the course of the sheath with resisted flexion (performed isometrically), and pain on stretching the tendon passively in extension, are common. Intermittent locking of the digit in flexion may also develop, particularly upon arising in the morning. Passive extension of the PIP joint of the finger or IP joint of the thumb may produce a crepitus and a popping sensation as the digit is straightened. Examination reveals tenderness over the area of the proximal pulley often associated with linear tenderness and swelling of the flexor tendon sheath, and limitation of digital flexion and extension. A nodule can often be palpated in the palm just proximal to the MCP joint as it moves during finger or thumb flexion and extension.

The most common cause of trigger finger or thumb is overuse trauma of the hands from repetitive gripping activities with increased pull and friction on the flexor tendons [9,14–17]. One digit is often affected, usually the thumb, middle or ring fingers in this order. Other causes of flexor digital tenosynovitis include RA [10], psoriatic arthritis, diabetes mellitus [18], amyloidosis, hypothyroidism, sarcoidosis, pigmented villonodular tenosynovitis and infections, including tuberculosis and sporotrichosis A [14].

Management consists of modification of hand activity, local heat treatment, gentle exercises and NSAIDs as required [9,12,15-17]. Extension splinting of the affected digit at night prevents painful flexion during sleep. One or more corticosteroid injections of the affected flexor tendon sheath are effective and often curative in the majority of patients [12,14-17,19,20]. Surgical transection of the fibrous annular pulley of the finger or thumb flexor sheath is rarely required for those with chronic symptoms not responding to medical treatment [12,15-17,19,20].

Dupuytren's Contracture

This is a relatively common condition characterized by nodular thickening and contraction of the palmar fascia drawing one or more fingers into flexion at the MCP joints [21–23]. In most patients, Dupuytren's contracture affects the ulnar side of both hands. The fourth finger is usually affected earliest, followed by the fifth, third, and second fingers in decreasing order of frequency. Fibrous nodules, resulting from contraction of proliferating fibroblasts in the superficial layers of the palmar fascia, are the earliest abnormality. The dermis is invaded by fibroblastic cells, resulting in puckering, dimpling and tethering of the overlying skin (Fig. 8.13) . There is usually little pain, and if no further progression occurs the hand function is preserved and no treatment is required. However, after a variable period of months or years, the aponeurotic thickening may extend distally to involve the digits. The fingers become flexed at the MCP joints by taut fibrous bands radiating from the palmar fascia, and the hand cannot be placed flat on a table (positive table top test) [21]. Although there is no direct involvement of the joints or tendons, progressive flexion deformity of the fingers can lead to severe functional impairment.

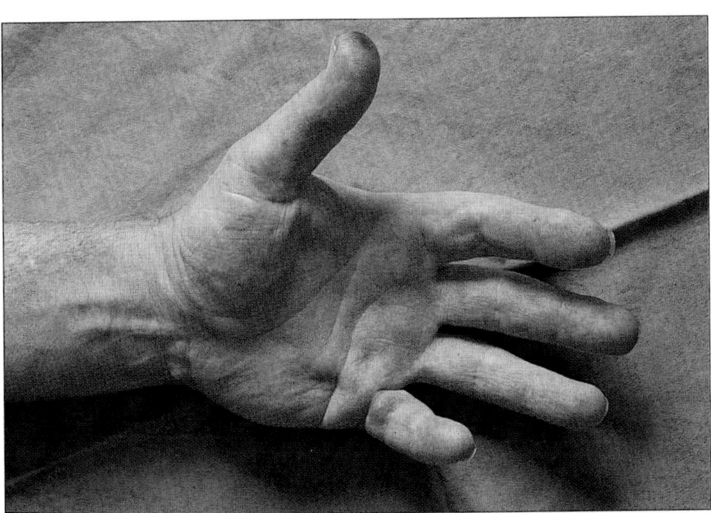

Fig. 8.13 Dupuytren's contracture of the palmar fascia.

The etiology of Dupuytren's contracture is poorly understood [21–23]. The disorder is rare in non-Caucasian individuals. Its incidence rises with increasing age, and the sex ratio is predominantly male (5:1). Familial predisposition is frequent, suggesting an autosomal dominant pattern with variable penetrance. Cytogenetic studies of Dupuytren's nodules have shown nonspecific chromosomal abnormalities, including numerical and structural clones and random aberrations, prophasing and premature centromere separation [24]. A pathogenetic role for local repetitive injury and occupational trauma remains unproven. A relationship to cigarette smoking, producing microvascular occlusion, has been suggested [25]. Dupuytren's contracture has been observed in association with idiopathic epilepsy, alcohol misuse, diabetes mellitus, chronic pulmonary disease and reflex sympathetic dystrophy syndrome [21-23]. No increased prevalance of the disorder has been found in patients with acquired immunodeficiency syndrome [26]. The association of Dupuytren's disease with other localized fibroses, such as nodular plantar fibromatosis, nodular fasciitis of popliteal fascia, Peyronie's disease and knuckle pads, has led to the concept of a 'Dupuytren's diathesis' [23,27]. The cause of these fibrosing diseases is unknown but seems to be determined by a dominant gene with high penetrance in males, usually middle aged white men of Celtic ancestry [23].

Pathologically, Dupuytren's disease is initially characterized by marked fibroblastic proliferation and vascular hyperplasia. This is followed by dense, disorderly collagen deposition with thickening of the palmar fascia and nodule formation [21–23,28,29]. The abnormal fascia demonstrates elevated total amounts of collagen with increased content of reducible cross links and hydroxylysine [28]. About 25% of the collagen is type III which is not normally present in the palmar fascia [28]. Ultrastructurally, contractile, smooth-muscle-like fibroblasts or myofibroblasts, surrounded by bundles of disarrayed collagenous fibrils and completely or partially occluded capillaries are present in the fibrotic nodules and cords [28,29]. Although myofibroblasts are not specific to Dupuytren's contracture, they are believed to be responsible for contraction of the palmar fascia and finger deformities [28]. The vasoactive prostaglandins, PGE_2 and $PGF_2\alpha$, are present in increased concentrations in Dupuytren's nodules, and are thought to influence myofibroblast contractility and contribute to the etiopathogenesis of the disorder [30]. Production of oxygen-derived free radicals may also be an important feature of the pathogenesis of Dupuytren's and other fibrotic conditions. Excessive formation of superoxide, hydrogen peroxide and hydroxyl radicals, resulting from microvascular occlusion and relative ischemia of the palmar fascia, can lead to tissue damage and enhanced fibroblastic proliferation [29,31].

Dupuytren's contracture runs a variable course: some patients show little change or incapacity over a period of many years, while in others fascial contraction progresses rapidly with severe deformity and impairment of hand function within a short period of time.

Treatment depends entirely on the rate of progression and severity of the lesions. In patients with mild disease, local heat, stretching exercises, and use of protective padded gloves during heavy manual grasping tasks, are often helpful [21-23]. Many patients learn the benign nature of the contracture, and adapt to the disorder. In more severe lesions with pain and inability to straighten the fingers, intralesional corticosteroid injections may be beneficial [21-23]. In those with advanced disease with progressive digital contracture of more than

30°, a positive table top test and functional impairment, surgical intervention (limited or total palmar fasciectomy with or without skin graft replacement), is indicated [21-23, 32, 33]. The risk of recurrence is increased in young patients with active bilateral disease, and in those with a strong family history and/or other ectopic fibrotic lesions [21,32,33].

REFERENCES

1. Markison RE, Kilgore ES. Hand. In:Davis JH, ed. Clinical Surgery. St. Louis: CV Mosby;1987:2292–353.
2. McMurtry RY, Little AH. The Wrist. In: Little AH, ed. The rheumatological physical examination. Orlando: Grune & Stratton; 1986:83–9.
3. Polley HF, Hunder GG. The wrist and carpal joints. In: Polley HF, Hunder GG, eds. Physical examination of the joints, 2E. Philadelphia: WB Saunders;1978;90–111.
4. McMurtry RY. The hand. In: Little AH. The rheumatological physical examination. Orlando: Grune & Stratton; 1986:91–100.
5. Polley HF, Hunder GG. The metacarpophalangeal, proximal and distal interphalangeal joints. In: Polley HF, Hunder GG, eds. Physical examination of the joints. Philadelphia:WB Saunders; 1978:112–48.
6. Strauch B, de Moura W. Digital flexor tendon sheath: an anatomic study. J Hand Surg. 1985;**10**(A):785–10.
7. Bluestone R: A practical approach to hand pain. J Musculoskel Med. 1989:**6**:75-85.
8. Field JH. De Quervain's disease. Am Fam Physician. 1979; **20**:103–4.
9. Thompson JS, Phelps TH. Repetitive strain injuries. How to deal with 'the epidemic of the l990's'. Postgrad Med. 1990;**88**:143–9.
10. Gray RG, Gottlieb NL. Hand flexor tenosynovitis in rheumatoid arthritis. Prevalence, distribution, and associated rheumatic features. Arthritis Rheum. 1977;**20**:1003–8.
11. Nygaard IE, Saltzman CL, Whitehouse MB, Hankin FM. Hand problems in pregnancy. Am Fam Physician. 1989;**39**:123–6.
12. Lapidus PW, Guidotti FP. Stenosing tenovaginitis of the wrist and fingers. Clin Orthop. 1972;**83**:87–90.
13. Harvey FJ, Harvey PM, Horsley MW. De Quervain's disease: surgical or nonsurgical treatment. J Hand Surg. 1990;**15**(A):83–7.
14. Canoso JJ. Bursitis, tenosynovitis, ganglions, and painful lesions of the wrist, elbow and hand. Curr Opinion Rheumatol. 1990;**2**:276–81.
15. Freiberg A, Mulholland RS, Levine R. Nonoperative treatment of trigger fingers and thumbs. J Hand Surg. 1989;**14**(A):553–8.
16. Kraemer BA, Young VL, Arfken C. Stenosing flexor tenosynovitis. South Med J. 1990;**83**:806–11.
17. Rhoades CE, Gelberman RH, Manjarris JF. Stenosing tenosynovitis of the fingers and thumb. Results of a prospective trial of steroid injection and splinting. Clin Orthop. 1984;**190**:236–8.
18. Yosipovitch G, Yosipovitch Z, Karp M, Mukamel M. Trigger finger in young patients with insulin dependent diabetes. J Rheumatol. 1990;**17**:951–2.
19. Marks MR, Gunther SF. Efficacy of cortisone injection in treatment of trigger fingers and thumbs. J Hand Surg. 1989;**14**(A):722–7.
20. Anderson B, Kaye S. Treatment of flexor tenosynovitis of the hand 'trigger finger' with corticosteroids. A prospective study of the response to local injection. Arch Intern Med. 1991;**151**:153–6.
21. Hueston JT. Dupuytren's contracture. In: Converse JM, McCarthy JG, Littler JW, eds. Reconstructive plastic surgery, 2E. Philadelphia: WB Saunders; 1977; 3403–27.
22. Lynch M, Jayson MIV. Fasciitis and fibrosis. Clin Rheum Dis. 1979;**5**:833–55.
23. Wooldridge WE. Four related fibrosing diseases. When you find one, look for another. Postgrad Med. 1988;**84**:269–74.
24. Wurster-Hill DH, Brown F, Park JP, Gibson SH. Cytogenetic studies in Dupuytren's contracture. Am J Hum Genet. 1988;**43**:285–92.
25. An HS, Southworth SR, Jackson WT, Russ B. Cigarette smoking and Dupuytren's contracture of the hand. J Hand Surg. 1988;**13**(A):872–4.
26. French PD, Kitchen VS, Harris JRW. Prevalence of Dupuytren's contracture in patients infected with HIV. Br Med J. 1990;**301**:967.
27. Wheeler ES, Meals RA. Dupuytren's diathesis: a broad spectrum disease. Plast Reconstr Surg. 1981;**68**:781–3.
28. Gelberman RH, Amiel D, Rudolph RM, Vance RM. Dupuytren's contracture. An electron microscopic, biochemical and clinical correlative study. J Bone Joint Surg. 1980;**62**(A):425–32.
29. Murrell GAC, Francis MJO, Howlett CR. Dupuytren's contracture. Fine structure in relation to aetiology. J Bone Joint Surg. 1989;**71**(B):367–3.
30. Badalamente MA, Hurst LC, Sampson SP. Prostaglandins influence myofibroblast contractility in Dupuytren's disease. J Hand Surg.1988;**13**(A):867–71.
31. Duthie RB, Francis MJO. Free radicals and Dupuytren's contracure. J Bone Joint Surg. 1988;**70**(B):689–91.
32. Ketchum LD, Hixson FP. Dermofasciectomy and full thickness grafts in the treatment of Dupuytren's contracture. J Hand Surg. 1987;**12**(A):659–63
33. Rombouts J-J, Noël H, Legrain Y, Munting E. Prediction of recurrence in the treatment of Dupuytren's disease: evaluation of a histologic classification. J Hand Surg. 1989;**14**(A):644–52.

REGIONAL PAIN PROBLEMS

9

THE KNEE

Geoffrey P Graham & John A Fairclough

FUNCTIONAL ANATOMY

The knee is the largest of the human joints in terms of the volume of its synovial cavity and the area of its articular cartilage. It actually consists of two joints, the tibiofemoral and the patellofemoral, which share a common synovial cavity. The synovial membrane of the joint is attached around the articular margins and the synovial cavity extends approximately one hand's breadth above the upper pole of the patella to form the suprapatellar pouch. Therefore, a collection of fluid in the joint or thickening of the synovium causes a characteristic swelling which extends above the patella.

The femoral and tibial condyles articulate with each other, with the fibrocartilaginous menisci interposed between them. The old name for the menisci was the semilunar cartilages, reflecting the fact that they are crescentic in shape. The lateral meniscus is nearly circular and the medial meniscus is semicircular. Their ends are attached to the intercondylar area of the tibia and their circumference to the meniscotibial and meniscofemoral ligaments, which are part of the capsule of the joint [1]. The lateral meniscus is attached to the femur posteriorly by the inconstant meniscofemoral ligaments of Wrisberg and Humphrey. The popliteus tendon enters the joint through a deficiency in the capsule adjacent to the lateral meniscus and may be attached to it [2,3]. The menisci transmit approximately 60% of the force through the normal tibiofemoral joint and play a role in lubrication. They alter shape in order to maintain congruity of the joint as the knee flexes and extends. The peripheral 10–30% of the meniscus and the anterior and posterior horns receive a blood supply from the geniculate vessels and have the potential for repair [4]. The rest of the meniscus is avascular and is nourished from the synovial fluid, thus there is little potential for healing in this area.

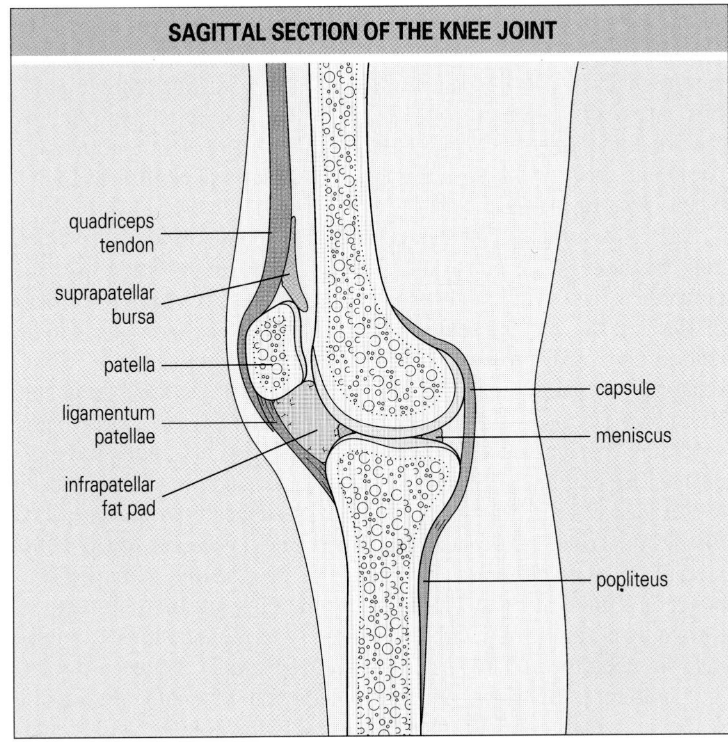

Fig. 9.1 Sagittal section showing the components of the knee joint.

The knee is capable of flexion, extension and rotation. However, it is not a simple hinge joint with a single axis: the movements which occur are complex and involve both rolling and gliding of the femur on the tibia. The axis of rotation alters as the knee is flexed and extended. The normal motion of the knee is controlled by the shape of the articular surfaces and menisci and by the tension in the ligaments and capsule. Alteration in the configuration of any of these structures due to injury or disease can cause abnormal motion to occur. As the knee approaches full extension the shape of the joint surfaces and the tension in the ligaments cause the femur to internally rotate on the tibia, into the 'screwed home' position. Any further attempt to extend the knee simply increases the tension in the ligaments. On standing, the center of gravity passes in front of the axis of rotation of the knee maintaining the ligaments in tension and the muscles can therefore relax. Standing requires very little energy expenditure due to this mechanism. No rotation is possible in the fully extended position; this can only occur in the flexed knee, when the ligaments are relaxed.

In health the center of the hip, the center of the knee and the center of the ankle lie in a straight line. Due to the medial inclination of the femur the long axes of the femur and tibia form a valgus angle of approximately 7°. Disease or an abnormality of growth may alter this angle – genu valgum represents an increase and genu varum a decrease.

The patella is a sesamoid bone lying in the quadriceps tendon (Fig. 9.1) and articulating with the trochlear groove of the femur. Its function is to increase the mechanical advantage of the quadriceps. It is triangular in section and has medial and lateral articular facets [5]. In full extension only the lower part of the patella is in contact with the articular cartilage of the femur. As the knee is flexed the patella enters the trochlea groove and sits centrally in it. A line drawn from the anterior superior iliac spine to the center of the patella represents the line of pull of the quadriceps which is lateral to the long axis of the femur. The angle formed by this line and a line drawn from the center of the patella to the tibial tubercle is called the Q angle (Fig. 9.2) [6]. The larger the Q angle, the larger is the force vector tending to pull the patella laterally. In a normal knee the Q angle measures approximately 15°, an angle exceeding 20° is abnormal. Genu valgum, persistent femoral anteversion and external tibial torsion

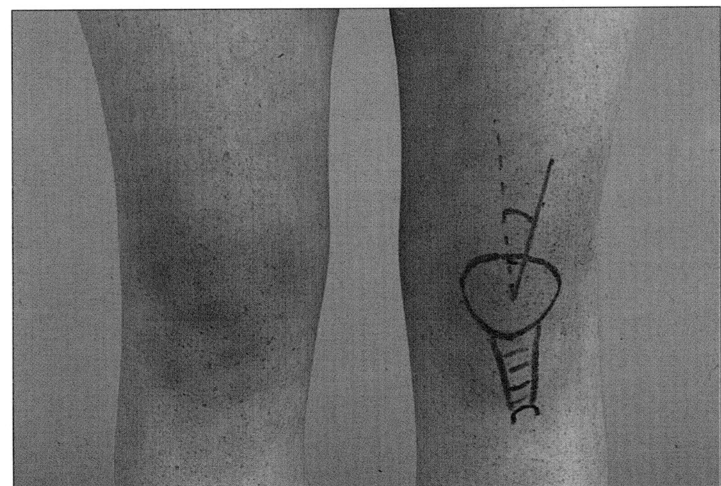

Fig. 9.2 The Q angle.

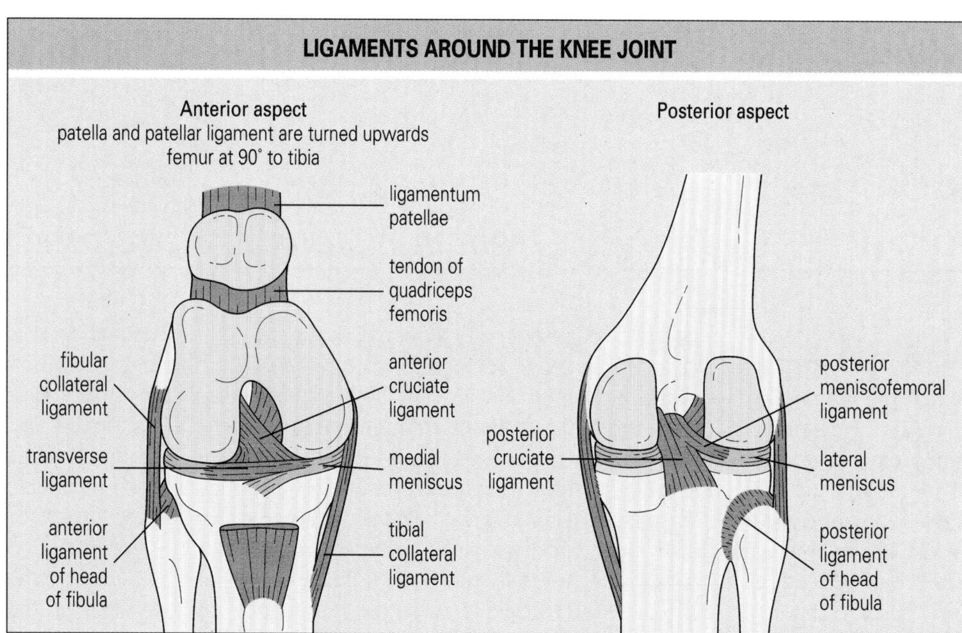

Fig. 9.3 Ligaments around the knee joint.

increase this angle and therefore increase the tendency for the patella to dislocate. The factors acting against dislocation are the lower fibers of the vastus medialis, the shape of the patello-femoral joint and the fact that the lateral condyle is higher than the medial. The action of the lower fibers of the vastus medialis (the vastus medialis obliquus) is the most important factor. They originate from the medial intermuscular septum and run horizontally to the patella, controlling its lateral motion.

The capsule of the knee joint is a complex structure, parts of which are thickened to form named ligaments. There are also four accessory ligaments which are the anterior and posterior cruciates and the medial and lateral collateral ligaments. The main capsular ligaments are the oblique popliteal ligament and the arcuate ligament. The oblique popliteal strengthens the posteromedial corner of the capsule and is formed by an expansion from the semimembranosus tendon. The arcuate ligament reinforces the posterolateral corner and arches across the popliteus tendon at its entry to the capsule.

The anterior cruciate ligament (ACL) runs forward from the medial aspect of the lateral femoral condyle in the intercondylar notch to the intercondylar eminence of the tibia in front of the tibial spines (Fig. 9.3). The posterior cruciate ligament (PCL) runs from the lateral aspect of the medial femoral condyle in the intercondylar notch to insert at the back of the intercondylar area of the tibia and on its posterior aspect. The cruciate ligaments are complex structures composed of bundles of fibers of different lengths which twist around a main axis. This arrangement allows part of the ligament to be under tension in all positions of the joint. For convenience the ACL is described as being composed of two bands; an anteromedial which is taut when the knee is flexed, and a posterolateral, which is taut when the knee is extended [7]. From the orientation of the cruciate ligaments it can be seen that they are the main stabilizers of the knee in an antero-posterior direction: the anterior cruciate prevents anterior translation of the tibia on the femur and the posterior cruciate prevents posterior translation of the tibia on the femur. A further important function is to help provide rotatory stability and in particular to act as a check to internal rotation of the tibia.

The medial collateral ligament runs forward and down from the medial femoral condyle to a broad insertion on the subcutaneous border of the tibia, deep to the pes anserinus. The ligament is a fan shaped structure. Its anterior border is straight and easily identifiable, but its posterior border blends with the capsule of the knee joint [8,9]. The lateral collateral ligament is cord-like and is attached to the lateral femoral condyle. It runs down and slightly backwards to insert into the styloid process of the fibula where it blends with the insertion of the biceps femoris tendon. The collateral ligaments, in association with the capsule and the cruciate ligaments, provide varus and valgus stability. They also provide some rotational stability and in particular help to prevent external rotation of the tibia.

The knee gains little stability from the shape of the articular surfaces. The main stabilizers of the joint are the ligaments and the muscles which provide dynamic stability.

The quadriceps muscle consists of the rectus femoris and the three vasti: intermedius, medialis and lateralis. It is the main extensor of the knee and inserts into the patella via the quadriceps tendon (Fig. 9.4). Fibrous expansions from the vastus medialis and lateralis run obliquely to insert into the sides of the patella, the patella tendon and the tibia to form the medial and lateral patellar retinacula [9,10]. The iliotibial band is a thickening of the fascia lata on the lateral aspect of the thigh [11]. Proximally, the tensor fascia lata muscle inserts into it. Its distal insertion is into Gerdy's tubercle on the tibia and more proximally by oblique fibers which blend with the lateral patellar retinaculum. It helps to stabilize the lateral side of the joint and acts as an extensor when the knee is already near full extension. As the knee is flexed the iliotibial band moves backwards behind the center of rotation of the knee and acts as a flexor. The hamstrings are the main flexors of the knee, helped by the gastrocnemius, sartorius and gracilis. Medial rotation of the flexed knee is controlled by the medial hamstrings (semimembranosus and semitendinosus), popliteus, sartorius and gracilis. Lateral rotation is controlled by the biceps femoris alone.

There are a number of bursae around the knee joint, all of which may become inflamed. The bursae in front of the knee are: the prepatellar bursa, which is subcutaneous and lies over the lower half of the patella; the infrapatellar bursa, which lies over the patella tendon and tibial tubercle; and the deep infrapatellar bursa, which separates the patella tendon from the upper tibia. On the medial side the anserine bursa is superficial to the medial collateral ligament and separates it from the tendons of sartorius, gracilis and semitendinosus. The common insertion of these three tendons lies superficial to the medial collateral ligament over the upper tibia and is called the pes anserinus. Other smaller bursae may be present deep to the medial collateral ligament [8]. Bursae lie deep to the semimembranosus and medial head of the gastrocnemius and may enlarge to form a swelling in the popliteal fossa [12]. On the lateral side, bursae may lie deep to the lateral head of gastrocnemius; between the lateral collateral ligament and the biceps femoris; and around the popliteus, separating it from the lateral femoral condyle and the lateral ligament.

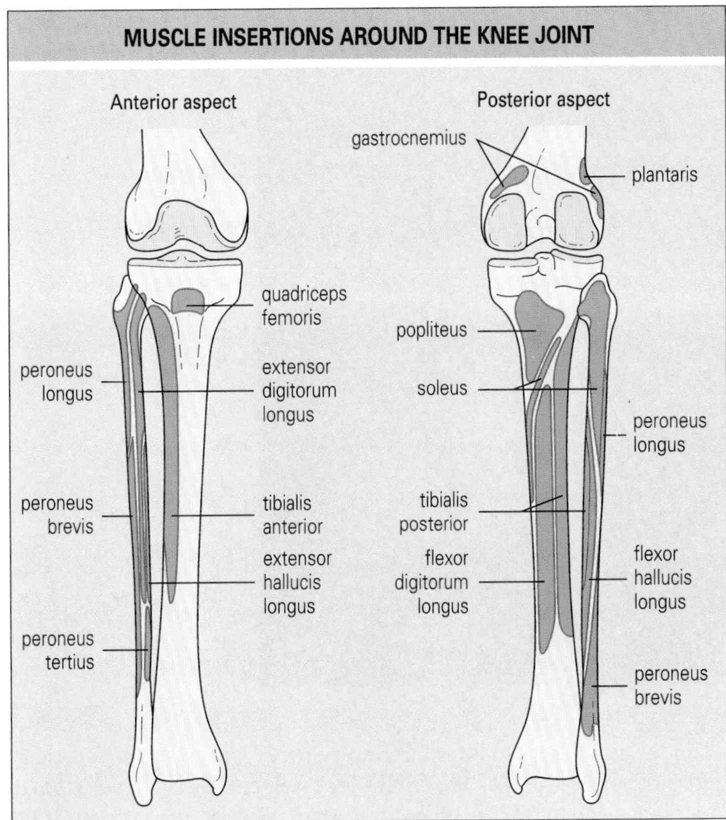

Fig. 9.4 Muscle insertions around the knee joint.

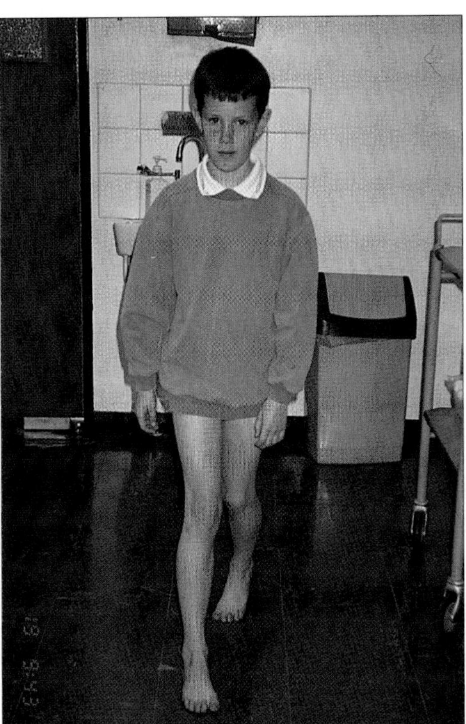

Fig. 9.5 Squinting of the patella caused by persistent femoral anteversion.

HISTORY AND EXAMINATION

The mechanism of the injury and the violence involved should be considered, as these give an indication of the type and severity of the disruption which may have occurred. The length of time an effusion takes to appear following injury is important – an intra-articular swelling that appears within an hour indicates a hemarthrosis, whereas swelling which appears over a period of a few hours indicates an effusion.

The examination of the knee follows the standard pattern of inspection, palpation, and movement [13]. Special tests for stability or meniscal pathology should be performed last. One of the most important aspects of examination of the knee which is often forgotten is to watch the patient standing and walking. It is important not to hurt the patient as this will increase muscle tone and make the rest of the examination more difficult. The examination should be modified in each individual case. Obviously the examination of a 75-year-old lady with rheumatoid arthritis differs from that of a 20-year-old who has a rugby injury.

Inspection

The patient should be asked to stand with the feet a few inches apart. The alignment of the knees and the presence of varus/valgus deformity on weight bearing should be noted. The degree of clinical varus is recorded by measuring the distance between the knees with the feet together and the degree of valgus is recorded by measuring the distance between the medial malleoli with the knees together. A recurvatum deformity is usually obvious on standing and persistent femoral anteversion causes 'squinting' of the patella (Fig. 9.5). The type of gait should be noted with and without aids.

Quadriceps wasting occurs very quickly with disuse, often within a few days. To assess this the patient should be asked to press the knees back into the couch to contract the quadriceps and the tone and bulk should be judged and compared to the other side. The vastus medialis obliquus is often the first part of the muscle to waste. The circumference of the thigh 10cm above the upper pole of the patella should be measured and compared to the other side; this gives an objective measure of thigh wasting. The presence of swellings around the knee should be noted. Swelling within the synovial cavity is seen above the patella and on either side of the patella and patella tendon (Fig. 9.6). A swelling which does not extend above the patella suggests local injury or an enlarged bursa. Inflammation of the pre- or infrapatellar bursae causes a characteristic swelling over the front of the knee. The presence of scars from previous surgery, injury or infection should be noted. Old scars fade and are easily missed, particularly arthroscopy scars which may be very small. They are usually situated on either side of the patella tendon, with another one superolateral to the patella. Bruising over the medial collateral ligament may indicate an injury to that structure and bruising in the calf may indicate rupture of the joint capsule. A swelling over the tibial tubercle in children indicates possible Osgood–Schlatter's disease. Tumors around the knee may present as a swelling particularly in children. Dilated veins over a swelling is an ominous sign, often indicating a neoplastic process.

Palpation

The temperature of the joint should be compared to the other side; a localized increase in temperature suggests an inflammatory process but may also be caused by a recently removed bandage.

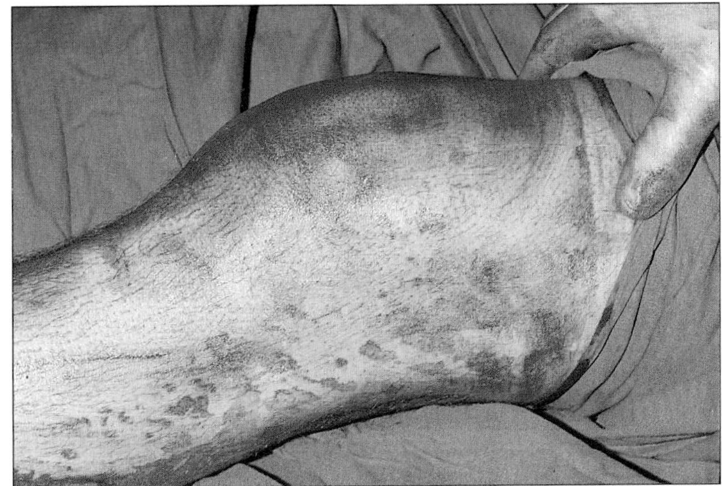

Fig. 9.6 Swelling within the synovial cavity.

With the knee straight the presence of a large effusion or synovial thickening is usually obvious. A large, tense swelling indicates a hemarthrosis or a pyarthrosis. A lax swelling is usually due to an effusion associated with synovitis. Pain may be caused by capsular distension. A small amount of fluid in the knee may be detected by stroking one side of the knee and noting the appearance of a bulge caused by the displaced fluid in the sulcus on the opposite side of the patella. The test can be made more sensitive by pressing over the suprapatellar pouch with one hand to push fluid from there into the joint. On inspection synovial thickening may look like an effusion and often the two coexist. Synovial thickening can be distinguished from an effusion by its characteristic feel: fluid may be displaced and balloted from one side of the joint to the other, while thickened synovium cannot. Although it is possible to aspirate one or two milliliters of fluid from a normal knee, a clinically obvious effusion is always significant. A popliteal cyst may be palpated at the back of the knee and is usually more prominent on extension.

With the knee flexed the following should be palpated: the medial and lateral femoral condyles; the lower pole of the patella; the tibial tubercle; the medial and lateral joint lines; and the course and insertions of the collateral ligaments. Tenderness elicited at these sites suggests different problems depending on the history and age of the patient. In a young patient, tenderness over the medial femoral condyle may indicate osteochondritis dissecans. Tenderness at the lower pole of the patella indicates Sinding-Larsen–Johansson syndrome in a young patient or patellar tendinitis (jumper's knee) in an older patient. Tibial tuberosity tenderness in a young patient suggests Osgood–Schlatter's disease and a tender ossicle may be palpable. Swelling over the lateral joint line may indicate a meniscal cyst or a discoid meniscus. Osteophytes are often palpable along the joint line in osteoarthritis. A tender swelling just below the joint line on the medial side may indicate an inflamed bursa deep to the medial collateral ligament. Tenderness over the joint line after injury suggests a meniscal tear.

Tenderness over the insertions or course of the medial collateral ligament after injury is suggestive of a medial collateral ligament sprain, particularly if associated with localized bruising. The lateral collateral ligament may be palpated in the flexed knee when a varus stress is applied. Swelling and tenderness over its course is suggestive of a sprain.

Movement

With the patient supine the examiner should pick up both legs under the heels. A fixed flexion deformity or hyperextension of the knee will be obvious. A solid block to full extension is usually due to degenerative change and contracture, while a 'springy' block is usually due to a bucket handle tear of the meniscus. In a conscious patient with a medial collateral ligament sprain a block to full extension may be due to pain. The range of active and passive movement should be assessed. The normal range is from zero to approximately 140°, although a little hyperextension is not uncommon, particularly in young girls. The range of movement is best measured with a goniometer. The extensor mechanism should be assessed by asking the patient to extend the knee against resistance. Rupture of the quadriceps or patellar tendons or fracture of the patella causes inability to extend the knee. The patient may still be able to straight leg raise due to the action of the iliotibial band and intact retinacular fibers; extension should therefore begin from a flexed position.

Sitting on the edge of the couch the patient should actively flex and extend the knee. Crepitus may be felt during this movement. Tracking of the patella may be assessed by placing the thumb and forefinger on the patella. It may be seen to subluxate laterally on flexion in a patient with recurrent dislocation or subluxation. A small high patella (patella alta) (Fig. 9.7) may be noted and predisposes to recurrent dislocation.

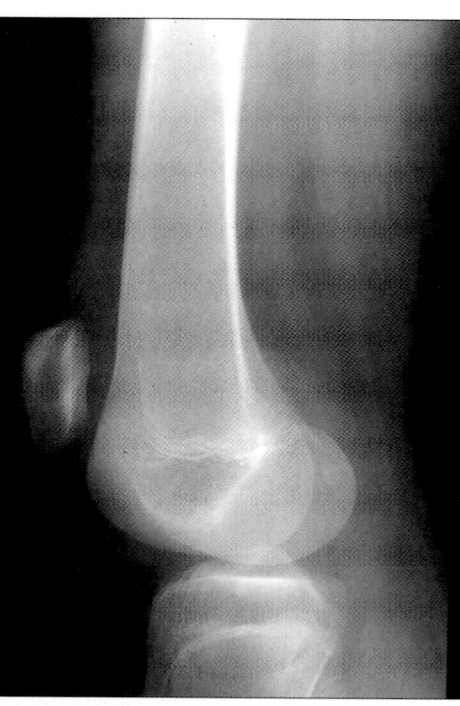

Fig. 9.7 Radiographic appearance of patella alta.

The foot pulses should be palpated routinely, particularly in a patient under consideration for knee joint replacement. Finally every knee examination should finish with examination of the hip, as it is common, particularly in children, for hip pathology to present with knee pain.

THE DIFFERENTIAL DIAGNOSIS OF KNEE PAIN

Pain is the commonest presenting symptom of knee pathology. It may arise from within the knee joint itself, from periarticular structures or be referred from a distant site – usually the hip. Pain may also be referred from a femoral tumor or from the spine. The causes of knee pain tend to be age related and one convenient way to classify them is by age group and whether the pain is intra-articular, periarticular or referred (Fig. 9.8).

Childhood

Pain in the knee in this age group (2–10 years) is uncommon but is always significant. Intra-articular causes include a torn discoid lateral meniscus and osteochondritis dissecans. Inflammatory causes include pauciarticular juvenile chronic arthritis and septic arthritis. Periarticular causes are osteomyelitis of the lower femur or upper tibia and, at the upper end of the age group, Osgood–Schlatter's disease and Sinding-Larsen–Johansson syndrome. Referred pain may come from the hip due to Perthe's disease.

Adolescence

Knee pain is common in adolescence (10–18 years). Intra-articular causes are usually related to osteochondritis dissecans or tears involving a discoid lateral meniscus. In girls the anterior knee pain syndrome and patellar maltracking are the most common causes of pain. Inflammatory causes are pauciarticular juvenile chronic arthritis and septic arthritis. Periarticular pain is usually due to traction apophysitis – Osgood–Schlatter's or Sinding-Larsen–Johansson syndrome. Tumors around the knee cause aching pain. Anteroposterior (AP) and lateral views of the femur and hip, and a bone scan, should be performed in cases of knee pain for which no cause can be found. Slipped upper femoral epiphysis in boys frequently presents with knee pain and a limp and is common in this age group. The hip should be carefully examined as loss of internal rotation is an early sign of slipped upper femoral epiphysis.

COMMON CAUSES OF KNEE PAIN IN DIFFERENT AGE GROUPS

Age group	Cause: Intra-articular	Periarticular	Referred
Childhood (2–10 years)	Juvenile chronic arthritis Osteochondritis dissecans Septic arthritis Torn discoid lateral meniscus	Osteomyelitis	Perthe's disease Transient synovitis of the hip
Adolescence (10–18 years)	Osteochondritis dissecans Torn meniscus Anterior knee pain syndrome Patellar malalignment	Osgood–Schlatter's disease Sinding-Larsen–Johansson syndrome Osteomyelitis Tumours	Slipped upper femoral epiphysis
Early adulthood (18–30 years)	Torn meniscus Instability Anteroir knee pain syndrome Inflammatory conditions	Overuse syndromes Bursitis	Rare
Adulthood (30–50 years)	Degenerate meniscal tears Early degeneration following injury or meniscectomy Inflammatory arthropathies	Bursitis Tendinitis	Degenerative hip disease secondary to hip dysplasia or injury
Older age (>50 years)	Osteoarthritis Inflammatory arthropathies	Bursitis Tendinitis	Osteoarthritis of the hip

Fig. 9.8 Common causes of knee pain in different age groups.

If this is suspected, AP and lateral radiographs of the hip should be performed.

Early Adulthood

The most common cause of knee pain in this age group (18–30 years) is injury. Intra-articular causes include meniscal tears and pain associated with instability following a ligamentous injury. In females the anterior knee pain syndrome is still frequent. Inflammatory joint conditions such as Reiter's disease and ankylosing spondylitis (see Chapter 19) may occur. Periarticular causes include the overuse syndromes such as jumper's knee. Referred pain in this age group is relatively rare.

Adulthood

In this age group (30–50 years) intra-articular causes of knee pain include degenerative meniscal lesions and post-traumatic degenerative change. Inflammatory conditions, such as rheumatoid arthritis and gout are relatively common. Periarticular causes include bursitis and tendinitis. Referred pain may be secondary to early degenerative disease in the hip due to untreated congenital dislocation, Perthe's disease or fracture.

Older age

Degenerative disease is the most common cause of knee pain in those aged over 50 years. The knee is affected by osteoarthritis more commonly than any other joint. The pain is associated with stiffness and swelling especially after activity. Loose bodies secondary to the degeneration may cause episodes of sharp pain associated with locking of the joint. Periarticular causes include bursitis and tendinitis. Referred pain in this age group is usually secondary to osteoarthritis of the hip.

SPECIFIC DISORDERS

Bursitis

Inflammation of the bursae around the knee is common and on occasion may cause diagnostic difficulty. An accurate knowledge of the anatomical sites of the bursae is helpful.

Prepatellar bursitis

Prepatellar bursitis is common. The condition is related to recurrent trauma and is seen most often in people who spend a lot of time kneeling, such as carpet fitters and, in earlier times, housemaids (hence the eponym, housemaid's knee). Diagnosis is usually obvious with a hot, red, well circumscribed and fluctuant swelling over the front of the patella. The skin in the area is often thickened. Although the bursa may look infected, in most cases it is not. The inflammation may be related to inflammatory arthritis or crystal arthropathy. The majority of cases settle with rest and avoidance of kneeling. Occasionally aspiration is necessary, in which case the aspirate should be sent for microscopy and culture. Re-accumulation is common and the process may have to be repeated. Recurrent episodes of inflammation may require surgical excision of the bursa. Infection may be secondary to a penetrating wound. Treatment is by rest, antibiotics and drainage if necessary.

Infrapatellar bursitis

The common term for this condition is Parson's knee. The presentation and treatment are the same as for prepatellar bursitis.

Anserine bursitis

The term anserine bursitis tends to be used loosely to describe pain over the medial aspect of the upper tibia in the region of the anserine bursa. While inflammation of the bursa may be the origin of the pain, it may also arise from the medial ligament or pes anserinus insertion, and the exact anatomical site may be impossible to identify. The conditions of anserine bursitis, medial ligament syndrome and pes anserinus tendinitis may therefore be impossible to separate. Treatment is initially by rest and nonsteroidal anti-inflammatory drugs (NSAIDs). In persistent cases injection of a small amount of steroid into the painful area is usually curative.

Bursae on the lateral side of the knee deep to the iliotibial band and the lateral ligament may occasionally become inflamed and cause symptoms.

Tendinitis

The insertions of the tendons around the knee may become inflamed due to overuse or in association with an inflammatory arthropathy. It may be difficult to differentiate tendinitis from the medial ligament syndrome and bursal inflammation.

Patellar tendinitis (Jumper's knee)

Patellar tendinitis [14] is a condition which most commonly affects young sportsmen but may also affect older patients. The symptoms are of pain at the inferior pole of the patella which is brought on by activity, particularly climbing stairs, running and jumping. The condition is due to mucoid degeneration of the patellar tendon at its insertion into the inferior pole of the patella. The majority of cases respond to rest and NSAIDs. For those that do not, injection of a small amount of steroid (0.2ml) into the tender area is usually helpful. A larger volume should not be injected, since necrosis of the tendon can occur. Occasionally, operative treatment to excise the involved portion of tendon is necessary.

Pes anserinus tendinitis

The pes anserinus insertion may become inflamed but this may be indistinguishable clinically from anserine bursitis and the medial ligament syndrome. In cases of overuse, rest is usually curative but in persistent cases a small amount of steroid injected into the point of maximum tenderness is usually curative.

Popliteus tendinitis

This is also an overuse injury which causes pain over the lateral aspect of the joint. It is caused by inflammation of the popliteus tendon and paratenon as it passes beneath the arcuate ligament complex. Symptoms usually settle with rest and NSAIDs.

Iliotibial Band Friction Syndrome (Runner's Knee)

This occurs in runners and is due to overuse [15]. It tends to occur in patients with genu varum and planus feet. The symptoms are of pain over the lateral epicondyle of the femur during running and are thought to be due to friction between the iliotibial band and the femur and may be due to an inflamed bursa. Tenderness is found over the lateral epicondyle. The symptoms usually settle with rest but in resistant cases a steroid injection into the tender site may help.

Medial Ligament Syndrome

This is an ill defined syndrome in which the patient complains of pain at the site of insertion of the medial ligament. Examination reveals tenderness over the insertion of the ligament, and valgus stress may exacerbate the pain. It is more common in females than males and is associated with valgus knees and the pain amplification syndrome. As stated previously it may be difficult to differentiate from anserine bursitis and pes anserinus tendinitis. The etiology is obscure but in some cases an inflammatory arthropathy, such as ankylosing spondylitis, is present. Treatment is initially conservative with rest and heat. Persistent symptoms usually settle following injection of a small amount of steroid into the painful area.

Pellegrini–Stieda Disease

Following an injury to the medial collateral ligament the patient presents with pain over the femoral insertion particularly on activity. The area is tender to palpation and pain is elicited on stressing the ligament. Radiographs reveal characteristic calcification at the ligament insertion [16] (Fig. 9.9). The condition is most likely due to calcification of a hematoma following injury to the femoral insertion of the medial collateral ligament. Treatment consists of rest and NSAIDs, since the condition is usually self-limiting. Occasionally a small amount of steroid injected into the area will help resolve persistent cases.

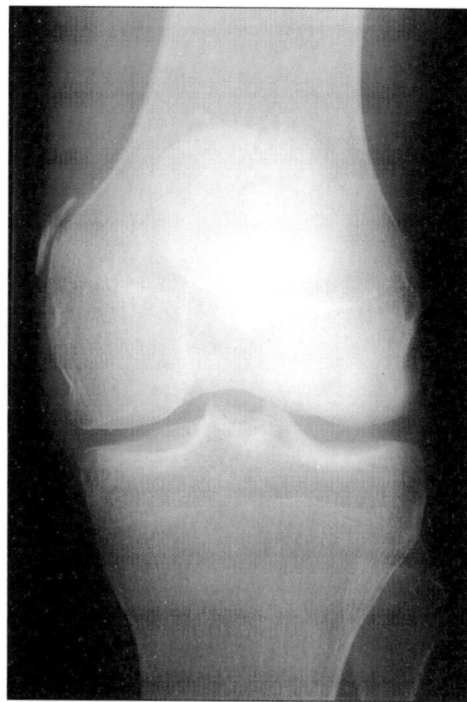

Fig. 9.9 Radiograph showing calcification of the insertion of the medial collateral ligament.

Popliteal Cysts and Swelling

Swellings occurring in the popliteal region are common and should be called popliteal cysts regardless of where they originate [12]. They may occur at any age from childhood onwards. They communicate with the knee joint in about two thirds of cases. Approximately 60% arise from bursae and 30% from synovial herniation through the posterior capsule of the joint. Approximately 10% are of indeterminate origin. The bursal cysts most commonly arise from the bursa deep to the semimembranosus on the medial side of the popliteal fossa. The hernial cysts arise most commonly from the medial side. The presenting complaint is usually of a swelling at the back of the knee. The swelling may be associated with aching and is more prominent when the knee is extended. The cysts often transilluminate. In children there is usually no other abnormality found on examination of the knee but in adults the cysts are associated with rheumatoid arthritis and osteoarthritis. Plain radiographs may show a soft tissue swelling, and double contrast arthrography will confirm the diagnosis in those that communicate with the joint. Ultrasound is a reliable method of differentiating cysts from aneurysms and solid swellings. Computer tomographic (CT) scanning is useful, particularly where the diagnosis is in doubt and for preoperative planning. The differential diagnosis includes popliteal artery aneurysm, and solid tumors such as osteochondroma. Occasionally a nerve sheath ganglion or a muscle tumor may cause difficulty with diagnosis. Popliteal cysts may become very large due to a valve effect of the opening into the joint, particularly in rheumatoid arthritis. If they burst they may simulate a deep vein thrombosis. The signs in the calf are similar but differentiation can usually be made due to a history of a swelling in the popliteal fossa and the sudden onset of pain, often with a sensation of water running down the leg. An arthrogram in the early stages will differentiate the two if there is doubt.

Treatment in children should be conservative, as the cysts commonly decrease in size spontaneously and those which are operated on have a high recurrence rate. Treatment in adults should be aimed at the underlying pathology. A large cyst which is causing pain or interfering with knee movement should be excised, although marsupialization and drainage into the calf is an alternative. Aspiration and injection of steroid solution may be performed but reaccumulation is frequent.

Synovial Chondromatosis

Synovial chondromatosis is a rare condition of unknown etiology in which multiple metaplastic foci of cartilage develop in joints, tendon sheaths and bursae. It occurs due to metaplasia in the subsynovial connective tissue. The cartilaginous bodies may become pedunculated or loose in the joint (Fig. 9.10). The knee is by far the most

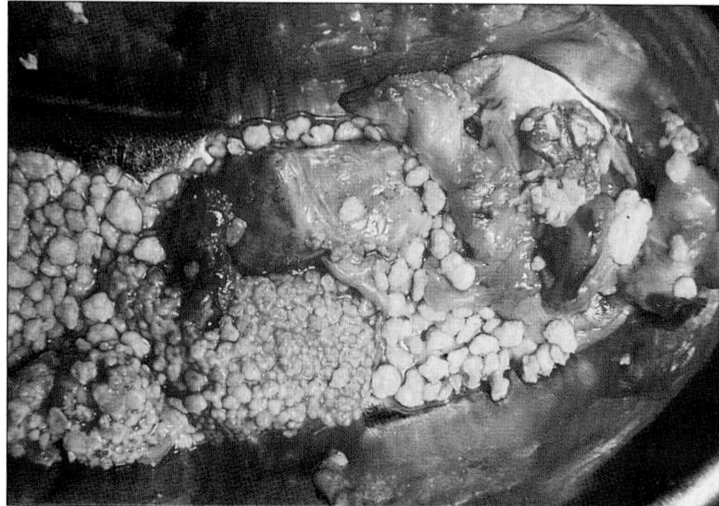

Fig. 9.10 Synovial chondromatosis. Cartilaginous bodies in the joint.

common joint affected by both intra-articular and extra-articular disease. Milgram [17] classified the disease into three phases: early, with active intrasynovial disease but no loose bodies; transitional, with active intrasynovial disease and loose bodies; and late, with multiple loose bodies but no synovial disease. The condition tends to occur in middle age but may present in the late teens. Pain is the usual presenting feature, commonly associated with swelling. Locking may be a feature when the lesions are loose or pedunculated. Examination reveals a swollen knee with thickened synovium, crepitus on movement and palpable loose bodies. In the later stages the range of motion may be decreased. Radiographs in the early stages may show multiple, stippled cartilaginous bodies. Double contrast arthrography is useful. In the later stages of the disease when the lesions have calcified they become more obvious on plain radiographs. Treatment of symptomatic disease involves arthroscopy or arthrotomy and removal of symptomatic loose bodies. In the first and second phases of disease the active synovium should be excised. Total synovectomy is impractical and unnecessary. Recurrence is only likely with generalized active disease, in which case a second arthrotomy may be necessary. The condition tends to resolve with time [17,18].

Pigmented Villonodular Synovitis

This condition, which tends to affect young adults, is characterized by a proliferative synovial reaction. The synovium becomes nodular and brown in color. The etiology of the condition is unknown. The knee joint is the most commonly affected joint. The presenting complaint is usually of pain and swelling. Locking may occur if the proliferative synovium becomes trapped between the joint surfaces. Examination reveals a swollen joint with thickened synovium and limitation of movement. Radiographs show lytic bone lesions and soft tissue swelling. Double contrast arthrography shows multiple filling defects in the synovium, which are diagnostic. On arthroscopy thickened nodular synovium which is reddish brown in color is seen. Histological examination shows a stroma of reticulin and collagen fibers with multinucleate giant cells, foam cells and hemosiderin deposits. Treatment is by synovectomy, preferably arthroscopic. This may need to be repeated as the disease is liable to recur. Marked bone destruction can occur and may require radiation therapy in extreme cases [19].

THE KNEE JOINT IN CHILDHOOD AND ADOLESCENCE

Children and adolescents experience a different spectrum of knee problems than adults. Knee pain is common and must be differentiated from pain arising in the hip from Perthe's disease or from slipped upper femoral epiphysis. It is therefore mandatory to examine the hip in every child with knee pain. Occasionally tumors of the femur may present with knee pain. If doubt exists, radiographs of the hip and femur should be obtained.

Osteochondritis Dissecans

Osteochondritis dissecans occurs most commonly in the knee joint. A fragment of cartilage with its underlying subchondral bone becomes detached and may become loose in the joint. Boys are affected more commonly than girls. The second decade is the usual time for presentation but it may occur earlier.

The symptoms are usually of an aching pain which occurs during and after activity. Clicking and giving way may occur. An antalgic gait may be present. There is often a mild effusion and tenderness over the site of the lesion. Wasting of the quadriceps is an early sign. If the fragment separates, symptoms of locking occur and a loose body may be palpable, usually in the suprapatellar pouch. Wilson's sign may be positive. The test involves straightening the internally rotated knee from a flexed position – pain at 30° of flexion which is relieved by externally rotating the tibia is said to be diagnostic of osteochondritis dissecans [20].

The etiology is unclear but the condition is associated with short stature, epiphyseal abnormalities and a positive family history. It is likely that vascular impairment, possibly associated with a traumatic initial event, is responsible for the lesions. Approximately 40% of patients give a history of injury [21,22]. The pathological changes which occur are avascular necrosis of the bone and degenerative changes in the overlying cartilage, with softening, fibrillation and fissuring.

The lesions occur most commonly on the lateral aspect of the medial femoral condyle but may also affect the posterior aspect of the lateral condyle, the trochlea and the patella. Abnormalities of ossification also occur in these sites and may be mistaken for osteochondritis dissecans.

Osteochondritic lesions of the condyles can often be seen on AP and lateral radiographs but are best seen on a tunnel view. The radiographic appearance is diagnostic, showing a well circumscribed fragment of subchondral bone (see Fig. 9.11). If the fragment has become detached an irregularity is seen at the site. CT scanning and magnetic resonance imaging (MRI) are useful to confirm the diagnosis and to define the extent of the lesion. In cases of doubt a bone scan may be useful to differentiate osteochondritis dissecans from abnormalities of ossification. A hot spot around the lesion confirms active disease, the uptake decreases with healing of the lesion [23].

Treatment of the undisplaced fragment in the younger child is rest and avoidance of activities which may injure the knee until the lesion is healed. Long term immobilization should be avoided and isometric quadriceps and hamstring exercises should be performed

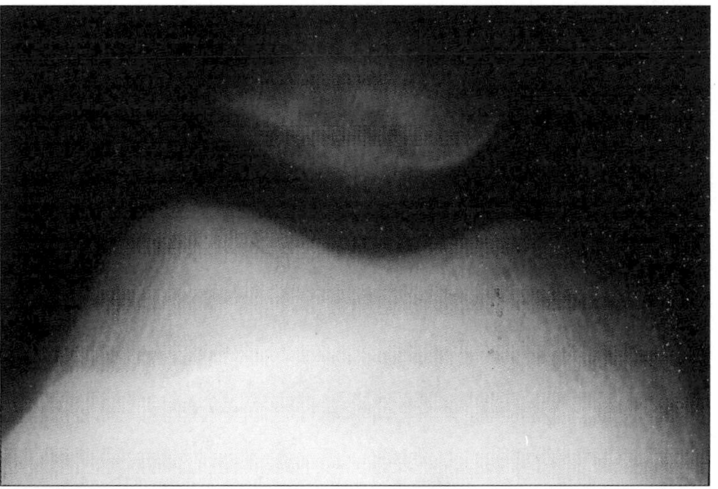

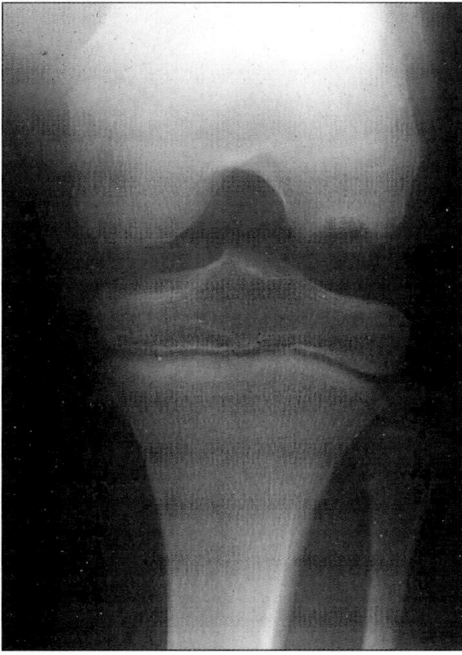

Fig. 9.11 Radiographic appearance of condylar osteochondritic lesions.

to prevent muscle wasting. Treatment of the older child follows the same lines but if the symptoms persist or if the fragment appears to be loosening, arthroscopic assessment should be undertaken and the fragment debrided and drilled if necessary. Loose fragments should be fixed if they are large. This may be performed open or arthroscopically using fine K-wires or Herbert screws. Smaller fragments loose in the joint should be removed arthroscopically. The defect which is left should be debrided and will fill with fibrocartilage. The prognosis is better in younger patients before skeletal maturity in whom the fragment does not separate.

Osgood–Schlatter's Disease

Osgood–Schlatter's disease is a traction apophysitis of the tibial tuberosity [24,25]. It occurs most commonly in those aged 10–14 years and is associated with overuse. The patients present complaining of pain over the tibial tuberosity particularly on activity. The clinical findings are of tenderness over the tibial tuberosity which is often enlarged (Fig. 9.12).

Lateral radiographs show characteristic fragmentation of the tibial tubercle, and there may be a loose ossicle. The symptoms usually respond to rest and disappear at the time of fusion of the tibial tuberosity. Occasionally a loose ossicle may remain and cause symptoms which necessitate removal (Fig. 9.13).

Sinding-Larsen–Johansson Syndrome

This is a condition similar to Osgood–Schlatter's disease occurring at the distal pole of the patella. It is a traction apophysitis and is related to overuse [26]. The patient complains of pain at the distal pole of the patella on activity. This area is tender and radiographs show fragmentation (Fig. 9.14). The condition responds to rest but may persist into adolescence as jumper's knee.

Patellofemoral Disorders

Disorders of the patellofemoral joint are common in children and adolescents.

Congenital dislocation

Congenital dislocation occurs in infancy and involves irreducible lateral displacement of the patella [27]. It is associated with genu valgum, a small patella, hypoplasia of the lateral femoral condyle and tethering of the lateral capsule. Treatment is surgical to release the tight lateral structures and realign the patella.

Habitual dislocation

In habitual dislocation lateral displacement of the patella occurs every time the knee is flexed. It is due to contracture of the vastus lateralis and iliotibial band with an abnormal insertion of the iliotibial band into the patella [28]. Because of this lateral contracture the patella must dislocate to allow the knee to flex. The constant physical sign is an inability to flex the knee when the patella is held reduced. Treatment is usually surgical and involves proximal realignment of the quadriceps mechanism by releasing the contracted lateral structures and if necessary lengthening the rectus femoris.

Recurrent dislocation and subluxation

Recurrent dislocation and subluxation of the patella are conditions in which intermittent episodes of dislocation or subluxation occur and may be grouped together under the heading of patella instability. It is common in adolescence, particularly in girls, but may also occur in younger children. It is associated with a variety of developmental abnormalities. These include generalized or localized joint laxity, patella alta and hypoplasia of the lateral femoral condyle. Genu-valgum, external tibial torsion and persistent femoral anteversion increase the Q angle and predispose to patella instability.

In adolescence patella instability may follow an acute traumatic dislocation or occur spontaneously [29]. In acute dislocation the patient describes the patella dislocating laterally and may reduce it by pushing it back. Examination in the acute phase reveals a painful swollen knee with obvious lateral dislocation of the patella. If the patella has already been reduced the chief findings are of tenderness over the torn medial retinaculum associated with knee swelling. Acute dislocation may be associated with an osteochondral fracture of the lateral femoral condyle. Treatment in the acute phase is by immobilization in a plaster cylinder for 4 weeks, which allows the torn retinacular fibers to heal, followed by an isometric exercise program to restore the power of the quadriceps, particularly the vastus medialis obliquus.

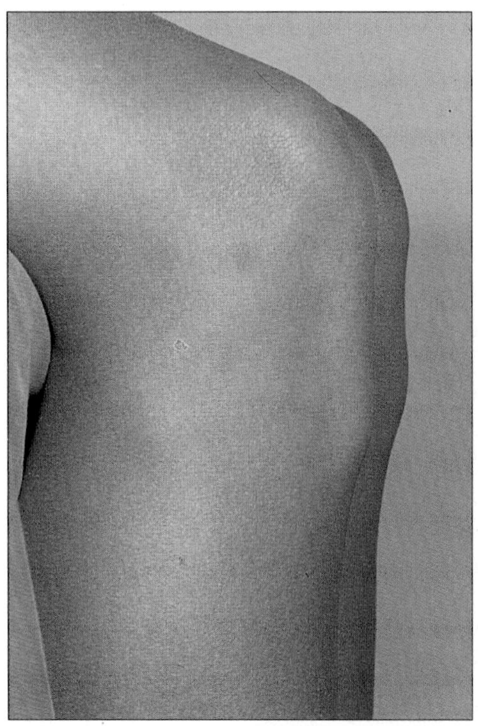

Fig. 9.12 Osgood–Schlatter's disease. Enlarged tibial tuberosity.

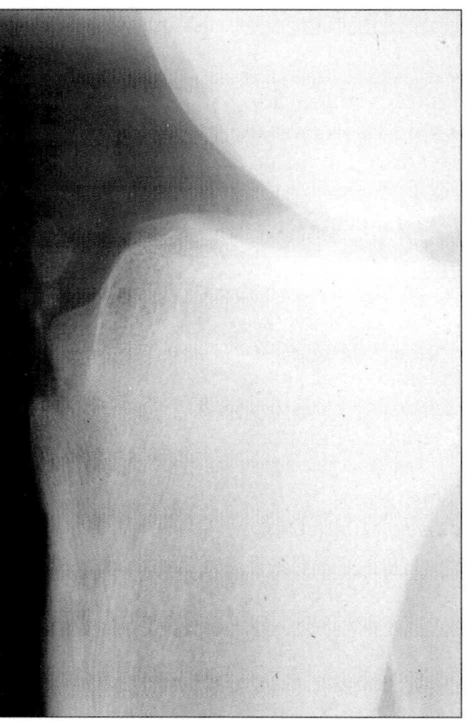

Fig. 9.13 Osgood–Schlatter's disease. Loose ossicle.

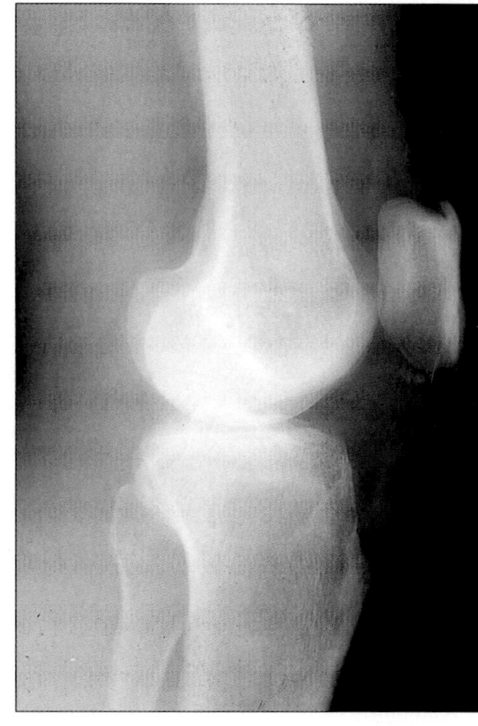

Fig. 9.14 Sinding-Larsen–Johansson syndrome. Radiograph showing fragmentation of the patella.

In the chronic phase the diagnosis of recurrent dislocation is straightforward. The patient is usually an adolescent girl describing episodes of lateral dislocation of the patella, which either reduce spontaneously or which she pushes back. The episodes usually occur during activities which involve knee flexion but in severe cases may occur during everyday activities.

Recurrent subluxation of the patella is more common than dislocation and is caused by the same factors, but the diagnosis may be more difficult to make. The patient often complains of a feeling of instability as the patella rides up on the lateral femoral condyle, and the knee may give way. Pain is due to compression of the lateral facet of the patella against the lateral femoral condyle. Pseudo-locking due to pain is common. The majority of cases are secondary to weakness of the vastus medialis obliquus associated with bony malalignment.

Examination may reveal any of the anatomical abnormalities mentioned above, and the patella may be found to track laterally on flexion of the knee. In the majority of adolescent girls with this condition there is poor muscle tone in the quadriceps, particularly the vastus medialis, and the Q angle may be increased due to the factors mentioned earlier [6]. Patellar tracking should be assessed clinically, as described in the section on examination. The apprehension test is usually positive in recurrent subluxation and dislocation. This is performed with the knee flexed to 30° and the examiner gently pushes the patella laterally. A positive test occurs when the patient feels as though the patella is going to dislocate and occasionally will push the examiner's hand away. In some girls with a small high patella the patella may be seen to sit laterally in full extension.

Lateral and AP views of the knee are useful to look for femorotibial malalignment, osteochondral fractures and patella alta. Patella alta is recognized on the lateral view by comparing the length of the patella to the length of the patella tendon. In normal knees the ratio is 1. In patella alta the patella is relatively short compared to the tendon and the ratio is less than 0.8 [30]. Sky-line views of the patella with the knee flexed 30–40° may show it to be tilted laterally and to ride high on the lateral femoral condyle. A variety of special views and measurements have been described to quantify the degree of subluxation or tilting. The patella should sit centrally in the trochlea with an equal joint space medially and laterally. The skyline views may show it to be tilted laterally with a narrower joint space on the lateral side. Occasionally, sclerosis may be seen in the subchondral bone of the lateral facet indicating increased stress through it. The angle formed by the lateral facet of the patella and a line drawn across the femoral condyles is called the lateral patellofemoral angle and should be open laterally. If the lines are parallel or the angle is open medially this suggests patella malalignment [31]. Unfortunately, radiographic findings such as these are common in the asymptomatic population and should only be taken as significant in conjunction with the clinical picture.

Recurrent dislocation or subluxation of the patella should initially be managed conservatively with isometric quadriceps and hamstring exercises [32]. Most patients will respond to conservative management provided they continue the exercises. Unfortunately many do not and the resultant weakening of the quadriceps may lead to recurrence. In the compliant patients who do not respond to conservative treatment, surgery is usually necessary as the condition can be disabling. An arthroscopic lateral release may be tried if there is a tight lateral tether but open surgery to realign the patella may be necessary.

Anterior Knee Pain Syndrome

Pain arising from the anterior aspect of the knee joint is common in adolescence. Specific conditions, such as patella malalignment, osteochondritis dissecans, Osgood–Schlatter's disease and trauma, may be responsible. However, there is a group of patients in whom no cause for the pain can be found, despite careful investigation. It is this idiopathic condition which should be called anterior knee pain syndrome. It usually occurs in adolescent girls and is commonly bilateral. The patient complains of pain in the anterior aspect of the joint around the patella. It may be present during sporting activity and necessitate its cessation. The pain is often present at night and may wake the patient from sleep. In the past these patients have been wrongly labelled as having 'chondromalacia patellae'.

Many adolescent girls with anterior knee pain tend to have an increased Q angle and poor quadriceps strength but no demonstrable patella instability or malalignment. Wearing high-heeled shoes may be a cause as the patient walks with a crouched gait, putting increased load on the patellofemoral joint. Tight hamstrings have been implicated for the same reason and some of these patients have limitation of straight leg raising. The condition is self limiting in the majority of cases and usually settles in early adulthood. Treatment is conservative and involves isometric quadriceps strengthening exercises and hamstring stretching exercises. Wearing high-heeled shoes should be avoided. Arthroscopy may occasionally be indicated to exclude intra-articular pathology. Empirical lateral release should be avoided.

Chondromalacia Patellae

A diagnosis of chondromalacia patellae means softening of the articular cartilage of the patella and can only be made at arthroscopy or arthrotomy. It is a pathological diagnosis and should not be used to describe the clinical syndrome of pain arising from the anterior knee joint. However, patients with anterior knee pain may be found to have chondromalacia patellae. It may be associated with patellar malalignment, in which case it is probably due to impact loading and shearing of the articular cartilage as the patella is compressed against the lateral femoral condyle. Articular cartilage is poor at resisting shear forces, and repetitive impact loading and shear may both be shown to produce cartilage softening. The majority of cases associated with malalignment respond to correction of the underlying abnormality provided cartilage loss has not occurred. Idiopathic chondromalacia patellae usually responds to the conservative measures of isometric quadriceps exercises and hamstring stretching.

Bipartite Patella

Bipartite patella occurs when the ossification centers of the patella fail to fuse. The defect is seen as a lucent line usually at the superolateral corner of the patella where it may be mistaken for a fracture. Occasionally the synchondrosis may fracture as a result of repetitive stress and cause pain and tenderness. Rest in a cricket pad splint is usually curative.

Plica Syndrome

Embryologically, the knee is divided into three synovial compartments which break down in the fourth intrauterine month. Failure of complete breakdown leaves synovial shelves or plicae. Pain arising from these is termed the plica syndrome. The infrapatellar plica (ligamentum mucosum) is the most common but does not usually become inflamed or cause pain. The suprapatellar plica is a remnant of the membrane which separates the suprapatellar pouch from the rest of the knee. This may be virtually complete, with only a small foramen or it may be seen as a crescentic fold [33]. It occasionally causes symptoms if it becomes inflamed. The medial patellar plica runs along the medial wall of the joint from the suprapatellar pouch to the infrapatellar fold. It is the most frequently symptomatic, becoming inflamed due to impingement as it passes over the medial femoral condyle. Occasionally it may be large and cover the medial femoral condyle. The medial patellar plica is the great imitator of symptoms in the knee and can be a diagnostic problem. It may present with pain, typically over the medial femoral condyle, but this may be generalized. A snapping sensation or giving way is also common. The diagnosis may be made clinically by palpating a tender thickened band over the medial femoral condyle, but commonly it is made at arthroscopy when an inflamed plica may be seen to impinge on the medial femoral condyle. If arthroscopy reveals a noninflamed plica the diagnosis of plica syndrome must then be in doubt but is often still made. Treatment is initially rest but the plica may need to be resected arthroscopically [34].

Meniscal Lesions and Discoid Meniscus in Children

Meniscal tears in children are uncommon due to the resilience of the fibrocartilage. When they occur they should be treated similarly to those in adults, leaving as much stable rim as possible. Cysts of the menisci usually arise from the lateral meniscus. Unlike cysts in adults they are rarely associated with a tear. They present as a swelling on the joint line, are of no functional consequence but may be removed for cosmetic reasons.

Discoid menisci usually occur on the lateral side of the joint and may affect both knees. They are normally asymptomatic unless they tear. However, a patient with an intact discoid meniscus can present with intermittent swelling over the lateral joint line or clicking in the knee. On examination the swelling may be palpated and a clunk felt on knee extension. The reasons for the formation of a discoid meniscus are unclear. It was initially thought to be due to persistence of the embryonic form but further studies have shown that this is unlikely, as the menisci are not discoid at any stage in development. No other theories satisfactorily explain their etiology. The diagnosis may be confirmed by double contrast arthrography or arthroscopy. Torn discoid menisci in children should be treated conservatively if possible, or by arthroscopic resection of the torn middle portion leaving a stable rim. A discoid meniscus found coincidentally at arthroscopy should be left.

Septic Arthritis and Osteomyelitis

Septic arthritis of the knee in children is relatively common. The infection is usually blood-borne but may occur after a puncture wound. The patient complains of severe pain on even the slightest movement and is generally unwell with a tensely swollen knee and a pyrexia. Treatment with appropriate antibiotics and thorough arthroscopic washout should be commenced as soon as the diagnosis is suspected. Aspiration of pus for culture should be performed at the same time to confirm the diagnosis. Arthroscopic washout is more efficient than arthrotomy and may need to be repeated. Arthrotomy is required if loculi have formed which cannot be broken down arthroscopically. The differential diagnosis includes other inflammatory processes such as juvenile chronic arthritis and nonspecific synovitis.

Acute hematogenous osteomyelitis commonly affects the lower femoral and upper tibial metaphyses. The diagnosis is clinical with tenderness over the area and is supported by an increased white cell count and ESR. Radiographic changes may take a number of days to appear. A sympathetic effusion may be present in the knee joint.

KNEE INJURIES

Meniscal Injuries

The meniscus in the young is a resilient fibrocartilaginous structure. With age and degenerative change it loses this resilience and becomes stiffer. Thus, different types of meniscal injury are seen in different age groups.

Meniscal injuries are common in young adults, usually occurring secondary to sporting trauma and often in combination with ligamentous injury (particularly ACL rupture). Meniscal injuries are also associated with chronic instability. The mechanism of the injury is usually a twisting force applied to the weight-bearing knee, causing entrapment of the meniscus between the tibial and femoral condyles. The resulting tear is usually longitudinal. If the tear is extensive the inner portion may displace into the joint causing the knee to lock (a bucket handle tear) (Fig. 9.15). This locking may be intermittent as the torn portion flips in and out of the joint. A tear may extend to the inner margin of the meniscus forming a 'parrot beak' tear. The flap formed can displace into the joint causing intermittent locking. Peripheral meniscal detachment may also occur. In the older age group, where the meniscus is less elastic, degenerative tears can occur [35]. These tears are usually horizontal cleavage tears or radial tears running into the substance of the meniscus.

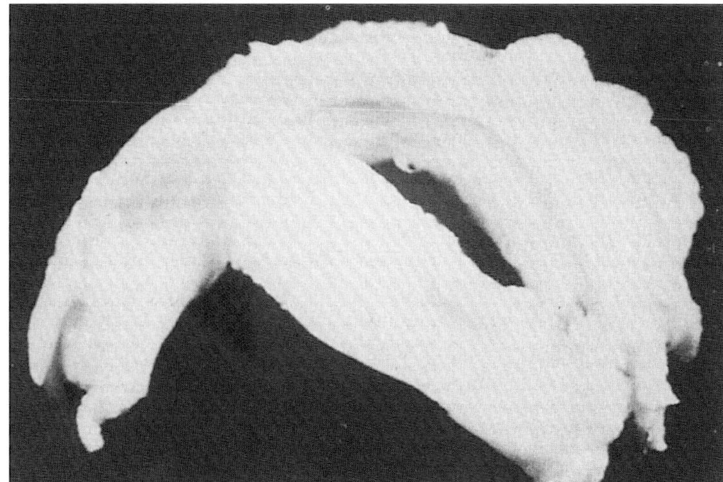

Fig. 9.15 Bucket handle tear of the meniscus.

The history of an acute meniscal tear in a young adult is often characteristic. A twisting injury occurs causing immediate severe pain. The patient is unable to weight bear and may be unable to fully extend the knee if a bucket handle tear has lodged in the joint. The knee swells within several hours. If a cruciate ligament rupture is also present a hemarthrosis will accumulate within an hour. The patient complains of pain well localized to the joint line. Examination reveals a painful knee with tenderness over the joint line adjacent to the tear. An effusion is virtually always present and if the torn portion has displaced into the joint, a springy block to full extension is felt.

In a chronic tear the patient may complain of pain over the joint line and a feeling of 'catching'. Joint line tenderness is usually present. True locking occurs when the torn portion of the meniscus displaces into the joint causing loss of full extension. Locking due to a meniscal tear always occurs with the knee flexed, although not necessarily weight bearing. Examination of a knee locked due to a meniscal tear reveals a springy block to extension; forced extension is painful. Flexion is usually full or only mildly reduced due to pain. Patients often confuse locking with stiffness and it is important to distinguish between the two. If the knee unlocks with a click or a clunk it is suggestive of a meniscal tear. McMurray's test [36] is widely used to diagnose meniscal tears. The test involves flexing and extending the knee while the tibia is first internally rotated and then externally rotated, with the thumb and fingers over the joint line. Pain and an associated click are said to be diagnostic of a meniscal tear. Apley's grinding test [37] is performed with the patient prone and the knee flexed. Downward pressure is exerted on the tibia while it is internally and externally rotated. Pain or a clicking sensation are said to be suggestive of a meniscal tear. However, these tests are not specific.

While the majority of acute and chronic meniscal injuries can be diagnosed on the history and examination, confirmation may be obtained by arthrography, MRI or arthroscopy (Fig. 9.16). Recently MRI has been found to be accurate, but, if the tear is symptomatic, arthroscopy is preferable as it can be excised at the same time (Fig. 9.17).

The treatment of a symptomatic meniscal tear in a young adult depends on the site of the tear. If the tear is peripheral, in the outer

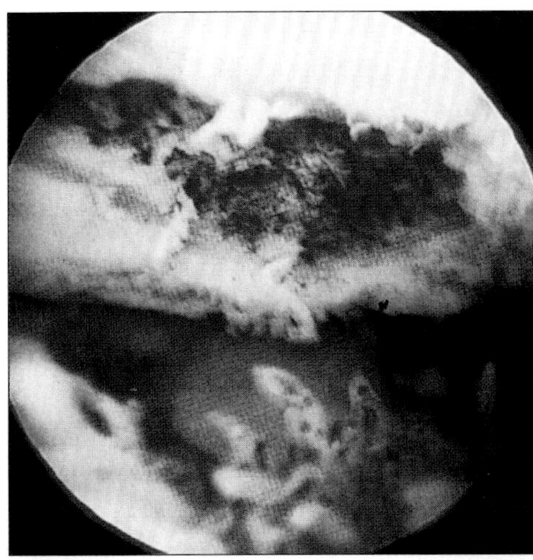

Fig. 9.16 Arthroscopic view of meniscal injury.

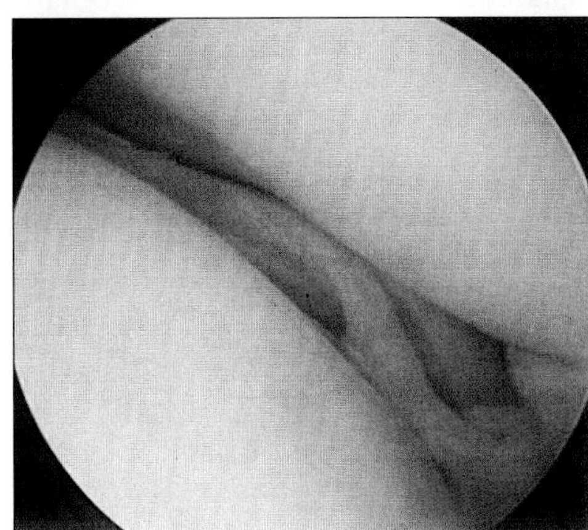

Fig. 9.17 Symptomatic arthroscopy of injured meniscus.

one third, there is potential for healing and surgical repair should be considered. If the tear involves the avascular inner two thirds, arthroscopic partial meniscectomy is the treatment of choice. The recovery following this is much quicker than following arthrotomy and total meniscectomy.

It is well recognized that total meniscectomy increases the risk of degenerative change [38]. Jackson found a 21% incidence of degeneration following total meniscectomy compared with a 5% incidence on the other side [39]. The effect of partial meniscectomy has not been determined but it is likely that the rate of degeneration will be less than with total meniscectomy. As much of the meniscus as possible should be retained to leave a 'balanced' stable rim.

In older patients with degenerative tears an initiating injury may not be remembered. The patient usually complains of acute well localized joint line pain which may wake him from sleep. Examination usually reveals joint line tenderness and a small effusion, although this is not a constant feature. Plain radiographs may reveal mild degenerative change and arthrography or MRI will confirm the diagnosis. Symptoms often settle with conservative treatment but arthroscopic resection of the torn portion of the meniscus may be required.

Ligamentous Injuries

Ligamentous injuries are common in young sportsmen. The diagnosis and treatment of knee ligament injuries has improved over the last 10 years. In the past the majority of knee injuries were diagnosed as meniscal tears and the coexisting ligamentous injury was either not recognized or ignored. The recognition of rotatory instability as a result of ligamentous injury and its effect on knee function has been an important advance. Arthroscopy has enabled accurate diagnosis of intra-articular pathology and recognition of the association between instability, meniscal tears and degeneration. Most of the ligaments of the knee have dual roles; the loss of one ligament may initially be masked by the secondary restraining structures. Over a period of time these secondary restraints may stretch and the instability become evident.

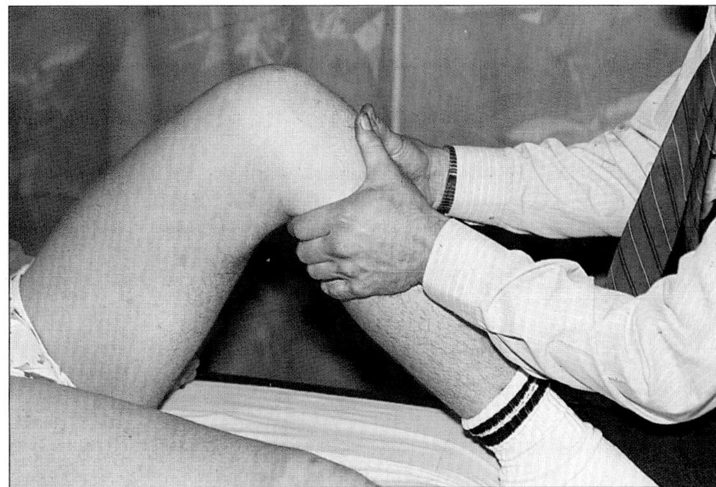

Fig. 9.18 Testing the integrity of the medial collateral ligament.

Instability may be functional and cause symptoms, or it may be found at examination. Instability demonstrated at examination is of little significance unless functional instability is also present. This is because the muscles control the instability during activity. Many sportsmen have pathologically lax ligaments on examination, but no functional disability. The examination of the unstable knee is sometimes considered difficult. However, accurate diagnosis of ligamentous injury can be made clinically in the vast majority of cases.

A ligament sprain is an injury in which the fibers are torn. In a first degree sprain there are torn fibers but unimpaired function. In a second degree sprain more fibers are torn with stretching of the ligament causing abnormal joint movement. A third degree sprain implies complete tearing and loss of function with marked abnormal motion. This is used synonymously with the term 'rupture' [40]. The degree of instability following a ligament injury is described by the amount of abnormal tibial movement which occurs in relation to the femur during testing. Hence: 1+ laxity is up to 5mm; 2+ is 5–10mm; and 3+ is 10–15mm. The pivot shift phenomenon is also scored on a 0–3 scale.

The examination of the unstable knee varies depending on the time from injury. In the acute phase, examination may be difficult due to pain and swelling. The knee should be examined for localized swelling, bruising and effusion or hemarthrosis. Seventy percent of hemarthroses are associated with an ACL tear. Examination and arthroscopy under general anesthetic may be necessary to define the extent of the damage if pain precludes an adequate clinical assessment. Radiographs should always be obtained to rule out associated fractures.

In chronic lesions the examination should take the following form. The knee is inspected and palpated in the usual way. An effusion is suggestive of instability or a meniscal tear. The range of movement is tested but is usually normal unless there is a meniscal tear.

Tests for cruciate ligament laxity

The integrity of the medial collateral ligament should be tested by applying a valgus stress with the knee held in 30° of flexion (Fig. 9.18). Opening of the joint compared to the other side suggests laxity or rupture of the medial collateral ligament and posteromedial capsule. The test should be repeated with the knee in full extension. If laxity is present it suggests a tear of the medial collateral ligament, medial capsule, posteromedial corner and the posterior cruciate ligament [41]. This is because in full extension all these structures act as a check to valgus movement. The same test should be repeated using a varus stress with the knee in 30° of flexion to test the lateral collateral ligament and posterolateral capsule. The test should be repeated in full extension to test these and the posterior cruciate ligament [42].

Tests for cruciate ligament laxity

With the knees flexed to 90° the profile of each knee should be examined. In PCL rupture the tibia sags back compared to the normal side, and when the tibia is pushed posteriorly no solid end point is felt. If this posterior sag is not recognized a PCL rupture may be mistaken for an ACL rupture as the tibia is reduced from its subluxated position during the anterior draw test. In ACL rupture the knee may be seen to hyperextend slightly, as the ACL helps to limit extension. The anterior draw test is performed with the knee flexed to 90° and the hamstrings relaxed. The tibia is pulled forward on the femur. An increase in anterior translation of the tibia on the femur compared to the other side is suggestive of an ACL tear. If the PCL is intact, on internal rotation of the foot the amount of anterior draw will be reduced. This is due to the PCL tightening and drawing the tibia onto the femur. With the foot in external rotation the anterior translation is often increased due to unwinding of the PCL.

The Lachman test is similar to the anterior draw test but the knee is held in 20° of flexion and the tibia is pulled forward on the femur [43]. An increase in this anterior translation suggests an ACL tear (Fig. 9.19). It can sometimes be difficult to perform the Lachman test if the examiner's hands are small or the patient has a large leg. In this case, in order to perform the test it often helps to rest the patient's knee on the examiner's thigh.

Anterolateral rotatory instability is the most common type to occur with ACL rupture. The ACL is the primary restraint to anterior translation and internal rotation of the tibia on the femur. When it is ruptured the tibia is able to move forward and internally rotate on the femur. This subluxation of the lateral tibial condyle occurs at between 15° and 20° of knee flexion, causing the pivot shift phenomenon [44]. The pivot shift is simply the term used to describe the phenomenon of subluxation or reduction of the tibia on the femur in a knee with anterolateral rotatory instability. This subluxation is what the patient describes as the knee 'giving way'. The secondary restraints of capsule, collateral ligaments and muscles may prevent subluxation during activity but if they have been damaged or become lax due to excessive loading and subsequent stretching, functional instability can occur.

A variety of tests have been described for the pivot shift phenomenon. The jerk test for anterolateral instability is performed with the examiner's upper hand over the tibia and the thumb behind the head of the fibula exerting a valgus force on the knee. The examiner's other hand internally rotates the foot (Fig. 9.20). As the knee is extended the lateral tibial condyle subluxates forward usually with a clunk, which the patient may recognize as the sensation experienced when the knee gives way. If the knee is then extended the tibial condyle will reduce again, often with a second clunk [45].

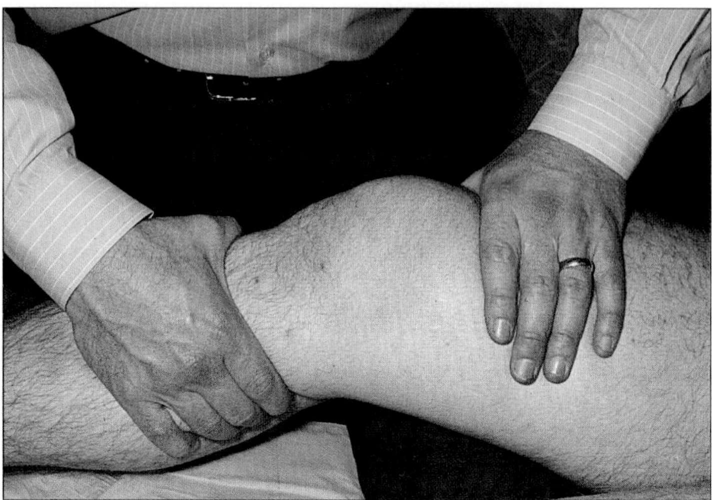

Fig. 9.19 The Lachman test for tears of the cruciate ligaments.

Anteromedial instability may also occur when the ACL is damaged in association with a lax medial collateral ligament and capsule. In this case the medial tibial condyle subluxates forward. Anteromedial and anterolateral instability may coexist.

The reverse pivot shift is the opposite of the pivot shift phenomenon and is due to posterior subluxation of the lateral tibial condyle due to an injury to the posterolateral corner of the knee and often the posterior cruciate ligament as well [46]. The reverse pivot shift test is essentially the reverse of the jerk test. The foot is held externally rotated while the upper hand applies a valgus force to the knee. As the knee is extended the lateral tibial condyle reduces at approximately 20° of flexion with a clunk.

Medial collateral ligament injuries

The medial collateral ligament is usually injured as a result of a valgus force, often associated with external rotation of the tibia. The classic example is a skiing injury where the ski moves laterally, causing a valgus external rotation force on the knee. In the acute phase the findings are of swelling and bruising over the course of the ligament with tenderness over the joint line or femoral insertion. Loss of full extension may be present in an incomplete tear due to pain as the ligament comes under tension in the last 20° of extension. Medial collateral ligament injuries may be associated with meniscal tears or peripheral detachment of the medial meniscus. An associated ACL injury may also be present. If doubt exists about the possibility of coexisting capsular or ACL damage an examination under anesthetic and arthroscopy should be performed. Treatment for isolated medial collateral ligament tears is conservative [47], consisting of 4 weeks in a cast brace with the range of motion set between 40° and 60° and then a further 4–6 weeks in a light brace to protect the ligament during rehabilitation.

Lateral collateral ligament injuries

The lateral collateral ligament is rarely injured in isolation but is usually torn in association with damage to the posterolateral ligament complex (lateral capsule, arcuate ligament and popliteus tendon). The cruciate ligaments may also be damaged. The mechanism of injury is usually a varus force on a flexed knee. The ligament usually ruptures at its fibular insertion or it may avulse the fibular styloid. A peroneal nerve palsy may be associated with a

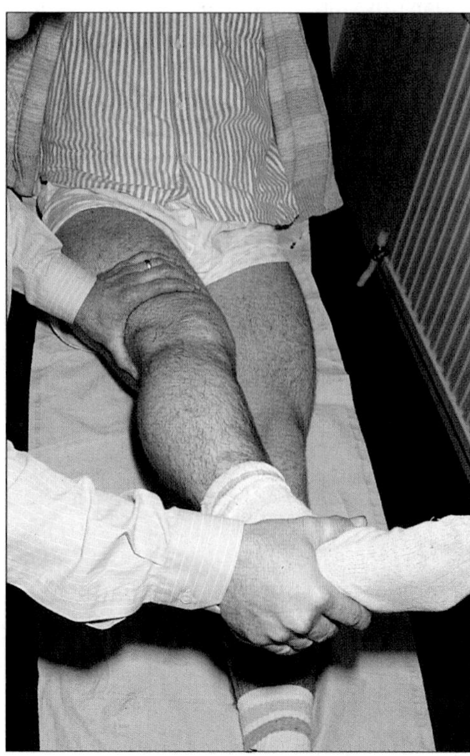

Fig. 9.20 The jerk test for anterolateral instability.

lateral collateral ligament tear and should be looked for at the time of the injury. Little functional instability arises from an isolated tear of the lateral collateral ligament, which therefore may be treated conservatively in a similar manner to the medial collateral ligament. Lesions of the lateral collateral ligament associated with capsular or cruciate ligament damage should be repaired acutely in active young sportsmen.

Anterior cruciate ligament injuries

The ACL is injured more frequently than previously thought, often with surprisingly little force. An acute tear of the ACL is usually associated with a hemarthrosis [48]. A pitfall occurs when an ACL tear is associated with capsular disruption when a tense hemarthrosis does not accumulate as the blood leaks out into the calf. Bruising and swelling in the calf is often an indication of serious knee disruption. The injury is usually a twisting injury. Two main mechanisms are recognized: a valgus external rotation injury to a flexed knee associated with damage to other structures; and a hyperextension internal rotation injury resulting in an isolated ACL tear. The patient usually feels the knee go out of joint and may hear a 'pop'. The ACL injury may be missed in the acute phase if other more obvious structures, such as the medial collateral ligament, are damaged. The Lachman test is a reliable indicator of ACL rupture and may be performed on an acutely injured knee without causing too much discomfort. In children, avulsion of the tibial spines tends to occur rather than a mid-substance tear.

Radiographs should be taken to look for avulsion injuries of the tibial spines and other associated fractures. A small flake of bone may be seen to be avulsed from the lateral aspect of the tibial condyle just above the fibula. This is called a Segond fracture and if present indicates a 60–70% chance of an ACL injury. If there is doubt about the diagnosis an examination under anesthetic and arthroscopy should be performed.

Approximately 60% of patients with an ACL rupture will have an associated meniscal tear and 20% will have an osteochondral fracture [49].

The symptoms of an ACL-deficient knee are giving way, swelling and pain. The patient experiences symptoms with twisting or jumping maneuvers. The symptoms are due to rotational instability rather than loss of anteroposterior stability. Symptoms of locking may occur, but these are usually due to a coexisting meniscal tear rather than to the ACL rupture itself. The incidence of meniscal tears in knees with functional anterolateral instability increases with time [50]. It is now generally agreed that recurrent episodes of subluxation will lead to early degeneration. The earliest degenerative changes occur on the medial femoral condyle in the area which is weight-bearing when subluxation occurs. This area acts as the fulcrum for the pivot shift and as articular cartilage is poor at withstanding shear stresses, breakdown occurs [51].

Treatment for acute ACL tears is controversial and beyond the scope of this chapter [52]. Most cases can be treated conservatively and any subsequent functional instability treated later. In athletes with ACL and associated ligamentous and meniscal damage, acute surgery is indicated.

Symptomatic chronic tears of the ACL in young patients which have not responded to conservative measures may be treated by intra-articular replacement of the ACL with autogenous tissue, such as patellar or semitendinosus tendon. In older patients extra-articular repair may control the instability.

Posterior cruciate ligament injury

This is much less common than are ACL tears and usually occurs due to road traffic accidents, when a blow to the anterior aspect of the tibia in a flexed knee forces the tibia posteriorly rupturing the PCL. Unless other structures have also been damaged the function of the knee following PCL rupture is usually good and reconstruction is not necessary [53]. Conservative treatment consists of a plaster cast for 6 weeks with the knee in 20° of flexion, followed by rehabilitation in a knee brace.

Tendon Injuries

The most common tendon injury around the knee occurs in the elderly and affects the extensor mechanism. Catching a foot against the edge of a pavement, or tripping, with contraction of the quadriceps, may be enough to cause rupture or avulsion of an already degenerate patellar or quadriceps tendon. On examination the patient is unable to extend the knee and there may be a high lying patella if the patella tendon has ruptured. If the quadriceps tendon has been avulsed a gap may be palpable above the patella. Fracture of the patella may be secondary to quadriceps contraction or a fall. It is associated with bruising, swelling and tenderness over the patella, and radiographs will confirm the diagnosis.

Injuries in Degenerative Knees

An effusion is relatively common following minor trauma in degenerative knees, presumably due to synovitis. Hemarthrosis may also occur secondary to hyperemia. A lipo-hemarthrosis however indicates an intra-articular fracture and should be investigated further.

The Relationship of Injury to Degeneration

It is well recognized that injury to the articular cartilage of a joint may lead to early degenerative changes. This relationship is important as it mainly affects young people. Prevention of joint degeneration following injury is therefore important particularly in the knee. Intra-articular fractures of the femoral condyles or tibial plateau may cause extensive hyaline cartilage damage. The treatment of these fractures by internal fixation with accurate reduction of the articular surfaces and early joint movement may minimize degeneration.

As already mentioned, total meniscectomy increases the likelihood of degenerative change and should not be performed unless absolutely necessary [39]. It is now generally accepted that a patient with anterolateral instability of the knee leading to repeated episodes of subluxation is at increased risk of degeneration at an early age [52,54] (Fig. 9.21). This process is accelerated if the patient has had a total meniscectomy. Thus, patients with instability should be advised to avoid activities which result in repeated episodes of subluxation. Alternatively, they may undergo surgical stabilization of the joint, although at present there is no clear evidence that this decreases the risk of degenerative change. Whether early changes in hyaline cartilage can be reversed by stabilizing the knee is also unclear. Both of these concepts are under investigation.

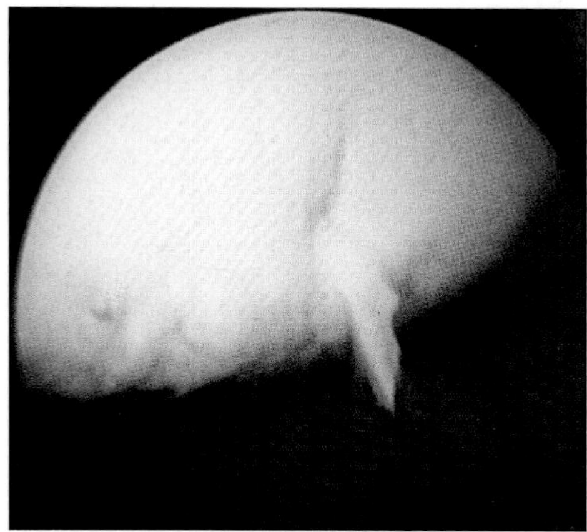

Fig. 9.21 Degeneration following repeated episodes of subluxation.

REFERENCES

1. Price CT, Allen WC. Ligament repair in the knee with preservation of the meniscus. J Bone Joint Surg. 1978;**60**(A):61–5.
2. Last RJ. Some anatomical details of the knee joint. J Bone Joint Surg. 1948;**30**(B):683–8.
3. Last RJ. The popliteus muscle and the lateral meniscus. J Bone Joint Surg. 1950;**32**(B):93–9.
4. Arnoczky SP, Warren RF. Microvasculature of the human meniscus. Am J Sports Med. 1982;**10**:90–5.
5. Goodfellow J, Hungerford DS, Zindel M. Patello-femoral mechanics and pathology I. Functional anatomy of the patello-femoral joint. J Bone Joint Surg. 1976;**58**(B):287–90.
6. Aglietti P, Insall JN, Cerulli G. Patellar pain and incongruence I: Measurements of incongruence. Clin Orthop. 1983;**176**:217–24.
7. Girgis FG, Marshall JL, Al Monajem ARS. The cruciate ligaments of the knee joint. Clin orthop. 1975;**106**:216–31.
8. Brantigan OC, Voshell AF. The tibial collateral ligament: Its function, its bursae and its relation to the medial meniscus. J Bone Joint Surg. 1943:**25**:121–31.
9. Warren LF, Marshall JL, Girgis FG. The prime static stabiliser of the medial side of the knee. J Bone Joint Surg. 1974;**56**(A):665–74.
10. Fulkerson JP, Gossling HR. Anatomy of the knee joint lateral retinaculum. Clin Orthop. 1980;**153**:183–8.
11. Kaplan EB. The iliotibial tract. Clinical and morphological significance. J Bone Joint Surg. 1985;**40**(A): 817–32.
12. Burleson RJ, Bickel WH, Dahlin DC. Popliteal cyst. A clinico-pathological survey. J Bone Joint Surg. 1956;**38**(A):1265–74.
13. Apley AG, Solomon L. The knee joint. In: Apley's system of orthopaedics and fractures, 6E. London: Butterworth;1982:277–305.
14. Blazina M. Jumper's knee. Orthop. Clin. North Am. 1973;**4**:665.
15. Renne JW. The iliotibial band friction syndrome. J Bone Joint Surg. 1975;**57**(A):1110–11.
16. Nachlas IW, Olpp JL. Para-articular calcification (Pellegrini-Stieda) in affectations of the knee. Surg Gynecol Obstet. 1945;**81**:206–12.
17. Milgram JW. Synovial osteochondromatosis: a histo-pathological study of thirty cases. J Bone Joint Surg. 1977;**59**(A):792–801.
18. Maurice H, Crone M, Watt I. Synovial chondromatosis. J Bone Joint Surg. 1988;**70**(B):807–11.
19. Flandry F, Hughston JC. Pigmented villonodular synovitis. J Bone Joint Surg. 1987;**69**(A):942–9.
20. Wilson JN. A diagnostic sign in osteochondritis dissecans of the knee. J Bone Joint Surg. 1967;**49**(B):440–7.
21. Aichroth P. Osteochondritis dissecans of the knee. A clinical survey. J Bone Joint Surg. 1971;**53**(B):440–7.
22. Green JP. Osteochondritis dissecans of the knee. J Bone Joint Surg. 1966;**48**(B):82–91.
23. Cahill B. The treatment of juvenile osteochondritis dissecans and osteochondritis dissecans of the knee. Clin Sports Med. 1985;**4**:367.
24. Osgood RB. Lesions of the tibial tubercle occurring during adolescence. Boston Med Surg J. 1903;**148**:114.
25. Ogden JA, Southwick WO. Osgood Schlatter's disease and tibial tuberosity development. Clin. Orthop. 1976:**116**:180–9.
26. Sinding-Larsen C. A hitherto unknown affection of the patella in children. Acta Radiol. 1921;171.
27. Jones RD, Fisher RL, Curtis BH. Congenital dislocation of the patella. Clin. Orthop. 1976;**119**:177–83.
28. Williams PF. Quadriceps contracture. J Bone Joint Surg. 1968;**50**(B):278–84.
29. McManus F, Rang M, Heslin DJ. Acute dislocations of the patella in children: the natural history. Clin Orthop. 1979;**139**:88–91.
30. Insall J, Salvati E. Patella position in the normal knee joint. Radiology. 1971;**101**:101–4.
31. Laurin CA, Levesque HP, Dussault R, Labelle H, Peides JP. The abnormal lateral patellofemoral angle: A diagnostic roentgenographic sign of recurrent patellar subluxation. J Bone Joint Surg. 1978;**60**(A):55–60.
32. Hungerford DS, Lennox DW. Rehabilitation of the knee in disorders of the patellofemoral joint: Relevant biomechanics. Orthop. Clin. North Am. 1983;**14**:397–402.
33. Hughston JC, Stone M, Andrews JR. The suprapatellar plica: Its role in internal derangement of the knee. J Bone Joint Surg. 1973;**55**(A):1318.
34. Patel D. Arthroscopy of the plicae: Synovial folds and their significance. Am J Sports Med. 1978;**6**:217.
35. Noble J, Hamblen DL. The pathology of the degenerate meniscus lesions. J Bone Joint Surg. 1975:**57**(B):180–6.
36. McMurray TP. The semilunar cartilages. Br J Surg. 1941;**29**:407.
37. Apley AG. The diagnosis of meniscus injuries. Some new clinical methods. J Bone Joint Surg. 1947;**29**:78–84.
38. Fairbank TJ. Knee joint changes after meniscectomy. J Bone Joint Surg. 1948;**30**(B):664–70.
39. Jackson JP. Degenerative changes in the knee after meniscectomy. Br Med J. 1968;**2**:525–7.
40. Noyes FR, Grood ES, Torzilli PA. The definitions of terms for motion and position of the knee and injuries of the ligaments. J Bone Joint Surg. 1989;**71**(A):465–71.
41. Hugston JC, Andrews JR, Cross MJ, Moschi A. Classification of knee ligament instabilities. Part 1. The medial compartment and cruciate ligaments. J Bone Joint Surg. 1976;**58**(A):159–72.
42. Hughston JC, Andrews JR, Cross MJ, Moschi A. Classification of knee ligament instabilities. Part 1. The lateral compartment. J Bone Joint Surg. 1976;**58**(A):173–9.
43. Torg JS, Conrad W, Kalen V. Clinical diagnosis of anterior cruciate ligament instability in the athlete. Am J Sports Med. 1976;**4**:84–93.
44. Galway RD, Beaupre A, Macintosh DL. Pivot shift: a clinical sign of symptomatic anterior cruciate insufficiency. J Bone Joint Surg. 1972;**54**(B):763.
45. Ireland J, Trickey EL. Macintosh tenodesis for anterolateral instability of the knee. J Bone Joint Surg. 1980;**62**(B):340–5.
46. Jakob RP, Hassler H, Staeubli HU. Observations on rotatory instability in the lateral compartment of the knee. Acta Orthop. Scand. 1981;**191**(Suppl):1–32.
47. Indelicato PA. Non operative treatment of complete tears of the medial colateral ligament of the knee. J Bone Joint Surg. 1983;**65**(A):323–9.
48. DeHaven KE. Diagnosis of acute knee injuries with hemarthrosis. Am J Sports Med. 1980;**8**:9–14.
49. Noyes FR, Basset RW, Grood ES, Butler DL. Arthroscopy in acute traumatic hemarthrosis of the knee. Incidence of anterior cruciate tears and other injuries. J Bone Joint Surg. 1980;**62**(A):687–95.
50. Indelicato PA, Bittar ES. A perspective of lesions associated with ACL insufficiency in the knee. A review of 100 cases. Clin Orthop. 1985;**198**:77–80.
51. Fairclough JA, Graham GP, Dent CM. Radiological sign of chronic anterior cruciate ligament deficiency. Injury. 190;**21**:401–2.
52. Noyes FR, McGinniss GH. Controversy about treatment of the knee with anterior cruciate laxity. Clin Orthop. 1985;**198**:61–76.
53. Cross MJ, Powell JF. The long term follow up of posterior cruciate ligament rupture: A study of 116 cases. Am J Sports Med. 1984;**12**:292–7.
54. Graham GP, Fairclough HA. Early osteoarthritis in young sportsmen with severe antero-lateral instability of the knee. Injury. 1988;**19**:247–8.

10

ASPIRATION AND INJECTION OF JOINTS AND PERIARTICULAR TISSUES

Joints and periarticular cavities such as bursae and tendon sheaths may need aspiration for diagnostic or therapeutic purposes. In addition, steroids and other drugs are often injected in and around soft tissue periarticular lesions to treat regional pain syndromes (Fig. 10. 1). The principles and practice of inserting a needle into either a joint cavity or periarticular lesion are very similar.

INDICATIONS FOR ASPIRATING OR INJECTING MUSCULOSKELETAL TISSUES

Aspirating Fluid for Diagnostic or Therapeutic Purposes

In patients in whom sepsis, crystal synovitis or bleeding is the suspected cause of a joint, bursal or tendon sheath lesion, aspiration and analysis of the fluid is essential for diagnosis. In addition, in patients who have poorly defined forms of arthritis, knowledge as to the nature of the synovial fluid, particularly the inflammatory cell content, will complement findings from the history and physical examination and help provide the basic framework for diagnosis and treatment. In patients with tense joint or bursal effusions, aspiration of synovial fluid provides prompt relief of pain and permits the patient to move or bear weight on the affected joint. Finally, in hemarthrosis or septic arthritis, the blood and pus within a synovial cavity may be toxic to the joint cartilage and synovial membrane, and evacuation of the fluid is necessary to avoid permanent joint damage.

Synovial fluid should be aspirated into sterile syringes, and either capped, or immediately aliquoted into sterile containers. Anticoagulants can help avoid the formation of fibrin clots, making the fluid easier to handle and assisting in analyses of the cellular content. If unusual or chronic infections are suspected it may be prudent to inoculate some of the fluid into appropriate growth media (such as chocolate agar for gonococcal infections) immediately after aspiration. The fluid should be inspected for the presence of blood and to see how opaque it is, which is a rough guide to cell content. Three laboratory investigations should then be carried out on all fluids aspirated for diagnostic purposes:

- the total and differential cell count,
- examination for organisms (Gram stain, culture, etc.),
- polarized light microscopy for the presence of urate or pyrophosphate crystals.

As crystal synovitis and infections can coexist it is never wise to rely on one of these investigations alone. The cellular content is indicative of the type of arthritis (Fig. 10.2). Other special investigations that can be of value include cytology, and the assay of a variety of biochemical markers of connective tissue turnover, such as products of the synthesis and degradation of cartilage aggrecan.

Injection of Steroids and Other Therapeutic Agents

Steroid injections are frequently used to achieve local anti-inflammatory activity. The indications for their use include the presence of persistent inflammation at a single site in the absence of a contraindication, such as suspicion of infection (see below). Synovial joints and other cavities should generally be injected with a long-acting, crystalline form of steroid such as triamcinolone hexacetonide or acetonide. These agents are taken up by the synovial lining

INDICATIONS FOR ASPIRATING OR INJECTING JOINTS	
Diagnosis	Mandatory if septic arthritis suspected Strongly advised if crystal arthritis or hemarthrosis suspected Differentiation of inflammatory from non-inflammatory arthritis Imaging studies – arthroscopy and arthrography Synovial biopsy
Therapy	To remove tense effusions to relieve pain and improve function To remove blood or pus from a joint For injection of steroids and other intra-articular therapies For tidal lavage of joints

Fig. 10.1 Indications for aspirating or injecting joints.

SYNOVIAL FLUID FINDINGS				
	Normal	Osteoarthritis	Rheumatoid and other inflammatory arthritis	Septic arthritis
Gross appearance	Clear	Clear	Opaque	Opaque
Volume (ml)	0–1	1–10	5–50	5–50
Viscosity	High	High	Low	Low
Total white cell count/mm^3	<200	200–10,000	5000–75,000	>50,000
% Polymorphonuclear cells	<25%	<50%	>50%	>75%

Fig. 10.2 Knee joint synovial fluid findings in common forms of arthritis.

cells, allowing continued local release into the targeted area. Only a relatively small proportion escapes into the general circulation but, during the first 24 hours after injection, patients may experience flushing or other evidence of a steroid 'pulse'. For periarticular injections, into entheses for example, a simple steroid such as hydrocortisone should be used, as long-acting preparations are likely to induce local fat atrophy. Local anesthetic is sometimes used mixed with steroids for such injections. In the case of some periarticular lesions, for example rotator cuff lesions around the shoulder, this can have the advantage of confirming the correct placement of the injection, as the local anesthetic should result in almost immediate relief of the problem if the injection is correctly placed.

A number of other agents have been used for intra-articular or periarticular therapy via injection. Examples include the radioactive colloids such as yttrium-90, which can irradiate the synovium to achieve a form of chemical synovectomy, other sclerosing agents, and long-acting local anesthetics, sometimes used alone to help sort out the origin of musculoskeletal pain.

CONTRAINDICATIONS AND COMPLICATIONS

Contraindications

There are few absolute contraindications to joint or soft tissue aspirations and injections; if infection is suspected then fluid should always be aspirated from a joint. In other indications, the procedures should probably be avoided if there is infection of the overlying skin or subcutaneous tissues or if bacteremia is suspected. The presence of a significant bleeding disorder or diathesis, such as a patient receiving anticoagulant therapy or with severe thrombocytopenia may also preclude joint aspiration. However, if it is deemed necessary for diagnosis or therapy, the procedure may be carried out after an injection of Factor VIII in a hemophiliac for example, or with other appropriate cover for the bleeding disorder. Aspiration of a joint with a prosthesis in it carries a particularly high risk of infection, and is often best left to surgeons using full aseptic techniques.

Lack of response to previous injections may be a relative contraindication to therapeutic injections and, if there is any suspicion of infection being the underlying cause of the musculoskeletal problem, steroids must not be injected, for fear of exacerbating the infection.

Complications

There are surprisingly few complications of these procedures. The most significant issue is the risk of infection, and care must always be taken to use sterile 'no-touch' techniques, as well as avoiding steroids in those who could have existing sepsis. It is estimated that the risk of a septic arthritis following aspiration or steroid injection is in the order of 1 per 15,000 procedures. Patients who have severe immunodeficiency problems, as well as those with implants, may be at greater risk. Depot steroid preparations, or large doses of any form of corticosteroid can result in fat atrophy following periarticular injections, or if there is leakage of an intra-articular injection, as well as depigmentation of overlying skin. Intra-articular steroids occasionally give rise to a significant systemic reaction, with flushing of skin and minor psychological change, and any periarticular or intra-articular injection of a crystalline form of steroid can occasionally cause a flare of inflammation before the therapeutic response. Minor hemorrhage occasionally occurs, either within joints or in the periarticular tissues. Leakage of other injected agents, such as radioactive colloids, can result in severe radiation burns and tissue atrophy, with a lot of pain.

Other complications can arise from misplaced injections. The best described problem is tendon rupture following steroid injections for tendinitis. The risk can be minimized by avoiding injection into the tendon itself, and no therapeutic agent should be injected against any unexpected resistance. Occasionally nerve damage can also result from a misplaced injection, for example median nerve atrophy following attempted injections for a carpal tunnel syndrome.

PRACTICAL PROCEDURE AND AFTERCARE

The Procedure

Aspiration or injection of joints or soft tissues is an outpatient procedure that does not require specialized equipment (Fig. 10.3). Universal precautions must be followed during the procedure; gloves are recommended and required by medical practice regulations in many countries.

EQUIPMENT REQUIRED FOR JOINT AND SOFT TISSUE INJECTIONS	
Skin preparation	Antiseptic solution (povidone iodine, merthiolate, chlorhexidine), alcohol swabs, 4 × 4 gauze pads
Local anesthetics	1% lidocaine, ethyl chloride spray
Needles	23–25 gauge needles for local anesthetic; 19 gauge for large to moderate size joints (knees, shoulders, ankles, etc.); 23 gauge for small joints (wrist, MCPs, etc.)
Syringes	3 or 5ml syringe for anesthetic/steroid injection and 10-50ml syringe for fluid aspiration
Miscellaneous	Gloves; forceps for removing needles from syringe; specimen tubes/plates for cultures and fluid studies

Fig. 10.3 Equipment required for joint and soft tissue injections.

The patient should be placed in a comfortable supine or recumbent position (in case of possible fainting, as well as to aid relaxation), and the procedure must be fully explained. Prior to cleaning the skin, bony and other landmarks need to be identified by palpation and the needle site marked in some way, such as with a thumbnail imprint in the skin. The skin must then be carefully cleaned with antiseptic agents. For local anesthesia, the skin and subcutaneous tissues can be infiltrated down to the level of the periarticular lesion or joint capsule, using 1% lidocaine without epinephrine, and a small-bore needle. However, physicians experienced with the procedure often prefer to use topical ethyl chloride or no anesthetic at all. This is often appropriate for joint aspiration, as it is difficult to anesthetize the capsule, and a single, simple, quick needle thrust may be much less painful than the local anesthesia. With the proper technique, the needle passes freely through the extra-articular tissues and a 'pop' is felt as the needle enters the joint. The ease with which fluid can be withdrawn depends on the needle size used, and the viscosity of the fluid, extent of synovitis, and presence of any fibrin clots or 'rice bodies' in the joint fluid. Free flow of fluid is often suddenly interrupted due to clogging of the needle end by the synovial membrane or debris. Rotating the needle, withdrawing it slightly, or even re-injecting a little of the fluid, will often help unclog the needle and allow additional fluid to be withdrawn. If corticosteroids or other substances are to be injected, this can be done through the same needle, but removing the aspirating syringe from the needle hub may be difficult and require forceps.

At the end of any procedure, the needle should be swiftly withdrawn, and light pressure put on the needle site of the skin. A simple Band-Aid for a few hours is all that is usually required thereafter.

Aftercare

There is a great deal of variation in the advice given to patients after aspiration or therapeutic injection of joints or soft tissues. Some doctors give no specific instructions, others recommend a prolonged period of rest to help facilitate the best possible therapeutic response. In most cases, it is sensible for patients to rest the affected joint for 24–48 hours after a therapeutic injection, to minimize leakage of the therapeutic agent, and improve the anti-inflammatory response. However, this advice must depend on the patient's circumstances.

ASSOCIATED PROCEDURES

There are a number of other procedures that may require joint puncture, they include:

- *Imaging joints with contrast agents:* injection of contrast agents with or without air can help image soft tissue and cartilage lesions in joints using radiography (arthrography).
- *Joint lavage:* tidal lavage of joints with saline, through a simple percutaneous cannula, or during arthroscopy can result in lasting relief of pain and inflammation in chronic arthritis.
- *Synovial biopsy:* synovial biopsy can be of diagnostic value, and is essential for the diagnosis of pigmented villonodular synovitis and other neoplastic lesions, as well as sometimes being necessary to diagnose chronic infections such as tuberculosis, and foreign body synovitis. This can be done percutaneously, using a 'Parker Pearson' needle, or through arthroscopy.
- *Needle arthroscopy and 'chondroscopy':* full arthroscopic examination and surgery is largely the province of the orthopedic surgeon. However, arthroscopic examination of some joints, especially the knee, can be carried out under local anesthesia, particularly if modern small-bore arthroscopes (needlescopes) are used. This can be of value in examining the synovium and cartilage (chondroscopy), as well as allowing biopsy under direct vision, and in joint lavage.

THE SHOULDER REGION

Seamus E Dalton

Injection of the shoulder region serves two purposes; firstly confirmation of the diagnosis, and secondly treatment of an inflammatory condition. Shoulder pain is often difficult to localize and the possibility of referred pain further complicates the issue. If the diagnosis is uncertain an injection of corticosteroid is inappropriate but injection of local anesthetic alone can help to localize the patient's symptoms. This is important when trying to confirm the presence of subacromial impingement. However, in the majority of cases clinical examination will provide a diagnosis or at least locate the source of inflammation. Corticosteroid injection around the shoulder is largely limited to intra-articular and intrabursal sites, and direct injection into a tendon should be avoided. Frequently a very painful procedure suggests that injection into the tissues and not the tissue spaces has taken place. The patient should be advised to rest the shoulder for at least 48 hours after the injection and to avoid aggravating activities, particularly overhead tasks, for 1–2 weeks.

Glenohumeral Joint

In inflammatory arthropathies where there is an effusion of the glenohumeral joint, injection is relatively simple, but in conditions such as adhesive capsulitis or degenerative arthritis, injection into the joint is difficult. Procedures such as arthrography have shown that placement of the needle into the joint cavity is not as simple as it appears, and many supposedly intra-articular injections are in fact periarticular. The posterior approach is easier and carries less risk of inadvertent damage to neurovascular structures. The posterior margin of the acromion is palpated and a point marked approximately 1cm below and 1cm medial to the posterior angle. The joint line can be felt in thinner individuals by gripping the humeral head and rotating the arm. The injection is then given from this point, directing the needle towards the coracoid process which is palpated anteriorly (Fig. 10.4). Once the needle hits bone the humerus can be gently rotated to establish where the needle is relative to the humeral head. Once placement is satisfactory, injection of the corticosteroid can be given using say 10mg of triamcinolone with 1% or 2% lidocaine made up to 5ml. Ease of flow indicates that injection into the tissues is not occurring.

The anterior approach is more difficult and careful placement is important. With the patient resting supine or semi-reclined the arm is rested in internal rotation with the forearm lying across the abdomen. The injection is given just lateral and inferior to the coracoid process aiming towards the joint line, which is identified by palpation and rotation of the arm (Fig. 10.5).

Subacromial Bursa

The subacromial space or bursa should be the site of injection in the treatment of impingement, rotator cuff tendinitis and subacromial bursitis. Although impingement usually occurs under the anterior margin of the acromion, access to the subacromial space is often easiest by a lateral or posterolateral approach. Adequate muscle relaxation is important and allows better palpation of the gap between the acromion and humeral head. Patient variation in acromial morphology, joint laxity and muscle bulk determines the ease with which this gap is felt. The needle is then aimed medially ensuring that it passes under the acromion (Fig. 10.6). It is important to avoid direct injection into the rotator cuff, and therefore directing the needle upwards once it is in the subacromial space will allow the

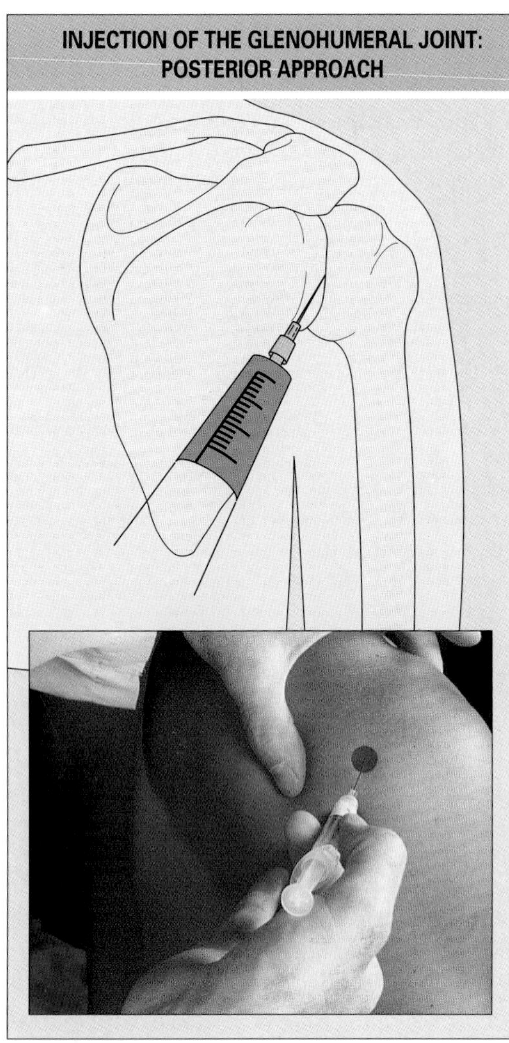

Fig. 10.4 Injection of the glenohumeral joint: posterior approach.

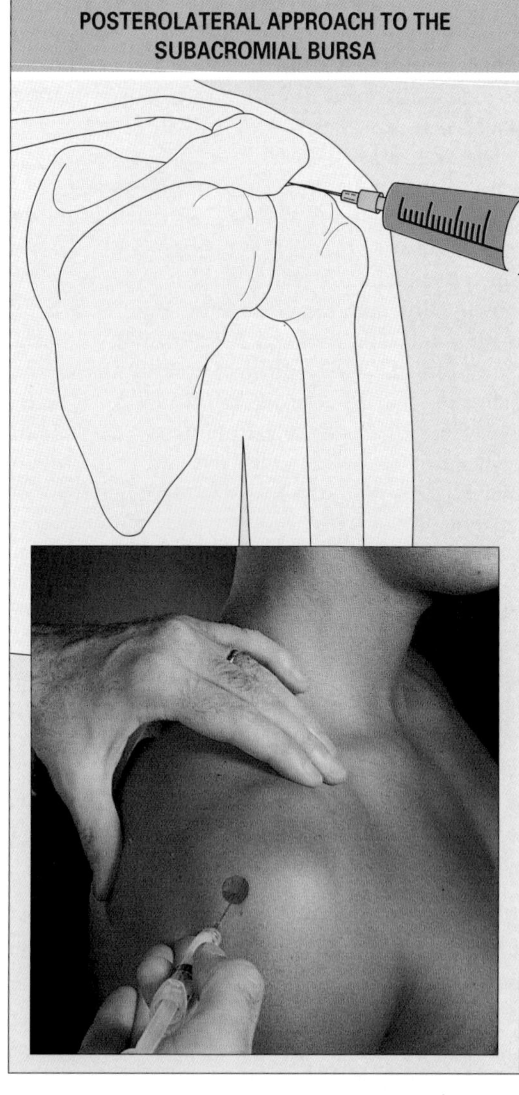

Fig. 10.6 Posterolateral approach to the subacromial bursa.

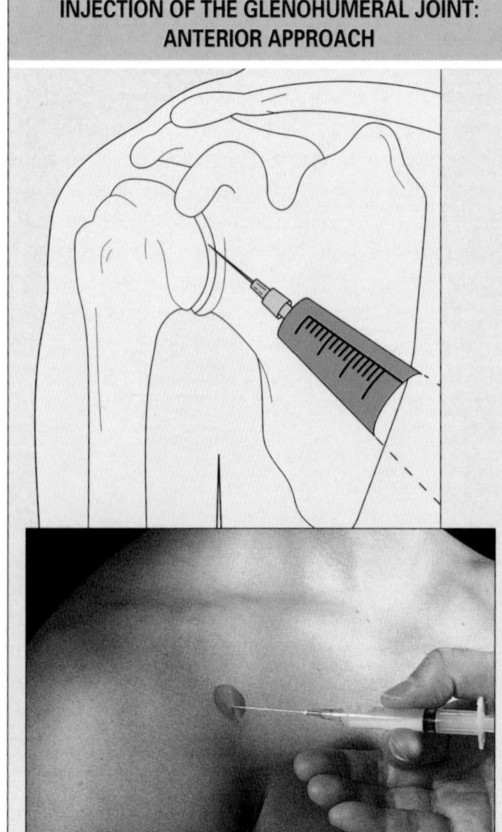

Fig. 10.5 Injection of the glenohumeral joint: anterior approach.

clinician to abutt the point of the needle against the undersurface of the acromion. Injection of 2–5ml of local anesthetic and 25–50mg of hydrocortisone acetate or 10mg of triamcinolone can now be given, ensuring that there is minimal resistance to flow. In some individuals there is localized tenderness under the anterior acromial margin and it may be preferable to enter the subacromial space at this point (Fig. 10.7). When injecting from a lateral or posterolateral approach it is important to direct the needle towards the anterior acromial margin.

Acromioclavicular Joint

In inflammatory or degenerative conditions of the acromioclavicular joint, injection of corticosteroid can be an effective means of settling symptoms. Palpation of the joint line is made easier by applying downward pressure on the end of the clavicle while moving the humerus up and down with the arm by the side. A small gauge needle is usually sufficient and is aimed perpendicular to the joint line either from a superior or anterosuperior direction. Injection is fairly straightforward when there is swelling or instability of the joint. However, access is more difficult in degenerative conditions with joint space narrowing and osteophyte formation. This is a small capacity joint and will seldom accept more than 0.5–1.0ml of fluid, usually with resistance. An appropriate dose is 2.5–5.0mg of triamcinolone in 1.0ml of 1% or 2% lidocaine. Occasionally, if there is rotator cuff tendinitis associated with acromioclavicular joint degeneration, an injection from above can be directed into the acromioclavicular joint cavity. Half the injection is given here before the needle is advanced through the inferior joint capsule into the underlying subacromial space, where the remainder of the syringe contents are deposited.

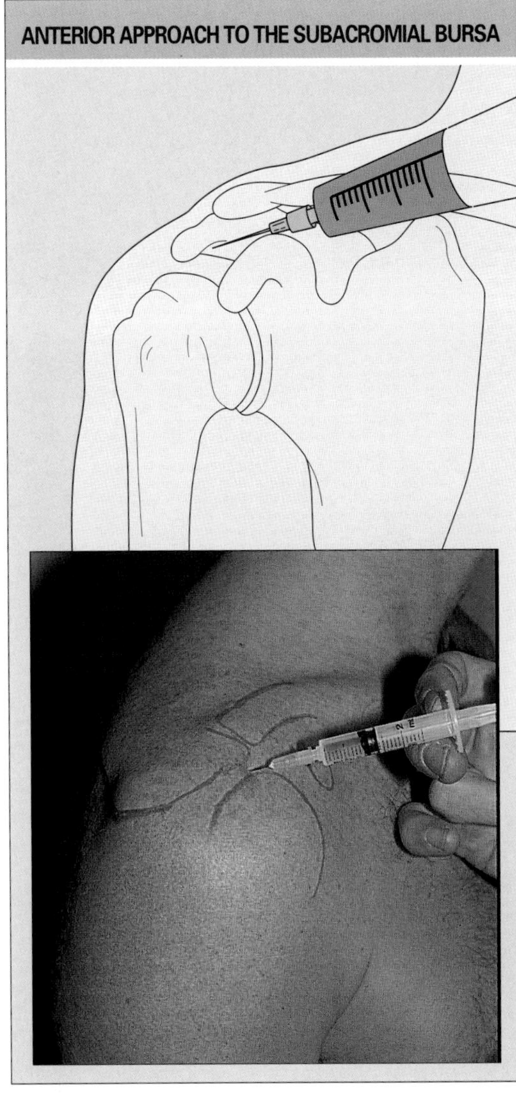

Fig. 10.7 Anterior approach to the subacromial bursa.

Bicipital Tendinitis

Often it is difficult to differentiate bicipital tendinitis from impingement or rotator cuff tendinitis (primary bicipital tendinitis is unusual in isolation), and selective injection with a local anesthetic is helpful. If injection into the subacromial joint fails to relieve pain and symptoms, injection of local anesthetic and 25mg hydrocortisone or 5mg triamcinolone can be given into the bicipital groove alongside the tendon, taking care not to inject the tendon itself. The patient is rested in the semi-reclined position with the elbow flexed, shoulder extended and the arm in a degree of external rotation. The bicipital tendon is palpated and a mark made on the skin. The needle is then directed somewhat superiorly and tangential to the tendon, ensuring easy flow of fluid (Fig. 10.8). A deeper injection into the groove is also safe if contact with bone is made and easy flow of fluid obtained.

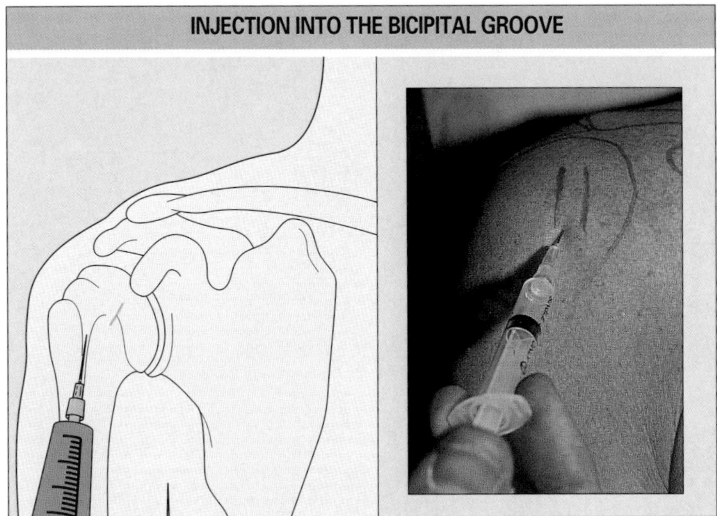

Fig. 10.8 Injection into the bicipital groove.

THE ELBOW REGION

Michael D Chard

Elbow Joint

Posterior approach

The elbow is flexed to 90° and the depression in the midline between the two halves of the triceps tendon is palpated at the back of the elbow. Injection is then performed by passing the needle just above the olecranon process perpendicular to the skin into the olecranon fossa (Fig. 10.9). Aspiration should be attempted since synovial fluid may be found when not clinically evident. It helps to confirm correct positioning but ease of injection is a more important sign. Where a lot of fluid is present it is useful to aspirate as much as possible of it before changing the syringe and giving an injection. The aspiration can both be therapeutic and enable synovial fluid examination. A variation on the posterior approach is to pass the needle into the infracondylar recess between the lateral epicondyle and olecranon process to enter the posterolateral aspect of the joint. Prior marking of the skin over the landmarks may aid positioning of the needle.

Lateral approach

With the patient's elbow fixed at 90° the head of the radius at the lateral radiohumeral part of the joint is felt with the thumb while rotating the patient's forearm with the other hand. This enables exact location of the joint line, which may be marked as a guide. The needle is then passed tangentially under the joint capsule rather than into the middle of the joint (Fig. 10.10). Aspiration is attempted before injection. Alternatively an injection may be performed with the elbow straight and the forearm fully supinated. The needle is passed into the joint vertically, just proximal to the radial head, but care must be taken to avoid contact between the needle and joint surface for risk of cartilage damage. Between 10mg and 25mg hydrocortisone acetate or 5–10mg triamcinolone (or equivalent) is usually enough.

Olecranon Bursa

Aspiration of fluid from the olecranon bursa is carried out with the elbow held at 90°. A 21- or 22-gauge needle attached to a 10ml syringe is inserted at a point lateral and posterior to the bony projection of the olecranon process into the center of the bursa. After the fluid has been aspirated the syringe may be changed and a local corticosteroid injection given (20mg methylprednisolone or equivalent) in the appropriate situation.

Lateral Epicondylitis

The aim is to inject the area of the tenoperiosteal junction of the common extensor tendon and lateral epicondyle. The favored patient posture is with the elbow supported at a right angle and the forearm

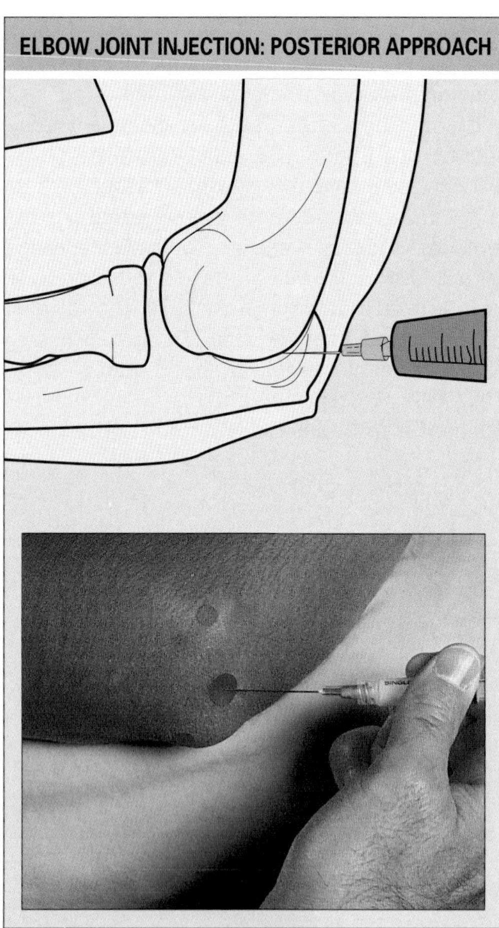

Fig. 10.9 Elbow joint injection: posterior approach.

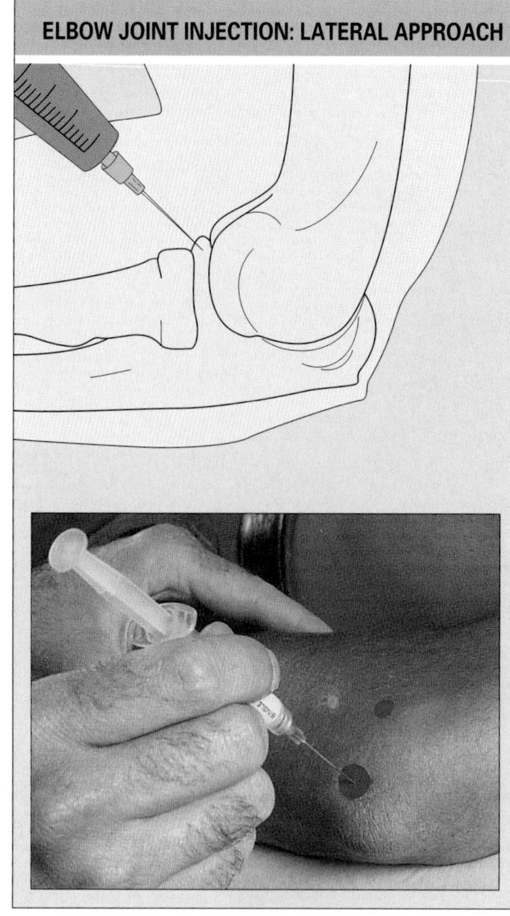

Fig. 10.10 Elbow joint injection: lateral approach.

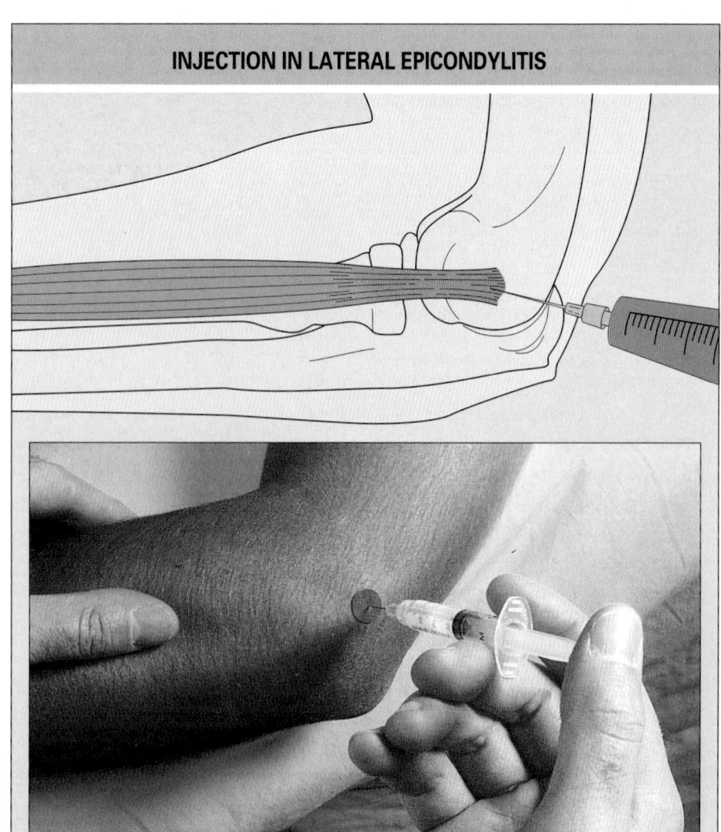

Fig. 10.11 Injection of corticosteroid and local anesthetic into the common extensor tendon origin at the lateral humeral epicondyle.

fully supinated. Injection is performed at the site of maximum tenderness to palpation (Fig. 10.11). This is normally a little distal to the epicondyle but is variable. After defining the site, marking the skin if necessary and cleansing the skin, the needle is passed down to the bone perpendicular to the skin. Injection is then performed as close to bone as possible. Since the site of injection is the tenoperiosteal junction, resistance to injection is experienced which may be considerable (make sure the needle hub is tight on the syringe) compared to the typical lack of resistance on injection of joint or bursa. Opinions vary, but a fan-shaped injection with partial withdrawal and reinsertion around the maximally tender site is probably the most beneficial. Usually 2–5ml of a combination of 10–25mg hydrocortisone acetate, 5-10mg triamcinolone or 10–20mg methylprednisolone with 1% lidocaine is used. The possible relative values of these types of corticosteroid have been discussed previously. The patient must be warned of at least a two in three chance of increased pain for up to 72 hours after injection. Failure of response within 2–4 weeks merits a repeat injection.

Medial Epicondylitis

The situation and injection technique are similar to those for lateral epicondylitis. Injection of the most tender site around the medial epicondyle is undertaken. The ulnar nerve lies in the groove just behind the medial epicondyle and particular care must be taken to avoid it.

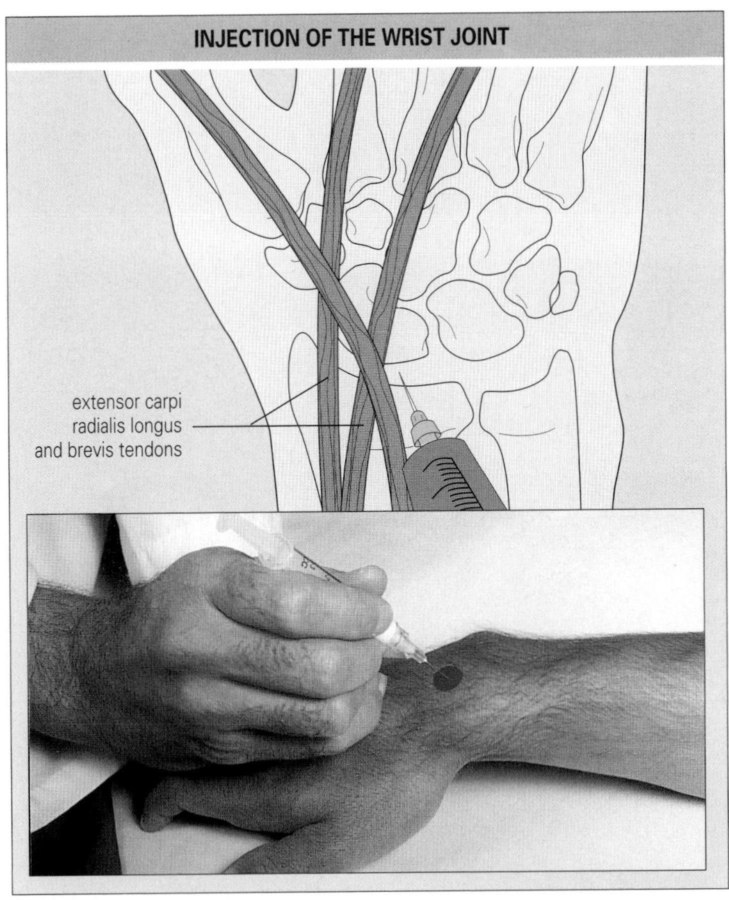

Fig. 10.12 Injection of the wrist joint.

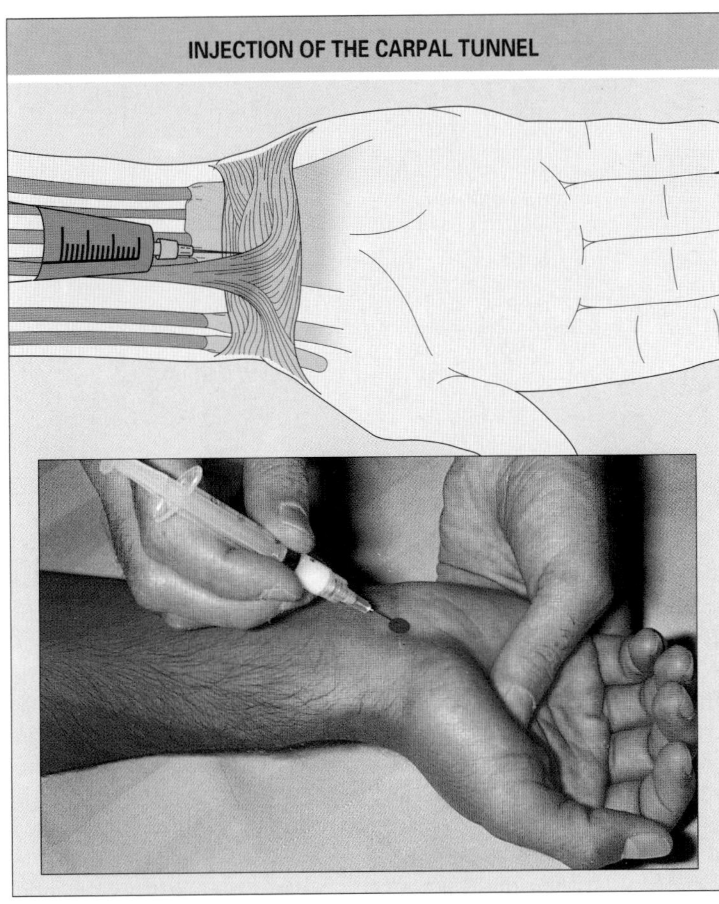

Fig. 10.13 Injection of the carpal tunnel.

The Wrist Joint

The radiocarpal joint can be aspirated and injected via a dorsoradial approach (Fig. 10.12). With the wrist slightly palmar flexed, the needle is inserted perpendicularly to a depth of 1–2cm at a point distal to Lister's tubercle of the radius and just ulnar to the extensor pollicis longus tendon.

The extensor tendon sheaths lie subcutaneous over the wrist and can be readily aspirated and injected with a small 27-gauge needle. In de Quervain's stenosing tenosynovitis, the tendon sheath of the abductor pollicis longus and extensor pollicis brevis can be injected through a dorsoradial approach. The needle is inserted tangentially into the distal end of the sheath. If correctly placed, injection of a local anesthetic distends the sheath and produces a swelling proximal to the extensor retinaculum.

The carpal tunnel and common flexor tendon sheath can be injected with a fine 27-gauge needle. The median nerve lies radial and underneath the palmaris longus tendon and should be avoided. The needle is inserted tangentially, directed towards the palm, just ulnar to the palmaris tendon and proximal to the distal wrist crease (Fig. 10.13). The needle is advanced to a depth of 3–6mm until the sheath is entered.

The First CMC Joint

This joint can be injected via a radial approach. The thumb is flexed across the palm towards the little finger. After feeling and localizing the joint line at the base of the first metacarpal, a small needle is inserted at an angle into the joint to a depth of 2–4mm, while avoiding the abductor pollicis longus and extensor pollicis brevis tendons.

The MCP, PIP, and DIP Joints

These joints can be readily entered via a dorsoradial or dorsoulnar approach using a 27-gauge needle (Figs 10.14 and 10.15). It is

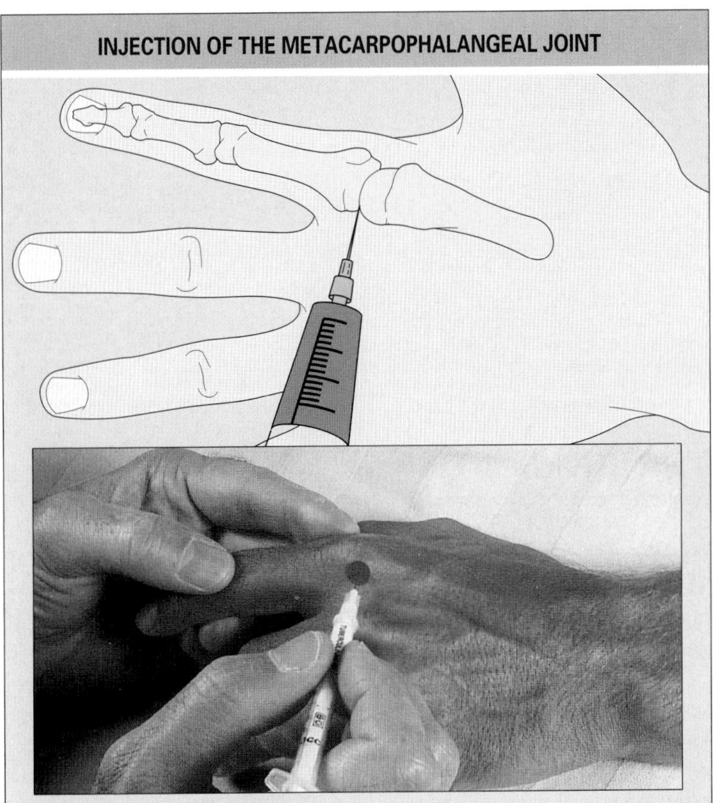

Fig. 10.14 Injection of the MCP joint.

sometimes necessary to tease the needle tip into the joint space while a slight traction is applied to the finger to pull the articulating surfaces apart. Synovial fluid is rarely obtained from these joints. Corticosteroid injection produces distension of the joint on all sides.

For injection of a trigger finger or a snapping thumb, a 27-gauge needle is inserted tangentially into the flexor sheath proximal to the first annular pulley, opposite the volar surface of the metacarpal head (Fig. 10.16). The needle is advanced until gentle passive movement of the finger (or thumb) makes a crepitant sensation indicating that the needle tip is rubbing against the surface of the tendon. When this occurs, the needle should be withdrawn 0.5–10.0mm before injecting the corticosteroid.

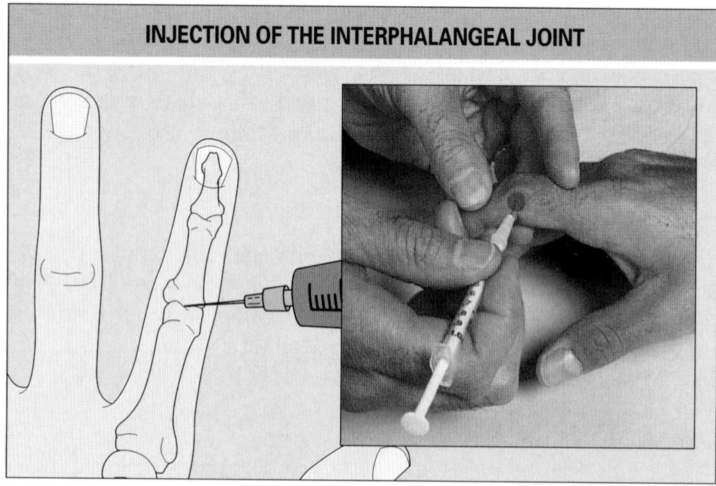

Fig. 10.15 Injection of the PIP joint.

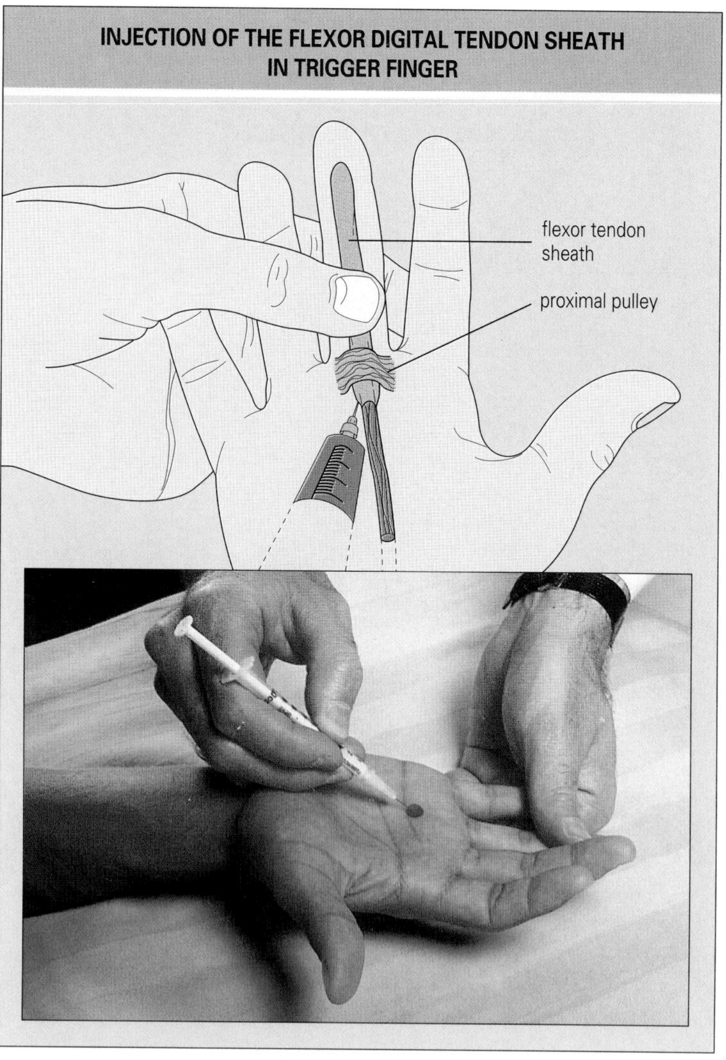

Fig. 10.16 Injection of the flexor digital tendon sheath in trigger finger.

THE HIP REGION

Bernard Mazières & Simon Carette

Hip Joint

The hip joint can best be aspirated and injected via an anterior approach. Fluoroscopic guidance is strongly advised. A 20-gauge needle should be used. With the patient lying supine, the hip slightly flexed and externally rotated, the needle will be inserted at the intersection of a vertical line drawn from the anterior superior iliac spine and a horizontal line drawn from the greater trochanter. The femoral vessels should be palpated one to two fingerbreadths lateral to the point of insertion of the needle. The needle is directed in a slightly upward and medial direction until it is felt to pass through the capsule (Fig. 10.17).

Trochanteric Bursa

With the patient lying on one side, the point of maximum tenderness is located (usually slighty posterior and superior to the greater trochanter). A 20-gauge needle may need to be used in obese patients. The needle is inserted vertically almost to the bone (Fig. 10.18), and a mixture of local anesthetic and corticosteroid (methylprednisolone acetate 40mg in 4–5ml of lidocaine) is injected while moving the tip of the needle in several directions to distribute the drugs over a wider area. After the needle is removed, a small massage of the area is recommended for the same purpose.

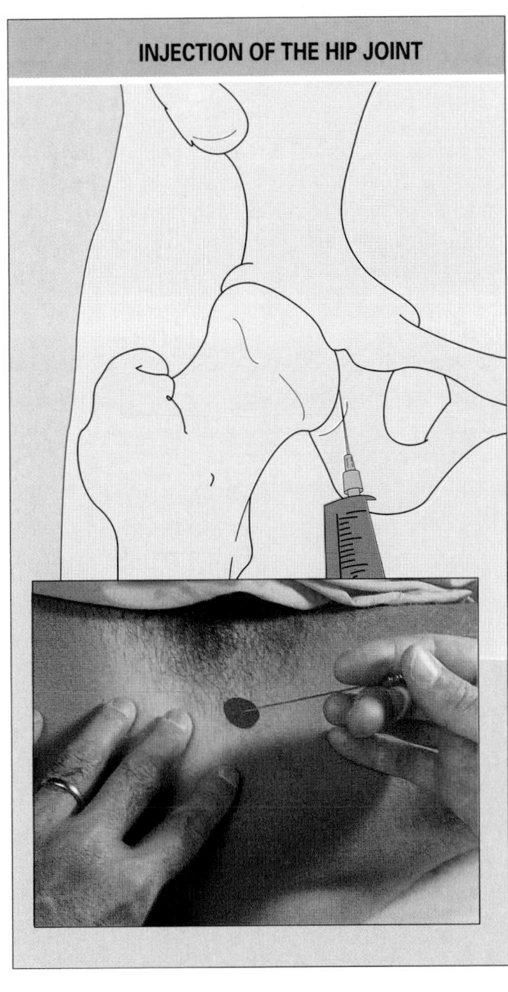

Fig. 10.17 Injection of the hip joint.

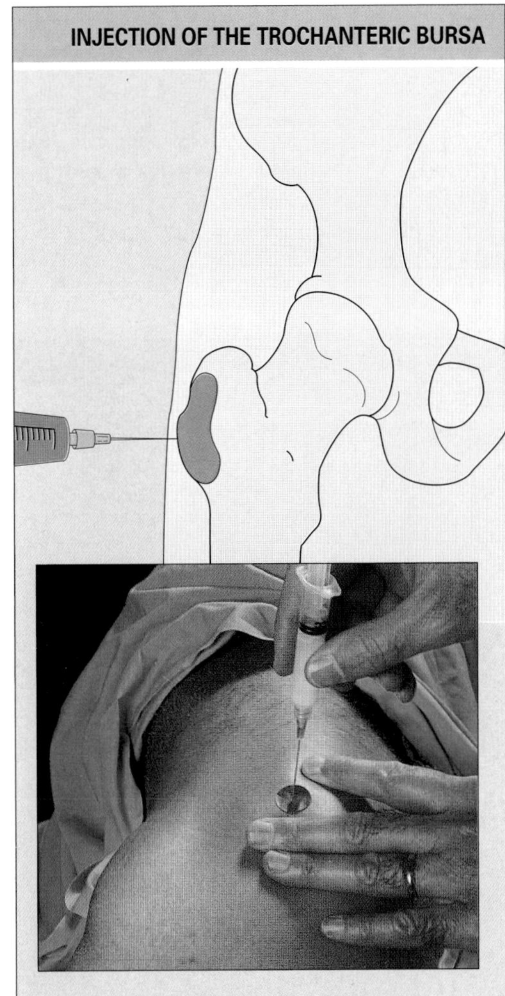

Fig. 10.18 Injection of the trochanteric bursa.

THE KNEE REGION

Geoffrey P Graham & John A Fairclough

Knee Joint

The knee joint is by far the easiest joint to inject. This can be done via lateral, medial or anterior approaches. For the lateral and medial approaches (see Fig. 10.19), the patient is supine with the knee fully extended. An 18- or 21-gauge needle is inserted perpendicular to the skin at a point slightly posterior to the lateral (or medial) upper border of the patella. An appropriate dose of corticosteroid for the knee joint is between 40 and 80mg methylprednisolone acetate or 20 and 40mg triamcinolone hexacetonide. For the anterior approach, the patient sits with the knee flexed at 90°. The needle is inserted just lateral to the patellar tendon in a slightly upward direction. It is usually difficult to obtain joint fluid from this approach.

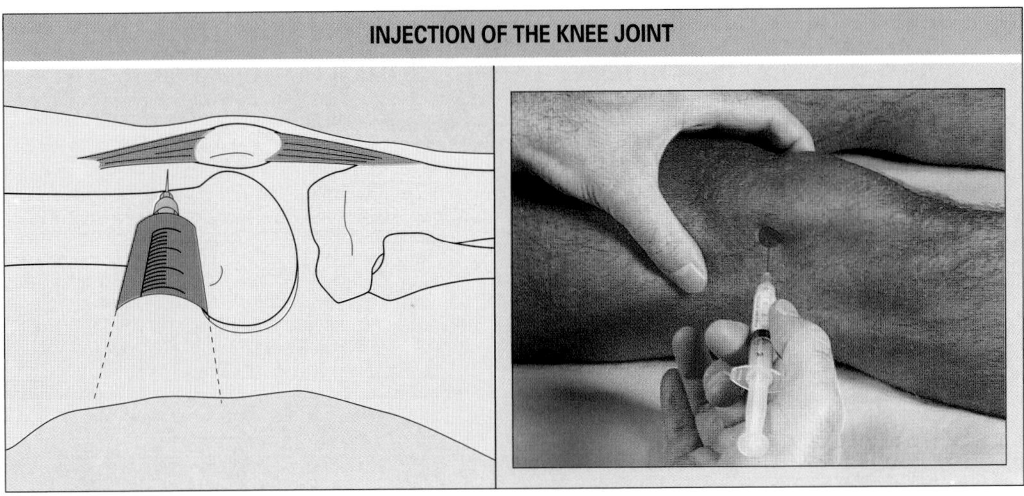

Fig. 10.19 Injection of the knee joint.

The Ankle Joint

The ankle joint can be injected via an anteromedial approach with the joint slightly plantar flexed. The needle is inserted at a point just medial to the tibialis anterior tendon and distal to the lower margin of the tibia. The needle is directed posteriorly and laterally to a depth of about 1–2cm (Fig. 10.20).

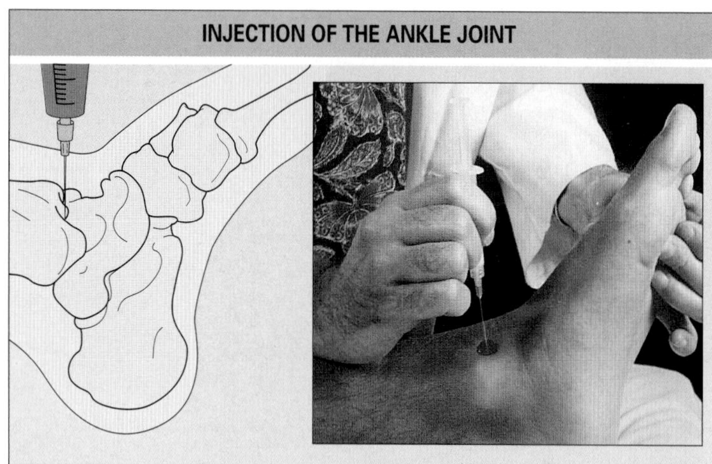

Fig. 10.20 Injection of the ankle joint.

Subtalar Joint

With the patient supine and the leg–foot angle at 90°, the needle is inserted horizontally into the subtalar joint just inferior to the tip of the lateral malleolus at a point just proximal to the sinus tarsi (Fig. 10.21). The other intertarsal and the tarsometatarsal joints cannot easily be injected without fluoroscopic guidance.

Metatarsophalangeal Joint

The MTP joint can be entered via a dorsomedial or dorsolateral route (Fig. 10.22). The joint space is first identified, then a 25-gauge needle is inserted on either side of the extensor tendon to a depth of 2-4mm. Slight traction on the appropriate toe facilitates entry. The PIP and DIP joints of the toes may be entered in a similar fashion via a dorsomedial or dorsolateral route.

Injection for Plantar Fasciitis

The injection is delivered from the medial side after carefully palpating the point of maximal tenderness under the heel. This point is marked with a ball-point pen, and after infiltration with lidocaine 1%, the needle is inserted through the thinner skin of the medial side of the heel and advanced in a lateral and slightly upward and posterior direction. The injection is made as close as possible to the plantar surface of the calcaneus. If the bone is struck, the needle is withdrawn slightly before injecting the corticosteroid-lidocaine mixture.

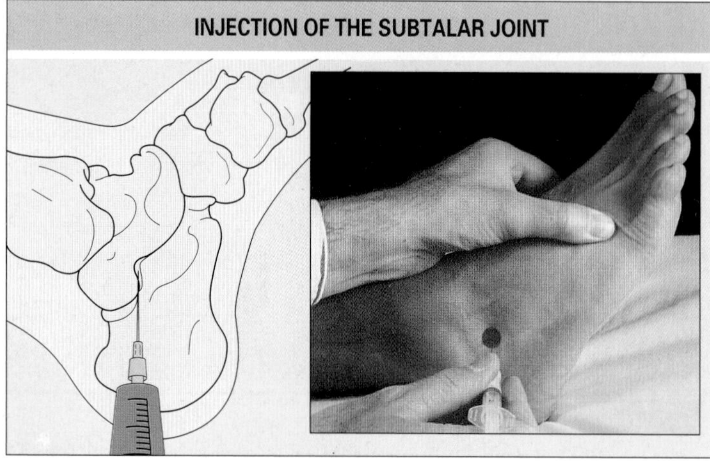

Fig. 10.21 Injection of the subtalar joint.

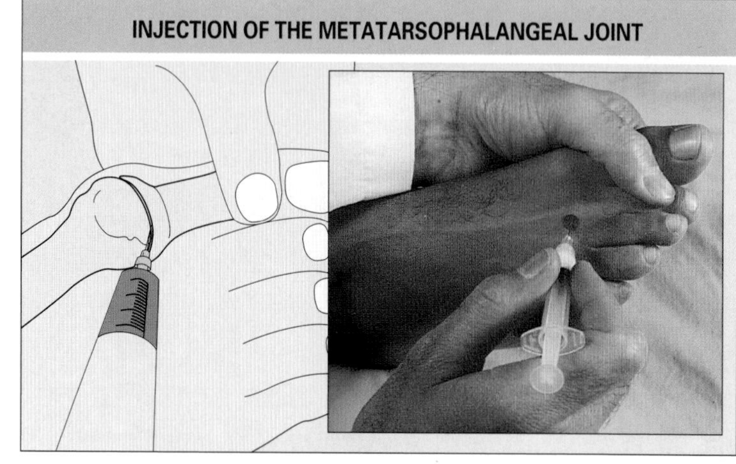

Fig. 10.22 Injection of the MTP joint.

REFERENCES

Blyth T, Hunter JA, Stirling A. Pain relief in the rheumatoid knee after steroid injection. A single-blind comparison of hydrocortisone succinate, and triamcinolone acetonide or hexacetonide. Br J Rheumatol 1994;**33**:461–3.

Cawley PJ, Morris IM. A study to compare the efficacy of two methods of skin preparation prior to joint injection. Br J Rheumatol 1992;**31**:847–8.

Chakravarty K, Pharoah PD, Scott DG. A randomized controlled study of post-injection rest following intra-articular steroid therapy for knee synovitis. Br J Rheumatol 1994;**33**:464–8.

Doherty M, Hazelman BL, Hutton CW, Maddison PJ, Perry JD, eds. Rheumatology examination and injection techniques. London: WB Saunders; 1992;121–7.

Freemont AJ, Denton J. Chuck A, et al. Diagnostic value of synovial fluid microscopy: a reassessment and rationalisation. Ann Rheum Dis 1991, **50**:101–7.

Gatter RA, Shcumacher HR. A practical handbook of joint fluid analysis, 2E. Philadelphia: Lea and Febiger, 1991.

Gray RG, Tenenbaum J, Gottlieb NL. Local corticosteroid injection treatment in rheumatic disorders. Semin Arthritis Rheum 1981;**10**:231–54.

Hasselbacher P. Arthrocentesis, synovial fluid analysis, and synovial biopsy. In: Schumacher HR, Klippel JH, Koopman WJ, eds. Primer on the rheumatic diseases, 9E. Atlanta: Arthritis Foundation; 1993;67–72.

Ike RW, Arnold WJ, Roschild EW,et al. Tidal irrigation versus conservative medical management in patients with osteoarthritis of the knee: a prospective randomized study. J Rheumatol 1992, **19**: 772–9.

Kaplan H. Therapeutic injection of joints and soft tissues. In: Schumacher HR, Klippel JH, Koopman WJ, eds. Primer on the rheumatic diseases, 9E. Atlanta: Arthritis Foundation; 1993;310–11.

McCarty DJ. A basic guide to arthrocentesis. Hosp Med 1968;**4**:778–8.

Pfenninzer J. Injection of joints and soft tissue: Part I. General guidelines. Am Fam Physician 1991;**44**:1196.

Pfenninzer J. Injection of joints and soft tissue: Part II. Guidelines for specific joints. Am Fam Physician 1991;**44**:1690.

Schaffer TC. Joint and soft-tissue arthrocentesis. Prim Care 1993;**20**:757–70.

Von Essen R, Savolainen H. Bacterial infection following intra-articular injections; A brief review. Scand J Rheumatol. 1989;**18**:7.

Zuckerman J, Meislin R, Rithenberg M. Injections for joint and soft tissue disorders : when and how to use them. Geriatrics 1990;**45**:45.

REGIONAL PAIN PROBLEMS

11

PRACTICAL PROBLEMS

CERVICAL ROOT IRRITATION

Cyrus Cooper

Definition of the Problem

It is important to consider rare but potentially serious syndromes such as atlantoaxial subluxation and cervical myelopathy. Thereafter, the major distinction lies between soft tissue cervical spine disorders (which do not usually cause brachial neuralgia) and cervical spondylosis. Both of these are stable conditions, and management consists of an algorithm of sequentially applied conservative measures.

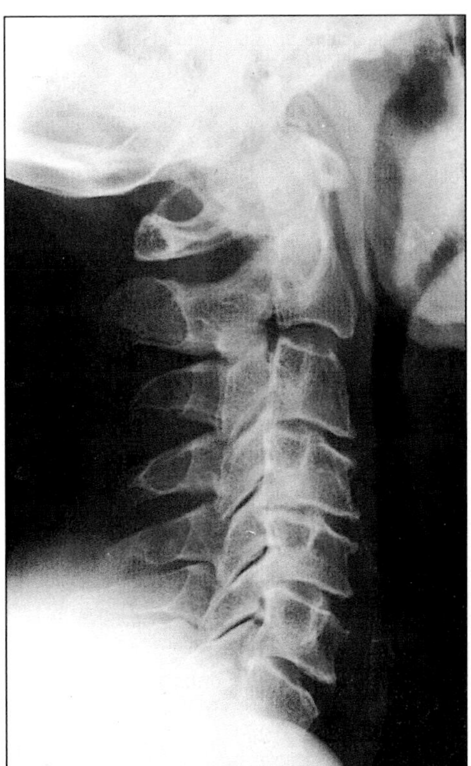

Fig. 11.1 Lateral cervical spine radiograph illustrating features of cervical spondylosis. There is loss of posterior disc height with irregularity of the disc margins at C4–C5 and C5–C6, with some subchondral sclerosis and osteophyte formation anteriorly and posteriorly at these levels.

The Typical Case

HD is a plump 62-year-old woman with a 5-year history of progressively worsening neck pain. This commenced after a fall while gardening and has had a remitting and relapsing course with exacerbations lasting 4–5 weeks in every 3 months. She presented with a 2-week history of severe pain radiating from her neck to the radial aspect of her left forearm and hand. This pain initially woke her from sleep, and had been continuous since. It was accompanied by numbness and tingling in the same area of the left arm, and she had noticed weakness in lifting objects such as a filled kettle. On examination, there was tenderness in the left paracervical region at the C5–C6 level, with a reduced left biceps tendon reflex. Neck movements were painful and restricted, especially right lateral flexion and rotation. Pain in the left arm was reproducible by vertical pressure on the head (Spurling's maneuver). The lateral cervical spine radiograph (Fig. 11.1) revealed disc-space narrowing at the C5–C6 level, with marginal osteophyte formation and subchondral sclerosis.

Diagnosis

The cervical spine is one of the most complex articular systems in the body, and numerous clinical syndromes have been associated with its dysfunction. The most frequent of these disorders is cervical spondylosis, a condition arising from a varying combination of cervical intervertebral disc degeneration and osteoarthritis affecting the apophyseal or intervertebral joints. The life-time prevalence of neck pain, the most frequent symptom, is greater than 35%, and radiological evidence of cervical spondylosis is almost universal above age 65 years.

Radiculopathy results from disc or osteophyte encroachment on one or several cervical nerve roots, especially C6 (C5–C6 disc) and C7 (C6–C7 disc). It may result in pain or paresthesias affecting the upper-limb dermatomes at the involved levels, with weakness and hyporeflexia (see Fig. 11.2).

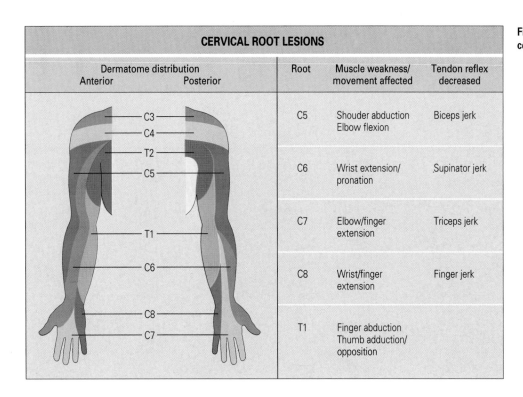

CERVICAL ROOT LESIONS

Dermatome distribution: Anterior / Posterior — C3, C4, T2, C5, T1, C6, C8, C7

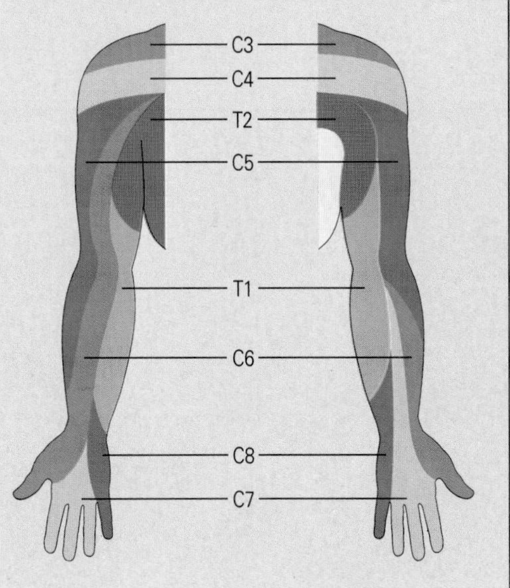

Root	Muscle weakness/ movement affected	Tendon reflex decreased
C5	Shouder abduction Elbow flexion	Biceps jerk
C6	Wrist extension/ pronation	Supinator jerk
C7	Elbow/finger extension	Triceps jerk
C8	Wrist/finger extension	Finger jerk
T1	Finger abduction Thumb adduction/ opposition	

Fig. 11.2 Sensory and motor distribution of the cervical roots.

Cervical cord or root involvement?

Cervical myelopathy must be distinguished from brachial root compression as a cause of neurologic features in the arm. Cervical myelopathy may arise from disc prolapse, as well as cervical spine instability. This latter cause is a potentially serious complication of inflammatory joint disorders such as rheumatoid arthritis, requiring urgent evaluation (most usefully by MRI) and assessment for surgical stabilization. Cervical myelopathy usually manifests with a combination of upper and lower limb sensory and motor signs. In contrast, brachial root signs are confined to the upper limb.

Inflammatory or mechanical?

Inflammatory arthritides, such as rheumatoid arthritis, ankylosing spondylitis and juvenile chronic arthritis commonly involve the cervical spine and enter the differential diagnosis of neck pain. It is extremely unusual for these disorders to result in brachial root irritation, so that neurologic symptoms and signs in the arm point towards a compressive lesion of spinal cord or roots.

MANAGEMENT OF CERVICAL SPONDYLOSIS WITH BRACHIAL ROOT IRRITATION
Education
Reassurance Rest/exercise Occupational changes Psychotherapy
Physiotherapy
Heat/cold Neck exercises Cervical collar Ultrasound/TENS/acupuncture Traction
Pharmacotherapy
Analgesics Muscle relaxants NSAIDs Local injection therapy

Fig. 11.3 Basic management program for cervical spondylosis with brachial root irritation.

Referred pain or root irritation?

Soft tissue disorders of the upper limb such as frozen shoulder and tennis elbow commonly result in referred pain and tenderness to more distant sites within the arm. The pattern of radiation may be difficult to distinguish from the dermatomal distribution in the arm, but it is not associated with neurologic signs in the upper limb.

Bony or soft tissue?

A large proportion of cervical spine syndromes arises through disruption of the soft tissues supporting the neck. These include acceleration and deceleration (whiplash) injuries, musculoligamentous strains, tension myositis and acute neck strain. While these disorders frequently result in pain and localized tenderness of the paraspinal tissues, they do not usually irritate the brachial nerve roots. Osteophytic or discal compression of roots, however, results in the neurologic picture already outlined.

Where is the neurologic lesion?

A number of investigations may aid in localizing the cause of neurologic symptoms and signs in the upper limb. Cervical spine radiography and MRI provide important structural information as outlined above. Isotope scintigraphy may be useful in excluding rarer intrinsic bone abnormalities such as infection or tumor. Finally, nerve conduction studies may help differentiate between a peripheral polyneuropathy, focal radiculopathy, and myopathy.

Therapeutic Options

Disorders of the cervical spine are best treated with a program incorporating multiple approaches, each individualized for the specific patient (Fig. 11.3). These include patient education, physiotherapeutic maneuvers to relieve pain and reduce nerve root compression, and drug therapy. While there is little controlled evidence by which to estimate the success of these measures, clinical experience supports their efficacy in certain groups of patients, and their widespread use is established. Surgery is only indicated in a few circumstances, and the outcome of surgical intervention is moderate at best.

Education
The more the patient understands about the mechanism of neck and arm symptoms, the more he or she is able to actively participate in the management program. Education must include postural training, the use of alternating rest (to diminish inflammation) and exercise (to maintain conditioning of muscles and ligaments), and advice about work and leisure activities.

Physiotherapy
The initial physiotherapeutic interventions in a patient with cervical spondylosis and brachial root irritation comprise the use of a cervical collar, local pain-relieving measures and traction.

The desired degree of immobilization dictates the type of collar used. When structural displacement of the cervical spine is a concern, only a rigid collar succeeds in limiting neck movements by over 50%. In most cases of cervical spondylosis, however, a soft collar will suffice. Patients with root irritation often find relief during and after wearing a soft collar, but those with disease at multiple levels do less well than those with single-level involvement.

The most usual local pain-relieving maneuvers adopted are hot and cold, with the aim of relieving muscle spasm, and ultrasound and short-wave diathermy. If these modalities are ineffective, it is worth a trial of transcutaneous electronic nerve stimulation (TENS) or acupuncture. The gate theory of pain provides a rational basis for the use of TENS or acupuncture in intractable musculoskeletal pain, but neither measure has been shown to predictably provide relief.

Studies of traction have shown that at least 10 kg is required to eliminate lordosis in the cervical spine. At this loading level, there is a 2–3mm increase in overall cervical length, which is preserved. Traction is reserved for situations where there are symptoms and signs of brachial root irritation.

In an otherwise healthy person, 10kg for 20 min after local application of heat to relieve muscle spasm is usually effective. This treatment is usually repeated daily for a fortnight. Traction is contraindicated in patients with atlantoaxial subluxation or those with vertebrobasilar insufficiency.

Manipulation of the cervical spine is used by those of its devotees who have intractable symptoms, but disasters have been documented, especially when performed by the poorly trained or in situations of diagnostic uncertainty.

Drug therapy
Analgesics, muscle relaxants and nonsteroidal anti-inflammatory drugs (NSAIDs) are useful in the management of cervical spine syndromes. Injection of local anesthetic and corticosteroid into areas of local tenderness about the lower neck, scapulae and shoulders may also be effective.

Surgery
As already stated, surgical intervention is rarely necessary. Indications include unremitting symptoms 4–6 months following documented disc prolapse, and clear progression of neurologic signs.

Conclusions
Brachial root irritation is a common rheumatologic problem that usually results from a combination of degenerative cervical disc disease and osteoarthritis of the intervertebral joints. Once cervical myelopathy is excluded, pain and neurologic dysfunction in the arm are usually alleviated with conservative measures as part of a graduated program. Surgical intervention is rarely necessary.

REFERENCES

Bland JH. Diagnosis and medical management of diseases and disorders of the cervical spine. Philadelphia: WB Saunders; 1987.

Holt L. Cervical, dorsal and lumbar spine syndromes. Acta Orthop Scand. 1954; (suppl 17):1–102.

Lawrence JS. Disc degeneration: Its frequency and relationship to symptoms. Ann Rheum Dis. 1969;**28**:121-38.

Spurling RG, Seperberg LH. Intervertebral disc lesions in the lower cervical region. JAMA 1953;**151**:354-9.

WHIPLASH INJURY

Maurice A Barry

Definition of the Problem
Whiplash injury, or acute hyperextension/flexion of the neck, is a common feature of motor accidents. The injuries sustained vary in severity from minor tearing of muscle fibers to vertebral fracture with spinal cord compression. The term 'whiplash' has passed into public usage because of the large numbers of these injuries, the frequent chronicity of symptoms and the association with financial compensation.

The Typical Case
JW, a 40-year-old female, was the driver of a car struck from behind by another vehicle. She was wearing a seatbelt and although thrown forward did not strike her head or lose consciousness. Initially dazed, over the next 2–3 hours she developed severe neck pain and stiffness, with radiation of pain to the head and upper back. Examination revealed neck muscle tenderness and marked restriction of movement; peripheral nerve examination was normal. Cervical spine radiographs demonstrated minor lower cervical degenerative changes only. Treatment consisted of oral analgesics, immobilization in a surgical collar and reassurance that symptoms should settle in a number of weeks. This was followed by physiotherapy with local pain-relieving measures and gentle mobilization.

At 1 month there had been no improvement in neck pain. She was unable to perform a number of normal housework and leisure activities. Further complaints included headache, pins and needles in the left arm, poor concentration and irritability. Neck and peripheral nervous system examination were unchanged. It was noted that she was in the process of pursuing a legal claim.

At 6 months there was some improvement in symptoms and signs; overall she felt only 10–20% improved despite treatment with a range of analgesics and further physiotherapy. Two years after the accident and 6 months after settlement of the legal case there had been considerable easing in symptoms, but overall she felt only 50% improved. She was reassured that symptoms should settle completely with time.

Diagnostic Problems
There are approximately 3.8 million rear-end motor accidents annually in the USA. Front, side and other accidents also give rise to whiplash injuries. The introduction of compulsory wearing of seatbelts in the UK was associated with a rise in the incidence of whiplash injuries, while head restraints reduce the incidence of injury in rear-end impacts by 15%. Between 38 and 60% of those injured develop neck pain and stiffness, with the majority settling completely in 3–6 months. A significant percentage, however (over

25% in one large retrospective series), have continuing neck pain often associated with other symptoms including headaches, poor sleep, paresthesiae, anxiety and depression. This group with what is termed 'late whiplash syndrome' (LWS) are difficult to manage as disabling symptoms continue despite what often appears to have been an initial minor injury.

Late Whiplash Syndrome

The persistence of neck pain and other symptoms beyond 6 months is a frustrating problem both for patient and physician. The clinical difficulty is in distinguishing the relative contribution, if any, of three important factors – unresolved injury, psychological influences and compensation neurosis. One school of thought proposes that all whiplash injuries heal within 6 months (in the absence of evidence of neurologic injuries), and that those with persisting symptoms exaggerate their symptoms for financial gain or else are of a 'neurotic' disposition and unable to cope with trivial injury. There is, however, gradually accumulating evidence that those with persistent symptoms may have unresolved and unrecognized injury. A recently published MRI study suggested avulsion of intervertebral disc from underlying end plate as a possible finding in LWS. A number of studies, some of them controlled, have demonstrated abnormalities in spinal and brainstem function in late whiplash without neurologic signs. Significant disturbances in trigeminal and oculomotor function and electronystagmographic abnormalities have been reported. The relevance of these changes is not known but supports the impression of many physicians that a balanced approach to the assessment of LWS is important.

Although the pathology of LWS is uncertain, a number of factors are associated with more severe injury or the persistence of symptoms and may be useful prognostically. High speed of impact, major damage to the vehicle and rapid onset or intense initial neck pain are associated with more severe injury, as is marked restriction of neck movement at initial presentation. Increasing age and the presence of paresthesiae or cervical spondylosis are associated with the persistence of symptoms, though not necessarily with more severe injury.

Psychological influences undoubtedly play an important role in LWS. Complaints of neck pain, paresthesiae, headaches, etc., are often out of proportion to the clinical findings. Associated symptoms of anxiety, irritability and fatigue are common, and many patients appear not to have returned to their former level of functioning socially or at work. It might be assumed that this group of patients would exhibit premorbid personality traits, such as neuroticism or a tendency to depression, and that the presence of these traits could predict a poor outcome. However, a recent study from Switzerland performed psychological profiles of patients within 1 week of injury and found no association between 'negative' personality traits and the persistence of symptoms. The only psychological trait which did predict persistence of symptoms was subjective cognitive impairment (forgetfulness, poor concentration, comprehension difficulties) at presentation. Rather than the presence of personality traits susceptible to reacting adversely to illness, a more probable influence on the clinical picture in some cases is post-traumatic stress disorder, a well recognized sequela of accidents. This can occur in any individual and shares many of the features of LWS, including headaches, paresthesiae, fatigue and depression. When combined with the natural frustration experienced by patients whose symptoms persist despite repeated assurances and numerous treatments, the psychological symptoms of many with LWS may be explained.

Those with whiplash injuries often are aggrieved at having suffered through no fault of their own. This anger and the prospect of financial compensation also plays a role in prolonging complaints in certain patients. Cases are seen where continuing but improbable symptoms are accompanied by inexplicable or inconsistent clinical signs. This represents only a small group of patients and the genuine disability (physical and psychological) of the majority is suggested by the similar numbers with LWS who are pursuing and not pursuing litigation, a tendency for the other injuries sustained in whiplash cases to heal in the expected time, and the strong tendency for symptoms to persist for long periods following compensation.

Therapeutic Options

Early whiplash

At presentation, features in the history suggesting more severe injury or the likelihood of persistence of symptoms (Fig. 11.4) should be noted. Changes on cervical spine radiographs should also be noted, most commonly prevertebral soft tissue swelling and angular deformity between vertebral bodies, although neither, surprisingly, is associated with the persistence of symptoms. The presence of fractures or cervical instability indicates serious injury and, as in those with neurologic signs, further investigation should be undertaken, particularly MRI.

Initial treatment of whiplash injury consists of rest and analgesics for 1–2 weeks. If symptoms are severe, a molded collar holding the neck in neutral or slight flexion appears to be superior to the standard soft collar. Subsequent outpatient physiotherapy is effective in improving severity of neck pain and cervical movement but in a number of trials has proved no better in this regard than merely a demonstration of home mobilization by a physiotherapist. Good communication between patient and doctor is important. Patients should be informed that they have suffered both physical injury and, in cases where this is suspected, a degree of psychological trauma as a result of the accident. It is best to state early on that recovery can be unpredictable, taking months or longer, but that complete resolution is expected. Confidant assurances of healing in a certain number of weeks only promotes uncertainty and frustration when this does not occur and can contribute significantly to prolongation of symptoms and reduce the effectiveness of the doctor. During the period of mobilization, further assurances can be given that neck pain related to reasonable activities is not perpetuating the injuries or causing a risk of permanent damage.

Patients should be reviewed 6–12 weeks following injury if still symptomatic. Neurologic signs and symptoms can first develop some weeks after injury and should be sought. Any treatment modalities, including physiotherapy, which are only minimally or

FACTORS ASSOCIATED WITH WHIPLASH INJURIES
Factors associated with more severe injury
High speed of impact
Major damage to the vehicle
Intense or rapid-onset initial neck pain
Severe restriction of neck movement at initial presentation
Abnormal neurologic signs
Bony injuries on cervical spine radiographs
Factors associated with persistence of symptoms
All of those above
Increasing age
Upper limb paresthesiae
Presence of cervical spondylosis on radiographs
Subjective cognitive impairment at presentation

Fig. 11.4 Factors associated with whiplash injuries.

temporarily effective are best discontinued. The limitations of current treatment should be explained and the patient encouraged towards a positive, self-help attitude.

Late whiplash syndrome

Where symptoms extend beyond 6 months the possibility of persisting injury must be accepted. This is of greater likelihood when factors associated with more severe injury are present. Flexion and extension radiographs of the cervical spine performed even months after injury occasionally reveals abnormal or restricted motion at one segment. This may not have been apparent on radiographs taken early on, when muscle spasm is often intense. These findings and possibly unremitting paresthesiae in the absence of signs are indications for further investigation. The role of electrophysiological studies is undetermined but they may be indicated in whiplash injuries associated with prolonged dizziness, vertigo or facial paresthesiae. Therapeutic trials in LWS are lacking but potent analgesics or hypnotics should be avoided. The temporary use of a collar or simple analgesics should be reserved for occasional exacerbations. The effects of TENS, manipulation or acupuncture have not been systematically studied.

Symptoms of psychological disturbance, including anxiety, irritability, poor sleep and depression, should be enquired after and dealt with in a sympathetic but positive manner. A dismissive or disbelieving attitude only adds to the patient's burden and can delay recovery. Psychiatric referral is rarely warranted.

The minority of patients with unconvincing physical and psychological symptoms or with inconsistent signs should be informed that their clinical picture is not that expected in whiplash injury and is unrelated to the accident. Previously bitter complaints such as muscle weakness, restricted movement and paresthesiae usually cease forthwith. The early settlement of legal cases would discourage malingering, and the common practice of awaiting the leveling off of symptoms before proceeding with the court case should be changed, as this only encourages the prolongation of complaints.

The current management of LWS in particular owes more to art than science. Much more information is needed to improve the management of these patients, and the results of a number of long-term prospective studies are keenly awaited.

REFERENCES

Davis SI, Teresi LM, Bradley WG, Ziemba MA, Bloze AE. Cervical spine hyperextension injuries: MR findings. Radiology. 1991;**180**:245–51.

MacNab I. Acceleration extension injuries of the cervical spine. In: Rothman R, Simeone F, eds. The spine, vol 2. Philadelphia: WB Saunders; 1975;515–28.

Miles KA, Maimaris C, Finley D, Barnes MR. The incidence and prognostic significance of radiological abnormalities in soft tissue injuries to the cervical spine. Skeletal Radiol. 1988;**17**:493–6.

Oosterveld WJ, Kortschot HW, Kingma GG, de long HAA, Saatcio MR. Electronystagmographic findings following cervical whiplash injuries. Acta Oteolaryngol (Stockh). 1991;**111**: 201–5.

Radanov BP, Di Stefano G, Schnidrig A, Ballinari P. Role of psychosocial stress in recovery from common whiplash. Lancet. 1991;**338**:712–15.

SPINAL STENOSIS

Joseph M Cash

Definition of the Problem

Lumbar spinal stenosis is the most important consequence of lumbar spinal degeneration. This disorder is common and has substantial economic impact, with approximately 0.1% of Americans over the age of 65 undergoing laminectomy surgery yearly. Many more patients suffer from chronic pain or develop significant disability.

The Typical Case

An 84-year-old woman presented with a 2-year history of slowly progressive lumbar, buttocks and leg pain. The pain was absent while lying in the flexed position, occurred when standing and gradually increased with walking. Initially she noticed the pain only after walking several blocks. However, over the preceding 6 months, pain limited her walking to less than 15 meters. She was otherwise in excellent health and was quite distressed by her limited ability to walk. She had no cardiac risk factors.

General physical examination including examination of joints and peripheral pulses was within normal limits for her age. Examination of the spine demonstrated decreased spinal motion in all planes. There was no spinal or paraspinal tenderness. Muscle tone, bulk and strength were normal. Neurologic examination was normal except for absent ankle reflexes. Electromyography was normal. Radiographs and MRI scans revealed extensive degenerative change and spinal stenosis (see Figs 11.5 & 11.6).

Initial treatment with enteric coated aspirin, 2000mg/day, and physical therapy was helpful for about 1 year. When symptoms worsened, intravenous and epidural corticosteroids were tried, with temporary relief only. She was then referred to an orthopedic spinal surgeon and underwent a multilevel decompressive laminectomy. Her postoperative course was unremarkable. At 1 year after surgery, she continued to have mild localized lumbar pain, especially with standing and walking. However, her leg pain had completely resolved and she was quite satisfied with her current ability to ambulate.

Diagnostic Evaluation

Spinal stenosis should be considered in any elderly patient presenting with leg or buttocks pain. Typically, patients complain of buttocks and leg pain that appears with standing, is increased with walking, and resolves with sitting or bending forward (pseudoclaudication). Lumbar pain secondary to associated disc and facet joint

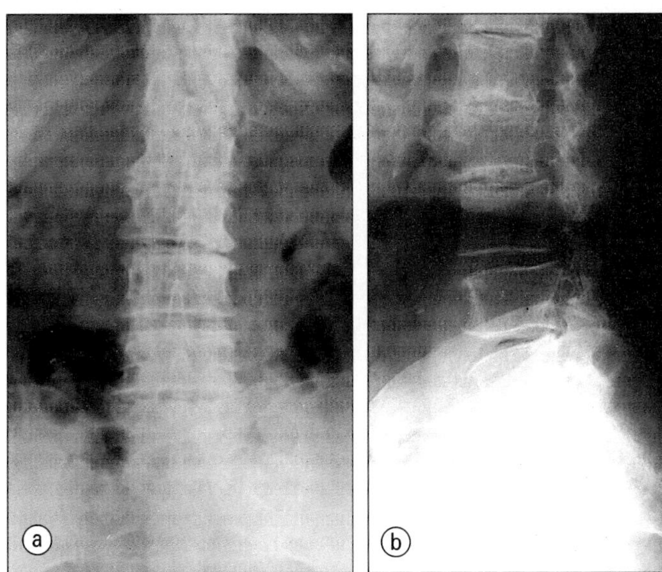

Fig. 11.5 Spinal stenosis. Anterior (a) and lateral (b) radiographs of the lumbar spine. Degenerative spondylolisthesis, disc degeneration with vacuum phenomenon, and facet joint hypertrophy are present.

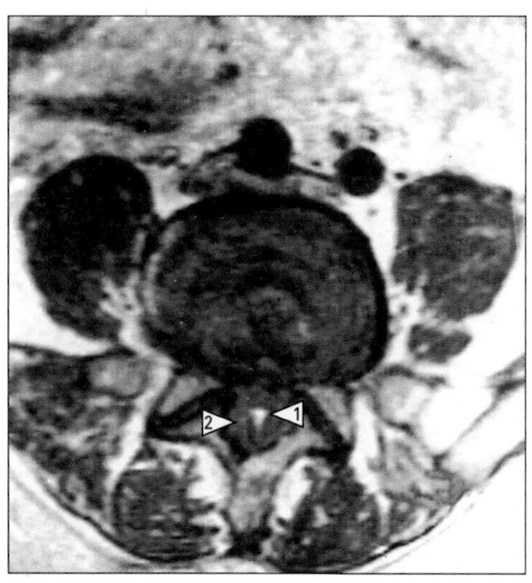

Fig. 11.6 Spinal stenosis. MRI scan at the L4–L5 interspace. The thecal sac (1) is severely constricted by hypertrophied ligamentum flavum (2).

degeneration is common but not universal. There are no consistent physical findings.

Lumbar spine radiographs characteristically show advanced degenerative changes. Typical findings include disc-space narrowing, traction osteophytes, facet-joint hypertrophy and low-grade spondylolisthesis. Pelvic radiographs should also be obtained to rule out hip disease and to check for evidence of Paget's disease – a treatable cause of spinal stenosis. MRI is rapidly replacing myelography and CT scanning as the diagnostic procedure of choice to precisely assess the dimensions of the spinal canal and thus confirm the diagnosis. However, MRI scanning is not mandatory unless the clinical presentation is confusing, spinal tumors are suspected or surgery is contemplated. Electromyography is rarely helpful in confirming the diagnosis or in guiding surgical therapy.

Pseudoclaudication is frequently confused with true vascular claudication. Nevertheless, several historical findings strongly suggest spinal stenosis. Standing alone frequently produces leg pain, in clear distinction from vascular claudication. In addition, pain is exacerbated with extending the spine. Weakness, numbness or paresthesias of the lower extremities may be seen. Patients with pseudoclaudication also may ride exercise bicycles without difficulty or walk in a flexed position behind shopping carts or walkers with a reduction in symptoms. Occasionally, patients will present with clinical evidence of both disorders. In this case, both possibilities should be evaluated. Correction of severe vascular insufficiency by angioplasty or by other means is the higher priority.

Therapeutic Options

The treatment of spinal stenosis is frustrating. No individual treatment is satisfactory in all patients. In addition, very little scientific data exists to guide therapy.

Conservative therapy

All patients initially presenting with spinal stenosis deserve a trial of conservative therapy. Initial medical options include aspirin, nonacetylated salicylates or NSAID therapy. Physical therapy should be directed at abdominal strengthening and improving spinal flexion. Lumbar supports are not helpful.

Empiric medical therapy

Calcitonin is the best studied agent and may improve pain control and walking distance – especially in patients with relatively mild stenosis. However, the high expense as well as generally poor patient acceptance of calcitonin may limit its applicability. Corticosteroids are commonly used, presumably to reduce edema surrounding neural elements. Prednisone, 40mg/day, is often used for 5 days in patients who fail to respond to initial conservative treatment. If oral corticosteroids fail, a course of in-patient intravenous corticosteroids may be tried next. A typical regimen would include dexamethasone 10mg i.v. initially, followed by 4mg i.v. every 8 hours for six doses and then 2mg i.v. every 8 hours for six doses. Epidural injections of corticosteroids are occasionally helpful as well.

Surgical therapy

Surgical referral for decompressive laminectomy and removal of hypertrophied ligamentum flavum should not be excessively delayed in patients who are good surgical candidates and have failed conservative therapy. The realistic goal of surgery is to relieve leg pain and thus allow for functional ambulation. Lumbar pain and lower extremity weakness may not improve. Outcome research suggests that patients with coexisting medical problems have worse results. Surgery should be avoided in patients with significant osteoarthritis of the knees, hips or ankles as they may not have significant functional improvement with surgery. Patients who receive single-level laminectomies may ultimately need repeat procedures. Fortunately, complications including infection, nerve-root injury, dural injury and symptomatic spinal instability are rare. Nevertheless, at least 50% of patients have excellent long-term symptomatic improvement following decompressive laminectomy. Even better results are possible if patients are carefully selected.

Conclusion

Spinal stenosis is a common cause of leg and low back pain in the elderly. This disorder is usually obvious after a careful history and physical examination and reviewing plain radiographs of the lumbar spine. All patients deserve a trial of physical therapy and analgesics. Calcitonin and corticosteroids are used as well, though without strong scientific support. Surgery should be reserved for those patients who do not have generalized osteoarthritis or serious coexistent medical problems. Surgical therapy offers the best hope of long-term symptomatic relief.

REFERENCES

Borenstein DG, Wiesel SW. Mechanical disorders of the lumbosacral spine. In: Low back pain. Medical diagnosis and comprehensive management. Philadelphia: WB Saunders; 1989:147–74.

Eskola A, Pohjolainen T, Alaranta H, Soini J, Tallroth K, Slatis P. Calcitonin treatment in lumbar spinal stenosis: a randomized, placebo-controlled, double-blind, cross-over study with one year follow-up. Calcif Tissue Int. 1992;**50**:400–3.

Katz JN, Lipson SJ, Larson MG, McInnes JM, Fossel AH, Liang MH. The outcome of decompressive laminectomy for degenerative lumbar stenosis. J Bone Joint Surg. 1991;**73A**:809–16.

Nasca RJ. Surgical management of lumbar spinal stenosis. Spine. 987;**12**:809–16.

Spengler, DM. Current concepts review. Degenerative stenosis of the lumbar spine. J Bone Joint Surg. 1987;**69A**:305–8.

'ARTHRITIS OR ARTHRALGIA?'

Paul A Dieppe

Definition of the Problem

Pain is the commonest presentation of arthritis. However, 'joint pain' is not well localized and there are many causes of musculoskeletal pain other than arthritis. The two main presentations are localized pain around a single joint site ('I have pain in my shoulder/hip/knee, etc.'), or more generalized pain ('all my joints and muscles hurt'). In each case, the physician must first distinguish articular from non-articular problems, as well as differentiating mechanical from inflammatory pathologies.

PAIN IN OR AROUND A JOINT

- The history helps define the pathology: *mechanical v inflammatory?*
- The examination helps define the anatomy: *articular v periarticular or referred?*

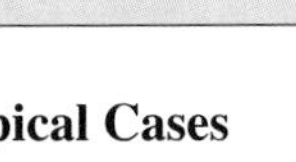

Fig. 11.7 Sorting out 'joint' pain.

Typical Cases

Case 1

FK, a 56-year-old female writer, presented with use-related pain of the right wrist, interfering with her extensive typing. The pain had come on gradually with no history of injury. The patient thought that there was some joint swelling and noted short-lasting early morning stiffness of the wrist. Her general practitioner had performed screening blood tests and a radiograph, both of which were normal, and prescribed a nonsteroidal anti-inflammatory agent, which had been ineffective, before referring her to a rheumatologist. On examination, there was a discrete area of tenderness and swelling around the radial border of the wrist, extending into the forearm, and passive full flexion of the thumb reproduced the patient's symptoms. A diagnosis of De Quervain's tenosynovitis was made. The tendon sheath was injected, relieving the inflammation. However, the patient still has to be careful not to overuse her computer keyboard, as this tends to exacerbate the problem.

Case 2

JF, a retired male lawyer, presented with a story of ill-defined proximal muscle and joint pain and stiffness. He noted that his exercise tolerance had decreased dramatically in recent months and he had lost 5 Kg in weight. His general practitioner had been unable to find any abnormal physical signs, and had initially diagnosed depression, prescribing anti-depressants. The patient returned for a further consultation 2 weeks later, complaining of increasing fatigue and night sweats, in addition to worsening back, shoulder and hip pain. Screening blood tests showed a high erythrocyte sedimentation rate (ESR), and the GP changed her diagnosis to one of polymyalgia rheumatica, prescribed prednisolone which caused some improvement, and referred the patient to a rheumatologist. On examination the patient looked ill and he had several areas of severe tenderness over the vertebrae of the spine. Further imaging, blood and urine tests were performed, and a diagnosis of multiple myeloma confirmed. The patient was started on therapy; his back pain has improved and he is doing well.

Diagnostic problems

A presentation with pain in or around one or more joints is extremely common, accounting for some 20% of all primary care consultations in many parts of the world. The commonest causes will be mechanical (often related to trauma) rather than inflammatory, and periarticular or referred pain, rather than being due to an articular disorder (arthritis). The first responsibility of the physician is to sort out these two issues (Fig. 11.7).

The *history* will help to define any predisposing trauma, either a single event, or, as in the first case, a repetitive usage problem. Furthermore, a mechanical disorder usually causes pain on certain movements, relieved by rest, and may be associated with locking or cracking of joints as well as inactivity gelling. In contrast, inflammatory disorders cause prolonged morning stiffness, swelling, heat over the joint and more persistent pain, exacerbated by any joint use. In addition, inflammatory diseases may be associated with systemic problems, such as weight loss or night sweats and a raised ESR, as in the second case. Because joint pain is poorly localized, the *examination* is the only way of defining the anatomical cause of the pain. Articular problems are associated with point tenderness, and pain

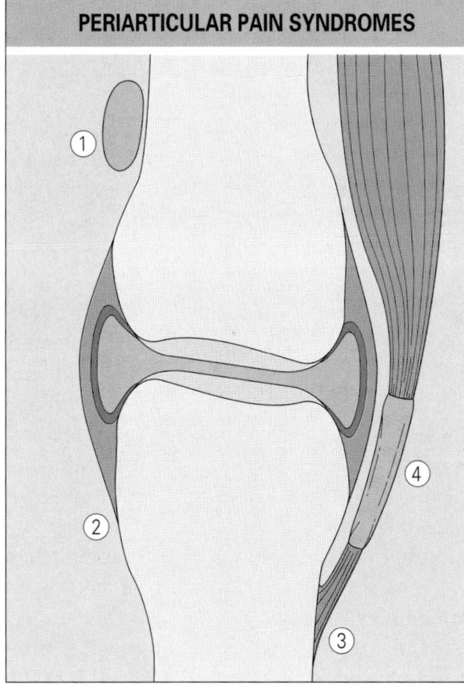

Fig. 11.8 Anatomical structures that can give rise to painful periarticular syndromes. (1) Bursitis is characterized by localized pain and swelling. (2) Capsular or ligament tears are characterized by pain on movements that stretch or produce tension of the affected ligament. (3) Tendon insertion (enthesis) problems are characterized by pain induced on isometric contraction of the muscle acting through the affected tendon. (4) Tendon sheath inflammation is characterized by pain and crepitus on movement of the affected ligament.

exacerbation with specific movements that may irritate the offending ligament or tendon (Fig. 11.8). This is well illustrated by the first case, in which the careful examination by the rheumatologist allowed the problem to be defined as a periarticular tendonitis, rather than the articular problem that had been diagnosed by the GP.

Conclusions

Most common presentations of musculoskeletal pain can be diagnosed from the history and examination alone, with few if any investigations being necessary. Figure 11.9 summarizes those features that help to distinguish an articular disorder (arthritis) from conditions due to periarticular or referred pain problems.

DISTINGUISHING ARTHRITIS FROM ARTHRALGIA

	Features suggesting arthritis	Non-specific features
History	Prolonged morning stiffness Joint swelling (or redness) Severe systemic symptoms	Site or severity of pain Short lasting stiffness Malaise or fatigue
Examination	Heat over joints Joint-line tenderness	Tender spots
Investigations	High ESR An acute-phase response	Positive rheumatoid factor/ANA (in low titre) High uric acid Normal radiographs

Fig. 11.9 Features that help to distinguish arthritis from periarticular syndromes, or from pain referred from other sites, or that due to systemic disease.

REFERENCES

Dieppe P, Cooper C, Kirwan J, McGill N. Arthritis and rheumatism in practice. London and New York: Gower Medical Publishing; 1991.

Doherty M, Doherty J. Clinical examination in rheumatology. London: Mosby–Wolfe; 1992.

Polley HF, Hunder GC. Rheumatological interviewing and physical examination of the joints. New York: WB Saunders Co.; 1978.

DIFFICULT FIBROMYALGIA

Geoffrey Littlejohn

Definition of the Problem

Fibromyalgia syndrome (FMS) is a common cause of musculoskeletal symptoms both in its generalized and localized forms. Generalized FMS may be mild and intermittent or severe and persistent, the latter presenting a difficult management problem.

The Typical Case

RP is a 40-year-old mother of three who presented with a 10-year history of variable musculoskeletal aching, pain, stiffness and fatigue. Her symptoms fluctuated according to activity, weather change or stress. While at times she was comfortable and without complaint, more usually she had episodes of distressing symptoms lasting weeks to months which resulted in a significant diminishment in her enjoyment of life and her ability to carry out a number of otherwise routine household, work-related or recreational activities. Her persisting symptoms have led to concern amongst her family members and have resulted in a large number of investigations and treatments over a number of years.

She recalled episodes, at the age of 13, of nocturnal myalgia, usually in the thigh and calf regions, which were often relieved by rubbing and simple analgesia. A jarring injury, at age 15, while playing netball resulted in 6 months of significant low back pain, which gradually subsided with modification of activity. Radiologic investigations at the time were unremarkable. In her early twenties she was a very active person, working full-time as a teacher, marrying at the age of 23 and subsequently having three children over the next 7 years. During these years she played tennis regularly, entertained friends, continued to work on a part-time basis and was busy 'always doing something'.

Without obvious reason, although she did have an upper respiratory tract infection that took longer than usual to throw off, she developed aching and discomfort around the neck and shoulder-girdle regions. This problem persisted and muscular aching was later prominent in thoracic, lumbar, buttock and leg regions. She noted that her sleep pattern, which had previously been good, had become disturbed, with fragmented shallow sleep and a feeling of unrefreshedness on awakening in the morning. Morning stiffness became prominent and nocturnal dysesthesia in the hands was noted.

She continued to do part-time work but had to cut it down in order to be able to cope with her domestic responsibilities. Even in the home, she required help to do all the day's chores.

The persistent distressing symptoms and disability led to review by medical practitioners who found that routine investigations for inflammatory disease, hormone dysfunction, biochemical disturbance and radiologic abnormality were all unremarkable. Various diagnostic labels had been attached to the symptoms as they persisted over the years, including 'postviral myalgia', 'seronegative arthritis', and similar nonspecific titles. Her local doctor became frustrated by the lack of resolution of the symptoms, having prescribed simple analgesics and, later, anti-inflammatory medication. Opinions followed from other health professionals including specialists in neurology, orthopedics and rheumatology, as well as other family physicians. She became upset when she was told 'there is nothing wrong with you'. Help from nonmedical sources included courses of acupuncture, naturopathy and physical treatments. Short-term help was obtained from some of these approaches, but expense precluded their continuation.

A thorough physical examination showed no abnormality in major organ systems. There was clearly defined abnormal tenderness to palpation in the tender points that characterize FMS. In addition, abnormal sensitivity to palpation of a fold of skin of the upper back, held between the thumb and forefinger, was prominent, together with exaggerated cutaneous wheal and flare on light stimulation of the same region with the finger nail. There was prominent paravertebral tightness and tenderness in the low cervical, mid-thoracic and low lumbar region. Her grip strengths were below the expected range for her body size and rings were tight at the time of examination.

Diagnostic Problems

In retrospect, such a history is typical of the difficult FMS patient, and anyone familiar with the syndrome will quickly predict the diagnosis prior to examination. However, as a syndrome may evolve over a long period of time, when there is no obvious precipitating cause, it may be necessary to consider a number of possibilities depending on the presenting symptoms and signs. The experienced clinician also recognizes that this is a syndrome, and not all features are present at one point in time. Important clues to the possibility of FMS are detailed in Figure 11.10. A recurring history of protracted painful episodes during adolescence may be noted. This is by no means invariable, and many have sudden onset of fibromyalgia more clearly associated with a triggering event. This might include an injury, usually 'soft tissue' in nature but often involving spinal regions such as 'whiplash' or a jarring low back injury.

Many patients develop FMS in the context of significant stress which is not perceived as such by themselves at the time. A history of coping extremely well with an extraordinarily large number of tasks only to begin, for no apparent reason, to cope poorly is also often seen. Many patients have seen numerous physiotherapists for mild and reasonably transient symptoms relating to neck, shoulder, back or buttocks. Initially there is reasonable improvement in symptoms with physiotherapy approaches, such as massage, mobilization, manipulation or similar treatments.

It is important to note that inflammatory joint diseases, such as RA or systemic lupus erythematosus, may present with myalgia. Objective signs of inflammatory joint disease and markers of inflammation and serologic abnormality need to be sought out. In contrast, it is common for patients with FMS to be extensively investigated and those younger females with low-titer, nonspecific antinuclear antibody levels are often mislabeled as having 'mild lupus'.

Other conditions that occur in the context of FMS include irritable bowel syndrome, 'tension' headaches, menstrual abnormality, fluid retention, pelvic pain problems, irritable bladder syndromes and chronic anxiety. A history of these conditions will also make the likelihood of FMS more apparent.

Management of Difficult Fibromyalgia Syndrome

Clearly, accurate diagnosis is the essential initial ingredient in appropriate management of even the most difficult case. Careful clinical examination and appropriate selected investigations will eliminate most of the common problems that might mimic the condition. The clinical features are usually straightforward, and the most useful ones are the abnormal pain threshold, most prominent in the tender point regions, paravertebral muscular tightness, limb-girdle co-contraction, dermatographia and allodynia. With accurate diagnosis comes appropriate explanation as to the nature of the syndrome and reassurance on the absence of other problems that may be worrying the patient, such as arthritis, cancer or other poorly perceived conditions such as multiple sclerosis. In milder cases, simple reassurance, explanation, a physical exercise program and attention to simple life stresses is usually most efficacious. If sleep disturbance is prominent, use of low-dose trycyclic medication in the mid-evening may be useful. Where there have been persisting and significant symptoms, and where life disruption is prominent, much more attention needs to be placed on the

CLUES TO THE POSSIBILITY OF FIBROMYALGIA SYNDROME

- Past/present prolonged localized pain complaint – important tests negative
- Often prior nonspecific label – 'lumbago', 'chronic fatigue' syndrome, 'restless legs' syndrome, 'whiplash', 'growing pains'
- Past/present tension headache, irritable bowel, fluid retention or similar syndromes
- Widespread joint/muscle pain
- Poor-quality sleep
- Background stress factors (may be subtle)

Fig. 11.10 Clues to the possibility of fibromyalgia syndrome.

psychological background of the patient, both from the point of view of chronic background stresses and the reaction of the patient to the chronic painful problem. This entails a careful clinical history, empathy and understanding on the part of the doctor, and often some time and return visits to identify the key factors that seem relevant. In many instances, this role can be better played by a clinical psychologist or someone particularly skilled in chronic pain management. Uncommonly is there a defined psychiatric illness in such patients; if there is, this will need to be treated appropriately. For instance, depression would require higher dose antidepressant medication and a severe chronic anxiety syndrome might require appropriate counseling.

More common to see is simple everyday background stresses building up in normal people in a subtle and additive fashion to the degree where some change in the central pain control pathways is effected. It is very helpful and appropriate to explain the nature of the condition in terms of a pain amplification syndrome altering pain threshold. The patient then realizes how physical activity initiates pain. The syndrome is expressed in terms of an abnormality of control of the pain pathways and they are reassured that there is no abnormality in the tissues within the body. This allows them to have confidence in participating in an exercise program to stretch tight areas, particularly in para-spinal regions which seem to be prominent in causing referred pain into more peripheral regions. It is also emphasized to the patient that any lively exercise program will by itself induce relaxation and hence better control of the amplified pain system.

Self-help is the key to management and this means aerobic exercise (pushing into the pain), stretching and strengthening paraspinal and abdominal musculature, as well as developing skills in stress and pain management, such as relaxation, meditation, yoga, tai-chi or similar activities. Each person will have to choose the modality that is best for them, and often several methods will need to be examined over time.

Patients such as the case described may need guidance in regard to time-management. Finding 'space' in the day's activities for themselves is important – it allows for relaxation, renewing of energy and better management of pain and fatigue. Exercise programs create time away from life-stresses. In addition, allocation of the day's tasks can be improved with advice, further diminishing

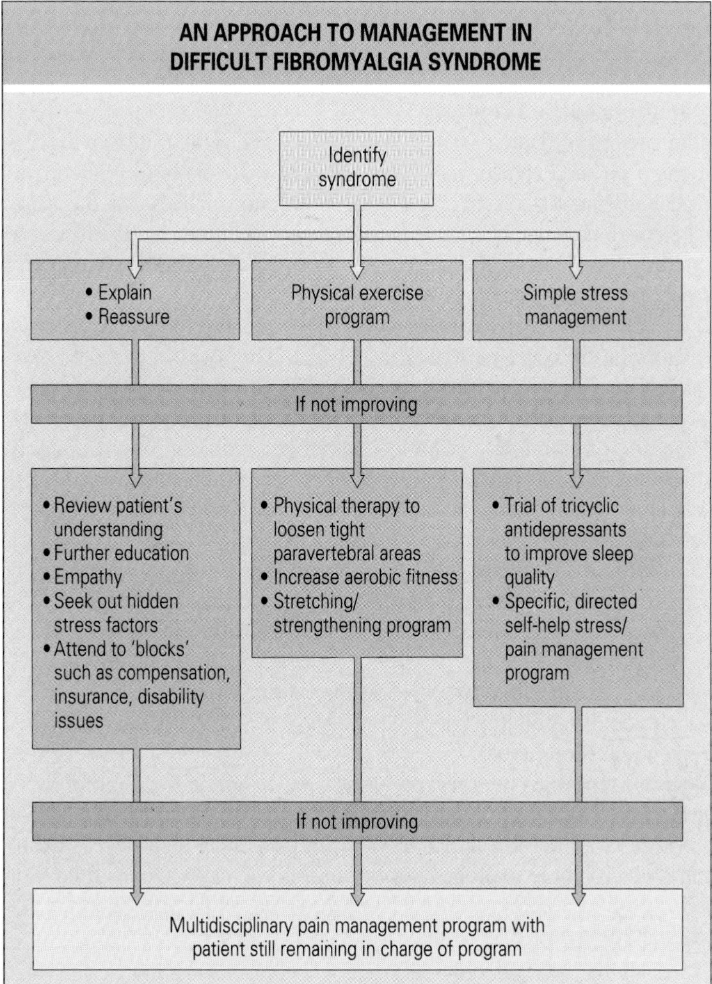

Fig. 11.11 An approach to management in difficult fibromyalgia syndrome.

everyday stresses. Stress management tactics are essential for pain management and need to be built into all everyday life activities.

Clinical psychological programs are usually straightforward, practical, nonthreatening and helpful to the patient. The patient with FMS is treated in the context of their total life, family and personal situation, and strategies to deal with the FMS are based on the premise that the patient does not have to 'learn to live with it' but that the pain syndrome will usually improve significantly with this understanding and approach.

Where there are blocks to this process through anger, resentment or other forces, which may often be of a medicolegal nature, such approaches will not work. The 'blocks' need specific and insightful attention. Finally, any new symptoms in such patients require careful independent assessment as other illnesses can co-exist with this syndrome. Figure 11.11 outlines the key management strategies in difficult FMS.

REFERENCES

Goldenberg DL. Treatment of fibromyalgia syndrome. Rheum Dis Clin North Am. 1989;**15**:61–72.

McCain GA. Nonmedicinal treatments in primary fibromyalgia. Rheum Dis Clin North Am. 1989;**15**:73–90.

OLECRANON BURSITIS

Gerald D Groff

Definition of the Problem

The olecranon bursa is a subcutaneous synovial pouch which is located on the extensor aspect of the elbow. It serves to reduce friction between tissues overlying the olecranon process of the ulna. The space between bone and skin is narrow with minimal soft tissue padding. As a result, the olecranon bursa is vulnerable to trauma and infection through puncture wounds or cellulitis.

Olecranon bursitis occurs when the bursa swells due to trauma, inflammation or infection (Fig. 11.12). The swelling can be secondary to synovial tissue hypertrophy or fibrosis, fluid accumulation, or nodular deposits (gouty tophi or rheumatoid nodules). Olecranon bursitis is a common outpatient problem (approximately three out of 1000 outpatient visits) and occasionally requires hospitalization when septic (about 1 in 1000 hospitalizations). It occurs most often in young males with recurrent elbow trauma due to work (automobile-mechanics, carpet layers, miners, book-keepers) or leisure activities (dart throwing, wrestling, gymnastics, gardening).

Olecranon bursitis can be classified clinically into three general categories (Fig. 11.13):

- traumatic (or idiopathic) noninflammatory,
- aseptic inflammatory or
- septic inflammatory.

Because appropriate therapy varies with bursitis category, it is important for the clinician to define the cause as soon as possible through examination and bursal aspiration. It is also necessary to recognize that the pathogenesis of bursitis can change over time. For example, a stable traumatic bursitis may become secondarily infected by a puncture wound or trivial abrasion.

The Typical Case

OB is a 43-year-old automobile mechanic in good health except for mild obesity and diet-controlled hyperglycemia. He frequently plays darts at the local pub on his way home from work. While attempting to remove a muffler, he repeatedly struck and rubbed his elbows. As he pulled his shirt on the next day, he noted swelling the size of a 'golf ball' at the end of his right elbow. The arm was stiff but not painful.

His initial presentation to the clinic revealed a healthy appearing man with olecranon bursal swelling. He was afebrile with firm thickening of the bursae and mild non-tender fluctuance. No warmth, erythema or adenopathy was noted. The elbow range of motion was normal and there was no joint effusion. No additional tests were performed and the patient was given a diagnosis of traumatic olecranon bursitis. Therapy included ibuprofen 600mg p.o. three times a day for 7 days and an elastic elbow pad.

The patient responded well. The swelling gradually reduced, leaving thickened tissue at the olecranon prominence but no pain or limitation. He stopped wearing the elbow pad. Six weeks later he scraped the same elbow on a sharp metal edge and swelling recurred over 48 hours. He did not present to clinic until 5 days later, when he noted warmth, redness and tenderness to touch.

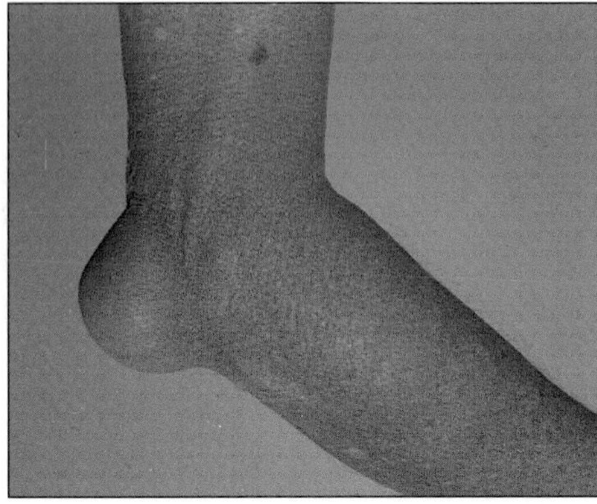

Fig. 11.12 Olecranon bursitis in early rheumatoid arthritis.

Repeat examination revealed fluctuant bursal swelling with erythema over the bursa but not the adjoining skin. A small abrasion was still present. The patient was again afebrile and nontoxic appearing. Bursal aspiration was performed with an 18-gauge sterile needle and produced 10ml of slightly yellow fluid. Gram stain demonstrated numerous white cells but no organisms. The patient was treated with dicloxacillin 500mg p.o. four times a day and cautioned to call if fever or further skin redness developed. Subsequent synovial analysis revealed a white blood cell count of 63,000/mm^3. No crystals were noted. The culture was eventually positive for *Staphylococcus aureus.* Close follow-up in the clinic with repeated aspiration demonstrated gradual improvement. Antibiotics were continued for 10 days, with resolution of erythema and swelling. He eventually gave up both automobile mechanics and dart throwing to pursue a career in politics.

Diagnostic Problems

The differentiation between septic and nonseptic olecranon bursitis represents the main diagnostic challenge. Septic bursitis has the greatest potential for morbidity and must be diagnosed as soon as possible. In addition, the source of nonseptic bursitis should be clarified, since the presence or absence of inflammation can determine appropriate therapy and outcome. Finally, the clinician should be aware of the potential for rapid change in the course of bursitis. As a result, a fresh diagnostic approach should be applied at each follow-up visit.

The history should include questions regarding occupation, duration of symptoms, and possible trauma or skin injury. Associated conditions such as rheumatoid arthritis (RA), gout or uremia may be primary causes of bursitis, while diabetes or immunosuppression may also increase the risk for sepsis. The physical examination should note the size, change in size, and turgor of the bursa. The presence of nodules, lymphadenopathy, warmth and erythema of bursa or skin are important clues. Effusion occasionally occurs in the adjacent elbow joint, but this is usually a noninflammatory, sympathetic process. Specific risk factors for bacterial infection include direct trauma, skin breakage and underlying illness (diabetes and immunosuppression) with the clinical findings of fever, erythema, tenderness or peribursal cellulitis.

Percutaneous diagnostic aspiration of the bursa should be performed whenever inflammation or infection is suspected. Patients with asymptomatic or obviously traumatic bursitis can be treated without aspiration but should be observed carefully. The aspiration technique is simple. A sterile 16- or 18-gauge needle with a syringe large enough to drain available fluid is used to enter the inferior aspect of the bursa. Fluid color and amount should be noted, with specimens sent for Gram stain, white blood cell count, crystal analysis, and bacterial culture. The majority of bacterial infections are caused by *S. aureus* followed by group A beta-hemolytic *Streptococcus*, *Staphylococcus epidermidis*, *Hemophilus influenzae* and *Pseudomonas* species. Special cultures for mycobacterium, fungi, or anaerobic bacteria may be necessary in immunocompromised patients. Elbow radiographs are rarely necessary and should only be used to rule out traumatic fracture or pre-existing joint injury. Diagnostic elements are summarized in Figure 11.13.

Therapeutic Options

Appropriate treatment of olecranon bursitis depends on the cause and duration of symptoms. Noninflammatory, traumatic (or idiopathic) bursitis usually responds to conservative therapy. Patients with limited symptoms should receive rest, elbow protection, and

DIFFERENTIAL DIAGNOSIS OF OLECRANON BURSITIS					
	Traumatic (idiopathic) noninflammatory	Aseptic inflammatory			Septic inflammatory
		Rheumatoid arthritis	Crystalline	Uremia	
Clinical symptoms					
Trauma	+++	+	+	0/+	+++
Tenderness	++	+	++	+	+++
Skin breakage	++	0	0	0	+++
Clinical signs					
Fever	0	0	0	0	++
Warmth	+	+	++	+	+++
Erythema	+	+	++	+	+++
Cellulitis	0	0	+	+	+++
Lymphadenopathy	0	0/+	0/+	0	++
Edema	0	0	0	0	++
Bursal fluid					
Color	C, S, H	C, S	S, H	S	S, H, P
White blood cells per mm^3	50–10,000 (mean 1,100)	1000–60,000 (mean 3000)	1000–50,000 (mean 2900)	1200	350–450,000 (mean 75,000)
Gram stain	Negative	Negative	Negative	Negative	Positive (70%)
Crystals	Negative	Rare cholesterol	Monosodium urate or pyrophosphate	Rare	Negative
Culture	Negative	Negative	Negative	Negative	Positive

Differential diagnosis: 0 usually absent; + rare; ++ occasional; +++ common. **Bursal fluid color:** C Clear; H Hemorrhagic; S Serosanguineous; P Purulent

Fig. 11.13 Differential diagnosis of olecranon bursitis.

possibly nonsteroidal anti-inflammatory drugs (NSAIDs). Padded elbow supports serve to avoid further trauma and skin abrasion. Percutaneous needle aspiration without injection should be considered for patients having stronger symptoms. Bursal aspiration reduces symptoms and allows delayed recovery with minimal complications. Intrabursal corticosteroid injection speeds recovery but can lead to complications (infection, skin atrophy, chronic pain) and should be avoided in traumatic bursitis.

Intrabursal corticosteroid injection is useful, however, in aseptic inflammatory olecranon bursitis related to RA, crystalline processes, or uremia. The initial approach is similar to traumatic bursitis except that all symptomatic patients should receive bursal aspiration for decompression and diagnosis. If bacterial cultures are negative, and symptoms recur despite rest and NSAIDs, repeat aspiration with corticosteroid injection is useful. Injection with 20mg triamcinolone hexacetonide or methylprednisolone acetate often leads to rapid recovery.

Septic inflammatory olecranon bursitis requires early recognition and immediate antibiotic therapy. Patients with clinical evidence for infection (fever, cellulitis, synovial fluid leukocytosis or positive Gram stain) should receive coverage for penicillin-resistant *S. aureus* while cultures are pending. Antibiotic therapy is modified as soon as culture results are available.

Oral antibiotic therapy results in adequate intrabursal drug levels. Patients with good general health, minimal cellulitis and limited systemic symptoms can be treated successfully as outpatients. They require close, often daily, follow-up.

Patients who fail to respond to outpatient therapy or who present with more severe initial infection should be hospitalized for intravenous antibiotic therapy. This would include patients with high fever, chills, prolonged duration of symptoms, and cellulitis. Hospitalization is also preferred in patients with complicating medical conditions (diabetes, uremia, RA) and immunosuppression (malignancy, HIV positivity, systemic corticosteroid therapy).

Drainage of the infected bursa is an essential part of therapy. This can be accomplished by daily percutaneous aspiration or percutaneous placement of a suction–irrigation system. Routine cell counts and culture of drainage fluid should be used to monitor response to therapy. The duration of therapy varies with the individual patient. Patients with symptoms for less than 1 week require an average of 4.4 days of antibiotic therapy to sterilize the bursa. Patients with symptoms for greater than 1 week require an average of 9.2 days. In general, antibiotic therapy should be continued for 10–14 days. Patients requiring initial intravenous antibiotic therapy can be switched to oral medication as soon as signs and symptoms show consistent improvement.

Surgical drainage or bursectomy is occasionally necessary in the management of olecranon bursitis. Recurrent traumatic olecranon bursitis can be approached by either arthroscopic or open resection. Persistent aseptic inflammatory bursitis usually requires open resection with careful dissection when symptoms result in dysfunction. Septic bursitis may require bursectomy if acute infection fails to improve or repeated infection occurs in a fibrotic, chronically inflamed bursa.

Conclusions

Olecranon bursitis is a common condition that is easily recognized. Careful use of history, physical examination, and percutaneous needle aspiration can differentiate the main categories of olecranon bursitis: traumatic noninflammatory, aseptic inflammatory and septic inflammatory bursitis. Appropriate management requires an understanding of these diagnostic categories and the corresponding treatment regimens.

Septic olecranon bursitis is the most serious potential complication, and requires early diagnosis and immediate antibiotic therapy. Initial therapy should include antibiotic coverage for penicillin-resistant *S. aureus* and regular bursal drainage.

REFERENCES

Ho G Jr, Su EY. Antibiotic therapy of septic bursitis. Its implication in the treatment of septic arthritis. Arthritis Rheum. 1981;**24**:905–11.

McAfee JH, Smith DL. Olecranon and prepatellar bursitis – diagnosis and treatment. West J Med. 1988;**149**:607–10.

Raddatz DA, Hoffman GS, Franck WA. Septic bursitis; presentation, treatment and prognosis. J Rheumatol. 1987;**14**:1160–3.

Roschmann RA, Bell CI. Septic bursitis in immunocompromised patients. Am J Med. 1987;**83**: 661–5.

Smith DL, McAfee JH, Lucas LM, Kumar KL, Romney DM. Treatment of nonseptic olecranon bursitis. A controlled, blinded prospective trial. Arch Intern Med. 1989;**149**:2527–30.

Weinstein PS, Canoso JJ, Wohlethan JR. Long-term follow-up of corticosteroid injection for traumatic olecranon bursitis. Ann Rheum Dis. 1984;**43**:44–6.

PAIN IN THE HIP

Paul A Dieppe

Definition of the Problem

Pain in the hip or buttock region is common. The most common causes are referred pain from the spine, trochanteric bursitis and osteoarthritis (OA) of the hip joint. However, there are many other possibile diagnoses, including several important conditions that can be difficult to diagnose, such as osteonecrosis of the head of the femur, or painful regional osteoporosis in pregnancy.

The Typical Case

AS is a 52-year-old female shop assistant, and a keen walker. She has suffered from asthma for many years, and has often been treated with systemic steroids. She presented with a history of gradually increasing pain in the right hip and buttock region, interfering with her leisure walks. The physician treating her for her asthma arranged for a radiograph of the hip, which was normal. However, the doctor remained concerned about the possibility of avascular necrosis and referred the patient to a rheumatologist.

The history suggested a mechanical cause, in that the pain was clearly related to activity, and patient also admitted to intermittent mild back pain for many years. On examination, there was no tenderness over the greater trochanter or in the groin (joint line and iliopsoas bursa), and the 'Patrick' or 'FABER' test (Fig. 11.14) was negative, suggesting that there was no pathology in or around the hip joint itself. Clinical tests for sacroiliac disease were also negative. On further examination, a 3cm discrepancy in leg length was detected, associated with a spinal scoliosis and decreased movements of the lumbar spine. Spinal radiographs confirmed the scoliosis and showed OA of the right-sided apophyseal joints from L1 to L3.

The patient was treated with physical therapy for her spine, and provided with a 2cm heel lift to partially correct the leg-length discrepancy, as well as shock absorbing insoles to help ease the discomfort with her walking. She still suffers from intermittent mild low back pain, but is otherwise well and has been able to return to long walks with her local rambling club.

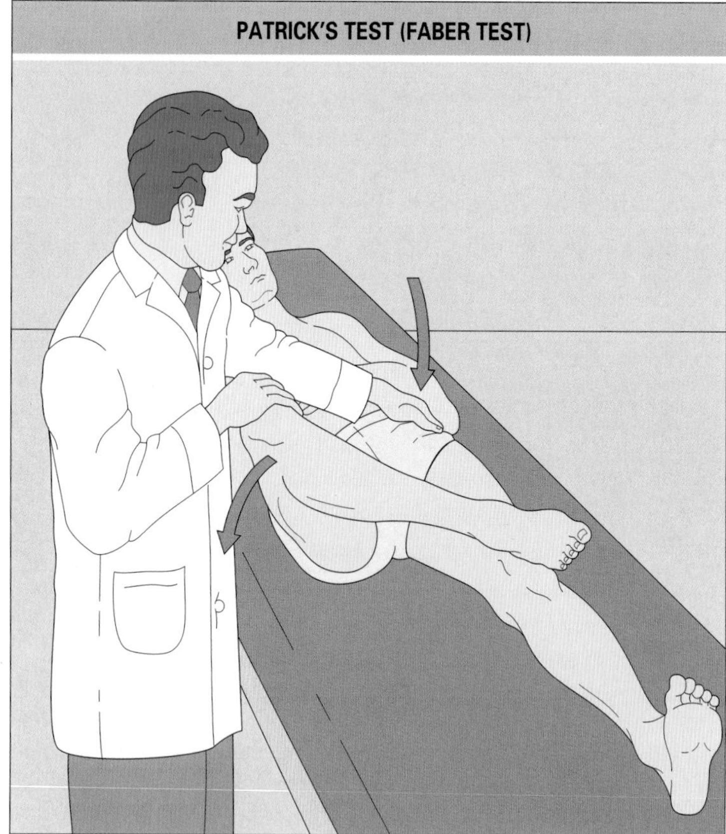

Fig. 11.14 Patrick's or FABER test. The contralateral iliac crest is stabilized with downward pressure while lowering the ipsilateral flexed, abducted, and rotated leg. Rapid lowering tests the sacroiliac joint, while slow lowering tests the hip joint.

The Diagnostic Problem

'Hip' pain must first be defined anatomically. Buttock pain is commonly called hip pain, and may be due to spinal or sacroiliac disorders, as well as ischiogluteal bursitis ('weaver's bottom'). Lateral pain may be due to trochanteric bursitis or the 'snapping hip' (the iliotibial band slips over the greater trochanter), as well as referred pain. Causes of anterior pain include iliopsoas bursitis in addition to hip disease and referred pain, but must be differentiated from inguinal or abdominal pathology.

Diagnosis is made more difficult by the fact that some important causes of hip pathology, such as avascular necrosis (considered in the case described) may not result in any radiographic changes in their early stages. However, pathology of the hip joint can usually be detected or excluded by careful physical examination. Most hip disease results in early loss of full internal rotation, with pain at the extreme of movement. The Patrick test (Fig. 11.14) combines abduction with internal rotation. The two sides should always be compared when using such tests, lack of symmetry being more important than the range of motion or discomfort induced. In addition to examining the hip itself, it is important to assess the spine, sacroiliac joints and abdomen.

Minor degrees of leg-length inequality (1cm or less) are common and usually asymptomatic. Larger discrepancies can cause, or be caused by hip disease. Deformities of the hip or a pelvic tilt can cause an 'apparent' leg-length discrepancy. 'True' leg-length inequalities can be caused by congenital or acquired disorders of the hip (dislocation, acetabular dysplasia, Perthes disease, slipped epiphyses, severe OA, poliomyelitis and others), as well as being an isolated finding. They result in a secondary, compensatory scoliosis. Leg-length inequalities can cause spinal disease due to the scoliosis, and numerous periarticular problems due to the abnormal mechanical loading of the legs and spine, as well as being associated with a higher prevalence of OA of both the hip and knee on the longer side ('long-leg arthropathy'). Leg-length inequalities are best detected with the patient lying supine and the legs some 20cm apart, using the superior iliac spine and lateral malleolus as landmarks (Fig. 11.15).

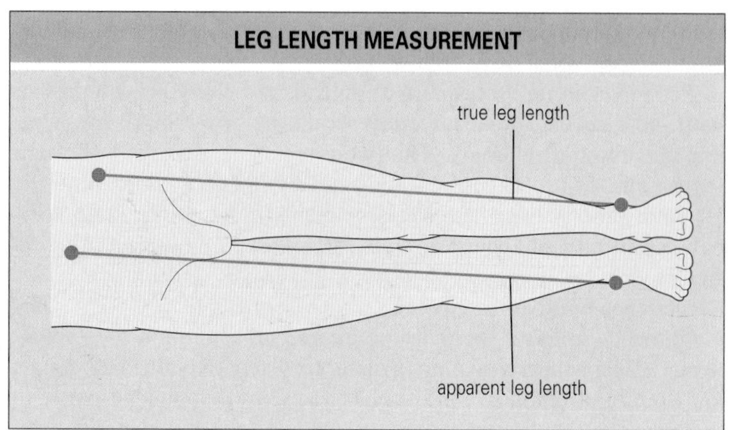

Fig. 11.15 Leg-length measurement. The measurement is best made from the anterior superior iliac spine to the lateral malleolus.

Conclusions

Hip or buttock pain has numerous causes. Diagnosis depends more on a careful history and examination than it does on radiographs. Hip radiographs can result in false positives (minor hip OA on the radiograph when the pain has another treatable cause, such as trochanteric bursitis) as well as false negatives (normal radiographs in the early stages of avascular necrosis, for example). Examination of the spine, sacroiliac joints and for leg-length inequalities are an essential part of the assessment of hip pain.

REFERENCES

Clarke GR. Unequal leg length: an accurate method of detection and some clinical results. Rheum Phys Med. 1982; 385–90.

Schapira D, Nahir M, Scharf Y. Trochanteric bursits: a common clinical problem. Arch Phys Med Rehabil. 1986; 815–7.

Underwood PL, McLeod RA, Ginsberg WW. The varied clinical manifestations of iliopsoas bursitis. J Rheumatol. 1988; **15**:1683–5.

Schaberg JE, Harper MC, Allen WC. The snapping hip syndrome. Am J Sports Med. 1984; **12**:361–5.

CHRONIC MONOARTHRITIS OF THE KNEE

Rodney A Hughes

Definition of the problem

It is not unusual for rheumatologists to encounter patients of either sex with synovitis confined to one knee and which has been present for longer than 3 months. These patients may have already received treatment with NSAIDs, oral antibiotics and intra-articular steroid injections to no avail. Chronic monoarthritis of the knee (Fig. 11.16) occurs in persons of all ages and can result from any disease that, under other circumstances, causes polyarthritis. In younger patients the etiology often remains obscure despite intensive investigation. Treatment of such 'undifferentiated seronegative arthritis' (USNA) has to be empirical.

The Typical Case

A 27-year-old male accountant developed monoarthritis of his left knee 6 months prior to consultation. He was single, heterosexual and, despite being sexually active, he denied any recent sexual contact with anyone other than his regular girlfriend. Previously he had been fully fit and active, had not traveled abroad recently, nor had he or any other member of his family suffered from significant joint, skin, eye or back problems. Clinical examination was unhelpful and genitourinary investigation negative. Cultures of stool, throat swab and midstream urine were sterile and he had absent or normal levels of antibody to parvovirus, *Yersinia, Chlamydia, Borrelia* and streptolysin O. Blood tests showed an acute phase response with ESR 72 mm/hr, CRP of 25 mmol/l and a polyclonal elevation of immunoglobulins. Tests for rheumatoid factor and antinuclear antibody (ANA) were negative and uric acid and liver function tests were normal. Joint aspiration yielded 35ml of sterile straw-colored synovial fluid with 35,000/mm leukocytes, which were predominantly lymphocytes. No crystals were visible under polarized light microscopy.

Arthroscopy was performed and examination of a synovial biopsy confirmed nonspecific synovitis. The knee was washed out with saline to good effect. Synovitis persisted for the next 4 years, despite several subsequent intra-articular hydrocortisone injections, and active physiotherapy helped to minimize loss of quadriceps muscle bulk. He has been reluctant to start treatment with any drug other than NSAIDs.

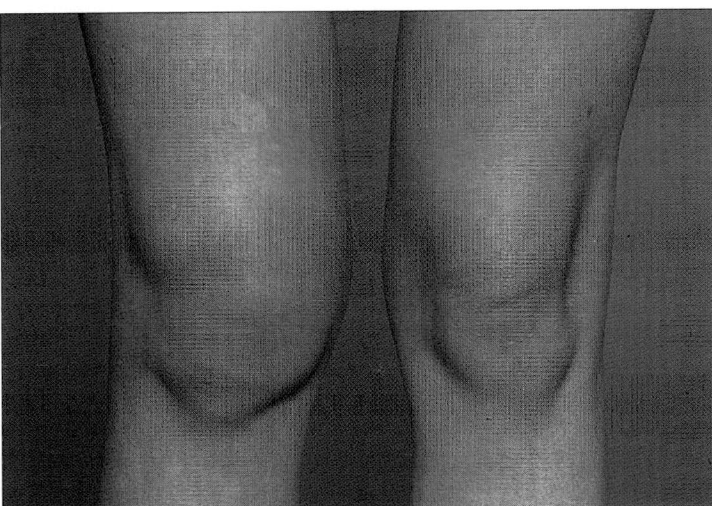

Fig. 11.16 Chronic monoarthritis of the knee.

Diagnostic Problems and Investigation

The differential diagnosis of a chronically inflamed knee is wide (Fig. 11.17). Infection must not be missed. Usually joint sepsis produces signs of severe inflammation, but these may be diminished or absent following antibiotic treatment or if the patient is immunosuppressed or elderly. Therefore joint aspiration and/or synovial biopsy are important investigations. It should be remembered that chronic infection may occur in a knee that has been damaged previously by chronic inflammatory arthritis, as well as in prosthetic joints. Crystal arthritis may cause chronic synovitis as well as the more usual acutely inflamed joint.

Careful history taking (Fig. 11.18) and examination may reveal occult genitourinary infection (for example gonorrhea), psoriatic plaques, nail pits or gouty tophi. Monoarthritis of the knee may be the

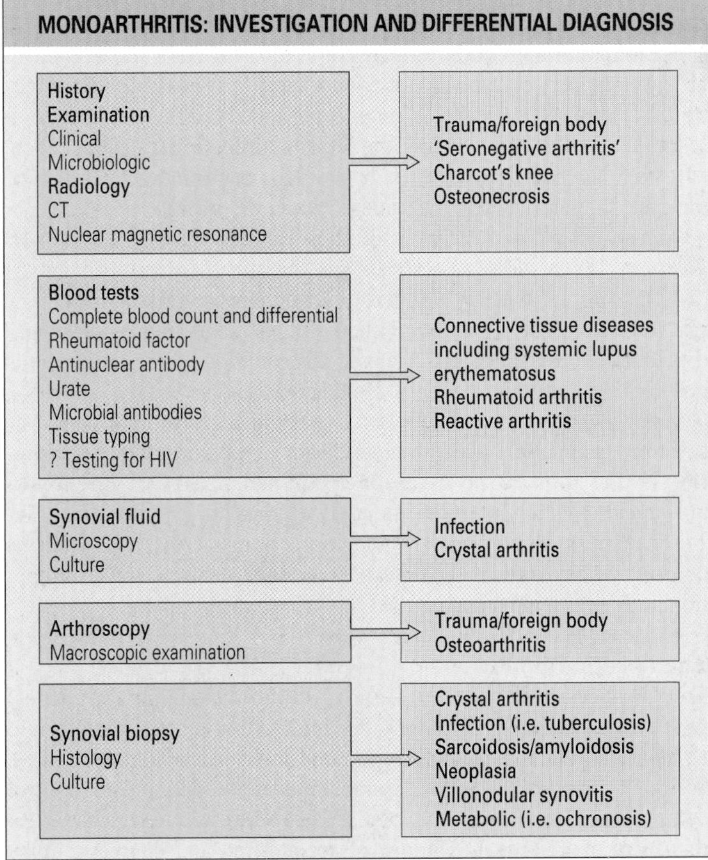

MONOARTHRITIS: INVESTIGATION AND DIFFERENTIAL DIAGNOSIS
History
Examination
Clinical
Microbiologic
Radiology
CT
Nuclear magnetic resonance
Trauma/foreign body
'Seronegative arthritis'
Charcot's knee
Osteonecrosis
Blood tests
Complete blood count and differential
Rheumatoid factor
Antinuclear antibody
Urate
Microbial antibodies
Tissue typing
? Testing for HIV
Connective tissue diseases including systemic lupus erythematosus
Rheumatoid arthritis
Reactive arthritis
Synovial fluid
Microscopy
Culture
Infection
Crystal arthritis
Arthroscopy
Macroscopic examination
Trauma/foreign body
Osteoarthritis
Synovial biopsy
Histology
Culture
Crystal arthritis
Infection (i.e. tuberculosis)
Sarcoidosis/amyloidosis
Neoplasia
Villonodular synovitis
Metabolic (i.e. ochronosis)

Fig. 11.17 Investigation and differential diagnosis of monoarthritis.

MONOARTHRITIS: HISTORY AND EXAMINATION
History taking: important history to elicit
• History of previous trauma to the knee • Past or family history of arthritis/connective tissue disease • History of past sexual contacts/genitourinary infections/risk • Gastrointestinal symptoms: bowel irregularity/diarrhea or blood protein/recent food poisoning • Symptoms of inflammation of the eyes/skin/spine or sacroiliac joints
• Genital examination (i.e. balanitis) and microbiologic examination of the urethra or cervix, even in asymptomatic patients if sexually active • Psoriasis (including nails and scalp); hair loss (systemic lupus erythematosus) or other skin rash • Tophi (ears, hands or feet) • Tendinitis; seen typically with gonococcal sepsis • Rheumatoid nodules over pressure points • Spine and sacroiliac joints, for evidence of spondylitis • Ophthalmologic examination: conjunctivitis, scleritis or uveitis • Metabolic conditions such as ochronosis or Wilson's disease may rarely present as monoarthritis • Microscopy and culture of stool, even when patients are asymptomatic

Fig. 11.18 History and examination in monoarthritis.

presenting feature of HIV infection and tell-tale lesions elsewhere may not always be apparent (Fig. 11.19). Standing radiographs of the knee may reveal erosions, degenerative changes or radio-opaque foreign bodies. It is worthwhile performing certain blood tests. Chronic infection may cause a neutrophilia; the serum uric acid level is often raised in patients with gout, and positive autoantibodies can help to confirm suspicions of a connective tissue disease such as SLE.

Examination and culture of a sample of synovial fluid is vital in all patients with chronically swollen knees. It is possible that infection may have been introduced into an acutely inflamed knee as a result of previous joint aspiration. Unusual infections, such as tuberculosis, brucellosis, viruses, fungi, protozoa or parasite infestation of the knee may not be detected unless awareness is high.

Measurement of serum antibodies to parvovirus, hepatitis B, *Yersinia, Chlamydia* and *Borrelia* may help to confirm a diagnosis of viral arthritis, reactive arthritis or Lyme disease. Tissue typing for HLA-B27 and DW4 may strengthen clinical suspicions of seronegative arthritis or rheumatoid disease, respectively, where diagnosis is unclear, but their presence is not diagnostic.

Arthroscopy is safe and relatively easy to perform, allowing synovial biopsies to be obtained under direct visual control and the interior of the joint to be carefully examined. Cases of previously unsuspected neoplasia, pigmented villonodular synovitis (Fig. 11.20), amyloid, sarcoidosis and more unusual diseases such as ochronosis have been diagnosed as a result of histologic examination of synovial biopsies.

Therapeutic Options

Treatment options are broadly similar to those available for patients with polyarthritis (Fig. 11.21). An intra-articular approach would appear to be the most logical treatment for monoarthritis of the knee. While intra-articular steroids are sometimes adequate to control symptoms, chronic synovitis of the knee often proves refractory to this form of treatment. The use of second-line antirheumatic drugs will be determined by the patient's response to NSAIDs and by the

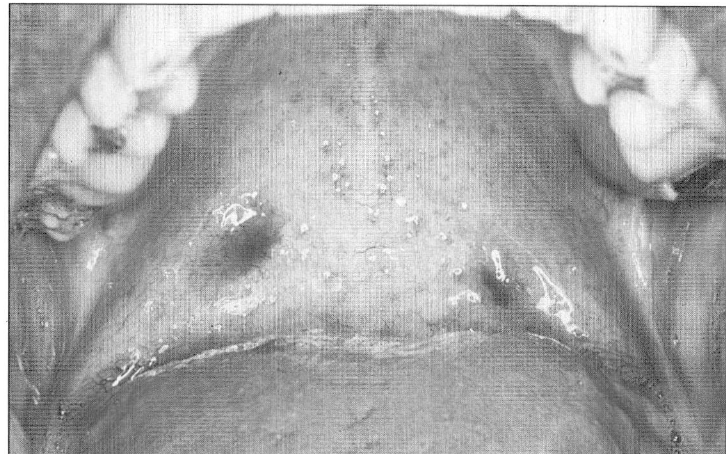

Fig. 11.19 Kaposi's sarcoma as the only other clinical feature of AIDS in a man presenting with sterile monoarthritis.

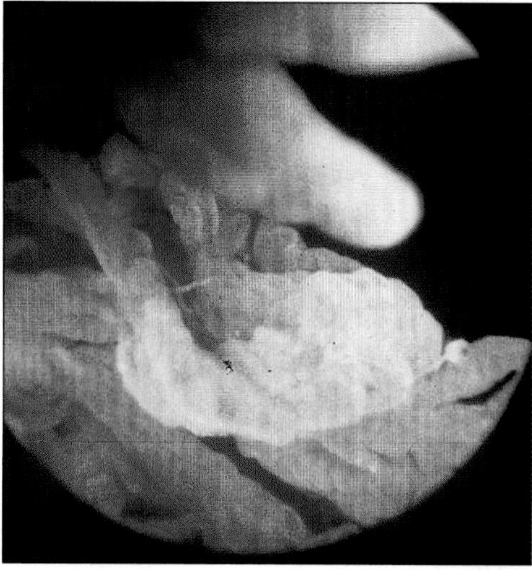

Fig. 11.20 Unsuspected pigmented villonodular synovitis seen in a patient with monoarthritis of the knee.

degree of disability; they are not an attractive choice in the treatment of chronic monoarthritis. In this setting, gold and penicillamine are rarely helpful, daily sulfasalazine and weekly methotrexate being more commonly used. Antibiotics may also have a place over and above their value in the treatment of septic arthritis; tetracyclines, including minocycline, have been given with some benefit to patients with reactive arthritis and USNA. This may reflect anti-inflammatory properties rather than antimicrobial activity.

The chronically swollen knee often responds well, albeit in the short term, to local saline wash-out performed at arthroscopy. Chemical or surgical synovectomy is still considered for refractory monoarthritis of the knee.

THERAPEUTIC OPTIONS IN CHRONIC MONOARTHRITIS	
Local injections	Intra-articular steroids Chemical synovectomy (yttrium, osmic acid)
Drug treatment	Nonsteroidal anti-inflammatory drugs and analgesics Second-line drugs (sulfasalazine, methotrexate) Antibiotics
Physiotherapy	Quadriceps strengthening
Surgery	Arthroscopic wash-out Synovectomy (arthroscopic, surgical)

Fig. 11.21 Therapeutic options in chronic monoarthritis.

The regular performance of active quadriceps exercises is essential to minimize the muscle loss that always accompanies arthritis of the knee.

Conclusions

In many cases, chronic arthritis of the knee remains undifferentiated; USNA should be a diagnosis of exclusion. Clinical history and examination alone can provide the most useful diagnostic information. It is vital to consider chronic infection or neoplasia as these may have drastic consequences. Remember that monoarthritis can be the presenting feature of AIDS. Joint aspiration should be performed in all patients with a joint effusion, and the wearing of gloves and careful aseptic technique should minimize the risk of infection for both patient and clinician. Arthroscopy under local anesthetic is a safe and well-tolerated procedure that has a place in the investigation and treatment of patients with a chronically inflamed knee joint.

REFERENCES

Curry HLF. Acute monoarthritis – differential diagnosis and management. Reports on Rheumatic Diseases Series 2, vol 10. Arthritis and Rheumatism Council; 1988.

Revell PA. The synovial biopsy. Recent Adv Histopathol. 1987;**13**:79–93.

Rowe IF, Forster SM, Seifert MH, et al. Rheumatological lesions in individuals with human immunodeficiency virus infection. Q J Med. 1989;**272**:1167–84.

ANTERIOR KNEE PAIN

Janet Cushnaghan, Conor McCarthy & Paul A Dieppe

Definition of the Problem

Anterior knee pain is a common symptom in young and middle-aged adults. It can present in both the presence and absence of OA. There is often a paucity of helpful physical signs, and diagnosing the cause of the pain can present major problems. Management is also difficult, many cases being relatively unresponsive to conventional analgesic and anti-inflammatory therapy.

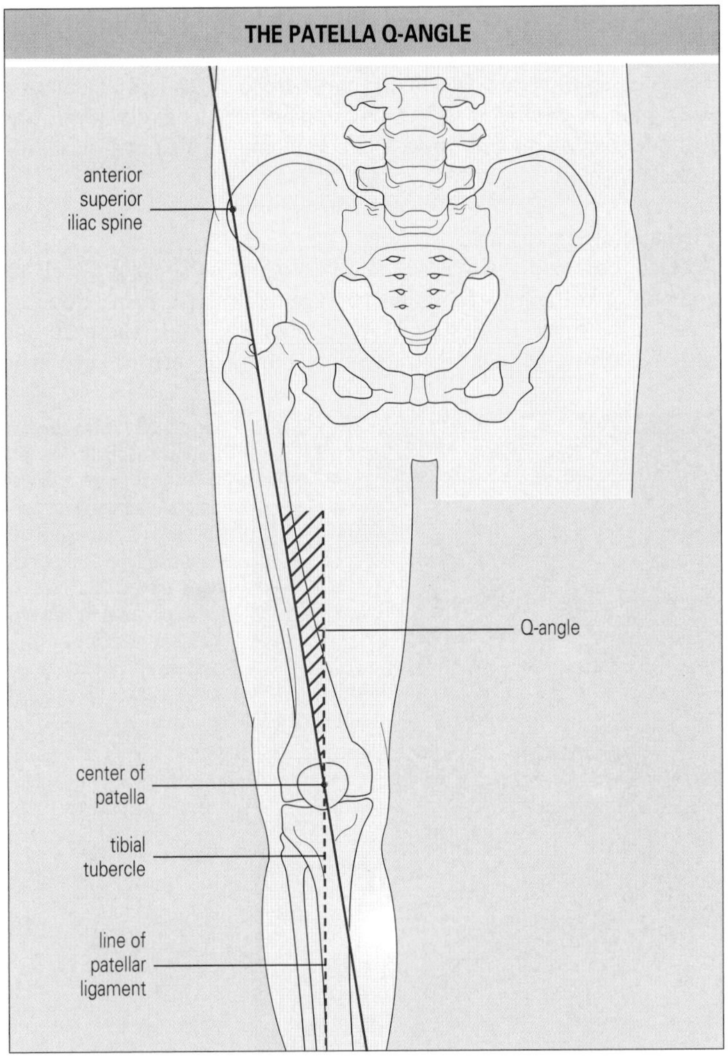

THE PATELLA Q-ANGLE

anterior superior iliac spine

Q-angle

center of patella

tibial tubercle

line of patellar ligament

Fig. 11.22 The patella Q-angle. The patella Q-angle is the angle between a line running from the anterior superior iliac spine through the center of the patella and the line of the patella ligament (patella center to tibial tubercule). The normal angle is less than 15 degrees.

Typical Cases

Case 1

SJ is a 28-year-old lady who had had anterior knee pain for the last 9 months, which had been stopping her from playing hockey for her country. She had no significant past history except for a possible patella dislocation about 10 years ago. On examination she had a positive patella pressure sign and some patellofemoral crepitus but no other physical signs except for a large 'Q angle' (Fig. 11.22). Her radiographs were normal, including skyline views; however, they confirmed the 'Q-angle'. Previous treatment had included quadriceps exercises and NSAIDs, but these were of little benefit.

Case 2

IT is a 52-year-old woman with a family history of OA. She presented with use-related knee pain for 2 years. On closer questioning it was apparent that most of the pain was felt in the front of the knee, and that climbing up stairs or sitting with her knees bent caused particular problems. On examination she had marked patellofemoral crepitus and tenderness on patella compression. Anteroposterior and lateral radiographs of the knee were considered normal, but on the skyline view there was obvious narrowing of the lateral facet of the patellofemoral joint (Fig. 11.23).

The Diagnostic Problem

There are many causes of pain felt at the front of the knee joint, including those listed in Figure 11.24. Any of these causes of anterior

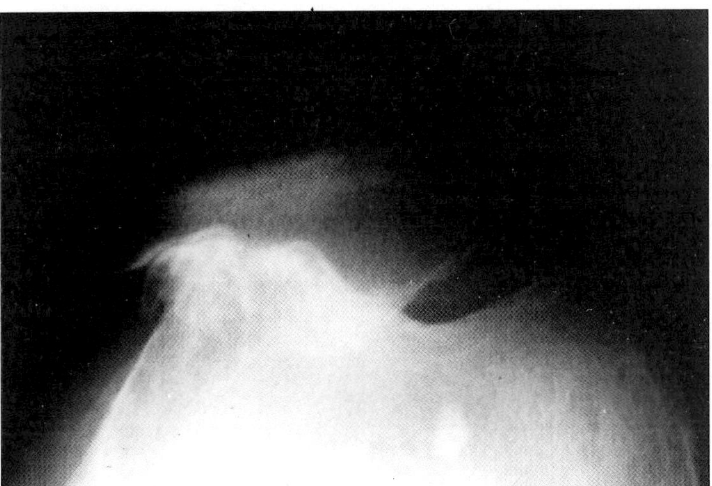

Fig. 11.23 Severe osteoarthritis of the patellofemoral joint. This skyline view shows osteoarthritis of the lateral facet, with loss of joint space, sclerosis and altered contour, resulting in ridges and grooves forming in the bones.

knee pain can cause diagnostic problems. However, it should be possible to eliminate many of the localized causes, such as Osgood–Schlatter disease, ligamentous injury and periarticular disorders, as well as inflammatory synovitis, on a careful examination, concentrating on signs of inflammation and the sites of severe tenderness. True patellofemoral disorders cause anterior knee pain associated with pain on compression of the patella and/or an 'apprehension sign' when the examiner tries to move the patella laterally. Pain occurs when the knee is flexed and under load, such as when climbing stairs. Prolonged sitting with the knee flexed causes increasing pain (the 'cinema' sign) and kneeling is often impossible. Due to abnormal biomechanics, quadriceps function may be compromised, leading to feelings of instability and possible giving way. Patellofemoral pain and dysfunction is a potentially very debilitating condition, common in young, active people, who often have great feelings of frustration and despair as a result.

Once the periarticular causes, referred pain syndromes, ligamentous injury and other possible causes of anterior knee pain have been excluded, further investigations may be necessary in order to delineate the type of patellofemoral disorder. The age, and any history of injury or previous dislocation (or hypermobility), will provide clues as to the likely cause. Careful examination of the knee to observe the quadriceps mechanism and patella alignment, patella tracking as the patient gets up out of a chair, and position of the patella on standing (any evidence of patella alta) and walking will help further. Further investigation revolves around imaging of the patellofemoral joint and quadriceps mechanism. An anteroposterior view of the knee will allow the 'Q-angle' to be measured (see Fig. 11.22). Lateral knee radiographs are of limited benefit, but will show patella alta and gross disease of the joint. Skyline views in varying degrees of flexion provide the best radiographic visualization of the joint, allowing both facets and any lateral subluxation of the patella to be seen. In diagnosing other soft tissue disorders, such as plicae, MRI may be useful. Scintigraphy can be useful if algodystrophy is suspected. Arthroscopy allows direct visualization of the joint, and can be used to diagnose the fibrillation and softening of the cartilage seen in chondromalacia. Although this is unlikely to change the approach to therapy, it is sometimes useful in providing a diagnostic label and because, if combined with joint lavage, it can provide symptomatic benefit.

SOME CAUSES OF ANTERIOR KNEE PAIN	
Diagnosis	**Features**
Patellofemoral pain syndrome	Younger patient
Patellofemoral osteoarthritis	Older patient
Overuse syndromes	Runners, athletes; osteochondral injuries
Malalignment	Increased Q-angle, knock knees, bow legs, rotation, quadriceps dysplasia
Tracking abnormalities	Patella dislocation, subluxation
Patellar disorders	Patella alta, chondromalacia, osteochondritis
Cruciate ligament injury	
Synovial disorders	Plicae, pigmented villonodular synovitis, inflammatory arthritis
Bursitis	Prepatellar, infrapatellar
Tendinitis	Prepatellar, infrapatellar
Fat pad syndrome	Infrapatellar fat pad hypertrophy
Nail-patella syndrome (Fong's syndrome)	
Algodystrophy	
Hypermobility syndrome	
Osgood–Schlatter disease	Pain at tibial tubercle, young boys
Referred pain	

Fig. 11.24 Some causes of anterior knee pain.

It is important to remember that in young people with anterior knee pain, there is a poor correlation between the evidence for pathology of the joint, as seen on images or arthroscopy, and the symptoms. Some cases present with severe pain but little or no cause can be found in spite of all investigations. In other instances, quite severe abnormalities of the quadriceps mechanism can be asymptomatic. The key to differentiating mechanical disorders of the patellofemoral apparatus from other causes of knee pain is a careful history and examination to detect pain arising from this structure. More diffuse pain, not clearly related to the use of the quadriceps apparatus and knee bending, may be due to other disorders, such as algodystrophy of the knee.

In the first of the cases described, all the radiographs were normal, but the history suggested patellofemoral disease, and on examination there was pain on patella pressure and a little patellofemoral crepitus, indicating a mechanical patellofemoral problem. The Q-angle was found to be increased, and this, plus the history of possible dislocation, indicated a patella malalignment and patella tracking problem. In the second case, there was marked patellofemoral crepitus and tenderness. Skyline radiographs revealed joint space narrowing and osteophytosis of the lateral facet of the patellofemoral joint, with consequent lateral shift of the patella (see Fig. 11.23). Isolated patellofemoral compartment OA was diagnosed. These cases illustrate two of the most frequent causes of anterior knee pain in younger and older patients, respectively; both are extremely common and cause a large amount of pain and disability in the community.

Therapeutic Problems

Specific problems such as prepatella bursitis will respond well to conventional local therapy, but most anterior knee pain is due to mechanical abnormalities of the patellofemoral joint. These do not respond well to most anti-arthritis drug therapy. Anterior knee pain

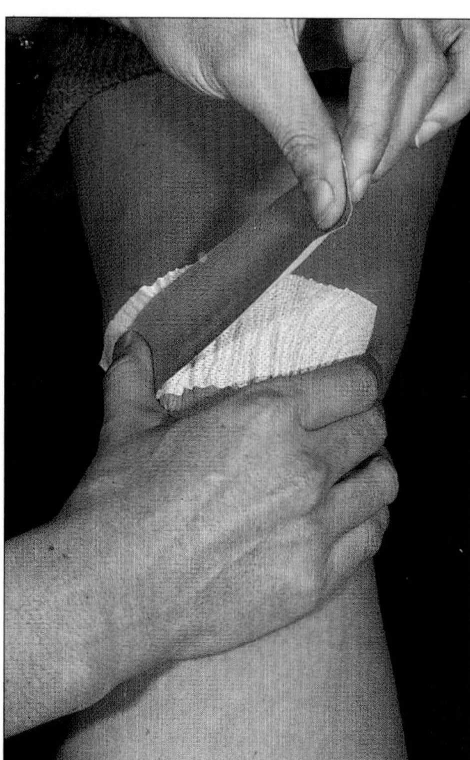

Fig. 11.25 Taping the patella medially. The operator is pushing the patella medially (with her thumb) and applying adhesive tape across the knee joint to hold the patella in a more medial position, reducing pressure on the lateral facet.

is often a difficult problem, lasting for years, and relatively unresponsive to conventional treatment.

In these cases, therapy should be directed at correcting any alignment and tracking abnormalities, to get the biomechanics of the quadriceps mechanism right, followed by specific exercises to train the quadriceps to hold the patella in the correct alignment. Competitive activities and overuse should be avoided. Prolonged sitting and kneeling should also be limited. Tracking and alignment of the patella can often be corrected by taping the patella; medial taping is particularly helpful in the common instances of a large Q-angle or lateral facet patellofemoral OA (Fig. 11.25). Specific exercises to re-educate the vastus medialis oblique muscle are vital in attempting to permanently realign the patella. These conditions are often unresponsive to drugs such as NSAIDs and local corticosteroid injections. A variety of surgical techniques have been used to try to realign the patella and stop dislocation, but surgery is a last resort and is not always successful .

The first of the cases described (a mechanical patellofemoral problem) improved considerably with taping and quadriceps work but had to give up her national hockey activities. Sporting activities were only possible when she wore a brace or a tape over the patella to pull it medially. The second case (patellofemoral compartment OA) had good symptomatic relief with medial taping and quadriceps exercises and was able to reduce her previously heavy consumption of drugs.

Conclusions

Anterior knee pain is common and has multiple causes, but the majority of protracted problems are due to mechanical abnormalities of the patellofemoral joint and quadriceps mechanism. A careful clinical assessment in conjunction with appropriate radiographs will allow the cause to be accurately diagnosed in most cases.

In most cases, attention to patella alignment and tracking problems, patella taping, and work on the quadriceps mechanism, will improve symptoms. Drugs are usually of little value, and surgery should be avoided if possible.

REFERENCES

Cushnaghan J, McCarthy C, Dieppe P. Taping the patella medially: a new treatment for osteoarthritis? Br J Rheumatol. 1993;**32**(suppl 1):105(abstract).

Fulkerson JP, Shea KP. Current concepts review: disorders of patellofemoral alignment. J Bone Joint Surg. 1990;**72A**:1425–9.

Imall J. Current concepts review: patella pain. J Bone Joint Surg. 1982;**64A**:147–52.

McAlindon TE, Snow S, Cooper C, Dieppe PA. Radiographic patterns of knee osteoarthritis in the community: the importance of the patellofemoral joint. Ann Rheum Dis. 1992;**51**:844–9.

McConnell JS. The management of chondromalacia patellae: a long term solution. Aust J Physiother. 1986;**32**:215–23.

Tria AJ, Palumbo RC, Alicea JA. Conservative care for patellofemoral pain. Orthop Clin N Am. 1992;**23**:545–54.

ANKLE SPRAIN

Gerald D Groff

Definition of the Problem

Ankle sprain results from the stretching or tearing of ankle ligaments following inversion or eversion foot injuries. It is the most common injury in athletics but can occur with trauma not related to sports in any age group. Although frequently self-limited, recovery can be complicated by ankle dysfunction, recurrence and acute or chronic instability. As a result, it is important for clinicians to be familiar with clinical evaluation maneuvers, potential diagnostic problems and basic therapies.

The Typical Case

Mrs M is a 64-year-old woman in good health except for mild knee OA. While rushing to catch a bus, she stepped on the edge of a curb, 'twisting' her right ankle. She noted immediate sharp pain located inferior and anterior to the right lateral ankle. She developed rapid swelling with moderate pain and insecurity with standing.

Medical review of the injury suggested inversion of the ankle, supination of the foot and external rotation of the tibia. Examination revealed soft tissue swelling, mild ecchymoses and tenderness just inferior to the right lateral malleolus. Tests for instability, including the anterior drawer sign, were negative. Because of pa n on weight-bearing and bony palpation, a plain radiograph was performed. This was normal. She was treated with ankle elevation and ice for 24 hours, and then NSAIDs plus an air splint for an additional 5 days. Thereafter, gentle range-of-motion and proprioceptive exercises, followed by muscle strengthening exercise, resulted in pain-free, stable ambulation after 3 weeks.

Diagnostic Problems

Although ankle sprain is common and often self-limited, clinicians should be aware of potential problems. Areas of particular concern include concomitant fracture, instability due to ligamentous rupture and conditions that mimic or complicate ankle sprain.

Ankle sprain can be classified into three groups depending on clinical signs and functional loss. Grade 1 sprain results in localized tenderness, minimal swelling or ecchymoses and normal range of motion without instability. Grade 2 sprain causes moderate to severe pain, swelling or ecchymoses and restricted range of motion. Mild instability may occur and weight-bearing is painful. Finally, grade 3 sprain is marked by severe pain, edema, hemorrhage, loss of motion and inability to ambulate. Ankle instability is common, with complete functional loss. The clinical grades reflect the degree of ligamentous injury, with stretching or minimal tearing in grade 1, partial tearing in grade 2, and complete tear in grade 3. Clinical classification is an important determinant of therapy and may require supportive radiographic studies.

The ankle ligaments are shown in Figures 11.26 and 11.27. Inversion ankle injury is much more common than eversion trauma. As a result, over 90% of sprains occur in the lateral complex, particularly the anterior talofibular ligament. Rupture of the talofibular ligament alone can cause mild lateral and moderate anterior ankle instability, with pain and swelling inferior to the lateral malleolus. Additional rupture of the calcaneofibular ligament occurs in 25% of lateral complex sprains and results in greater lateral instability. The posterior talofibular ligament is rarely injured. The medial deltoid ligament is involved in 5% or less of all sprains and is frequently complicated by fracture. Inferior tibiofibular (syndesmotic) ligament injury can complicate ankle ligament damage during high-energy trauma. In this case, tenderness is present over the ligament, just above the line of the ankle joint.

The most common fractures during ankle sprain are avulsions of the malleoli or tarsal bones. Other sites include the anterior process of the calcaneus, the base of the 5th metatarsal (insertion of the peroneus brevis tendon), the talar neck, the cuboid and the bony epiphyses in children. The strength of the deltoid ligament makes it an uncommon site for injury, but when it occurs malleolar fracture or concomitant sprains of the syndesmosis are more likely. Standard radiographs should be considered following a history of high-energy injury, pain with weight-bearing, moderate to severe pain with bony palpation, and for any medial sprain. In addition, for children with

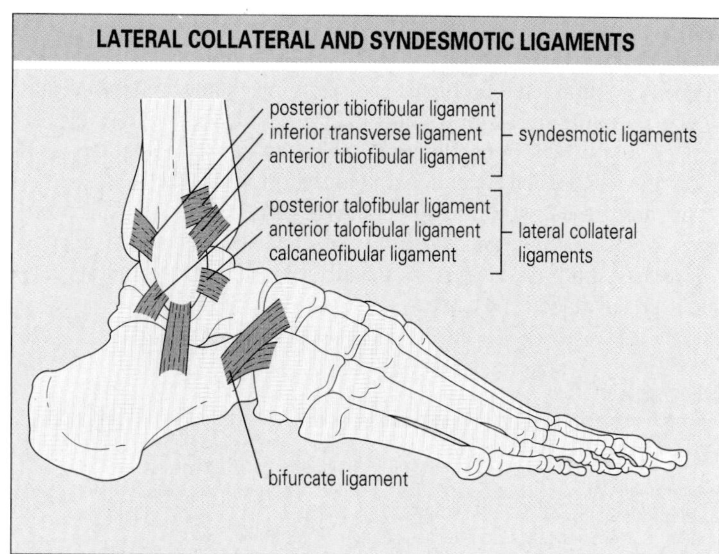

Fig. 11.26 Lateral collateral ligaments and syndesmotic ligaments of the ankle.

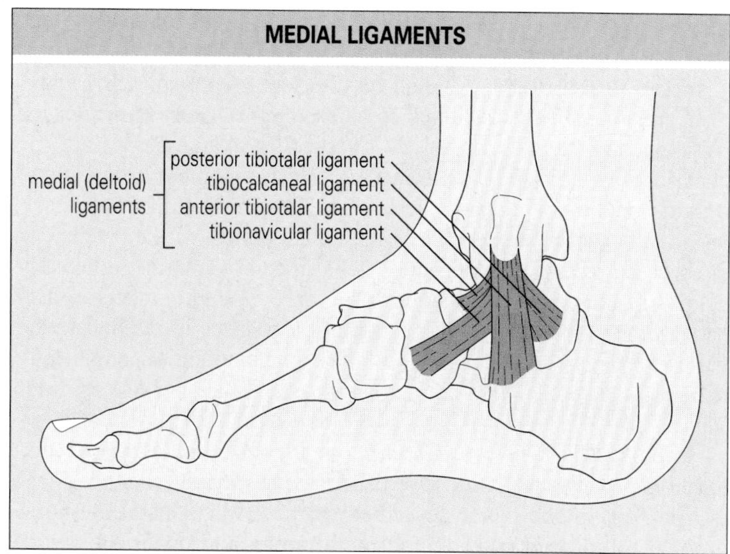

Fig. 11.27 Medial ligaments of the ankle.

open epiphyses and elderly patients with osteoporosis risk factors, radiographs should be obtained.

Ankle instability due to lateral ligament rupture is an important condition which must be considered during the initial evaluation. Unrecognized and untreated acute instability can lead to functional insecurity and recurrent ankle sprain. Chronic ankle instability has been linked to the development of OA. The clinical assessment of stability includes attempted active ankle inversion (Fig. 11.28) and the anterior drawer test (Fig. 11.29). Instability can be estimated by comparing the degree of laxity with the uninjured ankle. The severity of sprain can usually be determined by physical examination. However, the examination may be limited by pain, swelling or muscle spasm. These patients, as well as those with demonstrable laxity, may require additional diagnostic studies. Stress radiography can be performed during the talar tilt and anterior drawer maneuvers. An opening of the posterior tibiotalar joint of 6mm or greater during the anterior drawer maneuver suggests anterior talofibular ligament rupture. However, the accuracy of these studies is limited by several factors, such as patient co-operation, the amount of force applied and the angle of ankle flexion. Arthrography is generally more accurate, although dye extravasation in as many as 25% of procedures can reduce the diagnostic value. Magnetic resonance imaging may prove to be the preferred procedure.

The differential diagnosis of 'ankle sprain' includes peroneal tendon subluxation or inflammation, Achilles tendon injury and sprain or rupture of the inferior tibiofibular syndesmosis. Syndesmotic ligament tears are unusual, but when involved can require prolonged recovery or cause chronic ankle instability. Subtalar or talonavicular subluxation and acute lateral ankle synovitis can rarely mimic ankle sprain. Posterior tibial tendon rupture may be difficult to differentiate from the uncommon medial ankle sprain.

Systemic conditions may complicate recovery. Patients with peripheral neuropathy and poor proprioception (especially diabetics) can develop secondary reflex sympathetic dystrophy or destructive

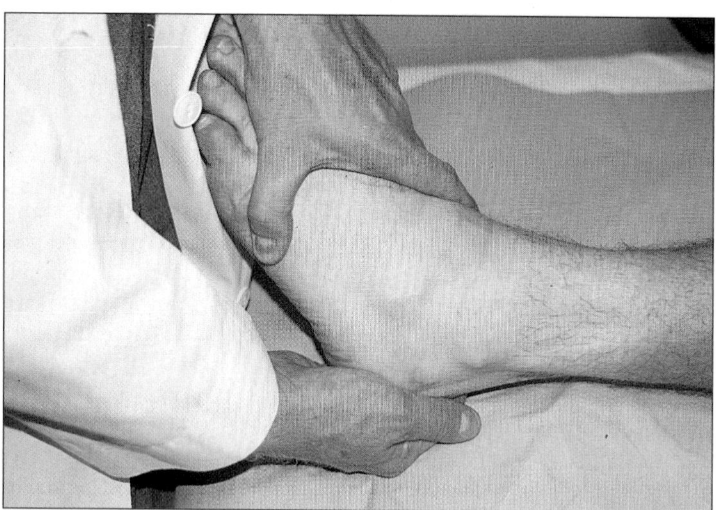

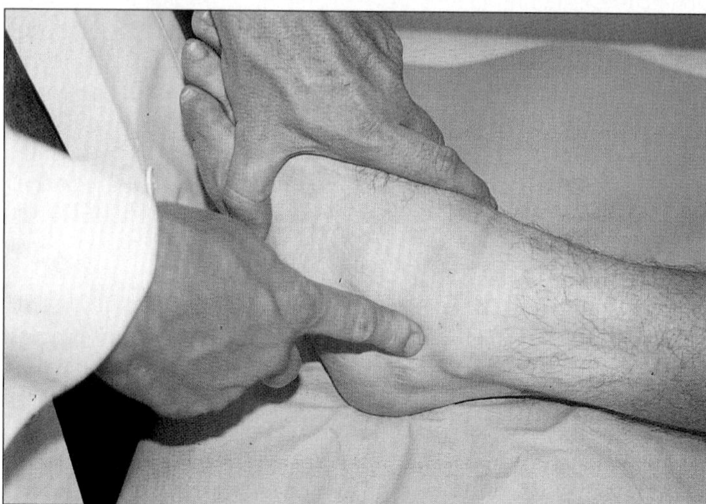

Fig. 11.28 Active ankle inversion. Gentle inversion of the foot with observation and palpations of the talofibular joint. Motion or laxity suggests ligamentous instability.

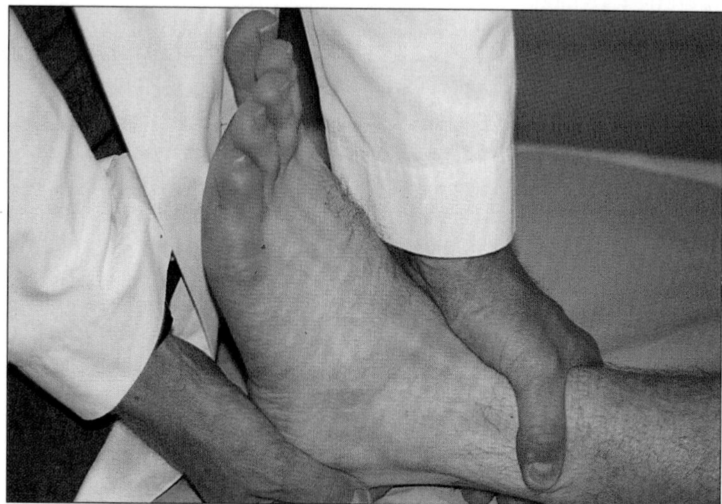

Fig. 11.29 The anterior drawer test. The distal leg is stabilized while upward pressure is applied to the heel. Anterior laxity of the ankle suggests ligamentous instability.

arthropathy. Patients with chronic hip or knee arthritis may have limitations to rehabilitation or may be at risk of recurrent sprain due to gait imbalance or chronic muscle weakness.

Therapeutic Options

The goals of acute ankle sprain management are reduction of pain and swelling and the prevention of chronic instability. Grade 1 and 2 sprains respond well to conservative therapy as long as treatment is begun as soon as possible after injury (Fig. 11.30). Acute instability or fracture should be ruled out by examination and radiography when indicated. Therapy over the initial 24–48 hours includes rest, elevation, and compression wrap. Cold packs may be applied for 15–20 minutes each hour as tolerated. NSAIDs may accelerate recovery if started within the initial 24 hours of treatment. Early use of NSAIDs permits return to sports sooner than when ankle support alone is utilized.

Depending on severity, healing may require 2–8 weeks. There is no precise information regarding the healing time of ligament injury. As a result, the guidelines for joint preservation and rehabilitation must be individualized. In general, grade 1 sprains can begin careful rehabilitation after 48 hours. This would include plantar and dorsiflexion range of motion, Achilles tendon stretching, and isometrics within the limits of discomfort.

After a few days, double- and single-leg toe raises with lateral ankle support helps to improve proprioception. Early mobilization with lateral ankle support is important. Grade 2 sprains may require a more prolonged period of immobilization during weight-bearing, utilizing a cast-brace or bivalved cast for 10–14 days. Rehabilitation may be more protracted with avoidance of ankle inversion. However, rehabilitation should be directed toward return to safe ambulation as soon as possible. The key to a successful outcome is a consistent, progressive rehabilitation program.

Ankle support with either adhesive taping or air-stirrup is a useful adjunct to rehabilitation. Supports serve to limit the extremes of ankle motion and increase ankle proprioception. Acutely, this allows early weight-bearing while reducing the risk of reinjury during the initial 3–4 weeks of recovery. Patients with mild functional instability or athletes at risk for recurrent injury may benefit by more prolonged use of ankle support. However, the goal is to make supports unnecessary by ankle strengthening through exercise. Taping techniques are described by Balduini *et al.* (1987). The air-stirrup consists of two segments of molded orthoplast with inflatable inner-lining air-bags connected by a heel strap (Air Cast Inc., Summit NJ, USA). The air-stirrup has the distinct advantages of being easily removable for rehabilitation and allowing dorsi and plantar flexion while limiting inversion.

The treatment of grade 3 sprain (complete ligamentous rupture and instability) is controversial. Management with rigid casting or primary surgical repair depends on a variety of factors, including the degree of subjective and objective instability, the number and position of ruptured ligaments, and the athletic goals of the patient. As a result, grade 3 sprains should be referred to an experienced orthopedic surgeon.

AN APPROACH TO THE MANAGEMENT OF ACUTE ANKLE SPRAIN (GRADES I AND II)
Immediate
• Rule out instability by examination • Radiography when indicated
Initial 24–48 hours
• Rest • Elevation • Ice • Compression • Nonsteroidal anti-inflammatory drugs (NSAIDs)
2–7 days
• NSAIDs • Modified weight-bearing with ankle support (adhesive taping or air-stirrup support) • Range of motion, proprioceptive exercise as tolerated
7–28 days
• Progressive mobilization with ankle support • Additional strengthening exercises
Chronic
• Ankle support if insecurity or mild stability • Resume athletic training when pain is minimal

Fig. 11.30 An approach to the management of acute ankle sprain.

Conclusions

Ankle sprain is a common injury, occurring in the geriatric population as well as in athletes. Appropriate initial management is essential in preserving long-term ankle function and avoidance of instability or recurrent injury. This should include clinical assessment of instability with supportive plain or stress radiographs when indicated. Grade 1 and 2 sprains respond well to conservative treatment and careful rehabilitation. Grade 3 sprains should be referred to an orthopedic surgeon for consideration of casting or surgical intervention.

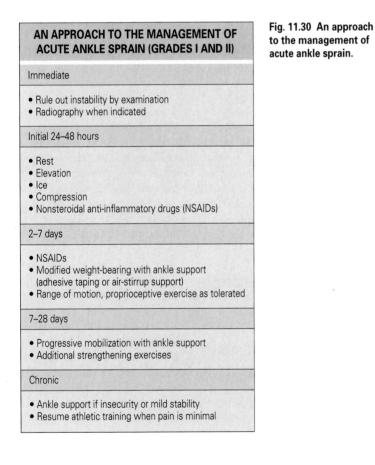

REFERENCES

Balduini F, Vesco J, Torg J, Torg E. Management and rehabilitation of ligamentous injuries to the ankle. Sports Med. 1987;**4**:364–80.

Cass J, Morrey B. Ankle instability: current concepts, diagnosis and treatment. Mayo Clin Proc. 1984:**59**:165–70.

Harrington K. Degenerative arthritis of the ankle secondary to long standing lateral ligament instability. J Bone Joint Surg. 1979; **61**(A):354–61.

Ouzounian T, Shereff M. Common ankle disorders of the elderly: Diagnosis and management. Geriatrics. 1988;**43**:73–80.

Raatikainen T, Putkonen M, Puranen J. Arthrography, clinical examination and stress radiograph in the diagnosis of acute injury to the lateral ligaments of the ankle. Am J Sports Med. 1992;**20**:2–6.

Stanley K. Ankle sprains are always more than 'just a sprain'. Postgrad Med. 1991;**89**:251–5.

PLANTAR HEEL PAIN

Shepard Hurwitz

Definition of the Problem

Plantar heel pain is common in the adult population at large and in seronegative arthropathy patients in particular. The most recalcitrant forms of plantar heel pain occur in those patients with radiographic enthesophyte formation and psoriatic arthritis, Reiter's syndrome and other spondyloarthropathies. These patients will commonly have posterior heel pain in addition to the plantar heel pain, a feature which is not commonly seen in plantar heel pain syndromes in the population at large.

The Typical Case

A 41-year-old woman has had multiple hand and foot surgeries for her arthritis. She has had psoriasis for 22 years and currently is treated aggressively by the dermatologist for lesions all over her body. She developed progressive stiffness and pain in the left ankle but complained most of painful right plantar heel discomfort. Her medications at this time included hydroxychloroquine sulfate, 200mg twice a day, and sulindac, 200mg twice a day. She has been wearing sneakers with cushioned insoles and will not walk with the assistance of a cane. Because of her dermatitis she was not allowed to use hydrotherapy, nor could she use frequent ice packs. She presented having been treated by her internist with several injections of steroids into the fat pad under the right calcaneus. Physical examination revealed a stiff ankle and hindfoot without signs of posterior tibial nerve entrapment or posterior tibial tendinitis. She was tender on the plantar and plantar medial aspect of the heel near the prominence of the calcaneus. There were no skin lesions on the sole of her foot. A radiograph was obtained (Fig. 11.31).

Differential Diagnosis

Evaluation of plantar heel pain should include careful physical examination which should differentiate between nerve pain, bone pain, soft tissue pain and the presence of any lesions such as tumor or infection. Tendinitis of the posterior tibial or flexor digitorum longus tendons may mimic plantar heel pain or may indirectly cause pain by exerting compression on the contents of the tarsal tunnel. Nerve entrapment of the posterior tibial nerve or its major branches may be caused by inflamed synovium, a ganglia, varicose veins or soft tissue encroachment of swollen muscle or fascia. Within the past 10 years, a syndrome involving entrapment of a specific nerve, the first branch of the lateral plantar nerve, has been described. Soft tissue pain may be the result of chronic or acute inflammation of the origin of the plantar fascia or any of the short muscles on the heel. Fibrosis of the plantar heel pad may lead to pain, as may disruption of the normal plantar architecture following trauma. Infection of the soft tissues may be overt, such as in the case of a skin ulcer, or occult, such as with a plantar abscess or osteomyelitis of the calcaneus. Bone pain may be due to stress fracture, enthesopathy of the plantar fascia or short flexor muscles originating on the calcaneus.

Primary tumors of the calcaneus are possible; metastatic lesions to the calcaneus are exceedingly rare.

Lateral and axial radiographs are the appropriate views. The soft tissues may be evaluated with an MRI scan and the bony architecture of the calcaneus is best evaluated with a CT scan. Radionuclide imaging of the calcaneus is a good screening examination when bone pain is suspected. However, this modality will not differentiate a periosteal process from an intraosseous process. Nerve conduction tests may detect slowing of transmission across the tarsal tunnel area and electrical studies may show denervation of group specific muscles, such as the abductor to the great toe for the medial plantar nerve and the abductor to the little toe for the lateral plantar nerve.

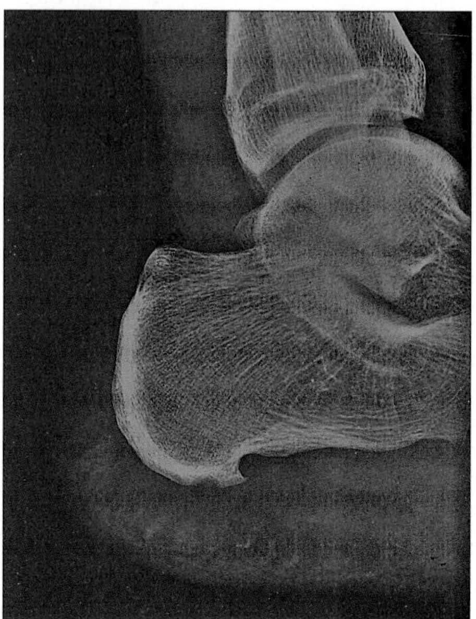

Fig. 11.31 Plantar heel pain in a patient with psoriasis. The radiograph shows erosive changes due to inflammation and proliferative bone change of the calcaneus.

Therapeutic Options

The painful plantar heel first needs a diagnosis. The pain of nerve entrapment may respond to a change in anti-inflammatory medication, including steroids, but in all likelihood will require infiltration with steroids at the point of entrapment. Physical therapy modalities such as iontophoresis with soluble steroid preparations may work as well as infiltration via injection. Limitation of activity is helpful as an adjunct, and this primarily involves reduction in weight-bearing activity. Entrapment neuropathy does not respond to vitamin therapy or exercises.

Sources of bone pain respond to rest and immobilization in the case of stress fracture. Tumors, such as Paget's disease of bone, require medical management or surgical treatment. The painful enthesopathy that is associated with proliferative bone change is a feature of the case with seronegative arthritis. Optimum management of the inflammatory component of the disease is helpful. The results of surgery are highly controversial and it is not one of the early treatment options. The initial treatment begins with analgesics (naproxen 375mg p.o. t.i.d.), and passive stretching of the plantar fascia and toe flexors in conjunction with a cushioned insole. This orthosis should provide softness for the heel, medial arch support and supination of the foot. The orthosis is designed to reduce the stretch on plantar fascia, the short muscles of the foot and the Achilles tendon. If the patient can tolerate pressure on the forefoot, then an elevation of the heel would be helpful to shunt some of the pressure up to the forefoot and away from the painful heel. Other physical therapy modalities including whirlpool, ultrasound, friction massage and assisted stretching exercises, all have their place in the nonsurgical management. Relief may be obtained under a tender area by removing contact with that area of the orthotic insole.

Patients without nerve entrapment or large plantar osteophytes constitute the majority of cases. This problem is best managed nonoperatively with the same shoe modifications, footwear inserts, physical therapy and modalities, and judicious use of injected corticosteroids. A word of caution about corticosteroid injections is that there is an incidence of plantar fascia rupture, which in the case of a flexible foot will lead to pes planus. Surgery for soft tissue pain on the sole of the foot is not very rewarding and involves creating an iatrogenic disruption of the plantar fascia. Patients with plantar fascia rupture or surgical excision should have an insole orthotic to try to control the hindfoot and support the arch, in an attempt to minimize mechanical collapse and pronation of the foot.

Conclusions

The patient with inflammatory seronegative arthritis and plantar heel pain presents a challenge to the clinician. The symptoms may be remarkably improved on a short-term basis by injection; however, this is probably not a long-term solution. Surgery is not very successful.

Currently, treatment recommendations include the use of appropriate well-fitting shoes and orthotic devices, stretching and judicious use of local injections. Treatment is often needed for protracted periods of time. The patient should be counseled against jogging and court sports during the acute phase.

REFERENCES

Capen D, Scheck M. Seronegative inflammation of the ankle and foot. Clin Orthop Rel Res. 1981;**155**:147–52.

Resnick D, Niwayama K. On the nature of bony proliferation in 'rheumatoid variant' disorder. Am J Roentgenol. 1977;**129**:275–81.

Solomon G. Inflammatory arthritis. In: Jahss MH, ed. Disorders of the foot and ankle. Philadelphia: WB Saunders. 1991:1681.

12

CLINICAL FEATURES AND DIAGNOSTIC PROBLEMS IN OSTEOARTHRITIS

Paul A Dieppe

Definition

- A heterogenous group of conditions sharing common pathologic and radiologic features.
- Focal loss of articular cartilage in part of a synovial joint is accompanied by a hypertrophic reaction in the subchondral bone and margin of the joint.
- Radiographic changes include joint space narrowing, subchondral sclerosis and cyst formation, and marginal osteophytosis.
- Extremely common and age-related, with a particular predilection for the knees, hips, hands and the apophyseal joints of the spine.
- Often accompanied by clinical manifestations which may include use-related joint pain, gelling of joints after inactivity, and loss of range of joint movement.

GENERAL FEATURES OF AN OSTEOARTHRITIC JOINT

OA is a heterogeneous condition with a variable presentation and a variety of patterns of expression. It is analogous to kidney or heart failure, in which similar pathologic and clinical features appear, irrespective of the cause(s) of the condition which may not be apparent. This section describes the clinical manifestations of OA which most affected joints have in common.

Onset

Many joints with pathologic or radiographic evidence of OA remain symptom free [1,2]. For those in whom the condition is expressed clinically, the onset is usually slow and insidious and patients are rarely able to pinpoint the exact nature or timing of the onset with any accuracy. The most frequent early features are a diffuse, intermittent ache or pain in the joint, usually related to, or immediately after use. A mild sensation of joint stiffness, associated with poorly localized aches in nearby muscles may also occur. Some patients notice the gradual development of a reduced range of movement of an affected joint. For example, they may slowly become aware of more difficulty in bending down to put their socks on because of stiffness in the hip. In a minority, the onset is more sudden, in which case it may be associated with joint trauma. For example, someone may be unaware of any problem with their knees until a minor injury takes place. Within days they may then develop some or all of the symptoms described. In a few such patients quite severe pain develops over the period of a few days or weeks. It is likely that pathologic OA was already present in the joints of these individuals, and that the trauma converts a previously asymptomatic OA joint into a symptomatic one.

THE MAIN SYMPTOMS AND SIGNS OF OSTEOARTHRITIS
Symptoms
Use-related pain (rest and night pain, tenderness) Stiffness ('gelling') after inactivity (early morning stiffness, usually <30min) Loss of movement (difficulty with certain tasks) Feelings of insecurity or instability Functional limitations and handicap
Signs
Tender spots around the joint margin (tenderness in nearby structures) Firm swellings of the joint margin Coarse crepitus (cracking or locking) Signs of mild inflammation (cool effusions) Restricted, painful movements 'Tightness' of the joint Instability (obvious severe bone/joint destruction)

Fig. 12.1 The main symptoms and signs of OA. The less common features are in brackets.

Clinical Presentation

Occasional muscle and joint pain or stiffness is a part of life for all of us. In most patients with OA, the clinical onset of the condition consists of little more than the gradual awareness of an intermittent increase in the frequency and severity of such problems, perhaps with their becoming increasingly localized to one joint site. Because of this, presentation to a doctor or therapist is often delayed by many months or even years after the onset. By the time most patients get to see a specialist, they have already developed the signs and symptoms of established OA described below.

SYMPTOMS AND SIGNS

The main symptoms and signs of an OA joint are listed in Figure 12.1. There has been relatively little scientific investigation of either the nature or the cause of these clinical features.

Pain and Tenderness

Clinical features

Pain is undoubtedly the most important symptom of OA [3]. Comparative studies of OA and RA have shown relatively little difference in either the quantity or quality of joint pain described by individuals, with the descriptions given varying enormously between different patients [4,5]. Longitudinal studies also indicate great variation in pain intensity over time. There is a discrepancy between radiographic grading and reporting of pain, which indicates further differences between the sexes and between different joint sites. As shown in Figure 12.2, for a given grading on radiography, the hip is most likely to be painful, and the hand least likely. This data taken from Lawrence's early studies [6] also indicates that women are more likely to report pain than men. More recent studies have investigated further the clinical associations of pain in OA (see Fig. 12.3). The severity of radiographic change is associated with an increase in the likelihood of pain, although severe joint damage can be asymptomatic [7]. The sex discrepancy, with women more likely to suffer pain than men, has also been confirmed [8]. The other main association reported is with psychological factors: in one study total pain has been correlated with anxiety, and the severity of pain with depression [9].

There have been relatively few studies of the pain experienced by OA sufferers, although Hart has described six different types, with an aching sensation associated with joint usage the commonest form [10]. In

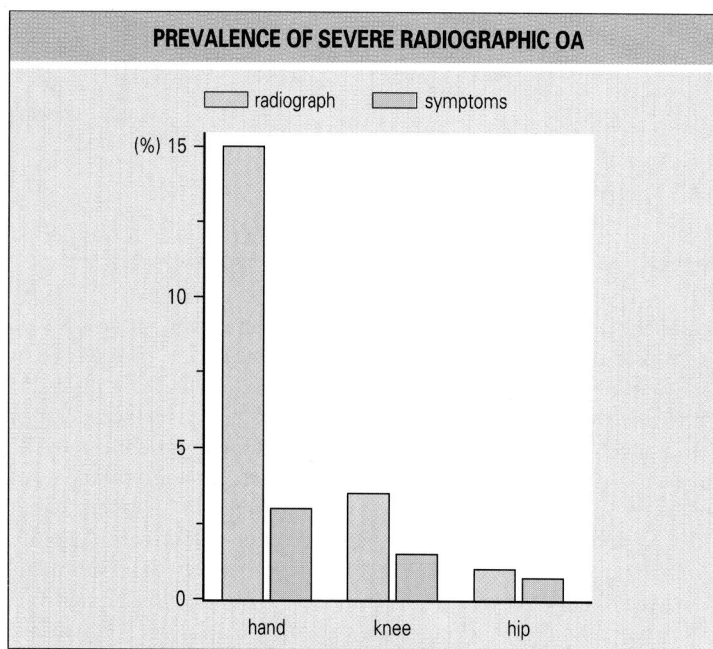

Fig. 12.2. Histogram illustrating rough estimates of the adult prevalence of severe radiographic OA (Kellgren and Lawrence grades 2–4) and of symptomatic OA of the three major peripheral joint sites involved. Note the discrepancy between radiographic changes and the symptomatic disease, which is more marked in women than in men.

a detailed study of pain reporting by 500 patients with peripheral joint OA, Cushnaghan confirmed previous reports that use-related pain was the most frequently described symptom [8]. This study also indicated that age and sex, as well as joint sites of involvement, influence the reporting of pain in OA. The pain related to activity usually starts within seconds or minutes of onset of joint use, but may continue for hours after the activity has ceased. Some patients describe discrete, stabbing pains coinciding precisely with certain movements or with weight bearing; others describe a poorly localized, constant ache or pain brought on by activity. Whereas nearly all symptomatic patients with OA have use-related pain, only some 50% or less describe rest pain, and about 30% report night pain [8]. A minority of patients develop severe pain which prevents any proper use of a joint, or keeps them awake at night. In these cases severe or rapidly progressive OA, often with destructive changes in bone, may be apparent on the radiograph.

The pain of OA is often accompanied by sensations of tenderness around the affected joint, which may be exquisitely painful if 'knocked' or injured. Both the patient and the examiner may be able to elicit a number of sites of tenderness around the joint margin and in surrounding muscles [11].

Pathogenesis

Several possible causes of pain and tenderness in OA have been investigated (Figs. 12.3 and 12.4). The data described above, including associations with both radiographic severity and psychological factors, would suggest that a combination of local, systemic and central neurologic factors are important.

Local mechanical factors

The alteration in the shape of an OA joint, the osteophytic lipping, and in advanced cases destruction and instability, can all cause abnormal mechanical forces to be applied to ligaments, capsule and other innervated structures, giving rise to pain and localized tender spots. This may account for local periarticular tenderness and sharp pains induced by activity.

Bone pain

There is good evidence that the intraosseous pressure in subchondral bone can be elevated in OA [14,15]. Furthermore, relief of this pressure, which is thought to result from obstruction of venous outflow, can relieve pain [18]. It has been suggested that this is the mechanism most responsible for severe prolonged, rest and night pain. Pain may also arise from the bony periosteum, which might become elevated as a result of chondrophytes or osteophytes [16].

ASSOCIATIONS AND POSSIBLE CAUSES OF PAIN IN OA

Associations	Possible causes
Severity of radiographic change	Raised intraosseous pressure
Sex (F>M)	Inflammatory synovitis
Age (less in the young or very old)	Periarticular problems
Joint site (less in hands)	Periosteal elevation
Psychological factors	Muscular changes
	Fibromyalgia/pain amplification
	Central neurogenic changes

Fig. 12.3 Associations and possible causes of pain in OA.

Synovitis

Mild synovitis is a feature of advanced OA [17,18] and may contribute to symptoms. The partial response of the pain to nonsteroidal anti-inflammatory drugs (NSAIDs) is often cited as evidence in favor of this mechanism. However, only a proportion of patients appear to respond to an anti-inflammatory agent [19], so it seems likely that synovitis is one of the contributory factors in some patients only.

Secondary periarticular syndromes

The abnormal biomechanics of the OA joint can contribute to the development of a secondary periarticular disorder, such as bursitis or tenosynovitis. It should be easy to distinguish this from true joint pain on examination, but the presence of signs and radiographic changes of OA can lead to the wrong diagnosis.

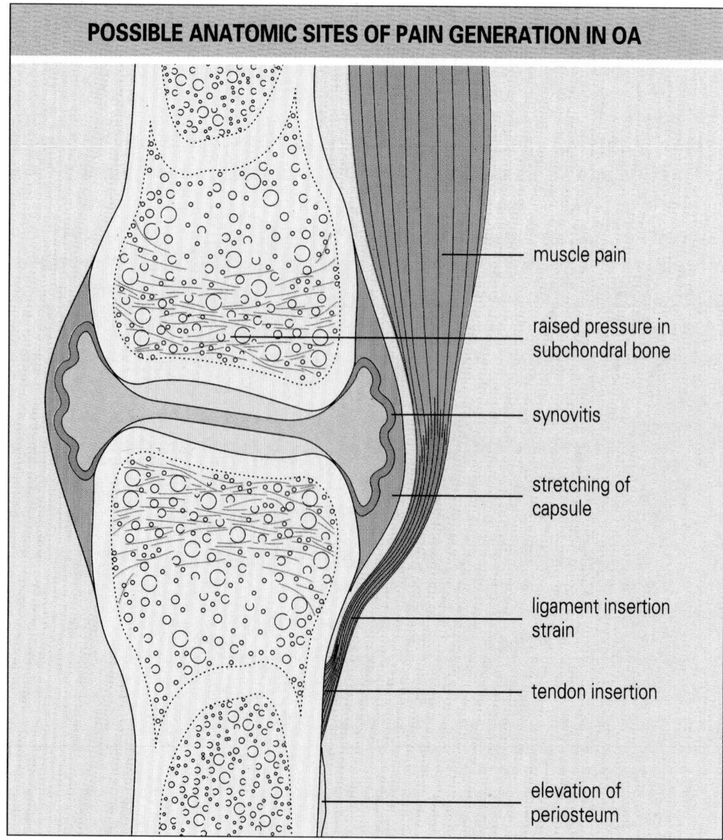

Fig. 12.4 Possible causes of pain in OA. The diagram shows some of the anatomic sites that might give rise to pain in OA, there being no nerve endings in the cartilage itself. The pathologic processes involved include degradation and repair of connective tissues leading to alterations in the anatomy of the joint and inflammation.

Muscular pain
Patients with OA often suffer from aching and tenderness in muscles which serve the affected joints. Muscle weakness is common, and muscle strengthening exercises may relieve pain [20]. This suggests that muscular dysfunction may be an important, independent cause of pain of the osteoarthritic 'joint'.

Referred pain
Kellgren and others have emphasized the importance of referral of both pain and tenderness from a damaged joint to the muscles that move the joint [21]. This may account for the frequent occurrence of pain and tenderness away from the immediate vicinity of an OA joint.

Central pain mechanisms
Patients with OA may have evidence of associated fibromyalgia or pain amplification [22]. In addition, the data of Summers and colleagues, associating OA pain with anxiety and depression [9], is indicative of an important central component.

The existence of a variety of different pain patterns and possible mechanisms for the generation of pain in and around the OA joint obviously has major implications for patient management, particularly in view of the fact that pain is the most important manifestation of the condition.

Stiffness
Clinical features
The sensation of 'stiffness' is reported by most OA patients. It may mean difficulty in the initiation of movement, problems in moving joints through a range of movement, or it may be used to describe an ache or pain on movement. The most characteristic feature of joint stiffness in OA is the phenomenon of 'gelling' after inactivity. This appears to be a problem of getting the joint to move after a period of rest, and although it may be severe, it usually only lasts for a few minutes. Patients may talk about having to 'work the joint in' after a rest period or first thing in the morning. Longer periods of stiffness in the morning occur in some patients, but in contrast to that of RA, it rarely lasts longer than about 30 minutes and is usually confined to a small number of affected joints.

Pathogenesis
The cause of joint stiffness in OA remains unknown. It is reasonable to speculate that the 'gelling' of a joint after inactivity has a simple mechanical explanation, perhaps relating to the capsular thickening and other periarticular changes that occur in OA, whereas the more prolonged morning stiffness experienced by some patients may be due to synovitis, and analogous to the morning stiffness of rheumatoid disease.

Loss of Movement
A reduction in the total range of movement of the affected joint usually occurs in OA. It is often accompanied by pain that is at its worst at the end of the reduced range. The likely explanation is that the chondrophytic and osteophytic lipping and remodeling of the joint, combined with the capsular thickening, is preventing a free range of movement. This might also explain the complaint of difficulty in moving the joint throughout the whole of the available range which occurs in some patients.

A Sensation of Insecurity or Instability
Many patients with OA complain of a sensation of insecurity or instability in the joints affected. Sometimes they will report that the joint 'gives way', or that they are afraid that it is going to give out on them. This symptom is not necessarily accompanied by any objective evidence of ligamentous instability or significant joint destruction. However, muscle wasting is usually apparent, and it seems likely that this symptom is due more to abnormal strength and functioning of the muscles than to mechanical abnormalities of the joints.

'Bony' Swelling and Crepitus
Firm swellings of the joint margin are often palpable, and may be tender. Course crepitations are usually felt on movement of an osteoarthritic joint. Along with 'bony' swelling of the affected joint, crepitus stands out as one of the best signs in the clinical differentiation of OA from other disorders [23]. In advanced OA the crepitus may be clearly audible, as well as palpable, loud cracks emanating from a hip or knee joint on walking, for example. The noise is probably due to the roughening of the joint surface and outgrowths at the rim of the joint interfering with the normally smooth movement between the joint surfaces. 'Cavitation', or the formation of gas bubbles within the synovial fluid may also contribute [24].

The crepitus of OA can usually be felt through much of the total range of movement, distinguishing it from the occasional 'cracking' of a normal joint. It also has a much coarser feel than the fine crepitus that can be caused by tenosynovitis and other inflammatory disorders.

Soft Tissue Swellings and Signs of Inflammation
The firm swellings around the margin of an OA joint are probably due to the soft tissue, cartilage and bony outgrowths at the rim of the joint. There may also be obvious soft tissue swelling, due to an effusion or synovitis. In some studies effusions, in addition to bony swelling, have been found in the majority of OA knee joints examined and interpreted as evidence of low grade inflammation [25]. Knee joints are frequently warm, and finger joints with OA may go through periods when there is obvious warmth and redness over them, providing further clinical evidence of the inflammatory component of OA [25]. 'Flare-ups', or episodes in which symptoms are unusually bad for a few days or weeks, may be accompanied by increased signs of inflammation in any affected joint.

Some OA joints develop relatively large effusions which are usually 'cool'. This may be due to an intercurrent attack of crystal synovitis (such as pseudogout), but if the fluid is aspirated it will frequently have a high viscosity, low cell count, and no crystals can be detected. The pathogenesis of these effusions remains obscure.

Evidence of Joint Destruction
In advanced OA there may be clear signs of destruction of the cartilage, bone and surrounding soft tissues. These may include deformities, such as a varus angulation of the knee joint due to damage confined to the medial compartment (Fig. 12.5), and ligamentous laxity

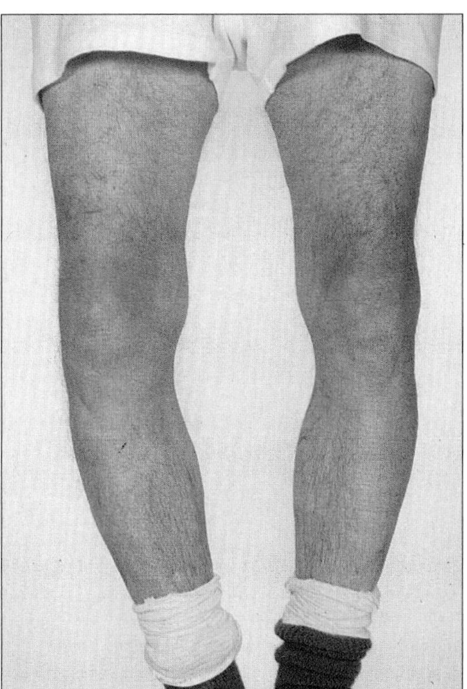

Fig. 12.5 A patient with typical OA of the knees. In the normal standing posture there is a mild varus angulation of the knee joints due to symmetrical OA of the medial tibiofemoral compartments.

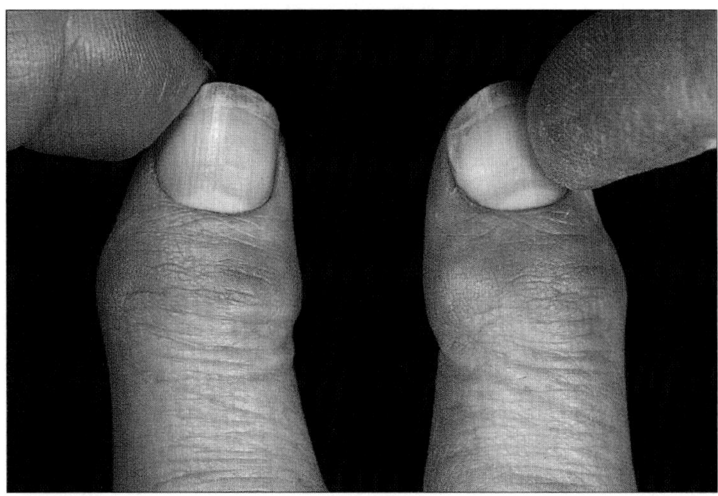

Fig. 12.6 Unstable distal interphalangeal joints in OA. The examiner is able to push the joint from side to side due to gross instability, a common finding in late interphalangeal joint OA.

or instability. Instability frequently develops in distal interphalangeal (DIP) joints (Fig. 12.6). Bone destruction may lead to leg shortening in hip disease and to gross deformities at other joint sites.

Loss of Function and Handicap

There is an enormous health burden resulting from OA that relates to the pain the disorder causes, as well as the muscle weakness and physical disabilities that result from OA.

The possible causes of functional loss, disability and handicap in relation to OA are shown schematically in Figure 12.7. The key factors will obviously vary in different patients and this should be explored when taking the history and carrying out a physical examination. Pain can be a major cause of reduced function, but other factors such as loss of power and a reduced range of movement may also prove important. For example, in some recent studies of knee OA, McAlindon and colleagues obtained evidence to suggest that decreased power in the quadriceps muscle correlated more strongly with functional problems assessed by the health assessment questionnaire (HAQ) score than did pain or the degree of radiographic change [26].

Natural History and Outcome

The natural history of OA differs enormously at different joint sites and in different patients, making it difficult to generalize. In addition, the relatively slow evolution of the condition in most cases makes the subject difficult to investigate, and there have been very few prospective studies of outcome.

In the majority of cases the condition takes years to evolve. During that time symptoms usually wax and wane and the natural history may be punctuated by 'flares' lasting days or months, in which symptoms are particularly severe. Conversely, some patients have periods of months, or even years, in which they are relatively free of trouble and the condition may appear stable for long periods of time [27]. Of the major peripheral joint sites involved, disease evolution tends to be fastest in the finger joints and slowest at the knee, with the hip being intermediate. 'Rapid' progression, meaning a major change in symptoms and radiographs over a period of months rather than years, occurs in a minority [28]. Bone destruction sometimes develops over a similar time period, especially in older females [29]. Conversely, hip and finger joints can show evidence of radiographic as well as symptomatic improvement [30,31].

There are several possible outcome measures and many different factors that may affect the natural history of OA (Fig. 12.8). Radiographic evidence of changes in the anatomy of the joint do not always correlate with changes in symptoms or disability and the choice of appropriate process and outcome measures is difficult [32,33].

Complications

OA is a condition that is confined to the involved joints; it has no systemic component. Any complications are related entirely to local changes or to the pain and disability caused by the damaged joints.

Local complications can include secondary periarticular syndromes and nerve entrapment problems resulting from the expanded joint margins and distorted anatomy. Severe disease and deformity can also cause secondary fractures or osteonecrosis of bone [34]. Other complications can arise as the result of falls or immobility caused by the pain and handicap.

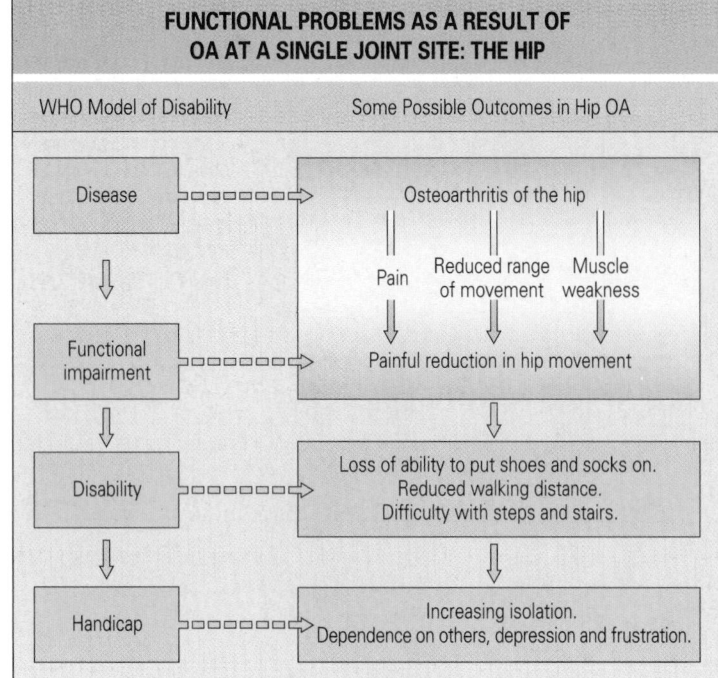

Fig. 12.7 Functional loss, disability and handicap as a result of OA. The chart uses the WHO model of disability and outlines an example of the way in which OA of the hip joint can lead to functional problems for the patient.

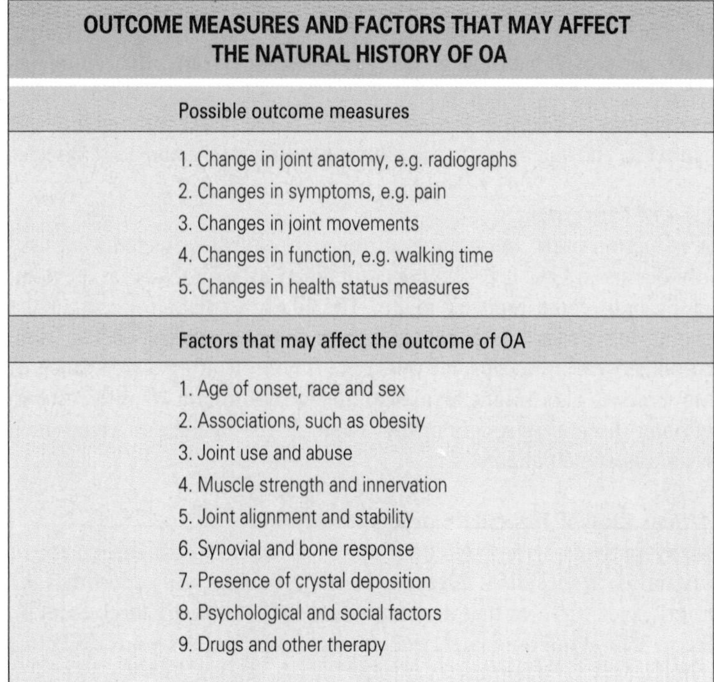

OUTCOME MEASURES AND FACTORS THAT MAY AFFECT THE NATURAL HISTORY OF OA
Possible outcome measures
1. Change in joint anatomy, e.g. radiographs 2. Changes in symptoms, e.g. pain 3. Changes in joint movements 4. Changes in function, e.g. walking time 5. Changes in health status measures
Factors that may affect the outcome of OA
1. Age of onset, race and sex 2. Associations, such as obesity 3. Joint use and abuse 4. Muscle strength and innervation 5. Joint alignment and stability 6. Synovial and bone response 7. Presence of crystal deposition 8. Psychological and social factors 9. Drugs and other therapy

Fig. 12.8 Outcome measures and factors that may affect the natural history of OA. Adapted from Felson DT [40].

SPECIFIC FEATURES OF OSTEOARTHRITIS AT DIFFERENT JOINT SITES

Introduction

The most frequent and important joint sites to be affected by OA include the knee, hand, hip and spinal facet joints. In this section, OA of each of these and other major sites will be discussed separately. Further discussion of distribution and the concept of 'subsets' based on sites of involvement is given in the next section.

OA of the Knee Joint

Anatomy, pathology and biomechanics

The knee is a complex joint, with three major compartments: the medial and lateral tibiofemoral joints and the patellofemoral joint. Each of these areas can be affected by OA separately, or in any combination [35]. Isolated medial compartment, or medial plus patellofemoral disease are the commonest combinations (Fig. 12.9).

Maximum evidence of cartilage damage is usually found on the lateral facet of the patella in patellofemoral OA, and on the tibial plateau area least well protected by the menisci in tibiofemoral disease. Arthroscopic and MRI studies indicate that meniscal damage is usually present alongside the damage to the articular cartilage [36]. A great deal of variation is seen in the distribution and extent of the accompanying osteophytosis and subchondral bone changes. Whereas the medial tibiofemoral compartment usually has the most loss of articular cartilage, osteophytosis is often more extensive in the lateral compartment.

The biomechanics of knee OA have been studied extensively [37]. In the normal knee joint the load-line passes through the center of the tibiofemoral joint. However, during activity, when loads of 2–3× body weight pass through the knee joint, the medial compartment takes the maximum force, whilst in knee flexion the loading on the patellofemoral joint can reach 7–8× that of body weight, perhaps explaining why these compartments are most often affected. Subtle alterations in load bearing may occur as a result of minor abnormalities of joint shape, perhaps contributing to the development of OA [38]. Meniscectomy and ligament damage alter both load transmission and contact areas of the knee joint, and are the major predisposing causes of 'secondary' OA of the knee. Finally, it should be appreciated that once the knee starts to develop varus or valgus angulation, the load will be transmitted predominantly to one compartment, adding significantly to the stresses and likely progression of damage in that area of the knee.

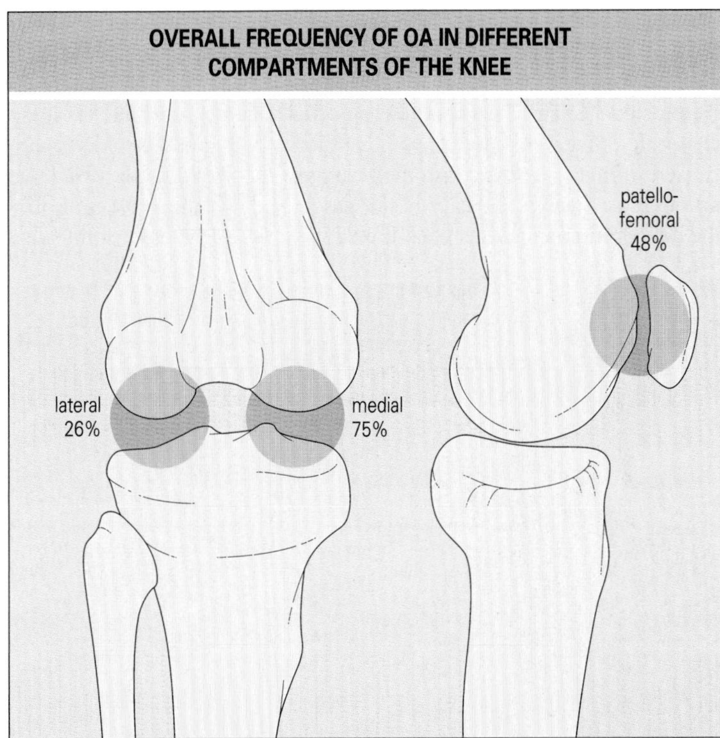

Fig. 12.9 Distribution of OA of the knee joint. OA of the knees can affect any combination of the three main compartments of each knee. It is usually symmetrical, and the compartments most frequently involved are the medial tibiofemoral and patellofemoral compartments. Data from McAlindon *et al.* [26]

Associations and clinical features

Patients presenting with knee OA fall into two major categories [1]: younger people, often men, with isolated knee disease that may be related to a previous injury or operation such as meniscectomy [2]; and middle-aged and older people, predominantly female, who often have OA of other joint sites, including the hands [39]. Obesity is very strongly associated with knee OA [40], particularly in the older, female group, which makes up the majority of cases in most series. However, in most patients no other obvious risk factors are discernible. It has recently been suggested that some cases are due to a mild dysplasia of the knee joint, which is difficult to discern without special radiographic techniques. Developmental abnormalities certainly can predispose to knee OA, as is apparent from cases of the rare African dysplasia, Blount's disease [41].

Pain on walking, stiffness of the joint and difficulty with steps and stairs are the major symptoms. The physical signs depend on the distribution and severity of the OA within the joint. Wasting of the quadriceps muscle, bony swelling, tenderness on and around the joint line, painful limitation of full flexion and course crepitus are the usual signs. Medial compartment disease often results in a varus deformity, a very common finding in knee OA (see Fig. 12.5). In patellofemoral OA, anterior crepitus, abnormal movement and tracking of the patella, and tenderness on patella compression occur. Predominant lateral compartment OA is the least common type, but can result in valgus deformities. In any type of knee OA a small effusion can usually be detected. In some cases the fluid build up is larger and associated with warmth of the joint. Ligament instability develops in severe cases.

Natural history and complications

The natural history of knee OA is not well described. Disease evolution is slow, usually taking many years. However, there is good evidence that once established the condition can remain relatively stable, both clinically and radiologically, for a further period of several years [27,42]. Symptomatic improvement sometimes occurs, at least for a period, but spontaneous improvement in radiographic changes is rare. The clinical presentation is often punctuated by symptomatic 'flares', lasting days or weeks, which may be associated with signs of increased inflammation. In a few cases (probably over-represented in hospital practice), the symptoms and signs get a lot worse over a period of a few weeks or months. This may be associated with the development of instability or subchondral bone collapse. A sudden, almost instantaneous increase in severe pain suggests the possibility of medial femoral bone necrosis. This is a rare but important complication of knee OA which can be detected by imaging studies. Other rare complications of severe disease include fractures through the tibia, as well as severe instability and gross angulation deformities. The development of a hemarthrosis, episodes of 'pseudogout', secondary joint sepsis, and damage to the lateral popliteal nerve can also occur.

OA of the Hip Joint

Anatomy, pathology and biomechanics

The hip is without doubt the joint that has been studied most extensively in relation to OA. On the basis of the radiograph, several different subsets have been described. However, as is the case in relation to other joint sites, and to OA in general, it is not clear to what extent these 'subsets' represent parts of a spectrum, rather than discrete entities.

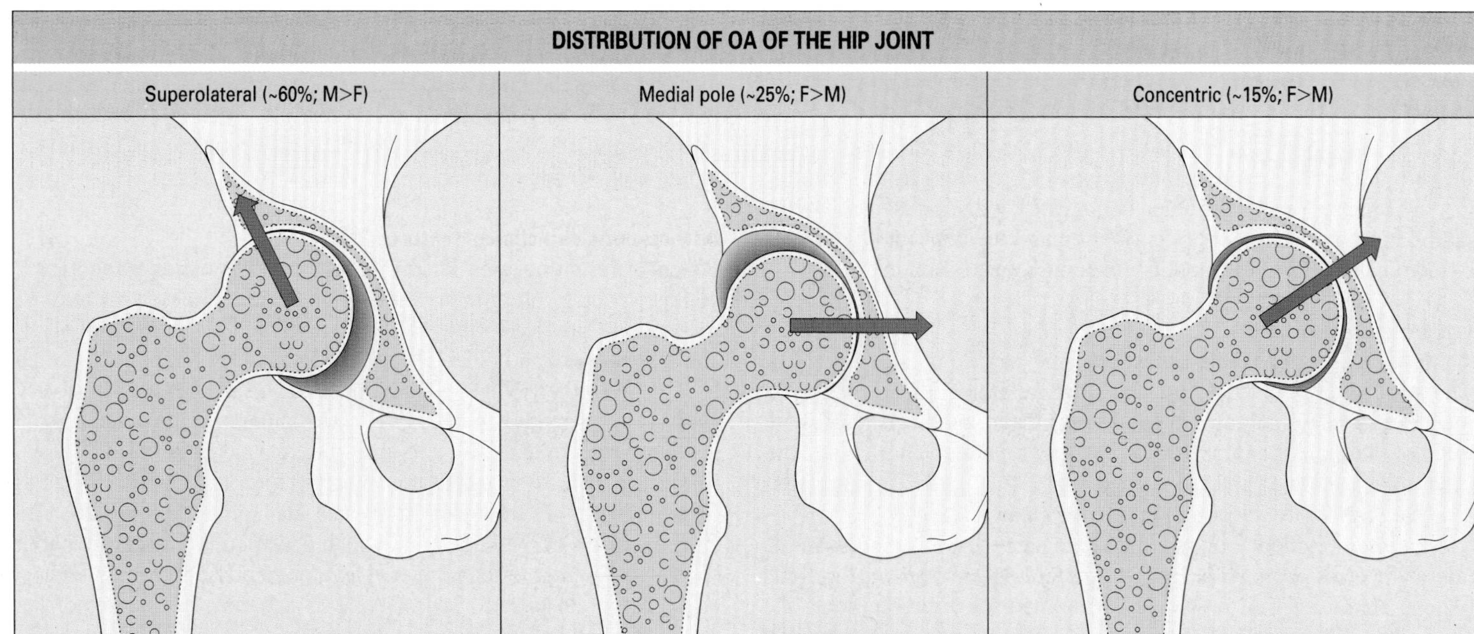

Fig. 12.10 Distribution of OA of the hip joint. OA can maximally affect the superior pole, inferior pole, posterior part or other segments of the hip joint. Superior pole involvement, with a tendency for the head of the femur to sublux superolaterally, is the commonest pattern. Involvement of the whole joint (concentric OA) is relatively

Three different patterns of distribution of OA of the hip joint are described [43] (Fig. 12.10). The superior pole pattern is commonest, and often results in superolateral migration of the femoral head. Medial pole disease is less common, but similarly, can sometimes result in medial migration and protrusio acetabulae. The concentric pattern, in which the whole of the joint appears to be involved, has been linked with the existence of OA at other joint sites more strongly than the other anatomic patterns [44]. Involvement of the postero-inferior portion of the joint can occur, and may be missed unless a lateral radiograph is taken.

On the basis of the radiograph, different pathologic patterns of hip OA are also described, although they appear to be less clear cut than the anatomic subsets. Solomon and colleagues have split the condition into two main types: the 'hypertrophic', in which there is extensive osteophytosis and subchondral bone sclerosis, and the 'atrophic' in which the bone response is deficient [45]. Several authors describe a separate entity of rapidly progressive hip OA in which there is evidence of accelerated loss of joint space and/or bone integrity over a period of a few months [46].

There have been many pathologic and biochemical studies of hip OA, mostly centered on resected femoral heads in advanced disease [47]. The focal nature of the cartilage changes and the important observation that not all cartilage fibrillation is progressive have been emphasized [48]. Extensive synovial changes and capsular thickening are frequently observed in advanced disease. Examination of material resected at the time of hip replacement also suggests that small areas of osteonecrosis of the femoral head are common.

Biomechanical studies have shown that the forces through the hip joint are a product of body weight and abduction forces [49]. The superior pole of the hip is the main area of contact on weight bearing, and the most susceptible area to OA. There is considerable debate about the extent to which minor changes in the shape of the hip joint can alter the biomechanics and predispose to OA [50].

Associations and clinical features

Hip OA develops over a wide age range, with a roughly equal sex incidence, and is frequently the only joint site affected. Several local predisposing causes are described, including congenital dislocation of the hip, Perthes disease, anomalies of leg length, and acetabular dysplasias [51]. The number of cases that can be ascribed to some anatomic defect is disputed. Some authors claim that the majority are caused in this way, whereas others suggest that only about 20% have an obvious 'cause'. Obesity is not associated with hip OA and only the concentric pattern has been linked with disease at other joint sites.

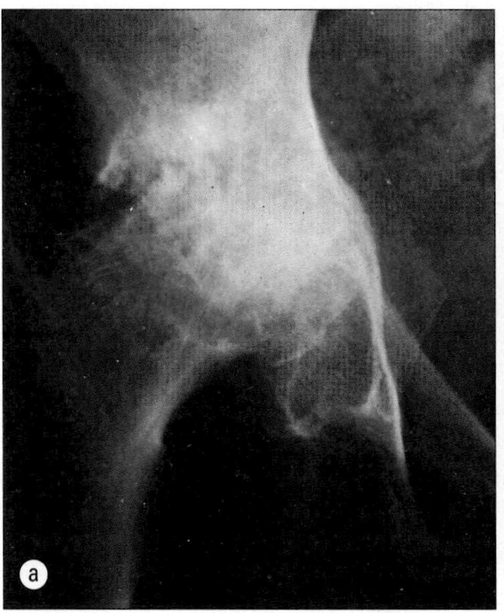

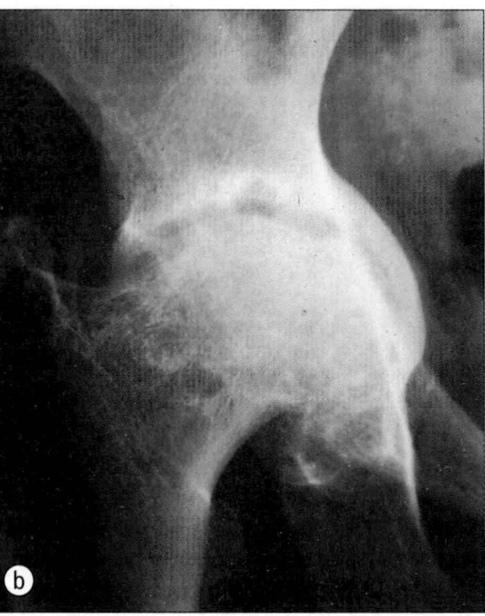

Fig. 12.11 Spontaneous healing of hip OA. These paired pelvic radiographs of the same patient were taken 30 months apart. The first film shows extensive OA with complete loss of the joint space in a concentric pattern and subchondral bone destruction (a). Two and a half years later the film shows reformation of a joint space, remodeling of the bone and extensive repair (b). The patient underwent no special therapy.

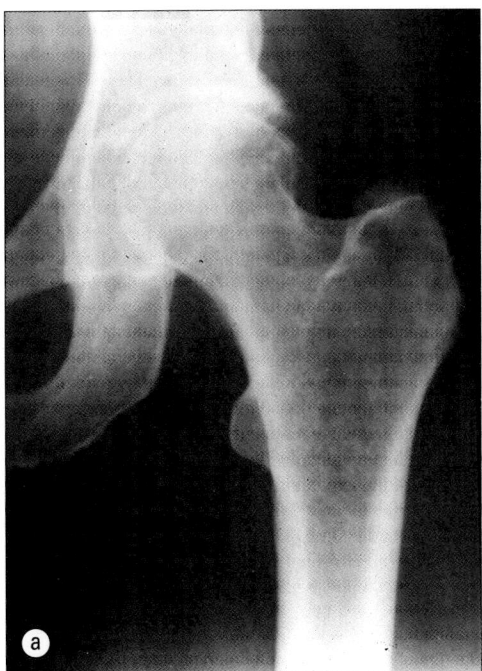

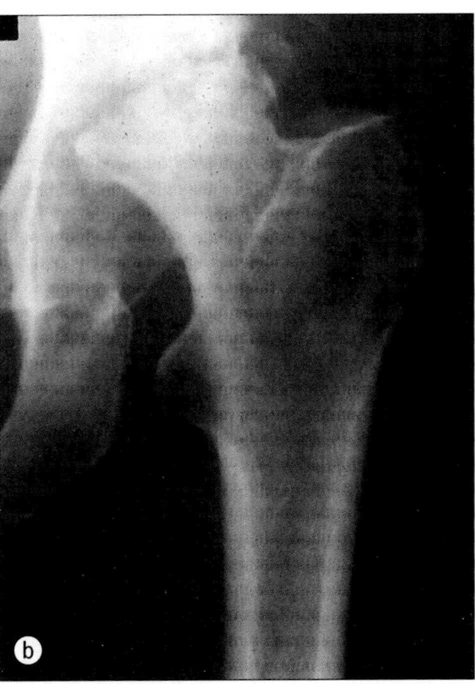

Fig. 12.12 Rapid progression of hip OA. Paired radiographs of the same patient taken 2 years apart showing rapid progression from early, superior pole hip OA (a) to total destruction of the femoral head (b). This pattern of radiographic change has been described as 'analgesic hip', but can occur, as in this patient, in the absence of consumption of significant quantities of analgesic or anti-inflammatory therapy.

There is good evidence that hip OA is negatively associated with osteoporosis, an association that has not been so well established for OA of other joint sites and may be singular for hip OA [52,53].

Pain on walking is the major symptom. It may be felt in the buttock region, in the groin, in the front of the thigh, or in the knee, causing potential problems with diagnosis. Inactivity stiffness and a reduced range of motion are common and patients frequently have difficulty bending to put shoes, socks and stockings on. On examination there is a reduced range of passive movement, with pain at the end of the range; internal rotation is usually the most compromised movement. Crepitus may be audible in severe cases, but cannot be palpated. Tenderness in the groin, over the front of the joint, is common, and there may be a secondary trochanteric bursitis causing lateral tenderness as well. In advanced cases leg shortening can develop due to the migration of the femoral head, referred to above. Muscle wasting around the joint is usually present. These features result in the typical 'antalgic' (coxalgic) gait and the 'Trendelenburg' sign in which the pelvis dips down when the patient tries to stand on the affected leg.

Natural history and complications

The natural history of hip OA is very variable. Many cases that come to surgery have a relatively short history of severe symptoms, suggesting that a progressive phase of perhaps between some 3 and 36 months may often precede the advanced stages of OA. The existence of a 'rapidly progressive' group, going from a near normal situation to being in need of a hip replacement in a matter of months, has already been mentioned. However, much longer periods of relatively mild problems are common. In one series, the disease often remained static over a period of a decade [32]. It may be that most hip OA develops very slowly and that a minority then develop a more progressive process at some stage. Spontaneous healing is an uncommon, but well described phenomenon, which may occur in as many as 5% of cases if surgery is delayed (Fig. 12.11). There is also some evidence that the different anatomic and pathologic subsets behave differently, concentric disease and the hypertrophic pattern having a more benign prognosis than other subsets [54].

Bone collapse is the major complication of hip OA. Osteonecrosis or collapse of the femoral head, as well as acetabular migration, collapse of cysts in the acetabulum and protrusio acetabulae occur. Rapidly progressive OA can lead to an unusual appearance in which there is extensive bone destruction, with a wide inter-bone distance. This appearance has been termed 'analgesic hip' but can occur in patients who ingest little or no anti-inflammatory or analgesic drugs (Fig. 12.12). Severe pain, at rest as well as with activity, may accompany this. Drugs have been implicated in the etiology of bone destruction in hip OA, but the case is far from proven [55]. Secondary problems with the ipsilateral or contralateral knee (including 'long-leg arthropathy') can develop [56]. Trochanteric bursitis is common, but other soft tissue problems or complications of surrounding tissues are rare.

OA of the Hand and Wrist

Anatomy, pathology and biomechanics

OA predominantly affects the distal (DIP) joint more than proximal (PIP), and the joints at the base of the thumb. The metacarpophalangeal joints and joints of the wrist are involved less often and less severely. This is a distribution that is practically the mirror image of RA [57]. Detailed studies of the distribution have been carried out and these are summarized in Figure 12.13.

The pathology has not been studied in the same detail as that of the hip or knee joint. However, it appears that the cartilage and bony changes are similar to those found at other joint sites, although the synovium can show extensive inflammatory changes [58]. Radin and

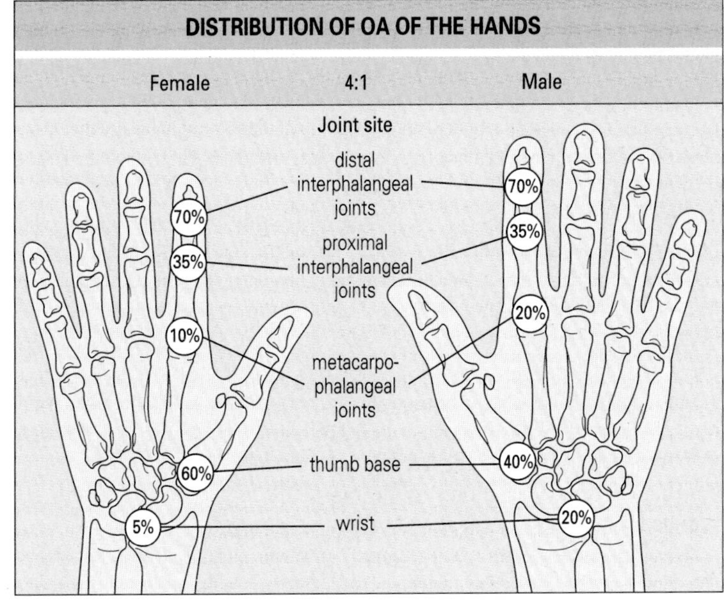

Fig. 12.13 Distribution of OA of the hands.

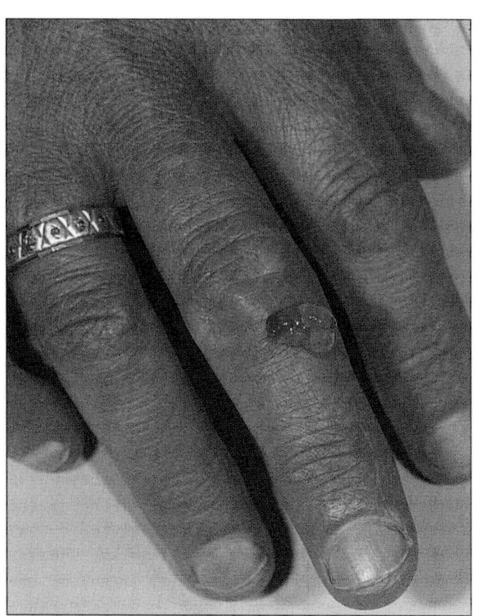

Fig. 12.14 Mucous cysts in OA of the hand. This patient has early interphalangeal joint OA. A mucous cyst, formed over the middle finger PIP joint, has been punctured and the hyaluronic acid contents of the cyst squeezed out. These cysts may form around the interphalangeal joints in the first few years of the evolution of OA and may be accompanied by clinical signs of inflammation and the subsequent development of erosions.

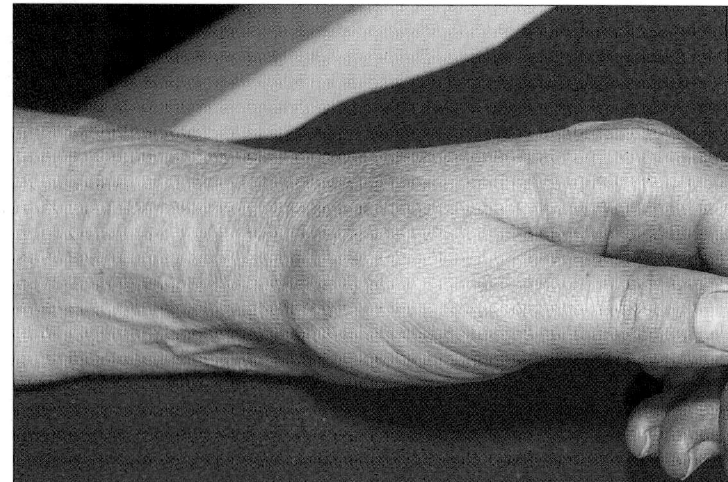

Fig. 12.15 OA of the base of the thumb. This condition results in subluxation of the carpometacarpal joint giving rise to the deformity shown. As with the interphalangeal joints, the thumb base may become inflamed with redness of the overlying skin shown prominently in this patient.

colleagues have suggested that the distribution of hand OA can be explained by biomechanics, there being evidence that the maximum forces go through the DIP joints [59].

Associations and clinical features

OA of the hand is far more common in women than in men [60]. Disease of the finger joints tends to start in middle age and an association with the menopause has been observed but remains unproven [61]. There is strong evidence of a major genetic predisposition and there is an association with knee disease and obesity. However, these associations may differ for the different joint sites within the hand. Wrist and metacarpophalangeal joint disease, which are relatively uncommon, have been reported to have a male preponderance in some studies. Isolated OA of the thumb base may not be as strongly related to knee OA and obesity as is interphalangeal joint OA. Isolated OA of one or two finger joints can be 'secondary' to some trauma, and wrist OA can be secondary to fractures and disorders such as Kienböch's disease (osteonecrosis of the lunate); however, a 'cause' is rarely apparent in hand OA.

The hallmarks of interphalangeal joint OA are the 'Heberden's (DIP joints) and Bouchard's (PIP joints) nodes'. These firm swellings, maximal on the superolateral aspect of the joints, are the most striking and characteristic clinical finding. They are often tender and sometimes red. Cysts may form as they first grow, and if punctured, these cysts exude a thick, colorless jelly, rich in hyaluronan (Fig. 12.14). Later in the evolution of the condition, lateral instability often develops (see Fig. 12.6). Loss of flexion also develops, with occasional interphalangeal joint fusion. Consequent disabilities can include difficulties with activities requiring fine finger movements [62].

Thumb base disease causes pain and tenderness which may be poorly localized 'around the wrist'. Tenderness over the base of the first metacarpal, with pain and crepitus on moving that bone, often occur. In more severe disease an adduction deformity of the metacarpal develops. Combined with the bony swelling this causes the classical appearance of 'squaring' of the thumb base (Fig. 12.15). It may be accompanied by hyperextension of the proximal phalanx. An effusion is occasionally palpable. Difficulty with pinch grip and bottle/jar tops are frequent complaints. Wrist OA can cause similar difficulties, along with classical signs of OA such as reduced, painful movement and crepitus.

Radiographs of thumb joint and interphalangeal joint OA show the typical features, including loss of joint space, osteophytosis, sclerosis and cysts. In addition, in severe cases there may be loss of cortical integrity over the surface of the joint, in which case the condition may be labeled 'erosive' OA [63].

Natural history and complications

The evolution of hand OA is usually complete after a period of a few years. It has been studied extensively with modern imaging techniques, as well as by clinical observation [64–66].

The condition usually starts with discomfort, aches, and sometimes an itching sensation in the interphalangeal joints and/or thumb base. During the first months and early years the condition waxes and wanes, often with clear evidence of inflammatory 'flares', in which individual joints become warm, the skin over them is red, and the pain and tenderness is at its worst. The swellings develop during this phase and cysts may form. After a variable time period, these flares and the pain tend to subside, the swellings become firm and fixed, the joint movement becomes reduced (unless instability develops) and the condition becomes stable.

Imaging studies show that this evolution of clinical change is accompanied by a sequential change in joint anatomy and physiology. However, each involved joint can go through the sequence at a different time, so that at any given point, some joints will be active, others stable, some may have completed the sequence, whereas others might just be starting it. The early radiographic changes may include soft tissue swelling followed by the formation of sclerosis, cysts and osteophytes. If 'erosions' develop, they usually subsequently heal, leaving a typical 'gull-wing' appearance (Fig. 12.16). Scintigraphic studies show that bone activity precedes the radiographic changes [66] and macroradiography indicates that juxta-articular radiolucencies are an early feature [67]. All of these studies indicate that interphalangeal joint OA is a phasic process in which each joint goes through a period of active change followed by stabilization. What controls the timing and distribution as different individual joints are switched on and then stop being active remains unknown.

There are very few complications of hand OA. Wrist disease can be accompanied by carpal tunnel syndrome and instability can develop at any joint. Interphalangeal joint fusion sometimes follows 'erosive' OA [68] which may be precipitated by corticosteroid injections [69]. Thumb base disease sometimes results in a severe destruction of the trapezium with disappearance of bone.

The Spine

Anatomy, pathology and biomechanics

OA of the spinal apophyseal (facet) joints and degeneration of the intervertebral discs are different processes, but they are closely

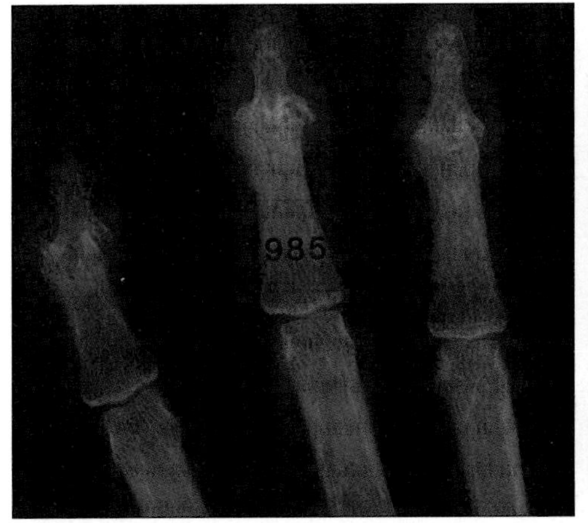

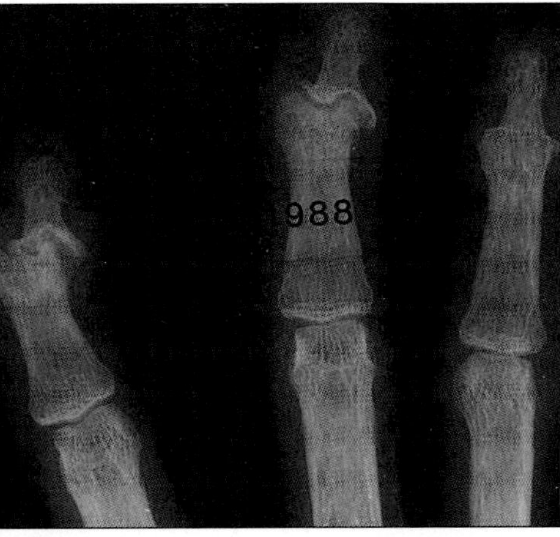

Fig. 12.16 Evolution of erosive OA of the interphalangeal joints. These paired radiographs from a middle-aged lady with erosive OA show the progression of three interphalangeal joints in one hand over a 3-year time interval. One joint has progressed, one has shown evidence of healing and one has fused. This indicates the whole range of changes that can occur and indicates that each individual joint follows its own course in the same patient.

linked together. There is good evidence that one can lead to the other [70], and they usually coexist in the same areas of the spine. The cervical spine (especially around C5) and lumbar spine (especially around L3–5) are the sites most often affected.

The pathology has been extensively studied [71]. Apophyseal joint OA is similar to OA elsewhere, and disc degeneration is accompanied by osteophytic lipping of the vertebrae. The variable degree of new bone formation is a major factor determining the consequences of spinal OA. The association between apophyseal joint OA and disc degeneration probably reflects their biomechanical relationship. Any change in the anatomy of one of these joints will put abnormal stresses on the other. The distribution of spinal osteophytes probably indicates where these stresses are maximal.

Associations and clinical features

Radiographic evidence of spinal OA is age-related and so common that almost everyone over the age of about 40 years will have some changes [6,72]. This raises the question as to whether it is a normal part of aging as opposed to a disease, a question made more pertinent by the fact that there is little or no relationship between radiographic change and symptoms. Solid associations are difficult to establish with such a common phenomenon in which clear radiographic end points are difficult to establish. However, it has been suggested that there may be links with 'generalized' OA in women and with premature hip OA in men [73]. There is little doubt that trauma and some anatomic abnormalities can precipitate premature and severe spinal OA and disc degeneration.

'Mechanical' low back pain, made worse by prolonged sitting or standing, and affected by movement, is the symptom most often associated with spinal OA. The pain may radiate into the buttocks and legs. Pain exacerbated by extension suggests facet joint disease; worsening on flexion is more common with disc disease. Spinal movements are often reduced and muscle spasm may be present.

Natural history and complications

The poor correlation between symptoms and radiographs makes this problem difficult to analyze. Radiographic changes appear to be generally progressive, although, as with OA elsewhere, long periods of stability can occur. Similarly, back pain is subject to exacerbations and remissions that are difficult to explain.

The main problem with spinal OA and disc disease is the potential for the development of severe complications, particularly neurologic problems. Pressure on nerve roots in the exit foramina and spinal stenosis are common consequences. Severe bone destruction and collapse can also occur, with neurologic sequelae.

OA of Other Joint Sites

The temporomandibular joint

The temporomandibular joint (TMJ) is a complex joint, subject to OA as well as the inflammatory arthropathies. OA is one of the causes of the TMJ pain/dysfunction syndrome [74,75].

Sternoclavicular and acromioclavicular joints

Radiographic changes of OA of the sternoclavicular joint are common, but this rarely causes problems. Painful subluxation of the joint can occur and OA may be associated with, or precede Freiberg's disease [76]. The acromioclavicular joint is more often a cause of problems. OA is again frequent at this joint site and a common cause of pain. The discomfort is not always well localized by patients, who may present with 'shoulder' pain. On examination there is point tenderness over the joint and superior osteophytes may be palpable as well as apparent on the radiograph.

The glenohumeral joint

OA of the shoulder joint is uncommon, except in elderly women. It is the joint site with the oldest age of onset in OA [39]. Apart from age and sex there are no obvious associations, except for the link with rotator cuff damage, which is also very common in the elderly [77].

Most OA of the shoulder presents with pain on movement and a restricted range of motion, especially external rotation and elevation. The radiograph shows evidence of OA, often with large inferior osteophytes on the glenoid (Fig. 12.17). This condition of 'uncomplicated shoulder OA' needs to be distinguished from capsulitis and

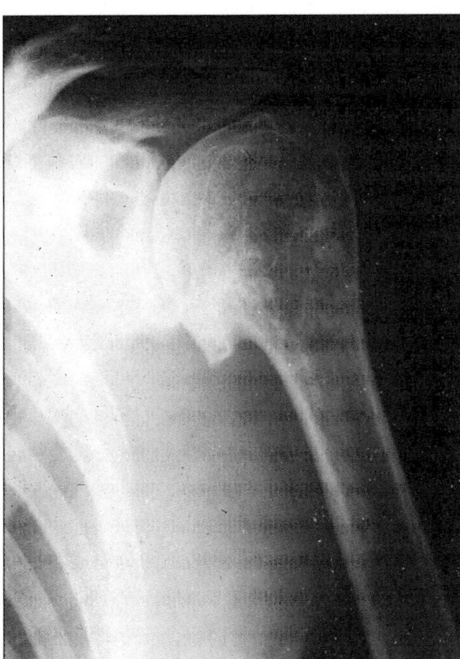

Fig. 12.17 OA of the shoulder. The radiograph shows all the features of a 'hypertrophic' form of OA of the glenohumeral joint, with joint space narrowing, subchondral sclerosis, large cysts in the glenoid and the massive inferior osteophytosis which is characteristic of this condition.

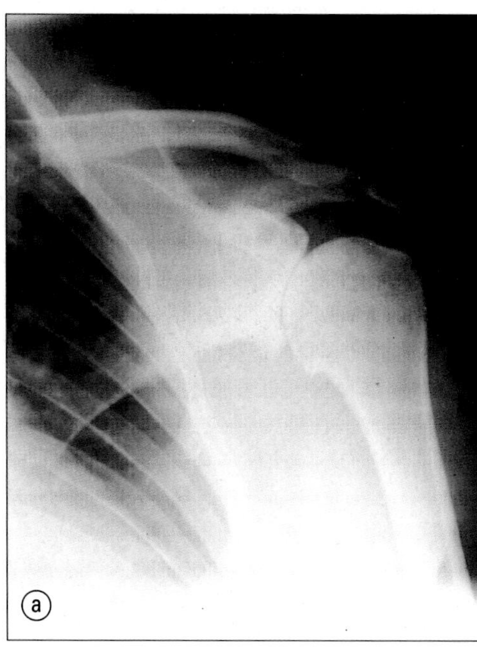

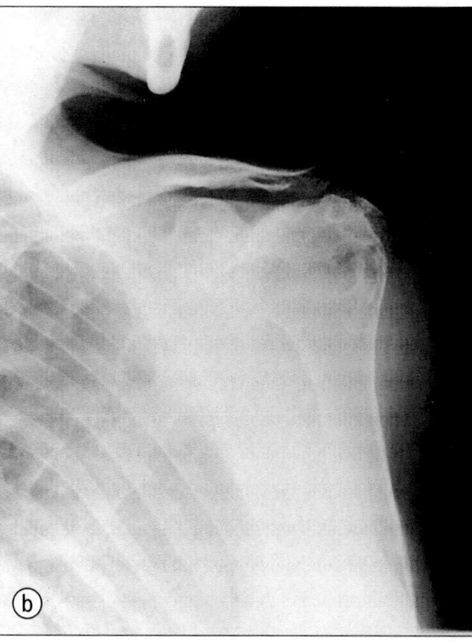

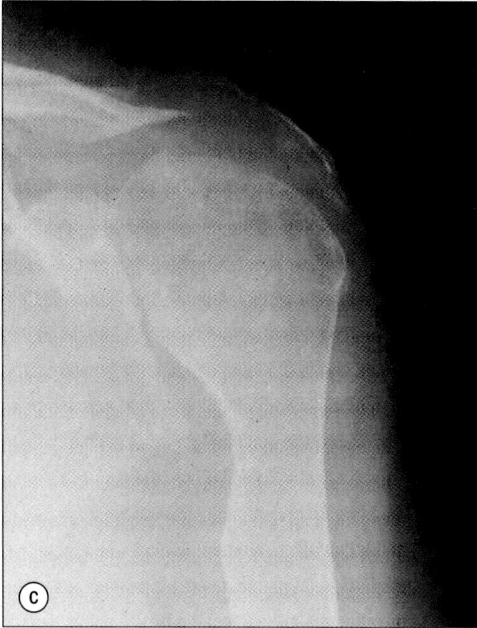

Fig. 12.18 Different types of shoulder disease resulting in destructive arthropathies. Osteoarthritis of the glenohumeral joint (a), cuff-tear arthropathy (b) and apatite-associated destructive arthropathy (c).

rotator cuff problems at the shoulder, and from two other conditions of the shoulder common in the elderly: 'cuff-tear arthropathy' and 'apatite-associated destructive arthritis' (AADA) (Fig. 12.18) [78,79].

Cuff-tear arthropathy

Damage to the rotator cuff is common in the elderly and can result in complete rupture, with consequent upward subluxation of the humeral head and impingement on the acromium, with formation of a pseudoarthrosis [78]. This results in problems in abducting or elevating the arm, although pain may be mild or absent.

AADA

This condition, also known as senile hemorrhagic arthritis of the elderly, or Milwaukee shoulder, is an uncommon but distinctive form of shoulder disease seen almost exclusively in very elderly women [79–81]. It may develop spontaneously or follow from a pre-existing arthritis or rotator cuff problem. A destructive arthritis of the glenohumeral joint develops over a period of a few months, associated with a large, cool, blood-stained effusion. Joint rupture can occur [82]. The synovial fluid contains numerous particles of basic calcium phosphates, some of which may come from the damaged bone. The pathogenesis of the condition is obscure, although it can be associated with a destructive OA of other joint sites, suggesting a possible inability to repair or adapt to OA in the elderly. Pain is variable and may subside after a period of a few months; the range of passive movement is often much greater than in shoulder OA or cuff-tear arthropathy, but active movement is usually very limited.

The elbow joint

The elbow is another relatively uncommon site for OA. Men are affected more than women and the humero-ulnar joint is usually the main site of the disease [83]. The development of a fixed flexion deformity is the commonest sign, with joint crepitus and reduced movement. Pain may be mild or absent, although severe pain on use can also occur.

The hindfoot

OA of the ankle joint is uncommon, in spite of its being one of the major weight-bearing joints susceptible to trauma. When it does occur it is often the sequel to some major injury or abnormality of the joint [84]. Subtalar joint OA is more frequent, but rarely presents major clinical problems. Radiographic evidence of OA, sometimes with big osteophytes, is often seen in the talonavicular, calcaneocuboid and midtarsal joints and may be associated with some discomfort and stiffness around the hindfoot. This stiffness is occasionally a source of major symptoms, with a lot of pain on walking and difficulty with balance on uneven surfaces.

The forefoot

The first metatarsophalangeal joint is the prime site of OA changes in the forefoot. However, the relationships between hallux valgus, hallux rigidus and 'simple OA' are obscure. Hallux valgus, an extremely common problem in women, seems to be dependent on primary metatarsal varus deformities and the use of modern footwear [85]. It results in radiographic evidence of OA like changes in the joint, in association with the deformity. The pathogenesis of hallux rigidus is more obscure; radiographs often show a small central defect in the head of the first metatarsal, followed by the development of 'OA' with the formation of large dorsal osteophytes that limit movement. Both conditions can result in pain on walking and secondary pressure problems.

OA can also develop in the other metatarsophalangeal joints and in the interphalangeal joints in association with OA of the hand. Interphalangeal 'inflammatory' OA of the foot is a poorly recognized problem, perhaps because it rarely presents clinically, but it can look very similar to the interphalangeal disease seen in the hand.

CLINICAL PATTERNS AND SUBSETS OF OA

Introduction to the Distribution and Patterns of OA

Studies of the epidemiology of OA have revealed differences in expression of OA in various racial groups and different parts of the world. The more comprehensive surveys have been largely confined to the mainly Caucasian populations studied in Europe and the US [40,86]. The data quoted on the prevalence of OA at different joint sites (Fig. 12.2), and on distribution patterns (Fig. 12.19) is based on these surveys.

In the comprehensive study of 500 symptomatic patients with peripheral joint OA of Cushnaghan and Dieppe, the relationship between age, sex and the number and site of involved joints was investigated [39]. A strong relationship between the number of involved sites and increasing age was established, and it was thought that this was more likely to be due to the slow addition of new joint

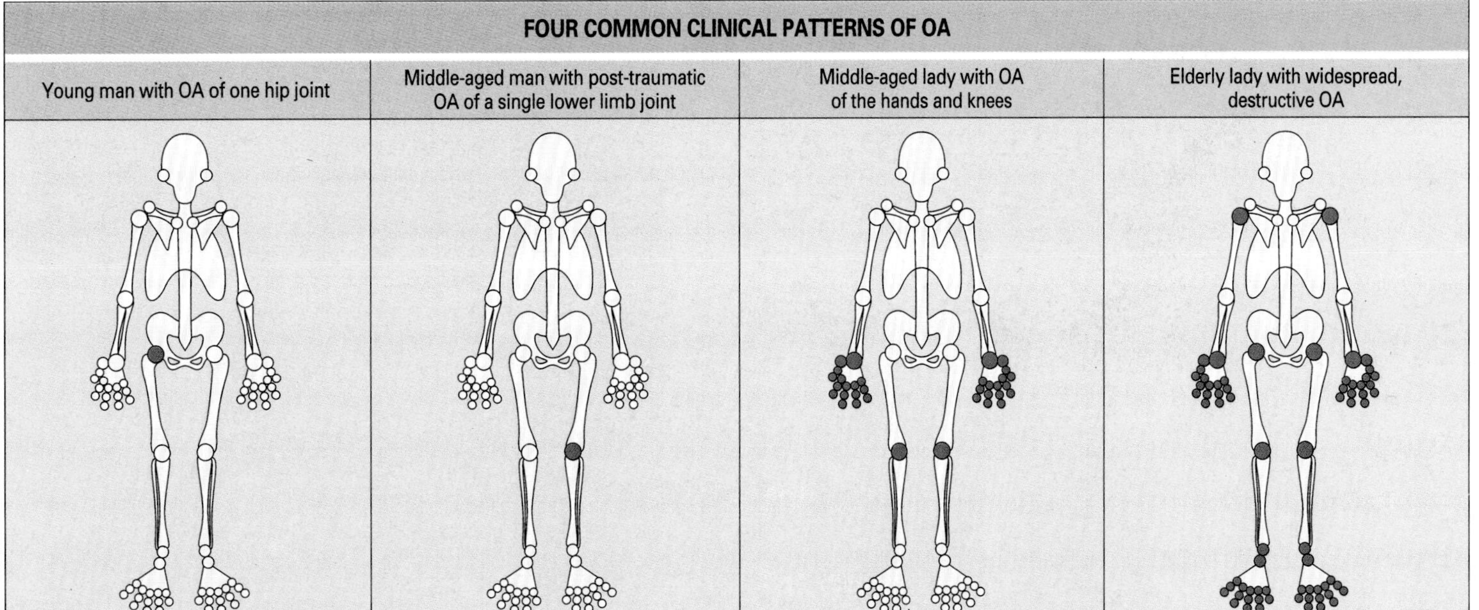

Fig. 12.19 Four common clinical patterns of OA.

sites with age, than to older people developing more polyarticular disease. The involvement of one site was more likely in men than in women, as well as in younger subjects, a few of whom had an obvious 'cause' of their secondary OA. As with other surveys, there was a female bias for clinical presentation of OA at most joint sites; the exceptions were the hip (male/female ratio approximately equal) and the ankle and elbow joints which showed a male preponderance. By far the commonest combination of joint sites in this survey was hand and knee disease in middle aged, often obese, women. Destructive changes were most frequently seen in elderly women.

Distinct 'subsets' of OA, or groups of patients with a clearly defined distribution or set of associations, did not emerge from this study. Furthermore, other attempts to establish a bi- or polymodal distribution of features in patients with OA have been largely unsuccessful [87], in spite of the epidemiologic and other evidence for different associations between joint sites, most notably the knee and hip. This is in accord with the suggestion that OA represents a heterogeneous disease process, rather than one or more specific disease entities. However, within the OA spectrum, a number of recognizable clinical clusters exist, even if they have blurred edges and should not be considered discrete entities. In this section, some of the common presenting patterns seen in rheumatology clinics will be discussed.

Premature 'Secondary' OA of a Single Joint

Osteoarthritis is generally classified into primary and secondary forms, although there are problems with that distinction. However, in clinical practice it is sometimes clear that a single joint has developed premature OA as a result of some previous problem, most commonly major trauma. Severe OA of a single joint site, particularly one of the less commonly affected areas such as an ankle joint, suggests 'secondary' OA. In most series of patients attending hospital clinics, the number of OA patients given this classification is relatively small [39,88]. It is not clear whether the prognosis is different from that of 'primary' OA.

Postmeniscectomy knee OA is probably the best studied human model of 'secondary' OA, and the extensive data indicates the overlap with 'primary' OA, and the variability in outcome in spite of a relatively uniform insult to the joint [89,90].

Premature Hip OA in Young Adults

Early OA confined to the hip joint presents a special case. As already mentioned, the extent to which this is a 'primary' as opposed to a 'secondary' form of OA is disputed. In practice, adults, men more than women, often present with OA of one or both hips, with a disease onset that may be from the 20s to 40s, and no obvious cause for their disease. They often manage for years without surgery, although most come to hip replacement at some stage. Minor forms of dysplasia may be responsible for some cases. Recent data has implicated genetic abnormalities of type II collagen in the pathogenesis of some of these dysplasias [91].

'Knee/Hand' OA

This is the commonest pattern of OA seen in Caucasian women, many of whom are obese and/or hypertensive. Interphalangeal disease of the hands, with nodes, and knee OA, predominantly in the medial and patello-femoral compartments, are the main features. Many have spinal disease, and a few have OA at other joint sites. The disease appears to stabilize in many cases and patients often manage well for long periods without major intervention. The presence of nodes and involvement of several joints in the hand often results in these patients being classified as having 'generalized' OA [91]. However, it may be that this is a genetically determined pattern with a specific predisposition, in which only two joint sites are at major risk [92].

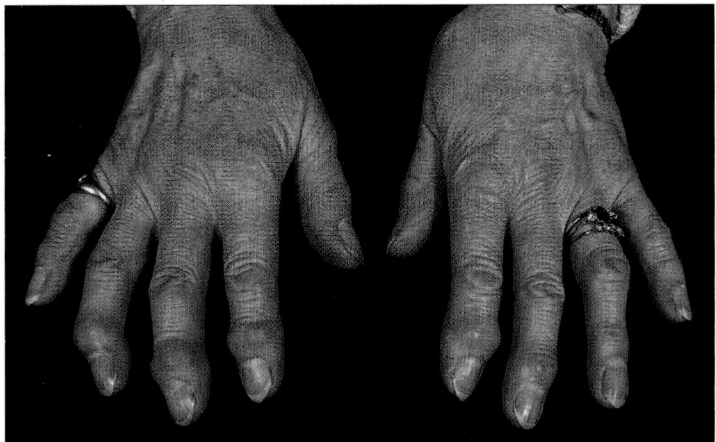

Fig. 12.20 Osteoarthritis of the DIP joints. This patient has the typical clinical findings of advanced OA of the DIP joints, including large firm swellings (Heberden's nodes), some of which are tender and red due to associated inflammation of the periarticular tissues as well as the joint.

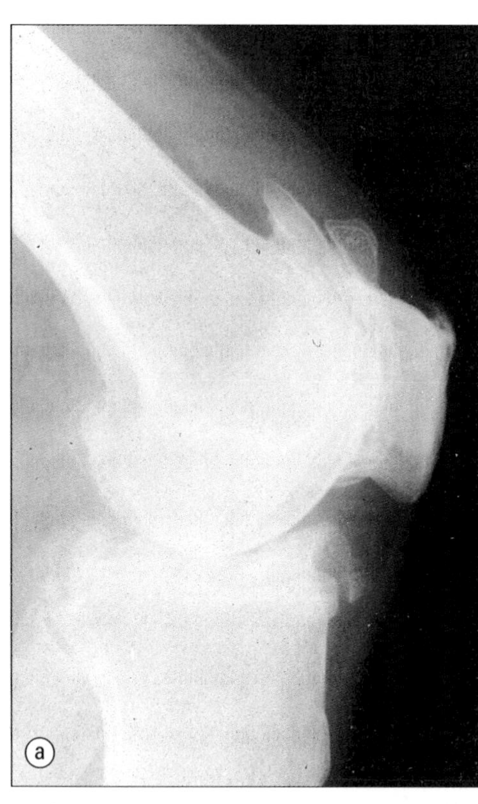

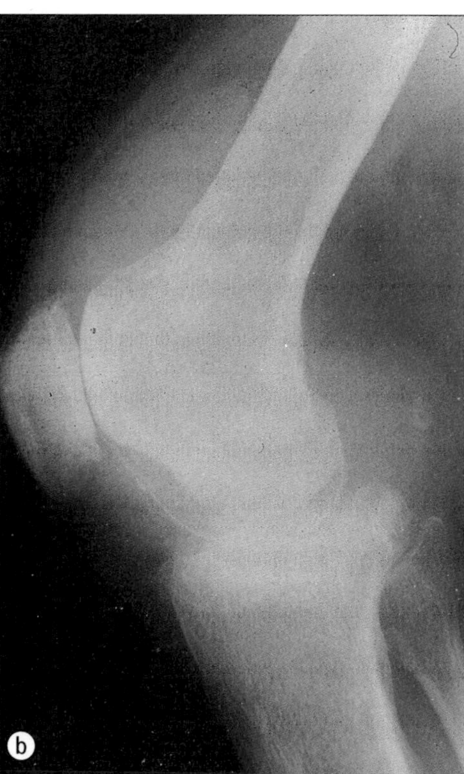

Fig. 12.21 Hypertrophic and atrophic forms of knee OA. These two lateral radiographs of the knee joint show the extreme ends of the spectrum of anatomic change seen in knee OA. The patient on the left has the 'hypertrophic' form of the disease, with massive osteophyte formation and extensive bone sclerosis; this pattern is often seen in association with chondrocalcinosis and pyrophosphate crystals (a). The patient on the right has the atrophic form of the disease with bone destruction and little or no evidence of a bone reaction (b); note the large effusion in the suprapatellar pouch – such effusions often contain numerous apatite crystals and particles.

'Inflammatory/Erosive' OA

A small minority of patients with interphalangeal OA of the hands develop striking inflammation in the joints (Fig. 12.20) and/or radiographic erosions. Very occasionally, other 'OA' joints show similar changes. The synovial histology in these cases has been reported to show extensive inflammatory changes, and in some series, a minor acute phase response and hypergammaglobulinemia have been reported. However, a recent controlled study failed to confirm any evidence of a systemic component to the condition [93]. The nature of inflammatory or erosive OA is not clear. It has variously been suggested that it is a distinct subset of OA, an 'overlap' condition, an intermediate phase between OA and inflammatory arthropathies such as RA, and simply a severe form of simple interphalangeal OA. In most cases the erosions seem to heal, although a link with connective tissue diseases and progression to typical RA have also been reported.

It is the author's current view that this condition is not a distinct entity, but merely the expression of severe OA of interphalangeal joints, perhaps akin to rapidly progressive or destructive OA of other joints.

Rapidly Progressive OA

The existence of a group of patients with hip OA, who develop severe pain and whose radiographs show evidence of 'rapid' loss of the joint space, has already been mentioned. The condition has been particularly well documented by Lequesne and others, who suggest that a loss of joint width of 2mm or more in less than 6 months can be taken as a criterion for designating OA as rapidly progressive [94]. Similarly rapid changes in joint space, without obvious bony destruction, are described at other joint sites. The pathogenesis of the process is unknown. Most cases come to early surgery so the long-term natural history is also unknown, although it has been suggested that the process can be halted by a period of nonweight-bearing.

'Hypertrophic' and 'Atrophic' OA

The amount of bone reaction seen on the radiograph of an OA joint varies enormously. Solomon and others have suggested that hip OA can be divided into hypertrophic and atrophic categories on this basis [45]. Other joint sites, particularly the knee, show similar variations in bony change (Fig. 12.21). There is a paucity of data to support the contention that this bony response separates distinct entities, but it does seem likely that the extent and type of response in subchondral and marginal bone will affect the symptom signs and outcome of OA. A hypertrophic bone response has been linked to OA with associated deposition of calcium pyrophosphate dihydrate (CPPD) crystals, and atrophic OA with the presence of basic calcium phosphates in the synovial fluid [95].

Destructive OA of the Elderly

Elderly people (generally over 75 and nearly always female) may develop a destructive form of joint disease, superimposed on preexisting 'simple' OA. The characteristics of this condition include severe destruction of subchondral bone on both sides of the joint space, and damage to soft tissues, as well as cartilage loss. Large cool effusions, which are often blood stained and may contain numerous bone fragments and calcium crystals, frequently occur. The condition has been described most often in the shoulder, but is also seen at the hip, knee and other joints, and may be present in several joints of the same individual (Fig. 12.22) [79].

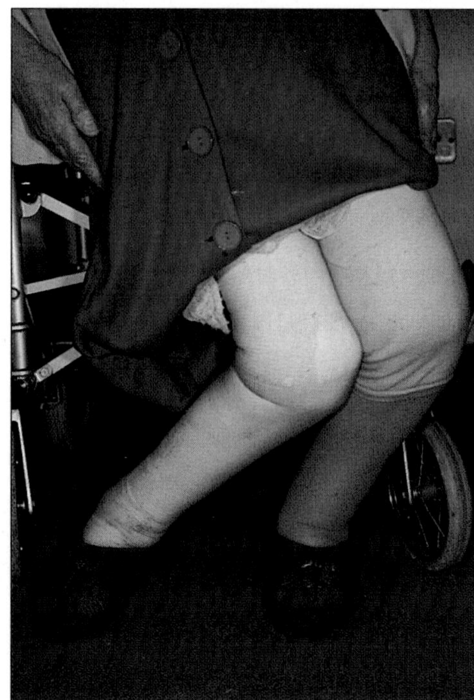

Fig. 12.22 A patient with atrophic destructive arthritis of the knee joints. She is an elderly lady with advanced destruction of the soft tissues as well as the bone, leading to total instability of the knee joints. They are also swollen due to large, cool effusions. Her radiograph shows similar features to those seen in Figure 12.21b.

DIFFERENTIAL DIAGNOSIS AND DIAGNOSTIC PROBLEMS

The Discrepancy between Radiographic OA and Clinical Problems

Radiographic OA has an age-related, high frequency in adults. Joint pain is less common and a clinical diagnosis of OA is made much less frequently. The relatively poor correlation between symptoms and radiographs has also been highlighted at the beginning of this chapter (see Fig. 12.2) [1,2].

This discrepancy between clinical problems and the clinician's surrogate for the pathology of OA means that caution must be exercised in diagnosing clinical OA, particularly in the elderly. The radiographic changes may be incidental to the clinical presentation. The problem is particularly severe in relation to spinal OA and back pain.

The Differential Diagnosis of an Individual Joint with OA

The diagnosis of established OA with the typical clinical features, such as bony swelling, crepitus and pain on movement, is not difficult. The radiograph will confirm the presence of severe joint pathology accompanying the clinical signs and symptoms. Other investigations will generally prove negative, and if synovial fluid is analyzed it will be viscous, clear, have a low cell count, and probably contain some cartilage fragments. Difficulties arise in early OA when the clinical presentation is atypical, or when the radiographic signs are not obvious (Fig. 12.23).

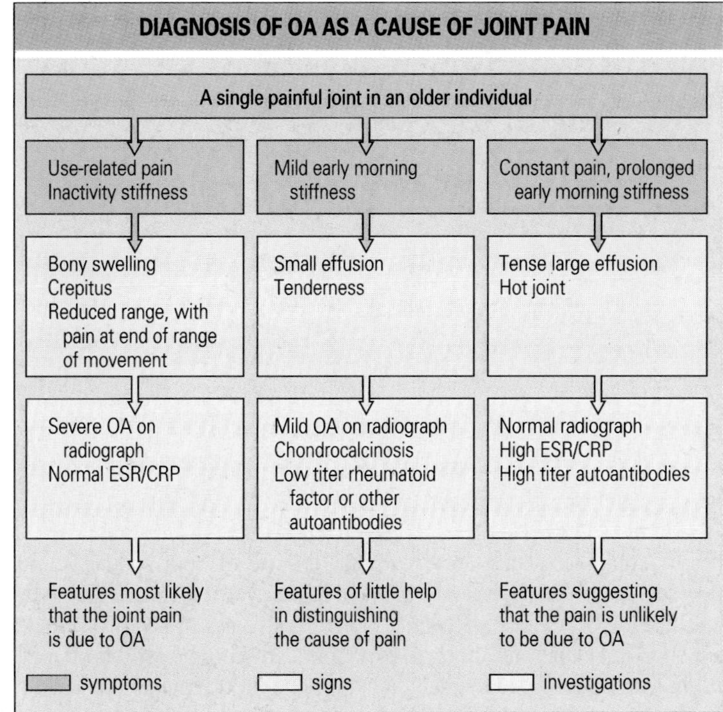

Fig. 12.23 A flow chart on the diagnosis of OA as a cause of joint pain. Note that radiographic features of OA are almost universal in the elderly and that one of the main diagnostic aims is to exclude other possible causes of pain.

'Early' OA

Patients may present with relatively mild discomfort, which heralds the clinical onset of OA. However, the classical signs may be absent at that stage, and the radiograph can be normal. Extensive cartilage damage and bony reaction is needed before joint space narrowing and bony change will be seen on a radiograph [96,97]; similarly, the changes probably need to be severe before firm swellings and crepitus will be palpable. In these circumstances the diagnosis of OA may be difficult, but is made more likely if the joint pain is use-related and accompanied by inactivity stiffness without prolonged morning stiffness, and if the joint distribution is typical of OA. Other clinical features and investigations may help to exclude other conditions.

An 'atypical' presentation

OA occasionally presents with the sudden onset of pain, which may be due to a complication such as a microfracture of subchondral bone or osteonecrosis of bone. Similarly, some patients present with symptoms related to a secondary periarticular problem rather than the joint itself. Clinical signs and the radiograph may reveal evidence of OA and the difficulty for the clinician is then deciding to what extent the current clinical problem relates to the OA.

An 'atypical' radiograph

It has already been noted that the radiograph may appear normal in early OA. Difficulty can also arise if there is extensive bone damage, when the question of primary OA, or of initial osteonecrosis or some other bone disease may arise. Similarly the presence of chondrocalcinosis or other atypical radiographic features can cause confusion (see below).

Diagnosing Polyarticular and Inflammatory OA

As outlined above, there is no clear definition of polyarticular OA and no distinctive subset. The term is usually applied to patients with nodal hand OA plus OA of some other joint site(s), usually the knee or spine. The disease distribution, clinical symptoms and signs, radiographs and other investigations should leave no doubt as to the diagnosis.

Greater difficulty arises in patients who have OA of some joints and another arthropathy as well. In view of the high frequency of OA, as well as other forms of joint disease, this is not an uncommon situation. Similarly, OA as a 'secondary' phenomenon resulting from an inflammatory arthropathy such as RA is a difficult diagnosis to make. The limited ways in which any joint can respond to injury means that some of the features of OA will often be present in association with a long-standing arthropathy of almost any sort.

The inflammatory features often present in early OA of the hands, as well as other joint sites, can make it difficult to distinguish early 'inflammatory OA' from another inflammatory arthropathy, such as RA.

OA with Crystal Deposition or a Crystal-Related Arthropathy?

Crystal deposition, as well as OA, is an extremely common phenomenon in older people [98]. Furthermore, the knee joint is the commonest site of both OA and chondrocalcinosis. It is therefore inevitable that there will be many patients with both OA and coincidental crystal deposition in their joints. However, it has also been suggested that crystals may contribute to OA, or be associated with a modification of the expression of the condition.

Currently, the presence of calcium crystal deposits in an OA joint will have little influence on management; it is therefore reasonable to take a pragmatic view in practice, simply describing and noting the presence or absence of obvious crystal deposits until research clarifies this association.

CLINICAL ASSESSMENT AND MEASUREMENT OF OA

OA is difficult to measure. Disease assessments can be divided into two categories: process measures that indicate the activity of a pathologic process in the joint, and health status measures that are concerned with the outcome of the disorder (see Fig. 12.24). The generally slow evolution of OA, its heterogeneity and lack of systemic effects are among the reasons that the measurement of either process or outcome is very difficult in OA. Furthermore, most of the process and outcome measures used in rheumatology have been designed for use in inflammatory disorders such as RA, and are often inappropriate in the OA patient.

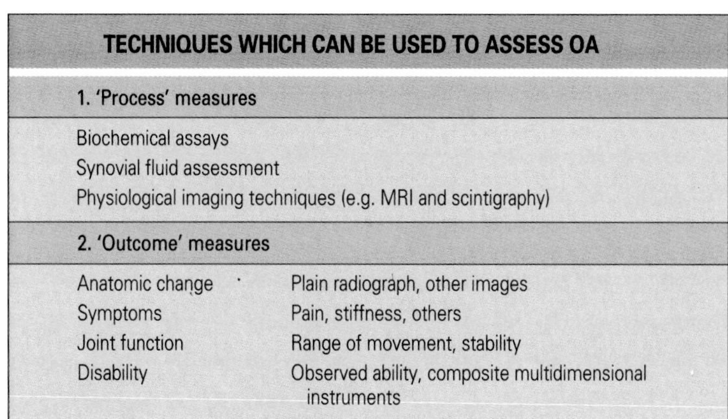

TECHNIQUES WHICH CAN BE USED TO ASSESS OA	
1. 'Process' measures	
Biochemical assays	
Synovial fluid assessment	
Physiological imaging techniques (e.g. MRI and scintigraphy)	
2. 'Outcome' measures	
Anatomic change	Plain radiograph, other images
Symptoms	Pain, stiffness, others
Joint function	Range of movement, stability
Disability	Observed ability, composite multidimensional instruments

Fig. 12.24 Techniques which can be used to assess OA.

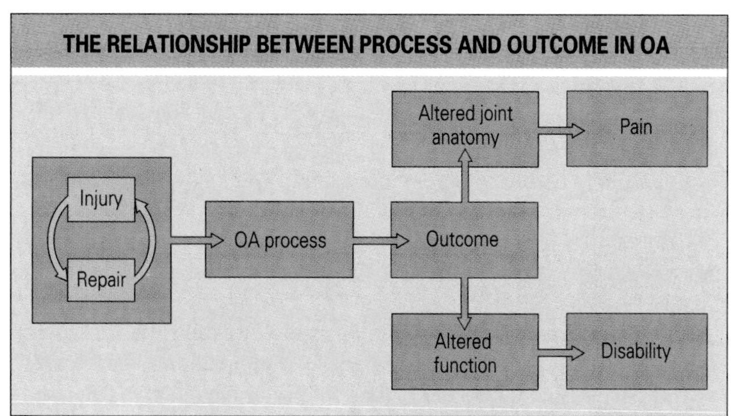

Fig. 12.25 The relationship between process and outcome in OA.

Measuring the OA Process

Biochemical and imaging techniques can give some insight into the processes going on within an OA joint. Products of both synthesis and degradation of cartilage can be assayed in the synovial fluid, and serum and other biochemical assays may give insight into the activity of the subchondral bone and other tissues. Joint physiology can be imaged using techniques such as scintigraphy, which reflect regional blood flow and bony activity, and MRI, which will reveal the water content of the tissues.

Measuring the Outcome of OA

The clinician sees the outcome of disease. By the time a patient presents, the OA process may already have been active for years and the clinical picture will reflect aspects of attempted repair as well as joint damage. Outcome measures used in OA can be divided into four main categories [33], as shown in Figures 12.24 and 12.25.

Anatomy

The anatomy of the joint is generally assessed by radiographs. Clinical assessments can include bony swelling, deformity and instability. The key radiologic features of OA are joint space narrowing, osteophytes, subchondral bone sclerosis and cysts. Composite scores of severity, such as the Kellgren and Lawrence five point scoring system, are widely used in epidemiological work, but have proved very insensitive in clinical studies [19,99,100]. Scoring systems which divide individual factors and measurements of joint space are now being used [101,102]. Techniques which improve the sensitivity and accuracy of measuring changes in joint anatomy are needed.

Pain and tenderness

Pain can be measured on descriptive scales or by visual analog scales. In OA, pain at rest, at night, or on joint use can be individually recorded. Pain at specific joint sites should be measured rather than 'global' pain, as often used in other arthropathies.

Tenderness is a widely used measure of the activity of rheumatoid and other arthropathies. A number of numerical indices of joint activity exist resting largely on tenderness. This is less valuable and of doubtful pathologic significance in OA. Attempts to assess the activity of joints by tenderness and swelling have been made [103], but are not widely used.

Joint function

Joint function can be measured by documenting the range of motion of the joint, the presence of joint laxity, and pain or crepitus during movement. However, many of these measurements, which are widely used in clinical trials, suffer from lack of reproducibility [104].

Disability

Disability can be assessed by using self-administered questionnaires, such as the HAQ [105], by observing a specific function, as in timed walking or seeing if the patient can climb stairs, or by use of a subjective clinical judgment, as in the Steinbrocker Index. There are now many instruments for measuring disability in rheumatic diseases, but very little work has been done on their value and validity in OA [33,106].

LEQUESNE INDICES OF SEVERITY OF HIP AND KNEE OA	
Hip OA	**Points score**
Feature	
1. Pain at night	
None	0
Only on movement	1
Without movement	2
2. Morning stiffness	
I minute or less	0
2–15 minutes	1
>15 minutes	2
3. Pain after standing for 30 minutes	0 or 1
4. Pain on walking	
None	0
Only after distance	1
Initially	2
5. Pain with prolonged sitting (2 hours)	0 or 1
6. Maximum walking distance	
Unlimited	0
More than 1km	1
About 1km in 15 minutes	2
500–900m	3
300–500m	4
100–300m	5
<100m	6
One stick or crutch	1
Two sticks or crutches	2
7. Activities of daily living (ADL) (Score 0–2: no difficulty, with difficulty, impossible)	
Put on socks	0–2
Pick an object off floor	0–2
Climb a flight of stairs	0–2
Get in and out of a car	0–2
8. Difficulty with sexual activity	0–2
Knee OA	**Point scores**
Feature (Scores exactly as for hip OA EXCEPT)	
5. Pain on getting up from a chair without help of arms	0 or 1
7. Activities of daily living (ADL)	0–2
Climb up stairs	0–2
Climb down stairs	0–2
Squatting	0–2
Walking on uneven ground	0–2
8. OMIT	

Fig. 12.26 Lequesne indices of severity of hip and knee OA.

Recording and Assessing OA in Clinical Practice

The key features noted in any system include: use-related pain and range of motion at the index joint site, inactivity stiffness, crepitus and bony swelling, and the main features on a current plain radiograph. Some simple measure of disability, such as the use of walking aids, should also be noted. It may also be helpful to record the features noted by the ACR in their classification criteria for OA of different joint sites [107].

Clinical Trials in OA

The inadequacy of the outcome measures used in most trials of OA have been highlighted by several authors and useful recommendations have been made [33,108]. It is clear that OA of different joint sites must be separated and that the reproducibility of both the clinical and radiographic assessments used need to be considered [109]. There are no agreed protocols, but the Lequesne indices for hip and knee OA [110], which have been approved by EULAR, are probably amongst the best available instruments at present (Fig. 12.26).

REFERENCES

1. Cobb S, Merchant WR, Rubin T. The relation of symptoms to osteoarthritis. J Chron Dis. 1957;**5**:197–204.
2. Bagge E, Bjelle A, Eden S, Svanborg A. Osteoarthritis in the elderly: clinical and radiological findings in 79- and 85-year-olds. Ann Rheum Dis. 1991;**50**:535–9.
3. Altman RD, Dean D, eds. Pain in osteoarthritis. Semin Arthritis Rheum. 1989;**18**(Suppl. 2):1–104.
4. Charter RA, Nehemkis AM, Keenan MA. The nature of arthritis pain. Br J Rheumatol. 1985;**24**:53–60.
5. Bellamy N, Buchanan WW. Outcome measurement in osteoarthritis clinical trials: the case for standardization. Clin Rheumatol. 1984;**3**:293–303.
6. Lawrence JS, Bremner JM, Bier F. Osteoarthritis: prevalence in the population and relationship between symptoms and X-ray changes. Ann Rheum Dis. 1966;**25**:1–24.
7. Hochberg MC, Lawrence RC, Everett DF, Cornoni-Huntley J. Epidemiologic associations of pain in osteoarthritis of the knee. Semin Arthritis Rheum. 1989;**18**(Suppl. 2):4–9.
8. Cushnaghan J. Osteoarthritis: a clinical and radiological study. MSc thesis, Bristol University; 1991.
9. Summers MN, Haley WE, Reveille JO, Alarcon GS. Radiographic assessment and psychological variables as predictors of pain and functional impairment in osteoarthritis of the knee or hip. Arthritis Rheum. 1988;**31**:204–9.
10. Hart FA. Pain in osteoarthritis. Practitioner. 1974;**212**:244–50.
11. Dixon A St J. Progress in clinical rheumatology. London: JA Churchill; 1965:313–29.
12. Dieppe PA, Harkness JAL, Higgs ER. Osteoarthritis. In: Wall PD, Melzack R, eds. Textbook of pain, 2E. Edinburgh: Churchill Livingstone; 1989:306–16.
13. Lynn B, Kellgren JH. Pain. In: Scott JT, ed. Copeman's textbook of the rheumatic diseases, 6E. Edinburgh: Churchill Livingstone; 1986:143–60.
14. Arnoldi CC, Djurhuus JC, Heerfordt J, Karte A. Intraosseous phlebography, intraosseous pressure measurements and ^{m}Tc-polyphosphate scintigraphy in patients with various painful conditions in the hip and knee. Acta Orthop Scand. 1980;**51**:19–28.
15. Arnoldi CC, Lempberg RK, Linderholm H. Immediate effect of osteotomy on the intramedullary pressure of the femoral head and neck in patients with degenerative osteoarthritis. Acta Orthop Scand. 1971;**42**:357–65.
16. Kellgren JH. Pain in osteoarthritis. J Rheumatol. 1983;**9**(Suppl.):108–10.
17. Dieppe PA. Inflammation in osteoarthritis. Rheumatol Rehabil. 1978;**17**(Suppl.):S9–63.
18. Revell PA, Mayston V, Lalor P. The synovial membrane in osteoarthritis. Ann Rheum Dis. 1988;**47**:300–7.
19. Dieppe PA, Cushnaghan J, Jasani MK, McCrae F, Watt I. A two-year placebo-controlled trial of non-steroidal anti-inflammatory therapy in osteoarthritis of the knee joint. Br J Rheumatol. 1993; **32**: 595–600.
20. Chamberlain MA, Care G, Harfield B. Physiotherapy in osteoarthritis of the knee: a controlled trial of hospital versus home exercises. Int Rehabil Med. 1982;**4**:191–206.
21. Kellgren JH. Some painful joint conditions and their relationship to osteoarthritis. Clin Sci. 1939–42;**4**:193–203.
22. Moldofsky H. Sleep influences on regional and diffuse pain syndromes associated with osteoarthritis. Semin Arthritis Rheum. 1989;**18**(Suppl. 2):18–21.
23. Altman R, Asch E, Bloch D. Development of criteria for classification and reporting of osteoarthritis: classification of osteoarthritis of the knee. Arthritis Rheum. 1986;**9**:1039–49.
24. Watson P, Kernohan WG, Mollan RAB. A study of the cracking sounds from the metacarpo-phalangeal joint. Proc Inst Mech Eng. 1989;**203**:109–18.
25. Huskisson EC, Dieppe PA, Tucker AK, Cannell LB. Another look at osteoarthritis. Ann Rheum Dis. 1979;**389**:423–8.
26. McAlindon TE, Cooper C, Kirwan JR, Dieppe PA. Determinants of disability in osteoarthritis of the knee. Ann Rheum Dis. 1993;**52**:258–62.
27. Massardo L, Watt I, Cushnaghan J, Dieppe PA. An eight year prospective study of osteoarthritis of the knee joint. Ann Rheum Dis. 1989;**48**:893–7.
28. Siefert MH, Whiteside CG, Savage O. A 5 year follow-up of 50 cases of idiopathic OA of the hip. Ann Rheum Dis. 1969;**28**:325–6.
29. Dieppe PA, Doherty M, Macfarlane DG, Hutton CW, Bradfield JW, Watt I. Apatite-associated destructive arthritis. Br J Rheumatol. 1984;**23**:884–91.
30. Perry GH, Smith MJG, Whiteside CG. Spontaneous recovery of the joint space in degenerative hip disease. Ann Rheum Dis. 1979;**31**:440–8.
31. Bland JH, Cooper SM. Osteoarthritis: a review of the cell biology involved and evidence for reversibility. Semin Arthritis Rheum. 1984;**14**:106–33.
32. Danielsson LG. Incidence and prognosis of coxarthrosis. Acta Orthop Scand. 1964;**66**(Suppl.):1–111.
33. Dieppe PA, Cushnaghan J. The natural course and prognosis of osteoarthritis. In: Moskowitz RW, Howell DS, Goldberg VM, Mankin HJ, eds. Osteoarthritis: diagnosis and management, 2E. Philadelphia: WB Saunders; 1991.
34. Bauer GCH. Osteonecrosis of the knee. Clin Orthop Rel Res. 1978;**130**:210–7.
35. Ahlback S. Osteoarthrosis of the knee. Acta Radiol. 1969;**277**(Suppl.):7–72.
36. McAlindon T, McCrae F, Watt I, Goddard P, Dieppe PA. Magnetic resonance imaging in osteoarthritis of the knee: correlation with clinical, radiographic and scintigraphic findings Ann Rheum Dis. 1991;**50**:14–19.
37. Maquet PGJ. Biomechanics of the knee. New York: Springer-Verlag; 1976
38. Cooke TDV. Pathogenetic mechanisms in polyarticular osteoarthritis. Clin Rheum Dis. 1985;**11**:203–38.
39. Cushnaghan J, Dieppe PA. Study of 500 patients with limb joint osteoarthritis. I. Analysis by age, sex and distribution of symptomatic joint sites. Ann Rheum Dis. 1991;**50**:8–13.
40. Felson DT. Epidemiology of hip and knee osteoarthritis. Epidemiol Rev. 1988;**10**:1–28.
41. Zayer M. Osteoarthritis following Blount's disease. Int Orthop. 1980;**4**:63–6.
42. Miller R, Kettelkamp DB, Lauberthal KN. Quantitative correlations in degenerative arthritis of the knee. J Bone Joint Surg. 1973;**55A**:956–62.
43. Solomon L. Patterns of osteoarthritis of the hip. J Bone Joint Surg. 1976;**58B**:176–83.
44. Marks JS, Stewart IM, Hardinge K. Primary osteoarthritis of the hip and Heberden's nodes. Ann Rheum Dis. 1979;**38**:107–11.
45. Solomon L, Schnitzker CM, Browett JP. Osteoarthritis of the hip: the patient behind the disease. Ann Rheum Dis. 1982;**41**:118–25
46. Edelman J, Owtn EJ. Acute progressive osteoarthropathy of large joints. J Rheumatol. 1981;**8**:482–5.
47. Meachim G, Whitehouse GH, Pedley RB. An investigation of radiological, clinical and pathological correlations in osteoarthritis of the hip. Clin Radiol. 1980;**31**:565–74.
48. Byers PD, Contemponi CA, Farkas TA. A post mortem study of the hip joint. Ann Rheum Dis. 1970;**29**:14.
49. Radin EL. Biomechanics of the human hip. Clin Orthop. 1980;**152**:28–34.
50. Stocker DJ. Osteoarthritis of the hip: one disease or many. Br J Radiol. 1977:**50**:81–3.
51. Harris W. Etiology of osteoarthritis of the hip. Clin Orthop. 1986;**213**:20–33.
52. Foss MVL, Byers PD. Bone density, osteoarthritis of the hip and fracture of the upper end of the femur. Ann Rheum Dis. 1972;**31**:259–64.
53. Dequeker J. The relationship between osteoporosis and osteoarthritis. Clin Rheum Dis. 1985;**11**:271–96.
54. Rueble M, Dubois JL. Interet pronostique d'une classification radioclinique des coxarthroses. In: Peyron JG. Epidemiology of osteoarthritis. Ciba-Geigy; 1981:215–9.
55. Rashad S, Revell P, Hemingway A, et al. Effect of non-steroidal anti-inflammatory drugs on the course of osteoarthritis. Lancet. 1989;**ii**:519–22.
56. Dixon A St J and Campbell-Smith S. Long leg arthropathy. Ann Rheum Dis. 1969;**38**:359–65.
57. Swanson AB, Swanson G de G. Osteoarthritis in the hand. Clin Rheum Dis. 1985;**11**:393–420.
58. Peter JB, Pearson CM, Marmor L. Erosive osteoarthritis in the hands. Arthritis Rheum. 1966;**9**:365–88.
59. Radin EL, Parker HG, Paul IL. Pattern of degenerative arthritis. Preferential involvement of distal finger joints. Lancet. 1971;**i**:377–9.
60. Acheson RM, Chan Y, Clemett AR. New Haven survey of joint diseases. XII. Distribution and symptoms of osteoarthosis in the hands with reference to handedness. Ann Rheum Dis. 1970;**29**:275–86.
61. Spector TD, Campion GD. Generalised osteoarthritis: a hormonally mediated disease. Ann Rheum Dis. 1989;**48**:523–7.
62. Pattrick M, Aldridge S, Hamilton E, Manhire A, Doherty M. Hand function in nodal and erosive osteoarthritis. Ann Rheum Dis. 1989;**16**:1637–42.
63. Utsinger PD, Resnick D, Shapino RF, Wiesner KB. Roentgenologic, immunologic and therapeutic study of erosive (inflammatory) osteoarthritis. Arch Intern Med. 1978;**138**:693–7.
64. Kellgren JH, Moore R. Generalised osteoarthritis and Heberden's nodes. Br Med J. 1952;**i**:181–7.

65. Ehrlich GE. Inflammatory osteoarthritis. I. The clinical syndrome. J Chron Dis. 1972;**25**:317–28.
66. Hutton CW, Higgs ER, Jackson PC, Watt I, Dieppe PA. ^{99m}Tc HMDP bone scanning in generalised nodal osteoarthritis. Ann Rheum Dis. 1986;**45**:6–621:622–6.
67. Buckland-Wright C, Macfarlane D, Lynch J. Quantitative microfocal radiographic assessment of disease and progression in osteoarthritis of the hand. J Rheumatol. 1991;**18**(Suppl. 27):40–41.
68. Crain DC. Interphalangeal osteoarthritis. JAMA. 1961;**175**:1049–53.
69. Gray RG, Tenenbaum J, Gottlieb NL. Local corticosteroid injection treatment in rheumatic disorders. Semin Arthritis Rheum. 1981;**10**:231–54.
70. Gotfried Y, Bradford DS, Oegema TR. Facet joint changes after chemonucleolysis-induced disc space narrowing. Spine. 1986;**11**:944–50.
71. Farfan HS. Mechanical disorders of the low back. Philadelphia: Lea & Febiger; 1973.
72. Frymoyer JW, Newberg A, Pope MH, et al. Spine radiographs in patients with low back pain: an epidemiological study in man. J Bone Joint Surg. 1984;**66A**:1049–55.
73. Brewerton DA. Degenerative joint disease of the spines of patients with osteoarthritis of the hips. J Rheumatol. 1983;**10**(Suppl. 9):34–5.
74. Guralnick W, Keith DA, Osteoarthritis of the temperomandibular joint. In: Moskowitz RW, Howell DS, Goldberg VM, Mankin HJ, eds. Osteoarthritis: diagnosis and management, 2E. Philadelphia: WB Saunders; 1991.
75. Zart GA, Carlsson GE. Temporomandibular joint function and dysfunction. St Louis: CV Mosby Co; 1979.
76. Cierboom MAC, Steinberg JDJ, Mooyaart EL, et al. Condensing osteitis of the clavicle. Ann Rheum Dis. 1992;**51:**539–41.
77. Chard M, Hazleman B. Shoulder disorders in the elderly. Ann Rheum Dis. 1987;**46**:684–9.
78. Neer CS, Craig EV, Fukada H, Cuff-tear arthropathy. J Bone Joint Surg. 1983;**65A**:1232–44.
79. Campion G, McCrae F, Alwan W, Watt I, Bradfield J, Dieppe PA. Idiopathic destructive arthritis of the shoulder. Semin Arthritis Rheum. 1988;**17**:232–45.
80. Lequesne M, Fallut M, Coulomb R. L'arthropathie destructrice rapide de l'epaule. Rev Rheum. 1982:**49**:427–37.
81. Halverson PB, McCarty DJ, Cheung HS. Milwaukee shoulder syndrome. Semin Arthritis Rheum. 1984;**14**:36–44.
82. Woolf AD, Cawston TE, Dieppe PA. Idiopathic haemorrhagic rupture of the shoulder in destructive disease of the elderly. Ann Rheum Dis. 1986;**45**:498–501.
83. Doherty M, Preston B. Primary osteoarthritis of the elbow. Ann Rheum Dis. 1989;**48**:743–7.
84. Mann RA. Osteoarthritis of the foot and ankle. In: Moskowitz RW, Howell DS, Goldberg VM, Mankin HJ, eds. Osteoarthritis: diagnosis and management, 2E. Philadelphia: WB Saunders; 1991:389–402.
85. Mann RA, Coughlin M, DuVries HL. Hallux rigidus. Clin Orthop. 1979;**142**:57–65.
86. Van Saase J, Van Romande L, Cats A, et al. Epidemiology of osteoarthritis. Zoetermeer survey. Ann Rheum Dis. 1989;**48**:271–80.
87. Wood PHN. Osteoarthritis in the community. Clin Rheum Dis. 1979;**2**:495–507.
88. Mitchell NS, Cruers RL. Classification of degenerative arthritis. Can Med Assoc. 1977;**117**:763–5.
89. Allen PR, Denham RA, Swan AV. Late degenerative changes after meniscectomy. J Bone Joint Surg. 1984;**66B**:666–71.
90. Doherty M, Watt I, Dieppe PA. Influence of primary generalised osteoarthritis on development of secondary osteoarthritis. Lancet 1983;**ii**:8–11.
91. Palotie A, Vaisanen P, Ott J, et al. Predisposition to familial osteoarthritis linked to type II collagen gene. Lancet. 1989;**i**:924–8.
92. Dieppe PA. Some recent clinical approaches to osteoarthritis research. Semin Arthritis Rheum. 1990;**20**(Suppl. 1):2–11.
93. Cobby M, Cushnaghan J, Creamer P, Dieppe PA, Watt I. Erosive osteoarthritis – is it a separate disease entity? Clin Radiol. 1990;**42**:258–63.
94. Lequesne M, Amouroux J. La coxarthrose destructrice rapide. Pr Med. 1970;**78**:1435–40.
95. Doherty M, Dieppe PA. Clinical aspects of calcium pyrophosphate dihydrate crystal deposition. Rheum Dis Clin North Am. 1988;**14**:395–414.
96. Rogers J, Watt I, Dieppe PA. Comparison of visual and radiographic detection of bony changes at the knee joint. Br Med J. 1990;**300**:367–8.
97. Brandt KD, Fife RS, Braunstein EM, Katz B. Radiographic grading of the severity of knee osteoarthritis. Arthritis Rheum. 1991;**34**:1381–6.
98. Dieppe PA, Watt I. Crystal deposition in osteoarthritis: an opportunistic event? Clin Rheum Dis. 1985;**11**:367–92.
99. Kellgren JH, Lawrence JS. Radiological assessment of osteoarthritis. Ann Rheum Dis. 1957;**16**:494–501.
100. Altman RD, Fries JF, Bloch DA, et al. Radiographic assessment of progression in osteoarthritis. Arthritis Rheum. 1989;**32**:1584–91.
101. Cooper C, Cushnaghan J, Kirwan J, et al. Radiographic assessment of the knee joint in osteoarthritis. Ann Rheum Dis. 1992;**51**:80–2.
102. Dacre JE, Huskisson EC. The use of digital image analysis for the assessment of radiographs in osteoarthritis. Br J Rheumatol. 1989;**28**:506–10.
103. Doyle DV, Dieppe PA, Scott J, et al. An articular index for the assessment of osteoarthritis. Ann Rheum Dis. 1981;**40**:75–8.
104. Bellamy N, Buchanan WW, Goldsmith CH, Campbell J, Duku E. Signal measurement strategies – are they feasible and do they offer any advantage in outcome measures in osteoarthritis? Arthritis Rheum. 1990;**33**:739–45.
105. Fries JF, Spilz P, Kraines RG, Holman HR. Measurement of patient outcome in arthritis. Arthritis Rheum. 1980;**23**:137–45.
106. Bellamy N. The clinical evaluation of osteoarthritis in the elderly. Clin Rheum Dis 1986;**12**:313–40.
107. Altman RD. Criteria for classification of clinical osteoarthritis. J Rheumatol. 1991;**18**(Suppl. 27):10–12.
108. Bellamy N, Carette S, Ford P, et al. Osteoarthritis antirheumatic drug trials. J Rheumatol. 1992;**19**:436–57.
109. Cushnaghan J, Cooper C, Dieppe PA, et al. Clinical assessment of osteoarthritis of the knee. Ann Rheum Dis. 1990;**49**:768–70.
110. Lequesne MG, Samson S. Indices of severity in osteoarthritis of weight bearing joints. J Rheumatol. 1991;**18**(Suppl. 27):16–18.

OSTEOARTHRITIS

13

MANAGEMENT OF OSTEOARTHRITIS

Paul A Dieppe

- Use a 'pyramidal' approach, starting with simple educational and physical modalities before considering drugs or surgery.
- Joints with osteoarthritis can be protected from excessive loading by weight loss, use of a cane, shock absorbing insoles and other simple measures.
- Maintain activity of the whole individual and affected joints, including range of movement and muscle strength.
- Reserve drugs for symptom flares and use as an adjunct to maintaining activity. NSAIDs and intra-articular therapy should be used sparingly.
- Surgery is available for patients with persistent symptoms.

INTRODUCTION

A wide variety of treatments are available for those who suffer from osteoarthritis (OA). They range from simple educational help to highly technical and skilled physical, medical or surgical procedures. Much can be done to relieve symptoms, optimize function and improve the quality of life.

To date, no 'specific' therapy has been proven to have efficacy in altering the disease process in humans. However, in animal models of the disease certain medical and biomechanical techniques do appear to be able to slow the progression of OA, and perhaps reverse the condition in some cases [1]. Furthermore, there is no doubt that a corrective osteotomy can stimulate 'healing' of an OA joint in some people [2]. These data, together with our increasing understanding of the nature of the process and its biomechanical and biochemical control, are cause for optimism. In the future it may be possible to provide specific 'anti-OA' therapy in addition to the measures already available.

'Therapy' covers many possibilities, including four quite different types of goal:

- prevention;
- screening of early asymptomatic disease to institute measures to prevent progression;
- therapy of an established condition, and
- salvage.

The epidemiology of OA suggests that prevention of some disease may become possible in the future. However, in this chapter only therapy of the established condition and salvage procedures will be discussed.

OBJECTIVES OF MANAGEMENT

The main objectives in the management of OA are listed in Figure 13.1. Several problems arise with any attempt to meet these objectives in current clinical practice, as outlined in the figure.

MANAGEMENT OF OSTEOARTHRITIS	
Objectives in management of osteoarthritis	
Education	The patient, relatives and carers should understand the condition and know what they themselves can do to help
Relieve symptoms	Pain, stiffness and other symptoms of the condition should be controlled as well as possible with minimum risk to the patient
Minimize handicap	Any consequences on function, and any disability or handicap, should be minimized through appropriate rehabilitative techniques
Limit progression	Any factors known to be likely to worsen the condition should be avoided, and any practices likely to reduce the risk of progression instituted, with minimum risk, if they do not conflict with the other objectives
Problems in realization of management objectives	
Widespread ignorance and misconceptions about the nature of OA	
Lack of understanding of the cause of symptoms	
Lack of understanding of disability and handicap in OA	
Inability to understand or control disease progression	

Fig. 13.1 Objectives and problems in the management of osteoarthritis.

Ignorance and Misconceptions

OA is still widely thought to be a degenerative disease caused by aging and excess use of joints (a 'wear-and-tear' disease). Evidence to the contrary is extensive but old concepts of OA are still very prevalent in the medical community as well as in the public domain. There is also extensive ignorance about the disorder, which receives much less publicity than many other common, age-related conditions, such as osteoporosis or ischemic heart disease.

Ignorance and misconceptions lead to negative attitudes. OA is easily dismissed as 'one of those things', an inevitable part of the aging process about which nothing can be done. Furthermore, patients and carers may believe that it is best to be inactive to protect joints – a policy which can have disastrous consequences.

The Causes of Symptoms in OA

Symptomatic relief is one of the primary aims in the management of OA. However, the symptoms are poorly understood. Pain, especially on joint use, is the most frequent complaint. However, this could have a number of causes, including raised intra-osseous pressure, periarticular strain, capsular stretching, periosteal elevation and synovitis [3]. Similarly, stiffness, and other forms of pain are ill-understood. It is difficult to institute rational therapy in the face of current ignorance as to the cause of symptoms. It therefore should come as no surprise that there is still debate about the value of drugs and many other treatment modalities in OA.

One of the prerequisites of good treatment is an examination to determine possible causes of pain (see Fig. 13.2). Patients with 'OA' may have joint pain not directly related to the disease.

Disability and Handicap in OA

The cause of disability and handicap is perhaps less obscure, it being self evident that pain, loss of motion and muscle weakness will be contributory. However, the extent and nature of the contribution of these and other factors is unclear and difficult to unravel in individual patients with OA. Ideally, each patient should be assessed with this in mind in an attempt to rationalize the treatment of their disability. However, this is a counsel of perfection that remains difficult to realize.

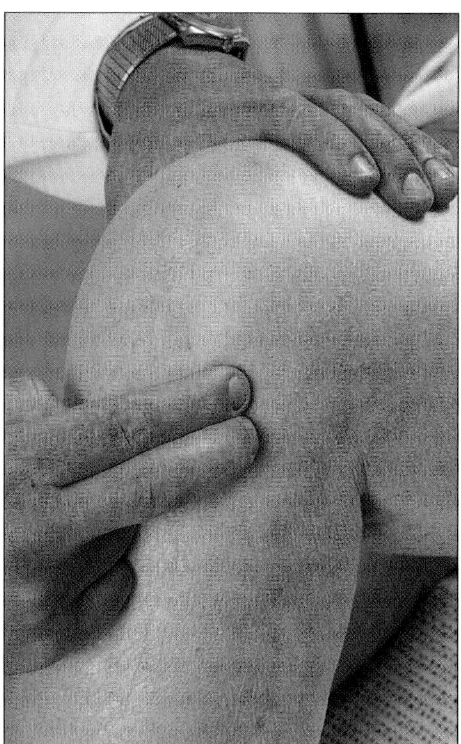

Fig. 13.2 Identifying the cause of pain in OA. One of the prerequisites to good therapy is to establish the cause of symptoms in a joint with 'OA'. This may be due to periarticular problems resulting in severe local tenderness rather than coming from the joint. In the case illustrated, this is due to anserine bursitis and stretching of the capsule at its insertion on the medial aspect of the knee. However, local pathology must be carefully distinguished from referred tender spots, which are commonly identifiable around damaged joints. True periarticular pathology results in severe point tenderness with other signs, such as reproduction of the pain on certain movements that stress the structures involved.

Progression of OA

The outcome of OA is very heterogeneous [4]. Phases of relative stability, apparent improvement and rapid worsening, as well as slow progression can all occur. An obvious management goal is to reduce the risk of progression and prevent phases of rapid worsening, although this assumes an understanding of what factors control the outcome. Mechanical factors almost certainly play a part; instability and malalignment of joints probably accelerate OA and should be corrected where possible. The role of various types of joint usage, normal and abnormal, is more controversial. Obesity may contribute and the disputed role of different medications is discussed below. Other factors, such as age and sex, remain largely beyond our control.

Conclusions on Management Objectives

Many texts, including much of what follows below, provide didactic advice on how to manage OA. Before reading or acting on such advice it is as well to be reminded of the lack of scientific foundation or of any firm rationale for it. It is easy enough to construct management goals, either globally or individually, but much more difficult to turn these into a rational, successful treatment program.

MODALITIES AVAILABLE FOR THE MANAGEMENT OF OA

There are many different forms of therapy that can be of value for patients with OA (Fig. 13.3).

THERAPY USED FOR PATIENTS WITH OA
Education
Exercise therapy
Hydrotherapy
Footwear and walking aids
Other aids and appliances
Other rehabilitation measures
Systemic drug therapy
Intra-articular drug therapy
Rubefacients and other local applications
Surgery
Complimentary techniques for pain relief

Fig. 13.3 Therapy used for patients with OA.

EDUCATION

The techniques available for the education of patients with OA are the same as for any other form of patient education; counselling can be supplemented with literature, videos, self-learning programs and other educational technology. Several groups have reported on the value of specific teaching programs for OA sufferers, in one case using telephone calls alone [5]. However, their content, format and outcome measures have varied extensively making it difficult to draw clear, general conclusions.

Opinions vary on the most appropriate content and priorities for such educational programs. Most include some simple explanation of what is going on in OA and the difference between a normal and an osteoarthritic synovial joint. Didactic advice on activity and exercises is often given, but the amount of activity that patients should be advised to take remains controversial. Tips on 'joint protection' and the use of simple aids such as a walking stick are usually included, and obese patients are generally advised to lose weight. Some attempts to answer common lay questions, such as the value of specific diets, are often added.

In the author's view the most important educational goal is to instil a positive attitude. Common negative thoughts about inevitable progression, a future life in a wheelchair, and having to avoid exercise in order to prevent joints from further damage, need to be countered by strong, positive advice to the contrary. Recent controlled data on the value of supervised fitness walking provides useful information to back up this advice [6]. The majority of patients with OA should be able to maintain a full active life, albeit with some discomfort, provided that they are allowed to, that their condition is not over 'medicalized', and they are not misled by negative advice and attitudes.

PHYSICAL THERAPY AND HYDROTHERAPY

Physical therapy and hydrotherapy have important roles, especially in the management of moderate or severe OA of large joints such as the hip and knee. The main indications for treatment and the objectives that can be realized by use of these modalities are summarized in Figure 13.4.

Physiotherapists have an important potential role in the education of patients as well as in realization of the specific goals listed in Figure 13.4. They are often able to instil a positive attitude and persuade patients that they can do more and enjoy a better quality of life than they might otherwise have thought. Isometric muscle strengthening exercises, gentle mobilization of stiff, 'stuck' joints and the re-education of patients in joint use are important techniques [7]. Local applications (e.g. heat, ultrasound, etc.) to relieve pain have a limited role, active work with the therapist being much more important. The main value of hydrotherapy is in helping pain relief and muscle

PHYSICAL THERAPY AND HYDROTHERAPY IN THE MANAGEMENT OF OA
Indications for use
Loss of joint motion without severe joint destruction Muscle weakness/wasting, and instability of joint(s) Malalignment of joint(s) and/or abnormal joint use (an abnormal gait for example) Severe symptoms not relieved by other measures
Objectives and role of treatment
Maintain/improve the range of joint motion Maintain/increase the strength of muscles acting on the affected joint(s), which also improves stability Optimize joint biomechanics to maintain/improve alignment, and reduce any abnormal or excess loading of the joint(s) Relieve pain, stiffness and other symptoms

Fig. 13.4 Physical therapy and hydrotherapy in the management of OA.

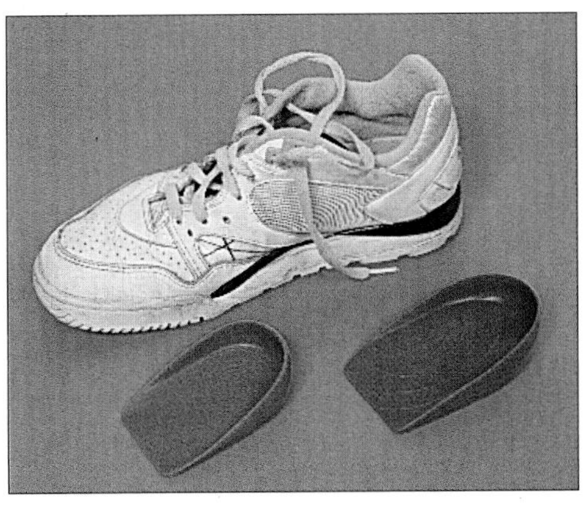

Fig. 13.5 The use of shoes and insoles to reduce impact loading on lower limb joints. Modern sports shoes ('trainers') often have appropriate insoles. Alternatively, special heel insoles of sorbithane or viscoelastic materials can be used. They may help relieve pain as well as reducing the peak impact load on the joints during walking.

relaxation, while reducing gravitational loading of joints; in OA it is of most value in the management of moderate or severe hip OA.

The main contraindications to physiotherapy are very severe pain on joint movement and severe or rapidly progressive joint destruction on the radiograph. In those situations, therapy is likely to be a miserable experience for the patient and just make matters worse.

OCCUPATIONAL THERAPY

The occupational therapist (OT), like the physiotherapist, may have an important role in education. Joint protection techniques may be of great help to the patient with OA, particularly if they are suffering from a lot of pain on joint use. Relaxation techniques and general coping strategies can also be valuable, particularly to anxious or elderly patients restricted and upset by their OA.

More specific indications for the use of the OT's skills include any significant disability or handicap due to OA. A destroyed, unstable joint, particularly in a patient who is unsuitable or having to wait for surgery, may present a special challenge. Other special forms of help and advice may be required and the OT may be amongst those best placed to provide information about issues such as the sexual difficulties that can arise from lower limb OA [8].

Aids and Appliances

A variety of splints, orthoses and walking aids may help patients with established OA, in addition to alterations to the home and lifestyle.

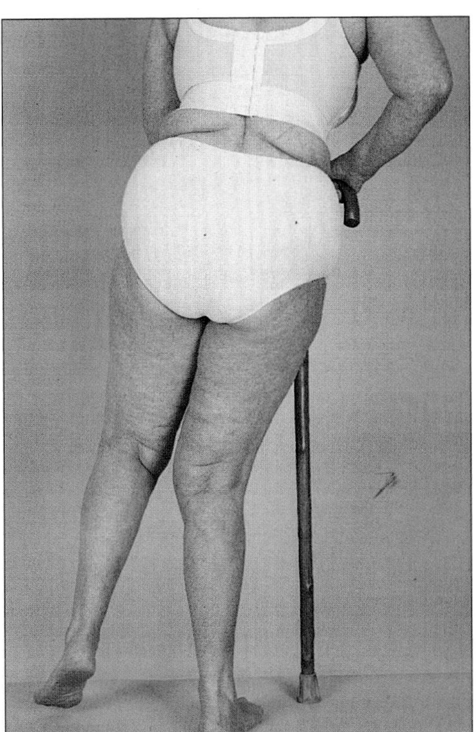

Fig. 13.6 Use of a cane, stick or other walking aid. This patient, who has hip OA, has found that she can reduce the pain in her damaged left hip by leaning on the stick in the right hand as she walks. The reduction in loading can be huge, and the effect on symptoms and confidence with walking very beneficial.

Shoes are particularly important in lower limb OA (Fig. 13.5). Cushioning of the heel to absorb impact loading may relieve symptoms on walking, and might in theory also help the joint. Recent work also suggests that heel wedges may help counteract the effects of varus and valgus deformities in OA of the knee [9]. Simple walking aids, such as a cane, reduce joint loading and relieve pain (Fig. 13.6). Other walking aids may be important to increase independence and walking distance. In more advanced OA, splints and orthoses to control instability may be required [10].

Disabled patients may also need a number of adaptations to the home. Lower limb OA may make it difficult to get on and off the toilet seat or in and out of a chair, and bathing may be difficult. Less commonly, upper limb OA can cause a significant disability with dressing and washing.

DRUGS

The use of drugs in the management of OA is currently a very unsatisfactory and controversial subject [11,12]. A huge number of medicines are prescribed for and consumed by OA patients, largely for relief of pain (Fig. 13.7). However, most of the agents used have been formulated for the treatment of other disorders. Their true value in OA has received very little attention, in spite of the volume of prescribing. During the last decade there has been increasing concern that some of the agents used may have either deleterious or beneficial effects on the OA joint, in addition to any symptomatic effects [13,14], although hard data in humans is lacking. In view of the potential toxicity of many of the drugs used, especially in the elderly, a very conservative attitude to the use of medication in OA seems to be appropriate at present.

Simple Analgesics

Simple analgesics such as paracetamol (acetaminophen), codeine, dextropropoxyphene, low dose salicylates and others are widely used for pain in OA. Combinations, such as paracetamol plus dextropropoxyphene are particularly popular in some countries. Mild to moderate osteoarthritic joint pain responds partially to these agents, and one recent study showed that many people with established knee OA can cope well with a small intake of paracetamol as their only drug therapy over a two year time period [15]. In another recent study no difference could be detected between paracetamol and ibuprofen in symptom relief for knee OA [16]. However, the relative efficacy of analgesics when compared to the nonsteroidal anti-inflammatory drugs (NSAIDs) has not been established. Two ways of using the simple analgesics have been recommended: an 'on demand' regime, and secondly, regular prescribing. 'On demand' analgesics can be taken when pain is particularly bad or before some activity that is likely to bring on more severe pain. Regular analgesia is used to suppress more constant pain. In the context of OA particular care needs to be taken in the elderly who may have compromised renal or hepatic function.

DRUGS USED IN THE MANAGEMENT OF OA	
Type of drug	Rationale/purpose
Simple analgesics	Pain relief
NSAIDs	Pain relief, reduction of other symptoms via anti-inflammatory effect
Intra-articular corticosteroids	Local relief of symptoms
Intra-articular radiocolloids and sclerosing agents	Symptomatic relief via obliteration of the synovium and synovitis
'Chondroprotectives'	Symptom relief and reduction in the progression of cartilage damage
Antidepressants and other agents	Relief of pain

Fig. 13.7 Drugs used in the management of OA.

Nonsteroidal Anti-inflammatory Drugs

In many parts of the world it has become fashionable to use NSAIDs, rather than simple analgesics, as first choice drugs for the routine medical treatment of pain and stiffness in OA. Many trials have indicated that NSAIDs are superior to placebos in OA in both the short term and over time periods of up to two years [15,17]. However, there have been very few comparative studies of NSAIDs and simple analgesics [16,18].

The stated indications for the use of NSAIDs in OA are pain and stiffness. The doses recommended are similar to those used for other, more overtly inflammatory disorders. Regular prescribing rather than 'on demand' usage is recommended. Some authors suggest that an NSAID should only be used for a short time period, perhaps a few weeks, with regular monitoring of the blood count and renal and hepatic function [19], although in practice many OA patients stay on them for months or years without any blood tests. The rationale for using NSAIDs in OA is the potential contribution of the inflammatory component of the disorder to symptoms. Unfortunately, in clinical practice it is difficult to assess how much inflammation is present in OA, and virtually impossible to know whether the symptoms result from it. In a recent survey of primary-care physicians in the US most used NSAIDs as the first-line drug for OA, although often in suboptimal doses for any anti-inflammatory effect [20].

Claims have been made that some of these agents accelerate joint damage in OA, whereas others might be 'chondroprotective' [13,14]. Almost all of these claims are based on in-vitro phenomena or animal models, and little or no hard evidence is available in the human disease. NSAIDs certainly have a variety of interesting effects on chondrocytes *in vitro* and on cartilage and bone in animal models of OA, which, if they also occur in humans, could affect the disease process. However, species differences occur and the complexity of the subject has been highlighted by Brandt and colleagues who have shown that the effects of NSAIDs on the cartilage of the dog depends on a wide variety of local factors [21]. Some evidence is available in human OA of the hip which suggests that some NSAIDs, particularly indomethacin, may accelerate the disease, perhaps via subchondral bone destruction [22,23].

NSAIDs are most likely to cause toxic side effects in elderly females [24]. However, elderly females are the group most in need of drug treatment for symptoms in OA. The prescriber therefore has to consider the balance of risk versus potential gain in the face of inadequate data (Fig. 13.8). Various ways of using NSAIDs in older patients are recommended, including close monitoring of the renal and hepatic function as well as the blood count, both before and at regular intervals after initiating therapy. However, the value of such regimes is unknown and further investigations are urgently needed to resolve the problem of NSAID usage in OA.

The recent introduction of a number of local applications of NSAIDs, in the form of gels and creams, offers an interesting alternative to systemic use in OA. The idea is particularly attractive for patients with predominantly monoarticular disease and those with involvement of a few hand joints. Clinical trials suggest that symptomatic relief is obtained [25] and there can be some penetration of these agents into the joints. However, more comparative trials including comparisons with simple rubefacients and other forms of medication would be helpful in the assessment of the role of these agents in OA.

Corticosteroids and Osteoarthritis

Systemic corticosteroids, like many of the NSAIDs, have interesting effects on chondrocytes and cartilage in culture, some of which could be interpreted as being of potential benefit in OA [14]. However, there is no evidence that they are of any value in human OA and their use cannot be justified at present.

In contrast, there may be a limited role for the use of intra-articular corticosteroids. Early uncontrolled, empirical observation suggested that an intra-articular injection of a short or long-acting corticosteroid into an OA joint caused great relief of symptoms. However, two placebo controlled trials of their use in knee OA indicate that the effect only lasts for a few weeks and that the corticosteroid is only marginally superior to placebo [26,27], suggesting that their regular use cannot be justified. All joint sites may not respond in the same way, however, and the base of the thumb is thought to respond better to this type of therapy than other joint sites (Fig. 13.9). In contrast, corticosteroid injections are contraindicated in OA finger joints where they may result in soft tissue calcification or joint fusion [28] and should be avoided in hip OA in view of reports of accelerated joint damage.

In practice, intra-articular corticosteroids are probably justified in three situations in the management of OA:

- when severe symptoms are arising from the thumb base,
- in a 'flare-up' of OA associated with a joint effusion, and
- as an adjunct to physical therapy.

The last indication is the most important. The injection should ideally be followed by a day or two of rest, followed by intensive physiotherapy to strengthen muscles and increase the range of motion of the joint. An effusion in a joint is known to result in loss of muscle strength ('arthrogenic muscle inhibition') so physiotherapy is unlikely to be successful unless any effusion is suppressed [29].

Medical Synovectomy

The intra-articular injection of agents which damage or obliterate the synovial lining of a joint are sometimes used in the treatment of inflammatory disorders such as rheumatoid arthritis (RA). The rationale is that the reduction in synovial tissue and synovitis which results from the injection will reduce local inflammation and thus symptoms. Symptomatic benefit, lasting a few months or years, may be observed [30]. The agents used have included radiocolloids such as yttrium-90 and sclerosing agents such as osmic acid.

Local synovitis may contribute to the symptoms of OA in some patients and it may be that those with extensive crystal deposition have more synovitis than most. With this in mind, Doherty and Dieppe carried out a small controlled trial of intra-articular yttrium-90 injections in knee OA associated with chondrocalcinosis [31]. The treated knees showed much more symptomatic improvement than control knees over a 6-month period. Subsequently, uncontrolled observations have suggested similar, lasting benefits from yttrium

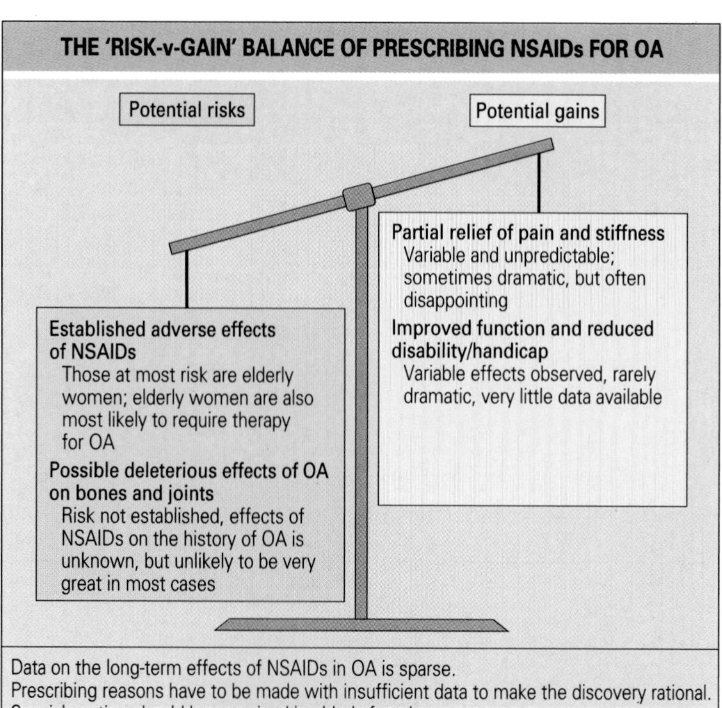

Fig. 13.8 The 'risk-versus-gain' balance with the prescribing of nonsteroidal anti-inflammatory agents for OA.

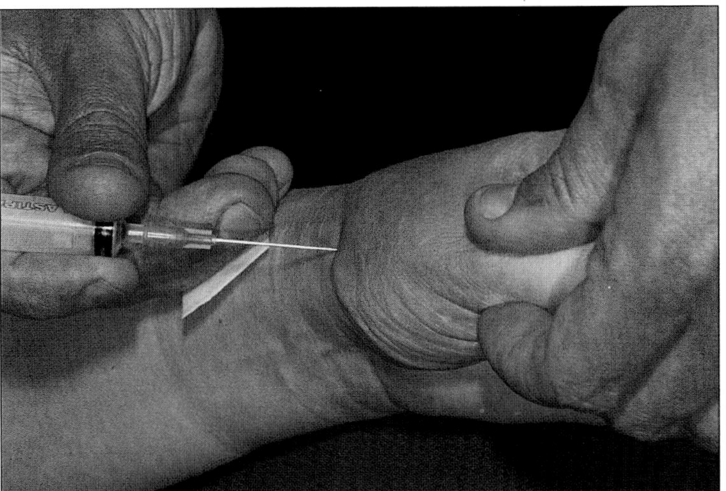

Fig. 13.9 A patient with OA of the carpometacarpal joint of the left thumb undergoing arthrocentesis for injection of a depot corticosteroid preparation. The operator is distracting the patient's thumb to open up the joint space.

SURGICAL PROCEDURES USED IN THE MANAGEMENT OF OA	
Procedure	**Indications**
Arthroscopic washout or 'tidal irrigation'	Moderate to severe symptoms without severe radiographic changes, useful in diagnosis, mainly used for the knee
Joint debridement	Moderate to severe symptoms, especially mechanical type, without advanced loss of articular cartilage
Bony decompression	Occasionally used in early osteonecrosis or to relieve severe pain
Osteotomy	Pain relief and realignment of joints with severe symptoms and focal damage, but without complete loss of cartilage
Arthroplasty	Severe symptoms with severe joint damage as well

Fig. 13.10 Surgical procedures used in the management of OA.

injections in simple OA of the knee. However, more controlled work is needed to establish both short and long-term effects of these agents in OA before their use could be recommended.

'Chondroprotective Agents'

In some parts of Europe a variety of agents have been available for use locally or systemically in OA, with the claim that they are able to benefit the joint as well as relieving symptoms. They include glycosaminoglycan polysulfate ester, glycosaminoglycan–peptide complex, pentosan polysulfate, hyaluronan and others. They have many potentially important in-vitro effects, including protease inhibition, and there is some evidence from animal models that these agents may be able to prevent disease progression or even reverse experimental OA [32]. However, well controlled trials in human OA are lacking. There is empirical data to suggest that they can relieve pain and the fact that this happens relatively quickly in the absence of any known analgesic activity of the agents has been interpreted as indicating some effect on the pathology of the condition. One study report suggests that some of these agents may have longer term benefits in human hip and knee OA [33], but these data have not been confirmed. Because of the lack of good objective data and concerns about the toxicity of these complex agents they are not available in most parts of the world. On present evidence their use cannot be recommended. The main importance of the agents mentioned is probably in the experimental laboratory and animal model situation, and in the further exploration of the potential for drug treatment of OA in the future.

Other Drugs

A variety of other agents have been used in attempts to relieve symptoms or improve the status of a damaged joint in OA [34,35].

Antidepressants and appetite suppressing agents have both been investigated for possible pain relieving activity. The antidepressants may have a minor role, particularly in patients who have 'fibromyalgia' with painful trigger points in addition to their OA, or in those with a significant sleep disturbance [36]. Low dose amitriptyline, (10–25mg at night) is an example of an agent of this class that seems to act as a useful adjunct to other therapy in some patients.

Recently, topical capsaicin has been reported to provide useful pain relief in OA [37]. Intra-articular use of the superoxide dismutase inhibitor orgotein has also been shown to relieve pain [38].

A huge number of other agents have been investigated for possible value in OA, ranging from hormones such as estrogen, and inhibitors such as tamoxifen, to chloroquine, ascorbic acid, silicone oil, *S*-adenosyl-L-methionine, and tetracyclines. Many such agents have shown some promise, either in experimental work or early human trials. However, the majority have not been fully investigated. One of the major problems with such work is the difficulty of long-term studies and of establishing any efficacy of drugs in OA given the current inadequate methods of disease assessment and poor outcome measures.

SURGERY

Several surgical procedures are available for the treatment of OA (Fig. 13.10). Most of the operations listed are only appropriate in advanced cases and the other measures outlined above should always be used before resorting to surgery. However, the judicious use of surgery in conjunction with medical and other measures increases the options for good management enormously. Arthroplasty in particular has transformed the lives of many OA sufferers, and the number of knee and hip replacements has increased dramatically over the last decade [39]. As with the management of RA, there is a good case for a team approach to the management of advanced OA in which physician, surgeon and therapists hold combined consultations with the patients. The timing of surgical procedures and their integration with all other aspects of management are of as much importance, if not more, than the choice of operation and technical skill with which it is performed.

Pain is the main indication for surgery in OA. If pain is continuing to disrupt life significantly, in spite of the use of the other treatment modalities outlined, then surgery can be considered. Persistent and severe night pain or rest pain are generally regarded as the most pressing reasons for operating. Disability must also be considered, although it is usually secondary when surgical decisions are taken for two reasons: first many of the available operations are better at relieving pain than improving function, and secondly, rehabilitative measures may be of much greater importance than surgery in the management of disability.

However, the criteria for surgery of any sort in OA, and of joint replacements in particular, needs to be considered further. Many arthroplasties have a limited life span, which may depend in part on the demands made by the patient's level of activity as well as their age. Revision surgery is on the increase. Furthermore, in some countries medical resources are insufficient to meet all of the potential demands for arthroplasty in OA. Some surgeons use rough criteria such as the presence of significant night pain, or the reduction of walking distance to a certain level, or loss of earnings ('cannot walk, cannot sleep or cannot work') to help decision making, but such criteria must vary according to the social and financial situations. More studies of the natural history of OA, and of the long-term benefits of surgery, as well as who benefits most, are urgently needed.

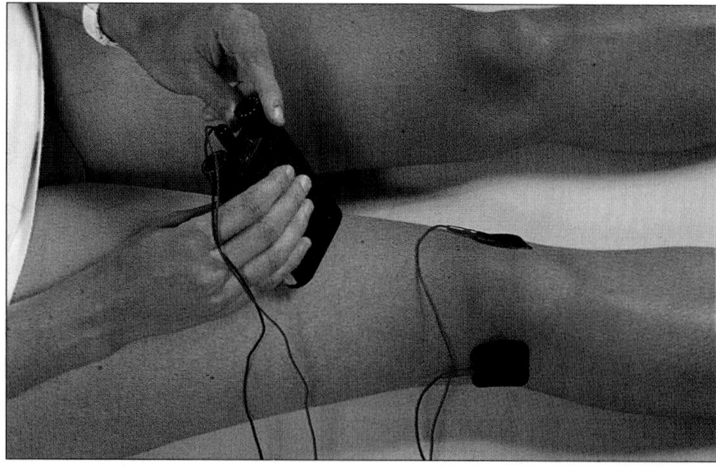

Fig. 13.11 Use of transcutaneous nerve stimulation (TENS) as an adjunct to other therapy for pain relief at the knee joint. The use of acupuncture, TENS and other local techniques to aid pain relief in difficult cases of OA is often worthwhile.

OTHER MODALITIES OF TREATMENT

Pain and disability are the major problems encountered in the management of OA. The symptoms are often progressive and the problems caused may be particularly intransigent in elderly people, who may have a number of confounding problems of a social or psychological type, as well as other medical problems. In view of this it is often valuable to consider the use of a number of other treatment modalities, including techniques coming under the umbrella term 'complimentary medicine'. Pain clinics can be helpful in severe pain, particularly in patients who may have a contraindication to the use of drugs or surgery. Acupuncture, transcutaneous nerve stimulation and other physical means of relieving pain can be used, although trials in OA have not produced particularly good results [40] (Fig. 13.11).

Social support and encouragement, self-help groups and other systems in the community can also be vital to the continuation of a reasonable quality of life for an elderly person weighed down by pain and difficulty moving around because of OA.

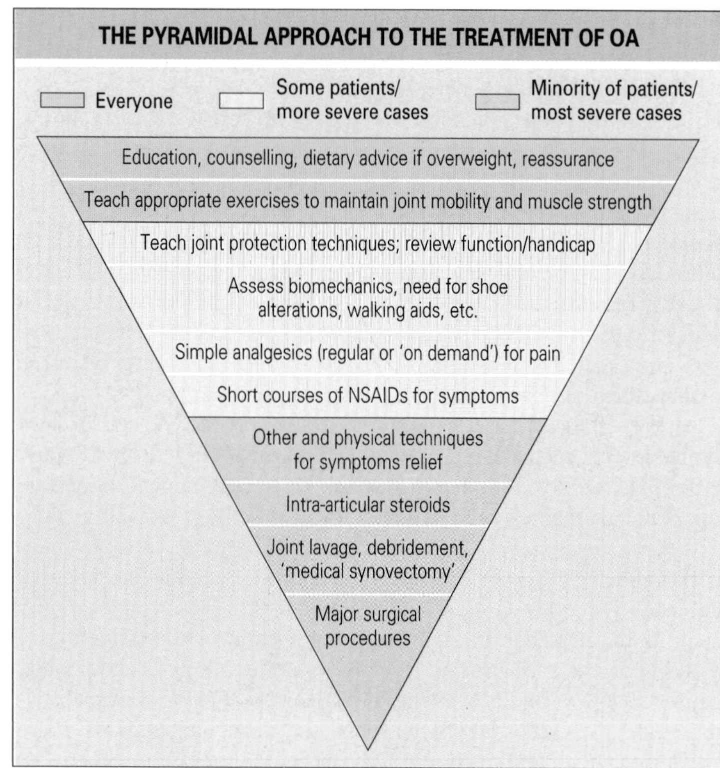

Fig. 13.12 The 'pyramidal' approach to the treatment of OA.

THE SPECIFIC MANAGEMENT OF JOINTS COMMONLY AFFECTED BY OA

In this section more didactic advice on the management of OA is provided. This should be read in the light of the first section of the chapter which highlighted the lack of understanding and controversies which surround the subject. In general, a 'pyramidal' approach to the treatment of OA is appropriate, moving from the most simple and least dangerous modalities, towards the more complex and invasive (Fig. 13.12).

OA of the Knee

Mild to moderate disease

Mild OA of the knee is extremely common, mainly affecting middle aged and elderly women [41]. The condition often remains relatively static for many years; progression to severe disease is probably uncommon. It is appropriate therefore to counsel patients with a cautious but relatively optimistic prognosis.

All patients with knee OA should be taught quadriceps exercises and encouraged to continue with them on a daily basis (Fig. 13.13). There is evidence that these exercises relieve symptoms as well as improving function and that some way of ensuring that patients continue with them is important [42,43]. Patients should also be encouraged to keep active, as a general fitness and walking program has been shown to be of benefit [6]. However, excessive activity, particularly if it involves a lot of high impact loading of the knee (running on hard surfaces for example), should be avoided. Many patients are able to organize their lives so that they avoid persistent activity likely to produce lasting or severe pain, keeping to a policy of 'little and often'. Shock absorbing insoles in shoes should be recommended and may be of immediate symptomatic value. In some cases, particularly in older people, a walking stick held in the contralateral hand to help reduce loading on the knee can also reduce pain and increase exercise tolerance. If an angulation deformity is present, adjustments to the footwear or orthoses to correct this can be considered [7,44]. Patients who are obese should be advised to lose weight, and this may reduce the risk of progression as well as relieving pain and increasing fitness [45].

Drugs should be used sparingly. Intermittent courses of a mild analgesic, or possibly an NSAID can be used when the condition is particularly painful, and 'on demand' analgesics can be provided for occasional use. Continuous drug administration should be avoided. Local rubefacients and other applications to relieve pain can be considered.

Severe knee OA

The measures outlined for mild to moderate disease are all appropriate

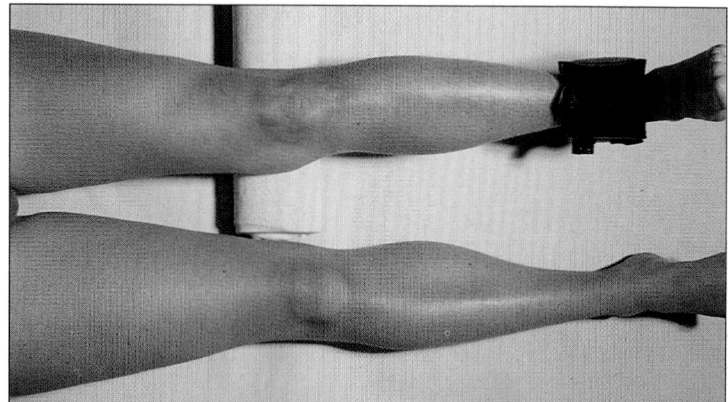

Fig. 13.13 Quadriceps exercises for knee OA. Quadriceps exercises are of proven value for pain relief and improving function, and everyone with knee OA should be taught the correct techniques and encouraged to make these exercises a lifetime habit. This patient is being shown how to fully straighten the knee, with the ankle dorsiflexed, and then practice straight leg raising, as well as the extension exercises, with a weight on the ankle.

for more severe cases. In addition, more attention may need to be paid to mechanical abnormalities of the joint, more drug therapy may be indicated, and surgical options should be considered. Any instability or severe angulation deformity of the joint probably accelerates progression as well as affecting symptoms. In addition to using footwear adjustments for angulation deformities, orthoses may be indicated if there is ligamentous instability [44]. Fixed flexion deformities and limitation of movement should be treated with vigorous physiotherapy. Some patients get considerable relief of symptoms from the use of an NSAID, although the value of continued prescription of these agents should be reviewed regularly. A 'flare-up' of symptoms associated with an effusion may respond to aspiration and injection of a long-acting corticosteroid preparation.

The surgical options include arthroscopic examination and washout (tidal lavage), or joint debridement, both of which can produce a temporary improvement [46,47]. These procedures also provide diagnostic information on the nature and extent of any confounding problems such as meniscal damage, which may be contributing to symptoms. More definitive surgical treatment involves corrective osteotomy or arthroplasty. Osteotomy may be indicated in younger patients (60s or less) with a stable joint in which the OA predominantly affects one compartment but a significant varus or valgus deformity exists. A variety of procedures are used, and long-term results appear to be good if the deformity is accurately corrected [48]. Arthroplasty is indicated in older patients, and in those with bi or tri-compartmental disease and/or ligamentous instability of the joint. The main indication for major surgery in knee joint OA is severe pain unresponsive to other measures.

OA of the Hip

OA of the hip is a common condition, spanning a wide age range with a roughly equal sex incidence [41]. Specific priorities in management will depend on the age, sex and circumstances of the patients, as well as disease severity.

Mild to moderate disease

Many patients with hip OA, particularly those in the younger, predominantly male group, manage well for many years in spite of quite marked disease. However, a significant proportion of all ages and both sexes come to surgery at some stage. When counselling patients and their relatives it is appropriate to take an optimistic approach, particularly in view of the relative simplicity and high success rate of modern arthroplasty operations for the hip, but the realities of the situation should be stated from the beginning.

The general approach is similar to that for knee OA. Patients should lose weight if they are obese, and be advised to wear shoes with shock absorbing insoles. All patients should be taught a simple regime of exercises to help maintain the range of movement of the hip, as reduced movement is responsible for many of the everyday problems encountered, such as difficulty putting on socks and shoes. Exercises to help keep the muscles around the hip strong are also valuable. In many cases, intermittent courses of formal physiotherapy are needed to maintain the status of the joint and muscles; hydrotherapy can be particularly beneficial in pain relief and mobilization of the joint. Any patient with significant symptoms from hip OA should probably be advised to use a walking stick. A correctly used stick, on the contralateral side (see Fig. 13.6), reduces loading on the joint by 20–30% [49], and also reduces activity-related pain in most cases. (If the muscles are very weak, and the joint feels 'unstable', the patient may prefer to use the stick on the ipsilateral side for security when walking.)

Drugs have a limited role in mild disease. 'On demand' analgesics used sparingly can be useful. Some patients experience 'flares', or episodes of days or weeks when symptoms are particularly bad, and these episodes may respond well to an NSAID. However, continuous or extensive use of NSAIDs cannot be recommended and indomethacin should be avoided. Injections should be avoided, with the exception of treatment for coexistent trochanteric bursitis, which may respond well to local corticosteroid injections.

Severe hip OA

Advanced disease of the hip is often accompanied by significant deformities including true shortening of the leg and fixed adduction, flexion and external rotation. Any leg length abnormality should be corrected, at least partially, by adjustment to footwear. Physiotherapy, including hydrotherapy, is useful to correct or minimize other deformities.

Severe disease may be accompanied by severe pain; this is often constant being present at night and at rest, as well as on joint use. Simple analgesics may not control the pain and an NSAID may have more efficacy. In these cases the use of NSAIDs would seem to be well justified, even if there is a greater risk of side effects and of accelerated hip damage than with simple analgesics.

Surgery is indicated in most cases of severe hip OA. Significant rest or night pain, activity tolerances of less than 15–20 minutes, and any major disability or handicap are general indications. Pain which remains uncontrolled by other measures is the most pressing reason for operating. The choice of operation depends on the patient's age and circumstances, and the surgeon. In general, younger patients and those with greater demands should be considered for an uncemented prosthesis whereas the older, less active patient is suitable for a standard prosthesis such as the Charnley. Osteotomy and other operations have very little place in the modern management of hip OA.

Sexual problems are common and important in patients with severe hip OA [8]. The responsible doctor should always endeavor to explore this area by raising the topic in a 'matter-of-fact' way and giving the patient 'permission' to discuss it further if they wish. Advice on less painful ways of having intercourse can be valuable. Severe sexual problems can be an indication for surgery.

OA of the Hand

Interphalangeal joint OA

OA of the distal and proximal interphalangeal joints is an extremely common problem, most prevalent in middle-aged women [50]. It carries a relatively benign prognosis. In most cases the joints become swollen and stiff over the course of a few years, during which episodes of pain are common. They subsequently stabilize, remaining swollen and stiff, but causing little pain and only modest disability. In the majority of cases no treatment is required. Making the correct diagnosis and reassuring the patient is usually all that is required. If inflammation of the joints is marked and accompanied by a lot of pain, a course of an NSAID may be indicated. Local applications of NSAID gels or creams, or other local analgesic preparations such as capsaicin, may be an excellent alternative to tablets for this condition. Injections should be avoided as they can precipitate calcification and ankylosis of the joints [28]. Prosthetic surgery is an occasional option for an individual joint that is particularly painful and stiff.

OA of the thumb base

OA frequently affects the carpometacarpal joint or other joints at the base of the thumb, with or without coexisting interphalangeal joint disease. Pain is often a persistent problem and disease at this site can cause more disability, as well as more protracted symptoms than OA of the finger joints. Analgesics or NSAIDs may provide partial relief of pain. Local injections of a long-acting corticosteroid preparation often appear to give an excellent response that can last for months [51]. Local NSAID creams and gels and other rubefacients may also provide some relief. In severe cases, orthoses to help patients who are having trouble with pinch grip can be valuable. Surgery is also an important option, with trapezectomy or use of an artificial plastic joint 'spacer', the favored procedures.

FUTURE PROSPECTS AND EXPERIMENTAL THERAPY

Recent developments in OA have led to a number of exciting new avenues of therapeutic exploration. To date, the majority of the available therapy has been aimed at relief of symptoms and disability in established disease. The hope for the future is that the condition might be either preventable, or curable in its earlier stages.

Strategies for Prevention

Delineation of the genetic predisposition to OA has begun [52]. In addition, there is increasing understanding of the environmental risk factors [53]. This combination could lead to prevention. It is already clear, for example, that a reduction in obesity would be likely to lead to a significant reduction in the prevalence of knee OA [45].

Strategies for Effective Treatment

New agents with disease-modifying activity are being sought. A huge number of different agents are already being investigated for possible activities in OA (Fig. 13.14).

In addition, a number of pharmaceutical companies and basic science units are exploring other ways of reducing connective tissue destruction, or increasing repair. In addition to strategies such as collagenase activity inhibition with tissue inhibitor metalloproteinase (TIMP) and blockade of cytokine activities such as interleukin-1 (IL-1), a number of enzymatic, cytokine and other pathways are being explored. It seems likely that there will be many agents available for trials of possible disease-modifying activity in OA. One of the new challenges in rheumatology will be the design and execution of appropriate trials to see if these agents are effective.

In the meantime a conservative pyramidal approach to the treatment of OA is appropriate (see Fig. 13.12).

SOME OF THE AGENTS BEING INVESTIGATED FOR POSSIBLE DISEASE-MODIFYING ACTIVITY IN OA	
Estrogens	Chloroquine
Tamoxifen	Glyvenol
Growth hormones	Diacetylrhein
Protease inhibitors	Tetracyclines
Cytokine inhibitors	Diphosphonates
Superoxide dismutase	Calcitonin
Ascorbic acid	*S*-adenosyl-L-methionine

Fig. 13.14 Some of the agents which have been or are currently being investigated for possible disease-modifying activity in OA.

REFERENCES

1. Bland JH, Cooper SM. Osteoarthritis: a review of the cell biology involved and evidence for reversibility. Semin Arthritis Rheum. 1984;**14**:106–33.
2. Radin EL, Burr D. Joints can heal. Semin Arthritis Rheum. 1984;**13**:293–308.
3. Altman RD. Pain in osteoarthritis. Semin Arthritis Rheum. 1989;**18**:1–104.
4. Dieppe P, Cushnaghan J. The natural course and prognosis of osteoarthritis. In: Moskowitz R, Howell D, Goldberg V, Mankin H, eds. Osteoarthritis, 2E. Philadelphia: WB Saunders; 1992:399–412.
5. Rene J, Weinberger M, Mazzuca SA, Brandt KD, Katz BP. Reduction of joint pain in patients with knee osteoarthritis who have received monthly telephone calls from lay personnel. Arthritis Rheum. 1992;**35**:511–5.
6. Kovar PA, Allegrante JP, MacKenzie R, Peterson MGER, Gutin B, Charlson ME. Supervised fitness walking in patients with osteoarthritis of the knee. Ann Intern Med. 1992;**116**:529–34.
7. Swezey RL. Essentials of physical management and rehabilitation in arthritis. Semin Arthritis Rheum. 1974;**3**:349.
8. Currey HLF. Osteoarthritis of the hip joint and sexual activity. Ann Rheum Dis. 1970;**29**:488–91.
9. Sasaki T, Yasuda K. Clinical evaluation of the treatment of osteoarthritis of the knee using a newly designed wedge insole. Clin Orthop. 1987;**221**:181–7.
10. Hicks JE, Gerber LH. Rehabilitation in the management of patients with osteoarthritis. In: Moskowitz R, Howell D, Goldberg V, Mankin H, eds. Osteoarthritis, 2E. Philadelphia: WB Saunders; 1992:427–64.
11. McAlindon T, Dieppe P. The medical management of osteoarthritis of the knee: an inflammatory issue? Br J Rheumatol. 1990;**29**:471–3.
12. Liang MH, Fortin P. Management of osteoarthritis of the hip and knee. N Engl J Med. 1991;**325**:125–7.
13. Doherty M. Chondroprotection by non-steroidal anti-inflammatory drugs. Ann Rheum Dis. 1989;**48**:521–619.
14. Ghosh P. Anti-rheumatic drugs and cartilage. Bailliere's Clin Rheumatol. 1988;**2**:309–38.
15. Dieppe P, Cushnaghan J, Jasani MK, McCrae F, Watt I. A two year placebo controlled trial of non-steroidal anti-inflammatory therapy in osteoarthritis of the knee. Br J Rheumatol. 1993;**35**:595–600.
16. Bradley JD, Brandt KD, Katz BP, Kalasinski LA, Ryan SI. Comparison of an anti-inflammatory dose of ibuprofen, an analgesic dose of ibuprofen and acetaminophen in the treatment of patients with osteoarthritis of the knee. N Engl J Med. 1991:**325**:87–91.
17. Bird H. The current treatment of osteoarthritis. In: Russell RGG, Dieppe PA, eds. Osteoarthritis – current research and prospects for pharmacological intervention. London: IBC Technical Services Ltd; 1991.
18. Brooks PM, Potter SR, Buchanan WW. NSAID and osteoarthritis – help or hindrance? J Rheumatol. 1982;**9**:3–5.
19. Batchelor EE, Paulus HE. Principles of drug therapy. In: Moskowitz R, Howell D, Goldberg V, Mankin H, eds. Osteoarthritis, 2E. Philadelphia: WB Saunders; 1992:465–92.
20. Mazzuca SA, Brandt KD, Anderson SL, Musick BS, Matz BP. The therapeutic approaches of community based primary care physicians to OA of the hip in an elderly patient. J Rheumatol. 1991;**18**:1593–600.
21. Brandt KD. Pain, inflammation and non-steroidal anti-inflammatory drugs. In: Russell RGG, Dieppe PA, eds. Osteoarthritis – current research and prospects for pharmacological intervention. London: IBC Technical Services Ltd; 1991.
22. Newman NM, Ling RSM. Acetabular bone destruction related to nonsteroidal anti-inflammatory drugs. Lancet. 1985;**2**:11–14
23. Rashid S, Revell P, Hemingway A, Low F, Rainsford K, Walker F. Effect of non-steroidal anti-inflammatory drugs on the course of osteoarthritis. Lancet. 1989;**2**:519–22.
24. Sommerville K, Faulkner G, Langman M. Non-steroidal anti-inflammatory drugs and bleeding peptic ulcer. Lancet. 1986;**1**:462–4.
25. Norris E, Guttadauna M. Piroxicam: new dosage forms. Eur J Rheumatol Inflamm. 1987;**8**:94–104.
26. Friedman DM, Moore ME. The efficacy of intra-articular steroids in OA: a double blind study. J Rheumatol. 1980;**7**:8850–56.
27. Dieppe PA, Sathapatayavongs B, Jones HE, et al. Intra-articular steroids in osteoarthritis. Rheumatol Rehabil. 1980;**19**:212–7.
28. Gray RG, Tenenbaum J, Gottlieb NL. Local corticosteroid injection treatment in rheumatic disorders. Semin Arthritis Rheum. 1981;**10**:231–54.
29. Faher H, Rentsch HV, Gerber NJ, et al. Knee effusion and reflex inhibition of the quadriceps. J Bone Joint Surg. 1988;**70B**:635–7.
30. Gumpel JM, Roles NC. A controlled trial of intra-articular radio-colloids versus surgical synovectomy in persistent synovitis. Lancet. 1975;**i**:488–9.
31. Doherty M, Dieppe PA. Effect of intra-articular yttrium 90 (^{90}Y) on chronic pyrophosphate arthropathy (CPA) of the knee. Lancet. 1981:1243–5.
32. Burkhardt D, Ghosh P. Laboratory evaluation of antiarthritic drugs as potential chondroprotective agents. Semin Arthritis Rheum. 1987:**17**(Suppl 1):3–34.
33. Rejholec V. Long-term studies of anti-osteoarthritic drugs: an assessment. Semin Arthritis Rheum 1987:**17**(Suppl 1):3–34
34. Fife R, Brandt KD. Other approaches to therapy. In: Moskowitz R, Howell D, Goldberg V, Mankin H, eds. Osteoarthritis, 2E. Philadelphia: WB Saunders; 1992.
35. Brooks P, Ghosh P. Chondroprotection: myth or reality? Bailliere's Clin Rheumatol. 1990;**4**:293–303.
36. Smythe HA. Fibrositis syndrome: a historical perspective. J Rheumatol. 1989;**15**:2–6.
37. Deal CL, Schnitzer TJ, Lipstein E, et al. Treatment of arthritis with topical capsaicin: a double-blind trial. Clin Ther. 1991;**13**:383–95.
38. Mazieres B, Masquelier A-M, Capron M-H. A French controlled multicentre study of intra-articular orgotein versus intra-articular corticosteroids in the treatment of knee osteoarthritis: a one year follow-up. J Rheumatol. 1991;**18**:134–7.
39. Frenkel S, Williams M, Nanchahal K, Coast J. Total hip and knee joint replacement. Report 2. DHA Project: Bristol; 1990.
40. Gaw AC, Chong LW, Shaw LC. Efficacy of acupuncture on osteoarthritis pain: a controlled double-blind study. N Engl J Med. 1975;**293**:375–8.
41. Felson DT. Epidemiology of hip and knee osteoarthritis. Epidemiol Rev. 1988;**10**:1–28.
42. Clark CR, Willis LA, Stenner L, Nicholls PJR. Evaluation of physiotherapy in the treatment of knee osteoarthritis. Rheumatol Rehabil. 1974;**13**:190–7.
43. Chamberlain MA, Care C, Harfield B. Physiotherapy in osteoarthritis of the knees. Int Rehab Med. 1982;**4**:101–6.
44. Jawad ASM, Goodwill CJ. TVS brace in patients with rheumatoid arthritis or osteoarthritis of the knee. Br J Rheumatol. 1986;**25**:416–7
45. Felson DT. The epidemiology of knee osteoarthritis: results from the Framingham osteoarthritis study. Semin Arthritis Rheum. 1990;**20**:42–50.
46. Dawes PT, Kirlew C, Haslock I. Saline washout for knee OA: results of a controlled study. Clin Rheumatol. 1987;**6**:61–3.
47. Bert JM, Maschka RN. The arthroscopic treatment of unicompartmental gonarthrosis. Arthroscopy. 1989;**5**:25–32.
48. Vainropaa S, Laike E, Kirvs P, Tinsanen P. Tibial osteotomy for osteoarthritis of the knee: a five to ten year follow-up study. J Bone Joint Surg. 1981;**62**:938–46.
49. Blount WP. Don't throw away the cane. J Bone Joint Surg. 1956;**38**:695–8.
50. Bergenudd H, Lingarde F, Nilsson B. Prevalence and coincidence of degenerative changes of the hands and feet in middle age. Clin Orthop. 1989;**239**:306–10.
51. Mayer JH. Carpometacarpal osteoarthritis of the thumb. Lancet. 1970:**ii**;270.
52. Ala Kokko L, Baldwin CT, Moskowitz RW, Prokop DJ. Single base mutation in the type II procollagen gene (Col 2AI) as a cause of primary osteoarthritis associated with a mild chondrodysplasia. Proc Natl Acad Sci USA. 1990;**87**:6565–8.
53. Lane N. Exercise and osteoarthritis. Bull Rheum Dis. 1991;**41**:5–7.

OSTEOARTHRITIS

14

PRACTICAL PROBLEMS

SUDDEN WORSENING OF PAIN IN KNEE OSTEOARTHRITIS

Paul A Dieppe

Definition of the Problem

Osteoarthritis (OA) of the knee is common. Symptoms vary in different patients but are generally relatively mild, and the evolution of the disease is usually slow. However, a sudden, severe increase in pain may occur, which should alert the physician to the possibility of a number of complications, some of which require prompt action.

The Typical Case

FF is an obese 68-year-old woman, with a 14-year history of use-related pain and inactivity stiffness in the knees. Clinical and radiographic findings have been consistent with moderate, bilateral knee OA, affecting the medial tibiofemoral and patellofemoral compartments. Her general health is good, and she takes mild analgesics only.

She presented with a history of a sudden onset of severe pain in the right knee 1 week ago. There was no history of trauma. She had pain at rest and at night and was unable to bear weight on the right knee. On examination there was severe tenderness over the medial femoral condyle and all movements were painful, but the knee was cool, with only a modest effusion, and was stable. The radiographs showed no obvious changes from previous films.

The synovial fluid was clear, had a low cell count, contained no crystals on polarized light microscopy, there were no organisms and it was culture negative. Scintigraphy revealed a suspicious area on the medial femoral condyle (Fig. 14.1), confirmed as osteonecrosis on MRI.

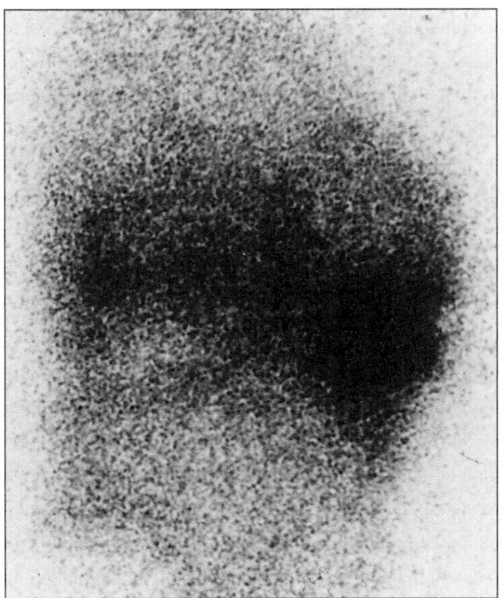

Fig. 14.1 Late-phase bone scan showing marked retention of isotope on both sides of the medial joint line, later confirmed as osteonecrosis on MRI.

Bed rest with static quadriceps exercises was followed by 6 weeks of nonweight-bearing (using crutches), and further quadriceps exercises, and then a gradual return to normal activity. Radiography 6 months later showed the typical flattening of the condyle but no significant bony collapse (Fig. 14.2). Symptoms are again controllable with analgesics alone, and the patient is fully active.

Steps in the Differential Diagnosis

Inflammatory or mechanical?

Sudden flares of knee OA can be caused by inflammation, typically a crystal-related synovitis. The effusion may be relatively small and 'cool', but a tight, warm knee is usual if pain is severe. A systemic reaction can occur. A drop of synovial fluid should be withdrawn and immediately examined for crystals and infections by well-trained, well-equipped observers. This will also exclude a hemarthrosis, which may complicate pseudogout or may occur alone.

Bony or soft tissue?

Disruption of soft tissue components of the joint can cause sudden increases in pain. Ligament ruptures, with consequent instability, can occur, and disruption and extrusion of the menisci is a common finding in knee OA. Anserine bursitis may produce local tenderness and pain, but rarely results in severe problems. Posterior joint rupture and other soft tissue problems also result in local tenderness and other characteristic physical signs. Physical examination should lead to the correct diagnosis, and examinations under anesthesia are rarely necessary.

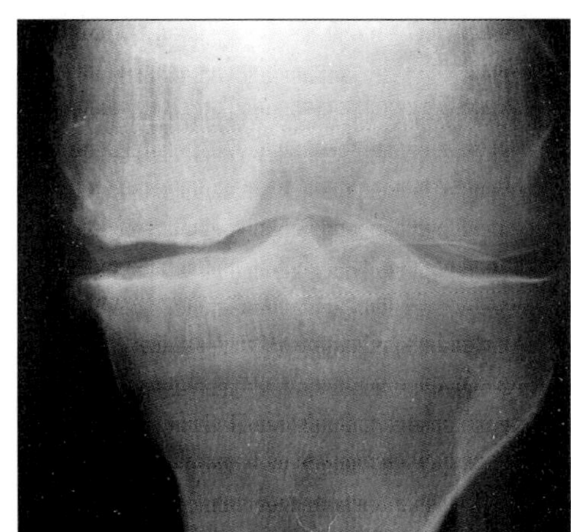

Fig. 14.2 Radiograph taken 1 year after presentation, showing a healed defect in the medial femoral condyle with sclerotic margins. Note the associated development of chondrocalcinosis and osteoarthritis.

What type of bony problem?

Several problems can arise in the subchondral bone, including stress fractures of the tibia, small trabecular fractures of subchondral bone, and osteonecrosis of either the medial femoral condyle (most commonly) or the tibial component (rarely). All of these complications may be invisible on plane radiographs in their early stages.

Bone scintigraphy may show evidence of fractures or indicate an area of abnormal perfusion in osteonecrosis. Magnetic resonance images are a very sensitive way of detecting osteonecrosis.

Obese middle-aged women are in the risk group for osteonecrosis, and a clinical picture of sudden severe pain at rest, made worse by weight-bearing, suggests this possibility.

Management

A period of nonweight-bearing may reduce the risk of femoral condyle collapse, and delay or prevent the need for a knee replacement or corrective osteotomy in the future. How long the patient should be nonweight-bearing and how much one should allow the patient to do at this stage is debatable. The value of bone decompression has not been established, and the place of surgery is unclear.

A period of rest with static quadriceps exercises only for 1 week is recommended, followed by ambulation on crutches to keep all weight off the knee for a further period of 6 weeks, by which time pain has usually subsided. This is followed by a graduated return to normal activity. Quadriceps exercises are maintained throughout.

Conclusions

Sudden increase in knee pain in patients with OA should be investigated promptly. It is particularly important to exclude osteonecrosis, which may be negative on radiographs in the early stage. Prompt treatment can prevent subsequent collapse of bone. This condition can occur spontaneously in patients with no preceding joint disease as well as in those with OA, and the diagnosis is often missed in the cure stage.

REFERENCES

Bauer CCI. Osteonecrosis of the knee. Clin Orthop Rel Res. 1978;**130**:210–17.

Lotke PA, Eker M, Alvi A. Painful knees in older patients. J Bone Joint Surg. 1977;**59A**:617–61.

INFLAMMATORY OSTEOARTHRITIS

Paul A Dieppe

Definition of the Problem

Osteoarthritis of the hand often presents relatively acutely in middle aged women, with evidence of inflammation in the affected joints. It may mimic an inflammatory arthropathy such as rheumatoid arthritis (RA) in its early stages. This diagnostic problem often causes confusion, and may lead to the use of inappropriate and dangerous medication.

The Typical Case

A 53-year-old lady presented to her primary care physician complaining of pain, stiffness and swelling of the joints of both hands. She was having trouble with her rings. The symptoms had started some 4 weeks prior to her presentation, and had got steadily worse during that time period. On examination she was noted to have firm swellings of the proximal interphalangeal (PIP) joints of both hands (Fig. 14.3), with some dusky redness over their dorsal surfaces. They were tender over the joint margins. No abnormality of the distal interphalangeal (DIP) joints was apparent, and the examination was otherwise unremarkable.

All blood tests were normal, including a normal erythrocyte sedimentation rate (ESR) and a negative test for rheumatoid factor. A presumptive diagnosis of an inflammatory polyarthritis, possibly early rheumatoid arthritis, was made, and the patient was given a course of a nonsteroidal anti-inflammatory drug (NSAID).The patient responded poorly to the drug, and appeared to have more pronounced changes in the joints when seen subsequently. By then it was apparent that the patient had nodal OA of the hands, as firm swellings of two DIP joints had appeared, and one of these developed a cyst, from which a thick, clear 'jelly' was aspirated. It took a lot of careful counseling to help the patient understand that she did not have RA, and that her condition was not going to be a crippling one.

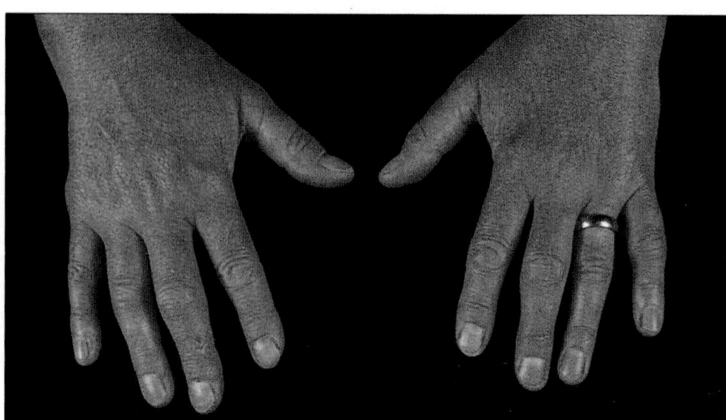

Fig. 14.3 Inflammatory osteoarthritis. Mild symmetric swellings of the PIPs at presentation.

The case subsequently evolved into one of 'erosive' interphalangeal joint OA (Fig. 14.4).

The Diagnostic Problem

Inflammatory polyarthritis or inflammatory osteoarthritis?

Perimenopausal women with a family history of arthritis are at risk of developing a number of arthropathies, including both OA and RA. Osteoarthritis usually affects a few DIP joints, rather than symmetric involvement of the proximal row, helping the differential diagnosis. However, OA can begin in the PIP joints. The absence of any signs or symptoms in the wrist, metacarpophalangeal or metatarsophalangeal joints should raise the suspicion that RA is not present, but the differential diagnosis can be difficult. Similarly, the absence of any positive tests should alert the physician to an atypical onset of interphalangeal OA. Although tests can be negative in the early stages of RA, some evidence of an acute-phase response, and some radiographic evidence of periarticular osteoporosis of affected joints is ususal. In contrast, normal tests are to be expected in OA, the early swelling of joints probably reflecting 'chondrophyte' formation at the joint margins; it is also difficult to detect on the radiograph.

Cases like the one described illustrate the need to wait for the diagnosis to reveal itself in cases of early polyarthritis when there is no clear diagnostic picture on clinical and laboratory evidence, and in the absence of obvious joint damage.

Erosive polyarthritis or erosive osteoarthritis?

Problems can also arise much later in the evolution of the disease. Some patients with interphalangeal OA develop erosions. Comparative studies have shown no great differences between such cases and others with nonerosive hand OA, except in disease severity. However, the appearance and reporting of 'erosions' – a charged term in rheumatology – can lead to the wrong diagnosis and errors of treatment of the sort that occured in the case illustrated. This need

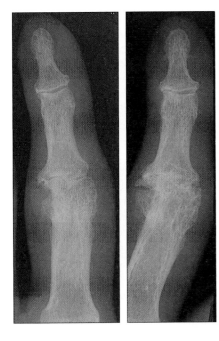

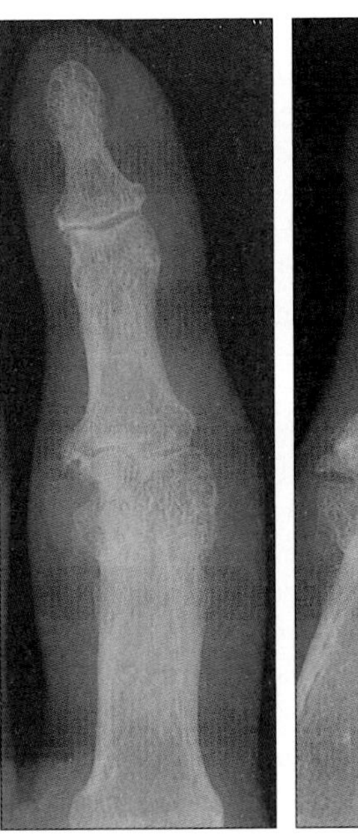

Fig. 14.4 Inflammatory osteoarthritis. Radiograph showing progression of disease, with the development of joint space narrowing, subchondral sclerosis and osteophytes (left) and subsequent typically erosive osteoarthritis (right).

not happen. The erosions of OA are quite different from those of RA or the seronegative spondyloarthropathies. The former occur in the central part of the articulating surface, rather than at the joint margin, and there is no associated osteoporosis or new bone growth, except for the marginal osteophytes of OA (see Fig. 14.4). Furthermore, the erosions of OA generally heal with time, and occasionally the joints fuse.

The Therapeutic Problem

The patient described was damaged in two ways by a misdiagnosis. Firstly, she suffered from bone marrow damage from sulfasalazine, a life-threatening event. Although this is extremely rare, there is always some risk accompanying the use of such agents in polyarthritis; they have not been shown to be of any value in interphalangeal joint OA, and should not be used when the diagnosis is in doubt. Secondly, this patient underwent a great deal of unnecessary psychological trauma from being told that she had RA.

Better management, while awaiting disease evolution to reveal the diagnosis, is to avoid a diagnostic label, or use the concept of 'polyarthritis', and to keep the therapy for pain and stiffness of the fingers as simple as possible. This may include the use of topical agents to rub onto the joints, as well as advice about how to keep the hands as supple as possible, by doing exercises in warm water for example.

Similar therapeutic errors can occur later in the disease evolution, when an erosive OA is misdiagnosed as RA.

Conclusions

- In cases of undiagnosed polyarthritis of the hands, one should await disease evolution, allowing a firm diagnosis to be made, before starting patients on potentially hazardous medication.
- Interphalangeal joint OA is frequently misdiagnosed as RA or psoriatic arthropathy. This can occur early in the condition, because of prominent clinical signs of inflammation, or later in the disease evolution, because of the appearance of erosions. Familiarity with the clinical, serologic and radiographic features of erosive OA should allow one to avoid this mistake.

REFERENCES

Bradley JD, Brandt KD, Katz BP, Kalanski LA, Ryan SI. Treatment of knee osteoarthritis: relationship of clinical features of joint inflammation to the response to a nonsteroidal anti-inflammatory drug or pure analgesic. J Rheumatol. 1992;**19**:1950–5.

Crain DC. Interphalangeal osteoarthritis characterised by painful anti-inflammatory episodes leading to deformity of the proximal and distal articulations. JAMA. 1961;**175**:1049–53.

Ehrlich GE. Inflammatory osteoarthritis. I. The clinical syndrome. J Chron Dis. 1972;**25**:317–28.

Kellgren JH, Moore R. Generalised osteoarthritis and Heberden's nodes. Br Med J. 1952;**1**:181–7.

DRUGS IN OSTEOARTHRITIS: TREATING THE ELDERLY PATIENT

Paul Creamer

Definition of the problem

Osteoarthritis is common, especially in the elderly. Such patients frequently have intercurrent medical problems that affect treatment options for their OA.

The Typical Case

Mrs BL is a 72-year-old lady with a 10-year history of painful knees. She was able to walk 100 yards but had to give up playing bowls and could no longer exercise her dog. She was occasionally woken at night by pain. She has a previous medical history of mild congestive cardiac failure, for which she takes diuretics (furosemide and amiloride), and type II diabetes, treated with glibenclamide. Ten years previously she had a duodenal ulcer diagnosed on endoscopy, following abdominal pain and indigestion; she is now symptom free. She was known to have mild renal impairment with a serum creatinine of 1.7mg/dl (150μmol/l) and, urea of 33.5mg/dl (12.0mmol/l).

Examination revealed bilateral osteoarthritic knees with quadriceps wasting and small effusions. Radiography confirmed moderate medial compartment and patellofemoral OA.

Her family practitioner had started treatment with simple analgesia, but symptoms persisted. Because of the renal failure and history of congestive heart failure, one of the most widely used classes of drugs for treatment of OA (NSAIDs) was relatively contraindicated. However, in view of the failure of simple analgesics, it was decided that a trial of an NSAID together with prophylactic anti-ulcer therapy was appropriate.

Therapeutic Problems

The fact that many patients are elderly in itself presents some therapeutic problems. The incidence of adverse drug reactions is increased in the elderly, as is the potential for medication errors. The elderly have more illnesses and take more intercurrent medication, including over-the-counter preparations; the potential for drug interactions is therefore increased.

The pain of advanced OA is always difficult to treat, and contraindications to NSAIDs compound the problem.

The most significant side effects of NSAIDs are gastrointestinal and renal, both mediated through inhibition of prostaglandin synthesis. NSAIDs are associated with a high incidence of acute gastric erosions, though the relation of such changes to more clinically relevant complications is uncertain. The elderly, particularly females, have an increased risk of ulceration, bleeding and perforation, and adverse reactions are more likely to be serious or fatal. Previous peptic ulceration constitutes another risk factor.

The effect of NSAIDs on the kidney is usually a reversible fall in renal function, though progression to acute renal failure is recognized. This may occur when circulating levels of angiotensin II are raised, resulting in renal vasoconstriction. In this situation, vasodilatory prostaglandins (PGE_2, prostacyclin) become essential to maintenance of adequate renal function. Inhibition of cyclo-oxygenase can then result in a catastrophic fall in renal blood flow and glomerular filtration rate. Risk factors include heart failure with reduced cardiac output, hepatic disease, diuretic-induced volume depletion and pre-existing renal disease.

Other NSAID side effects on the kidney, including interstitial nephritis and hyperkalemia, are also more common in the elderly.

Therapeutic Options

Nonpharmacologic treatments should be attempted first. Exercise programs, specifically quadriceps exercises, may improve walking time and decrease pain. Local treatments, including heat, cold and ultrasound, are widely used and some patients derive benefit from such measures. Hydrotherapy may be helpful, especially in hip disease. A walking aid can be supplied and suitable footwear, including insoles, given with the aim of reducing impact forces and reducing load through painful joints. Leg-length inequality can be corrected with suitable heel raises. Simple adjustments to the home may make a large difference to the patient's quality of life.

Simple analgesics should be the first-line drug therapy. Paracetamol is safe but may not be sufficiently potent. Compound preparations, including dextropropoxyphene or codeine phosphate with paracetamol, are often helpful. Major side effects include central nervous system depression and constipation; these may limit use in the elderly.

Given transcutaneously, NSAIDs are safe and well tolerated and appear to act as more than simple rubefacients. They also permit a degree of control by the patient over their disease.

Intra-articular injection of corticosteroid often produces symptomatic relief, though part of this effect may be placebo or related to removal of synovial fluid. It is a procedure with remarkably few complications, and even repeated injections do not seem to be detrimental. Patients may benefit from intra-articular corticosteroids prior to a course of physiotherapy. Other intra-articular therapies such as radiosynovectomy (e.g. yttrium-90) may help, particularly if persistent, large effusions are present.

All the foregoing should be attempted before considering use of NSAIDs. It should also be remembered that evidence for a superior effect of NSAIDs over analgesics in OA is largely lacking. They have potentially dangerous side effects even though, statistically, the chance of a major problem is small: perhaps only 1 in 6000 NSAID prescriptions result in a major gastrointestinal bleed in the elderly.

AN APPROACH TO THE MANAGEMENT OF OSTEOARTHRITIS IN THE ELDERLY
Initial approaches
• Physiotherapy and exercise • Local treatments: heat, cold and ultrasound • Analgesics • Aids to daily living • Intra-articular corticosteroid • Topical nonsteroidal anti-inflammatory drug (NSAID)
If initial approaches fail
• Trial of NSAID: Consider prophylaxis with misoprostil (800mg/day) or ranitidine (150mg b.i.d.) Check renal function at 7–10 days Endoscopy if gastrointestinal symptoms persist • Consider surgery

Fig.14.5 An approach to the mangement of osteoarthritis in the elderly.

There is little to suggest that one NSAID is preferable to another; in general, the less expensive, older drugs should be used first. Azapropazone may enhance the antidiabetic effect of sulfonylureas; indomethacin may be poorly tolerated in the elderly. General principles should include using the smallest effective dose and titrating gradually against symptom relief, regularly re-assessing for beneficial effect. 'Intelligent non-compliance' should be encouraged: if the patient can manage on a lower or less frequent dose than that prescribed she should be allowed to do so. Patients should be reminded to report any side effects, particularly indigestion.

Data to support rational use is limited because dyspepsia is common with NSAIDs and is often not related to ulceration, while bleeding or perforating ulcers are often painless. Acute erosions are common but often heal. In terms of gastrointestinal safety, no one drug is clearly better than others. There are theoretical reasons why a prodrug (nabumetone, fenbufen) are preferable, however. Similarly, there are no convincing data on renal side effects; it has been suggested that sulindac does not impair renal function, but these findings have not been confirmed.

For an elderly patient with proven previous peptic ulceration, use of an NSAID should be combined with prophylactic anti-ulcer treatment. Options include the prostaglandin analogue misoprostil or the H_2-blockers ranitidine or cimetidine. Misoprostil has a beneficial effect on the gastric as well as the duodenal mucosa and has the potential to protect against small-bowel NSAID enteropathy. If dyspeptic symptoms recur on this combination then, ideally, the patient should undergo endoscopy. If an ulcer is found, the NSAID should be stopped and standard anti-ulcer therapy given. If endoscopy is normal and the NSAID is helping symptoms, it may be continued, perhaps with simple antacids as an additional measure. If endoscopy is impractical, gastric pathology should be assumed to exist and the NSAID stopped.

Renal function and serum potassium should be checked 7–10 days after starting NSAID therapy. Deteriorating renal function is an indication to cease NSAIDs.

Conclusions

Elderly patients with OA and intercurrent medical problems are seen frequently in rheumatologic practice. There are many approaches to tackling the pain, all of which should be attempted before considering NSAIDs. Undoubtedly some patients do benefit from NSAIDs and, if all else has failed, they may warrant a trial. The decision to treat with these potentially harmful drugs should be constantly reviewed.

The approach to managment of OA in the elderly is summarized in Figure 14.5.

REFERENCES

Beardon PHG, Brown SV, McDevitt DG. Gastro-intestinal events in patients prescribed non-steroidal anti-inflammatory drugs: a controlled study using record linkage. Tayside Q J Med. 1989;**266**:497–505

Doogan P. Topical non-steroidal anti-inflammatory drugs. Lancet. 1989;**ii**:1270–1

Hopkinson N, Doherty M. NSAID-associated gastropathy – a role for misoprostil? Br J Rheumatol. 1990;**29**:133–6

Which NSAID? Drug Ther Bull. 1987;**25**:81–4.

RHEUMATOID ARTHRITIS

CLINICAL FEATURES OF RHEUMATOID ARTHRITIS: EARLY, PROGRESSIVE AND LATE DISEASE

15

Duncan A Gordon
& David E Hastings

INTRODUCTION

Rheumatoid arthritis (RA) is a disease that affects at least twice as many women as men. Although it may begin at any age its peak onset is in the fourth and fifth decades of life, rising sharply with age thereafter. The onset of RA appears to be more frequent in the winter than the summer months [1,2]. Its diagnosis is compatible with a variety of presentations and a clinical course that can last from a few weeks or months of discomfort to many years of profound disability. Although diagnostic criteria [3,4] may be helpful in diagnosis, in a given case they may not be definitive since the diagnosis may only become obvious with the passage of time.

Although we know a good deal about the epidemiology and immunologic and genetic aspects of RA, it is a sporadic condition of unknown cause and we have no idea what initiates or perpetuates the process. Until the cause of RA becomes known it cannot be precisely defined. It may be one disease with more than one cause or more than one disease with a single cause. At present, RA is best defined by a clinical description such as the 1987 criteria of the American Rheumatism Association (ARA) (Fig. 15.1) [3].

These criteria were presented in two forms, a traditional one (see Fig. 15.1) and a classification tree (Fig. 15.2). In the first, a patient fulfilling four of seven criteria is said to have RA. In the second scheme criteria 1 and 5 were deleted so that arthritis of three or more joints for 6 weeks or more with radiographic joint erosions or the presence of rheumatoid factor meets criteria for the diagnosis of RA. The entire criteria set strongly separates patients with RA from those with other conditions. Moreover, unlike the previous 1958 criteria the classification tree format shows better accuracy in patients with disease duration of one year or less [3,4]. These new criteria include objective features seen in a majority of patients with RA, but unlike the former set there are no exclusions [3,4].

When faced with a patient with polyarthritis, many other conditions resembling RA must be kept in mind. Moreover, it is important

AMERICAN RHEUMATISM ASSOCIATION REVISED CRITERIA FOR RHEUMATOID ARTHRITIS CLASSIFICATION

Criterion	Definition
1. Morning stiffness	Morning stiffness in and around the joints, lasting at least 1 hour before maximal improvement
2. Arthritis of 3 or more joint areas	At least 3 joint areas (out of 14 possible areas: right or left PIP, MCP, wrist, elbow, knee, ankle, MTP joints) simultaneously have had soft-tissue swelling or fluid (not bony overgrowth alone) as observed by a physician
3. Arthritis of hand joints	At least one area swollen (as defined above) in a wrist, MCP or PIP joint
4. Symmetric arthritis	Simultaneous involvement of the same joint areas (as defined in 2) on both sides of the body (bilateral involvement of PIPs, MCPs or MTPs, without absolute symmetry is acceptable)
5. Rheumatoid nodules	Subcutaneous nodules over bony prominences or extensor surfaces, or in juxta-articular regions as observed by a physician
6. Serum rheumatoid factor	Demonstration of abnormal amounts of serum rheumatoid factor by any method for which the result has been positive in less than 5% of normal control subjects
7. Radiographic changes	Radiographic changes typical of rheumatoid arthritis on posteroanterior hand and wrist radiographs, which must include erosions or unequivocal bony decalcification localized in, or most marked adjacent to, the involved joints (osteoarthritis changes alone do not qualify)

Note: For classification purposes, a patient has RA if at least 4 of these criteria are satisfied (criteria 1–4 must have been present for at least 6 weeks)

Fig. 15.1 The 1987 American Rheumatism Association revised criteria for the classification of RA [3]. If at least four of these criteria are satisfied (1–4 for at least 6 weeks), the patient has RA. Patients should not be designated as having classic definite or probable RA.

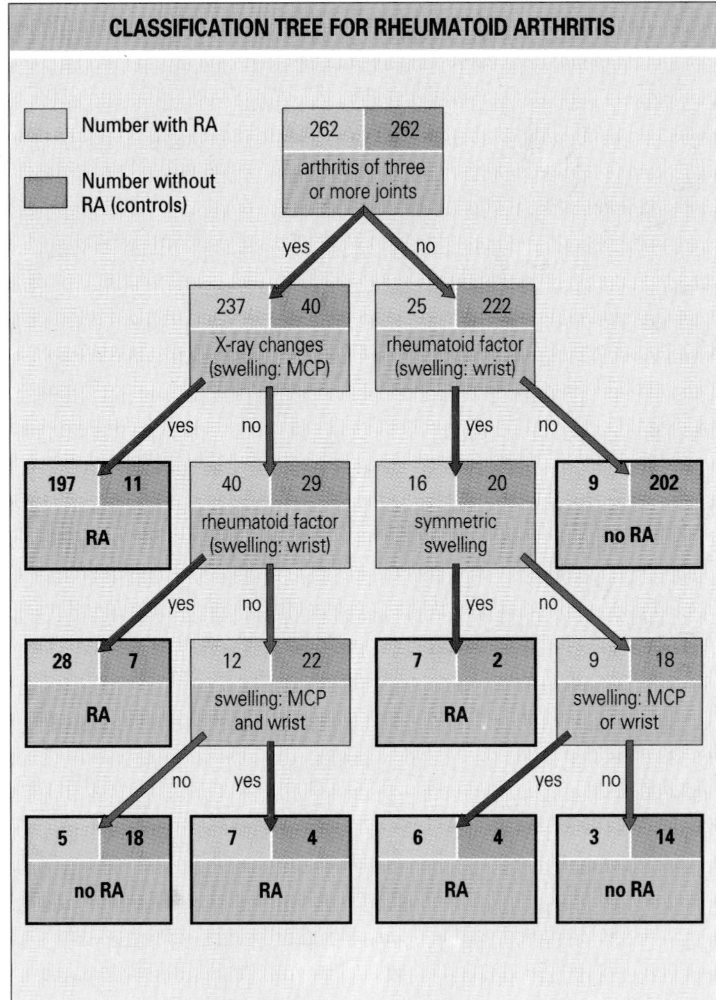

Fig. 15.2 A modified classification tree for RA [3]. The clinical criteria must have been observed by a physician and been present for at least 6 weeks. Subjects can be classified as having or as not having RA (no RA). In parentheses are indicated surrogate variables that can be used when another variable (radiograph or rheumatoid factor test result) is not available.

CLINICAL EVALUATION OF RHEUMATOID ARTHRITIS – HISTORY OF PRESENT ILLNESS
Chronological account of illness from the onset
Onset: acute or gradual, with details
Location of pain (local or referred): precise anatomy, presence/absence of swelling
Pattern of joint involvement: axial, peripheral, symmetrical
Type of pain: quality and character
Severity: pain threshold effects, interference with activities of daily living, range of joint movement
Radiation of pain: local or deep referred type
Clinical course: duration, frequency, periodicity, persistence
Modifying factors: aggravating, relieving, medication effects
Associated symptoms: fatigue, other systemic symptoms
Duration of morning stiffness: nonrestorative sleep pattern
Present status: regional review of joints, extra-articular features, functional class, activities of daily living, psychological state

Fig. 15.3 Clinical evaluation of RA: details required from the history of present illness [5].

to distinguish such disorders from RA as soon as possible, because the correct diagnosis of RA is fundamental to the application of good management (see Chapter 17).

CLINICAL EVALUATION

A careful clinical evaluation is the first step towards winning the patient's confidence and cooperation. And it is the most important step in the successful management of RA [5].

History

Making a diagnosis of RA depends on an accurate description of the patient's illness, obtained from a careful history (Fig. 15.3). Success in this endeavor requires effective communication with the patient and family, and this takes time. Diffuse symmetrical joint pain and swelling affecting the small peripheral joints are the commonest presenting symptoms. These symptoms are often associated with difficulty making a fist and morning stiffness of variable duration.

A history of non-restorative sleep pattern may be informative in understanding the patient's morning stiffness and other diffuse aching. The symptoms should be interpreted in terms of the patient's functional ability to perform self-care and other daily home, work or sports activities (Fig. 15.4). It must be remembered that RA affects the patient's body as a whole, not just the articular system, and invariably has an impact on every aspect of the patient's physical and psychosocial life. In men (or the elderly), the disease may pursue a much more severe course [6,7]. RA in teenage girls may also show an adverse course.

A history of RA in other members of the family should trigger suspicion of hereditary influences and heighten suspicion that the patient's symptoms could be an expression of early RA. It can be the case, however, that this knowledge has heightened the patient's anxiety about the symptoms, regardless of whether RA is the correct diagnosis.

It might be assumed that anxiety and depression would correlate with continuing disease activity, but it appears that socioeconomic factors may be greater determinants of depression than physical factors [8,9]. In other instances, patients who exhibit increased diffuse pain at a time when they exhibit decreased joint activity may show features of fibromyalgia, which explain this paradoxical reaction [10,11]. The role of physical trauma as a cause of RA is unproven, but physical trauma in someone with RA may be a significant aggravating factor delaying recovery. A history of psychological trauma or stress preceding the onset of RA should be sought, although the relevance of psychological factors in the cause of RA is uncertain. A retrospective study of a group of twins discordant for RA examined this aspect of their disease [12]. In each case the twin affected by arthritis had a background of psychological entrapment not seen in the unaffected twin.

Hormones have an important influence in women with RA. The manifestations of RA subside in about 70% of women during pregnancy and recur in the early postpartum period [13]. A decreased risk of RA has been reported in women with previous pregnancies [14] and a reduced incidence in women taking oral contraceptives [15]. Postmenopausal use of estrogen replacement therapy may protect against the subsequent development of RA [16]. It appears paradoxical that although women are more prone to RA, female hormones may modify its severity. Thus, hormones seem to affect severity of disease more than its frequency. Moreover, there is evidence that the incidence of new cases of RA in women has been falling in recent decades [17, 18].

The patient's educational background and occupation may affect management and outcome and should be carefully documented. Notwithstanding genetic and sex factors, patients with more years of education seem to develop less severe disease [19]. Current cigarette smokers may be at increased risk of RA, and miners exposed to mineral dusts may be at risk not only of RA [20] but also, once it has developed, at increased risk of developing associated pneumonoconiosis, Caplan's syndrome [21], through the inhalation of dust. Persons whose occupations are associated with less physical stress, however, show a better functional outcome.

Functional Disability Indices

A number of self-report questionnaires, such as the Stanford Health Assessment Questionnaire (HAQ), Functional Disability Index (FDI), Arthritis Impact Measurement Scales (AIMS), and modifications of these, have been developed for ongoing evaluation of patients with RA (Fig. 15.5) [22–25]. These provide clinically useful information not available by conventional means. They can be used to document the patient's functional status with results similar to many traditional measures of RA activity, including joint-count score, radiographic score, sedimentation rate and walking time. It is questionable, however, whether they can reliably assess problems of anxiety or depression in the patient with RA [25]. The value of these scales is attested by many rheumatologists who have incorporated them into their practice routines. Basic demographic variables are also part of this documentation.

CLINICAL EVALUATION OF RHEUMATOID ARTHRITIS – FUNCTIONAL CAPACITY AND ACTIVITIES OF DAILY LIVING
Classification of functional capacity
Normal function without or despite symptoms
Some disability, but adequate for normal activity without special devices or assistance
Activities restricted, requires special devices or personal assistance
Totally dependent
Classification of activities of daily living
Mobility: walking, climbing, use of transport, bed–chair transfers
Personal care: eating, dressing, washing, grooming, use of toilet
Special hand functions: door handles, keys, coins, jar tops, carrying, pen, scissors
Work and play activities: work outside home, light and heavy work in house, hobbies, sports

Fig. 15.4 Clinical evaluation: functional capacity and activities of daily living [5].

SELF-REPORT QUESTIONNAIRE FOR RHEUMATOID ARTHRITIS				
Please check (✓) the ONE best answer for your abilities.				
At this moment, are you able to:	Without any difficulty	With some difficulty	With much difficulty	Unable to do
a. Dress yourself, including tying shoelaces and doing buttons?				
b. Get in and out of bed?				
c. Lift a full cup or glass to your mouth?				
d. Walk outdoors on flat ground?				
e. Wash and dry your entire body?				
f. Bend down to pick up clothing from the floor?				
g. Turn regular faucets (taps) on and off?				
h. Get in and out of a car?				

Fig. 15.5 Self-report questionnaire for RA. The questionnaire is used to assess quantitatively the functional capacity of the patient to carry out the tasks of daily living. [24].

Examination

As RA is a systemic condition, the clinical evaluation should include a complete physical examination that also documents the presence or absence of a number of extra-articular features. These include subcutaneous nodules, digital vasculitis and the other systemic features described in Chapter 16. Any one of these may be mistaken for a nonrheumatoid condition and their presence indicates a more ominous form of the disease [6]. Various systemic features may also be the result of an adverse drug reaction. The joints shown in Figure 15.6 should be examined systematically, as described in the next three sections of this chapter, to determine which ones are inflamed or damaged [5]. The pattern of joint involvement, whether symmetrical, axial or peripheral, should be recorded.

JOINT INFLAMMATION

The key signs of joint inflammation in RA are those of tenderness and swelling. These may be associated with local heat, but erythema is not a feature of rheumatoid inflammation. Heat and erythema may be seen with coincidental septic or gouty arthritis, however.

A joint is considered 'active' if it is tender on pressure or painful on passive movement with stress and/or swelling other than bony proliferation. The presence/absence of pain and swelling are recorded separately. Joint swelling may be periarticular or intra-articular. Intra-articular swelling is associated with the detection of a joint effusion, described below.

A diagram depicting the joints (Fig. 15.6) may be used at each assessment to record signs of disease activity or tender joint count. Joint effusions are recorded separately, because although the presence of an effusion usually indicates inflammation, this is not always the case. In any event, if fluid is detected the matter can be settled by aspirating and examining it to see whether leukocytosis or other signs of rheumatoid joint inflammation are present. At this juncture it is useful to mention the distinction between a tender 'joint count' and a tender 'point count'. Patients with RA or fibromyalgia may have widespread pain, and sometimes both conditions coexist. In the case of RA, however, tenderness is related to one or more joints specifically, whereas fibromyalgia is defined as present in a patient if 11 or more of 18 specific tender point sites are found that are not articular. It is also helpful to use a diagram to record tender points. The number of minutes of morning stiffness and measurements of grip strength using a blood-pressure cuff manometer are other commonly used indices of disease activity.

Tenderness

This is elicited by direct palpation pressure over the joint. Firmer pressure on the tissues between or remote from the joints should not be tender with the exception of the fibrositic tender points (see above). Testing for joint tenderness is particularly useful for detecting disease activity in wrist, finger and toe joints. Pain during the arc of movement however may be due to bare bone rubbing on bare bone from loss of articular cartilage, and is not a reliable indication of the presence of inflammation. For this reason, the hips should be excluded from the routine simple joint count.

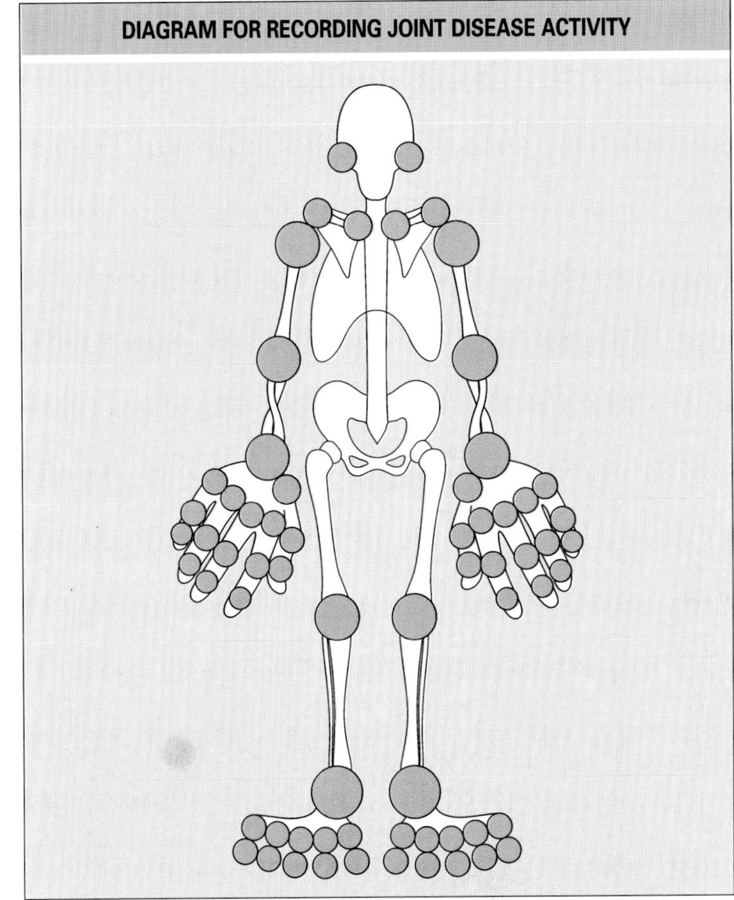

Fig. 15.6 Pictorial method for indicating joint disease activity or destruction. The figure may be used on a printed form or rubber stamp to chart which joints are active or deformed at the time of each assessment. The joints circled here should always be assessed.

Stress Pain

Stress pain is produced when a joint at the limit of its range of movement is nudged a little further. It is an especially useful symptom in the shoulder (limit of internal and external rotation), wrists, metacarpophalangeals, and joints in the ankle region. To determine how hard to press in testing for stress pain, the general level of tenderness can be assessed by squeezing control sites in the midtrapezius and lower calf, and by pressing over manubrium, metacarpals and proximal phalanges. Pressure on joints should be about 20% less than that required to reach the pain threshold over the control sites. When in doubt, it is best to record the joint as inactive.

Synovial Effusion

The most reliable general sign of a synovial effusion is the demonstration of fluctuation: the hydraulic effect of an increase in fluid tension produced by pressure in one direction is transmitted equally in all three planes (Fig. 15.7). This is the four-finger technique – relatively easy to learn, but applicable only when the joint can be surrounded. For most joints, a two-finger or two-thumb technique must be used, one pressing downward, the other feeling an upward lift. These techniques can be practiced on a slightly softened grape. In the latter technique, the direction of pressure should differ slightly from the sensor finger to prevent false-positive scorings due to lateral shifts of fat or tendons. Fat, being fluid at body temperature, may fluctuate. If it is subcutaneous, it can be pinched up in a way impossible with effusions; if deep, it is rarely exactly coextensive with the synovial space. Muscle will also fluctuate across the direction of the fibers, but not parallel with them. In the knee joint, the 'bulge' sign (Fig. 15.8) is a sensitive and dramatic indication of a small effusion. The pouch of synovium medial to the patella is emptied of fluid by a gentle upward stroke, and refilled by a downward stroke on the lateral side. Similarly, a sudden bulge can be detected when a mildly affected elbow is gently moved to 90° of extension.

JOINT DAMAGE AND DESTRUCTION

Joint destruction may be assessed clinically or radiologically (Fig. 15.9). Common clinical observations associated with joint disruption include a reduction in the range of movement, collateral instability, malalignment, subluxation or loss of articular cartilage causing bone-on-bone crepitus. No simple method of describing these often complicated changes has yet achieved international acceptance. A separate, simple count of damaged joints is recommended.

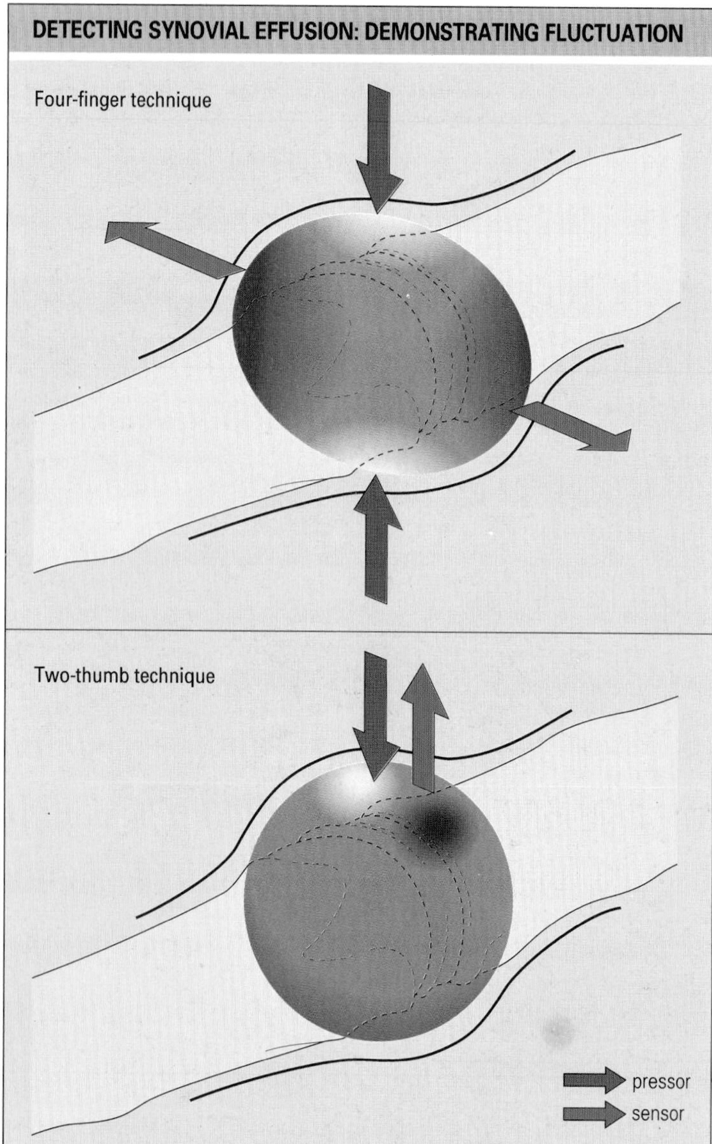

Fig. 15.7 Demonstration of fluctuation for the detection of a synovial effusion. An increase in fluid tension induced by finger pressure in one area is transmitted so that the sensor finger(s) can detect it elsewhere. In the two-thumb (or two-finger) technique the pressure should be in a slightly different direction to the sensor finger, to avoid false positive results.

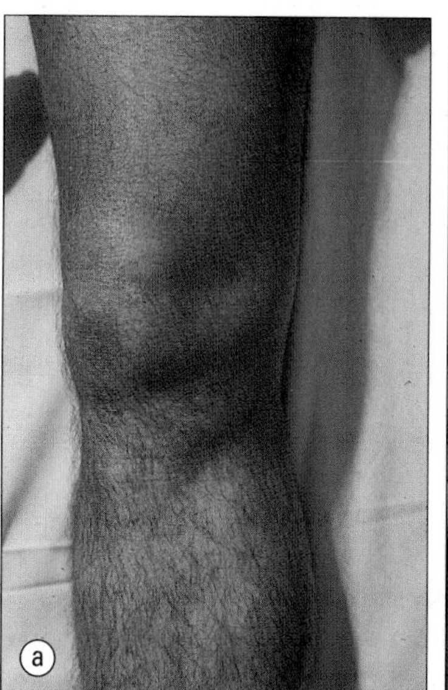

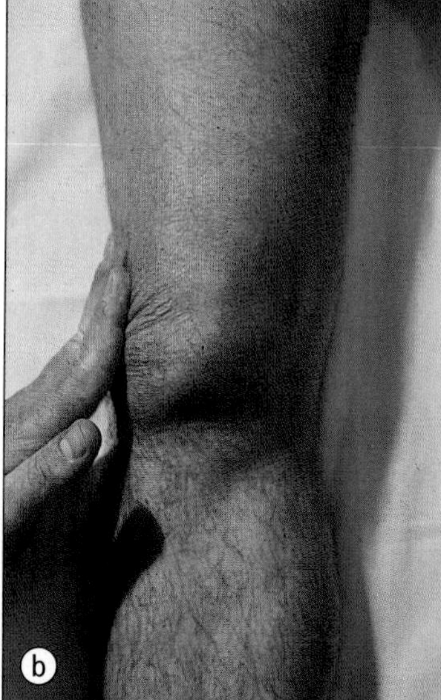

Fig. 15.8 The fluid 'bulge' sign for the demonstration of small synovial effusions of the knee. Anterior view of the relaxed right knee in a recumbent position. A gentle upward stroke with the palm of the examiner's right hand depresses the medial synovial pouch (a). A downward stoke with the palm of the examiner's left had is then followed by the appearance of a synovial fluid bulge in the previously depressed area (b).

CLINICAL EVALUATION OF RHEUMATOID ARTHRITIS - EXAMINATION
Extra-articular features
Record presence of nodules, Raynaud's phenomenon, digital infarcts, episcleritis, peripheral neuropathy, palmar erythema, leg ulcers
Note tendon sheath involvement, or tendon nodules, subluxation or rupture
Check for anemia, splenomegaly, leukopenia, pleuritis or pericarditis, the sicca syndrome or renal involvement
Articular: measures of inflammatory activity
Check for tenderness, stress pain, synovial effusion, grip strength and duration of morning stiffness
Articular: measures of destruction and deformity
Check for lax collaterals, subluxation, malalignment, metatarsal prolapse, hammer toes and bone-on-bone crepitus

Fig. 15.9 Clinical evaluation of RA examination [5].

The information obtained from clinical evaluation will reveal which joint structures are affected by inflammation, which are damaged and to what extent function is impaired. Nevertheless, even with training, standardization and refinement of these methods, a good deal of interobserver variability exists when they are applied to clinical trials [26]. For this reason, it is a customary requirement for trials that sequential measurements in the same patient should be performed by the same examiner.

After the foregoing baseline evaluations have been accomplished, the diagnosis of RA can usually be confirmed and the patient can be categorized as having early, progressive or late disease.

Early Disease

This describes patients who as yet exhibit no clinical evidence of joint damage or radiologic signs of cartilage loss or bone erosion. Our use of the term 'early disease' is synonymous with 'mild disease' activity. It is not meant to have any particular prognostic significance. Although it is unpredictable whether patients with early disease will eventually run a benign or malignant course, most exhibit an intermediate, smoldering activity [2]. Spontaneous remission may occur, especially where the onset of polyarthritis has been quite sudden [1]. Even though patients are categorized as having 'early disease', a number of prognostic factors should be sought (Fig. 15.10). These factors when present suggest a more unfavorable outlook and may indicate a need for more aggressive therapy.

Often the diagnosis of RA is obvious, but frequently there are too few definite features and the diagnosis can only be tentative, in which case the patient may be placed in this early category. The ARA criteria for classification of RA may not always be helpful in diagnosis of patients at the earliest stage of disease. Over time, developments may show that a presumptive diagnosis of early RA was incorrect and features of another diffuse connective tissue disorder – such as SLE, scleroderma, or psoriatic arthritis – may evolve. Thus, it may be a mistake to apply the RA 'label' to a patient too soon, because when new symptoms arise other diagnostic possibilities or unrelated complications may not be considered soon enough to effect better treatment.

Progressive Disease

Some patients show a more progressive course from the outset. They have unrelenting, continuous disease activity despite treatment. In addition to persistent polyarthritis, these individuals usually have an elevated erythrocyte sedimentation rate (ESR), positive rheumatoid factor test and early radiographic evidence of joint erosions. They may also have one or more of the systemic features of RA.

Late Disease

This category is used to describe patients whose disease has led to definite joint damage with all its attendant complications. In most cases, the disease is of many years' duration and its damaging effects are a reflection of its severity. Typically these patients have been resistant to various disease-suppressive medications, though in some patients the disease may have 'burned itself out', leaving only residual joint damage.

INDIVIDUAL JOINTS – A REGIONAL APPROACH

Joint involvement in RA is symmetrical, and while wrists, fingers, knees and feet are the most commonly affected joints, severe disease is associated with larger joints that contain more synovium, such as the shoulders, elbows and knees. In fact, articular indices weighted for size and amount of synovium, such as the historical Lansbury index [27], have been found to correlate better with the amount of inflammation than simple joint counts [28]. The simultaneous presence of joint tenderness and swelling also show a higher correlation with joint inflammation than either variable alone [28]. Eventually, if unchecked, persistent inflammation leads to destruction of soft tissue with ligamentous laxity and deformity.

FACTORS IN RHEUMATOID ARTHRITIS INDICATING AN UNFAVORABLE PROGNOSIS
High accumulated joint damage rate Uncontrolled polyarthritis Structural damage and deformity Functional disability
Presence of extra-articular features Local and/or systemic – nodules, vasculitis, etc.
Psychosocial problems (adverse reaction by the patient)
Rheumatoid factor at high level, presence of immune complexes

Fig. 15.10 Clinical evaluation of RA – prognostic factors. The presence of these factors suggests a more unfavorable outlook [5].

The Hands

Examination of the hands is important because the features they exhibit are frequently a reflection of the patient's overall disease, whether early, late or progressive. Symmetrical swelling of the metacarpophalangeal (MCP) and proximal interphalangeal (PIP) joints, with fusiform swelling of the latter, are typical of RA (Fig. 15.11). Distal interphalangeal (DIP) involvement may be seen, but should be distinguished from coincidental osteoarthritis. Tenderness on palpation will determine which of these joints are to be noted as 'active'. Effusion should be sought using the four-finger technique (see Fig. 15.7). Hand assessment is incomplete without recording grip strength, but it is worth noting that poor grip strength may be as much a reflection of tendon involvement as of joint disease affecting wrists and fingers.

Although local swellings of the MCP and PIP joints are characteristic of RA, massive diffuse swelling of both hands with a 'flipper' or 'boxing glove' appearance may be associated with an acute onset. Pitting edema is characteristic of this swelling, and if a seronegative elderly person is affected, a more likely diagnosis is that of benign polyarthritis of the aged [29]. If diffuse swelling of one or both hands is associated with signs of sympathetic overactivity and shoulder stiffness, then reflex dystrophy may be a better explanation than RA. However, reflex dystrophy may coexist with RA or contribute to its

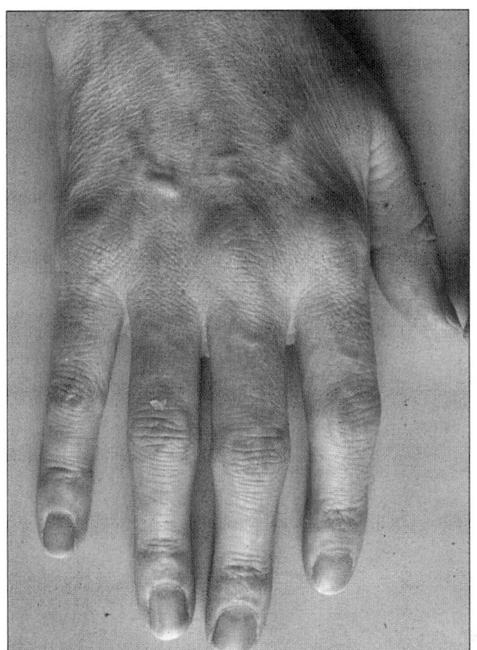

Fig. 15.11 The hand in early RA. View of the right hand, showing swelling of the MCP and PIP joints. Fusiform swelling of the PIP joints is typical of RA and associated with morning stiffness, difficulty making a fist, reduced grip strength and tenderness of the affected joints. The left hand showed similar changes. Reproduced with permission from Dieppe PA, *et al.* Slide Atlas of Clinical Rheumatology. London: Gower Medical Publishing; 1983.

HASTING'S CLASSIFICATION OF RHEUMATOID HAND		
Joint involvement	MCP joints	Synovitis Passively correctible ulnar drift Fixed volar subluxation, ulnar drift
	PIP joints	Synovitis Boutonnière deformity Swan-neck deformity Flail IP joint
	Thumb	Flail IP joint Boutonnière deformity Duckbill thumb (CMC) dislocation
	Wrist	Synovitis Carpal supination–subluxation Radiocarpal dislocation
Tendon involvement	Flexor tendon disease	Loss of active flexion Triggering Tendon rupture Median nerve involvement
	Extensor tendon disease	Synovitis – dorsal mass Extensor tendon rupture Extensor tendon dislocation

Fig. 15.12 Hasting's classification of rheumatoid hand deformities. Data from Hastings DE, pp147–179 in Gordon [5].

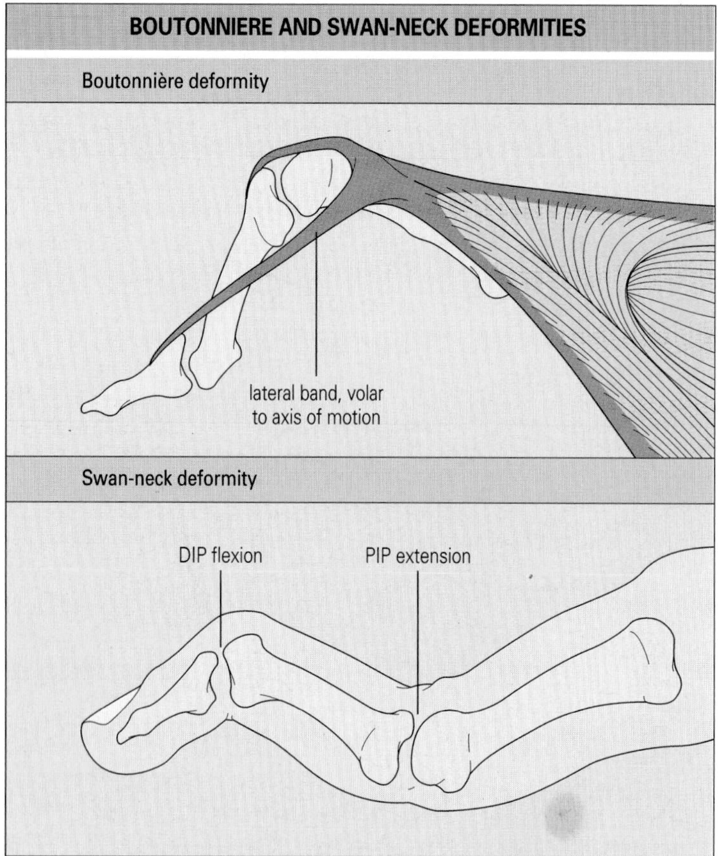

Fig. 15.13 PIP joints deformities in RA. The boutonnière deformity – PIP flexion and DIP hyperextension – results from relaxation of the central slip, with 'button-holing' of the PIP joint between the lateral bands. The swan-neck deformity – MCP flexion, PIP hyperextension and DIP flexion – may be mobile, snapping or fixed. Its pathogenesis may be related primarily to PIP or MCP involvement. Combinations of MCP and PIP involvement are less frequent. Adapted with permission from Hastings DE, Welsh RP, Surgical reconstruction of the rheumatoid hand, Toronto: Orthopaedic Medical Management Corporation; 1979.

disease expression. Interestingly, articular signs may be absent when RA develops in a patient with pre-existing hemiparesis [30]. The greater the paralysis the less the degree of joint inflammation.

Inspection of the hands may reveal other extra-articular features. Raynaud's phenomenon may be seen in a minority of patients, and palmar erythema in more. Digital and nailfold infarcts indicate rheumatoid vasculitis and a more severe form of arthritis [6].

A more detailed examination of joints and tendons is required to monitor progressive hand deformity in RA. Hasting's classification and description is helpful in identifying these problems (Fig. 15.12) [5].

Metacarpophalangeal joints

MCP involvement, with the development of volar subluxation and ulnar drift, is a characteristic deformity of RA. A number of factors favor its occurrence and progression [31]. Synovitis within the MCP joints tends to weaken the dorsal and radial structures and relatively lengthen the collateral ligaments. Inherent mechanical factors then favor ulnar drift of the fingers. The power of hand grip pulls the tendons ulnarwards as the fifth metacarpal descends. The ulnar collateral ligaments are shorter and less oblique than the radial counterparts, and thus the elongation is greater on the radial than the ulnar side. The firm attachment of the volar plate also fixes the pull of the long flexors to the proximal phalanx and tends to displace the proximal phalanx in both an ulnar and volar direction. The transverse linkage of the extensor tendons functions much like a clothes-line, so that anything pulling the extensor tendon of the fifth finger in a ulnar direction will pull the other fingers the same way. An effect of radial deviation of the wrist must also be considered. In the presence of ulnar drift, a normal wrist will tend to radially deviate to compensate for that deformity. Moreover, any wrist involvement that produces radial deviation will tend to aggravate the tendency to ulnar drift of the fingers.

Proximal interphalangeal joints

Three deformities due to lack of collateral ligament support characterize PIP joint involvement – the boutonnière, the swan-neck (Fig. 15.13) and the unstable PIP joint. Synovitis in the PIP joint can produce any of these deformities. As noted, synovitis with joint effusion in early RA causes fusiform swelling. Synovitis may appear as a bulge on the dorsal aspect, often on each side of the extensor tendon.

A boutonnière deformity develops when there is relative laxity or attenuation of the central slip and the lateral bands move in a volar direction. This destroys the extensor balance of the fingers and extension is concentrated on the terminal phalanx while the lateral bands actually become flexors of the PIP joints. The lack of passive flexion of the terminal IP joint with the PIP joint in extension is the earliest sign of this complication. It may be rapidly progressive. A swan-neck deformity represents the reverse of the boutonnière deformity and exists when the main extensor forces focus on the base of the proximal phalanx and the lateral bands sublux to a dorsal position. It may be a physiological deformity, the result of trauma, secondary to PIP joint disease or a result of MCP joint disease with secondary intrinsic contracture. In the early stages, the deformity seems relatively reversible, but as the lateral bands displace to the dorsal position, flexion becomes increasingly difficult. Often the movement is only accomplished by a snap as the lateral bands move from the dorsal to the normal dorsal–lateral position. Once the lateral bands become fixed in a dorsal position, then flexion of the PIP joint is no longer possible.

Distal interphalangeal joints

Involvement of the DIP joint is not characteristic of RA but probably occurs more frequently than appreciated [32]. It is never an initial or isolated manifestation of RA, and it is usually episodic and more likely to occur in seropositive RA. DIP disease must be distinguished from coincidental osteoarthritis that at times may also show inflammatory features.

The rheumatoid thumb

Three deformities affect the thumb: the flail IP joint, the boutonnière thumb and the relatively rare duckbill thumb. The flail IP joint results from synovitis leading to the destruction of the collateral ligaments. Pinching pushes the terminal phalanx away and the patient begins to pinch against the proximal phalanx. The boutonnière thumb is the same deformity as that described earlier for the other fingers. MCP synovitis weakens the insertion of the extensor pollicis brevis to the base of the proximal phalanx and results in an MCP flexion deformity and a secondary IP hyperextension due to the unbalanced action of extensor pollicis longus. The duckbill thumb develops when the primary pathology is at the first carpometacarpal joint. This is a dislocation accompanied by an adduction deformity of the first metacarpal. The MCP joint is hyperextended and the IP joint flexed; the deformity is similar to a swan-neck deformity of the finger.

Flexor tendon involvement

Tendons, as well as joints, are sheathed with synovium and when inflamed the condition is known as tenosynovitis. Flexor tenosynovitis can take many different forms.

Loss of active flexion

If passive flexion of a finger exceeds active flexion, tenosynovitis is present. Crepitus can be felt in the palm as the fingers are extended and flexed. Adhesions between the superficial and deep tendons may limit the excursion of the profundus tendon and the patient will not be able to make a full fist. A trigger finger is a frequent feature of flexor tenosynovitis. The pathology is a thickening of the tendon (often by a rheumatoid nodule within the tendon) rather than stenosis of the tendon sheath.

Ruptures of flexor tendons occur but are much less common than extensor rupture. The tendon most likely to rupture is the flexor pollicis longus. The cause is usually synovitis in the carpal tunnel and wrist disease, with encroachment of a spicule of carpal bone from the floor of the carpal tunnel.

Florid flexor tenosynovitis of the carpal tunnel leads to compression of the median nerve. Volar wrist pain may be confused with articular disease, but the weakness, finger tingling and thenar wasting point to nerve involvement that can be confirmed by electromyographic studies. RA can actually present with a carpal tunnel syndrome as the sole feature before polyarthritis becomes apparent [33]. Occasionally, triggering may develop in the carpal tunnel.

Extensor tendon involvement

Extensor tenosynovitis is evident by swelling over the dorsum of the wrist, below the extensor retinaculum. Asking the patient to extend the fingers will accentuate the swelling – the 'tuck' sign (Fig. 15.14). This mass on the back of the wrist is usually only a painless cosmetic deformity. Painful finger extension, however, may indicate active tendon erosion. There may be a triggering effect, and with further erosion tendon rupture follows. This is usually the result of carpal supination–subluxation and attrition of the tendons over the distal ulna. It is important to differentiate an extensor tendon rupture from an extensor tendon dislocation at the MCP joints. At first, the latter is passively correctable, but it soon becomes fixed. Examination will reveal the intact extensor tendon over the dorsum of the hand. Another rare complication is the loss of finger extension caused by an entrapment neuropathy of the posterior interosseous branch of the radial nerve, due to rheumatoid synovitis about the elbow [34].

The Wrist

Symmetrical disease of the wrists is almost invariably present in RA [31]. Ulnar styloid swelling and loss of wrist extension indicate early involvement. Synovitis commonly affects the weakest support of the wrist on the ulnar side: where attenuation of the weak triangular ligament allows displacement of the wrist in a volar direction. The wrist also tends to rotate around the stronger radial dorsal ligament, promoting a deformity known as carpal supination–subluxation. This subluxation is responsible for the prominence of the distal ulna, causing erosion of the floor of the extensor compartments and extensor tendon rupture. As the wrist rotates into supination, subluxation of the extensor carpi ulnaris occurs so that this tendon no longer functions as a dorsiflexor. Contracture of the extensor carpi radialis longus and brevis leads to unopposed radial dorsiflexion with ulnar translocation of the carpus. With disease progression, the volar and ulnar aspect of the radius erodes, with the carpus moving in a volar and ulnar direction. This strains the extensor carpi radialis brevis and if this tendon ruptures, the wrist goes on to volar dislocation. The intercarpal ligaments may also be affected, with wrist collapse. This accentuates the instability. Rarely, synovitis appears to promote fibrous and then bony ankylosis of the carpal bones. Then stiffness, rather than instability, becomes the problem.

The Elbow

This joint is frequently involved in RA, with loss of extension as an early sign. Even with extensive involvement, elbow function is usually well maintained. When loss of flexion occurs, however, this can become a great problem as it interferes with the patient's self-care activities. Elbow effusions are visible and palpable in the dimple between the tip of the olecranon and the head of the radius. When small effusions are not visible, gentle extension to 90° may show a sudden bulge. Periarticular cysts may be associated with elbow effusion and, as in the knee, may rupture (into the forearm) with inflammatory swelling. With persistent synovitis, erosive changes first develop in the humeroulnar joint. Because the radius is linked to the ulna by an interosseous membrane, the two move as a unit. When the cartilage between the humerus and the ulna is lost, the head of the radius moves proximal to the capitellum, blocking flexion and extension. Loss of elbow extension precedes loss of flexion. Constant abutment of the radial head produces typical lateral pain, limited supination and crepitus with pronation and supination. Medial swelling of the elbow joint with damage and destruction may be associated with an ulnar entrapment neuropathy. As well, synovitis of the lateral elbow joint may cause entrapment of the posterior interosseous branch of the radial nerve [34].

Subcutaneous nodules

Subcutaneous nodules overlying the extensor aspect of the proximal ulna are present in about 30% of patients with RA. Not only is the nodule a cardinal diagnostic feature of RA, but it may break down

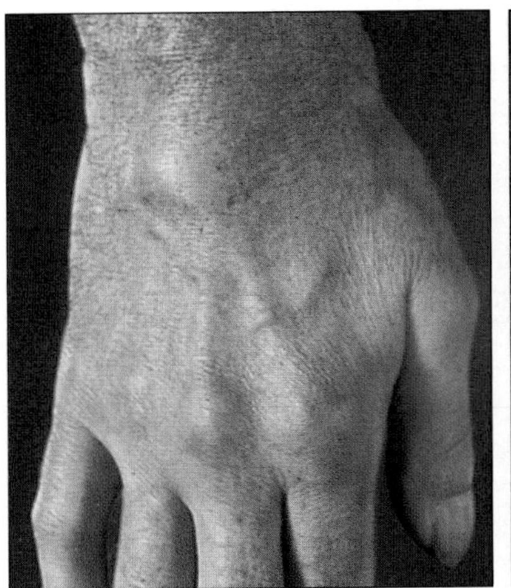
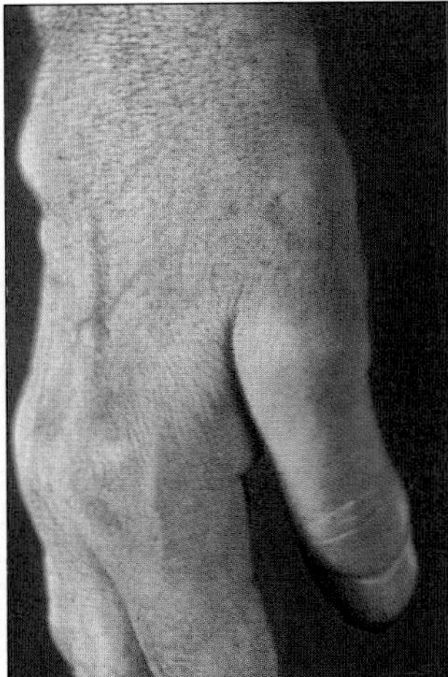

Fig. 15.14 Tenosynovial swelling from tenosynovitis – the 'tuck' sign. Tenosynovial swelling overlies the metacarpals of the right hand. Bulging becomes accentuated with full extension of all the fingers of the hand. Persistent tenosynovitis over the dorsal wrist may lead to extensor tendon erosion and rupture, particularly of the tendons of the fourth and fifth fingers.

forming a cyst and serving as a site for local infection (Fig. 15.15) or as a portal for complicating systemic infection causing septic arthritis. Vasculitis of the skin overlying the nodule may also contribute to these complications. Subcutaneous nodules form over other pressure locations, such as the occiput, sacrum or Achilles tendon, and may become infected (see Chapter 16). They should be sought in any RA patient who has septic complications.

Bursae

Bursae should not be overlooked in the evaluation of any joint region since they may be a site of rheumatoid activity [35]. There are about 80 bursae on each side of the body and they are lined by a synovial membrane that secretes synovial fluid and may develop rheumatoid synovitis. Only occasionally do they communicate with an adjacent joint space. Involvement of the olecranon bursa by RA is an obvious example of bursitis. Pain and swelling may be manifestations of synovitis or infection (see Fig. 15.15). While septic arthritis is almost invariably the result of hematogenous spread of bacteria, septic olecranon bursitis is always a consequence of a skin break with direct entry from outside. Skin vasculitis overlying bursal swelling can contribute to this septic complication. Occasionally the bursa ruptures and causes diffuse forearm edema.

Other bursae that may be similarly affected include the subacromial, trochanteric, iliopsoas, gastrocnemius, semimembranosus, sub-Achilles and posterior calcaneal. Sometimes multiple bursae may be affected by rheumatoid granulomas [36].

The Shoulder

Involvement of the shoulder joint in RA is variable but is usually only a feature in patients who have progressive disease. Often shoulder symptoms do not arise until joint destruction has become advanced. This is because adaptive mechanisms – the hands, wrists and elbows – are sufficiently good for daily self-care activities to be maintained for a long time.

Synovitis leads to erosion and damage of both the humeral head and the glenoid fossa. When shoulder effusions develop they appear anteriorally below the acromion. Subacromial bursal swelling may also appear as a pouch independent of the glenohumeral joint. The bursa may also rupture. The long head of the biceps may also rupture in patients with RA. This can be detected as a biceps bulge when the patient flexes the elbow against resistance.

The rotator cuff is also lined with synovium and may show inflammation and destruction, with monoarticular pain and limitation sufficiently acute to mimic septic arthritis. Frequently, there is weakening and loss of attachment of the rotator cuff, with secondary upward migration of the humeral head.

Acromioclavicular joint disease is frequently found in RA and may be the prime source of shoulder pain. Acromioclavicular involvement also correlates with the degree of glenohumeral disease.

The Temporomandibular Joint

This joint is commonly involved, with tenderness and painful limitation of mouth opening. It may eventually become associated with a receding or 'gump jaw' deformity.

The Cricoarytenoid Joint

Involvement of this joint is commonly associated with hoarseness. Superimposed upper respiratory infections may lead to upper airway obstruction with respiratory stridor requiring life-saving tracheostomy [37]. Limitation of cricoarytenoid movement may also be associated with lung aspiration and attendant complications.

Ossicles of the Ear

Ankylosis of these joints may be associated with hearing loss independent of a medication-induced effect.

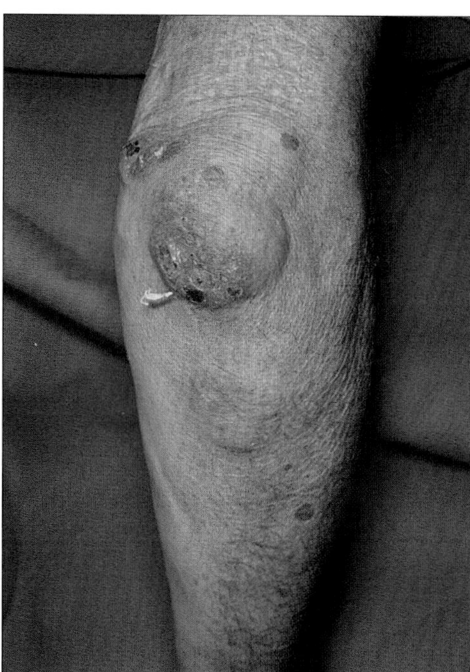

Fig. 15.15 Olecranon bursitis and subcutaneous nodule. Olecranon swelling with erythema from septic bursitis after incision and drainage. A subcutaneous nodule appears distal to the olecranon bursa. Either of these lesions may serve as a portal for systemic infection.

Sternoclavicular and Manubriosternal Joints

These joints possess synovial and cartilage portions and are more commonly affected than appreciated. Subluxation and actual dislocation of the manubriosternal joint may occur [38].

The Cervical Spine

The neck is an important target in RA, particularly at the C1–2 level [39]. The space between the odontoid process and the arch of the atlas normally measures 3mm or less. If this space exceeds 3mm this is defined as atlantoaxial subluxation (AAS). It can often exceed

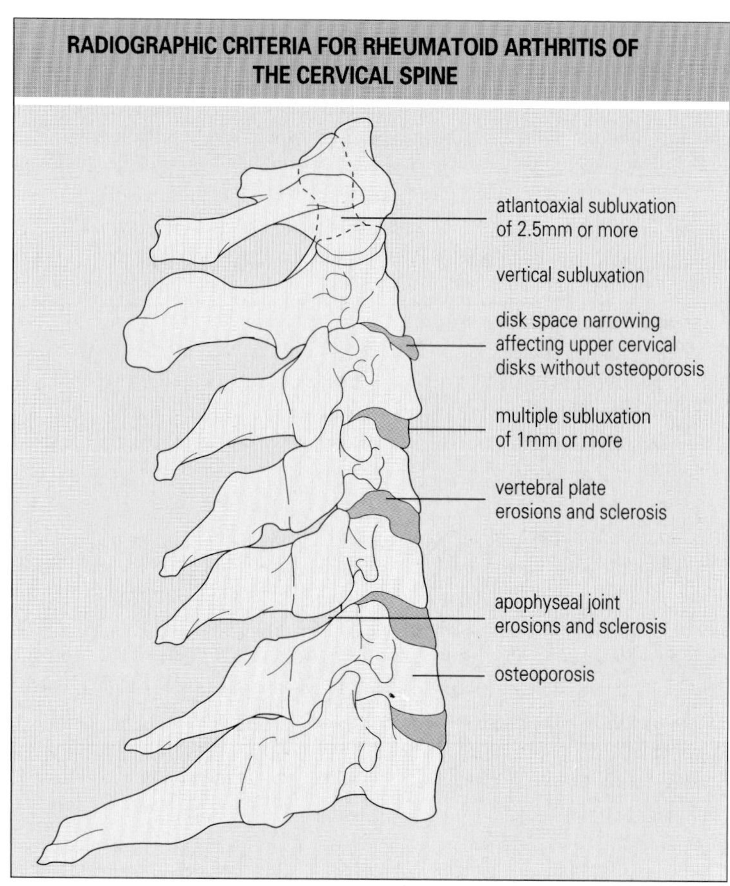

Fig. 15.16 The cervical spine in RA. These radiographic criteria for RA of the cervical spine are modified after Winfield, *et al.* [40].

10mm. Cervical subluxation at any level is common in severe erosive RA and may be found in 30% of patients in this category [40]. Although neck stiffness is common in RA, the majority of patients with AAS are not much affected by severe neck pain. When neck pain occurs it is usually high in the cervical spine, with radiation into the occiput or occasionally into temporal and retro-orbital regions. Sometimes AAS is associated with a frightening 'clunking' sensation on neck extension.

When considering the cervical spine at the C1–2 level, it is helpful to divide the space through the arch of the atlas into thirds; one-third for the odontoid process, one-third for the spinal cord and one-third free. If a C1–2 slip exceeds 10mm, the free third is lost and cervical cord damage becomes a risk (Figs 15.16 & 15.17). There is a synovial articulation between the transverse ligament of the atlas and the posterior aspect of the odontoid. This transverse ligament prevents a forward slip of C1 on C2, and continuing synovitis in this articulation compromises the ligament and may produce erosions of the dens. Synovial involvement may also affect the apophyseal joints in the occipitoatlantal area. If this causes loss of bone and change in shape, the odontoid may move up through the foramen magnum, producing basilar invagination and threatening the upper cervical cord and medulla. In these patients sudden death may occur after unexpected vomiting or physical trauma. Basilar–vertebral vascular insufficiency may also occur in these cases, with syncope after downward gaze. The usual indication for neurosurgical intervention in these cases is either intractable neck pain or pyramidal tract weakness of the arms and legs. RA of the apophyseal joints and disk spaces may cause subluxation at other levels, which may slowly lead to quadriparesis [41]. Fortunately, these complications are rare.

When a patient with RA requires surgery, the presence of cervical subluxation presents a general anesthetic risk. Preoperative assessment by lateral flexion cervical radiographs is essential to exclude this possibility. If cervical involvement is detected, then special precautions are required perioperatively to prevent cervical cord damage.

The Thoracic and Lumbar Spine

Involvement of these regions is very uncommon in RA. Apophyseal synovitis may rarely present as an epidural mass, and lumbar spinal stenosis has been reported. Compression fractures secondary to the osteoporosis of RA aggravated by corticosteroids are common in the thoracic region. Compression fractures in the lumbar region are not characteristic of RA and suggest that other underlying causes, such as osteomyelitis or cancer, should be considered and excluded.

The Sacroiliac Joints

Radiographic changes of the sacroiliac joints may be seen in advanced RA; usually they consist of erosions and osteopenia. However, ankylosing spondylitis and RA may occasionally coexist, usually in men, just as RA may be seen in patients with psoriasis, gout or osteoarthritis [42].

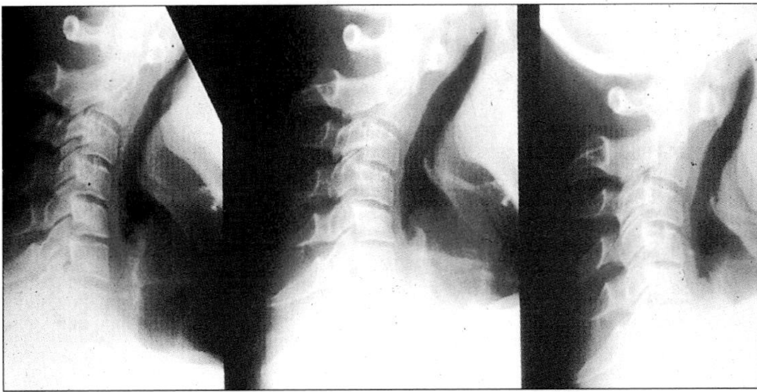

Fig. 15.17 The cervical spine in RA. Serial radiographs of the cervical spine show progression after the appearance of subluxation within 2 years of disease onset. (By courtesy of Dr John Winfield.)

The Hip

Early symptoms of hip involvement may be an abnormal gait or groin discomfort. Even with progressive RA, however, the hips are often spared. Moreover, the onset of hip disease in patients with RA is subtle, because patients maintain a pain-free range of hip movement until synovitis causes a progressive loss of cartilage space. Once this symmetric erosive process becomes established, bilateral protrusion of the acetabulae is inevitable [43]. Alternatively, with collapse of the femoral head from avascular necrosis, the deformity is lateral migration rather than protrusion into the pelvis. Once these complications arise, stiffness and pain interfere with the patient's ability to walk. A previous history of glucocorticosteroid use is often noted in these cases.

Iliopsoas bursa

Synovitis and effusion of the iliopsoas bursa (Fig. 15.18) may present with a unilateral or bilateral inguinal mass, or with lower extremity swelling without obvious relationship to the hip [44]. The bursa lies between the capsule of the hip and the iliopsoas muscle lateral to the femoral vessels. It rarely communicates with the hip joint and it is the largest bursa around the hip. Symptoms that may be mistaken for a hernia, lymphadenopathy or aneurysm arise from the inguinal mass. Femoral vein compression may lead to lower limb edema and a picture resembling deep-vein thrombosis.

Trochanteric and ischial bursae

Bursitis of the trochanteric bursa is more common than that of the ischial bursa. Either may be mistaken for true hip joint involvement (see Fig. 15.18).

The Knee

Involvement of the knee is common in RA and usually is obvious. Sometimes, however, meniscal surgery has been performed in patients before the diagnosis of RA became apparent. Small effusions of the knee joint are detectable in early disease by means of the 'bulge' sign (see Fig. 15.8). Although this sign is useful for detecting small amounts of fluid, it does not necessarily confirm an inflammatory process unless the results of synovial fluid analysis show changes consistent with RA. The normal skin temperature of the knee is significantly lower than that of the thigh or tibia. This is the basis of the 'cool patella' sign [45]. In the case of knee inflammation, palpation over the thigh, patella and calf with the back of the hand shows the temperature over the patella to be equal to the heat over the thigh and tibia (i.e. a loss of the cool patella sign).

With an increase in the amount of the knee effusion, the fluid bulge sign disappears and positive ballottement or the patellar tap

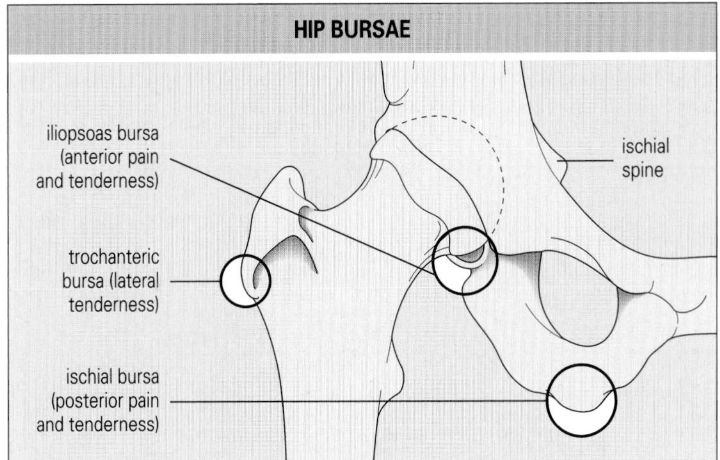

Fig. 15.18 Hip bursae that may be affected by rheumatoid granuloma. Involvement of the iliopsoas bursa is associated with an inguinal mass that may be mistaken for a hernia, lymphadenopathy or an aneurysm [44].

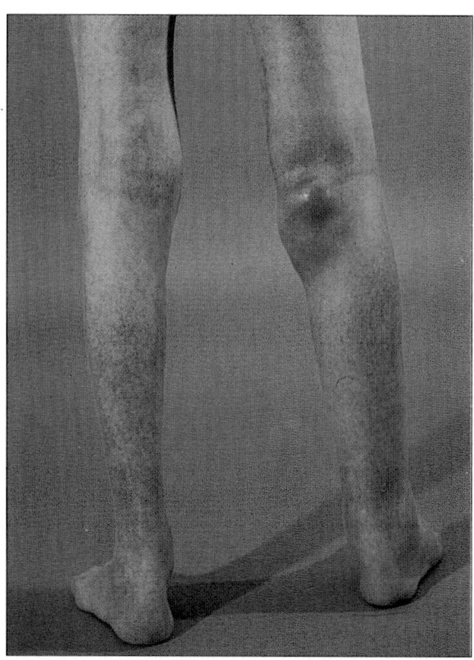

Fig. 15.19 Baker's popliteal cyst. Posterior view showing rheumatoid swelling behind the right knee. Swelling of the lower limb was related to venous compression by popliteal synovitis.

sign develops. The patient tends to assume a more comfortable position with the knee flexed and, if this becomes a habit, a loss of full knee extension eventually results. In full extension, the recumbent patient will be unable to push the popliteal surface of the knee into the examiner's hand.

Popliteal (Baker's) cysts

Knee extension lag may be associated with popliteal fullness caused by a Baker's cyst. The cyst can extend from its location in the gastrocnemius bursa down into the medial aspect of the calf. This is seen best by observing the standing patient from behind (Fig. 15.19). Sometimes these cysts extend into the medial ankle region. The Baker's popliteal cyst arises as an extension from the joint cavity; synovial tissue acts as a ball-valve allowing fluid accumulation without means for decompression [46]. Exertion sufficient to raise the intra-articular knee joint pressure can lead to rupture of the synovial cyst, with extravasation of inflammatory synovial fluid into the calf presenting a picture that mimics acute thrombophlebitis [46]. A hemorrhagic 'crescent' sign in the skin about the ankle below the malleoli is characteristic of synovial rupture and is not a feature of thrombophlebitis [47]. Rarely, after inflammation from a rupture into the calf has subsided, another rupture may cause posterior thigh extravasation and hemorrhage (Fig. 15.20). Anterolateral joint cysts may also extend below the knee, but this is a very rare occurrence [48].

Knee instability

Eventually destruction of the knee by RA leads to limitation in walking similar to the disability seen with the rheumatoid hip. With loss of cartilage comes laxity of the collateral and cruciate ligaments. This is detected by stressing the knee joint for lateral and medial collateral stability with the knee cradled in the arms of the examiner at 15° of flexion. Cruciate anterior–posterior instability is detectable by means of the 'drawer' sign. A special problem arises in women with physiological valgus. This produces increasing loading on the lateral compartment of the knee joint with erosion of the tibial plateau and progressive valgus deformity. As the valgus increases so does the loading, so that a vicious cycle is produced. Less common is the same set of circumstances in a varus position. With varus there is often collapse or fracture of the medial plateau and even more severe deformity.

Occasionally, inflammation results in binding of the collateral ligaments to the side of the femoral condyle. This destroys the normal anteroposterior gliding motion of the tibia on the femur and leads to a relative posterior subluxation of the tibia. The resultant deformity is usually associated with fixed flexion of the knee, and as the tibia tries to extend it digs into the femoral condyle producing a bony block anteriorly.

The Ankle

The ankle joint (tibial–talar articulation) is not as frequently involved as the subtalar and midtarsal joints of the hind foot. Persistent synovitis of the ankle joint leads to loss of cartilage and bone-on-bone contact. However, ankle involvement is not usually a cause of great disability because the joint remains quite stable.

The Foot

Hindfoot involvement

The subtalar and talonavicular joints are commonly affected in RA, but this is not always appreciated. Synovitis of these joints causes pain and stiffness and sometimes subtalar dislocation. Secondary peroneal muscle spasm develops and tends to immobilize the subtalar joint. The spasm promotes a valgus deformity and causes a peroneal spastic flat foot. As cartilage loss and bone erosion develop, valgus deformity increases, with progressive flattening of the longitudinal arch. Eventually the os calcis abuts against the lateral malleolus with collapse through the midfoot, producing pressure points over the head of the talus. At this stage the joint may spontaneously fuse without further progression.

Although heel pain is a characteristic of the spondyloarthropathies it can be a particular problem in RA. It can arise with development of a subachilles or retrocalcaneal bursitis that may be associated with nodule formation in the Achilles tendon. Rupture of the Achilles tendon may also complicate the picture [49]. Persistent

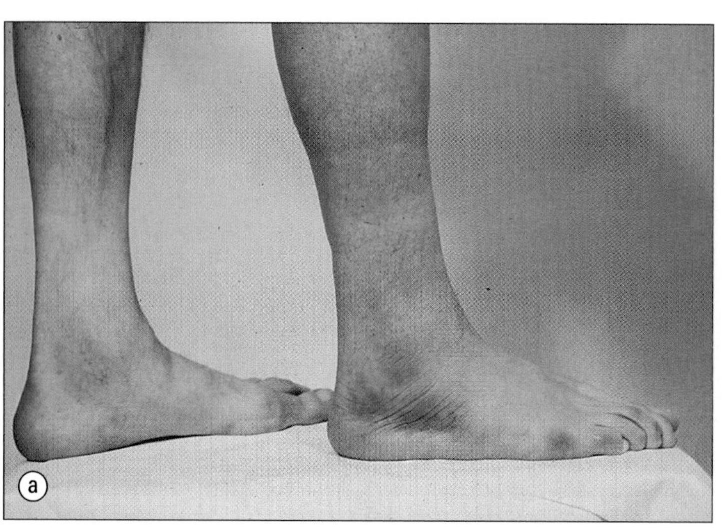

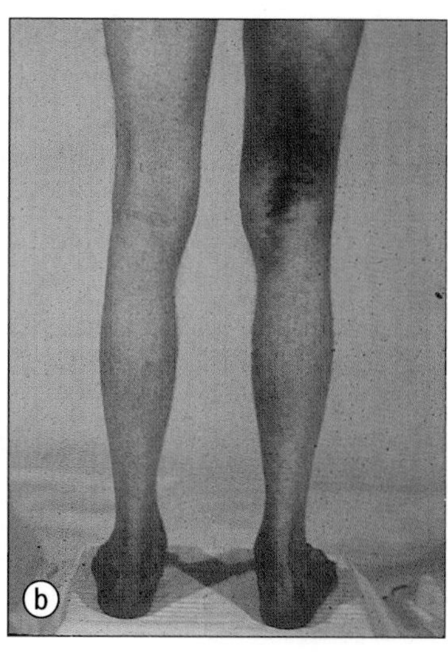

Fig. 15.20 Acute synovial rupture. A 51-year-old man with RA of 3 years' duration developed a right knee effusion after an evening of square dancing. Two days later he noted progressive pain and swelling of the right calf and 6 days later bluish discoloration of both sides of the ankle (a). A few weeks later, after more dancing, he noted posterior thigh pain and swelling that soon became associated with purple discoloration of his right posterior thigh (b) [47].

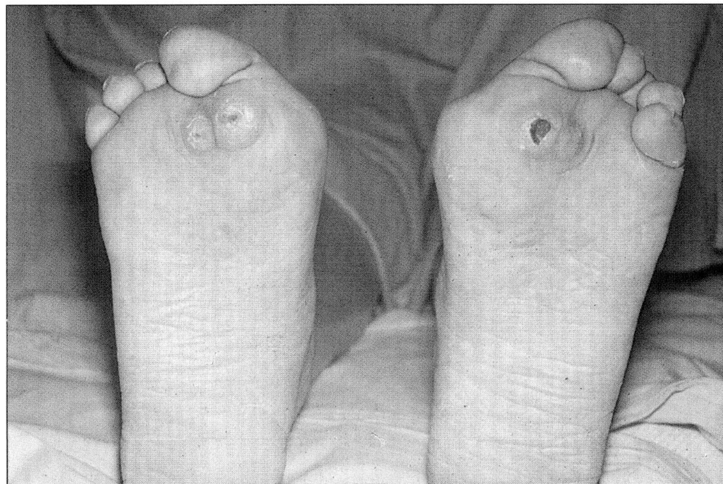

Fig. 15.21 Rheumatoid forefoot. Plantar view of the feet in a patient with RA. Hallux valgus, MTP subluxation and bursal swelling under weight-bearing areas are seen. Subluxation of the metatarsal head is associated with clawing of the toes, cock-up digital deformities and over-riding of the toes. The ulcerated bursae under the left metatarsal head may become associated with a chronic synovial fistula and secondary infection [56].

heel pain caused by a calcaneal stress fracture is sometimes misinterpreted as subtalar or ankle synovitis [50].

The forefoot

Disease of the metatarsal heads is common in RA, causing much pain and disability. Forefoot deformity usually starts with synovitis of the metatarsophalangeal (MTP) joints and involvement of the flexor tendons within their sheath. Because of volar pain, the patient tends to walk on the heels with maximum dorsiflexion. This leads to reactivity of the extensor digitorum longus, with clawing of the toes and the eventual dorsal dislocation of the MTP joint (Fig. 15.21). With this comes a secondary depression and erosion of the metatarsal heads and widening of the entire forefoot. Metatarsus primus varus is commonly seen in women with RA and this leads to a severe hallux valgus deformity.

Forefoot fistulae

Chronic synovitis of the metatarsal heads may be associated with severe erosive changes and the formation of bony cysts known as geodes. Spread of the synovial granuloma and bony breakdown causes calluses or bunions to form over these areas. Further breakdown of tissue leads to a chronic cutaneous fistula as synovial fluid tracks from the MTP joint to the dorsal or plantar surface of the foot [51]. Secondary infection along this fistulous track is a hazard that may require surgery extending back into the MTP joint. Although chronic fistulous rheumatism is seen most often with metatarsal synovitis, chronic cutaneous fistulae may develop in relation to any rheumatoid joint. Diffuse pitting edema of the feet may be due to local venous insufficiency, obstruction of lymphatics or veins from a swollen ankle, knee or hip, or it may even relate to cardiac disease, sometimes associated with RA, such as pericarditis. Numbness of the medial aspect of the forefoot may result from a tarsal tunnel entrapment neuropathy of the medial peroneal nerve.

NATURAL HISTORY

Disease Onset

The clinical course of RA follows an onset of disease that may be either abrupt and acute, or gradual and insidious, or subacute between these extremes [1,2]. A gradual onset is most common (at least 50% of cases), whereas a sudden onset is much less common (10–25%) [1,2]. RA begins predominantly as an articular disease and one or many joints may be affected. It may also start with an extra-articular or non-articular presentation, such as a local bursitis or tenosynovitis, or as a systemic presentation with diffuse polyarthralgia or polymyalgia. Although the onset is predominantly articular, it is frequently associated with a variety of extra-articular features, including generalized weakness, anorexia, weight loss or fever. In some cases, fatigue alone or diffuse nonspecific aching with other extra-articular features, such as pulmonary disease, may herald by weeks or months the onset of polyarthritis [2].

Pattern of Presentation

Gradual onset

The commonest presentation at onset is a gradual or insidious one affecting small peripheral joints such as the wrists, MCP, PIP, ankles or MTPs. A gradual onset is defined as one that the patient can only date to the nearest month. This gradual onset is usually symmetrical with considerable morning stiffness and the patient complaining of difficulty making a fist and poor grip strength. The morning stiffness may last minutes to hours.

Slow, monoarticular presentation

Less common is a slow monoarticular presentation affecting larger joints such as shoulders or knees. The symptoms may remain confined to one or two joints, but frequently spread over the ensuing days and weeks additively to affect wrists, fingers, ankles or feet in a widespread fashion.

Abrupt, acute polyarthritis

Less frequently RA presents as an abrupt acute polyarthritis of the shoulders, elbows, wrists, fingers, hips, knees, ankles and feet, with intense joint pain, diffuse swelling and limitation leading to incapacitation. A sudden onset is defined as one for which the patient can give a specific date. This type of onset may affect patients at any age but has particular significance in the elderly. Aged males especially may develop a syndrome of 'remitting, seronegative, symmetric, synovitis with pitting edema (RS3PE syndrome)' [29] that may be confused with RA. A similar subgroup of elderly British males showed an acute 'stormy' onset with resolution usually within a year– 'benign RA of the aged' [52]. However, a prospective controlled study of 71 Dutch patients over 60 years of age, mostly with an acute onset, showed after 2 years a more progressive course than their younger counterparts [7].

Acute monoarthritis

An acute monoarthritis of a knee, shoulder or hip can present a picture suggesting a septic, pseudogout, or gouty process, though this presentation is rare. Joint pain more severe than that found in RA is characteristic of the latter conditions, which may resemble or even complicate RA. The results of synovial fluid analysis should settle any diagnostic confusion in these cases. An acute monoarticular presentation may proceed to more widespread involvement with any of the preceding patterns.

Tenosynovitis or bursitis may also be associated with mono- or polyarthritis and subcutaneous nodules over extensor surfaces, such as the elbow, sacrum or Achilles tendon, may appear.

Palindromic rheumatism

Another variation of the abrupt onset of polyarthritis is known as palindromic rheumatism [53]. Here, variable episodes of polyarthritis suddenly affect one or more large and/or peripheral joints, last a few hours or a few days, and then spontaneously subside, with complete clearing of all rheumatic signs between attacks. These short-lived episodes may recur over weeks or months, with increasing frequency and severity, and may herald the onset of persistent polyarthritis. At least one-third of these palindromic cases evolve into typical RA.

ACR CRITERIA FOR CLINICAL REMISSION OF RHEUMATOID ARTHRITIS

A minimum of five of the following for at least 2 consecutive months:

1. Morning stiffness not to exceed 15 minutes
2. No fatigue
3. No joint pain
4. No joint tenderness or pain on motion
5. No soft tissue swelling in joints or tendon sheaths
6. ESR (Westergren's method) less than 30mm/hour (females) or 20mm/hour (males)

Exclusions prohibiting a designation of complete clinical remission:

Clinical manifestations of active vasculitis,
Pericarditis,
Pleuritis,
Or myositis
And/or unexplained recent weight loss or fever secondary to RA

Fig. 15.22 The ACR preliminary criteria for complete clinical remission of RA. In a patient with a definite or classical RA, at least five of these must be fulfilled for at least 2 consecutive months [55].

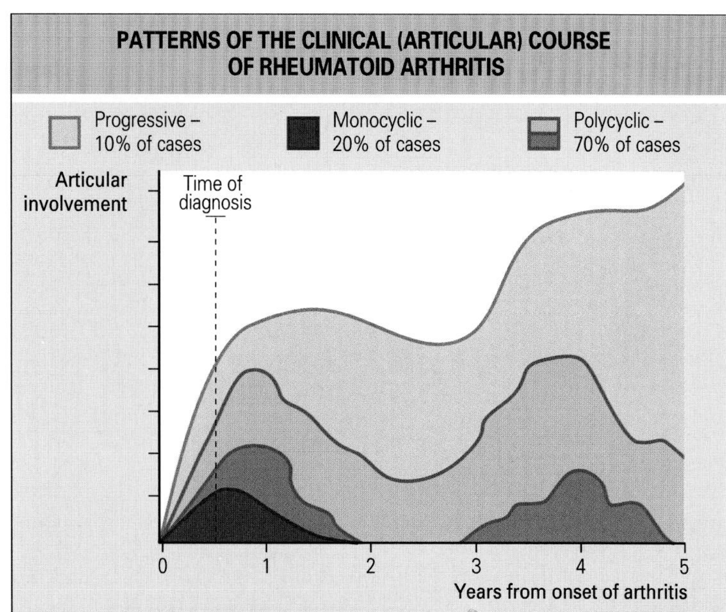

Fig. 15.23 Clinical (articular) course patterns in RA: articular patterns in 50 patients with RA. Data from Masi *et al.* [56].

Local extra-articular features

As noted, bursitis and tenosynovitis may be associated with RA. Sometimes, however, the earliest manifestation and presentation of RA may be a median nerve compression (carpal tunnel syndrome) from volar wrist tenosynovitis [33]. Similarly, other local extra-articular features may be the presenting feature.

Systemic extra-articular features

Elderly patients, in particular, may present with polyarthralgias and polymyalgias affecting the neck and shoulders or hips and knees, with associated profound fatigue. Although these features, especially in association with fever and high ESR lasting several weeks, suggest a diagnosis of polymyalgia rheumatica, this picture may be a forerunner of full-blown RA. Moreover, some investigators have advanced the notion that seronegative RA in the elderly has more in common with polymyalgia rheumatica than typical seropositive erosive RA [54].

Pattern of Progression

No matter what the onset or presentation, the patient's subsequent progress may follow several different patterns. It may be a course that is brief or episodic, prolonged and progressive, or something intermediate. The severity may vary from mild to intense. Attacks may be prolonged and smoldering or prolonged and progressive. With continuing disease activity, the patient's daily activities and functional capacity are affected to a greater or lesser extent. Although disability is usually proportional to the amount of painful joint involvement, in men who do physically hard work there is sometimes progressive joint dysfunction and disability without much pain. The physical abilities of patients who have this 'neuropathic' picture may dwindle insidiously before the seriousness of the situation becomes apparent. This highlights the importance of careful evaluation and re-evaluation of the patient's condition. For this reason, good records are essential to document the patient's progress and response to therapy, and these records should incorporate the features contained in the ACR criteria for clinical remission in RA (Fig. 15.22) [55]. The criteria include features thought to predict a favorable outcome and are mostly inflammatory articular characteristics of RA. Unlike the self-report questionnaires these criteria do not take into account the patient's present functional state. The latter is frequently a better predictor of the patient's future condition [22]. Moreover, when a patient is not responding to therapy as expected, it is important to be aware of all the factors that may adversely affect outcome. The patient's systemic reaction and extra-articular features and serologic status may in fact be more important than the articular features and their complications [6]. Alternatively, the patient may be showing an adverse reaction to one or more medications. Contrary to many patients' belief, weather conditions do not appear to influence symptoms of arthritis.

Few studies have examined the natural history of a group of patients with a well-defined RA over a long period of time. One such representative study is that by Masi *et al.* who followed 50 patients with early RA for almost 6 years and described three articular patterns (Fig. 15.23) [56]:

- Monocyclic pattern: a single cycle with remission for at least 1 year, seen in 20% of patients.
- Polycyclic pattern: seen in 70% of patients with either intermittent or continuing subtypes. The latter group showed smouldering activity with incomplete remission or progression.
- Progressive pattern: with increasing joint involvement seen in about 10% of patients.

Patients with malignant RA would fall under this last category. Most authorities would agree with these general observations, but many current ideas on the natural history of RA must remain speculative until the results of modern, long-term clinical population studies become available.

CLINICAL COURSE – MORBIDITY AND MORTALITY

Studies of the natural history of RA provide insights into outcome variables and prognosis. Understanding prognosis helps us to evaluate better the medicolegal or psychosocial implications for estimating work disability in RA, and social implications, such as health-service planning and costs. It is worthwhile considering whether the type of disease onset and patterns of presentation previously outlined can be used to predict the subsequent course of RA. A generally held view is that an acute onset forecasts a favorable prognosis whereas an insidious onset heralds a worse outlook.

Acute Onset Pattern

In a series of 102 early cases of adult RA, Fleming *et al.* reported that 11 cases with sudden onset showed after 5 years a better functional outcome than 69 patients with a slow onset of disease [1]. However, in a later series of 100 patients, Jacoby *et al.* observed that after an 11-year follow up, there was no difference in functional class whether disease onset was acute, subacute or gradual [2]. In the past, a favorable prognosis may have been ascribed to cases of acute onset RA because they had not yet evolved into a different, more benign condition. For example, cases with acute onset due to a reactive or viral polyarthritis may have been mistaken for RA. Another explanation of why patients with acute onset may have had a better outcome is that they were more likely to seek prompt medical attention than were patients with a gradual onset of disease. The favorable course of mild or transient RA, however, has not attracted much attention, because rheumatologists are mostly concerned with progressive RA.

Gradual Onset Pattern

In Fleming's report [57] a worse prognosis was found in patients who had disease that was gradual in onset and associated with large joint involvement (shoulders, elbows, wrists, knees) as well as involvement of the first and second MTPs. In the Jacoby series [2], the type of onset was not predictive of functional status after 11 years; moreover, in a later Finnish study of 235 RA patients, radiographically evident damage after 7 years was the same whether the onset had been acute (69), subacute (55) or gradual (111) [58].

General Variables

A number of variables are thought to have prognostic implications (see Fig. 15.10). In a large Finnish population survey of 7217 adults, the detection of rheumatoid factor in 15 of 21 patients with seropositive RA antedated the onset of RA usually by 5 years [59]. Unfortunately, however, the presence of these risk factors often only confirms continuing disease activity rather than predicting it. And in any of these high-risk patients, sudden severe persistent pain worse in one joint, such as the shoulder, hip or knee, may signify a complicating septic arthritis or avascular necrosis. Thus, in spite of the validity of the factors listed in Figure 15.10, better markers are needed for detecting early disease and identifying at an early stage patients who are likely to pursue a progressive course. Ideally, some of the newer immunogenetic, synovial or imaging methods may fulfill these needs.

Health Status Questionnaire Assessments

In assessing prognosis, a number of health status self-report questionnaires have been developed and found valuable for routine and research use [22–25]. Data obtained by rheumatologists using these suggests that the overall prognosis in patients with RA may be much worse than previously estimated. Wolfe and Cathey assessed functional disability using the Stanford HAQ and functional disability index in 1274 patients with RA followed up longitudinally for up to 12 years [60]. Half of the patients showed loss of function that was moderate within 1–2 years, severe in 2–6 years and very severe in 10 years. The progression of disability was most rapid in the early years and then tapered off. Simple demographic and clinical assessment showed that disease worsened more quickly in women and was associated with a longer duration of disease, decreased grip strength, and worse pain, global severity and psychologic scores. Older patients also showed more systemic features associated with greater functional loss [7].

In another longitudinal study, from Santa Clara County, California, patients with disease for more than 20 years deteriorated more rapidly than those with disease of a shorter duration [61]. The Stanford HAQ disability index also showed more rapid deterioration in women, in patients with fewer years of education and with increased age. The same investigators showed that the Stanford HAQ disability index is a useful prognosticator of length of survival [62]. Patients with more severe disease are more likely to receive prednisone, and its long-term use was a risk factor associated with greater disability and premature death [62].

A loss of function measured by these prognostic methods may predict not only morbidity but also an increased mortality that is comparable to malignant conditions such as Hodgkin's disease or chronic heart disease [63,64]. Moreover, these prognostic analyses confirm that RA is a marker for the development of many co-morbid chronic conditions [65], particularly in older patients, such as bacterial infections and renal disease. Their proponents believe that estimates of functional status using these questionnaires may provide a better estimate of long-term prognosis than radiographic or serologic measures [64].

Although self-report questionnaires have proved valuable, patients with limited education find them difficult to use and rheumatologists are reluctant to rely on questionnaire data alone. Pincus *et al.* [66] studied three simple measures of functional status – grip strength, walking time and a button test. Their results were comparable to laboratory measures, showed reliable reproducibility, and were similar to self-report questionnaires in their capacity to predict outcome [67] (Fig. 15.24). While patients with poor long-term outlook have attracted the attention of hospital-based rheumatologists, these severely affected patients may not be representative of RA as a whole. This is because, as has been suggested recently, RA may currently be a milder disease than in the past or may even be disappearing [68, 69].

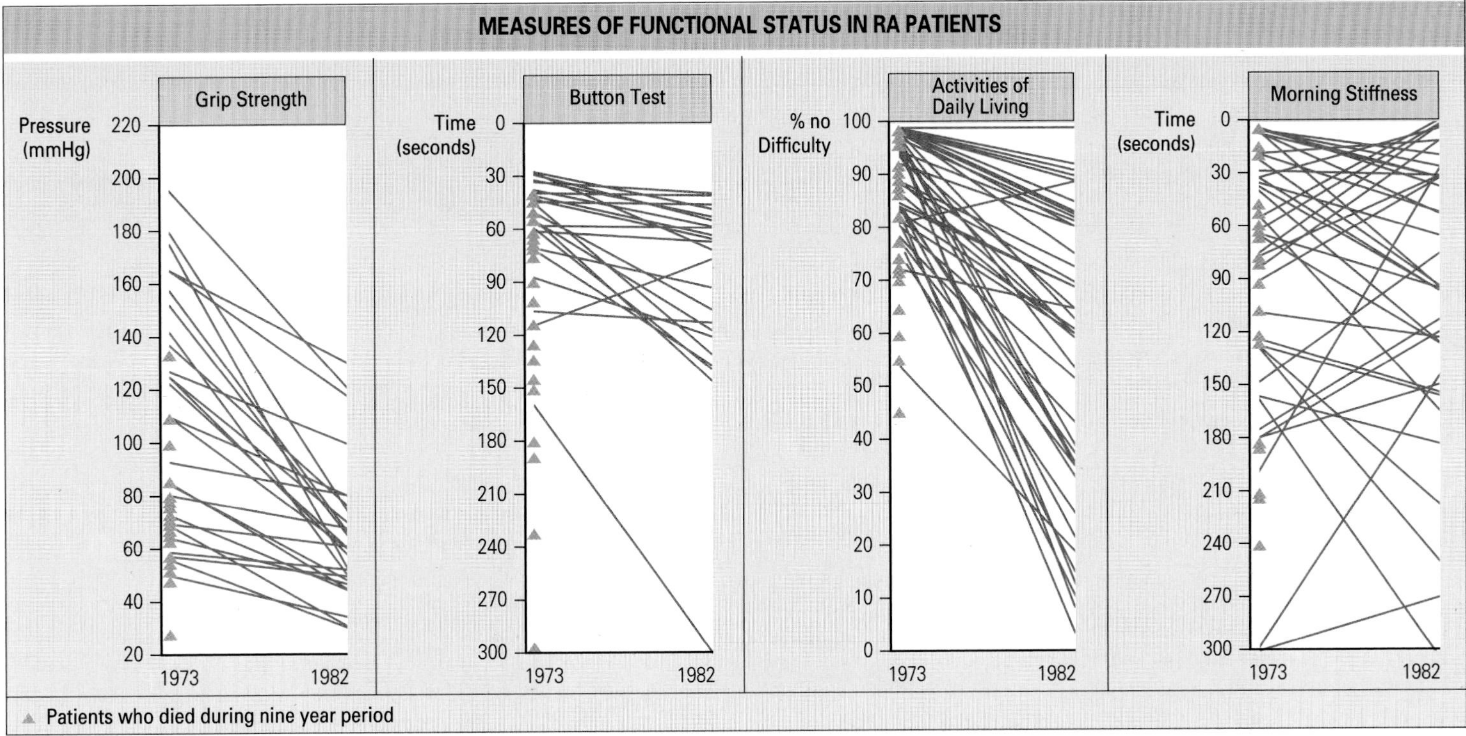

Fig. 15.24 Morbidity in RA patients. Data from Pincus T, et al.[66] and Pincus T, Callahan LF [67].

REFERENCES

1. Fleming A, Crown JM, Corbett M. Early rheumatoid disease. 1. Onset. Ann Rheum Dis. 1976;**35**:357–60.
2. Jacoby RK, Jayson MIV, Cosh JA. Onset, early stages and prognosis of rheumatoid arthritis: a clinical study of 100 patients with 11 year follow-up. Br Med J. 1973;**2**:96–100.
3. Arnett FC, Edworthy SM, Bloch DA, et al. The American Rheumatism Association 1987 revised criteria for the classification of rheumatoid arthritis. Arthritis Rheum. 1988;**31**:315–24.
4. Ropes MW, Bennett EA, Cobbs S, et al. 1958 Revision of diagnostic criteria for rheumatoid arthritis. Bull Rheum Dis. 1958;**9**:175–6.
5. Gordon DA, ed. Rheumatoid arthritis – contemporary patient management series. 2nd ed. New York: Medical Examination Publishing; 1985.
6. Gordon DA, Stein JL, Broder I. The extra-articular features of rheumatoid arthritis. A systematic analysis of 127 cases. Am J Med. 1973;**54**:445–52.
7. Desiree MFM, van der Heijde, Piet LCM, et al. Older versus younger onset rheumatoid arthritis: results at onset and after 2 years of a prospective follow-up study of early rheumatoid arthritis. J Rheumatol. 1991;**18**:1285–9.
8. Hawley DJ, Wolfe F. Anxiety and depression in patients with rheumatoid arthritis: a prospective study of 400 Patients. J Rheumatol. 1988;**15**:932–41.
9. McFarlane AC, Brooks PM. Determinants of disability in rheumatoid arthritis. Br J Rheumatol. 1988;**27**:7–14.
10. Moldofsky H, Chester W J. Pain and mood patterns in patients with rheumatoid arthritis. Psychosom Med. 1970;**32**:309–18.
11. Wolfe F, Cathey, MA, Kleinkeksel SM, et al. Psychological status in primary fibrositis and fibrositis associated with rheumatoid arthritis. J Rheumatol. 1984;**11**:500–6.
12. Meyerowitz S, Jacox RF, Hess DW. Monozygotic twins discordant for rheumatoid arthritis. Arthritis Rheum. 1968;**11**:1–21.
13. Nicholas NS, Panayi GS. Rheumatoid arthritis and pregnancy. Clin Exp Rheumatol. 1988;**6**:179–82.
14. Hazes JMW, Dijkmans AC, Vandenbroucke JP, et al. Pregnancy and the risk of developing rheumatoid arthritis. Arthritis Rheum. 1990;**33**:1770–75.
15. Spector D, Brennan P, Harris P, et al. Does estrogen replacement therapy protect against rheumatoid arthritis? J Rheumatol. 1991;**18**:1473–6.
16. Carette S, Marcoux S, Gingras S. Postmemopausal hormones and the incidence of rheumatoid arthritis. J Rheumatol. 1989;**16**:911–13.
17. Linos A, Worthington JW, O'Fallon, W, Kurland LT. The epidemiology of rheumatoid arthritis in Rochester, Minnesota: a study of incidence, prevalence and mortality. Am J Epidemiol. 1980;**111**:87–98.
18. Wicks IP, Moore J, Fleming A. Australian mortality statistics for rheumatoid arthritis 1950–81: analysis of death certificate data. Ann Rheum Dis. 1988;**47**:563–69.
19. Leigh JP, Fries JF. Education level and rheumatoid arthritis: evidence from five data centers. J Rheumatol. 1991;**18**:24–34.
20. Hernandez-Avila M, Liang MH, Willett WC, et al. Reproductive factors, smoking, and the risk for rheumatoid arthritis. Epidemiology. 1990:**1**:285–91.
21. Gordon DA, Hyland RH, Broder I. Rheumatoid arthritis. In: Cannon GW, Zimmerman GA, eds. The lung in rheumatic diseases. New York: Marcel Dekker; 1990;229–59.
22. Wolfe F, Kleinheksel SM, Cathey MA, et al. The clinical value of the Stanford Health Assessment Questionnaire Functional Disability Index in patients with rheumatoid arthritis. J Rheumatol. 1988;**15**:1480–8.
23. Anderson JJ, Felson DT, Meenan RF, Williams HJ. Which traditional measures should be used in rheumatoid arthritis clinical trials? Arthritis Rheum. 1989;**32**:1093–9.
24. Pincus T, Callahan LF, Brooks RH, et al. Self-report questionnaire scores in rheumatoid arthritis compared with traditional physical, radiographic, and laboratory measures. Ann Intern Med. 1989;**110**:259–66.
25. Hagglund KJ, Roth DL, Haley WE, Alarcon GS. Discriminant and convergent validity of self-report measures of affective distress in patients with rheumatoid arthritis. J Rheumatol. 1989;**16**:1428–32.
26. Klinkhoff AV, Bellamy N, Bombardier C, et al. An experiment in reducing interobserver variability of the examination for joint tenderness. J Rheumatol. 1988;**15**:492–4.
27. Lansbury J, Haut DD. Quantitation of the manifestations of rheumatoid arthritis. Area of joint surfaces as an index to total joint inflammation and deformity. Am J Med Sci. 1956;**232**:150–5.
28. Thompson PW, Silman AJ, Kirwan JR, Currey HLF. Articular indices of joint inflammation in rheumatoid arthritis. Correlation with the acute phase response. Arthritis Rheum. 1987;**30**:618–23.
29. McCarty DJ, O'Duffy JD, Pearson L, Hunter JB. Remitting seronegative symmetrical synovitis with pitting edema. (RS3PE) syndrome. JAMA. 1985;**2545**:3763–276.
30. Thompson M, Bywaters EGL. Unilateral rheumatoid arthritis following hemiplegia. Ann Rheum Dis. 1961;**21**:370–7.
31. Hastings DE, Evans JA. Rheumatoid wrist deformities and their relation to ulnar drift. J Bone Joint Surg. 1975;**57A**:930–4.
32. Jacob J, Sartorius D, Kursunoglu S, et al. Distal interphalangeal joint involvement in rheumatoid arthritis. Arthritis Rheum. 1986;**29**:10–15.
33. Chamberlain A, Corbett M. Carpal tunnel syndrome in early rheumatoid arthritis. Ann Rheum Dis. 1970;**29**:149–52.
34. Chang LW, Gowans JDC, Granger CV, et al. Entrapment neuropathy of the posterior interosseous nerve. Arthritis Rheum. 1972;**15**:350–2.
35. Bywaters EGL. The bursae of the body. Ann Rheum Dis. 1965;**24**:215–18.
36. Yasuda M, Ono M, Naono T, Nobunaga M. Multiple rheumatoid bursal cysts. J Rheumatol. 1989;**16**:1986–8.
37. Polisar I, Burbank B, Levitt LM, et al. Bilateral midline fixation of cricoarytenoid joints as a serious medical emergency. JAMA. 1960;**172**:901–6.
38. Khong TK, Rooney PJ. Manubriosternal joint subluxation in rheumatoid arthritis. J Rheumatol. 1982;**9**:712–15.
39. Martel W. Pathogenesis of cervical discovertebral destruction in rheumatoid arthritis. Arthritis Rheum. 1977;**20**:1217–25.
40. Winfield J, Young A, Williams P, et al. A prospective study of the radiological changes in the cervical spine in early rheumatoid disease. Ann Rheum Dis. 1981;**40**:109–14.
41. Nakano KK, Schoene WC, Baker RA, Dawson DM. The cervical myelopathy associated with rheumatoid arthritis: an analysis of 32 patients, with 2 postmortem cases. Ann Neurol. 1978;**3**:144-51.
42. Fallet GH, Barnes CG, Berry H, et al. Coexisting rheumatoid arthritis and ankylosing spondylitis. J Rheumatol. 1987;**14**:1135–8.
43. Hastings DE, Parker SM. Protrusio acetabuli in rheumatoid arthritis. Clin Orthop. 1975;**108**:76–83.
44. Underwood PL, McLeod RA, Ginsburg WW. The varied clinical manifestations of iliopsoas bursitis. J Rheumatol. 1988;**15**:1683–5.
45. Menard HA, Paquette D. Skin temperature of the knee: and unrecognized physical sign of inflammatory disease of the knee. Can Med Assoc J. 1980;**122**:439–40.
46. Gerber NJ, Dixon AStJ. Synovial cysts and juxta-articular bone cysts. Semin Arthritis Rheum. 1974;**3**:323–48.
47. Kraag G, Thevathasan EM, Gordon DA, Walker IH. The hemorrhage crescent sign of acute synovial rupture. Ann Intern Med. 1976;**85**:477–8.
48. Thevenon A, Hardouin P, Duquesnoy B. Popliteal cyst presenting as an anterior tibial mass. Arthritis Rheum. 1985;**28**:477–8.
49. Rask MR. Achilles tendon rupture owing to rheumatoid disease. JAMA. 1978;**239**:435–6.
50. Semba CP, Mitchell MJ, Sartoris DJ, Resnick D. Multiple stress fractures in the hindfoot in rheumatoid arthritis. J Rheumatol. 1989;**16**:671–6.
51. Shapiro RF, Resnick D, Castles JJ, et al. Fistulization of rheumatoid joints. Spectrum of identifiable syndromes. Ann Rheum Dis. 1975;**34**:489–98.
52. Corrigan AB, Robinson RG, Terenty TR, et al. Benign rheumatoid arthritis of the aged. Br Med J. 1974;**1**:444–6.
53. Schumacher HR. Palindromic onset of rheumatoid arthritis. Clinical, synovial fluid and biopsy studies. Arthritis Rheum. 1982;**25**:361–9.
54. Healey LA, Sheets PK. Polymyalgia rheumatica and seronegative rheumatoid arthritis may be the same entity. J Rheumatol. 1992; **19**:270–2.
55. Pinals RS, Masi AF, Larsen RA, et al. Preliminary criteria for clinical remission in rheumatoid arthritis. Bull Rheum Dis. 1982;**32**:7–10.
56. Masi AT, Feigenbaum SL, Kaplan SB. Articular patterns in the early course of rheumatoid arthritis. Am J Med 1983;**75**(suppl 6A):16–26.
57. Fleming A, Benn RT, Corbett M, Wood PHN. Early rheumatoid disease. II. Patterns of joint involvement. Ann Rheum Dis. 1976;**35**:361–3.
58. Luukkainen R, Isomaki H, Kajander A: Prognostic value of the type of onset of rheumatoid arthritis. Ann Rheum Dis. 1983;**42**:274–5.
59. Aho K, Heliovaara M, Maatela J, et al. Rheumatoid factors antedating clinical rheumatoid arthritis. J Rheumatol. 1991;**18**:1282–4.
60. Wolfe F, Cathey MA. The assessment and prediction of functional disability in rheumatoid arthritis. J Rheumatol. 1991;**18**:1298–1306.
61. Leigh JP, Fries JF, Parikh N. Severity of disability and duration of disease in rheumatoid arthritis. J Rheumatol. 1992;**19**:1906–11.
62. Leigh JP, Fries J. Mortality predictors among 263 patients with rheumatoid arthritis. J Rheumatol. 1991;18:1307–12.
63. Pincus T, Callahan LF. Taking mortality in rheumatoid arthritis seriously – predictive markers, socioeconomic status and co-morbidity. J Rheumatol. 1986;**13**:841–5.
64. Kazis LE, Anderson JJ, Meenan RF. Health status as a predictor of mortality in rheumatoid arthritis: a five-year study. J Rheumatol. 1990;**17**:609–13.
65. Berkanovic E, Hurwicz M-L. Rheumatoid arthritis and comorbidity. J Rheumatol. 1990;**17**:888–92.
66. Pincus T, Brooks RH, Callahan LF. Reliability of grip strength, walking time and button test performed according to a standard protocol. J Rheumatol. 1991;**18**:997–1000.
67 Pincus T, Callahan LF. Predictive value of quantitative physical and questionnaire measures of functional status for 9-year morbidity in rheumatoid arthritis. J Rheumatol. 1992;**19**:1051–7.
68. Silman AJ. Has the incidence of rheumatoid arthritis declined in the United Kingdom? Br J Rheumatol. 1988;**27**:77–9.
69. Aho, K, Tuomi T, Palosuo T, et al. Is seropositive rheumatoid arthritis becoming less severe? Clin Exp Rheumatol. 1989;**7**:287–90.

CLINICAL FEATURES OF RHEUMATOID ARTHRITIS: SYSTEMIC INVOLVEMENT

16

Eric L Matteson,
Marc D Cohen & Doyt L Conn

INTRODUCTION

Constitutional features of rheumatoid arthritis (RA), such as fatigue and weight loss, may occur early in the course of the disease and may predominate, overshadowing the joint manifestations. At times inflammation may extend beyond the joints and involve other organs. Laboratory abnormalities that accompany systemic involvement include elevated erythrocyte sedimentation rate, anemia, thrombocytosis and elevation of certain liver function tests (Fig. 16.1).

NODULES

Subcutaneous nodules occur in 20% of RA patients with positive tests for blood rheumatoid factors and rarely in seronegative patients (Fig. 16.2). The nodules reflect the level of rheumatoid disease activity and accompany severe disease. Multiple, widespread nodules (rheumatoid nodulosis) occasionally presents as a separate condition, usually in men, with a low-grade and sometimes barely detectable synovitis [1].

Nodules develop most commonly on pressure areas, including the elbows, finger joints, ischial and sacral prominences, occipital scalp, and Achilles tendon. Rheumatoid nodules are firm and frequently adherent to the underlying periosteum. Histologically there is a focal central fibrinoid necrosis with surrounding fibroblasts. This is thought to occur as a result of small vessel vasculitis with fibrinoid necrosis which forms the center of the nodule, and surrounding fibroblastic proliferation [2].

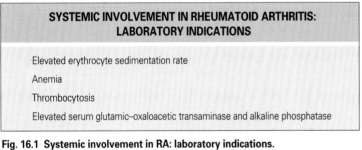

SYSTEMIC INVOLVEMENT IN RHEUMATOID ARTHRITIS: LABORATORY INDICATIONS
Elevated erythrocyte sedimentation rate
Anemia
Thrombocytosis
Elevated serum glutamic–oxaloacetic transaminase and alkaline phosphatase

Fig. 16.1 Systemic involvement in RA: laboratory indications.

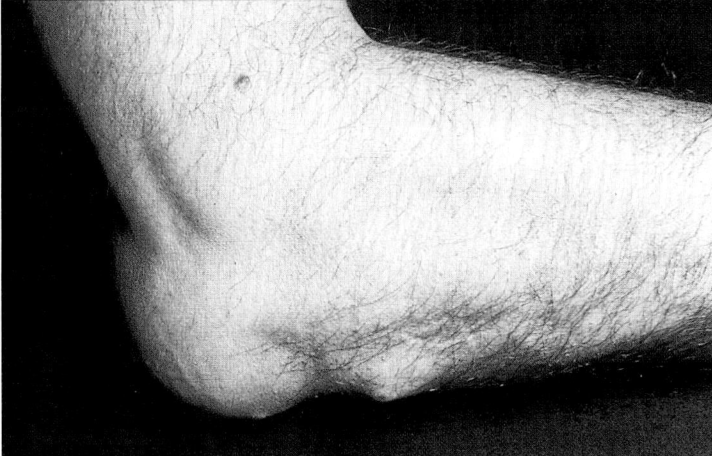

Fig. 16.2 Olecranon bursitis, rheumatoid nodule.

Subcutaneous nodules may regress during treatment with disease-modifying drugs, usually as the RA improves. Methotrexate treatment paradoxically may result in an increase in nodules, particularly over finger tendons, despite improvement in the overall disease activity [3].

HEMATOLOGICAL ABNORMALITIES

The cause of anemia in RA is multifactorial [4]. Iron utilization is impaired, as reflected by decreased serum iron and transferrin concentrations. As with other forms of chronic inflammation, there is an increased synthesis of ferritin and hemosiderin, abnormal retention of iron from senescent red blood cells by the reticuloendothelial system, and increased lactoferrin which contributes to the binding and lowering of serum iron [5,6]. Also contributing to the anemia of RA are reduced erythropoietin levels and a slightly depressed response of the bone marrow to erythropoietin. Ineffective erythropoiesis occurs with premature destruction of red blood cells and inhibition of production of red blood cell precursors [7]. Red blood cell life span may be reduced [8]. Additional factors include an increased phagocytosis of red blood cells by lymph nodes and even the synovium.

The degree of anemia in RA correlates with the activity of the underlying disease, particularly the degree of articular inflammation. It is commonly normochromic and normocytic unless complicated by concomitant conditions, such as blood loss, poor nutrition, hemodilution, intercurrent infections, autoimmune hemolytic anemia, or bone marrow suppression secondary to drug treatment.

While various medications used to treat RA can contribute to the anemia, that caused by rheumatoid inflammation can improve with therapy that treats the disease successfully. The administration of erythropoietin to patients with RA has been shown to improve red blood cell counts without influencing disease activity [9]. Iron deficiency may complicate the anemia associated with RA, but repletion of iron may fail since the anemia is due to inhibition of hemoglobin synthesis caused by inflammation.

Thrombocytosis is a frequent finding in active RA [10]. The degree of thrombocytosis may correlate with the number of joints involved with active synovitis, and may be associated with extra-articular features. The mechanism of thrombocytosis is uncertain. Increased intravascular coagulation with a compensatory increase in platelet production has been suggested. The thrombocytosis does not predispose to an increase in thrombotic events and is not correlated with bone marrow neoplastic changes.

Thrombocytopenia is rare in RA, except when related to drug treatment or Felty's syndrome. Drug-induced platelet dysfunction may be seen. Coagulation inhibitors may be produced in RA [11]. Hyperviscosity has rarely been reported [12]. It occurs in association with high titers of rheumatoid factor and may cause neurological and vascular occlusive symptoms.

Eosinophilia accompanying RA is sometimes associated with extra-articular manifestations [13,14]. The pathogenesis is not known. Immune complexes may be chemotactic for eosinophils and cytokines known to stimulate eosinophil production could be important. Eosinophilia has been associated with high titers of blood rheumatoid factor, elevation of serum gamma globulins, and diminished serum complement levels. Pulmonary complications may be associated with eosinophilia [15]. A number of drugs used to treat RA, especially gold, may cause eosinophilia.

Lymphadenopathy is frequent in patients with active RA [16]. Palpable lymph nodes are generally detected in the axillary, inguinal, and epitrochlear areas. These lymph nodes are usually mobile and nontender. The presence of lymphadenopathy has no bearing on the outcome of the disease. As the RA is controlled, the lymphadenopathy will decrease. Histological examination reveals follicular hyperplasia occasionally prominent enough to suggest lymphoma. The reported increased incidence of lymph node neoplasia has not been confirmed [17,18], but concomitant Sjögren's syndrome may confer an increased risk of lymphoma [19].

FELTY'S SYNDROME

Felty's syndrome is defined as RA in combination with splenomegaly and leukopenia. The syndrome characteristically occurs in patients with longstanding, seropositive, nodular, deforming RA. Approximately one-third of this group of patients have no active synovitis at the time Felty's syndrome develops. Many of these patients have lower extremity ulcerations, hyperpigmentation, and antinuclear antibodies.

Bacterial infections are common in Felty's syndrome, correlate with a polymorphonuclear leukocyte count of less than $100/mm^3$, and account for most deaths in this syndrome [20]. Other factors associated with an increased incidence of infections are skin ulcers, glucocorticoid dose, hypocomplementemia, and high levels of immune complexes [21]. Immune complexes coat granulocytes, which results in their sequestration and reduced survival, and specific antibodies directed against white blood cell surface antigens (granulocyte-specific antinuclear antibodies) may contribute to the leukopenia. In some patients, the bone marrow does not respond appropriately to the degree of leukopenia, perhaps because of inhibitors which suppress myelopoiesis. Thrombocytopenia also occurs in Felty's syndrome.

Treatment of the rheumatoid disease with disease-modifying drugs, such as parenteral gold, frequently improves the cytopenias, cutaneous vasculitis, and may decrease susceptibility to infection [22]. Splenectomy may improve the hematological abnormalities and may be indicated for recurrent serious infections caused by the neutropenia which has been unresponsive to disease-modifying drugs. Splenectomy rarely helps the underlying disease process, although it might improve leg ulcers. Despite splenectomy, granulocytopenia may recur and persist. Glucocorticoids transiently improve the granulocytopenia but may predispose to infections. Parenteral testosterone, lithium and other treatments such as granulocyte colony stimulating factor have been used with success in selected patients, but large studies using such agents are not available.

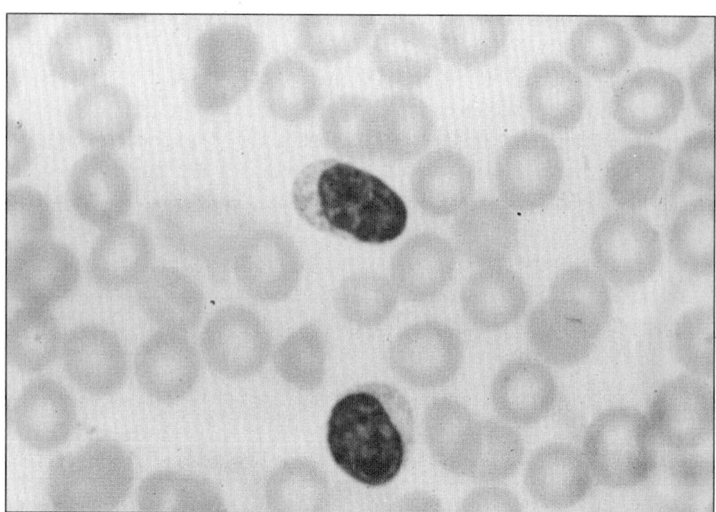

Fig. 16.3 Large granular lymphocyte.

A recently recognized variant of Felty's syndrome has been described [23]. These patients have neutropenia and an increase in the number of large granular lymphocytes in blood and bone marrow (Fig. 16.3). The actual white blood count may be normal or increased. Such patients may also have thrombocytopenia, anemia, and splenomegaly. This syndrome occurs in older patients and early in the course of the arthritis. In patients with symptoms related to neutropenia, improvement may occur with treatment with glucocorticoids and/or immunosuppressive treatment [23].

HEPATIC DISORDERS

Active RA may be associated with an elevation of liver enzymes (especially serum glutamic oxaloacetic transaminase and alkaline phosphatase) [24]. Liver function abnormalities may parallel the anemia, thrombocytosis, and increased erythrocyte sedimentation rate. With control of the rheumatoid inflammation the liver function abnormalities return to normal. Examination of liver histology at the time of liver function abnormality reveals only minimal nonspecific changes with some periportal mononuclear cell infiltration.

Nonsteroidal anti-inflammatory drugs (NSAIDs) may induce liver enzyme abnormalities and it may be difficult to differentiate between drug effects and disease activity. However, if the liver function abnormalities are due to NSAIDs, enzyme levels will improve with their discontinuation. NSAIDs seldom cause serious liver deterioration.

Liver involvement may be present in up to 65% of patients with Felty's syndrome [25]. There may be histological abnormalities, even when liver function tests are normal. The liver pathology varies from portal fibrosis and abnormal lobular architecture to nodular regenerative hyperplasia (Fig. 16.4). The nodular regenerative hyperplasia may be secondary to inflammation of small portal veins, possibly immune complex induced. Frequently a liver wedge biopsy (an open biopsy) is necessary to establish the diagnosis. These patients can develop portal hypertension, esophageal varices, and variceal bleeding.

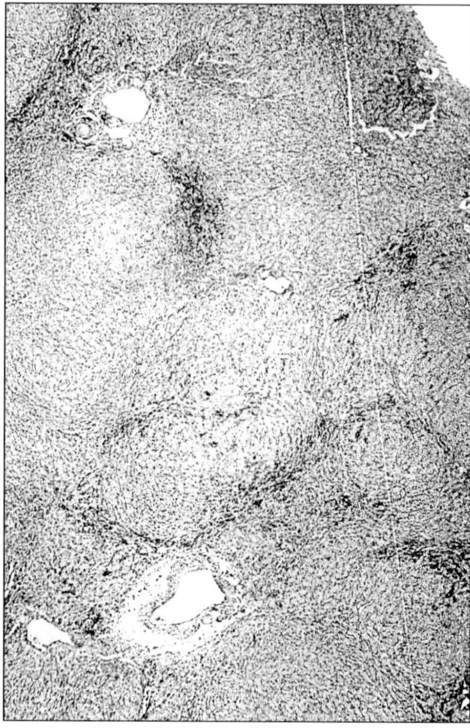

Fig. 16.4 Nodular regenerative hyperplasia of the liver in a patient with Felty's syndrome. (Original magnification ×40.)

PLEURAL FLUID IN RHEUMATOID ARTHRITIS	
Color	Green-yellow to clear yellow
WBC	Variable – low to very high
Glucose	Low (<25 mg/dl, <1.4mmol/l)
Complement:	Low
Protein	High (4 gm/dl)
Lipid and cholesterol	High
Pleural biopsy	Nonspecific

Fig. 16.5 Pleural fluid in RA.

PULMONARY DISORDERS

Pulmonary involvement in RA is frequent, although the clinical features may be subtle. Diffuse interstitial pulmonary fibrosis was first described in RA in 1948 [26]. An incidence of 28% has been reported, although the true figure is probably less [27].

In autopsy studies, involvement of the pleura is reported in up to 50% of patients with RA [28]. Pleural effusions are transudates with low cell counts, predominately lymphocytes (Fig. 16.5) [29]. Glucose levels are often less than 25 mg/dl (1.4mmol/l). The low glucose in rheumatoid pleural effusions are a result of impaired transport across an inflamed pleura [30]. Pleural fluid hemolytic complement levels are low, rheumatoid factor is present, and the leukocytes have inclusions containing rheumatoid factor. Pleurisy and pleural effusions may improve spontaneously or may require treatment. Persistent effusions can lead to fibrosis.

Parenchymal pulmonary nodules (Fig. 16.6) are generally asymptomatic and are found in seropositive RA patients who have widespread synovitis and usually nodules elsewhere. The pulmonary nodules tend to be peripheral in location, and can measure less than 1cm or up to 6–8cm in diameter [31]. They can cavitate and cause pleural effusions and bronchopleural fistulas. The differential diagnosis of pulmonary rheumatoid nodules includes neoplasms, tuberculosis, and fungal infections. In the case of a solitary rheumatoid nodule in the lung, an excisional biopsy may be necessary to confirm the diagnosis. Treatment of the underlying rheumatoid disease frequently results in improvement of the pulmonary nodules.

Pneumoconiosis in patients with RA (Caplan's syndrome) is characterized by multiple nodules greater than 1cm in diameter scattered throughout the peripheral lung field (Fig. 16.7) [32]. This condition is seen in individuals with extensive exposure to coal dust. The pulmonary nodules may appear suddenly, often accompanied by an exacerbation of the arthritis. The nodules may cavititate. Histologic examination of these nodules reveals a central necrotic zone that contains varying amounts of coal dust and collagen tissue, surrounded by a cellular area of proliferating fibroblasts typical of a rheumatoid nodule [33].

Obliterative bronchiolitis has been reported in patients with RA [34]. Whether this pulmonary manifestation is a consequence of the rheumatoid inflammatory process, a concomitant condition, or due to medications, remains uncertain. Airway obstruction may develop in patients with RA; however, this may not necessarily be caused by the disease itself but rather by other factors known to predispose to obstructive pulmonary disease.

Isolated pulmonary arteritis is a rare complication of RA. It is frequently associated with other manifestations of rheumatoid lung disease, such as interstitial fibrosis and nodulosis [35].

CARDIAC DISORDERS

Pericarditis is the most common cardiac manifestation of RA. Although symptomatic pericarditis is relatively uncommon, both random electrocardiographic evaluation of RA patients and autopsy studies reveal evidence of pericardial inflammation in 50% of patients [36]. Pericarditis occurs in seropositive patients with nodules [37]. An analysis of pericardial fluid reveals changes similar to those found in rheumatoid pleural effusions (see Fig. 16.5), including a variable white blood cell count, high protein levels, decreased complement, decreased glucose concentrations, the presence of rheumatoid factor and immune complexes [38]. Commonly the pericarditis resolves as the rheumatoid disease is controlled. Symptomatic patients generally respond to NSAIDs. Occasionally glucocorticoids

Fig. 16.6 Radiograph of pleural effusion and rheumatoid nodule in RA.

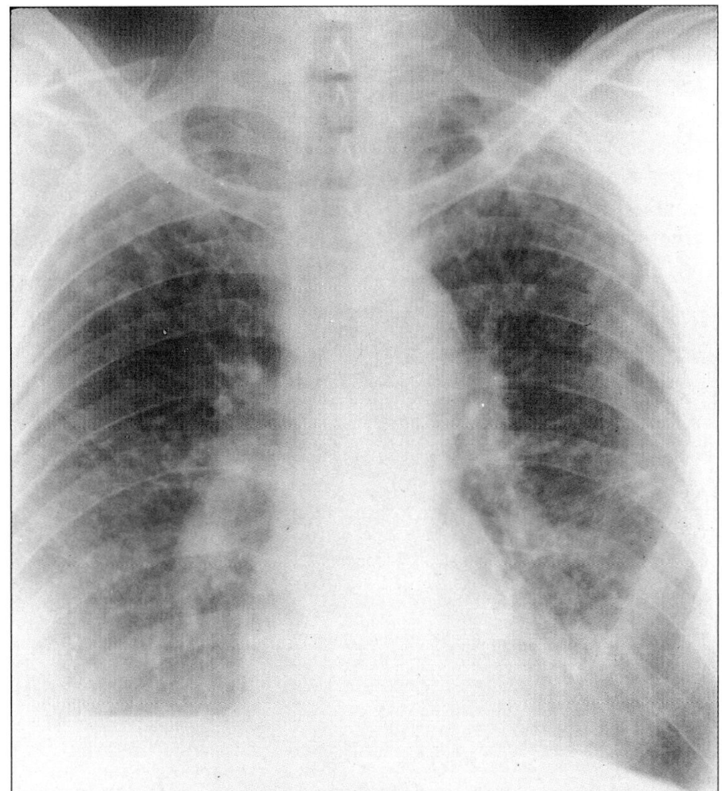

Fig. 16.7 Radiograph of Caplan's syndrome.

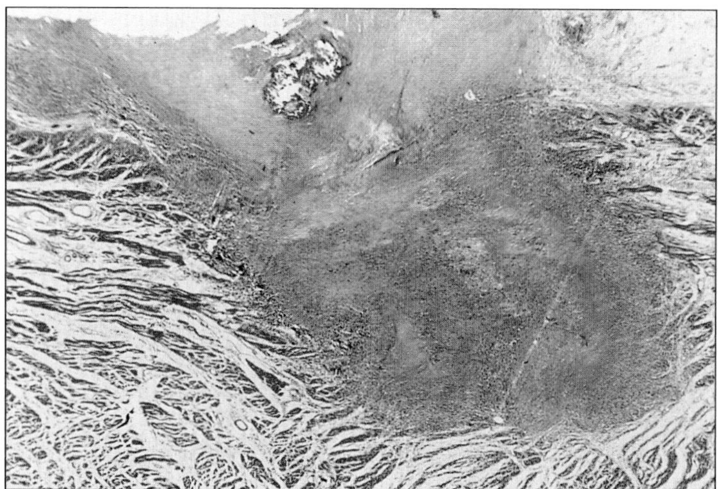

Fig. 16.8 Rheumatoid myoepicarditis with inflammatory cellular and rheumatoid nodular infiltrate of the epicardium and myocardium. (Hematoxylin and eosin stain, original magnification ×5.)

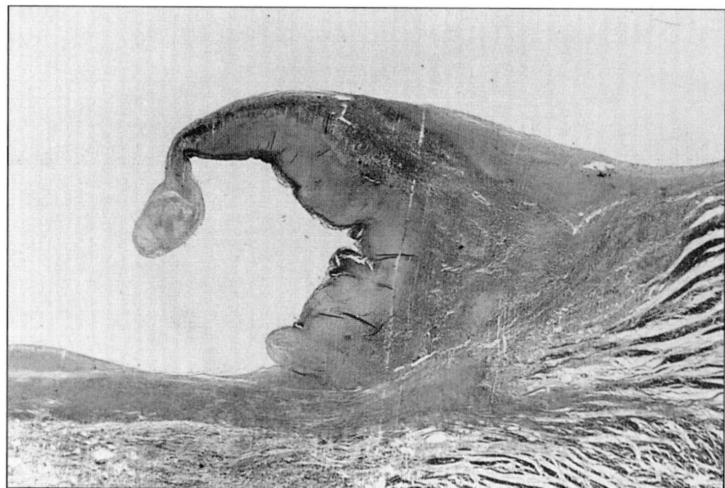

Fig. 16.9 Rheumatoid nodule in the aortic valve cusp in a 54-year-old woman. The cusp is seen as a finger-like projection to the left. At the base of the cusp, a rheumatoid nodule is noted. The muscle tissue in the lower right corner is of the left ventricle. (Hematoxylin and eosin stain, original magnification ×2.5.)

are required if the symptoms are severe and recalcitrant to the usual management. Chronic, constrictive pericarditis is an infrequent sequela. In these cases, pericardiectomy may be required [39].

Myocardial disease resulting from nodular granulomatous lesions or more diffuse fibrosing lesions has been seen in RA (Fig. 16.8) [40]. Nonspecific myocarditis is usually asymptomatic and rarely effects cardiac size or function. Abnormalities in the conduction pathways have been described. Endocardial involvement may be diffuse, but is rarely clinically significant.

Echocardiographic evidence for some degree of valve involvement can be detected in about 30% of patients, but is usually hemodynamically insignificant [41]. However, a few patients develop valvular incompetence (Fig. 16.9) [42]. Coronary arteritis can occur as part of systemic rheumatoid vasculitis (Fig. 16.10) [40]. Because myocardial and endocardial disease associated with RA is usually a result of vasculitis and nodule formation, appropriate treatment of the underlying disease is necessary.

OCULAR DISORDERS

The most common ocular involvement in RA is keratoconjunctivitis sicca which affects between 10 and 35% of patients [43]. The severity of the symptoms may not be correlated with that of the arthritis. Some patients have only dry eyes, while others have the classical symptoms of the sicca syndrome, which include burning, foreign body sensation, and a mucoid discharge. Tear production may be assessed by the Schirmer's test or by corneal staining with fluorescein or Rose-Bengal dye. Treatment of keratoconjunctivitis sicca remains symptomatic and is generally unsatisfactory.

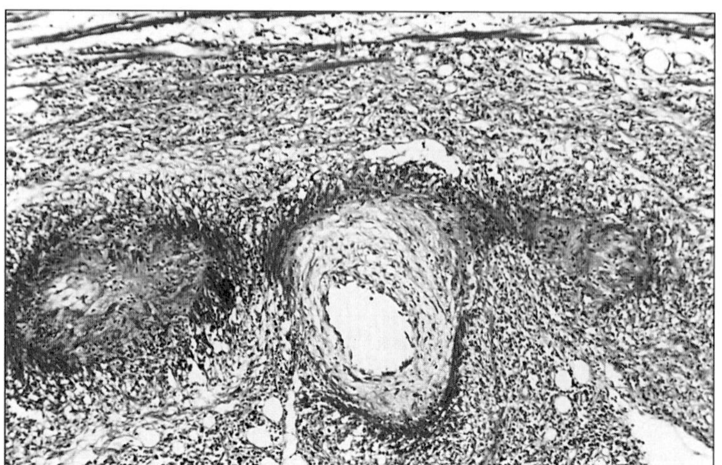

Fig. 16.10 Coronary arteritis. Two arteries are seen. There is a dense inflammatory infiltrate in the adventitia with some intimal luminal narrowing and destruction of the media of one artery. (Hematoxylin and eosin stain, original magnification ×25.)

Episcleritis usually correlates with the activity of RA (Fig. 16.11). This process, which may be either nodular or diffuse, appears acutely and causes eye redness and pain, but only rarely changes in visual acuity [43]. Scleritis is less common than episcleritis but is more obviously correlated with vasculitis, longstanding arthritis, and active joint inflammation [44]. Untreated scleritis may progress to scleromalacia (Fig. 16.12). Control of the RA may not improve the episcleritis or scleritis. The avascular nature of the sclera contributes to its resistence to treatment [45]. Other rare ocular findings in RA include uveitis, episcleral nodulosis, and corneal melt.

Drugs used to treat RA can also affect the eyes. Glucocorticoids may cause cataracts and glaucoma, gold may result in conjunctival and corneal deposition, and chloroquine derivatives cause both a keratopathy and a retinopathy [46,47].

An uncommon ocular complication of RA is Brown's syndrome, which is defined as diplopia upon upward and inward gaze and is thought to be due to inflammation and thickening of the superior oblique tendons [48].

NEUROLOGIC DISORDERS

Nerve compression is a common cause of neurologic impairment in RA. Peripheral entrapment neuropathies tend to correlate with the

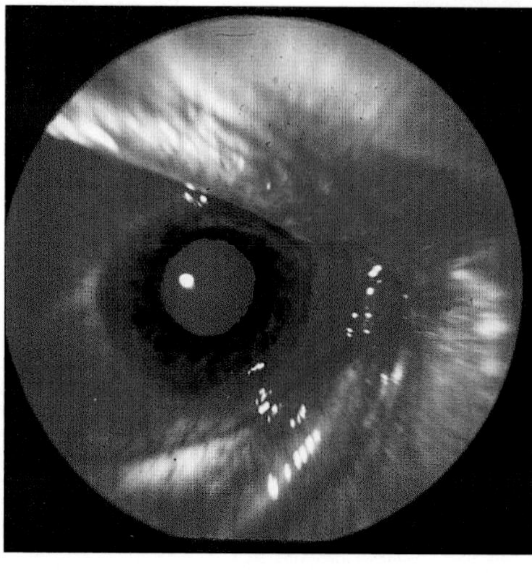

Fig. 16.11 Episcleritis.

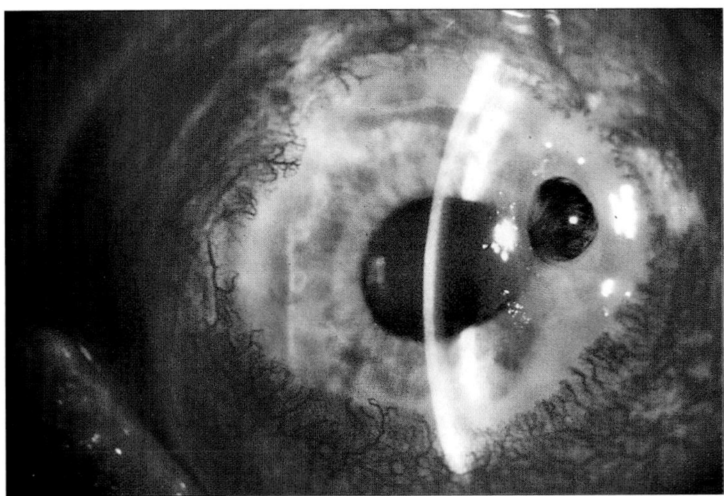

Fig. 16.12 Scleromalacia.

degree and severity of local synovitis, but are not related to duration, level of activity, or severity of extra-articular manifestations of RA. They generally occur when the nerve is compressed by the inflamed synovium against a fixed structure. The median, ulnar, posterior tibial, and the posterior interosseous branch of the radial nerves are the most commonly involved nerves. The diagnosis is suggested by clinical symptoms and neurologic findings. Percussions over the carpal tunnel and tarsal tunnel may elicit symptoms (Tinel's sign). The pain and paresthesias from the affected nerves often have a nocturnal accentuation and may radiate from the site of compression. Medical treatment may be effective, particularly if the synovitis can be controlled, but surgical release may be necessary to prevent permanent muscle atrophy.

Atlantoaxial subluxation caused by erosion of the odontoid process and/or the transverse ligament of Cl may allow the odontoid process to slip posteriorly and cause a cervical myelopathy (Fig. 16.13) [49]. Basilar invagination, with upward impingement of the odontoid process into the foramen magnum can also result in cord compression (Fig. 16.14) [50]. The presence of cord compression is indicated by a postive Babinski sign, hyperreflexia, and weakness. This may require surgical stabilization. These complications are seen in association with severe progressive, destructive, longstanding rheumatoid disease.

MUSCULAR DISORDERS

Muscle weakness in RA is usually due to muscle atrophy secondary to joint inflammation. Occasionally nutritional problems, medication, and neurologic dysfunction also contribute. A rare inflammatory myopathy has been described in RA and includes a patchy cellular infiltration in muscle fibers resulting in some fiber degeneration [51].

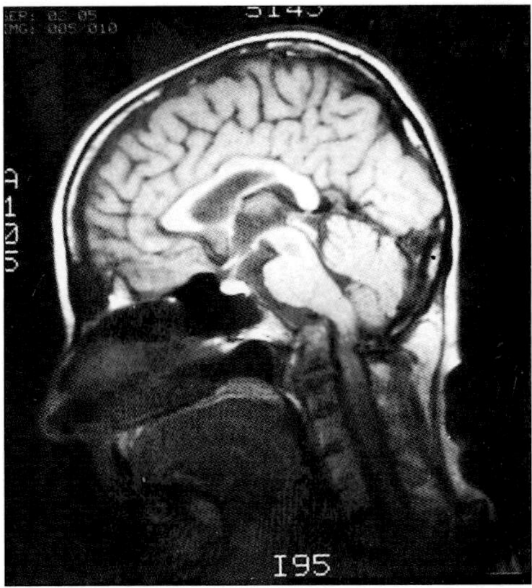

Fig. 16. I4 MRI of the cervical spine showing basilar invagination.

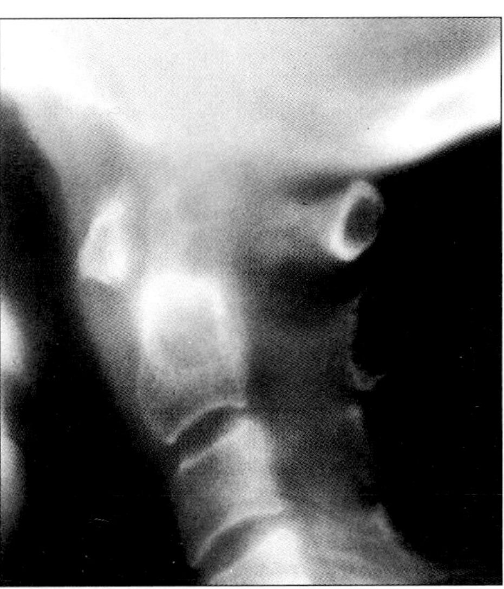

Fig. 16.13 CT of cervical spine showing erosion of the odontoid.

Similar changes have been seen in other systemic inflammatory conditions. Usually, such patients have normal or only modestly elevated levels of serum creatine phosphokinase.

Other forms of secondary muscle involvement in RA include a diffuse polymyositis caused by D-penicillamine or a neuromyopathy with hydroxychloroquine. The muscle atrophy of chronic steroid use is common and leads to further debility.

RENAL DISORDERS

The kidneys are usually spared in RA, although a low-grade membranous nephropathy [52], glomerulitis, vasculitis, or secondary amyloidosis have all been described [53]. More commonly, renal abnormalities result from the agents used in treating RA, notably gold, D-penicillamine, cyclosporine and NSAIDs [54,55].

AMYLOIDOSIS

Amyloidosis may rarely complicate longstanding RA [56]. Its true incidence varies widely. Amyloidosis may be primary, associated with myeloma and related disorders, or secondary, as in RA, and develops as a result of longstanding active inflammation. Proteinuria is a frequent finding in the amyloidosis associated with RA. Virtually every organ system may be involved in secondary amyloidosis that complicates RA, including the heart, kidney, liver, spleen, intestines, and skin. The diagnosis of amyloidosis is confirmed by biopsy of involved tissue (Fig. 16.15). The presence of secondary amyloidosis in patients with RA portends a poor outcome and there is no satisfactory treatment.

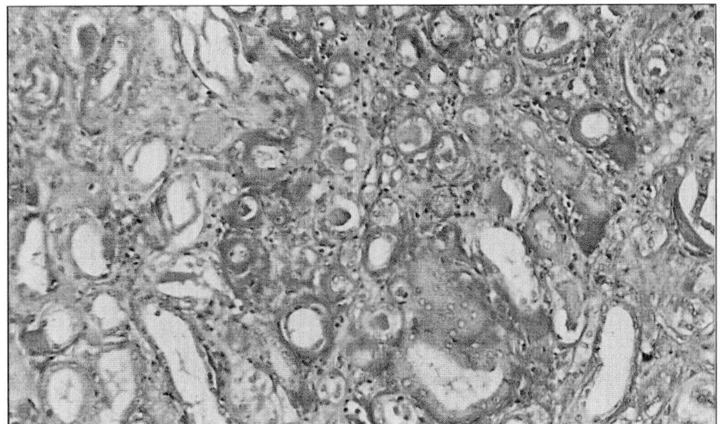

Fig. 16.15 Renal amyloidosis in RA (secondary AA). There is diffuse amyloid deposition throughout the renal parenchyma, with deposition in blood vessel walls. Amyloid deposits are green colored. (Sulfated Alcian blue stain ×40.)

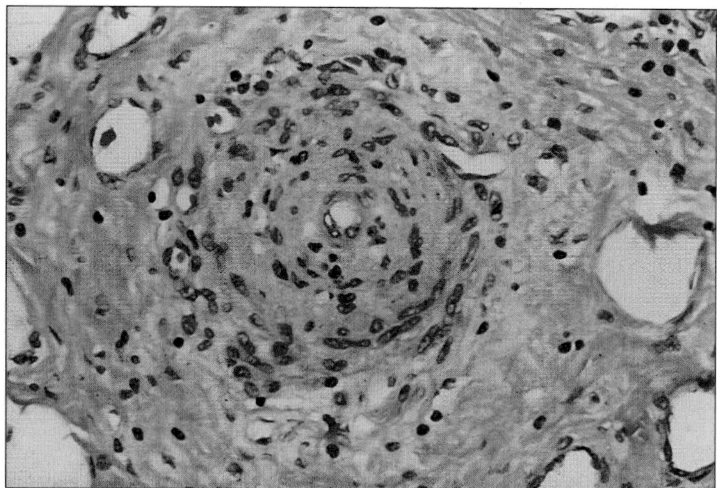

Fig. 16.16 Artery with intimal proliferation and luminal occlusion. (Hematoxylin and eosin stain, original magnification ×312.)

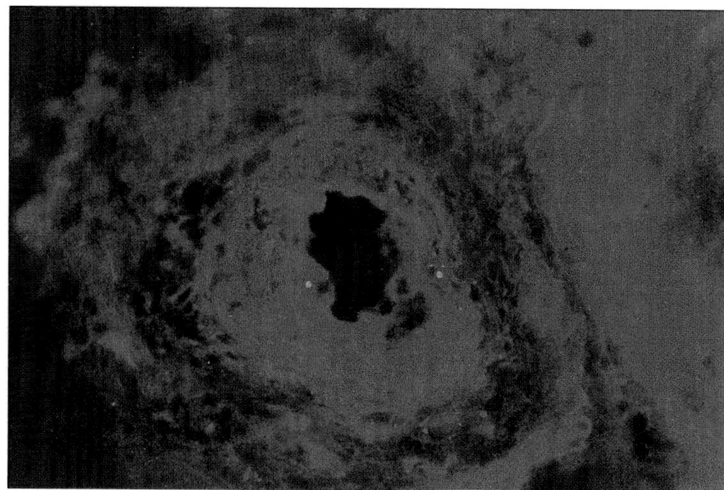

Fig. 16.17 IgM in artery with fibrinoid necrosis. (IgM by immunofluorescence, original magnification ×312.)

RHEUMATOID VASCULITIS

A small vessel vasculitis is intimately associated with many of the clinical manifestations seen in RA. The earliest events in the development of the rheumatoid nodule are a small-vessel vasculitis. Inflammation of the small- and medium-sized arteries in the extremities, peripheral nerves, and occasionally other organs may complicate RA. Patients with this form of rheumatoid vasculitis have a higher frequency of HLA-DR4 than those with uncomplicated RA, suggesting an inherited susceptibility to this complication [57].

Study of involved vessels from patients with rheumatoid vasculitis reveals a pathologic picture and distribution similar to that seen in polyarteritis, but renal involvement is rare [58]. Early lesions show fibrinoid necrosis of the vessel wall with an inflammatory cell infiltrate. Chronic changes with artery wall fibrosis, occlusion, and recanalization may be seen (Fig. 16.16). One pathologic difference from polyarteritis is the finding of small- and medium-sized arteries involved with an occlusive intimal proliferation with little inflammation [59]. The acute arterial lesions are immune complex-mediated, as indicated by the finding of immunoglobulins and complement in the involved arteries (Fig. 16.17) [60]. Immune deposits are not detected in the more chronic lesions, rather, fibrinogen is found (Fig. 16.18).

The systemic vasculitis that complicates RA is uncommon. It usually occurs in rheumatoid patients who have longstanding disease, usually of 10 years or more. Rarely, a systemic vasculitis is present at the onset of RA, and in such cases the outcome is poor [61]. Men are afflicted as commonly as women. These patients have more severe RA with destructive joint disease, rheumatoid nodules, and higher titers of blood rheumatoid factor [57]. Patients with Felty's syndrome are more likely to develop vasculitic complications. Rheumatoid synovitis may not be active when the features of the systemic vasculitis are present. Small vessel vasculitis commonly involves the skin and causes nailfold infarcts (Fig. 16.19), digital gangrene (Fig. 16.20) and leg ulcers (Fig. 16.21). Patients with nailfold infarcts and leg ulcers usually do not develop more widespread vascular involvement. Distal sensory neuropathy is another manifestation seen in small vessel vasculitis that also may occur alone without progressing to widespread vascular involvement.

The more ominous manifestations of vasculitis are the appearance of infarcts of the fingertips and a sensorimotor neuropathy [62]. Rapid, progressive, and widespread appearance of new areas of involvement indicates systemic arterial disease and a poorer outcome. In some patients, the vasculitis may extend to involve mesenteric, coronary, and cerebral arteries.

It is likely that other factors, in addition to the vasculitis, influence the final vascular outcome. In the pathogenesis of leg ulcers there is usually an underlying vasculitis which initiates the lesions, but ulcer expansion and its chronicity may be influenced by other features, including concomitant venous insufficiency, arterial insufficiency, dependent edema, trauma, and chronic glucocorticoid use (Fig. 16.22).

Patients with rheumatoid vasculitis have high serum titers of rheumatoid factor, low serum complement, cryoglobulins, and

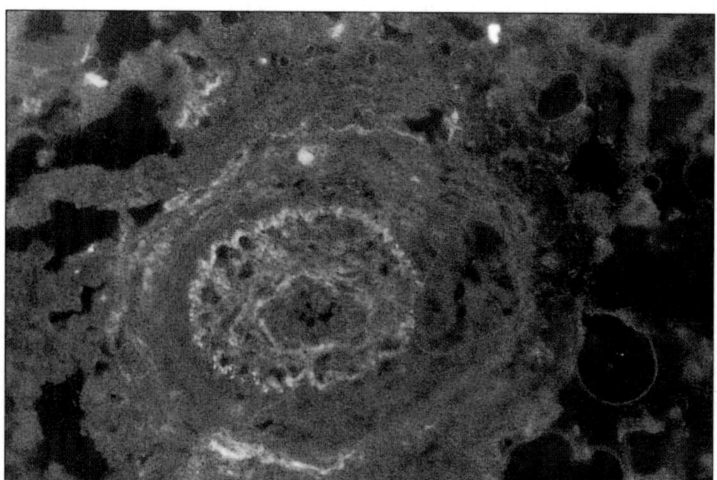

Fig. 16.18 Fibrinogen in artery with intimal proliferation. (Fibrinogen by immunofluorescence, original magnification x 312.)

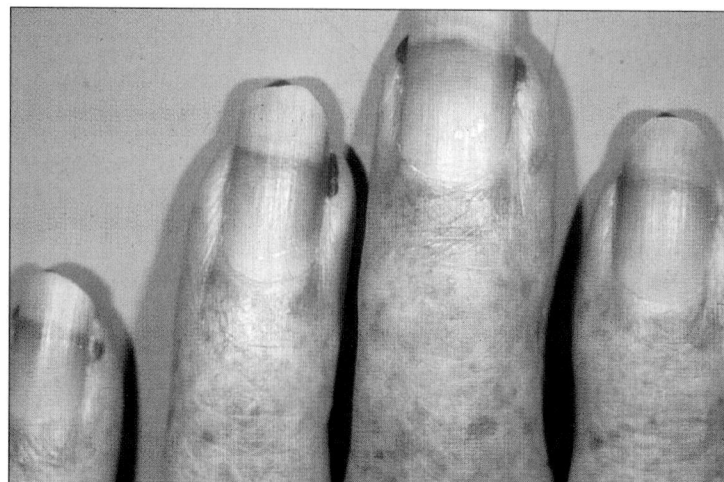

Fig. 16.19 Nailfold infarcts.

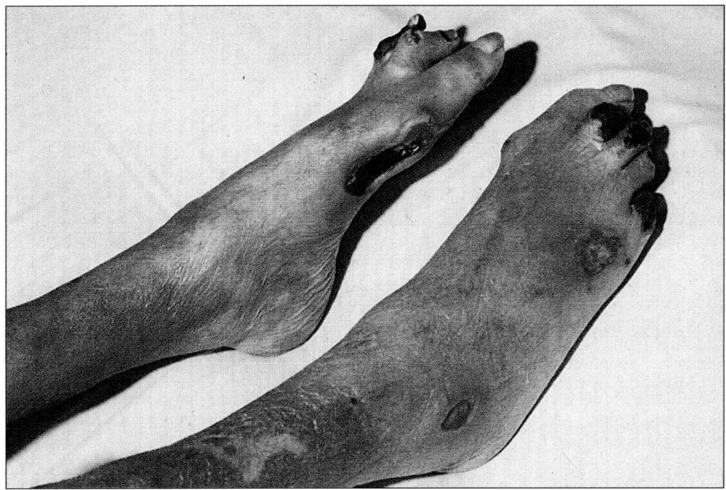

Fig. 16.20 Digital tip infarcts.

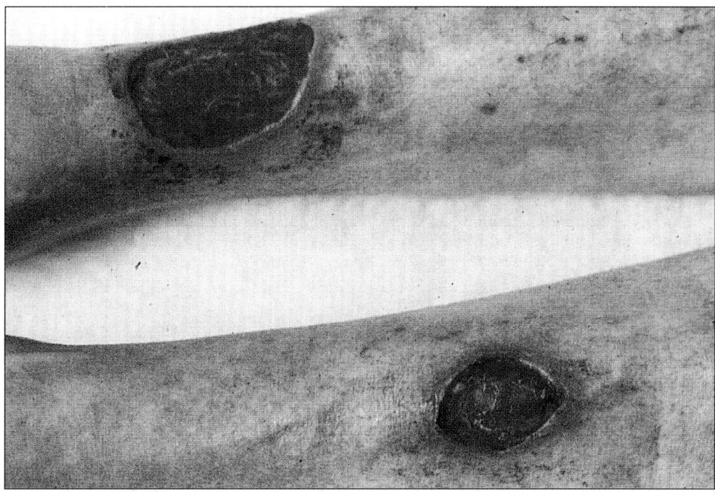

Fig. 16.21 Leg ulcers.

circulatory immune complexes [63]. In addition, they will usually have an elevated erythrocyte sedimentation rate, anemia, thrombocytosis, and a diminished serum albumin.

Despite the belief that the widespread vasculitis which complicates RA is caused by glucocorticoids, patients who have never taken glucocorticoids may develop vasculitis. However, wide fluctuations in glucocorticoid dose, such as those caused by abruptly stopping the drug, seem to allow an underlying vasculitis to blossom [64].

The chronic use of glucocorticoids to treat RA predisposes to atherosclerosis and may permit the transformation from vasculitis to an occlusive vasculopathy [65]. Conversely, NSAIDs may modify and lessen the vasculopathic changes. A study of survival in rheumatoid vasculitis has failed to show any single clinical feature that was associated with a worse outcome [66]. A poor prognosis is influenced by older age, concomitant atherosclerosis, and the severity of vascular involvement.

LEG ULCERS IN RHEUMATOID ARTHRITIS
Triggered by small vessel vasculitis
Perpetuated by
Relative arterial insufficiency
Venous insufficiency
Dependent edema
Chronic glucocorticosteroid use
Repeated trauma

Fig. 16.22 Leg ulcers in RA.

REFERENCES

1. Wisnieski JJ, Askari AD. Rheumatoid nodulosis. A relatively benign rheumatoid variant. Arch Intern Med. 1981;**141**:615.
2. Sokoloff L, McCluskey RT, Bunim JJ. Vascularity of the early subcutaneous nodules of RA. Arch Pathol. 1953;**55**:475.
3. Segal R, Caspi D, Tisher M, et al. Accelerated nodulosis and vasculitis during methotrexate therapy for RA. Arthritis Rheum. 1988;**31**:1182.
4. Bently DP. Anaemia and chronic disease. Clin Haematol. 1982;**11**:465.
5. Aisen P, Listowski I. Iron transport and storage proteins. Ann Rev Biochem. 1980;**49**:357.
6. Smith RJ, Davis P, Thomson ABR, et al. Serum ferritin levels in the anemia of RA. J Rheumatol. 1977;**4**:389.
7. Samson D, Halliday D, Gumpel JM. Role of ineffective erythropoiesis in the anaemia of RA. Ann Rheum Dis. 1977;**36**:181.
8. Dinant HJ, DeMatt CEM. Erythropoiesis and mean red-cell lifespan in normal subjects and in patients with anaemia of active RA. Br J Haematol. 1978;**39**:437.
9. Pincus T, Olsen NJ, Russell JI, et al. Multicenter study of recombinant human erythropoietin in correction of anemia in rheumatoid arthritis. Am J Med. 1990;**89**:161.
10. Hernandez LA, Rowan RM, Kennedy AC, et al. Thrombocytosis in RA: A clinical study of 200 patients. Arthritis Rheum. 1975;**6**:635.
11. Green D, Schuette PT, Wallace WH. Factor VIII antibodies in RA: Effect of cyclophosphamide. Arch Intern Med. 1980;**140**:1232.
12. Pope RM, Mannik M, Gilliland BC, et al. The hyperviscosity syndrome in RA due to intermediate complexes formed by self-association of IgG-rheumatoid factors. Arthritis Rheum. 1975;**18**:97.
13. Winchester RJ, Litwin SD, Koffler D, et al. Observations on the eosinophilia of certain patients with RA. Arthritis Rheum. 1971;**14**:650.
14. Panush RS, Franco AE, Schur PH. Rheumatoid arthritis associated with eosinophilia. Ann Intern Med. 1971;**75**:199.
15. Crisp AJ, Armstrong RD, Grahame R, et al. Rheumatoid lung disease, pneumothorax, and eosinophilia. Ann Rheum Dis. 1982;**41**;137.
16. Motulsky AG, Weinberg S, Saphir 0, et al. Lymph nodes in RA. Arch Intern Med. 1952;**90**:660.
17. Goldenberg GJ, Paraskevas F, Israels LG. Lymphocyte and plasma cell neoplasm associated with autoimmune diseases. Semin Arthritis Rheum. 1971;**1**:174.
18. Lewis RB, Castro CW, Knisley RE, et al. Frequency of neoplasia in systemic lupus erythematosus and RA. Arthritis Rheum. 1976;**19**:1254.
19. Kassan SS, Chused TL, Moutsopoulos HM, et al. Increased risk of lymphoma in Sicca syndrome. Ann Intern Med. 1978;**89**:888.
20. Breedveld FC, Fibbe WE, Hermans, et al. Factors influencing the incidence of infections in Felty's syndrome. Arch Intern Med. 1987;**147**:915.
21. Weisman M, Zvaifler N. Cryoimmunoglobulinemia in RA. Significance in serum of patients with rheumatoid vasculitis. J Clin Invest. 1975;**56**:725.
22. Dillon AM, Luthra HS, Conn DL, et al. Parenteral gold therapy in the Felty syndrome: Experience with 20 patients. Medicine. 1986;**65:**107.
23. Barton JC, Prasthofer EF, Egan ML. Rheumatoid arthritis associated with expanded populations of granular lymphocytes. Ann Intern Med. 1986:**104**:314.
24. Fernandes L, Sullivan S, McFarlane JG, et al. Studies on the frequency and pathogenesis of liver involvement in RA. Ann Rheum Dis. 1979;**38**:501.
25. Thorne C, Urowitz MB, Wanless I, et al. Liver disease in Felty's syndrome. Am J Med. 1982;**73**:35.
26. Ellman P, Ball RE. 'Rheumatoid disease' with joint and pulmonary manifestations. Br Med J. 1948;**2**:816.
27. Walker WC, Wright V. Diffuse interstitial pulmonary fibrosis and RA. Ann Rheum Dis. 1969;**28**:252.

28. Walker WC, Wright V. Pulmonary lesions and RA. Medicine. 1968;**47**:501.
29. Dieppe PA. Empyema in RA. Ann Rheum Dis. 1975;**34**:181.
30. Dodson WH, Hollingsworth JW. Pleural effusion in RA: Impaired transport of glucose. N Engl J Med. 1966;**275**:1337.
31. Portner MM, Gracie WA. Rheumatoid lung disease with cavitary nodules, pneumothorax and eosinophilia. N Engl J Med. 1966;**275**:697.
32. Caplan A. Certain unusual radiological appearances in the chest of coal-miners suffering from RA. Thorax. 1953;**8**:29.
33. Gough J, Rivers D, Seal RME. Pathological studies of modified pneumoconiosis in coal-miners with RA (Caplan's syndrome). Thorax. 1955;**10**:9.
34. Penny WJ, Knight RK, Rees AM, et al. Obliterative bronchiolitis in RA. Ann Rheum Dis. 1982;**41**:469.
35. Gardner DL, Duthie JR, MacLeod J, et al. Pulmonary hypertension in RA: Report of a case with intimal sclerosis of pulmonary and digital arteries. Scott Med J. 1957;**2**:183.
36. Bonfiglio T, Atwater EC. Heart disease in patients with seropositive RA. Arch Intern Med. 1969;**124**:714.
37. Hara KS, Ballard DJ, Ilstrum DM, et al. Rheumatoid pericarditis: Clinical features and survival. Medicine. 1990;**69**:81.
38. Franco AE, Levine HD, Hall AP. Rheumatoid pericarditis: Report of 17 cases diagnosed clinically. Ann Intern Med. 1972;**77**:837.
39. Thadani U, Iveson JMI, Wright V. Cardiac tamponade, constrictive pericarditis and pericardial resection in RA. Medicine. 1975;**54**:261.
40. Lebowitz WB. The heart in RA (rheumatoid disease): A clinical and pathological study of 62 cases. Ann Intern Med. 1963;**58**:102.
41. MacDonald WJ Jr, Crawford MH, Klippel JH, et al. Echocardiographic assessment of cardiac structure and function in patients with RA. Am J Med. 1977;**63**:890.
42. Roberts WC, Kehoe JA, Carpenter DF, et al. Cardiac valvular lesions in RA. Arch Intern Med. 1968;**122**:141.
43. Duke-Elder S, Soley RE. Summary of systemic ophthalmology. In Duke-Elder S, ed. System of Ophthalmology Vol XV. St. Louis: CV Mosby; 1976: 139.
44. Jayson MIV, Jones DEP. Scleritis and RA. Ann Rheum Dis. 1971;**30**:343.
45. Smoleroff JW. Scleral disease in RA: Report of three cases in one of which both eyes were studied postmortem. Arch Ophthalmol. 1943;**29**:98.
46. Henkind P. Ocular complications of drug treatment of rheumatic disorders. Ann Physical Med. 1963;**7**:258.
47. Scherbel AL, MacKenzie AH, Nousek JE, et al. Ocular lesions in RA and related disorders with particular reference to retinopathy: A study of 741 patients treated with and without chloroquine drugs. N Engl J Med. 1965;**273**;360.
48. Cooper C, Kirwan JR, McGill NW, et al. Brown's syndrome: an unusual ocular complication of RA. Rheum Dis. 1990;**49**:188.
49. Lipson SJ. Rheumatoid arthritis of the cervical spine. Clin Orthop. 1984;**182**:143.
50. Menezes AH, Van Gilder JC, Clark CR, et al. Odontoid upward migration in RA. J Neurosurg. 1985;**63**:500.
51. Sokoloff L, Wilens SL, Bunim JJ. Arteritis of striated muscle in RA. Am J Pathol. 1951;**27**:157.
52. Via CS, Hasbargen JA, Moore J, et al. Rheumatoid arthritis and membranous glomerulonephritis: A role for immune complex dissociative techniques. J Rheumatol. 1984;**11**:342.
53. Brandt K, Cathcart ES, Cohen AS. A clinical analysis of the course and prognosis of forty-two patients with amyloidosis. Am J Med. 1968;**44**:955.
54. Samuels B, Lee JC, Engleman EP, et al. Membranous nephropathy in patients with RA: Relationship to gold therapy. Medicine. 1977;**57**:319.
55. Lawson AAH, MacLean N. Renal disease and drug therapy in RA. Ann Rheum Dis. 1966;**25**:441.
56. Husby G. Amyloidosis in RA. Ann Clin Res. 1975;**7**:154.
57. Scott DGI, Bacon PA, Tribe CR. Systemic rheumatoid vasculitis: A clinical and laboratory study of 50 cases. Medicine. 1981;**60**:288.
58. Sokoloff L, Bunim JJ. Vascular lesions in RA. J Chron Dis.1957;**5**:668.
59. Bywaters EGL. Peripheral vascular obstruction in RA and its relationship to other vascular lesions. Ann Rheum Dis. 1975;**16**:84.
60. Conn DL, McOuffie FC, Dyck PJ. Immunopathologic study of sural nerves in RA. Arthritis Rheum. 1972;**15**:135.
61. Lakhanpal S, Conn DL, Lie JT. Clinical and prognostic significance of vasculitis as an early manifestation of connective tissue disease syndromes. Ann Intern Med. 1984;**101**:743.
62. Conn DL, McDuffie FC. Neuropathy: The pathogenesis of rheumatoid neuropathy (Session III). In: Symposium Hernstein. Organic manifestations and complications in RA. Stuttgart: Schattauer; November 2-5 1975.
63. Scott DGI, Bacon PA, Allen C, et al. IgG rheumatoid factor, complement, and immune complexes in rheumatoid synovitis and vasculitis: Comparative and serial studies during cytotoxic therapy. Clin Exp Immunol. 1981;**43**:54.
64. Kemper JW, Baggenstoss AH, Slocumb CH. The relationship of therapy with cortisone to the incidence of vascular lesions in RA. Ann Intern Med. 1957;**46**:831.
65. Baggenstoss AH, Shick RM, Polley HF. The effect of cortisone on the lesions of periarteritis nodosa. Am J Pathol. 1951;**27**:537.
66. Vollertsen RS, Conn DL, Ballard DJ, et al. Rheumatoid vasculitis: Survival and associated risk factors. Medicine. 1986;**65**:365.

17

EVALUATION AND MANAGEMENT OF EARLY AND ESTABLISHED RHEUMATOID ARTHRITIS

Pascel Hilliquin & Charles-Joël Menkes

- The principal elements of management of rheumatoid arthritis include education, physical and occupational therapy, drug therapy, and surgical intervention.
- Key early decisions are to distinguish rheumatoid arthritis from other causes of symmetrical polyarthritis and to determine prognosis.
- Disease activity and functional assessment must be carefully monitored during treatment.

PATIENT EDUCATION

Most patients are interested in learning more about their illness, and this interest does not appear to decrease with time. Silvers *et al.* surveyed 101 patients with RA of average duration of 14 years; 92% indicated that they wanted to learn more about their disease [1]. Patient education can produce improved knowledge of the disease and behavior, including better self-control, compliance with therapy, practice of exercise and joint protection. Informed patients are also better able to communicate with their families about the problems and restrictions of chronic disease. Education programs to increase patient knowledge have been developed in many centers [2,3].

Assessing the Need for Patient Education

It is important to identify patients' educational requirements and their basic knowledge of the disease. Questionnaires have been developed to assess patients' understanding of the causes, the evolution and the treatments of RA.

Hill *et al.* [4] studied 70 RA patients, using a multiple-choice Patient Knowledge Questionnaire (PKQ). The questionnaire was self-administered and investigated four major topics, including general knowledge of RA, drugs, exercise regimens and joint protection. Overall, this study demonstrated a lack of knowledge about RA and its treatments. Many patients knew something about their symptoms; however, there was a widespread ignorance about biological surveillance, etiology and drug therapy. There was some confusion between NSAIDs and the SAARDs. Patients also had difficulty in distinguishing between joint protection and energy conservation. The PKQ demonstrated a wide variation in patient knowledge, with total scores ranging from 3 to 28 out of a maximum of 30. This variation would be expected from a nonhomogeneous population of people from different social and educational backgrounds.

In Kay's and Punchak's study [5], a questionnaire was designed to study 100 patients with RA of more than 6 months' duration. Only 46 patients said they had received information about their disease from health-care professionals. Patients' beliefs about factors that cause RA and cause disease flare-ups were numerous, including injury to joints, stress, diet, infections, climate or the natural aging process. Fifty-eight patients had tried nonprescribed remedies for RA and 55 claimed to be totally compliant with their medication regimens. Sixty-seven patients wanted more information about their disease, especially about disease management, prognosis, causes of disease and disease course.

There is conflicting evidence about the relationship between knowledge and the duration of RA or the age of the patient [6,7]. The one variable that better correlates with patients' knowledge is the number of years of general education that patients have received .

Patient education is now accepted as an important component of management in RA, and the lack of knowledge exhibited by many patients supports the role of educational programs. However, patients' perceived needs for education and support vary widely. Buckley *et al.* [8] surveyed RA patients about the importance of psychosocial and educational issues, and asked patients from what source they preferred to get help with these issues. The issues rated most important by patients were communication with the doctor, understanding of medications, and, after physical therapy, diet and causes of arthritis. Four educational issues (occupational therapy, physical therapy, understanding medication, surgery for arthritis) were correlated with the severity of the disease. Most patients preferred to seek help from their physicians, but a great number of them also wanted to attend groups or to see individual counselors for some issues.

There are several ways to improve patients' knowledge about their disease. Education is time-consuming and can be difficult for the individual doctor to provide singlehandedly. A multidisciplinary team for patient education may be one method of providing information. This approach requires the participation of several members, such as nurses and therapists. The development of programs to educate physicians about the concerns of patients with chronic illness may be helpful, and physicians' education should include reinforcement of the team approach to patient care. Physicians who have received such training may be more effective providers of information, and may also direct patients to other sources of help.

Methods of Patient Education

There are a number of methods available to educate patients about arthritis. In Kay's study, the principal sources of education used by patients were television, followed by books, booklets and leaflets, magazines, radio and newspapers [5]. Most patients considered written leaflets as the best method of receiving information. The advantages of leaflets over verbal instruction include patients reading at their own pace, with the possibility to refer back to written material. Alternatives include videos and audiocassettes, which patients could use at home. Some authors advocate self-help education taught by trained lay people [9]. This would be low in cost and avoids dependence on the expensive and limited time of health professionals. The teachers could be patients who had previously received training and a teaching manual, or retired health professionals. Participants could also include family members.

Lorig *et al.* [10] conducted such an educational program, with a 4-month randomized experiment and a 20-month follow-up longitudinal study. At 4 months, in comparison with control subjects, the educated patients had a better knowledge of their disease (measured by questionnaire), had reduced pain and also had improved their practice of self-management behaviors. These improvements remained significant at 20 months. There was also a socioeconomic impact, with a reduction of the number of visits to physicians. Other studies have shown the persistence of acquired knowledge several months after an educational program [2,3]. Some educational programs, in addition to increasing knowledge of RA and the lifestyle dimensions of arthritis, have focused upon topics such as stress management, self-awareness, communication skills and the availability of community resources [3]. Education of patients with RA should be more widely developed in therapeutic programs, as it has been shown to improve physical disability, pain and psychosocial impacts. No conclusions can be drawn, however, about the clinical significance of these programs because there is no evidence of improvement of clinical outcomes.

Patients should be given information on their drug therapy (Fig. 17.1). Iatrogenic complications from drugs represent a great part of the socioeconomic impact of RA and some of them could be avoided if patients were better informed. Typically patients often know of the digestive troubles caused by NSAIDs, but they are less aware of the side effects of slow-acting drugs.

Education programs could also improve compliance with therapy and help patients to cope better with their disease. Patients with chronic diseases such as RA often try nonprescribed treatments, most often without asking their doctor about the utility and the innocuousness of such treatments.

The development of support groups for RA patients may also be very useful in an attempt to improve patients' education, and this form of 'group therapy' may also be developed during hospitalization. Education of RA patients encourages self-management behavior and better adaptation to the disease, with psychologically, socially, financially and perhaps clinically favorable consequences.

DRUG THERAPY IN RHEUMATOID ARTHRITIS: INFORMATION TO GIVE TO PATIENTS

- The purpose of the drug
- Indications: when and how to take it
- What to do if a dose is missed
- The expected duration of the treatment (important for immunosuppressive and cytotoxic agents)
- The mechanism of action
- Information about side effects and what to do if they occur

Fig. 17.1 Drug therapy in RA: information to give to patients.

GLOBAL MANAGEMENT OF PATIENTS: NONPHARMACOLOGIC ASPECTS OF THERAPY

A Multidisciplinary Approach

Multidisciplinary programs are aimed at preserving the patients' quality of life by improving functional ability, mental and social health, vocational status, and disease activity. The comprehensive management of RA should include a variety of nonpharmacologic interventions to improve and maintain function, such as physical therapies, psychological interventions and energy conservation behavior (Fig. 17.2). Although rheumatologists are familiar with the principles of RA rehabilitation, many of them believe that medication accounts for most improvements. However, rehabilitation therapy and pharmacologic therapy can be mutually enhancing.

The professionals included in a rehabilitation team are physicians (rheumatologists, orthopedic surgeons, psychiatrists), nurses, physiotherapists and occupational therapists, social workers, psychologists, dieticians, patient educators, podiatrists and vocational counselors. The actions of the different members of this team must be closely coordinated; the physicians must be aware of the services provided by allied health professionals, and the coworkers have to meet at regular intervals to discuss the therapeutic modalities for individual patients. Although all the rehabilitative therapeutic modalities are usually available during hospitalization in referral centers or rehabilitation units, a multidisciplinary care system should also be made possible for outpatients, via home nursing or therapist visits and coordinated care using out-patient multidisciplinary management conferences.

The goals of physical therapy are relief of pain, reduction of inflammation, and preservation of joint integrity and function. The physical rehabilitative therapies are polymodal and require the same application and monitoring as medications. The major therapeutic interventions are relief of pain, joint protective modalities such as splinting and rest, and exercise therapy [11]. The relative contributions of these therapies to the program will have to be adapted to the patient, taking into account disease stage. The joint protection modalities will be very different for a patient with early RA and for one with longstanding disease and progressive deformities. Advice must be realistic and practical; after an initial period of help from the therapist, therapeutic regimens will be performed at home, often on a daily basis, and a program that is too demanding will not be completed by patients.

Pain Relief

Pain relieving modalities include the use of heat or cold, which provide a transient relief. Ultrasound has no advantage over simple heating modalities, and transcutaneous nerve stimulation is not justified for control of peripheral joint pain. Phonophoresis (use of ultrasound to drive certain drugs through the skin) and iontophoresis (use of electrical stimulation to drive ionized substances in solution through the dermal–epidermal barrier) could be an alternative treatment to local injections in superficial joints, bursae and tendon sheaths.

Rest, Relaxation and Correct Use of Joints

Rest improves synovitis in RA and is recommended during the acute flares of the disease. Patients with RA are often tired, and energy conservation behaviors, consisting of interspersing physically active periods with short rest periods once or twice daily, have been shown to be effective in increasing total amounts of physical activity as compared with standard occupational therapy [12] without tiring the patient. Some patients find it helpful to integrate various relaxation techniques into their daily routine, and balancing work and rest could permit RA patients to go on working for longer periods. The amount of rest necessary must be determined individually and depends on the stage and the activity of RA. Such behavior-changing interventions are easier for outpatients, and could favor a better adaptation to the disease.

Joint protection methods are aimed at performing daily activities with a minimal amount of stress to the joints in order to reduce pain and preserve joint structures. These techniques must integrate the disease process with the patient's lifestyle. Some basic principles are taught to the patient. It is important for the patient to learn to monitor his or her activities, and to stop when discomfort occurs. The patient should be instructed to avoid positions that could ultimately lead to or hasten joint deformities, and correct positioning of the joints during activities is important. Patients must use stronger and larger joints when possible, as the larger joints can more easily tolerate the stress of daily activities than the smaller joints. For example, the patient

MODES OF NONPHARMACOLOGIC THERAPY AVAILABLE FOR RHEUMATOID ARTHRITIS

Pain relief (heat, cold, phonophoresis, iontophoresis)
Rest and relaxation
Advice on correct/appropriate use of joints in daily life
Aids to daily living, splints
Exercise programs
Psychotherapy and counseling

Fig. 17.2 Modes of nonpharmacologic therapy available for RA.

should carry a bag either on the shoulder or the forearm to reduce the stress on the small joints of the hands. Patients must avoid being in one position for a prolonged period of time, and their activities should be altered to facilitate positional changes. Patients must also plan their activities to minimize prolonged or excessive joint use.

Aids to Daily Living, Splints and Surgery

It sometimes becomes necessary to use adaptive equipment to allow the patient to maintain independence while protecting the joints. This is particularly true for hand function; normal functional hand patterns, such as power grip, pulp pinch and strong lateral pinch, place stress on the joints of the wrist and hand. Some adaptive methods can reduce stresses on the joints and improve overall function [13]. Instruments can be used to open bottles or jars or doors. The use of large-handled utensils will help to reduce stress on the small joints of the hands.

Splints and braces are a part of the rehabilitation treatment of RA patients [13]. There are, however, conflicting views about the use of splints in RA, with regard to indications and evidence that they are efficacious [11]. Splints can be used to reduce swelling and inflammation in an acute phase of the disease. They help to properly position joints, and protect them from excessive or painfully forceful motion, making possible functional activities that would otherwise be precluded. Splints are also used to correct or prevent joint deformity, such as ulnar deviation and boutonnière or swan-neck deformities of the fingers. Splinting at night and during rest periods is often better tolerated, and can help prevent contractures and maintain the joints in more functional positions. Splints are indicated for the wrist, the metacarpophalangeal and the interphalangeal joints. Postoperative splinting with either static or dynamic splints is also an integral part of the management of RA patients. The therapist plays an important role in the surgical management of these patients, both in the preoperative phase, in patient evaluation and education, and after surgery. For example, in the case of metacarpophalangeal arthroplasty, proper postoperative splinting is crucial in the development of the new capsular–ligamentous system.

Exercise

Patients with RA may for a short or a longer time be forced into muscular inactivity, resulting in weakness and wasting of muscles. Muscle wasting can develop very rapidly, and it is important for RA patients to maintain physical activity. The low muscle strength found in arthritic patients is a source of disability and handicap. Exercise therapy in RA has many objectives, such as preserving or restoring joint motion, and increasing muscle strength and endurance [11]. It also has psychological goals, as it can enhance a feeling of well-being and provide active recreation.

Each joint must be individually assessed and appropriate exercise judiciously prescribed. A joint that is normal or has undergone bony fusion does not need exercise. Moving swollen or unstable arthritic joints against resistance such as lifting a weight, is painful and potentially aggravating, and isometric strengthening is often an excellent method of re-education for arthritic muscles. Benefits from water exercise therapy have also been described for RA patients [14]. Exercise therapy is also of great importance in the post-operative management of RA patients; after hand surgery or large-joint prosthetic replacement, a careful rehabilitation program will increase the chances of a favorable outcome and shorten the period for recovery.

Training and information programs have been developed for physiotherapists and occupational therapists for the assessment of patients with RA [15].

Psychotherapy and Counseling

Psychological interventions can be integrated into management of RA patients. Psychological factors are implicated in pain perception, and the intensity of pain is in part related to patients' beliefs in their ability to cope with or control the effects of their disease. Cognitive behavioral therapies can produce significant reductions in RA patients' self-reported pain, functional disabilities or joint involvement. A randomized clinical trial was conducted by Bradley *et al.* [16] to evaluate a psychological treatment intervention, compared with a control group. The psychological therapy produced significant reductions in patients' pain-related behavior, disease activity and anxiety post-treatment. Psychological therapy can improve patients' self-esteem and social behavior.

Counseling about employment is also an important aspect in the overall management of RA patients, and is frequently overlooked. Patients with RA are often limited in their options for work; therefore, a consultation with a vocational counselor or a social worker regarding the outlook for continued employment or for advice on vocational training may be helpful. Arthritic patients may take advantage of some possibilities, such as working at home. Patient's self-esteem often depends on the maintenance of useful and purposeful work, and the utilization of available resources for the patient's rehabilitation may prevent the loss of self-esteem and yet help the person to accept the realities of his or her functional abilities.

Evaluation of Rehabilitation Programs

Several studies have evaluated the benefits of rehabilitation programs [17]. Both inpatients [18–20] and outpatients [21,22] experienced significant improvement of functional ability and employment status. In a 9-year study, Duthie *et al.* [18] reported that severe restriction in functional capacity was present in 60% of the 307 patients at baseline, but in only 40% at follow-up, most improvement taking place in the first 2 years after hospitalization. At 4 years, the percentage of patients employed or able to do at least light housework had increased from 6% on admission to 68%.

Further studies are needed to evaluate the effects of rehabilitation programs; comparison of treated groups with control groups is necessary, because of the known variability in the course of RA and the occurrence sometimes of spontaneous remissions. The development of multifunctional care units for RA patients would be the ideal system, but the economic costs make this possible only in referral centers.

Nutrition

Nutritional status in RA is often inadequately evaluated. In a recent study in which no control subjects had evidence of malnutrition, 13 out of 50 RA patients were malnourished, five of them severely affected [23]. Anthropometric measurements showed that the body-mass index and the triceps skinfold thickness values in men and women were significantly lower in RA patients than in controls. In addition, levels of serum albumin, transferrin, retinol-binding protein, thyroxine-binding prealbumin, zinc and folic acid were significantly lower in RA patients. Among the RA patients, the malnourished patients had more active disease, with higher ESRs and levels of CRP. Diet did not differ between RA patients and controls, and the best interpretation is that, in RA, the severity of disease adversely influences the nutritional state. It has not been determined, however, whether efforts to correct malnutrition in RA patients can positively affect the outcome of RA.

Many arthritis patients, unbeknown to their physicians, follow diets to treat their arthritis [24]. Diets and supplements are recommended in popular books and articles readily available to the public. The authors of unproven regimens suggest diet regimens and mineral and vitamin supplements, often without any rationale and without any indication of suggested or safe dosages [25]. In some cases, the regimens are harmless; however, others, especially if followed over a long period, may be dangerous. Dieticians and other health workers need to be aware of these problems and to inform their patients about them. Some 'treatments', for example, prohibit entire food groups, such as meat or fruit or all milk products. Even fasting has been considered as being able to improve arthritis symptoms [26]. Some patients may stop taking medications and substitute diet as the sole therapy. This is harmful as RA patients, especially those receiving a daily dose of corticosteroids, must have a sufficient intake of calcium, and often supplemental calcium and vitamin D is needed.

DRUG THERAPY IN RHEUMATOID ARTHRITIS

The traditional treatment of RA is represented by a pyramid starting with NSAIDs and progressing to slow acting antirheumatic drugs (SAARDs) including antimalarials, gold, D-penicillamine, methotrexate, azathioprine and immunosuppressive cytotoxic agents; oral corticosteroids can then be used as a 'bridge therapy' between NSAIDs and SAARDs.

Most rheumatologists advocate the use of a slow-acting drug, typically early in the disease course, while continuing NSAIDs. However, the full response of these drugs is obtained after a period ranging from 6 weeks for methotrexate to 3 or 4 months for the other drugs. In most of the cases, it is necessary to obtain a rapid control of the inflammatory process while waiting for a response to the remittive agents. If a limited number of joints is involved, intra-articular corticosteroids can be given, using long-acting products. High-dose intravenous boluses of methylprednisolone also have an indication in early RA in case of polyarticular active disease, in an attempt to stop the flare (see Chapter 18).

A pharmacologic approach to early and established RA is summarized in Figure 17.3.

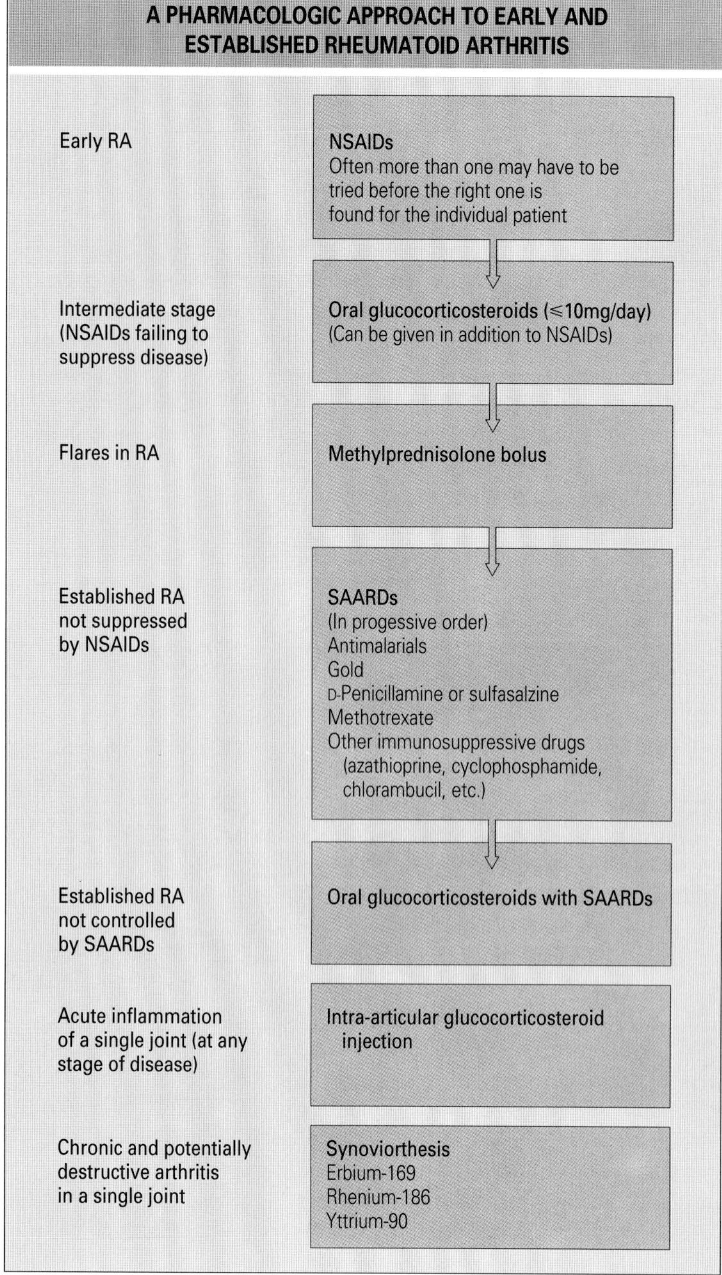

Fig. 17.3 A pharmacologic approach to early and established RA.

Nonsteroidal Anti-Inflammatory Drugs

In the traditional approach, NSAIDs are the only therapeutic option at the early stages of RA. Patients are most often improved by NSAIDs and it is entirely appropriate to use them in early RA.

Aspirin, the foundation of drug therapy in RA, has been widely used. Compliance can be measured objectively by serum salicylate levels. The drug is inexpensive and serum salicylate levels correlate well with reversible toxic symptoms. Many patients tolerate aspirin without gastric toxicity, particularly when an enteric-coated preparation is used [27]; modern preparations are absorbed efficiently. Salicylates are less well tolerated in the elderly patients; bleeding from gastritis or colonic diverticuli may occur without warning, and renal excretion can fluctuate in response to other drugs.

Non-salicylate NSAIDs are more commonly used than aspirin. There are many of these compounds, with similarities of action and side effects. The choice of drug should be based on awareness of dosage schedules, as well as specific side effects. It is difficult to predict which drug will be more effective in individual patients. If one NSAID is not effective, it should be replaced by another one from a different chemical class, after a trial at full dosage. For patients who wake with symptoms in the night, a bedtime dose may be useful. Physicians must remember that all the currently available cyclo-oxygenase inhibitors may diminish the glomerular filtration rate, and produce edema or hypertension.

Glucocorticosteroids

Oral glucocorticosteroids

Precise guidelines for prescribing oral glucocorticosteroids in RA are lacking. Glucocorticosteroids are given in conjunction with a SAARD in patients with active RA. Daily doses of more than 10mg prednisone have been avoided by most rheumatologists because of side effects, particularly the diminution of bone mineral content. However, a low dose (5–10mg/day) seems often to be effective in patients with established RA, with little risk of morbidity [28–30]. Alternate-day therapy is not helpful at these low doses; a dose in the evening may be useful to alleviate morning stiffness.

Glucocorticosteroids at these low doses do not appear as a risk factor for the development of generalized osteoporosis. Sambrook and colleagues evaluated the risk of osteoporosis using low-dose prednisone (mean dose 8mg/day) over a mean period of 9 years [29]. Using dual photon absorbtiometry, they showed a reduced axial bone mass in the corticosteroid-treated group, when compared to noncorticosteroid-treated patients, a finding which did not reach statistical levels of significance however. Postmenopausal-induced osteopenia can be a particularly severe problem in the rheumatoid patient treated with glucocorticosteroids. Some measures recommended to retard bone loss may be effective, such as supplementation with vitamin D and calcium salts. Over long periods of time, even low doses of corticosteroids may have adverse sequelae, such as Cushingoid habitus and suppression of the hypothalamic–pituitary–adrenal axis. However, elderly patients or those who have features indicating progression of RA are likely to benefit from carefully controlled doses of prednisone.

Pulse methylprednisolone therapy

Pulse methylprednisolone therapy is used along the course of the disease to obtain rapid control of the inflammatory process. Three consecutive boluses are usually prescribed, with a daily dose ranging from 200mg to 1g. Minipulses of 100mg have also been shown to be effective in the treatment of RA flares [31]. A single dose can also be given, and repeated if necessary. Methylprednisolone pulse therapy has no disease remission properties on its own, but it can be combined with the initiation of a SAARD. The clinical response has a rapid onset and can have a prolonged duration, sometimes for 3–4 months.

This therapy is well tolerated with few minor and self-limiting side effects such as flushing, psychological disturbance, palpitations and taste disturbance. Some serious side effects – myocardial infarction, severe infection, cardiovascular collapse – have been reported in patients with failing cardiovascular or immune systems [32]. Intermittent pulse therapy has none of the adverse effects resulting from long-term use of oral glucocorticoids; also it has no prolonged suppressive effects on the hypothalamic–pituitary axis, and it does not seriously affect bone metabolism in the short term.

Intra-articular injections

Intra-articular corticosteroid injections are an alternative method of controlling acute inflammation in joints that are inflamed out of proportion with others. Injection of corticosteroids can provide prolonged relief and markedly improve function. Other than suppressing synovitis, there is no evidence that these injections can retard progression of erosive disease. The duration of action varies with the product being used. Injection of triamcinolone hexacetonide can suppress inflammation in RA for up to 3 months. This therapy should not be abused, and a single joint should not have more than three or four injections before more definitive procedures are carried out.

SAARDs in RA

Over the past decade there has been an increasing use of SAARDs, especially early in the RA course. It is reasonable to begin with drugs that have the least toxicity, hydroxychloroquine being a good example. Another possibility is to use gold as the first SAARD. Patients must stop the drug if mucous membrane or cutaneous side effects occur.

Methotrexate

Methotrexate is currently considered by many as the drug of choice after NSAIDs; this is appropriate if rapid action is needed, or if the disease is aggressive with unexpected development of early joint destruction [33]. Methotrexate works quickly, and most patients experience significant improvement within the first 4–6 weeks of therapy. Numerous studies, both open and closed, double-blind, have established the effectiveness of methotrexate. Methotrexate is easy to administer by a weekly pulse regimen, either oral or intramuscular. A wide dose range is effective, from 7.5–25.0mg/week.

As with most SAARDs, the major limiting factor for long-term use of methotrexate is the development of toxic reactions. Pulmonary toxicity is not predictable: opportunistic infections and hypersensitivity pneumonitis may occur. Several studies have documented that acute pulmonary toxicity from methotrexate occurs with a prevalence of 2–6%, even at low doses [34–36]. This toxicity, sometimes leading to severe hypoxemia and acute respiratory distress syndrome, can be life-threatening. *P. carinii* or fungal infection may also occur, even in the absence of concomitant prednisone use; cases of cryptococcosis [37], histoplasmosis [38] and aspergillosis [38] have been documented. There are recent reports of diffuse fungal infections. These side effects can also lead to death.

Hepatic effects do not appear to limit the use of methotrexate in RA; however, there are are several reports of progressive hepatic fibrosis in RA patients treated with methotrexate [39–41]. A potentially dangerous hepatic side effect is sudden-onset, acute hepatic failure [42]. Some cases of leukopenia [43–45], thrombocytopenia [45,46] and aplasia [47–49] have also been reported.

D-Penicillamine and Sulfasalazine

D-Penicillamine is generally considered to be as beneficial as parenteral gold therapy; few patients remain on long-term treatment because of its toxicity, but prolonged remissions are observed with D-penicillamine. The active dose is between 600 and 900mg/day. The side effects include gastrointestinal distress, altered taste, stomatitis, pruritis, cutaneous reactions, renal effects with proteinuria, hematologic effects, myositis, and autoimmune-induced diseases such as SLE, pemphigus or myasthenia.

Sulfasalazine also has a disease-modifying action in RA; the mode of action is unknown but is likely to be due to sulfapyridine. Sulfasalazine is less frequently effective than gold or D-penicillamine [50–53]. However, its safety profile is superior, and patient dropout because of adverse side effects is less common. Dyspepsia, nausea and abdominal discomfort are the most common reactions; rashes and hematologic and hepatic side effects may also occur, and continual monitoring is necessary during long-term therapy [54].

Other Immunosuppressive Drugs

Immunosuppressive drugs are used in progressive and resistant RA, or in cases of vasculitis. They include azathioprine, a purine analogue, and alkylating agents, such as cyclophosphamide and chlorambucil.

Combination SAARDs

Combinations of SAARDs are sometimes used in established RA, in an attempt to obtain better control of disease progression [55]. The rationale behind combination therapy is that selected SAARDs have different sites of action. When one SAARD fails, it is possible to add a second drug to the first, while carefully monitoring for adverse effects. Combination therapy appears in some cases to be effective, especially if it includes cyclophosphamide or methotrexate. There is, nevertheless, no evidence that the efficacy of combinations of SAARDs is synergistic or even additive, despite a potential risk of increased toxicity.

Synoviorthesis

The intra-articular injection of radioisotopes should be considered after long-acting steroids have failed, especially when a limited number of joints is involved. Synoviorthesis can be used alone, without long-acting treatment, when a chronic monoarthritis is the only expression of the disease. The injection must be performed under arthrographic control, to detect and avoid extra-articular leaks. For the treatment of knee and hip synovitis, osmic acid is usually used [56,57]. Osmic acid is preferred to isotope products for hip arthritis in young adults, because of the risk of irradiating the gonads. It is not used in small joints because of its toxicity to skin and subcutaneous tissues. It can be followed by an acute inflammatory reaction, despite the concomitant injection of a corticosteroid agent.

Erbium-169 is a β-emitting agent used for the treatment of rheumatoid digital joints. Rhenium-186 is a β-emitter with a half-life of 3.7 days and a maximum tissue penetration of 3.7mm; it is used for the treatment of wrists, elbows, shoulders and ankles. Yttrium-90, another radioactive compound, is reserved for larger joints.

Synoviorthesis can be repeated in the same joint; but the total cumulative dose must not exceed approximately 15mCi. The injections do not impair the results of later surgical treatment. Synoviorthesis can locally complement the benefits of an otherwise active systemic treatment.

Some complications may occur, such as sepsis, subcutaneous sclerosis or radiation dermatitis; these can be avoided if elementary precautions are taken during injection. The major disadvantage of synoviorthesis is the extra-articular migration of the product, with the theoretical risk of chromosome alteration. Nevertheless, synoviorthesis can provide a prolonged remission of synovitis, sometimes over several years, and retard joint destruction. The best results are obtained when synoviorthesis is used before the onset of joint destruction.

Other Therapies and Prospects for the Future

Cyclosporine A can provide significant joint improvement, but it has the problem of potential nephrotoxicity; however, significant clinical benefit can be obtained at doses that cause minimal damage to the kidneys [58–60]. New directions in RA therapy include immunoregulatory interventions such as anti-CD4 antibodies [61] and anti-IL-2 receptor antibodies [62], which have been used successfully in patients with RA. Inhibitors of IL-1 have been given with limited benefit [63]. Future therapies may use cytokine inhibitors or antagonists directed against specific components implicated in RA, such as T-cell receptors, class II major hisocompatibility complex proteins, or one or more relevant antigens.

With the ongoing progression of DNA biotechnology, one can hope for the development of molecules acting on the transcription of cytokines or proteins pathogenetically relevant in RA. The goals of future therapeutic interventions will be to block, soon after the onset of the disease, the cascade of events that leads to established synovitis and progressive joint destruction.

DO PHARMACOLOGIC TREATMENTS AFFECT LONG-TERM OUTCOME?

Studies of RA patients receiving slow-acting drugs show that only a small minority remain on these drugs for long, therapy often being stopped because of adverse reactions or loss of effect. In an English study of 317 RA patients [50], fewer than 20% of patients who started gold, penicillamine or sulfasalazine were still taking any of these drugs 5 years later. After 2 years of therapy, 60–70% of patients were no longer taking these drugs. A study of methotrexate therapy in RA showed that less than 30% of patients remained on the drug after 5 years [64].

Can these drugs affect the long-term progression of RA if they are not taken over long periods? There is in fact no firm evidence that any of the so-called remittive agents used in RA halt the progression of the disease. In an English study [65], the authors determined outcome prospectively in 112 patients with RA treated for 20 years at one center, where a policy of active treatment was pursued with the use of gold, chloroquine, steroids and, in resistant cases, penicillamine or cytotoxic drugs. Function improved in the early years of treatment but declined considerably between 10 and 20 years. After 20 years of treatment, 37% of the patients were dead, and 20% were in functional classes IV or V; radiographs showed evidence of increasing joint destruction. A study by Amor *et al.* [66] determined the outcome after 10 or 15 years of therapy in 100 patients and compared the findings with patients treated one generation earlier. The functional status of the patients in the later time period was better than in the earlier. However, the major factor responsible for improvement in the late stages of the disease was surgery rather than drugs.

Studies to determine the influence of second-line agents on radiologic progression in RA have yielded contradictory results [67,68]. Sigler *et al.* [69] carried out a 2-year follow-up of 13 placebo-treated patients, who showed significantly more radiographic changes than 15 patients treated with intramuscular gold. Gofton and O'Brien reported that a 12-month treatment with auranofin could slow radiologic progression in RA [70]. These results have not been confirmed by other studies, which have failed to demonstrate significant slowing of radiologic damage in gold-treated patients [71,72]. A controlled trial of cyclophosphamide [73] reported that radiologic deterioration was more frequent in the placebo group than in the treated group, but the differences were not significant. Scott *et al.* [74] evaluated the overall changes of peripheral joint damage in 50 RA patients followed for 10 years. Patients were treated with NSAIDs, slow-acting drugs and corticosteroids, often in combination. In 48 cases, the total joint score deteriorated, and there was no difference in the pattern of progression in any of the patients; approximately half of the initially normal joints were damaged by the end of the study. Several other studies have shown no effect of second-line drugs on radiologic progression of disease. In a study from Glasgow on 67 patients followed for 2 years [75], there was a significant deterioration of hand radiograph scores in three groups treated either with gold, penicillamine or levamisole. Studies of the effects of methotrexate on the radiographic course of RA have yielded contradictory results [76–79]. In a controlled prospective study, on 18 patients with an average of 30 months of methotrexate therapy, Nordstrom *et al.* showed that, despite prolonged clinical improvement, the mean rate of development of erosions and joint-space narrowing during methotrexate therapy was not significantly different from that observed before therapy [76]. These data differ, however, from those reported in another long-term clinical trial of methotrexate [78], in which there was no progression in radiographic erosions in a select group of 11 patients during the first 2 years of methotrexate therapy.

SUMMARY

Treatment of RA is a complex procedure. The chronicity of the disease, its variable expression, with remissions and exacerbations, and its implications for the patient's life must be taken into account, and the therapeutic decisions must be adapted to the *individual patient* at any particular time.

The goals of management are to relieve patients from pain and other articular symptoms, to improve mobility and function, but also to alter the long-term progression of the disease. Patients have very individual preferences in the values that they place upon one outcome dimension relative to others. The setting of goals must logically precede the development of the individual management strategy. In some instances, a limited goal, such as regaining the ability to walk by hip or knee prosthesis, may be more useful for the patient than a modest reduction in the general severity of the disease. The goals of management for a patient must be adapted to their age, gender and the duration and severity of their RA, and the associated morbidity. Management strategies are designed to provide the most favorable outcomes throughout the duration of the disease. The patient must be aware of the duration and impacts of RA; and, in a young patient, the expectation for outcome must be integrated over 20–40 years. The physician must establish a long-term strategy, shared and negotiated with the patient. A hierarchy of treatments can be suggested, being modified according to the evolution of the disease.

REFERENCES

1. Silvers IJ, Hovel MF, Weisman MH, Mueller MR. Assessing physician–patient perceptions in rheumatoid arthritis: A vital component in patient education. Arthritis Rheum. 1985;**28**:300–7.
2. Spiegel TM, Knutzen KL, Spiegel JS. Evaluation of an impatient rheumatoid arthritis patient education program. Clin Rheumatol. 1987;**16**:412–6.
3. Lindroth Y, Bauman A, Barnes C, McCredie M, Brooks PM. A controlled evaluation of arthritis education. Br J Rheumatol. 1989;**28**:7–12.
4. Hill J, Bird HA, Hopkins R, Lawton C, Wright V. The development and use of a patient knowledge questionnaire in rheumatoid arthritis. Br J Rheumatol. 1991;**30**:45–9.
5. Kay EA, Punchak SS. Patient understanding of the causes and medical treatment of rheumatoid arthritis. Br J Rheumatol. 1988;**27**:396–8.
6. Vignos PJ, Parker WT, Thompson HN. Evaluation of a clinic education program for patients with rheumatoid arthritis. J Rheumatol. 1976;**3**:155–65.
7. Moll JMH. Doctor–patient communication in rheumatology studies of visual and verbal perception using educational booklets and other graphic materials. Ann Rheum Dis. 1986;**45**:198–209.
8. Buckley LM, Vacek P, Cooper SM. Educational and psychosocial needs of patients with chronic disease. A survey of preferences of patients with rheumatoid arthritis. Arthritis Care Res. 1990;**3**:5–10.
9. Cohen JL, Sauter S, Devellis R, Devellis B. Evaluation of arthritis self-management courses led by lay persons and by professionals. Arthritis Rheum. 1986;**29**:388–93.
10. Lorig K, Lubeck D, Kraines RG, Seleznick M, Holman HR. Outcomes of self-help education for patients with arthritis. Arthritis Rheum. 1985;**28**:680–5.
11. Swezey RL. Rheumatoid arthritis: the role of the kinder and gentler therapies. J Rheumatol. 1990;**17**(Suppl 25):8–13.
12. Gerber L, Furst G, Shulman B, et al. Patient education program to teach energy conservation behaviors to patients with rheumatoid arthritis: a pilot study. Arch Phys Med Rehabil. 1987;**68**:442–5.
13. Philips CA. Management of the patient with rheumatoid arthritis. The role of the hand therapist. Hand Clin. 1989;**5**:291–309.
14. Danneskiold-Samsoe B, Lyngberg K, Risum T, Telling M. The effect of water exercise therapy given to patients with rheumatoid arthritis. Scand J Rehab Med. 1987;**19**:31–5.
15. Helewa A, Smiythe HA, Goldsmith CH, Groh J, Thomas MC. The total assessment of rheumatoid polyarthritis. Evaluation of a training program for physiotherapists and occupational therapists. J Rheumatol. 1987;**14**:87–92.
16. Bradley LA, Young LD, Anderson KO. Effects of psychological therapy on pain behavior of rheumatoid arthritis patients. Treatment outcome and six-month follow-up. Arthritis Rheum. 1987;**30**:1105–14.
17. Spiegel JS, Spiegel TM, Ward NB. Are rehabilitation programs for rheumatoid arthritis patients effective? Semin Arthritis Rheum. 1987,**16**:260–70.
18. Duthie JJR, Brown PE, Truelove LH, Baragar FD, Lawrie AJ. Course and prognosis of rheumatoid arthritis: a further report. Ann Rheum Dis. 1964;**23**:193–204.
19. Conaty JP, Nickel VL. Functional incapacitation in rheumatoid arthritis: a rehabilitation challenge. J Bone Joint Surg. 1973;**53A**:624–37.
20. Barraclough D, Alderman WW, Popert AJ. Rehabilitation of non-walkers in rheumatoid arthritis. Rheumatol Rehab. 1976,**15**:287–91.
21. Katz S, Vignos PJ Jr, Moskowitz RW, et al. Comprehensive outpatient care in rheumatoid arthritis. A controlled study. JAMA. 1968;**206**:1249–54.
22. Vignos PJ Jr, Thompson HM, Katz S, et al. Comprehensive care and psycho-social factors in rehabilitation in chronic rheumatoid arthritis. A controlled trial. J Chronic Dis. 1972;**25**:457–67.
23. Helliwell M, Coombes EJ, Moody BJ, Batstone GF, Robertson JC. Nutritional status in patients with rheumatoid arthritis. Ann Rheum Dis. 1984;**43**:386–90.
24. Subcommittee on Health and long-term care, Select Committee on aging, House of Representatives, 98th Congress. Quackery. A $10 Billion scandal. House document 98-262. Comm. Publ. No 98-435. Washington, DC: Government Printing Office; 1984.
25. Wolman PG. Management of patients using unproven regimens for arthritis. J Am Dietetic Assoc. 1987;**87**:1211–14.
26. Skoldstam L, Larsson L, Lindstrom FD. Effects of fasting and lactovegetarian diet on rheumatoid arthritis. Scand J Rheumatol. 1979,**8**:249–55.
27. Orozco-Alcala JJ, Baum J. Regular and enteric coated aspirin: a re-evaluation. Arthritis Rheum. 1979;**22**:1034–7.
28. Harris ED Jr, Emkey RD, Nichols JE, Newberg A. Low dose prednisone therapy in rheumatoid arthritis: a double blind study. J Rheumatol. 1983;**10**:713–21.
29. Sambrook PN, Eisman JA, Yeates MG, Pocock NA, Eberl S, Champion GD. Osteoporosis in rheumatoid arthritis: safety of low dose corticosteroids. Ann Rheum Dis. 1986;**45**:950–3.
30. Verstraeten A, Dequeker J. Vertebral and peripheral bone mineral content and fracture incidence in postmenopausal patients with rheumatoid arthritis: effect of low dose corticosteroids. Ann Rheum Dis. 1986;**45**:852–7.
31. Iglehart IW, Sutton JD, Bender JC, et al. Intravenous pulsed steroids in rheumatoid arthritis: a comparative dose study. J Rheumatol. 1990;**17**:159–62.
32. Smith MD, Ahern MJ, Roberts-Thomson PJ. Pulse methylprednisolone therapy in rheumatoid arthritis: Unproved therapy, unjustified therapy, or effective adjunctive treatment? Ann Rheum Dis. 1990;**49**:265–7.
33. Willkens RF. Resolve: methotrexate is the drug of choice after NSAIDs in rheumatoid arthritis. Semin Arthritis Rheum. 1990;**20**:76–80.
34. Alarcon GS, Tracy IC, Blackburn WD. MTX in rheumatoid arthritis. Toxic effects as the major factor in limiting long-term treatment. Arthritis Rheum. 1989;**32**:671–6.
35. Cannon GW, Clegg DO, Samuelson CO JR, Ward JR. Pulmonary toxicity during treatment of rheumatoid arthritis with methotrexate: prevalence, clinical features, treatment and follow-up. Arthritis Rheum. 1984;**27**(suppl):S6.
36. Carson CW, Cannon GW, Egger MJ, et al. Pulmonary disease during the treatment of rheumatoid arthritis with low dose pulse methotrexate. Semin Arthritis Rheum. 1987;**16**:186–95.
37. Altz-Smith M, Kendall JR LG, Stamm AL. Cryptococcosis associated with low-dose methotrexate for arthritis. Am J Med. 1987;**83**:179–81.
38. Erikson N, Fursyt DE. Significant methotrexate (MTX) toxicity in RA patients: Results of an ongoing long-term prospective trial. Arthritis Rheum. 1987;**30**(suppl):S9.
39. Tolman KG, Lee RG, Clegg DO, et al. Hepatic fibrosis is the only lesion characteristic of methotrexate treatment in rheumatoid arthritis. Gastroenterology. 1986;**90**(suppl):1776.
40. Lundberg MS, Leonard PA, Clegg DO, et al. Methotrexate associated hepato-toxicity with long term treatment of rheumatoid arthritis. Arthritis Rheum. 1989;**32**(suppl):S128.
41. Shergy WJ, Polisson RP, Caldwell DS, Rice JR, Pisetsky DS, Allen NB. Methotrexate-associated hepatotoxicity retrospective analysis of 210 patients with rheumatoid arthritis. Am J Med. 1988;**85**;771–4.
42. Clegg DO, Furst DE, Tolman KG, et al. Acute reversible hepatic failure associated with methotrexate treatment of rheumatoid arthritis J Rheum. 1989;**16**:1123–6.
43. Scully CJ, Anderson CJ, Cannon GW. Long-term methotrexate therapy for rheumatoid arthritis. Semin Arthritis Rheum. 1991;**20**:317–31.
44. Groff GD, Shenberger KN, Wilke WS, et al. Low dose oral methotrexate in rheumatoid arthritis: An uncontrolled trial and review of the literature. Semin Arthritis Rheum. 1983;**12**:333–47.
45. Thompson RM, Watts C, Edelman J, et al. A controlled two centre trial of parenteral methotrexate therapy for refractory rheumatoid arthritis. J Rheumatol. 1984;**11**:760–3.
46. Steinsson K, Weinstein A, Korn J, et al. Low dose methotrexate in rheumatoid arthritis. J Rheumatol. 1982;**9**:860–6.
47. Anderson PA, West SG, O'Dell JR. Weekly pulse methotrexate in rheumatoid arthritis, clinical and immunologic effects in a randomized, double blind study. Ann Intern Med. 1985;**103**:489–96.
48. Gispen JG, Alarcon GS, Johnson JJ, et al. Toxicity to methotrexate in rheumatoid arthritis. J Rheumatol. 1987;**14**:74–9.
49. Mackinnon SK, Starkebaum G, Willkens RF. Pancytopenia associated with low dose pulse methotrexate in the treatment of rheumatoid arthritis. Semin Arthritis Rheum. 1985;**15**:119–26.
50. Situnayake RD, Grindulis KA, McConkey B. Long term treatment of rheumatoid arthritis with sulphasalazine, gold, or penicillamine: a comparison using life-table methods. Ann Rheum Dis. 1987;**46**:177–83.
51. Bax DE, Amos RS. Sulphasalazine: a safe, effective agent for prolonged control of rheumatoid arthritis. A comparison with sodium aurothiomalate. Ann Rheum Dis. 1985:**44**;194–8.
52. Farr M, Tunn E, Crockson AP, Bacon PA. The long term effects of sulphasalazine in the treatment of rheumatoid arthritis and a comparative study with penicillamine. Clin Rheumatol. 1984:**3**;473–82.
53. Grindulis KA, McConkey B. Outcome of attempts to treat rheumatoid arthritis with gold, penicillamine, sulphasalazine, or dapsone. Ann Rheum Dis. 1984;**43**:398–401.
54. Hilliquin P, Munoz A, Menkes CJ. Traitement de la polyarthrite rhumatoïde par la salazosulfapyridine. Rev Rhum Mal Ostéoart. 1991;**58**:535–41.
55. Paulus HE. The use of combinations of disease-modifying antirheumatic agents in rheumatoid arthritis. Arthritis Rheum. 1990;**33**:113–20.
56. Nissila M. Use of osmic acid in the topical treatment of exudative synovitis of the knee joint. Scand J Rheumatol. 1979;**29**(suppl):3–44.
57. Menkes CJ. Is there a place for chemical and radiation synovectomy in rheumatic diseases? Rheumatol Rehabil. 1979;**2**:65-77.
58. Yocum DE, Klippel JH, Wilder RL, et al. Cyclosporin A in severe, treatment-refractory rheumatoid arthritis: a randomized study. Ann Intern Med. 1988;**109**:863–9.
59. Dougados M, Awada H, Amor B. Cyclosporin in rheumatoid arthritis: a double blind placebo controlled study in 52 patients. Ann Rheum Dis. 1988;**47**:127–33.
60. Dougados M, Duchesne L, Awada H, Amor B. Assessment of efficacy and acceptability of low dose cyclosporin in patients with rheumatoid arthritis. Ann Rheum Dis. 1989;**48**:550–6.
61. Herzog C, Walker C, Muller W, Riethmuller G, Muller W, Pichler WJ. Anti-CD4 antibody treatment of patients with rheumatoid arthritis. I. Effect on clinical course and circulating T cells. J Autoimmun. 1989,**2**:627–42.
62. Kyle V, Coughlan RJ, Tighe H, Walkmann H, Hazleman BL. Beneficial effect of monoclonal antibody to interleukin-2 receptor on activated T cells in rheumatoid arthritis. Ann Rheum Dis. 1989;**48**:428–9.

63. Herzog C, Walker C, Pichler WJ. New therapeutic approaches in rheumatoid arthritis. Concepts Immunopathol. 1989;**7**:79–105.
64. Hilliquin P, Laoussadi S, Menkes CJ. Traitement de la polyarthrite rhumatoïde par le Méthotrexate. Rev Rhum Mal Ostéoart. 1991;**58**:419–26.
65. Scott DL, Symmons DPM, Coulton BL, Popert AJ. Long-term outcome of treating rheumatoid arthritis: results after 20 years. Lancet. 1987:1108–11.
66. Amor B, Herson D, Cherot A, Delbarre F. Polyarthrites rhumatoïdes évoluant depuis plus de 10 ans (1966–1978). Analyse de l'évolution et des traitements de 100 cas. Ann Méd Interne. 1981;**132**:168–73.
67. Sharp JT. Radiographic evaluation of the course of articular disease. Clin Rheum Dis. 1983;**9**:541–57.
68. Gabriel SE, Luthra HS. Rheumatoid arthritis: Can the long-term outcome be altered? Mayo Clin Proc. 1988;**63**:58–68.
69. Sigler JW, Bluhm GB, Duncan H, et al. Gold salts in the treatment of rheumatoid arthritis. Ann Intern Med. 1974;**80**:21–6.
70. Gofton JP, O'Brien WN. Effects of auranofin on the radiological progression in rheumatoid arthritis. J Rheumatol. 1982;**9**:169–72.
71. Empire Rheumatism Council Subcommittee. Multi-centre controlled trial comparing cortisone acetate and acetyl salicylic acid in the long-term treatment of rheumatoid arthritis. Results of three years' treatment. Ann Rheum Dis. 1957;**16**:277–89.
72. Cooperating Clinics Committee of the American Rheumatism Association. A controlled trial of gold salt therapy in rheumatoid arthritis. Arthritis Rheum. 1973;**16**:353–8.
73. Cooperating Clinics Committee of the American Rheumatism Association. A controlled trial of cyclophosphamide in rheumatoid arthritis. N Engl J Med. 1970;**183**:883–9.
74. Scott DL, Coulton BL, Popert AJ. Long term progression of joint damage in rheumatoid arthritis. Ann Rheum Dis. 1986;**45**:373–8.
75. Pullar T, Hunter JA Capell HA. Does second-line therapy affect the radiological progression of rheumatoid arthritis. Ann Rheum Dis. 1984;**43**:18–23.
76. Nordstrom DM, West SG, Andersen PA, Sharp JT. Pulse methotrexate therapy in rheumatoid arthritis. A controlled prospective roentgenographic study. Ann Intern Med. 1987;**107**:797–801.
77. Sany J, Kaliski S, Couret M, Cuchacovich M, Daures JP. Radiologic progression during intramuscular methotrexate treatment of rheumatoid arthritis. J Rheumatol. 1990;**17**:1636–41.
78. Kremer JM, Lee KJ. The safety and efficacy of the use of methotrexate in long-term therapy for rheumatoid arthritis. Arthritis Rheum. 1986;**29**:822–31.
79. Drosos AA, Karantanas AH, Phsychos D, Tsampoulas C, Moutsopoulos HM. Can treatment with methotrexate influence the radiological progression of rheumatoid arthritis? Clin Rheumatol. 1990;**9**:342–5.

RHEUMATOID ARTHRITIS

18

PRACTICAL PROBLEMS

RHEUMATOID FLARE

David L Scott

Definition of the Problem

Rheumatoid arthritis (RA) has a variable clinical course characterized by intermittent flares in disease activity. These involve increased inflammatory synovitis together with increased systemic features of inflammation; there are variable constitutional symptoms.

The Typical Case

A 39-year-old woman, had presented with RA 1 year previously. Her disease had been controlled with anti-inflammatory medication (ibuprofen, 400mg q.d.) and intermittent analgesic (paracetamol, one or two tablets p.r.n.). For 1 month she had increasing joint pain and swelling and was stiff for several hours each morning. She felt tired and unwell and had anorexia. Her peripheral joints were swollen and tender, she had large bilateral knee effusions, and she walked slowly and with difficulty. Her hemoglobin was 9.6g/dl with a normocytic film, platelet count 608 $\times 10^9$/l, ESR 98mm/hour, C-reactive protein 120g/dl, and rheumatoid factor titer (RA hemagglutination assay) 1:1024.

Medical treatment was changed to naproxen 500mg b.i.d. and co-proxamol 2 tablets q.d. Intramuscular gold (50mg weekly) was started. She was advised to rest at home for 2 weeks and was given advice on the nature of her medical treatment, the monitoring required and the likely course of her arthritis.

After 3 weeks her condition had still not settled. She was therefore admitted to a specialist rheumatology ward, put on bed rest for a week, and given prednisolone acetate (100mg, intramuscularly) and she gradually improved. After discharge, the gold injections, naproxen and co-proxamol were continued without adverse effects. She continued an exercise program and planned rehabilitation.

Diagnostic Problems

The diagnosis of RA is usually well established and the flare in disease activity is self evident, although intercurrent illnesses and sepsis can be difficult to differentiate. Rheumatoid disease follows a variable clinical course and disease activity waxes and wanes; it is sometimes debatable when current treatment has failed and a flare developed.

There are no absolute criteria for a disease flare; key points are given in Figure 18.1. Most will have more active disease. Extra-articular features, such as an increased number of subcutaneous nodules, can accompany a flare.

Although most flares are polyarticular, sometimes they are more restricted, involving a smaller number of joints, such as both knees. A related problem is when a flare occurs in late disease; there may be considerable joint destruction in longstanding RA and it can be problematic to differentiate a generalized disease flare from the pain and associated factors of end-stage joint failure. Another feature important to separate from a flare is the onset of extra-articular disease, especially vasculitis. Patients with systemic rheumatoid vasculitis usually develop this late in their disease and many have inactive synovitis. It is as if systemic vasculitis is at the opposite end of the spectrum of disease pathogenesis from active synovitis and its treatment is somewhat different. However, in both circumstances there are raised serum acute-phase reactants, and constitutional symptoms such as fever, weight loss and malaise can occur.

Therapeutic Options

Patients require a variety of antirheumatic drugs together with rest and subsequent rehabilitation. They will normally need therapy with both a slow-acting antirheumatic drug (SAARD) and a nonsteroidal anti-inflammatory drug (NSAID). There is no evidence that specific

RHEUMATOID FLARE: THE KEY POINTS
Characterized by increased activity of synovitis with variable systemic and constitutional symptoms
Clinically many tender swollen joints (six or more), prolonged morning stiffness (more than 1 hour), and marked joint pain
Elevated acute phase reactants with high ESR (>30mm/hour or equivalent) and C-reactive protein.
A period of bed rest may be sufficient treatment to settle flares in some patients
Principal drug treatment is a slow-acting antirheumatic drug together with a nonsteroidal anti-inflammatory drug
Occasionally a short course (about 1 month) of steroids is needed
Local intra-articular steroids may be of benefit in the worst affected joints

Fig. 18.1 Rheumatoid flare: the key points.

drugs in either category are especially effective for treating a disease flare, though auranofin (oral gold) and the antimalarials (chloroquine and hydroxychloroquine) are less effective SAARDs in such cases. Sodium aurothiomalate (injectable gold), penicillamine, sulfasalazine and methotrexate can all be used to treat a flare. Analgesics have a smaller role; paracetamol alone or in a compound formulation (co-proxamol or co-codamol) usually suffices.

The response to a SAARD such as injectable gold or sulfasalazine is not immediate, and it may take 6–8 weeks for an effect to occur. Sometimes a response is delayed for 3 months or more. There is anecdotal evidence that some SAARDs have a more rapid onset of activity; this has been suggested for sulfalazine and methotrexate, though the evidence is not strong in either case. During this time, symptomatic treatment with NSAIDs and analgesics helps control the activity of the synovitis. It is often worthwhile changing the NSAID used at the onset of the flare, though there are no special advantages of one drug over another in this situation.

There is uncertainty about the relative benefits of hospitalization for RA. The balance of evidence suggests some time in a specialist unit as an in-patient helps control disease activity; in very active arthritis, bed rest is advantageous.

Local corticosteroid injections into active joints are useful in controlling the extent of the synovitis and are frequently used. The place of systemic steroids is more contentious. Short courses of oral prednisolone or a depot injection are often used in active disease when commencing therapy with a SAARD in an attempt to control symptoms before the SAARD has an appreciable effect. However, it is important to restrict these to short courses. Steroids are not the first choice of treatment and should not be continued for much longer than a month. Pulse therapy with intravenous steroids remains an experimental treatment.

Supportive measures such as patient education, the provision of simple aids, splinting of active joints, and mobilizing physiotherapy are all helpful adjuncts to medical treatment.

Conclusions

Rheumatoid patients with a flare in disease require assessment of disease severity, the introduction of a SAARD or changing to a new SAARD, modification of their treatment with NSAIDs, and a period of rest. Education about their disease is important. Hospitalization and the use of corticosteroids are controversial, and systemic steroids should only be given for a short course.

REFERENCES

Hansen TM, Kryger P, Elling H, Haar D, et al. Double blind placebo controlled trial of pulse treatment with methylprednisolone combined with disease modifying drugs in rheumatoid arthritis. Br Med J. 1990;**301**:268–70.

Anderson RB, Needleman RD, Gatter RA, Andrews RP, Scarola JA. Patient outcome following inpatient vs outpatient treatment of rheumatoid arthritis. Rheumatol. 1988;**15**:556–60.

Murphy NG, Zurier RB. Treatment of rheumatoid arthritis. Curr Opin Rheumatol. 1991;**3**:441–8.

Corkill MM, Kirkham BW, Chikanza IC, Gibson T, Panayi GS. Intramuscular depot methylprednisolone induction of chrysotherapy in rheumatoid arthritis: a 24 week randomized controlled trial. Br J Rheumatol. 1990;**29**:274–9.

INSTABILITY OF THE CERVICAL SPINE

Arnold Cats

Definition of the Problem

Destructive lesions of the cervical spine in RA are the result of chronic, nonspecific inflammation of the synovial tissue leading to the destruction of cartilage, bone and ligaments. Postmortem studies have frequently shown synovitis in the odontoid–atlas joints, in the uncovertebral joints (joints of Luschka) and in the interlaminar joints. The pathologic changes give rise to instability of the cervical spine. Abnormal mobility is most commonly found in the Cl–C2 region, but may also occur at lower levels. Like the arthritis of the peripheral joints, involvement of the cervical spine can cause pain and impaired mobility. The instability leads to nontraumatic dislocations that may occasionally cause neurologic disturbances.

The Typical Case

A 63-year-old housewife with a 17-year history of seropositive RA was seen for evaluation of occipital headaches, heaviness of the arms and tingling and numbness in the hands. She had noted muscle weakness in the arms and intermittent, spontaneous jumping legs when recumbent. Micturition was not impaired. A global reduction in head movements of about 50% had been present for several years. Neurologic examination revealed a spastic paresis of both arms and the right leg with a positive Babinski's sign and impaired vibration sense in both lower arms, hands and legs. Radiographs of the cervical spine showed a subluxation of C1 on C2 of 15mm in flexion and 2mm in extension (Fig. 18.2). Magnetic resonance imaging of the cervical spine revealed an anteroposterior slip of C1 on C2, obliteration of the subarachnoid space and compression of the cervical cord by the posterior arch of Cl (see Fig. 18.3). Lying supine as much as possible during a week, followed by nearly 1 week's skull traction relieved the symptoms in the hands. She gained strength in her arms. Neurologic examination disclosed normal vibration sense in both legs and flexor plantar responses. At operation, fusion was performed of the occiput down to C4, using two autogenous bone grafts from the iliac crest fixed by steel wire (Fig. 18.4). After the operation, the patient received continuous skull traction applied through a Blackburn caliper and was nursed on a Strijker circoelectric bed for a period of 3 months. After removal of the traction the patient was provided with a soft collar.

Diagnostic Problems

The prevalence of radiologically established instability of the atlantoaxial vertebrae in patients with RA has been estimated to be 6.4% in patients with clinical evidence of RA and 19% in RA patients admitted to a hospital. Other hospital studies have confirmed these figures, and percentages as high as 23–32% have been reported.

Motor power testing in these patients is often unreliable due to severe joint deformities and muscle wasting. It may be impossible to elicit reflexes. Sensory disturbances in the extremities are major

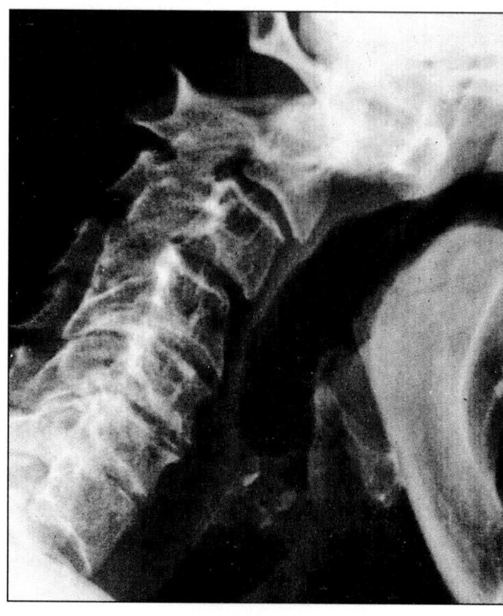

Fig. 18.2 Instability of the cervical spine. The slip of C1–C2 distance between atlas and ventral side odontoid process exceeds 15mm.

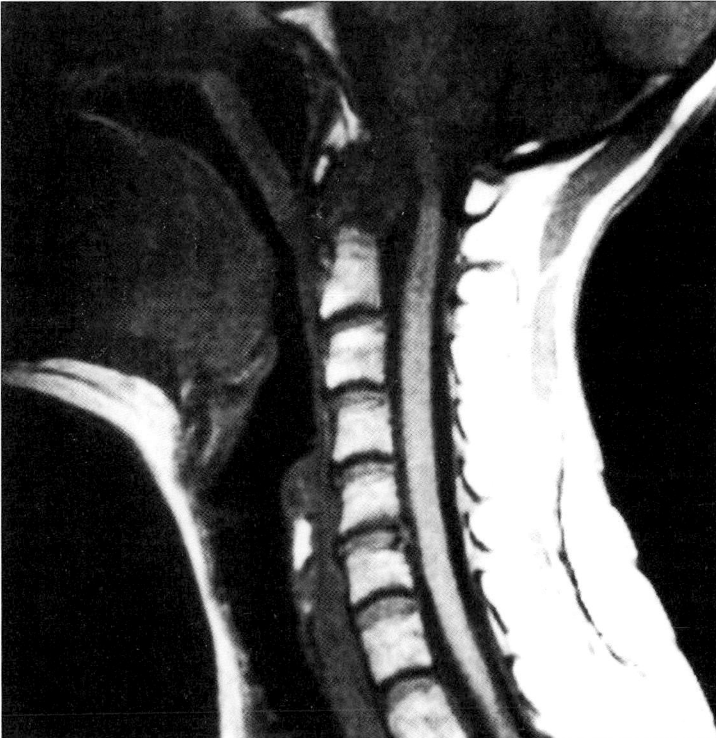

Fig. 18.3 MRI of the unstable cervical spine (TI-weighted). There is compression of the cervical cord by the posterior arch of C1. Courtesy of John L Sherman, Washington Imaging Center, Washington DC.

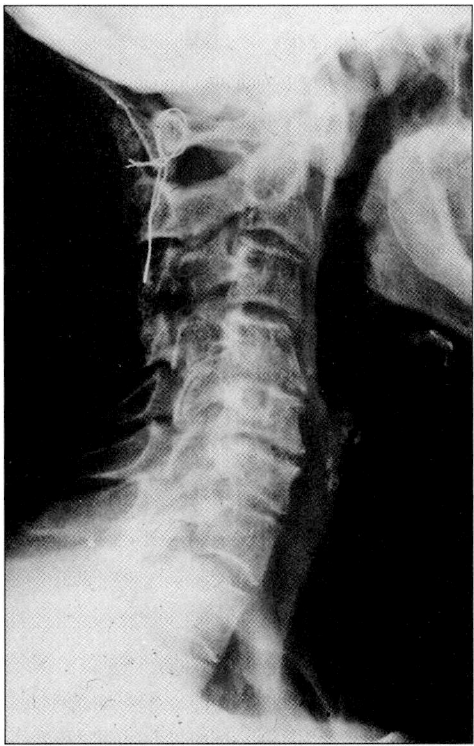

Fig. 18.4 Status of the cervical spine shortly after surgical procedure (bone graft and wiring).

ALARM SIGNS OF SPINAL CORD DAMAGE IN RHEUMATOID ARTHRITIS
Severe neck pain, often radiating to the occiput
Diminished motor power in arms and legs
Tingling of the fingers and feet, or only numbness
A 'marble' sensation in the limbs and trunk
Jumping legs, as a consequence of spinal automatism
Disturbed bladder function, varying from incontinence to urinary retention

Fig. 18.5 Alarm signs of spinal cord damage in RA.

pointers to a spinal cord lesion. Because the sensory loss in these patients may frequently be symmetrical, other neurologic disorders such as carpal tunnel syndrome and polyneuropathy as a result of vasculitis or nutritional deficiency should be considered. It is striking that, just as in other cervical myelopathies and syringomyelia, the vibration sense is lost and the position sense retained in the majority of patients with rheumatoid cervical myelopathy. Painful arthritis of the knee(s) may mask jumping legs; the latter is a consequence of spinal automatism. Involvement of the cervical spine by the rheumatoid process is often accompanied by neck pain radiating to the occiput, even in the absence of spinal cord lesions. Occipital headache may occur in the absence of any visible radiologic spinal abnormality, but the reverse is also true: severe lesions can be seen in patients without any complaints.

However, severe neck pain, often radiating to the occiput, is one of the main features alerting the physician to the possibility of spinal cord damage. Clinical signs and symptoms as a result of vertebral artery dysfunction (vestibular features and diplopia) occur in only a minority of these patients. Additional alarm signs of spinal cord damage in RA are recognized (Fig. 18.5).

Collapse of the lateral mass of C1 may result in characteristic tilting of the head towards the affected side. A C1–C2 slip (or horizontal atlantoaxial dislocation) is the result of laxity or destruction by pannus of the transverse ligament of the atlas. This ligament connects the lateral masses of the atlas, keeping the odontoid process in close apposition to the anterior arch of the atlas. A C1–C2 subluxation can be visualized on a lateral radiograph of the upper cervical spine in maximal flexion (Fig. 18.6). The distance between the posterior rim of the anterior arch of the atlas and the anterior margin of the dens is abnormal if it exceeds 4mm. Destruction of the odontoid process by rheumatoid granulomatous inflammation may also produce a Cl–C2 slip. Vertical dislocations, also visible on lateral views, are caused by destruction or collapse of the lateral part of the atlas and axis. The odontoid process can then penetrate the foramen magnum, putting pressure on the brainstem, which may be fatal (basilar invagination). Destruction of the dens by the rheumatoid process may be life-saving in both vertical and horizontal dislocations.

Myelography is a relatively difficult and hazardous procedure for establishing cord compression in patients with severe deformity. MRI appears to be a valuable addition in the assessment of spinal cord damage.

Therapeutic Options

The presence of neurologic symptoms and signs and cord compression confirmed by MRI is a very strong indication for neurosurgery.

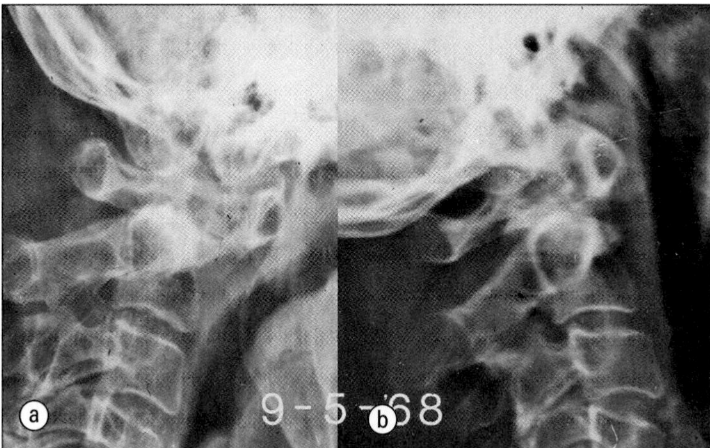

Fig. 18.6 Lateral views of the cervical spine. Lateral view in extension (a): the distance between the dorsal side frontal bow C1 and ventral side of the odontoid process is 2mm (a). Lateral view cervical spine in flexion (b): there is a slip of at least 8mm (distance between frontal bow C1 and odontoid process)(b).

A single horizontal or vertical spinal dislocation without significant neurologic features and no visible spinal cord damage on MRI requires no surgical intervention. Occipital headache may often be the only symptom present in these patients; for this a neck collar may suffice and, if necessary, NSAIDs and simple neck traction. This conservative approach is in contrast to that of others who advocate surgical treatment for intractable neck pain and instability without neurologic deficit. An operation is inevitable if a patient has cord compression and neurologic abnormalities. If an operation can not be performed because of bad general health (involving too great an operative risk) or because of refusal, neurologic progression is to be expected and the 1-year prognosis is very poor. As most patients with this neurologic complication of RA are already severely crippled, ambulant postoperative treatment with halo traction and brace is not a practical alternative. Skull traction using a Blackburn caliper should be started a few days before operation, and the patient is continued on a Strijker circoelectric frame for about 3 months postoperatively. The aim of the operation is fusion of Cl and C2 spinous processes with the occiput and some lower vertebrae by means of a bone graft and wiring. Different surgical techniques are now being developed which allow removal of the odontoid peg and/or fusion without the need for such long periods of immobilization.

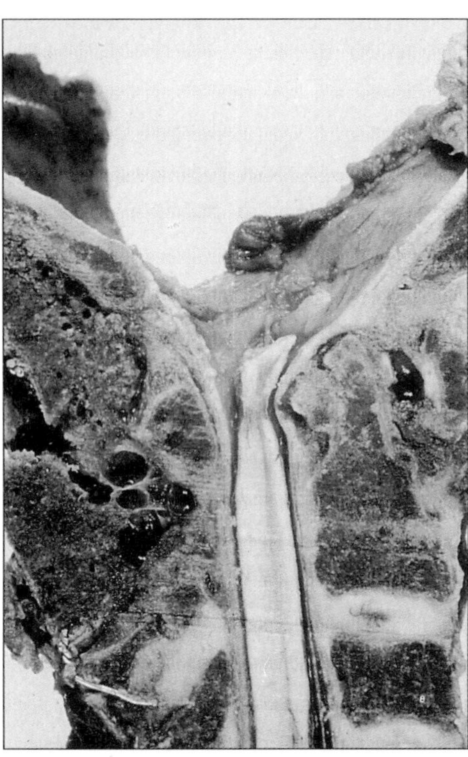

Fig. 18.7 Median saw cut of the cervical spine in RA. There is compression of medullary cord and forward dislocation of the atlas with respect to the axis.

Recurrent subluxation has been observed after some years, often at subaxial levels. About 10% of the patients in whom the diagnosis of Cl–C2 slip has been established die pre- and shortly postoperatively. Half of the patients operated upon have a life expectancy of approximately 5 years; in this latter group, death is not the direct result of cord compression (Fig. 18.7).

Conclusions

RA patients are at risk of developing instability of the cervical spine. These patients should be carefully assessed because neurologic symptoms may develop. MRI is the preferred technique for establishing the site of the cord compression. Surgical intervention is indicated in the presence of neurologic deficits and a neuroanatomic lesion.

REFERENCES

Agarwal AK, Peppelman WC Jr, Kraus DR, Eisenbeis CH Jr. The cervical spine in rheumatoid arthritis (editorial). Br Med J. 1993;**306**:79–80.

Breedveld FC, Algra PR, Vielvoye CJ, Cats A. Magnetic resonance imaging in the evaluation of patients with rheumatoid arthritis and subluxation of the cervical spine. Arthritis Rheum. 1987;**6**: 624–9.

Horst-Bruinsma van der IE, Markusse HM, Macfarlane JD, Vielvoye CJ. Rheumatoid discitis with cord compression at the thoracic level. Br J Rheumatol. 1990;**29**:65–8.

Marks JS, Sharp J. Rheumatoid cervical myelopathy. Q J Med. 1980:**199**(new series):307–19.

CARPAL TUNNEL SYNDROME

Michael H Weisman

Definition of the Problem

Carpal tunnel syndrome is an entrapment neuropathy caused by compression of the median nerve at the wrist in the carpal canal. Initially, the median nerve appears normal when examined microscopically but as the process proceeds and becomes chronic, focal demyelination or Wallerian degeneration may take place. In late stages, frank axonal atrophy can occur both proximal and distal to the site of compression, and functional impairment of the thumb and hand is the inevitable consequence of untreated disease.

The Typical Case

A 74-year-old man was referred for evaluation of the abrupt onset of polyarthritis of his hands, wrists and shoulders. He had noted marked limitation in mobility of his wrists as well as his shoulders and had been entirely overcome by this illness such that he became almost nonfunctional. He was having difficulty even getting up out of bed or a chair. On detailed questioning it became clear that he was waking in the middle of the night with quite severe pain in his hands, described as 'being like burning' and associated with a loss of feeling. He felt 'as if he had gloves on his hands' and could not feel fine objects. He found that rubbing his hands together and shaking them 'gets the circulation back' and this improved the symptoms.

Sensory testing for light touch and pin-prick was normal in both hands and wrists. Testing for thenar motor power was limited by pain in the thumb joints. Thenar muscle bulk appeared to be normal bilaterally. Phalen's sign was negative, although the patient was unable to complete the maneuver because of wrist pain. Tinel's sign was negative bilaterally.

Diagnostic Problems

The diagnosis of carpal tunnel syndrome (CTS) is clinical and based upon the proper interpretation of symptoms and signs with confirmation by electrodiagnostic testing. The earliest signs of CTS are sensory, and late findings are motor. Pain and paresthesias may occur in either the $3^1/_2$ finger distribution or sometimes the whole hand. Forearm pain is not uncommon. Patients almost always experience the pain at night and give a typical history of awakening with their hands asleep, rubbing them together, shaking them to get the normal feeling back. When motor compromise occurs later, attention should be drawn to atrophy of the thenar eminence with selective weakness of abductor pollicis brevis and opponens pollicis.

The time-honored noninvasive tests are simple to do but are either nonspecific, in the case of Phalen's sign, or insensitive, for example Tinel's sign. Electromyography and nerve conduction tests are more sensitive and have the virtue of providing quantification of the deficit, especially if there is motor involvement of the thumb. However, even these examinations are not 100% accurate.

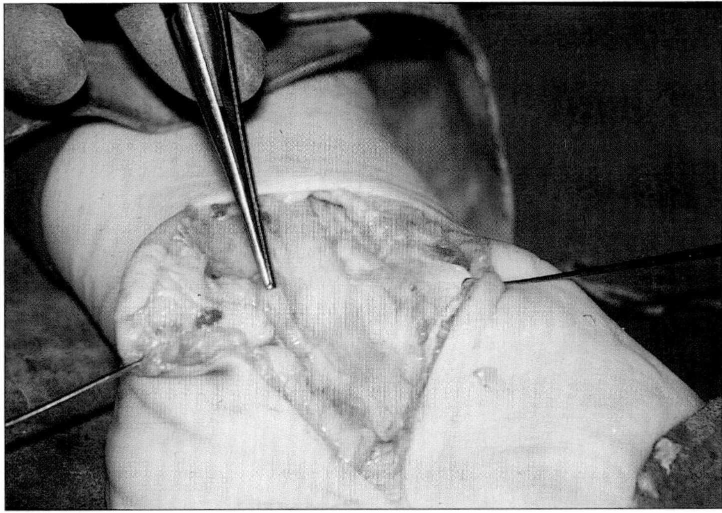

Fig. 18.8 Compression of the median nerve in carpal tunnel syndrome in RA. In this surgical decompression of the median nerve, the carpal tunnel is exposed from the palmar aspect and inflamed synovial tissue and the compressed median nerve are seen. Courtesy of Mr J Browett.

Differential diagnosis

It is not difficult to see why CTS occurs frequently in RA – dramatic swelling of the hands is a common early finding in the disease; later, synovial hypertrophy and tenosynovial thickening are responsible for compressing the median nerve (Fig. 18.8). Not uncommonly older patients with seronegative arthritis present with swollen hands and paresthesias due to median nerve compression. In early stages of seropositive RA, pain and stiffness in the joints may overshadow the sensory symptoms of carpal tunnel syndrome.

Several conditions that occur in patients with RA can mimic CTS (Fig. 18.9). Treatment for each of these conditions is highly specific, and distinction of one from another is required. Mononeuritis multiplex from vasculitis of the vaso nervorum can cause a mononeuropathy of the median nerve. The setting is usually (but not always) in longstanding RA and in patients seropositive for rheumatoid factor in high titer with evidence of other systemic manifestations. In the case of mononeuropathy, nerve conduction velocity will be slowed at different points, not just limited to the carpal canal.

Physical examination will usually distinguish between tendon rupture and weakness of the small abductor and opponens of the thumb associated with atrophy of the outer aspects of the thenar muscle bulk. A more difficult problem arises (discussed below) in differentiating extensor tendon rupture from radial nerve entrapment.

Cervical spine radiculopathy involving C6 may cause a sensory and motor neuropathy that could be confused with carpal tunnel syndrome. However, the sensory loss is in a C6 dermatome distribution with findings on the dorsal surface of the hand extending up the arm to the elbow. Diminished biceps and brachioradialis reflexes are usually associated with the weakness of the biceps and brachioradialis muscles.

The use of crutches by a RA patient can lead to radial nerve compression in the axilla and a brachial plexus compression neuropathy.

Ulnar nerve compression at the elbow, caused by rheumatoid inflammation and/or joint destruction, can produce ulnar nerve symptoms that range from minor irritating paraesthesias to weakness of the intrinsic muscles of the hand. Sensory loss involves the fifth finger and part of the fourth finger, the hypothenar eminence and part of the dorsum of the hand.

A posterior interosseous nerve syndrome, or compression of the pure motor branch of the radial nerve at several possible locations near the elbow, may be caused by rheumatoid disease and lead to some variability in physical findings. However, pain and paresthesias are always absent, pointing to the correct diagnosis. Inability to extend the four digits at the MCP joints while maintaining wrist extension is the cardinal sign of this syndrome.

DIFFERENTIAL DIAGNOSIS OF CARPAL TUNNEL SYNDROME IN RHEUMATOID ARTHRITIS
Mononeuritis multiplex due to vasculitis
Tendon rupture
Cervical spine radiculopathy
Brachial plexus compression neuropathy
Ulnar nerve compression at the elbow
Posterior interosseous nerve syndrome

Fig. 18.9 Differential diagnosis of carpal tunnel syndrome in RA.

Therapeutic Options

The first principle for treatment is to make an accurate diagnosis and differentiate CTS from other neuropathies.

In the recent-onset RA patient, treatment is usually not directed at the CTS *per se* but at the active synovitis. Once the swelling in the hands is reduced, the symptoms of median nerve compression will almost always abate. RA treatments such as NSAIDs, corticosteroids, and the early introduction of disease modifying agents should be sufficient. An important adjunct not only for the arthritis of the hands and wrists but also to control symptoms of CTS is the liberal use of resting hand and wrist splints in this early stage disease. Optimally, the splints should be individually fashioned from lightweight materials for each patient and extend from the upper forearm to include the hand and all of the digits. They should be worn at night and as much as possible during the day.

The development of CTS symptoms in established RA under optimum treatment requires a different approach. When symptoms are minor and intermittent, empirical use of splints should be tried. If symptoms are not eliminated, then electrodiagnostic studies should be performed. If electrodiagnostic studies reveal prolonged median nerve distal motor latency, or if there is evidence of denervation of the thumb muscles innervated by the median nerve, further conservative treatment is likely to fail, and the patient should be referred to an experienced hand surgeon for carpal tunnel release.

There is no convincing evidence that steroid injections have a long-term benefit. Indications for tenosynovectomy are the same as in any other joint; they are synovitis and pain in one joint out of proportion to that in the rest of the joints in the body and producing significant important disability beyond that which can be controlled with systemic medications.

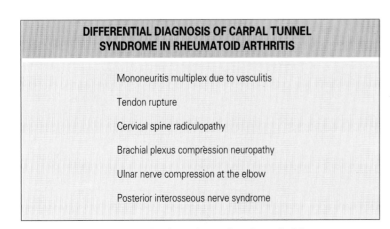

REFERENCES

Chamberlain MA, Corbett M. Carpal tunnel syndrome in early rheumatoid arthritis. Ann Rheum Dis. 1970;**29**:149–52.

Hadler N. The carpal tunnel syndrome. In: Medical management of the regional musculoskeletal diseases. Orlando: Grune & Stratton; 1984:143–55.

Katz JN, Stirrat CS. A self-administered hand diagram for the diagnosis of carpal tunnel syndrome. J Hand Surg (Am). 1990; **15**:360–3.

Katz JN. Carpal tunnel syndrome and other workplace-related upper extremity pain disorders. Postgrad Adv Rheumatol. 1991;**IV–IX**:16.

Kritchevsky M. Disease of peripheral and cranial nerves. In: Wiederholt W, ed. Neurology for non-neurologists. Philadelphia: Grune & Stratton; 1988:223–38.

DIAGNOSIS AND MANAGEMENT OF ACUTE SYNOVIAL RUPTURE OF THE KNEE (RUPTURED BAKER'S CYST, PSEUDOTHROMBOPHLEBITIS SYNDROME)

Allan StJ Dixon

Definition of the Problem

Joints distended with synovial fluid under pressure may rupture, releasing the fluid into the surrounding tissue spaces. When the fluid contains mediators of inflammation, as in RA, it causes widespread inflammation and edema. Noninflammatory fluid, as in some forms of osteoarthritis, causes little reaction other than transient swelling of the surrounding tissues.

The Typical Case

A 42-year-old woman had recently developed RA and her right knee was swollen. She sat on a bench watching her son playing football. When the game was over she stood up but felt a sharp pain at the back of the knee. Later the calf began to swell painfully and she had difficulty in walking home. When examined, a deep vein thrombosis was suspected and she was sent to hospital where it was noted that the right calf was 2cm greater in girth than the left and that there was edema of the foot and calf (Fig. 18.10). A contrast arthrogram showed acute synovial rupture (Fig. 18.11).

Diagnostic Problems

The joint that most commonly ruptures in RA is the knee, usually via the interconnection with the semimembranosus–gastrocnemius bursa in the popliteal fossa. Vectors of the forces of contraction of the quadriceps muscle acting over the swollen knee are responsible for compressing the fluid; the pressure may rise to over 1000mmHg. The moment of the rupture may be felt as a sharp pain in the popliteal fossa or upper aspect of the calf: the subsequent swelling of the calf closely resembles that caused by deep crural vein thrombosis. The synovial membrane and capsule rupture where they are weakest. In longstanding RA the joint capsule thickens and scars, resisting rupture. Thus it is usually in early RA, when the muscles are still strong and the capsules of the joint and bursa thin, that acute synovial rupture is most likely to occur. The severity of the reaction also reflects the amount of fluid extravasated. Small leakages can be missed unless the calf muscles are inspected from behind and the girth of the calves routinely measured.

Typical features are early inflammatory arthritis, pain at the back of the knee on powered extension from the flexed position, and redness and tenderness maximal in the upper medial part of the posterior aspect of the calf. Sometimes the knee becomes less swollen as the calf swells. Pitting edema may spread both to the foot and above the knee. Fever and leukocytosis occur in some patients. Passive dorsiflexion of the ankle increases calf pain (positive Homan's sign). A palpable popliteal cyst is usually absent although ultrasonic scanning may reveal one. Diagnosis is confirmed by a positive contrast arthrogram and, if necessary, a negative contrast venogram. The clinical resemblance to acute deep vein thrombosis in the calf is very strong. If in doubt, remember that, in the presence of arthritis of the knee, acute synovial rupture is much more common than deep vein thrombosis. Misdiagnosis can be hazardous as anticoagulation can turn the synovial fluid extravasation into a tense hematoma in the posterior muscular compartment of the calf, with the danger of muscle compression and necrosis.

The differential diagnosis includes rupture of the plantaris muscle, rupture of the medial head of the gastrocnemius (usually a football or skiing injury) and, rarely, a leaking popliteal artery aneurysm.

Arthography of the knee

The patient lies supine on the radiography table, with a small cushion under the knee if full extension is too painful. Some fluid is aspirated by the lateral approach to ensure that the needle is in the synovial cavity. It is only necessary to remove about 5ml for diagnostic investigations unless the joint is very tense, when up to 20ml can be removed. Twenty milliliters of a suitable contrast material, such as meglumine iothalamate, mixed with 5ml of 1% lidocaine is injected into the joint. The patient gets down off the couch, walks a few steps and then climbs back on. This allows the contrast material to outline the complete distribution of the synovial fluid. The radiographs taken are anteroposterior with the knee extended, and lateral with the knee in 45° flexion, covering from the lower third of the femur to the lower third of the tibia.

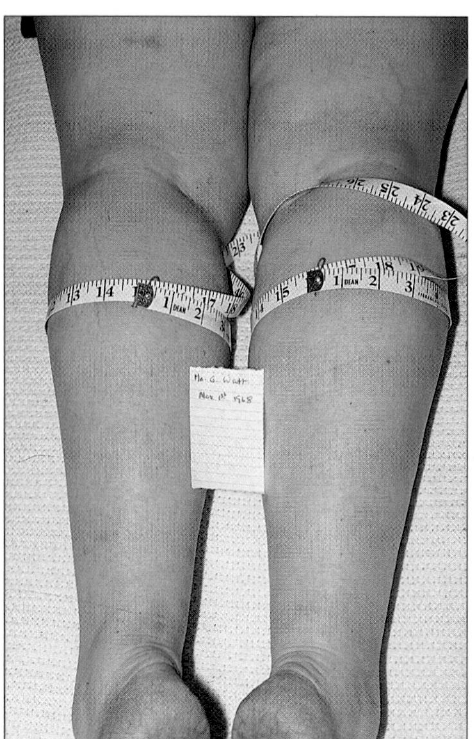

Fig. 18.10 Swelling of calf following acute synovial rupture of the knee in early inflammatory arthritis.

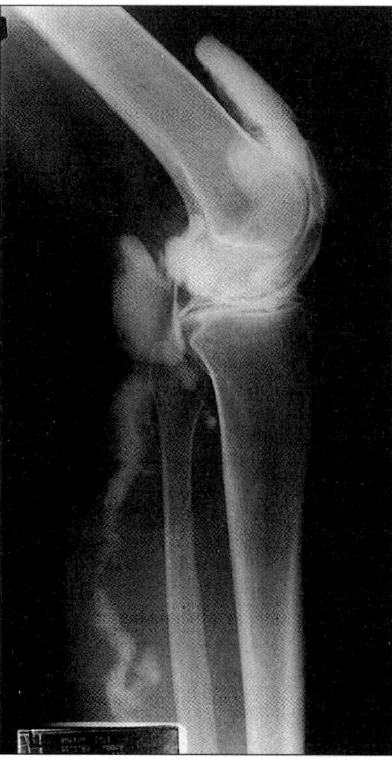

Fig. 18.11 Contrast arthrogram following acute synovial rupture of the knee.

Repeat films after 10 and 20 minutes can follow the diffusion of the synovial fluid. A locally active corticosteroid, such as a suspension of 20mg of triamcinolone hexacetonide or methylprednisolone acetate, can be injected to control inflammation before the needle is withdrawn from the joint.

In acute synovial rupture, the contrast dye tracks down the back of the calf, most commonly along the course of the neurovascular bundle, and may outline the feathery appearance of the fibers of the soleus muscle. Occasionally one sees a pre-existing enlarged popliteal cyst which has ruptured, and sometimes the contrast spreads upwards into the lower thigh.

Therapy

Treatment is directed at decompressing the knee with bed rest, elevation of the limb and intra-articular corticosteroid injections as above (Fig. 18.12). These may need to be repeated after a week if the calf is still tense; diuretics are unnecessary and on no account should anticoagulants be given. If the calf muscle is very tense and painful, it may be helpful to needle it in several places under aseptic conditions. It will not be possible to aspirate fluid, but the puncture sites will continue to drain synovial fluid and edema as long as the calf is under pressure. If the synovial rupture has followed a persistent noninflammatory hydrarthrosis, decompression can be done by repeated aspiration of the knee. Follow-up after a severe episode of synovial rupture has shown that some calf swelling persists for at least 3 years, presumably from residual stretching of the fascial envelopes of the calf.

AN APPROACH TO DIAGNOSIS OF A SWOLLEN CALF IN RHEUMATOID ARTHRITIS

- There must have been previous swelling of the knee, which may have decreased as the calf swelling increased
- Other features are: onset after powered extension of the knee, relatively early arthritis, a popliteal cyst which is often not palpable, redness maximal in the upper posteromedial aspect of the calf, Homan's sign positive, edema may spread above the knee
- Complications include fever and leukocytosis and sometimes posterior compartment compression with danger of muscle necrosis
- An arthrogram is diagnostic
- Treatment is by decompression of the knee by aspiration, bed rest and injection of a locally active corticosteroid
- Recovery within a week is usual

Fig. 18.12 An approach to diagnosis of a swollen calf in RA.

REFERENCE

Dixon A StJ, Emery P. Local injection therapy in rheumatic diseases, 4E. Basle: EULAR; 1992.

Dixon A StJ, Grant G. Acute synovial rupture in rheumatoid arthritis. Lancet. 1964;**1**:742–4.

AN INFECTED RHEUMATOID ARTHRITIS JOINT

John R Ward

Definition of the Problem

While the exact frequency of bacterial joint infection in RA patients is unknown, these patients are at greater risk for joint infection. Usually, the patient is older and has longstanding seropositive disease. Almost half of the patients are receiving systemic corticosteroids and essentially all are receiving NSAIDs, which may mask signs of infection such as fever, leukocytosis and joint findings. While usually a monoarticular disease involving large joints, septic arthritis in patients with RA may be polyarticular.

The Typical Case

A 64-year-old woman with RA of 10 years' duration was receiving prednisone 5mg daily, sulindac 200mg b.i.d. and methotrexate 7.5mg weekly. She presented with a 36-hour history of redness, heat, and increased swelling and pain in her left knee. There was no history of any infections at other sites, fever or chills. On physical examination, she had mild synovitis of several joints and subcutaneous nodules over both extensor surfaces of the forearms. Her right knee was swollen, warm, and had a palpable effusion (Fig. 18.13). While the joint was only moderately tender, there was marked pain on flexion and extension. There was no evidence of associated infection on physical examination and the skin was intact throughout. Her oral temperature was 37.3°C, the rheumatoid factor was 1:1280, Westergren ESR 56mm/hour, and blood leukocyte count 13,000/mm^3 with 80% neutrophils and 8% bands. She was admitted to the hospital and blood cultures were obtained. The synovial fluid had 92,000 nucleated cells per cubic millimeter with 88% neutrophils. Examination for crystals was negative. No organisms were seen on the Gram stain of centrifuged synovial fluid. Cultures were obtained for *Neisseria*, aerobic and anaerobic bacteria, mycobacteria, and fungi. Radiographs of the knee showed mild joint space narrowing. Because the Gram stain of the synovial fluid was negative, and in view of the absence of an identifiable portal of entry, concomitant infection, or features of bacterial sepsis, no antibiotic treatment was initiated.

The following day, reaspiration of the left knee revealed similar findings as those on admission except that the Gram stain revealed Gram-positive cocci. Nafcillin, 2g given intravenously (i.v.) 6-hourly, was started. The next day, synovial fluid cultures grew *Staphylococcus aureus,* which was sensitive to penicillin. Blood cultures yielded no growth. Antibiotic therapy was changed to 1.2 million units of penicillin G, i.v. 6-hourly.

Daily joint aspirations were done and cultures became negative after 2 days. By day 7, the synovial fluid cell count had fallen to 20,000/mm^3 and the joint examination revealed only minimal effusion. The patient was then placed on oral penicillin V with serum bactericidal levels of over 1:16. The patient was discharged, to continue on oral penicillin for 3 weeks.

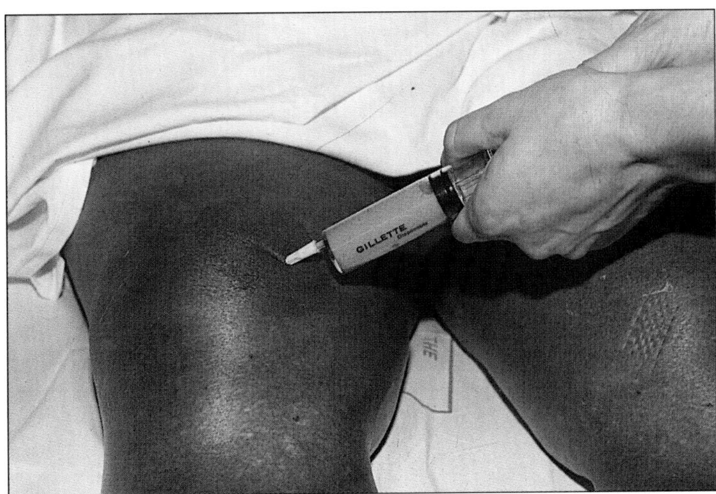

Fig. 18.13 An infected rheumatoid arthritis joint. A high degree of clinical suspicion of infection in patients with rheumatoid arthritis is essential. Pus may be present as in this case.

Diagnostic Problems

Monoarticular flare of rheumatoid arthritis?

In the absence of trauma or unusual use to a joint, a monarticular flare in RA is unusual. Laboratory data, such as an elevated ESR, are not helpful. Mild leukocytosis is sometimes observed in RA, and prednisone may increase the absolute number of mature granulocytes in the circulation. The degree of pain on motion in the knee would be unusual. While synovial fluid nucleated cell counts above 50,000/mm^3 can infrequently be seen in RA, a high proportion of neutrophils would be more consistent with a bacterial infection.

Bacterial joint infection?

Concomitant corticosteroids and NSAIDs can minimize the early systemic and articular findings of infection. Care must be taken to exclude bacterial infection by repeated synovial fluid analysis and Gram stain and cultures.

Crystal-induced arthritis in a patient with rheumatoid arthritis?

Gout and pseudogout can uncommonly occur, but even if crystals are seen infection, which can be catastrophic if untreated, must be excluded to make certain that there is no infection.

Pseudoseptic arthritis?

An entity termed 'pseudoseptic arthritis' in RA patients who present with clinical and laboratory findings that are highly suggestive of bacterial infection of the joints can mimic bacterial infection. However, cultures are negative and attacks only last 12–48 hours and do not require antibiotic treatment.

Identifying the infection

The usual approach to suspected bacterial infection of a joint in the patient with RA is to look for an associated infection such as urinary tract infection or a skin ulcer and to culture all suspected joints as indicated by clinical findings. Also, cultures of blood and asymptomatic sites such as the cervix are obtained. Synovial fluid analysis for total nucleated and differential cell counts, crystals, glucose content, and cultures for *Neisseria gonorrhoeae* and aerobic and anaerobic bacteria are done. Cultures for mycobacteria and fungi are considered. A Gram stain on the centrifuged fluid specimen is examined, and appropriate antibiotics are given immediately based on the most likely infecting organism.

Therapeutic Options

When there is no evident portal of entry or concomitant systemic bacterial infection, and a gram stain of the synovial fluid is negative, antibiotic therapy is nevertheless implemented if the synovial fluid nucleated cell count is high and there are greater than 90% neutrophils. Since *S. aureus* is the most likely infecting organism, a penicillinase-resistant penicillin (or vancomycin, third-generation cephalosporin or a fluoroquinolone) is given parenterally and joint drainage is begun. If infection with a Gram-negative bacillus is suspected, treatment with a third-generation cephalosporin and an aminoglycoside can be given. Antibiotic therapy is then adjusted once culture results and sensitivities are known.

The best indicator of response to treatment is for a positive synovial fluid culture to revert to negative and this should occur within 24–72 hours. A decrease in arthritis, total nucleated cell count and neutrophil count may not be observed for up to 7 or more days.

At its inception, bacterial infection of joints most often results from hematogenous seeding of the synovium and ultimately spreads to the joint space. If antibiotics are started at this stage, before extension to the joint space, synovial fluid cultures will be negative. Thus, the initial synovial fluid culture may yield no growth, and subsequent cultures ultimately become positive. The decision on when to initiate antibiotic therapy is often difficult and must be individualized to the patient. If the gram stain is positive, antibiotics should be initiated to cover the identified organism and selection of antibiotics reviewed after the organism is recovered on culture and sensitivities are determined. If initial gram stain and culture are negative, broad-spectrum antibiotics may be given pending final culture results. An alternative approach is to delay treatment pending recovery of the infecting organism from the synovial fluid or blood so that specific antibiotic treatment can be prescribed. Thus, the physician will be able to selectively administer antibacterial therapy and monitor the response by observing synovial fluid cultures showing no growth within 1–4 days of treatment. The problem of long-term antibiotic treatment without a known organism can be avoided by delaying treatment until culture results are positive. Also, patients with 'pseudoseptic arthritis' will be recognized by their spontaneous improvement without antibiotic therapy. Based on the available data, a delay of 2–5 weeks early in the course of bacterial infection of joints would not influence successful results.

In addition to appropriate antibacterial therapy, complete aspiration of the joint should be done whenever fluid reaccumulates. This can often be done successfully by needle aspiration but may require surgical drainage for joints in which needle aspiration is difficult, such as the hip, or when fluid appears to be loculated. Range-of-motion exercises are implemented as tolerated by the patient.

Conclusion

Patients with RA have an increased susceptibility to bacterial infection of joints. The typical signs of septic arthritis may not be present and the disease may be polyarticular (Fig. 18.14). Appropriate antibiotic therapy and complete joint drainage will generally produce excellent results. 'Pseudoseptic arthritis' can mimic a true bacterial infection and does not require antibacterial treatment.

DIAGNOSIS AND MANAGEMENT OF AN INFECTED JOINT IN RHEUMATOID ARTHRITIS

- Onset may be insidious
- May be polyarticular
- Confirm diagnosis by appropriate synovial fluid examination and cultures
- Monitor response to antibacterial therapy by repeated synovial fluid examination and cultures
- Adequately drain infected joint
- Start early range of motion
- Be aware of possible 'pseudoseptic arthritis'

Fig. 18.14 Diagnosis and management of an infected rheumatoid arthritis joint.

REFERENCES

Atcheson SG, Ward JR. Acute hematogenous osteomyelitis progressing to septic synovitis and eventual pyarthrosis—the vascuiar pathway. Arthritis Rheum. 1978;**21**:968–71.

Call RS, Ward JR, Samuelson Jr CO. Pseudoseptic arthritis in patients with rheumatoid arthritis. Western J Med. 1985;**143**:471–3.

Goldenberg DL. Infectious arthritis complicating rheumatoid arthritis and other chronic rheumatic disorders. Arthritis Rheum. 1989;**32**:496-502.

Rheumatologists frequently encounter the management dilemma of rheumatic disease during pregnancy. Issues that need to be addressed include an awareness of the possible effects medication might have on a developing fetus and advising patients of the potential impact should pregnancy occur. An appreciation of the effect of prescribed medication on both fetal physiology is also important. The influence the rheumatic disease may have on pregnancy and vice versa needs to be considered, and the impact of the disease on female fertility is also important.

The Typical Case

A 32-year-old nulliparous medical secretary had a 2-year history of seropositive and erosive RA. At the onset of disease her hemoglobin was 114g/l, ESR 68mm/hour, rheumatoid factor 126IU/ml. Antibodies to Ro(SS-A) and phospholipids were negative. Initial disease activity was such that weekly intramuscular sodium aurothiomalate was introduced, with piroxicam 20mg/day. After 16 weeks of therapy, early morning stiffness was reduced to less than 5min, and the patient remained on piroxicam in a reduced dose (10mg/daily). Radiologic evaluation 18 months later demonstrated several erosions in the right 3rd and 4th metatarsophalangeal joints. At this stage, she noted an increase in her morning stiffness, had some difficulty in walking and had pain in her wrists. At the time of consultation, she was 6 weeks pregnant while still receiving 50mg aurothiomalate each week and taking daily piroxicam. Investigations at this time showed an ESR of 26mm/hour, a hemoglobin of 126g/l and a rheumatoid factor of 250IU/ml.

This woman is already experiencing erosive disease affecting her feet and wrists and will have increasing difficult in the years to come coping with a growing child if the disease is not suppressed.

After discussion with the patient, it was decided to use 20mg injections of gold aurothiomalate every 2 weeks during the pregnancy and to increase these to weekly 50mg injections for the first 6 weeks after birth. Ibuprofen was continued on an as-needed basis but suspended at 28 weeks, as further analgesia was not required. Joint swelling began to recur 4 weeks postpartum and ibuprofen was reintroduced in a dose of 400mg every 6 hours, timed to coincide with the beginning of breast-feeding (see later). Paracetamol was also required during the immediate postpartum period for pain relief.

Management Problems

What effect does the pregnancy have on rheumatoid disease?

Some 70% of women with RA will have some amelioration of their disease during pregnancy. Most of those will show improvement in the first 3 months. Even though improvement occurs, there are likely to be fluctuations during the pregnancy and thus there will be need for continuing analgesia.

PROBLEMS ASSOCIATED WITH NONSTEROIDAL ANTI-INFLAMMATORY DRUGS DURING PREGNANCY
Prolonged gestation
Prolonged labor
Increased risk of intracranial hemorrhage in premature infants receiving aspirin
Postpartum hemorrhage
Premature ductus arteriosus closure leading to pulmonary hypertension

Fig. 18.15 Problems associated with nonsteroidal anti-inflammatory drugs during pregnancy.

Unfortunately, the vast majority of women in whom disease stabilizes during pregnancy are likely to have a significant relapse in the postpartum period, usually in the first 8 weeks. Such recurrences are not influenced by breast-feeding or the return of menstruation. This makes it important that suppression of disease activity is maintained as much as possible during pregnancy, so that the risk of postpartum flare is reduced. It also means that almost all women with RA will at least need full-dose NSAID therapy in the postpartum period.

There has been no evidence to suggest that RA alone will have an adverse effect on the outcome of pregnancy, although infants with mothers who have Sjögrens syndrome with antibodies to Ro(SS-A) are at increased risk of neonatal lupus syndrome.

What effect will NSAIDs have on the developing infant?

Firstly, there is potential for teratogenicity during the first 8 weeks and, secondly, there is potential to influence fetal physiology. In general, no consistent teratogenic effects have been reported in humans taking NSAID. However, in animal models using higher than normal pharmacologic doses, various developmental abnormalities have been reported. The physiologic effects relate to the antagonism of the prostaglandins involved in the regulation of systemic and pulmonary blood vessels. Premature closure of the ductus arteriosus has been reported in both humans and animals taking NSAID prior to delivery. Thus, NSAID use in the third trimester should be restricted. Other considerations regarding NSAID use in pregnancy include the effect on platelet aggregation and uterine muscle tone at the time of birth (Fig. 18.15). From a practical point of view, it would seem reasonable to continue NSAID, if required, throughout the pregnancy but to restrict their use as much as possible in the last month and to use drugs that have a relatively short half-life.

What effect do gold compounds have on the developing infant?

In rats and rabbits, central nervous system malformations have been reported with gold or aurothiomalate. Gold has been demonstrated to cross the placenta; indeed, therapeutic concentrations have been detected in umbilical blood samples of a developmentally normal infant at the time of delivery. There have been no adverse effects reported in a retrospective follow-up of seven pregnancies receiving gold treatment. In these particular patients, at least one intramuscular gold injection had been given after the pregnancy commenced. In the

FACTORS INFLUENCING DRUG CONCENTRATION IN BREAST-FED INFANTS
Maternal
Milk composition (fat, protein, water) and pH Mammary blood flow Maternal drug metabolism Time and frequency of feeding in relation to maternal dosing
Drug
Molecular weight p*Ka* Lipid solubility Pharmacokinetics Dose and dosage interval
Infant
Volume of milk consumed Absorptive capacity of infant Deconjugating ability of infant

Fig. 18.16 Factors influencing drug concentration in breast-fed infants.

ELIMINATION HALF-LIVES OF COMMONLY USED NONSTEROIDAL ANTI-INFLAMMATORY DRUGS	
Drug	Half life (hours)
Diclofenac	3
Diflunisal	10
Fenoprofen	2
Ibuprofen	2
Indomethacin	8
Ketoprofen	2
Naproxen	12
Piroxicam	26
Salicylate	4–15*
Sulindac	16
Tenoxicam	36
*dose dependant kinetics	

Fig. 18.17 Elimination half-lives of commonly used nonsteroidal anti-inflammatory drugs.

patient described earlier, it would seem that the gold had controlled the RA to a certain extent but the disease still had some activity. There is no reason why gold should not be continued in a slightly lower dose throughout the pregnancy, but if the disease shows any increase in activity then this would be a good argument to return to full-dose gold treatment, at least during the last 6 months.

Can NSAIDs be used during breast-feeding?

Given the clinical setting of using NSAIDs in the postpartum period, only indomethacin has been reported to produce an adverse reaction. As most medications will enter breast milk to some extent, the aim is to use medication that achieves subtherapeutic milk concentration. Basic drugs accumulate in milk compared to acidic compounds. Additional medication factors that need to be considered, in deciding on appropriate agents to be used during lactation, include the propensity of the infant to release active medication from metabolites (Fig. 18.16). Glucuronide metabolites may be cleaved by the infant to release free drugs. The presence of active metabolites with a longer half-life than parent compounds may expose the infant to pharmacologic effects.

There are theoretical concerns with the use in the postpartum period of sulindac and phenylbutazone as well as diflusinal because of their long half-lives. Diclofenac has active metabolites that have a longer half-life than the parent compound, although clinical studies indicate that the amount of diclofenac present in the breast is subtherapeutic.

When taking into account the above considerations, it would seem appropriate to use ibuprofen or ketoprofen (not in sustained-release form). The ideal situation would be to use the NSAID at the beginning of each breast-feeding. Assuming that breast-feeding is not going to be repeated in under 4 hours and each feeding lasts an average of 20 min, minimal infant exposure to the medication will be achieved.

Can antirheumatic medication be used while breast-feeding?

No adverse effects have been reported in the breast-fed babies of mothers taking corticosteroids or sulfasalazine. Although there are theoretical risks with antimalarial drugs, babies are exposed to very small amounts in the breast milk (less than 2%). Gold is excreted in breast milk and has been detected in breast-fed babies. There are no data on D-penicillamine excretion in breast milk, but it is likely to be low.

Therapeutic Options

Erosive disease is likely to flare in the postpartum period, and this should weigh heavily in deciding the management option during the pregnancy itself. It may be safer in such women to reduce the dosage and frequency of gold during the pregnancy in order to avoid a postpartum flare in disease activity, rather than stopping gold altogether.

In order to reduce the physiologic impact of NSAIDs on the fetus, the use of medications with short half-lives is more appropriate. If an anti-inflammatory drug is required during the pregnancy, one of the short half-life propionic acid derivatives used intermittently should achieve the dual purpose of adequate pain relief with minimal effect on fetal pulmonary arterial musculature. Figure 18.17 lists the elimination half-lives of commonly available NSAIDs.

Likewise, in considering NSAIDs to be used in the postpartum period, short half-life agents are ideal. If used, infant exposure to medication is minimized when the dosing is timed to coincide with the beginning of breast-feeding. Given the average feeding time of 20min with the medication having a half-life of 4–6 hours, minimum drug concentration would be present within the breast milk at 5–6 hours after the last oral dose. Gold compounds have been detected in breast milk but cannot be absorbed by the infant. As such, exposure of the infant to gold compounds is minimal, and lactation itself does not pose a contraindication to the continued use of gold aurothiomalate.

Conclusions

Where possible, all medication should be withdrawn during pregnancy and avoided during the postpartum period. However, given adverse prognostic factors at the onset and the risk to the mother's and the child's physical and psychological wellbeing, a disease-suppressive agent is often required. This situation also reinforces the need to be vigilant of prescribed medications in all women of child-bearing age. Appropriate counseling as to the possible adverse effect of medication on the developing child is desirable.

REFERENCES

Ostensen M. Husby G. A prospective clinical study of pregnancy on rheumatoid arthritis and ankylosing spondylitis. Arthritis Rheum. 1983;**26**:1155–9.

Needs C, Brooks P. Anti-rheumatoid medication during pregnancy. Br J Rheumatol. 1984;**24**:282–90.

Tarp V, Graudal H. A. Follow-up study of children exposed to gold *in vitro*. Arthritis Rheum. 1985:**28**;235–6.

Preston S, Needs C. Guidelines on the use of antirheumatic drugs in women during pregnancy and child-bearing age. Clin Rheumatol. 1990;**4**:687–98.

NONSTEROIDAL ANTI-INFLAMMATORY DRUGS AND PEPTIC ULCERATION

Peter M Brooks, Ric Day & Neville Yeomans

Definition of the Problem

Nonsteroidal anti-inflammatory drugs are among the most commonly prescribed drugs, reflecting the high prevalence of chronic musculoskeletal disease in the community. However, there is now overwhelming evidence that NSAID use is associated with gastric ulceration and with complications of both gastric and duodenal ulcers (Fig. 18.18). Peptic ulcer complications in association with NSAID use are much more common in the elderly but may be a result of the increased frequency of gastrointestinal adverse events with age rather than a specific effect of NSAIDs on the aged stomach. As NSAIDs are an important 'background' therapy for a whole range of rheumatic complaints, the question of arthritis treatment in the face of peptic ulceration has to be faced frequently.

The Typical Case

A 67-year-old woman with a 20-year history of erosive rheumatoid arthritis (RA) presented following a small hematemesis. Her hemoglobin had dropped from 11 to 8.5g over a period of 2 days, and endoscopy revealed a chronic gastric ulcer with no evidence of malignancy. Her treatment was regular NSAIDs, prednisolone 7.5mg daily, and methotrexate 10mg once a week together with folic acid. Examination of her joints revealed active synovitis involving her metacarpophalangeal (MCP) joints, wrists, shoulders and knees. Over the preceding 2 months her ESR had been 36mm/hour. Initial treatment involved bed rest, stopping NSAIDs and increasing the prednisolone to 10mg daily. Full-dose ranitidine (H_2-blocker) was commenced, and she was mobilized after 3 days. While mobilizing, she found she was very restricted because of pain in her knees and her shoulders.

Therapeutic Options

When ulceration occurs, it is very important to treat both the ulceration and the RA (Fig. 18.19).

Therapy for the rheumatoid arthritis

The NSAIDs should be ceased but this will often lead to an exacerbation of synovitis, leading to difficulty in mobilization. As patients have active synovitis, an attempt should be made to suppress this in the following ways:

- Local corticosteroid injection can be given to painful joints, such as the knees and shoulders.
- Oral prednisolone dose may be increased slightly, i.e. to 15mg/day but fairly rapid reduction (lmg/week) should be attempted down to the pretreatment regimen. Another option would be to give an intramuscular injection of methyl prednisolone (100–200mg).
- Regular analgesia in the form of paracetamol should be provided, i.e. up to 4g daily. Liver function tests should be done as there is the potential for increased toxicity in association with slow-acting antirheumatic drug treatment, especially methotrexate.

Therapy for the ulcer

Between 60 and 70% of NSAID-associated gastric ulcers will be healed by 8 weeks even if NSAIDs are continued. This is substantially less than the mean healing rate in most studies of gastric ulceration not associated with NSAID use. One study randomized patients with gastric and duodenal ulcers into two groups, one continuing and one ceasing NSAIDs, both groups continuing with ranitidine. After 4 weeks, regardless of ulcer type, of those who stopped the NSAID, 20% more had healed than was the case in the group continuing the NSAID. Prostaglandins have also been shown to accelerate ulcer healing, although the mean 8-week healing rate is still only about 70%. A significantly higher rate of healing (85%) at 8 weeks has been demonstrated with omeprazole, an acid-pump inhibitor.

Ranitidine, at full dose (600mg b.d.), should be prescribed to combat ulceration. If at 8 weeks endoscopy shows the ulcer to be healed, the question of whether to continue the H_2-blocker is an interesting one. There are no data available to clearly answer this question but, on first principles, it would seem sensible to continue the ranitidine for at least a further 3 months and then reduce it slowly, remembering that a significant number of patients develop NSAID-associated peptic ulceration without symptoms.

Peptic ulcer prophylaxis

The epidemiology of NSAID-associated peptic ulceration is difficult to interpret because approximately 10% of the general population will experience frank peptic ulcer disease at some time. However, the best estimate of absolute risk of severe upper gastrointestinal adverse reactions seems to be approximately two cases of NSAID-induced reaction per 10,000 person-months of prescription. Using a variety of techniques, relative risks for perforated ulcer or hemorrhage as a result of NSAID therapy would seem to be of the order of

PEPTIC ULCER RISKS AND USE OF NONSTEROIDAL ANTI-INFLAMMATORY DRUGS

	Relative risk of ulceration	95% confidence interval
Occurrence		
Gastric ulcer	5.0	1.4–26.9
Duodenal ulcer	1.1	0.4–3.7
Ulcer complication		
Bleeding:		
Gastric ulcer	2.8	1.5–5.4
Duodenal ulcer	2.7	1.3–5.8
Perforation:		
Peptic ulcer	7.3	4.4–11.8
	1.6	0.7–3.7
Death		
Gastric ulcer	4.2	1.9–9.0
Duodenal ulcer	7.9	3.7–16.8

Fig. 18.18 Peptic ulcer risks and use of nonsteroidal anti-inflammatory drugs. Data from Langman *et al.* (1991).

AN APPROACH TO THE MANAGEMENT OF A PATIENT WITH A PEPTIC ULCER WHO IS DEPENDENT ON A NONSTEROIDAL ANTI-INFLAMMATORY DRUG (NSAID)

- Try to stop/reduce NSAID
- Provide symptomatic local pain relief:
  Physiotherapy
  Intra-articular steroid
- Increase or change suppressive therapy:
  Increase oral steroid
  Intramuscular depot steroid
- Treat peptic ulcer on its merits:
  H_2 antagonist
  Omeprazole
  Prostaglandin

Fig. 18.19 An approach to the management of a patient with a peptic ulcer who is dependent on nonsteroidal anti-inflammatory drugs.

3/7. Given the relatively high rate of prescription of these drugs in the community, the most important way to reduce the number of NSAID-associated gastrointestinal problems is to reduce the overall prescribing of NSAIDs. However, given that they do provide symptomatic relief for a variety of rheumatic complaints, the issue of prophylaxis is an important one. The histamine H_2-receptor antagonists, such as ranitidine, appear to prevent duodenal but not gastric ulceration, while misoprostol prevents gastric ulceration and possibly duodenal ulceration. It is not known whether these drugs reduce the complications of peptic ulceration – the important factor producing hospitalization and death.

However, important in any discussion of ulcer prophylaxis is the subject of costs. Although the data are conflicting, it seems reasonable to provide prophylaxis with prostaglandins (misoprostol) for those NSAID-dependent patients over the age of 60 years who have a history of peptic ulcer disease or who are receiving corticosteroid therapy. In view of the fact that gastric adaptation to NSAIDs seems to occur, there are good arguments to be raised against long-term prophylaxis, and this may even be the case in the high-risk group.

REFERENCES

Barrison I. Prophylaxis against non-steroidal induced upper gastrointestinal side effects. Ann Rheum Dis. 1991;**50**:207–9.

Lancaster-Smith MJ, Jaderberg ME, Jackson DA. Ranitidine in the treatment of NSAID-associated gastric and duodenal ulcers. Gut. 1991;**32**:252–55.

Langman MJS, Brooks P, Hawkey CJ, Silverstein F, Yeomans N. Non-steroidal anti-inflammatory drug associated ulcer: Epidemiology, causation and treatment. J Gastroenterol Hepatol. 1991;**6**:442–9.

Kurata JH. Ulcer epidemiology: An overview and proposed research framework. Gastroenterology. 1989;**96**:569–80.

Roth SH, Fries JH, Abadi IA, Hubscher O, Mintz G, Samara AM. Prophylaxis of non-steroidal anti-inflammatory drug gastropathy: A clinical opinion. J Rheumatol. 1991;**18**:958–61.

Walan A, Bader JP, Glassen M, Lamaers CB, Piper DW. Effect of omeprazole and ranitidine on ulcer healing and relapse rates in patients with benign gastric ulcer. N Engl J Med. 1989;**320**:69–7.

ANKYLOSING SPONDYLITIS

19

CLINICAL FEATURES OF ANKYLOSING SPONDYLITIS

Muhammad Asim Khan

INTRODUCTION

Ankylosing spondylitis (AS) is a chronic systemic inflammatory rheumatic disorder that primarily affects the axial skeleton (spine and sacroiliac joints) (Fig. 19.1). Sacroiliac (SI) joint involvement (sacroiliitis) is its hallmark [1–6]. Hip and shoulder joints may be involved in some patients, but the involvement of the more peripheral limb joints is uncommon. The name is derived from the Greek roots angkylos – meaning 'bent' (the word ankylosis means joint stiffening or fusion) – and spondylos – meaning spinal vertebra. However, spinal ankylosis appears only in very late stages of the disease and may not occur at all in some patients with mild disease. There has been a renewed interest in this disease since 1973, when a remarkably strong association with a histocompatibility antigen, HLA-B27, was first discovered [7,8].

The earliest and most typical and consistent findings are seen in the SI joints; the other sites characteristically affected include discovertebral, apophyseal, costovertebral, and costotransverse joints of the spine, and the paravertebral ligamentous structures [1-6]. A striking feature of the disease is the high frequency of inflammation at entheses. This enthesitis frequently results in fibrous and bony ankylosis, perhaps as a secondary consequence of the primary inflammatory process.

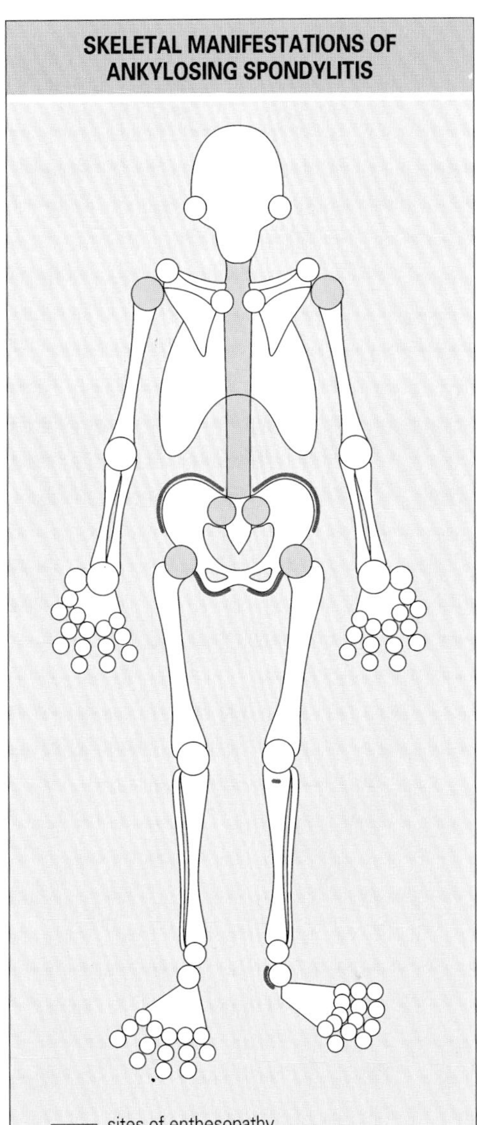

Fig. 19.1 Skeletal manifestations of AS.

Ankylosing spondylitis may occur in association with reactive arthritis (Reiter's syndrome), psoriasis, ulcerative colitis or Crohn's disease; these forms of AS may be called 'secondary' AS [1–3]. However, most patients have no evidence of these associated diseases and are best classified as suffering from 'primary', or 'uncomplicated' or 'pure' AS [3-7]. These disorders are frequently referred to collectively as spondyloarthropathies because spondylitis and inflammatory peripheral arthritis are frequent manifestations of these diseases [3–5]. Sometimes a prefix 'seronegative' is added to the name because of lack of association with serum IgM rheumatoid factor [5].

The major clinical features of AS can be divided into skeletal and extraskeletal manifestations (Fig. 19.2). The first internationally accepted diagnostic criteria were proposed in Rome in 1961, and were revised 5 years later in New York, when the presence of radiographic evidence of sacroiliitis was proposed to be necessary for the diagnosis. These criteria were revised further in light of the recent progress in our understanding of the broader spectrum of the disease. It now appears likely that AS has a wider clinical spectrum than is represented by its current definition [9–11].

CLINICAL FEATURES

Clinical manifestations of AS usually begin in late adolescence or early adulthood (the average age of onset is 26 years); onset after age 40 is very uncommon. The disease is three times more common in men than women, and the clinical and radiographic features of the disease probably evolve more slowly in women [9,11].

CLINICAL FEATURES OF ANKYLOSING SPONDYLITIS	
Skeletal	Axial arthritis, such as sacroiliitis and spondylitis Arthritis of 'girdle joints' (hips and shoulders) Peripheral arthritis uncommon Others: enthesopathy, osteoporosis, vertebral fractures, spondylodiscitis, pseudoarthrosis
Extraskeletal	Acute anterior uveitis Cardiovascular involvement Pulmonary involvement Cauda equina syndrome Enteric mucosal lesions Amyloidosis, miscellaneous

Fig. 19.2 Clinical features of AS.

The most common and characteristic initial symptom is chronic low back pain of insidious onset. The inflammatory back pain due to AS has some special features that help differentiate it from the other, vastly more common, noninflammatory variety [12]. The presence of inflammatory back pain is strongly suggested when the following items of clinical history are present:

- onset of back discomfort before the age of 40 years;
- insidious onset;
- persistence for at least 3 months;
- association with morning back stiffness;
- improvement with exercise.

The low backache of AS is usually of insidious onset, dull in character, and difficult to localize. It is usually felt deep in the gluteal area or the sacroiliac region. The pain can be quite severe at this early stage, and may be accentuated on coughing, sneezing, or maneuvers that cause a sudden twist of the back. The pain may be unilateral or intermittent at first; however, within a few months it generally becomes persistent and bilateral, and the lower lumbar area becomes stiff and painful. In some patients pain in the lumbar area, rather than the more typical buttock-ache, may be the initial symptom.

The second common early symptom is back stiffness that is worse in the morning after sleeping. This morning stiffness tends to be eased by a hot shower, by moving about ('limbering up') and other mild activity, or by exercise. Back pain and stiffness worsen after prolonged periods of inactivity. At times the pain may wake the patient from sleep; some patients have difficulty sleeping well or find it necessary to wake up at night to exercise or move about for a few minutes before returning to bed. The patient often experiences considerable difficulty in getting out of bed because of pain and stiffness and may roll sideways out of bed, trying not to flex or rotate the spine.

Back complaints are the first clinical manifestations in approximately 75% of patients. Occasionally, back pain may be absent or too mild to impel patients to seek medical care. Some may complain only of back stiffness, fleeting muscle aches, or musculotendinous tender spots. These symptoms become worse on exposure to cold or dampness, and such patients are often diagnosed as having 'rheumatism' or 'fibrositis' [11]. Pain in the buttocks or down the back of the thigh can be misdiagnosed as 'lumbago' or 'sciatica', although neurologic examination is within normal limits.

Mild constitutional symptoms, such as anorexia, malaise, weight loss, and mild fever, may occur in some patients in the early stages of their disease, and are relatively more common among patients with juvenile onset, especially in developing countries [3].

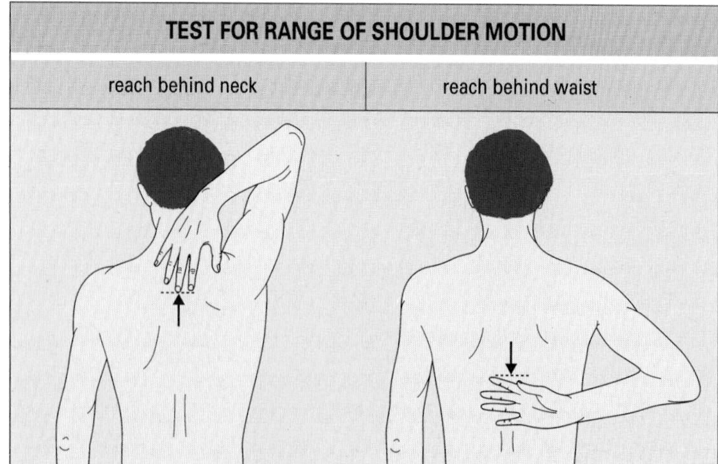

Fig. 19.3 Relatively subtle limitation of motion of the shoulder joint can easily be detected. The patient is asked to bring the arm behind the waist (to test internal rotation) and reach up along the spine as high as possible, then to bring the arm behind the neck and reach down along the spine as far as possible (to test external rotation). In individuals with the normal range of motion of the shoulder joints, these reaches overlap, but in patients with limited range of motion there is a gap between these reaches.

Extra-articular or juxta-articular bony tenderness can be a major or presenting complaint in some patients. Enthesitis causes tenderness of costosternal junctions, spinous processes, iliac crests, greater trochanters, ischial tuberosities, tibial tubercles, or heels.

Involvement of the thoracic spine (including the costovertebral joints) and enthesitis at costosternal areas and manubriosternal joints, may cause chest pain. The pain may be accentuated on coughing or sneezing, and at times the chest pain mimics atypical angina or pericarditis. Many AS patients give a history of having complained of chest pain to a physician before AS had been diagnosed. Some patients notice an inability to expand the chest fully on inspiration. Stiffness and pain in the cervical spine generally tend to develop after some years, but occasionally occur in the early stages of the disease. Some patients may get recurrent episodes of stiff neck (torticollis).

Sometimes the first symptoms may result from involvement of 'root' or 'girdle' joints (the hips and the shoulders). These joints may be involved at some stage of disease in one third of the patients [11]. An accurate assessment of range of motion of these joints should be recorded (Fig. 19.3), because their involvement can result in severe clinical limitation and disability. Hip disease as a presenting manifestation is relatively more common when the disease begins in childhood or adolescence, and can result in limitation of motion, muscle atrophy, and flexion contractures. The frequency of hip joint involvement varies from 17–38%; this might reflect, at least in part, the study of patients at different stages of their disease, because it has been shown that if hip involvement has not occurred in the first 10 years, it is very unlikely to occur later [13].

Hip disease is usually bilateral, insidious in onset and potentially more crippling than involvement of any other joint of the extremities. Some degree of flexion contractures at the hip joints is common in most AS patients at later stages of the disease (Fig. 19.4), and it gives rise to a characteristic, rigid gait with some flexion at the knees to maintain erect posture.

Involvement of peripheral joints, other than hips and shoulders, is infrequent in primary AS. When present it is usually mild and transient, tends to resolve without any residual joint deformity in most patients, and is rarely persistent or erosive. Peripheral joint involvement occasionally can occur after the axial disease has become inactive [14]. Intermittent knee hydroarthrosis is occasionally the presenting manifestation of juvenile onset AS.

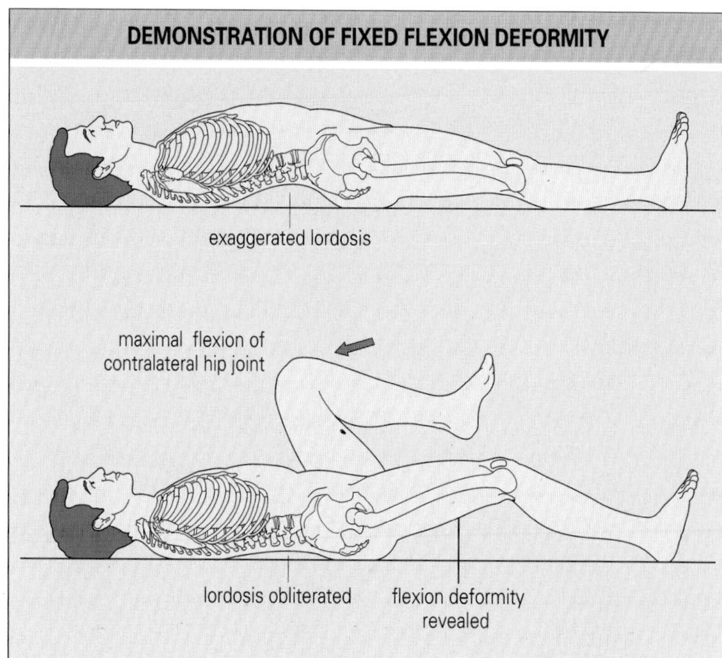

Fig. 19.4 Fixed flexion deformity of the hip joint can be revealed as the contralateral hip joint is maximally flexed to obliterate the exaggerated compensatory lumbar lordosis.

Temporomandibular joint pain and local tenderness may occur in about 10% of patients, sometimes resulting in decreased range of motion of this joint.

A thorough physical examination, particularly of the spine, is critical in making an early diagnosis of AS. As in other diseases where the etiology is not clearly defined, the diagnosis of AS is based on clinical (including radiographic) features. Clinical signs are sometimes minimal in the early stages of the disease; however, SI joint involvement may be evident from palpation of these joints and there is often some limitation of motion of the lumbar spine, most easily recognized on hyperextension or lateral flexion. Associated tenderness of paraspinal muscles is common, and the initial loss of spinal mobility is usually due to pain and muscle spasm rather than ankylosis. Therefore, marked improvement in spinal mobility can occur after treatment with nonsteroidal anti-inflammatory drugs (NSAIDs) and proper physical therapy at an early stage of the disease. With progression, there is a gradual loss of the normal lumbar lordosis.

The loss of mobility of the lumbar spine is best assessed by checking lateral flexion, hyperextension, forward flexion, and rotation. The ability of a patient to touch the floor with fingertips, keeping the knees fully extended (Fig. 19.5), should not solely be relied on for evaluation of spinal mobility, since a good range of motion of the hip joints can compensate for considerable loss of mobility of lumbar spine, and vice versa. To detect limitation of forward flexion of the lumbar spine, the Schober test is quite useful (Fig. 19. 6). This is performed by having the patient stand erect. Then, one mark is placed with a marking pencil on the skin overlying the fifth lumbar spinous process (usually at the level of the posterior superior iliac spine or the dimple of Venus) and another 10cm above in the midline. The patient is then asked to bend the spine forward maximally without bending the knees. In normal healthy individuals the distance between the two marks on the skin should increase due to stretching of the skin overlying the lumbar spine. If the distance between the two marks does not reach 15cm, this indicates diminished lumbar spine mobility. Decreased spinal mobility may also be detected readily by checking lateral flexion or hyperextension. Recently, more refined techniques for assessment of lumbar spine mobility have been proposed [3].

Direct pressure over the SI joints frequently, but not always, elicits pain (Fig. 19.5). Sometimes SI pain may be elicited by pressure over the anterior superior iliac spines, and by compressing the two iliac bones of the pelvis towards each other, or forcing them away from each other, while the patient is lying supine (Fig. 19. 7). The pain can also be elicited by maximal flexion of one hip and hyperextension of the other. Maximal flexion, abduction and external rotation of the hip joints, or compression of the pelvis with the patient lying on the side (see Fig. 19.8), or pressing the sacrum forcefully forward when the patient is lying prone can also cause pain if the SI joints are inflamed. If two or more of these maneuvers elicit pain in the region of the SI joints, the likelihood of the presence of sacroiliitis will be quite

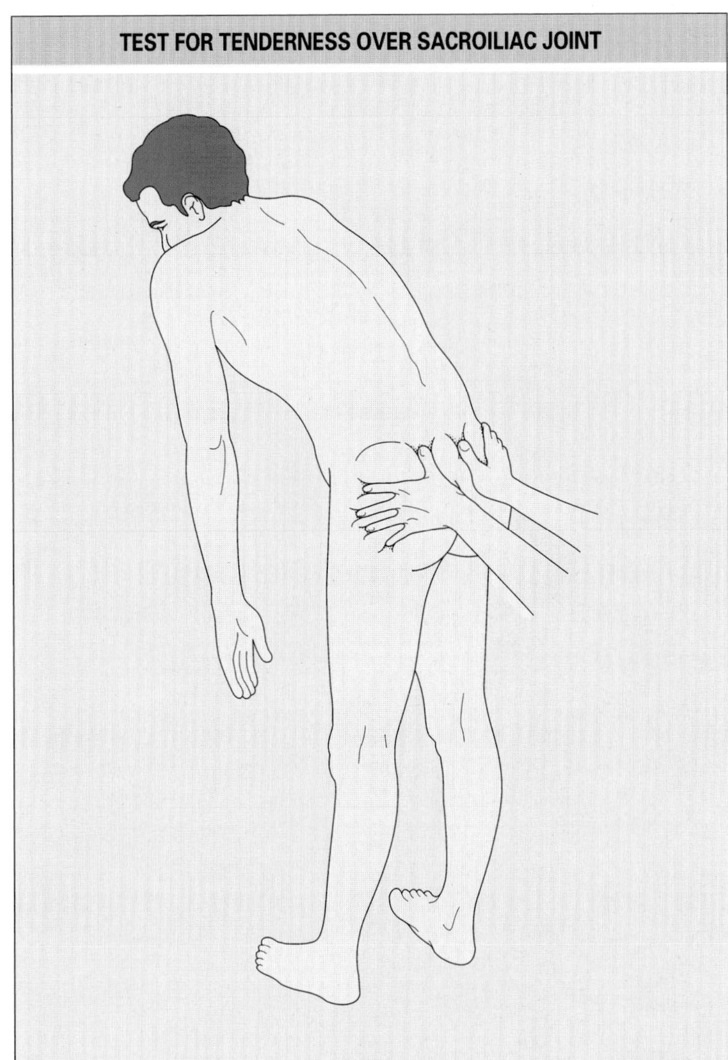

Fig. 19.5 Application of direct pressure by thumbs over the SI joints to elicit tenderness. The figure also illustrates the patient's inability to touch the floor. The decrease in spinal mobility is often more readily recognized on hyperextension (dorsiflexion) or lateral flexion of the spine.

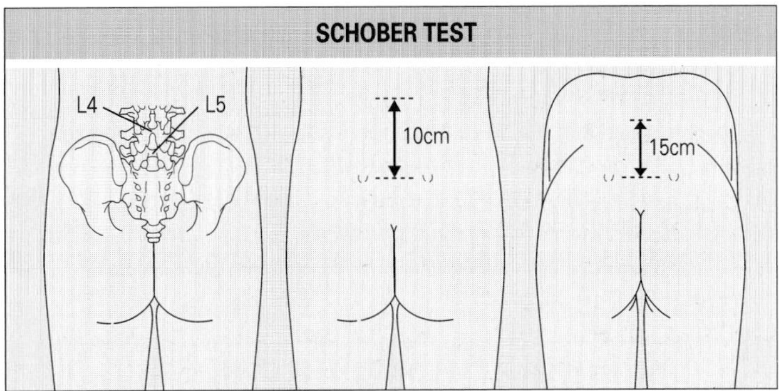

Fig. 19.6 Schober test to measure ability to flex the lumbar spine.

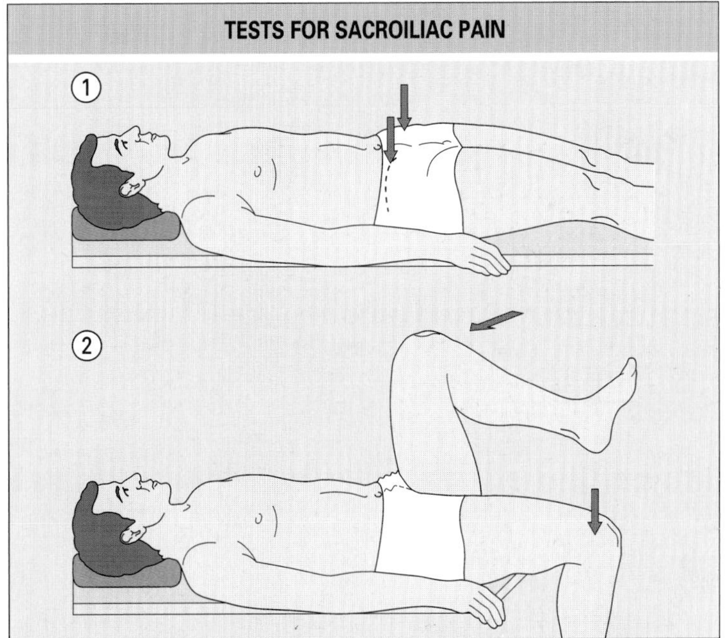

Fig. 19.7 Two procedures that may cause pain in the sacroiliac area in patients with sacroiliitis. Application of direct pressure on the anterior superior iliac spines, along with attempts to force the iliac spines laterally apart (1); and forced flexion of one hip maximally towards the opposite shoulder, with hyperextension of the contralateral hip joint (2).

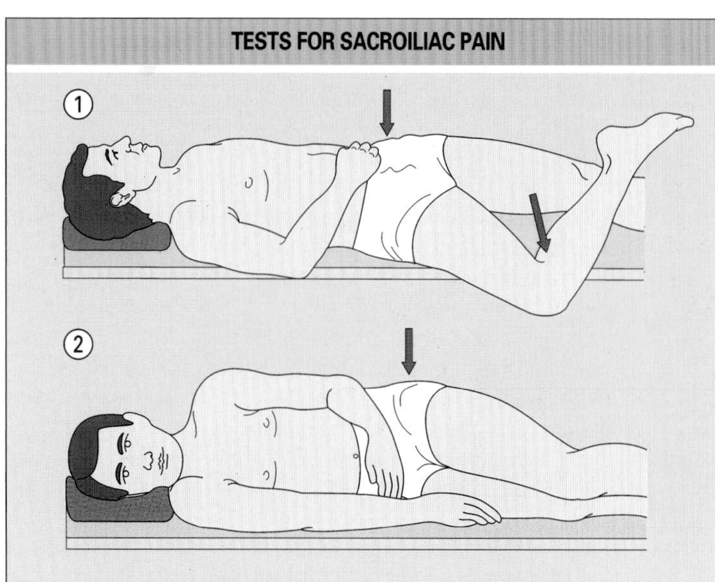

Fig. 19.8 Two procedures that may cause pain in the sacroiliac area in patients with sacroiliitis. Application of downward pressure on the flexed knee, with hip flexed, abducted and externally rotated (1); and compression of the pelvis with the patient lying on one side (2).

strong. These signs may be absent in some patients despite sacroiliitis because the SI joints are surrounded by strong ligaments that limit motion. In addition, these signs become negative in late stages of the disease, as inflammation is replaced by fibrosis and bony ankylosis.

Involvement of costovertebral and costotransverse joints results in restriction of respiratory excursion, and therefore most patients with AS breathe primarily by using their diaphragms [2,15]. The normal chest expansion is 5cm or greater, although it is age- and sex-dependent. It is measured at the fourth intercostal space (or just below the breast in females) on maximal inspiration after forced maximal expiration. Mild to moderate reduction of chest expansion is often detectable at an early stage of AS and should not be considered a late physical finding. Limited chest expansion in an individual with insidious onset of chronic low back pain and without a chest disease such as emphysema or scoliosis should strongly raise the possibility of AS.

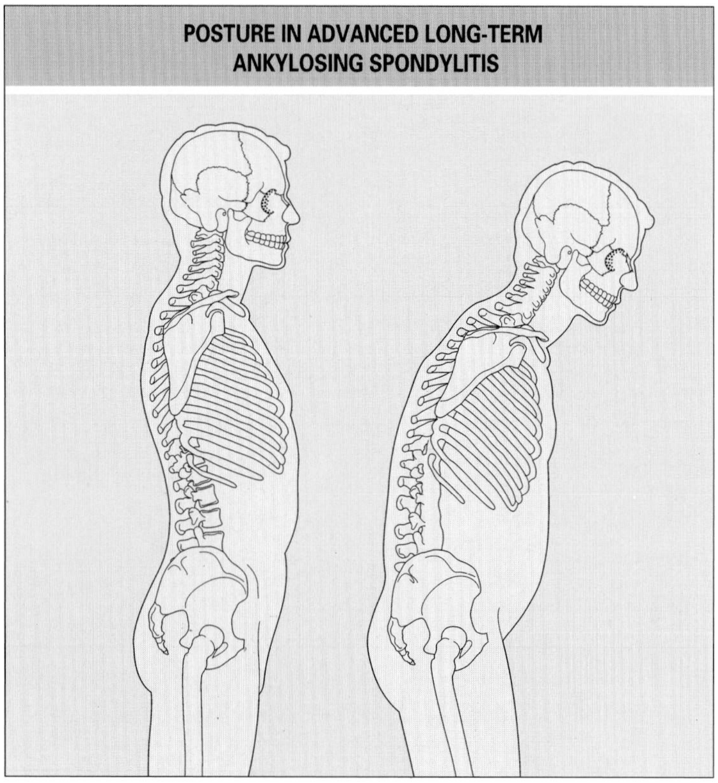

Because of the presence of enthesopathy, an important additional early physical finding (which is often overlooked) is tenderness over ischial tuberosities, greater trochanters, costochondral or manubriosternal junctions, anterior-superior iliac spines or the iliac crest, and sometimes even over calcaneii, tibial tubercle or pubic symphysis. There is often tenderness in the mid-line over the vertebral spinous processes due to enthesitis at those sites.

The entire spine becomes increasingly stiff after many years of disease progression, and the patient loses normal posture because of flattening of the lumbar spine and development of gentle thoracic kyphosis (Fig. 19.9).

The anterior chest becomes flattened, the abdomen becomes protuberant, and the breathing becomes increasingly diaphragmatic. Finally, involvement of the cervical spine results in progressive limitation of neck motion, and a forward stoop of the neck gradually develops (Fig. 19.9), which can be measured by the occiput to wall test (Fig. 19.10). The diagnosis is readily apparent at this advanced stage because of the characteristic gait and posture, and the way the patient sits or rises from the examining table. At this stage the pain from spinal involvement diminishes and there is less morning stiffness, but some degree of inflammatory pain is usually present.

Spinal ankylosis develops at a variable rate and pattern; occasionally the disease may remain confined to one part of the spine. Typical deformities usually evolve after 10 or more years of the disease [13]. In extreme cases, the entire spine may be fused in a flexed position and the field of vision become limited, making it difficult for some patients to look ahead as they walk. Similarly, the hips and shoulders may become ankylosed. Such patients may injure them-

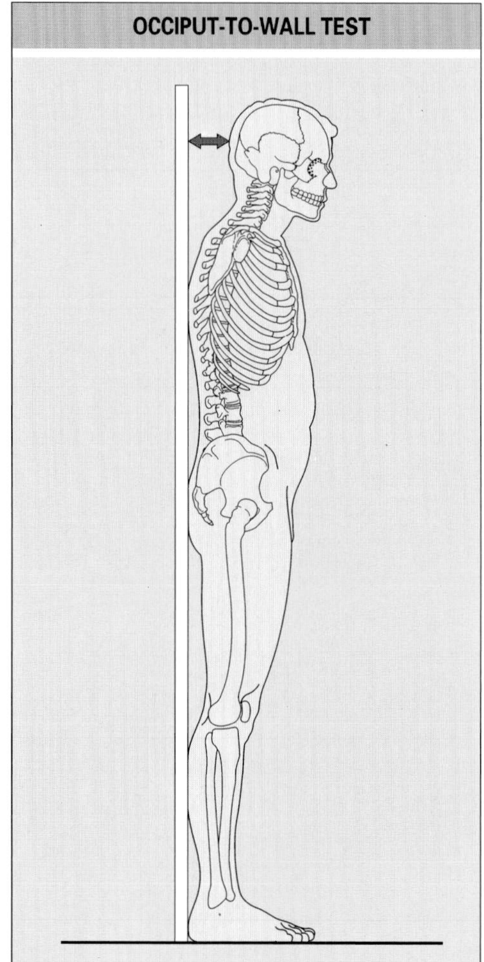

Fig. 19.10 Demonstration of occiput-to-wall test.

POSTURE IN ADVANCED LONG-TERM ANKYLOSING SPONDYLITIS

Fig. 19.9 Posture in advanced long-term ankylosing spondylitis. Progressive flattening of lumbar spine and forward stooping of the thoracic and cervical spine, along with prominence of the abdomen, mild flexion contracture of the hip joints, and diminution of vertical height after many years of the disease process.

selves more readily because of the rigid spine that impairs their ability to balance themselves after sudden changes of position.

Extraskeletal Manifestations

Acute anterior uveitis (also called acute iritis or iridocyclitis) is the most common extraskeletal involvement in patients with AS. It occurs in 25–30% of patients at some time in the course of their disease[16], and is relatively more common in HLA-B27$^+$ than HLA-B27$^-$ patients with AS [9]. The uveitis is virtually always unilateral. The symptoms usually begin acutely and include pain, increased lacrimation, photophobia and blurred vision. There is circumcorneal congestion (Fig. 19.11), the iris is edematous and appears discolored compared to the contralateral side, and the pupil is small but may become irregular if posterior synechiae form. There is copious exudate in the anterior chamber of the eye, which can be seen on slit-lamp examination. The inflammation is 'non-granulomatous', i.e., the inflammatory cells adhering to the endothelial lining cells of the cornea form aggregates called keratitic precipitates, which are small, in contrast to what is usually seen in granulomatous disorders of the uveal tract, such as tuberculosis or sarcoidosis [16]. Individual attacks of uveitis usually subside within 2–3 months, and usually without any sequelae. The uveitis has a strong tendency to recur, not infrequently in the contralateral eye. Residual visual impairment is very rare; it may occur if treatment is inadequate or delayed. Occasionally acute iritis may be the presenting symptom which draws attention to the diagnosis of AS or related spondyloarthropathy [16].

Cardiovascular involvement is a relatively rare feature of AS. Ascending aortitis, aortic valve incompetence, cardiac conduction abnormalities, cardiomegaly, and pericarditis have been observed [17,18]. The aortitis can range from chronic, hemodynamically unimportant fibrosis accompanying severe and long-standing AS, to acute aortic (and rarely even mitral) insufficiency with rapid deterioration of cardiac function in relatively young patients with minimal spondylitis. The risk of occurrence of aortic insufficiency increases with the age of the patient, the duration of AS, and the presence of arthritis of peripheral joints other than the hips and shoulders [17,18]. Aortic incompetence has been observed in 3.5% of patients who had AS for 15 years, and in 10% after 30 years. Cardiac conduction disturbances also occur with increasing frequency with the passage of time, occurring in 2.7% of those with disease of 15 years' duration, and in 8.5% after 30 years. As in the case of aortic incompetence, prevalence of cardiac conduction disturbances is twice as common in AS patients with peripheral joint involvement. Complete heart block causing Stokes-Adam's attacks may supervene in some patients, necessitating implantation of cardiac pacemakers.

An HLA-B27-associated inflammatory disease process may be the underlying cause in 14–20% of patients with lone aortic incompetence [17]. Studies in Sweden have shown that in men the occurrence of complete heart block without spondyloarthropathy and the cardiac syndrome of 'lone aortic incompetence and pacemaker-requiring bradycardia' are HLA-B27-associated inflammatory disease processes, because an increased frequency of HLA-B27 has been observed among such patients. There is no association between HLA-B27 and lone aortic incompetence in the absence of spondyloarthropathy and heart block.

Rigidity of the chest wall in patients with AS results in inability to expand the chest fully on inspiration. However, this inability does not usually result in ventilatory insufficiency because of increased diaphragmatic contribution. Pleuropulmonary involvement can occur as a rare and late extraskeletal manifestation; a review of 2080 AS patients at the Mayo Clinic disclosed 28 who had this manifestation, an incidence of 1.3% [15]. The most common abnormality is characterized by a slowly progressive fibrosis of the upper lobes of the lungs, appearing on average two decades after onset of AS. It is usually bilateral and appears as linear or patchy opacities on chest X-ray, eventually becoming cystic. These cavities may subsequently be colonized by Aspergillus species with the formation of mycetoma. The patient may complain of cough, increasing dyspnea, and occasionally hemoptysis.

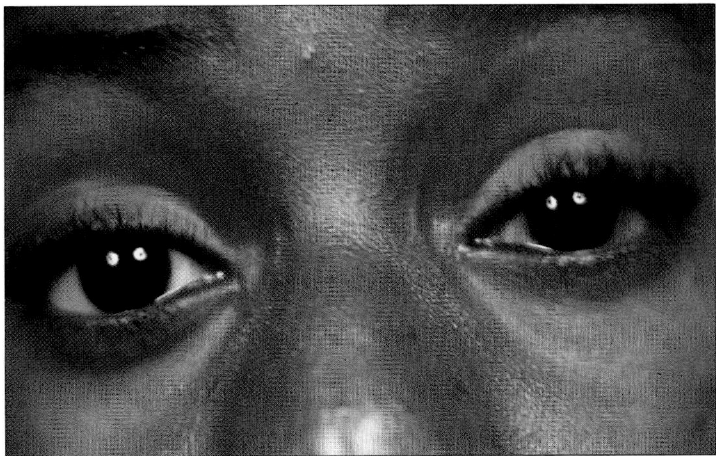

Fig. 19.11 Untreated acute anterior uveitis. Note the circumcorneal congestion, the edematous and discolored iris and the small pupil.

Neurological involvement may occur in patients with AS and is most often related to fracture dislocation of the spine, atlantoaxial subluxations, or cauda equina syndrome. The fracture usually occurs in the cervical spine and the resultant quadriplegia is the most dreaded complication, with a high mortality [19].

Spontaneous anterior atlantoaxial subluxation is a well-recognized complication of AS, presenting as occipital pain with or without signs of spinal cord compression. It occurs in about 2% of patients with AS, and is much less frequent in AS than in RA. It is observed more commonly in those with peripheral joint involvement, and generally occurs in the later stages of the disease, although in rare cases it may be an early manifestation. Vertical, rotatory, or posterior atlantoaxial subluxation, as well as subaxial subluxation, are extremely uncommon.

A slowly progressive cauda equina syndrome have been reported in patients with long-standing AS [20]. This syndrome is a rare but significant complication of long-standing AS. Recently it has been suggested that multiple sclerosis, or a neurologic disease closely resembling it, may occur more commonly in patients with AS than would be expected by chance alone. However, proper epidemiologic studies are needed to establish an association [3].

Amyloidosis (secondary type) is a very rare complication of AS, especially in the USA. However, amyloidosis should be considered in the differential diagnosis of proteinuria with or without progressive azotemia in a patient with AS or a related spondyloarthropathy.

An IgA nephropathy has been reported in AS patients and is of interest because elevation of serum IgA is frequently observed in AS [21]. The presence of renal abnormalities on electron microscopy and immunofluorescent studies, as well as proteinuria, impairment of renal function, and renal papillary necrosis induced by analgesics and NSAIDs have also been occasionally noted [3]. There may be a modestly increased incidence of chronic prostatitis among patients with AS.

Convincing evidence for involvement of skeletal muscles in AS is lacking. The marked muscle wasting seen in some patients with advanced disease probably results from disuse, although some ultrastructural changes in muscle and a raised level of serum creatine phosphokinase have occasionally been observed.

Clinically 'silent' (asymptomatic) enteric mucosal lesions in terminal ileum and colon have been detected on ileocolonoscopic studies in 30–60% of patients with AS and reactive arthritis, suggesting that gastrointestinal inflammation may have a role in the pathogenesis of even 'primary' AS unassociated with clinical inflammatory bowel disease [4,22].

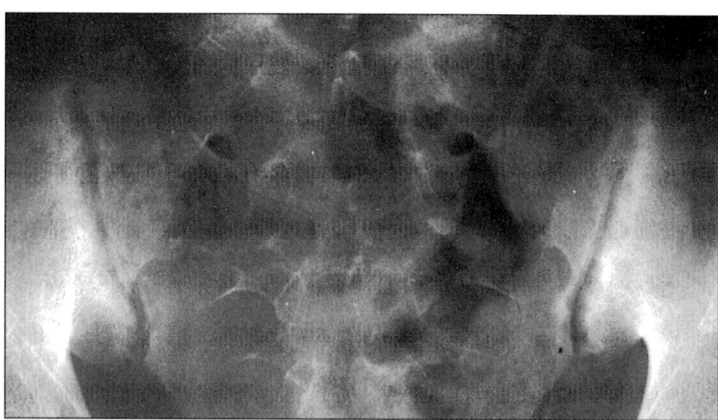

Fig. 19.12 Early radiographic changes of sacroiliitis in AS consist of bony erosions ('postage stamp serrations') and adjacent bony sclerosis. These changes are typically seen first, and tend to be more prominent, on the iliac side of the SI joints.

INVESTIGATIONS

An elevated erythrocyte sedimentation rate (ESR) is present in up to 75% of patients with AS, but it may show lack of correlation with clinical disease activity [11]. Serum C-reactive protein (CRP) may be a better marker of disease activity. In general, the finding of an elevated ESR or serum CRP in a person with 'inflammatory back pain' suggests the likelihood of inflammatory disease (in this context, AS). A normal ESR has been noted in patients with clinically active AS in the presence of elevated levels of serum CRP. Possibly, ESR and CRP relate more to the peripheral than to the axial arthropathy of AS. Mild to moderate elevations of serum concentration of IgA are frequently observed in AS, and the serum IgA level correlates with acute phase reactants: serum CRP, alpha-l-antitrypsin, alpha-l-acid glycoprotein, and haptoglobin [3]. Serum complement levels are normal or elevated. Some investigators have detected circulating immune complexes in the serum of patients with AS, while others have not confirmed these findings. Positive tests for rheumatoid factor and antinuclear antibodies do not occur more frequently in AS than in healthy controls [1–3].

A mild normocytic normochromic anemia is present in 15% of patients. Modest elevations of serum alkaline phosphatase (primarily derived from bone) are seen in some patients but are unrelated to the activity or the duration of the disease [3]. The synovial fluid in AS patients does not show markedly distinctive features compared to other inflammatory arthropathies. Mild elevation of cerebrospinal fluid protein has been noted in some patients, perhaps as a result of mild arachnoiditis.

Mild but persistent elevation of serum creatine phosphokinase (CPK) of muscle origin (confirmed by CPK isoenzyme testing) in the presence of normal levels of serum aldolase has been reported in 15% of patients with AS or related spondyloarthropathies. This CPK elevation does not correlate with disease activity, therapy, ESR, or presence or absence of HLA-B27. Moreover, these patients do not develop any muscle weakness and do not require any treatment for their CPK elevation.

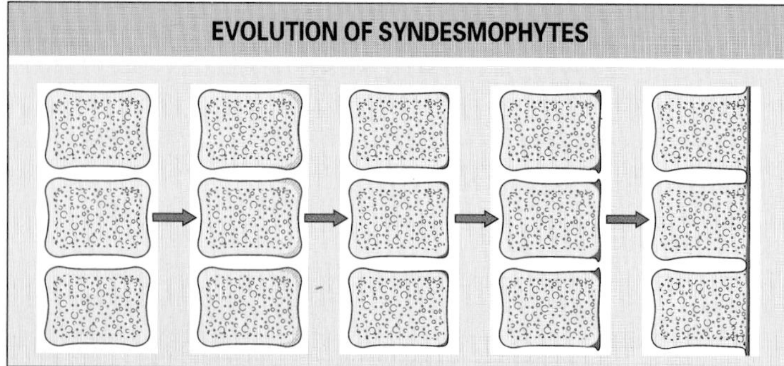

Fig. 19.13 Evolution of syndesmophytes, lateral view of the spine. Osteitis of the corners of the vertebral bodies anteriorly, causing reactive sclerosis ('shiny corners') leads to subsequent erosions and resultant 'squared' vertebral bodies. This is followed by vertical bony 'bridges' (syndesmophytes) between vertebral bodies, resulting from ossification of the superficial layers of the annulus fibrosus. Modified from Khan MA. Ankylosing spondylitis. In: Calin A, ed. Spondyloarthropathies. Orlando: Grune & Stratton; 1984.

Pulmonary function tests show no ventilatory insufficiency even in advanced cases of AS; an increased diaphragmatic contribution helps to compensate for the rigidity of the chest wall. Vital capacity and total lung capacity are moderately reduced, reflecting the restricted chest wall movement; residual lung volume and functional residual capacity are usually, but not always, increased; and airflow measurements are normal.

Characteristically, the radiographic changes of AS are seen in the axial skeleton, especially in the SI, discovertebral, apophyseal, costovertebral, and costotransverse joints [6]. They evolve over many years, and the earliest, most consistent and most characteristic findings are seen in the SI joints. The radiographic findings of sacroiliitis are usually symmetric, and consist of blurring of the subchondral bone plate, followed by erosions and sclerosis of the adjacent bone (Fig. 19. 12). Erosions of the SI joints resemble postage stamp serrations, and are very helpful in radiographic diagnosis of sacroiliitis.

The changes observed in the synovial portion of the SI joint (i.e., the lower two-thirds of the joint) result from inflammatory chondritis and osteitis of the adjacent subchondral bone. The cartilage covering the iliac side of the joint is much thinner than that covering the sacral side, therefore the erosions and subchondral sclerosis are typically seen first, and tend to be more prominent, on the iliac side (Fig. 19.12). In the upper one-third of the SI joint, where the bones are held together by strong intra-articular ligaments, the inflammatory process may lead to similar radiographic abnormalities.

Progression of the subchondral bone erosions can lead to 'pseudowidening' of the SI joint space. With time there is gradual fibrosis, calcification, interosseous bridging, and ossification. Erosions become less obvious, but the subchondral sclerosis persists, or becomes more prominent. Ultimately (usually after several years) there may be complete bony ankylosis of the SI joints, with resolution of bony sclerosis. Bony erosions and osteitis ('whiskering') at sites of osseous attachment of tendons and ligaments are frequently observed [6]. These radiographic findings result from enthesopathic lesions, and are seen particularly at the ischial tuberosities, iliac crest, calcaneii, femoral trochanters, and spinous processes of the vertebrae.

The inflammatory lesions in the vertebral column affect the superficial layers of the annulus fibrosus, at their attachment to corners of vertebral bodies. There is reactive bone sclerosis, seen radiographically as highlighting of the corners, and subsequent bone resorption (erosions). This combination of a destructive osteitis and repair leads to 'squaring' of the vertebral bodies (Fig. 19.13). This squaring is associated with gradual ossification of the superficial layers of the annulus fibrosus and eventual 'bridging' between verte-

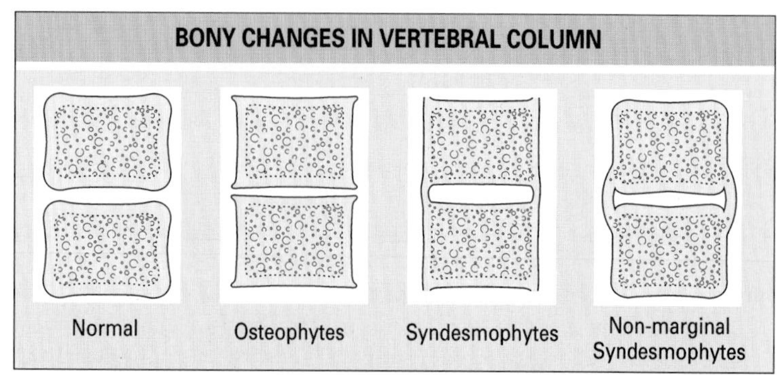

Fig. 19.14 Bony changes observed in degenerative disc disease (osteophytes), AS (syndesmophytes), and psoriatic spondylitis (non-marginal syndesmophytes and paraspinal ossification).

brae; these vertical bony bridges are called syndesmophytes (Figs 19.13 and 19.14). There are often concomitant inflammatory changes and resultant ankylosis in the apophyseal joints, and ossification of some of the spinal ligaments. These processes ultimately result in virtually complete fusion of the vertebral column ('bamboo spine') in many patients with severe AS of long duration.

Spinal osteoporosis is frequently observed in patients with severe AS of long duration, as a result of ankylosis and lack of mobility. However, presence of a marked reduction in bone mineral density of the lumbar spine and femoral neck has been reported in a group of young patients with early AS [23]. There is also an increased prevalence of vertebral compression fractures due to osteoporosis in AS.

Hip joint involvement leads to symmetric concentric joint space narrowing, irregularity of the subchondral bone plate with subchondral sclerosis, osteophyte formation at the outer margins of the articular surfaces (both the acetabulum and the femoral head), and ultimate bony ankylosis. Shoulder joint involvement causes concentric joint space narrowing, with erosions primarily at the superolateral aspect of the humeral head [6].

The evaluation of SI joints and the spine by infrared thermography, radionuclide scintigraphy, and computerized tomography (CT) has been attempted in patients with early disease in whom standard radiography of the SI joints may show normal or equivocal changes [11]. Infrared thermography is not useful in the diagnosis of early sacroiliitis. SI quantitative scintigraphy has generally been found to be too sensitive and too nonspecific to be of much clinical value. CT of the SI joint has recently been claimed to be more sensitive and equally specific in the recognition of sacroiliitis when compared with conventional radiography. However, CT needs to be used only in those patients who have radiographs with normal or equivocal results and in whom AS is highly suspected; it should not be applied to the routine evaluation of SI joints. Magnetic resonance imaging (MRI) produces excellent computer-generated imaging without ionizing radiation, and is also very useful in visualizing arachnoid diverticuli associated with cauda equina syndrome in AS [20].

Use of HLA-B27 Typing as an Aid to Diagnosis

The best clues to diagnosis are offered by the patient's symptoms, the family history, and the articular and extra-articular physical findings. The most widely used diagnostic criteria for AS greatly depend on radiographic evidence of bilateral sacroiliitis, which is the best nonclinical indicator of the disease presence. However, the status of the SI joints on routine pelvic radiographs may not always be easy to interpret in the early phase of the disease, especially in adolescent patients. In such situations, or where a clinical suspicion of AS presenting in an unusual or an atypical manner is raised, there is a need for a laboratory test that could further minimize the degree of uncertainty of the diagnosis.

The HLA allele, HLA-B27, shows strong association with AS, although the strength of this association differs appreciably among various ethnic and racial groups. Although the HLA-B27 test can be used as an aid to diagnosis of AS, it should not be thought of as a 'routine', 'diagnostic', 'confirmatory' or 'screening' test for AS in patients with back pain, (even though among Whites of Northern extraction the test is highly sensitive (92% sensitivity) and highly specific (92% specificity) for AS). An overwhelming majority of patients with AS can be readily diagnosed clinically on the basis of history, physical examination and radiographic findings, and they do not need to be tested for HLA-B27.

In general, the usefulness of a test depends on the clinical setting in which it is performed. A test that is very valuable in a particular clinical setting might be useless if performed on a random population. The predictive value of a test in a particular clinical setting depends on the pre-test estimate that the disease is present. The test's predictive value reflects the magnitude of decrease in the degree of uncertainty about the diagnosis, after the test result becomes known. The same test may have a great predictive value in one individual and very little value in another; this depends on the *a priori* estimate of disease before the test in question (in this case HLA-B27 typing) is done (Fig. 19.15). Therefore, the pre-test probability estimate of the presence of disease has to be sought prior to and independent of the test, in order to properly discern the probability that the disease is present once the test result is known (Fig. 19.15).

A useful 'rule of thumb' to remember is that: if one is dealing with a test with reasonably high degrees of sensitivity and specificity (such as the HLA-B27 test for AS), which is only ordered when there is a 'toss-up' situation (i.e., the pre-test estimate of disease likelihood is close to 50%), then if the test result is positive, the probability that the patient has the disease roughly approximates the specificity of the test. On the other hand, if the test result is negative in this clinical situation, the probability that the patient does not have the disease roughly approximates the sensitivity of the test [24]. As a rule, in those patients in whom history and physical examination suggest AS, but whose X-ray findings do not permit this diagnosis to be made, the HLA-B27 test may allow the presumptive diagnosis of AS to be accepted or rejected with greater certainty. In patients with back pain in whom AS is suggested by neither history nor physical examination, HLA-B27 testing is inappropriate; a positive result would still not permit the diagnosis of AS to be made.

Although HLA-B27 typing can define the population at a higher risk for AS and related spondyloarthropathies, it is of very limited practical value for that purpose because no effective means of prevention is currently available. Moreover, most HLA-B27$^+$ persons never develop AS or related diseases. The test is not a useful indicator of prognosis of AS, although familial aggregation and acute iritis are more common in HLA-B27$^+$ patients, nor does it help distinguish between AS, Reiter's syndrome and other spondyloarthropathies, because all these diseases are associated with HLA-B27 (although the strength of the association varies). Differentiation between these diseases is based primarily on clinical grounds (see Fig. 19. 16).

The current state of the clinical and functional assessment of AS has recently been reviewed [3]. Clinical assessment of disease activity in patients with AS is difficult, especially in uncomplicated disease confined to the SI joints and spine. Pain and tenderness of enthesis (enthesopathy index), and mobility of the spine and the peripheral joints (articular index) provide useful clinical parameters. A functional index has also been proposed that correlates reasonably well with the overall (global) assessment by the patient and the physician.

POST-TEST PROBABILITIES OF ANKYLOSING SPONDYLITIS IN WHITES

Pre-test probability	Probability given positive test result	Probability given negative test result
0.01	0.100	0.001
0.05	0.380	0.005
0.10	0.560	0.010
0.20	0.740	0.020
0.30	0.830	0.030
0.40	0.880	0.050
0.50	0.920	0.080
0.60	0.950	0.120
0.70	0.960	0.170
0.80	0.980	0.260
0.90	0.990	0.440
0.95	0.995	0.620
0.99	0.999	0.900

Fig. 19.15 Post-test probabilities of AS in Whites. (Data from Khan and Khan [24].)

COMPARISON OF ANKYLOSING SPONDYLITIS AND RELATED DISORDERS					
Characteristic	Disorder				
	Ankylosing spondylitis	Reactive arthritis (Reiter's syndrome)	Juvenile spondyloarthropathy	Psoriatic arthropathy*	Enteropathic arthropathy†
Usual age at onset	Young adult age <40	Young to middle age adult	Childhood onset, ages 8–16 years	Young to middle age adult	Young to middle age adult
Sex ratio	Three times more common in males	Predominantly males	Predominantly males	Equally distributed	Equally distributed
Usual type of onset	Gradual	Acute	Variable	Variable	Gradual
Sacroiliitis or spondylitis	Virtually 100%	<50%	<50%	~20%	<20%
Symmetry of sacroiliitis	Symmetric	Asymmetric	Variable	Asymmetric	Symmetric
Peripheral joint involvement	~25%	~90%	~90%	~95%	15–20%
HLA–B27 (in Whites)	~90%	~75%	~85%	<50%§	~50%§
Eye involvement**	25–30%	~50%	~20%	~20%	≤15%
Cardiac involvement	1–4%	5–10%	Rare	Rare	Rare
Skin or nail involvement	None	<40%	Uncommon	Virtually 100%	Uncommon
Role of infectious agents as triggers	Unknown	Yes	Unknown	Unknown	Unknown

* About 5–7% of patients with psoriasis develop arthritis, and psoriatic spondylitis accounts for about 10% of all patients with psoriatic arthritis.
† Associated with chronic inflammatory bowel disease.
§ B27 prevalence is higher in those with spondylitis or sacroiliitis.
** Predominantly conjunctivitis in reactive and psoriatic arthritis, and acute anterior uveitis in the other three disorders listed above.

Fig. 19.16 Comparison of AS and related disorders. (Adapted from Arnett FC, Khan MA, Wilkens RF. A new look at ankylosing spondylitis. Patient Care. 1989:82–101.)

DIFFERENTIAL DIAGNOSIS

The clinical diagnosis of AS depends primarily on history and physical examination, and is confirmed by radiographic examination. Low back pain with stiffness is the most common presenting symptom in patients with AS, although a variety of other presentations may antedate back symptoms in many patients. Low back pain, however, is very prevalent in the general population, and AS is not its most common cause [12] (see Chapter 6). Acute and chronic lumbar strains are the most frequent causes of back pain.

The various causes of back pain may be divided into two main subtypes:

- spondylogenic: traumatic, structural (degenerative and discogenic), inflammatory, metabolic, infective, and neoplastic or other bone lesions;
- non-spondylogenic: neurologic, vascular, viscerogenic, psychogenic.

The back pain from many of the noninflammatory spondylogenic causes is generally aggravated by activity and relieved by rest; there is no limitation of chest expansion; lateral flexion of the lumbar spine is usually within normal limits; and the ESR is frequently normal.

On initial evaluation of a patient, certain features of the patient's history and physical examination raise the index of suspicion, and the probability of AS is markedly heightened by finding radiographic evidence of bilateral sacroiliitis. It needs to be emphasized, however, that sacroiliitis is not unique to AS, and it does occur in other spondyloarthropathies. However, radiography of the pelvis is a useful screening test for differentiating AS from other causes of back pain. Various methods have been used to examine the SI joints radiographically; none is ideal because of the complex configuration and individual variations of these joints

Radiographic changes identical to those seen in primary AS are seen in some patients with secondary AS, i.e., those with ulcerative colitis and Crohn's disease [3,6,11]. Spondylitis that accompanies psoriasis or Reiter's syndrome also demonstrates fundamentally similar radiographic features; however, there are usually subtle differences. For example, in primary AS, syndesmophytes usually form in an ascending fashion, initially forming in the lower thoracic and the adjacent lumbar spine and then appearing in the upper thoracic and, ultimately, the cervical spine. Conversely, syndesmophyte formation in psoriatic spondylitis tends to be more random and usually does not have this ascending order of formation. Some physicians have used the term 'marginal' to indicate the classical syndesmophyte seen in primary AS, i.e., syndesmophytes beginning at the angles of vertebral bodies. In contrast, patients with spondylitis in association with reactive arthritis and psoriasis tend to develop more bulky 'non-marginal' syndesmophytes that do not just extend from one vertebral angle to the other but may start from the middle of one vertebral body and extend to the same area of the adjacent vertebral body (see Fig. 19.14). In the end, of course, differentiation of these diseases is based on accompanying clinical features rather than any radiographic differences (Fig. 19.16).

The osteoarticular manifestations of a collection of unusual skin conditions, including acne conglobata, acne fulminans, hidradentitis suppurativa, palmo-plantar pustulosis, sterno-costo-clavicular hyperostosis, and chronic recurrent multifocal osteomyelitis, include several spondyloarthropathic features. These include seronegative asymmetrical oligoarthritis, sacroiliitis, syndesmophytes, enthesopathies, anterior chest wall involvement, and a possible weak association with HLA-B27. A new name has been suggested for this syndrome – synovitis-acne-pustulosis-hyperostosis-osteomyelitis (SAPHO) syndrome.

At times, other diseases can be confused radiologically with AS, particularly degenerative joint disease and ankylosing hyperostosis. In degenerative disc disease, changes are seen in discovertebral junctions and apophyseal joints, with adjacent osteophytes. The SI joints are usually normal or show only mild degenerative changes; erosions and subchondral sclerosis typical of sacroiliitis are absent. In some elderly patients severe degenerative changes of the SI joint, such as joint space narrowing, subchondral bone sclerosis, and bridging osteophytes in the lower part of the joints may erroneously suggest sacroiliitis.

Ankylosing hyperostosis, also called Forestier's disease or diffuse idiopathic skeletal hyperostosis (DISH) is a condition usually seen in elderly individuals and characterized by hyperostosis affecting the anterior longitudinal ligament and bony attachments of tendons and ligaments [3]. It may be radiographically confused with AS. There is no association between HLA-B27 and DISH. The differentiating features of the two diseases are listed in Figure 19.17. Occasionally, in some patients with DISH, severe degenerative and hyperostotic changes of the SI joints, such as joint space narrowing, subchondral bone sclerosis, and capsular ossifications give a radiographic appearance superficially resembling that of sacroiliitis on anteroposterior view of the pelvis. The syndesmophytes in AS patients who have concomitant degenerative disc disease at the time syndesmophytes are forming may also lead to some diagnostic confusion.

Miscellaneous conditions that might be confused with AS because of SI joint involvement or syndesmophyte-like appearance of the spine include fluorosis, chondrocalcinosis, ochronosis, hypoparathyroidism, and Paget's disease. Others that can be confused with AS include tuberculous spondylitis, Scheuermann's disease, congenital kyphoscoliosis, and chronic brucellosis. Malignancies should also be considered in the differential diagnosis of back pain, in both young and old individuals. Other causes of back pain include pelvic inflammatory diseases, septic (pyogenic) sacroiliitis or discitis, axial osteomalacia or osteoporosis, and sacral insufficiency fractures.

Primary and secondary hyperparathyroidism can lead to irregularity of the SI joint surfaces, particularly on the iliac side, as a result of subchondral resorption and adjacent bony sclerosis; however, narrowing and ankylosis of the joint space do not occur. Occurrence of destructive spondyloarthropathy of a noninfectious nature, resembling erosive discovertebral lesions and spinal pseudoarthrosis of AS has been observed in some patients on chronic hemodialysis. This is not HLA-B27-associated and may result from secondary hyperparathyroidism, deposition of hydroxyapatite and calcium oxalate crystals, or amyloid deposition associated with β_2-microglobulin [19].

SI joint changes suggesting sacroiliitis, and even complete fusion of these joints, can be observed in paraplegics and quadriplegics. Although these changes superficially resemble those seen in AS, they most likely do not result from an inflammatory process but may be a consequence of immobility. These abnormalities appear to be related to the duration and level of disease. Ankylosing spondylitis very rarely develops after 50 years of age, although ten such cases, all HLA-B27$^+$, have recently been described [26]. At onset of the disease, the patients had little or no clinical involvement of the axial skeleton, but instead had peripheral oligoarthritis with relatively low cell counts in the synovial fluid. Pitting edema of the lower limbs, constitutional symptoms or an elevated ESR occurred frequently. Five of these ten patients later showed bilateral sacroiliitis and four of them developed AS. This late-onset peripheral spondyloarthropathy syndrome could represent up to 10% of seronegative polyarthritis in males over 50 years of age, and its recognition might prove helpful in the management of these patients. This arthropathy resembles somewhat the syndrome of Remitting Seronegative Symmetrical Syndrome with Pitting Edema (RS3PE syndrome). Patients with RS3PE are predominantly male, over 50 years of age, and have polyarthritis, pitting edema, and low numbers of cells in the synovial fluid. These patients are frequently HLA-B7$^+$ in contrast to HLA-B27$^+$ late-onset spondyloarthropathy patients. In addition, RS3PE patients all had symmetrical involvement of the hands which was absent among the late-onset spondyloarthropathy patients.

FEATURES DIFFERENTIATING BETWEEN ANKYLOSING HYPEROSTOSIS AND ANKYLOSING SPONDYLITIS		
Feature	Ankylosing hyperostosis	Ankylosing spondylitis
Usual age of onset (years)	>50	<40
Thoracolumbar kyphosis	±	++
Limitation of spinal mobility	±	++
Pain	±	++
Limitation of chest expansion	±	++
Radiographic features		
Hyperostosis	++	+
SI joint erosion	−−	++
SI joint (synovial) obliteration	±	++
SI joint (ligamentous) obliteration	+	++
Apophyseal joint obliteration	−−	++
Anterior longitudinal ligament ossification	++	±
Posterior longitudinal ligament ossification	+	?
Syndesmophytes	−−	++
Enthesopathies (whiskerings) with erosions	−−	++
Enthesopathies (whiskerings) without erosions	++	+

Fig. 19.17 Features differentiating between ankylosing hyperostosis and AS. Adapted from Yagan R, Khan MA. Confusion of roentgenographic differential diagnosis of ankylosing hyperostosis (Forestier's disease) and ankylosing spondylitis. Spine: State of the Art Reviews. 1990;**4**:561–75.

Osteitis condensans ilii [27], a disorder seen primarily in young multiparous women and quite often asymptomatic, is characterized by radiographic evidence of a triangular area of dense sclerotic bone in the iliac bones of the pelvis adjacent to the lower half of the SI joints; the joints themselves are normal. It is a self-limiting condition that shows no association with HLA-B27, and there is no evidence to indicate that it is a form of AS.

The distinction of AS from RA is usually not difficult. Patients with RA usually have polyarthritis which is symmetric in distribution and affects small and large joints of the extremities; involvement of the SI, apophyseal, and costovertebral joints is very rare. In AS on the other hand, any involvement of peripheral joints (other than hip and shoulder joints) is oligoarticular and asymmetric, affecting more often the larger joints of lower extremities; serologic tests for rheumatoid factor are negative; and subcutaneous nodules are absent. There are rare instances of concurrent AS and RA.

NATURAL HISTORY

The course of AS is highly variable and can be characterized by spontaneous remissions and exacerbations, particularly in early disease. The outcome is generally favorable because the disease is often relatively mild or self-limited, and the majority of the patients remain fully employed [3,9,13]. Only rarely does AS show persistent disease activity that results in early and severe disability. Earlier studies suggesting a generally unremitting course of AS primarily involved severe disease studied in hospitals or clinics.

Good functional capacity and the ability to work are maintained in most patients, even in cases of protracted disease, especially if the patient can avoid carrying heavy loads, prolonged standing, and excessive bending, jarring, and twisting. Although it is difficult to predict the ultimate prognosis for an individual patient, some factors that influence the overall prognosis include severity in early disease, development of extra-articular complications, stage of disease at the time of diagnosis and start of therapy, quality of management, and degree of patient compliance with suggested treatment. Those patients with hip joint involvement or completely ankylosed cervical spine with kyphosis are more likely to be disabled [13]. The results of total hip arthroplasty in recent years are very gratifying in preventing partial or total disability in many such patients.

Excess mortality of AS patients, primarily ascribed to complications of radiotherapy and amyloidosis, has been reported in the past. In subsequent studies an excess mortality has also been observed among nonirradiated patients with AS, but these studies consisted of patients with disease severe enough to both impel the patients to seek specialized care and be correctly diagnosed at a time when AS was felt to be a rare disease. It is quite likely that the survival of those patients with mild disease, who form the majority of patients with AS, is comparable to the general population. However, complications of treatment with NSAIDs, spinal fracture, surgery, as well as associated medical conditions such as ulcerative colitis or Crohn's disease may contribute to premature mortality in some patients.

The rigid (ankylosed) osteoporotic spine is unduly susceptible to fracture even after a relatively minor trauma, including events that may not be remembered or recalled by the patient. The ankylosed spine breaks like a long bone, and the fracture line is usually transverse. Fractures in the cervical spine are the most common [6,19], usually at the C5-6 or C6-7 level. Cervical fracture dislocation, with resultant quadriplegia, is a very serious complication with a high mortality. One should exclude the possibility of spinal fracture in any patient with advanced AS who complains of neck or back pain after even a mild trauma. Sometimes the undiagnosed or improperly treated fracture results in spondylodiscitis and pseudoarthrosis.

There is ample evidence to suggest disease heterogeneity of AS, best exemplified by the difference between the HLA-B27$^+$ versus HLA-B27$^-$ disease [9,28,29]. Even though there are a lot of similarities, generally speaking, HLA-B27$^-$ AS is somewhat later in its onset, significantly less frequently complicated by acute anterior uveitis and more frequently accompanied by psoriasis, ulcerative colitis and Crohn's disease, and less often shows familial aggregation. In fact, it is unusual among people of Northern European extraction to observe families with two or more first-degree relatives affected with HLA-B27$^-$ primary AS in the absence of psoriasis or chronic inflammatory bowel disease in the family. There is over representation in HLA-B27$^-$ AS patients of the B7 cross-reacting group (CREG) of HLA antigens (HLA-B7, -B22, -B40 and -Bw42), Bw62, Bw35 CREG, the Bw38 split of HLA-Bw16, and the psoriasis associated HLA alleles HLA-B13, -B17 and -B37.

If AS is defined as low back pain in the presence of early radiographic sacroiliitis and one looks at individuals with only these two features, then there are no differences between HLA-B27$^+$ and HLA-B27$^-$ patients. But if one looks at the core classical AS with limitation of motion of the lumbar spine, one finds that more typical spinal radiographic features, such as bamboo spine, seem to occur primarily in HLA-B27$^+$ patients. These data strongly suggest that AS represents a heterogeneous group of phenotypically similar diseases, and that the pathogenic mechanism in HLA-B27$^+$ disease may differ from that in HLA-B27$^-$ AS [29].

HLA-B27 homozygous individuals seem not to be more susceptible to getting AS, or to having more severe disease, than HLA-B27 heterozygotes. Recent findings in Euro-caucasians suggest that among HLA-B27 heterozygous individuals, the other (i.e., non-HLA-B27) HLA-B allele may sometimes influence disease occurrence. For example, the susceptibility to AS in HLA-B27$^+$ individuals is further increased by a factor of three when Bw60, (which is a split of HLA-B40), is also present; and patients with HLA-B27, B44 phenotype have a higher risk for concurrent Crohn's disease and AS [9,29].

Clinically diagnosable AS may be three times more common in males than in females in the general population, but the prevalence rates of sacroiliitis may be equal in both sexes [9]. The disease expression may be different in males and females; however, the results of several studies are conflicting, and no consistent picture has yet emerged [9,30]. The clinical features of AS may not differ between males and females with regard to spinal symptoms, chest expansion, peripheral arthritis, and extra-articular features, except that males show more pronounced radiological changes and demonstrate radiographically detectable sacroiliitis earlier then females. Although axial disease is more severe in males, the overall pattern seems to be similar in both sexes.

Pregnancy does not improve the symptoms of AS; mostly, women with AS have either no change or only temporary aggravation of activity during pregnancy. Hormonal status, fertility, course of pregnancy and childbirth have been reported to be normal [30]. However, a recent study suggests presence of ovarian dysfunction in Mexican women with AS that is characterized by low levels of estradiol and progesterone during the late secretory phase of the menstrual cycle. Moreover, this dysfunction was found to correlate with clinical activity of the disease. A possible imbalance in the androgen/estrogen ratio in some male patients with AS has also been reported from the same medical center. There is a need for additional and properly controlled studies, in the light of prior reports of normal gonadal function in AS.

REFERENCES

1. Moll JMH, Haslock I, Macrae IF, et al. Associations between ankylosing spondylitis, psoriatic arthritis, Reiter's disease, the intestinal arthropathies and Behcet's syndrome. Medicine (Baltimore). 1974;**53**:343–64.
2. Moll JMH (ed.) Ankylosing spondylitis. Edinburgh: Churchill Livingstone; 1980.
3. Khan MA (ed.). Ankylosing spondylitis and related spondyloarthropathies. Spine: State of the Art Reviews, Philadelphia: Hanley & Belfus; 1990.
4. Khan MA (ed.) Spondyloarthropathies. Rheum Dis Clin North Am. 1992;**18**:1–276..
5. Arnett FC: Seronegative spondylarthropathies. Bull Rheum Dis.1987;**37**:l–8.
6. Resnick D, Niwayama G. Ankylosing spondylitis. In: Resnick D, Niwayama G (eds.). Diagnosis of bone and joint disorders. Philadelphia: WB Saunders;1981:1040–102.
7. Brewerton DA, Hart FD, Nicholls A, et al. Ankylosing spondylitis and HL-A 27. Lancet. 1973;**1**:904-7.
8. Schlosstein L, Terasaki PI, Bluestone R, et al. High association of an HL-A antigen, W27, with ankylosing spondylitis. N Engl J Med. 1973;**288**:704–6.
9. Khan MA, van der Linden SM. Ankylosing spondylitis and associated diseases. Rheum Dis Clin North Am. 1990;**16**:551–79.
10. Khan MA, van der Linden SM. A wider spectrum of spondyloarthropathies. Semin Arthritis Rheum. 1990;**20**:107–13.
11. Khan MA, Kushner I. Diagnosis of ankylosing spondylitis. In: Cohen AS (ed.). Progress in clinical rheumatology, vol. 1. Orlando: Grune and Stratton;1984:145–78.
12. Brown MD: The source of low back pain. Semin Arthritis Rheum. 1989;**18**(Suppl. 2):67–72.
13. Carette S, Graham DC, Little H, et al. The natural disease course of ankylosing spondylitis. Arthritis Rheum. 1983;**26**:186–90.
14. Cohen MD, Ginsburg WW. Late-onset peripheral joint disease in ankylosing spondylitis. Ann Rheum Dis. 1982;**41**:574-8.
15. Rosenow EC III, Strimlan CV, Muhm JR, et al. Pleuropulmonary manifestations of ankylosing spondylitis. Mayo Clin Proc. 1977;**52**:641–9.
16. Rosenbaum JT: Acute anterior uveitis and spondyloarthropathies. Rheum Dis Clin North Am. 1992;**18**:143–51.
17. Bergfeldt L, Insulander P, Lindblom D, et al. HLA-B27: an important genetic risk factor for lone aortic regurgitation and severe conduction system abnormalities. Am J Med. 1988;**85**:12–18.
18. Graham DC, Smythe HA. The carditis and aortitis of ankylosing spondylitis. Bull Rheum Dis. 1958;**9**:171–4
19. Murray GC, Persellin RH. Cervical fracture complicating ankylosing spondylitis. A report of eight cases and review of the literature. Am J Med. 1981;**70**:1033–41.
20. Tullous MW, Skerhut HEI, Story JL, et al. Cauda equina syndrome of long-standing ankylosing spondylitis. Case report and review of the literature. J Neurosurg. 1990;**73**:441–7.
21. Bruneau C, Villiaumey J, Avouac B, et al. Seronegative spondyloarthropathies and IgA glomerulonephritis: A report of four cases and a review of the literature. Semin Arthritis Rheum. 1986;**15**:179–84.
22. De Vos M, Cuvelier C, Mielants H, et al. Ileocolonoscopy in seronegative spondylarthropathy. Gastroenterology. 1989;**96**:339–44.
23. Will R, Palmer R, Bhalla AK, et al. Osteoporosis in early ankylosing spondylitis: a primary pathological event? Lancet. 1989;**2**:1483–5.
24. Khan MA, Khan MK. Diagnostic value of HLA-B27 testing in ankylosing spondylitis and Reiter's syndrome. Ann Intern Med. 1982;**96**:70–6.
25. Kessler M, Netter P, Azoulay E, et al. Dialysis-associated arthropathy: A multicenter survey of 171 patients receiving hemodialysis for over 10 years. Br J Rheumatol. 1992;**31**:157–62.
26. Dubost JJ, Sauvezie B. Late onset peripheral spondyloarthropathy. J Rheumatol. 1998;**16**:1214–17.
27. De Bosset P, Gordon DA, Smythe HA, et al. Comparison of osteitis condensans ilei and ankylosing spondylitis in female patients: Clinical, radiological and HLA typing characteristics. J Chron Dis. 1978;**31**:171–81.
28. Woodrow JC. Genetics of the spondylarthropathies. Baillières Clin Rheumatol. 1988;**2**:603–22.
29. Khan MA, Kellner H. Immunogenetics of spondyloarthropathies. Rheum Dis Clin North Am. 1992;**18**:837–64.
30. Gran JT, Husby G. Ankylosing spondylitis in women. Semin Arthritis Rheum. 1990;**19**:303–12.

20

MANAGEMENT OF ANKYLOSING SPONDYLITIS

Ian Haslock

- Early diagnosis, patient education, and physiotherapy are essential for the successful management of ankylosing spondylitis.
- The goals of physiotherapy are to restore and maintain posture and movement as near normal as possible.
- Nonsteroidal anti-inflammatory drugs relieve pain and stiffness and facilitate physiotherapy.
- Sulfasalazine appears to be the most effective of the second-line drugs.

INTRODUCTION

The cornerstones of treatment of all rheumatic diseases are early, accurate diagnosis and effective patient education. These are probably more important in ankylosing spondylosis (AS) than in any other condition. Early diagnosis enables treatment before permanent rigidity and deformity have taken place. It also enables patients to develop an appropriate lifestyle as early as possible. The patients' long-term cooperation is the single most crucial factor leading to successful management of AS. It is unlikely that the degree of long-term cooperation and commitment needed to develop a therapeutic lifestyle will be achieved unless the patient has a thorough understanding of the disease and the rationale behind its management.

MANAGEMENT TECHNIQUES

Drug Treatment

Simple analgesics are usually considered to have a limited role in treating inflammatory rheumatic diseases. They are, however, quite widely used, about one-third of patients taking them, often as over-the-counter rather than prescribed medication. This reflects the patients' desire for pain relief as their most important objective of drug treatment [1]. Patients also desire their medication to be as risk-free as possible [2], and the extensive publicity regarding NSAID-induced gastrointestinal bleeding seems to have had a considerable effect on patients' perceptions, of these drugs which enhances the desire to stick with simple analgesics, or no drugs at all, whenever possible.

Nonsteroidal anti-inflammatory drugs (NSAIDs) are used extensively to provide symptom relief to patients with AS. Overall the objective of NSAIDs is to relieve pain sufficiently to allow free movement, especially the exercise program essential to the spondylitic patient. During early stages of the disease they are often used in full dosage to cover the entire day. This schedule is particularly important when initial physiotherapy is being used to maximize movement. This phase of treatment may cause discomfort as lost movement is regained. The importance of these exercises is such that adequate analgesia to enable them is a necessity. Subsequently, morning stiffness is often the only symptom, or the most prominent one, and a single sustained release or long-acting night-time dose is often the preparation of choice, allowing freedom of movement in the morning. Many patients find that even this level of medication is only needed on an occasional basis provided they maintain their regular exercises. Some will require either prolonged night-time medication or the continued use of divided doses to give more sustained symptom relief.

Choice of NSAID

The traditional 'best' NSAID is phenylbutazone, which has been claimed for many years to have additional benefits in patients with AS. For this reason, although phenylbutazone has been banned for general use in many countries, it is still permitted for prescription, by hospital consultants only, specifically in the treatment of AS. Despite continuing availability of this medication for AS, it is now little used in the UK and there is no convincing evidence that its special efficacy has been missed. This view is not shared in much of continental Europe, where it remains the treatment of choice in AS for many physicians and where its efficacy is still considered outstanding. The intriguing possibility, derived from a retrospective analysis of a small number of patients, that phenylbutazone actually inhibits the calcification of syndesmophytes [3] has never been explored by prospective, controlled evaluation.

Indomethacin is probably the most widely used NSAID in AS, and does appear subjectively to have assumed the mantle of phenylbutazone as being especially valuable for patients with seronegative arthritis. A large study of more than 1,300 British AS patients showed that indomethacin was both the most used NSAID and the one that was most likely to be continuously useful over a prolonged period [4]. As with phenylbutazone, indomethacin has been suggested as a cause of diminished radiological progression of AS [5]. Again no prospective evaluation of this suggestion has been made. Indomethacin has the advantage of several dosage forms and sizes, making it flexible in use. Single sustained-release 75mg doses at night are an effective way of diminishing morning stiffness. Suppositories have been used for this purpose in the mistaken belief that they deliver a sustained action by virtue of slower absorption; this is untrue, the morning activity being related to the higher dose in the suppositories (100mg) rather than to differences in absorption rate. Indomethacin has a reputation as a drug with a high incidence of side effects. CNS toxicity, especially headaches, do limit its use. These appear to be associated with peak plasma levels and are reduced by sustained-release preparations. The belief that indomethacin is particularly toxic as far as the upper gastrointestinal tract is concerned is not borne out by endoscopic studies, and in any case spondylitic patients are usually in a younger age group, with less risk of serious side-effects on the gut, at their time of maximal NSAID need.

Naproxen was found to be the second most popular NSAID in a large study of AS patients [4]. It has an intrinsically long half-life, giving relief of morning stiffness from a 500mg night-time dose, or whole-day symptom relief from twice-daily dosage. The dose may be increased to 1.5g daily to relieve symptoms from acute exacerbations.

Almost all other NSAIDs are also used in treating AS. Selection is always a balance of effectiveness and tolerance. Patients' responses, both positive and adverse, are highly individual and far exceed the overall statistical differences between drugs. It has been suggested that summation of these apparently idiosyncratic differences can result in an overall 'pecking order' of NSAIDs being constructed which might give guidance for selection taking into account factors such as age and sex as well as individual diagnoses [6]. Although the methodology of this and similar studies offends scientific purists, its similarity to the reality of everyday practice is attractive to practicing clinicians, and there is increasing interest in harnessing the subjective risk–benefit analysis made by rheumatological patients into indices of effectiveness measured as persistence rates with different drugs [7,8].

Two aspects of NSAID use in AS deserve particular attention. First, their proven action is restricted to relief of symptoms such as pain and stiffness. Any increase in spinal movement is related to an increased ability to exercise because of this symptom relief rather than to any intrinsic action of the drug. No drug is a substitute for exercise therapy - pain-free patients have just as great a capacity to fuse their spines as those with continuing discomfort. Second, clinical trials of NSAIDs in AS must be studied with considerable attention to the details of the trial protocols. Many trials allow physiotherapy to continue during drug treatment if the patient was being treated with it on entry to the study. Physical therapy is such an important part of AS management that the results of any study which allows inconsistent physiotherapeutic input should be rejected.

The effects of NSAIDs on the upper gastrointestinal tract are well recognized, but recent work has highlighted effects in the small bowel and has given rise to suggestions that these might be both common and important [9,10]. When these observations are coupled with the observation of silent lesions in the same area observed by ileocolonoscopy of patients with seronegative spondyloarthropathies, the potential for NSAIDs to have an adverse effect on the disease, even contributing to disease perpetuation, must be considered. At present this remains an area of speculation, but more structured observation of the effect of NSAIDs on intestinal lesions and the differences, if any, between different drugs and different types of formulation will need to be undertaken to clarify thinking and rationalize therapy.

Second line treatment

In contrast to RA, no drugs have yet been claimed to have a disease modifying effect on AS. However, several of the second line drugs used to treat and possibly modify the course of RA have also been used in AS with at least symptomatic benefit. In general, the progress for AS treated with a vigorous exercise regime is said to be excellent [7]. While many patients do have a good response to physical treatment and simple medication, in others the disease causes severe symptoms and severe incapacity, often involving peripheral as well as spinal joints. It is these patients who are at present being treated with second line agents and in whom some success, at least on a short-term basis, has been achieved.

Almost all the second line drugs used in the management of RA have been tried at some time in AS. The majority have been disappointing, gold, penicillamine and antimalarials proving ineffective. Sulfasalazine has an additional property commanding attention. Despite becoming 'unfashionable' as a treatment for RA in the 1960s and 1970s, it continued to enjoy widespread use in the treatment of inflammatory bowel disease. Although it was generally accepted that AS is an hereditary accompaniment to inflammatory bowel disease [11], rather than being caused by it, as is the case with enteropathic arthritis, this view received challenge from the work of Mielants and colleagues. They undertook colonoscopy and visual examination of the terminal ileum, initially in patients with reactive arthritis following enteric infection. They observed inflammatory lesions in the small bowel, and later extended their observations to idiopathic AS, when similar lesions were again demonstrated [12]. Although clinically silent, these lesions bear a striking histological similarity to Crohn's disease, and their relationship to etiology became a source of speculation. Under these circumstances, use of sulfasalazine combined the serendipidous logic of extrapolation from RA to AS with scientific logic suggested by these observations.

Several studies of sulfasalazine have now been undertaken both in patients with peripheral joint synovitis and those with spinal disease alone. The results have been variable, but meta-analysis does confirm both effectiveness and safety in short-term treatment of AS [13]. There is some evidence that the effect is greater in those with early disease than those in whom disease is more advanced, this being defined by the presence of fixed or bony deformity [14]. There is also some evidence that clinical improvement is accompanied by lowering of CRP and ESR, a combination of events which, in RA, is considered indicative of disease modifying action. As sulfasalazine is a drug of which there is considerable clinical experience, including its safe use over many years, it would seem reasonable to introduce it early in treating patients whose disease shows signs of poor control by physical treatment coupled with NSAIDs, given the proviso that the results at present are suggestive rather than proved and that the possibility of long-term benefit is entirely speculative. Incremental doses to 1.5g b.i.d. have been used in studies to date, although slightly higher doses are sometimes used to treat inflammatory bowel disease and are logical if partial response occurs.

Methotrexate has been used to treat psoriatic arthritis and reactive arthritis. It has been given to patients with AS in similar low-dosages, 7.5–15mg oral or intramuscular weekly pulsed doses, as those used in RA and appears to have a beneficial effect on both peripheral joints and spinal disease, although no controlled studies have yet been published. Many of the patients to whom methotrexate might be of particular value are young people with severe, active disease which is unremittingly progressive despite cooperation with an exercise regime. Some of these patients wish to start a family, and the potentially teratogenic effect in both males and females taking this drug has proved a significant practical problem.

Intravenous cyclophosphamide, 200mg alternate days for 3 weeks, followed by a 100mg oral dose weekly for 3 months, has also been used successfully on an open basis, producing reduction in peripheral joint synovitis and spinal pain although not spinal movement [15]. This was accompanied by a significant fall in ESR, but no controlled studies have been undertaken.

In summary, there is evidence that second line drugs have a significant effect on the symptoms of AS under circumstances where NSAIDs have proved inadequate. It seems likely that, as in RA, they will be used earlier in the course of the disease in the future. It would be logical for their early use to be restricted to those patients who have a poor prognosis, but no sufficiently accurate prognostic factors as yet exist to make this judgement before clinical deterioration has actually taken place. At present uncontrolled disease activity is the indication for their use. Whether their effect will be long-lasting and whether they will prove to be truly disease modifying, are at present unanswered questions. Logically the proof of disease modification would require not only symptomatic benefit but also some more objective hallmarks of disease control. In this context, prevention of syndesmophyte formation might occupy the same place in relation to AS disease modification as prevention of erosions does in RA.

Corticosteroids

Long-term systemic corticosteroids have little part to play in the management of AS, although rare patients exist in whom no other form of treatment proves effective. Despite its appearance of over-ossification, the spine in AS contains vertebrae which are significantly osteoporotic, possibly due to diversion of mechanical stress from the vertebral bodies to the surrounding syndesmophyte bridges. The effect of long-term corticosteroids on this osteoporosis is unproved, but on theoretical grounds might be expected to increase it. Parenteral low dose corticotrophin proved ineffective when added to an in-patient rehabilitation regime [16]. Intravenous pulsed methylprednisolone is undoubtedly effective in reducing severe symptoms. The indications for its use are poorly defined but experience suggests it is an extremely effective way of controlling symptoms on a short-term basis. The period of reduced symptoms produced by this therapy should always be utilized for intensive physiotherapy in order to maximize movement and correct posture as much as possible. Local corticosteroid injections are useful both for peripheral joint disease and for local treatment of enthesopathy.

Radioactive Isotopes

Radioactive synovectomy, using yttrium especially, is a useful treatment for chronic synovitis, particularly in the knee. This treatment should be reserved for those who have completed their family, due to the small risk of chromosome damage through irradiation of the groin lymphatics.

Non-locomotor Disease

Eye disease is the most common extra-articular complication of AS with at least 20% of patients suffering isolated or repeated attacks of iritis (anterior uveitis). As there is no close temporal relationship between severity of iritis and spondylitis, the eye disease is treated as a separate entity. The most important aspect of treatment is to ensure that the patient seeks immediate medical advice on developing a painful red eye. They should not 'give it the benefit of the doubt' and wait to see if the symptoms settle, or assume they are due to some alternative cause such as a foreign body; it is safer to seek unnecessary advice immediately than to delay treatment. The consequences of delayed or inadequate treatment are the formation of synechiae, which are adhesions from the back of the iris. Secondary glaucoma may then supervene.

Anterior uveitis associated with AS is usually unilateral. In most cases topical therapy with corticosteroid eye-drops and mydriatics is all that is required. The eye may need to be protected from the light to ensure comfort during the period of pupillary dilatation. Administration of steroids orally or by intra-ocular injection is required when local treatment fails to relieve the inflammation.

Iritis is, on occasions, the presenting symptom of AS, especially where back pain is mild or stiffness has occurred insidiously. Those treating apparently idiopathic anterior uveitis, especially when unilateral, should always consider the possibility of this diagnosis.

The two major internal organs involved in AS are the heart and the lungs. Disease such as aortic valve disease is treated identically to similar disease in nonspondylitic patients. Extra precautions may be needed at the time of any surgery as neck rigidity can produce anesthetic difficulties. Long-term anticoagulation following valve surgery complicates the therapy of the joint disease because of interactions with NSAIDs, which displace warfarin from protein binding and thus alter anticoagulant need. Also, patients who are in need of cardiac surgery and hence anticoagulation are usually older and so come into the age group where the risk of major bleeding produced by NSAIDs is increased. It is prudent in these patients to avoid NSAIDs if at all possible, and if symptom relief cannot be obtained in any other way, to protect the patient by co-prescribing H_2 receptor antagonists, prostaglandins or proton-pump inhibitors.

Ankylosing Spondylitis Associated with other Diseases

As the central member of the seronegative spondyloarthropathies, AS may be associated with other group members, particularly psoriasis and inflammatory bowel disease. The treatment of the skin and joint components of AS associated with psoriasis are separate, except that methotrexate might have a beneficial effect on both aspects of the disease. When AS is associated with inflammatory bowel disease it must be remembered that NSAIDs may cause exacerbation of the bowel disease [17] and must be used with care. The propensity for fenamates to cause diarrhea makes them particularly unsuitable. There is speculation that sustained release formulations which are designed to release small quantities of drug throughout the length of the gut might be particularly problematic, although presently this is unproved. The effect of sulfasalazine on both gut and joints makes it a particularly good choice under these circumstances although the salicylate-only medications such as mesalizine which are now being used to treat inflammatory bowel disease have no effect on joint disease.

Physiotherapy

Physiotherapy is widely recognized as the single most important aspect of management of AS. There is some evidence that exercise alone can produce adequate symptom relief in many patients with AS, with 178 of the 236 patients from the armed forces followed long-term by Wynn Parry achieving symptom control by this means alone [18] . Controlled studies of physiotherapy are rare, although significant benefit from exercise and education can be demonstrated over relatively short periods [19] and manipulative therapy has also been shown to increase range of movement in the short-term [20]. Physical therapy takes two forms; that provided within the physiotherapy department, and the patients' own home exercise regimes.

At the time of diagnosis of AS, patients should have an immediate referral to a physiotherapist whose aims will be to restore posture and movement to as near normal as possible. Hydrotherapy is particularly valuable in producing the appropriate environment in which movement can be maximized (Fig. 20.1). A variety of pain relief methods such as pulsed short-wave therapy, local heat or cold, interferential therapy, local ultrasound (Fig. 20.2) or transcutaneous nerve stimulation [21] may be useful in facilitating movement. NSAIDs in high doses may also be needed during this phase of treatment, again with the objective of diminishing pain to a sufficient degree to allow full mobilization. Regaining lost movement at this time may cause discomfort, and this causes apprehension to many patients especially those who have been previously misdiagnosed and instructed to rest if pain increases. The attending physician must be sensitive to the patients' anxieties and willing to produce the greatest possible degree of analgesia to facilitate increased range of movement. Chest expansion and breathing exercises are also important. Local enthesopathy may need systemic drug treatment, local steroid injection or local treatment by the physiotherapist using modalities such as ultrasound.

The initial period of treatment must be combined with an intensive educational program. The patient must be told repeatedly that long-term success in disease management is dependent on the regularity of their home exercise regime. Extra discomfort must be seen as a need for extra exercise not extra rest. In teaching the patients their home exercise regime, it is essential that therapists recognize that doing regular exercises is time-consuming and boring. It is therefore essential to try to incorporate as much appropriate exercise as possible into the patients' lifestyle encouraging recreational exercise such as swimming and badminton. Postural correction often involves undoing ingrained habits, particularly sitting in slouched positions. Good chest movement and breathing technique have to be taught, not assumed, and all spondylitics should be strongly advised not to smoke.

The initial period of physical therapy is a time of intense activity for the therapist and the patient. If treatment has been started before a significant amount of fixed deformity has occurred, and if the patient has proved cooperative with the treatment program, both therapist and patient will be rewarded by improved movement and decreased symptoms. The fact that this period of disease management is short and that the gains made are often quite dramatic, makes it a popular time for all concerned. However, unless the instant gratification of this exciting treatment can be translated into commitment to a long-term management program, the progress made is likely to be transient.

The patients' own efforts are the key to long-term success. Persuading all spondylitics that a daily exercise program must become as automatic a part of their day as cleaning their teeth or combing their hair calls for a major educational effort and constant reinforcement. The program which the therapist teaches must be realistic physically, taking into account the degree of deformity which has already become fixed, and must have a time commitment which can be accommodated within the patients everyday life (Fig. 20.3). Unrealistic expectations produce negative reactions which sabotage the entire program. The exercise and lifestyle program should also aim at cardiovascular fitness, as this has been shown to be important in maintaining work capacity even if chest wall rigidity occurs [22].

Reinforcement of the exercise program is the responsibility of all health professionals coming into contact with the patient. The understanding, help and support of family members is also important, and securing this cooperation is a vital part of the educational process. Every consultation, for whatever purpose, should include the questions, 'Are you still doing your exercises? How often are you doing them? Are you doing all the exercises the physiotherapist showed you?' Any deterioration in posture should also be noted and commented on, with an attempt made to find the cause and remedy the problem.

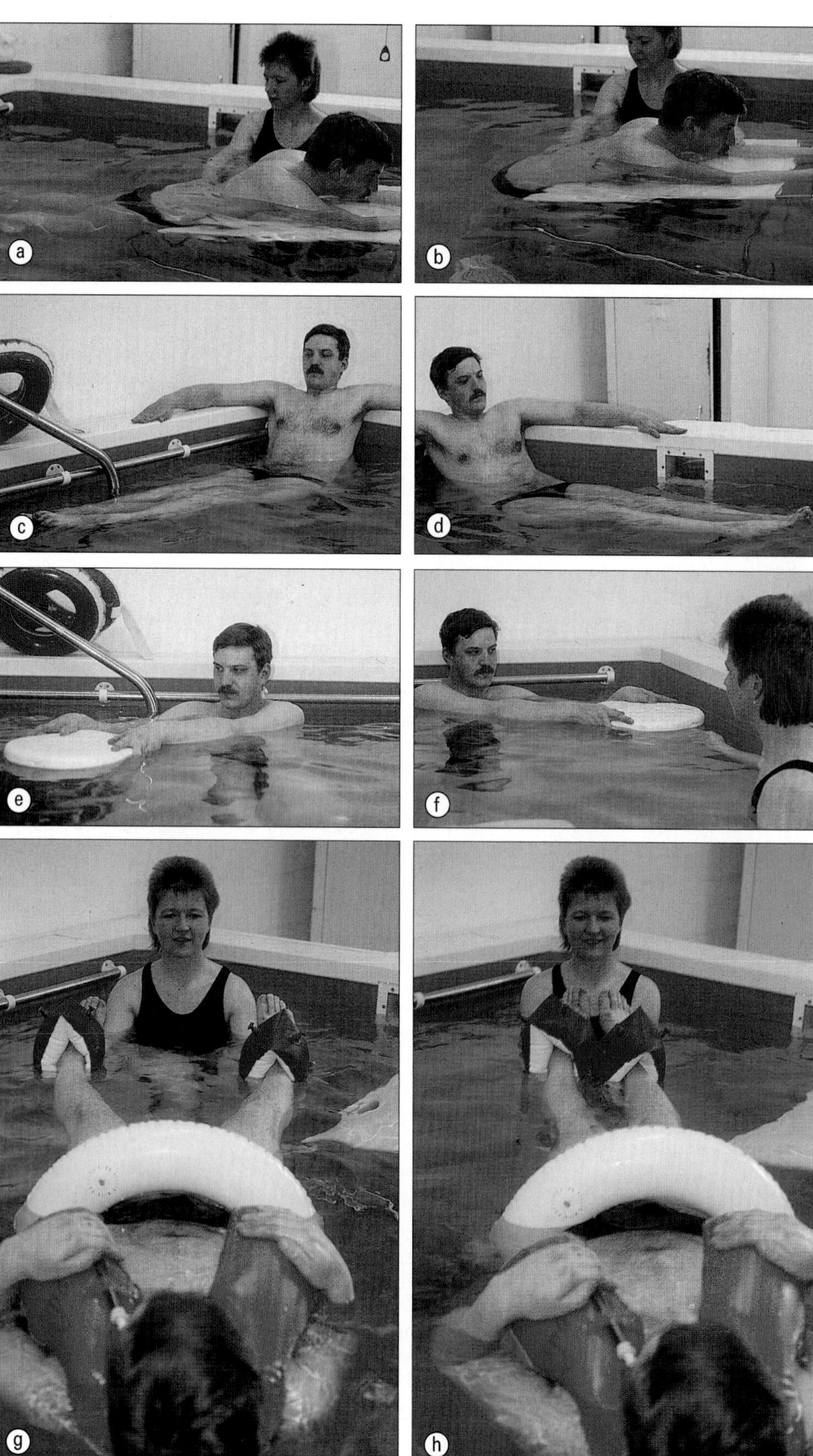

Fig 20.1 Hydrotherapy is valuable in restoring and maintaining movement. This can include spinal movements (a,b), hip and trunk (c, d) and shoulder movements (e, f). The therapist is often able to gain considerably more movement by stretching in the pool (g, h) than is possible on dry land.

Many patients with AS do not require regular prescriptions or sick-notes, and some mechanism must exist to ensure that they are seen and assessed regularly by their physiotherapist, family doctor or hospital consultant. A chart showing progressive change in objective measurements, which the patient keeps, is a good method of documenting progression for both the patient and the medical team. Although the patients' own efforts are of paramount importance in maintaining mobility, physiotherapy interventions may be necessary either regularly or where problems have been noted. Even patients with late disease benefit from techniques such as passive stretching appropriately applied [23] , and once demonstrated to be effective, techniques such as this can be taught to the patient for use with the assistance of a helper. Supervised training periods, including sessions in a hydrotherapy pool, undertaken at weekly intervals have also been shown to maintain mobility and function over prolonged periods, although no untreated control group was available for comparison [24]. However, the measured retention of movement and posture over a five-year period using this regime provides a useful benchmark for alternative treatment strategies.

A particularly intensive approach to physical treatment has been described by the unit at Bath, England [25]. These patients were admitted to hospital each year for an intensive three-week period of physiotherapy and hydrotherapy, accompanied by an educational program and reinforcement of their home exercise regime. Benefit was found short-term by comparing measurements made at the beginning with those at the end of each in-patient period. It was concluded that even in advanced disease small but worthwhile benefit could be achieved. Whether such a highly expensive use of resources is justified, especially in comparison with intensive out-patient regimes, remains open to question. For more everyday practice, one reliable way of reinforcing exercises and lifestyle is through a patient-run group such as the National Ankylosing Spondylitis Society (NASS). NASS was founded in England but now has branches, or similar societies, in many parts of the world. Most branches have arrangements for regular assessment and exercise sessions, usually staffed by volunteer physiotherapists. Each session incorporates a warm-up and stretching period followed by exercise sessions, including hydrotherapy where available, and often culminating in light-heartedly competitive games. They give the opportunity for discussion of problems with the therapist and more formal educational sessions to improve self-knowledge of the disease and its management. NASS is also a rich source of knowledge and opinion and a focus of pressure for better diagnostic and treatment facilities.

The end product of these efforts should be knowledgeable, active patients with a postural and exercise program built in to their daily lives enabling them to be fit and active with minimal symptoms.

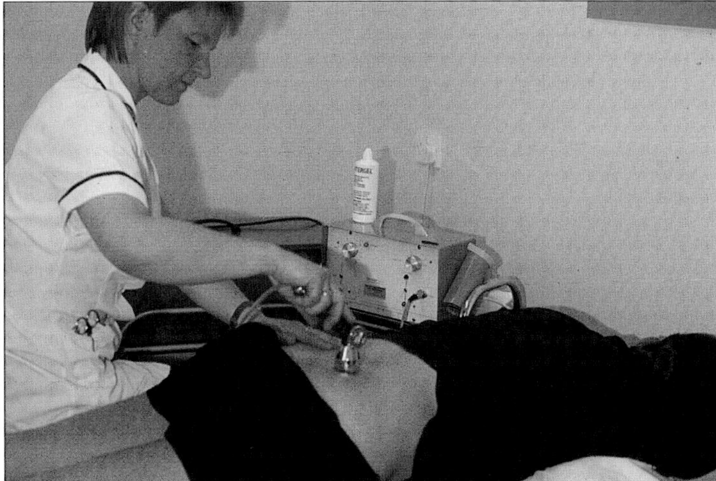

Fig 20.2 Local application of ultrasound over the sacroiliac joint.

Occupational Therapy

In the case of patients with early disease, occupational therapists will probably limit their interventions to the educational part of patient management. This will particularly involve advice about posture, especially appropriate seating, and recreation. The psychological training of occupational therapists often makes them the appropriate team member to lead in developing pain control strategies with the patients [26].

Where disease is more advanced, assessment of activities of daily living and ergonomic assessment of the work place become more prominent, including the provision of aids where deformity produces significant practical problems. Patients with spondylitis often find that their decreased bending causes problems with dressing, and items such as elastic laces and stocking aides are often essential for independence. Mobility is vital to all patients with arthritis, and car adaptations including wide-view mirrors and modified controls may be required by the more advanced spondylitic. For patients with very severe fixed spinal deformity, prismatic spectacles may be the only method of achieving an adequate amount of forward vision.

Other members of the multidisciplinary team, such as chiropodists and social workers, will also become involved with any patient whose disease progresses. Where continued active disease requires long-term complex medication, the rheumatology clinical nurse specialist will have a greater part to play in patient management, and will in some cases take over from the physiotherapist the role of prime manager of the patient's problems.

Work is an area of particular importance to patients with AS, as many are on the thresholds of their careers when the diagnosis is made and a realistic discussion about the possibility of disease progression must be an important part of career choice. Those in employment may need skilled career advice to facilitate changing to more suitable occupations, but for most this can be achieved without a significant diminution in their job satisfaction or income [27].

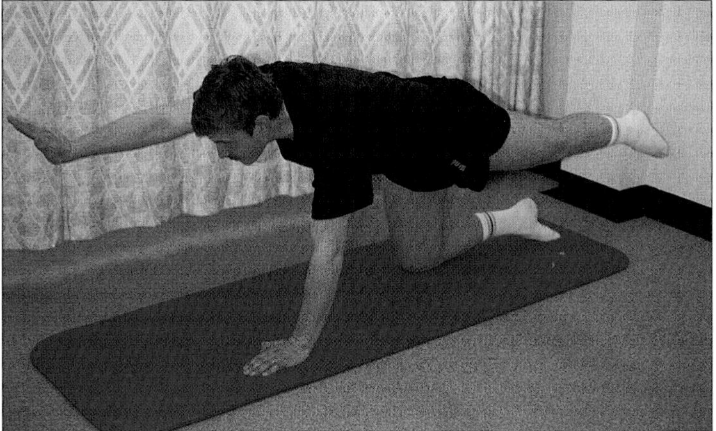

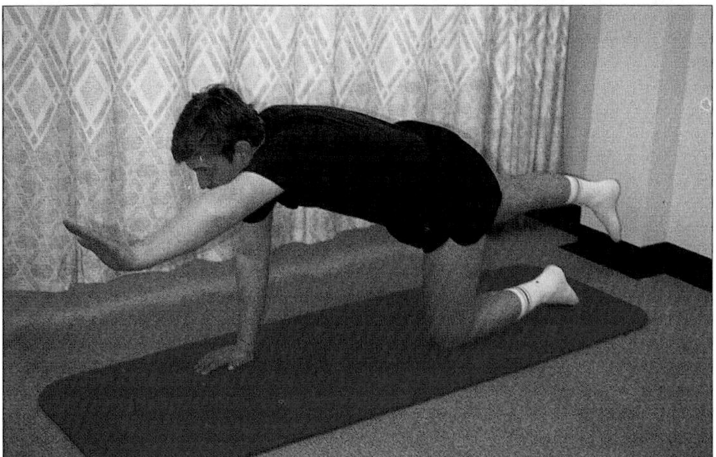

Fig 20.3 A home exercise regime. This must be individually devised taking into account the patient's social circumstances and the severity of the disease.

Studies undertaken in the armed forces demonstrate the ability of fit, active, well motivated people to follow a physically demanding career despite AS. Unfortunately, the persuasive talents of the Regimental Sergeant Major regarding regular exercise has no equal in civilian lifestyle. In general, the greatest problems to AS patients lie in jobs involving prolonged work in a single posture, especially desk-work. Work posture is vital here, as is the need to change posture regularly and, preferably, undertake some form of exercise such as a brisk walk during the lunch-break.

Surgery

The rigid flexed cervical spine and immobile chest wall of the patient with AS may produce significant technical difficulties for the anesthetist and a need for immaculate perioperative management by the physiotherapist. Despite this, surgery can be an extremely valuable part of the management of a patient with AS.

Spinal surgery involves two areas particularly: the cervical spine, where atlanto-axial subluxation may take place; and the dorsolumbar spine where the paradoxical operation of spinal fusion may be needed for a 'last joint' problem, or where osteotomy may be used to improve spinal posture.

Atlanto-axial subluxation is less common in AS than in RA. Patients with RA can have significant degrees of atlanto-axial slip with no symptoms because of the general ligamentous laxity and erosion of bones which accompany this pathology. In contrast, the bone and ligaments in AS are rigid and unyielding with neurological sequalae being consequently more common. In such patients cervical fusion may be necessary in order to retain neurological integrity and control symptoms such as referred occipital pain (Fig. 20.4).

The 'last joint' syndrome, in which bridging ossification of syndesmophytes has taken place at every level except one, presents a cruel dilemma. On the one hand, exercise continues to be important in maintaining posture, even where extensive fusion has taken place. On the other, the sole mobile segment is exposed to considerable stresses during exercise with pain, which may be severe, and sometimes the development of discitis. Treatment is initially by rest, sometimes by the use of a corset or brace [28]. Surgical fusion is required where the pain is unrelieved by conservative means, or where discitis is so severe that healing under external immobilization fails to occur.

Spinal surgery may also be indicated when the posture of a fixed spondylitic spine is so extreme that forward vision can only be achieved with prismatic spectacles. A wedge osteotomy produces a less stooped posture with a consequent ability to see ahead. This surgery is accompanied by a risk of neurological damage which must be balanced against the potential improvement in lifestyle produced by postural correction and enhanced forward vision. In this and all surgery to AS patients, the period of postoperative immobilization should be kept to a minimum and the physiotherapist should ensure that the patient maintains the fullest possible range of movements compatible with any necessary postoperative fixation.

The root joints, particularly the hips, are frequently involved in AS, and total hip replacement is indicated where severe pain or severe limitation of movement occur. Loss of range at the hips may reveal a greater than expected degree of disability caused by spinal fusion, forward flexion especially being entirely dependent on hip movement in some patients.

Two anxieties have been expressed regarding hip replacement in patients with AS. As many are young and active, it has been suggested that mechanical failure produced by high use might be a major problem. There is also anxiety that AS patients might be particularly prone to extra-articular ossification causing loss of movement in the replaced joint. Long-term follow-up suggests that these are not common problems, with a high degree of short-term and long-term value accruing from the operation [29]. It should be noted too that patients followed long-term in these studies had replacement with conventional cemented hips rather than the cementless ones which are now selected for younger, more active patients.

CONCLUSION

Epidemiological studies of AS have suggested that the disease is becoming milder and its age of onset later [30]. In contrast, our experience in a generalist rheumatology department suggests that an increasing number of people have severe, aggressive disease which is failing to respond to the simple NSAID plus exercise programs which have appeared to be so successful in the past. The team approach to treatment, often utilizing the physiotherapist as the focal point for the patient, remains a valid way of delivering care. However, there is a need to develop better prognostic markers early in the course of the disease so that intensive drug therapy can be started early in those patients for whom it is appropriate. Development of strategies based on this need, while maintaining the primacy of physical treatment and patient education, will be a priority for the development of AS treatment.

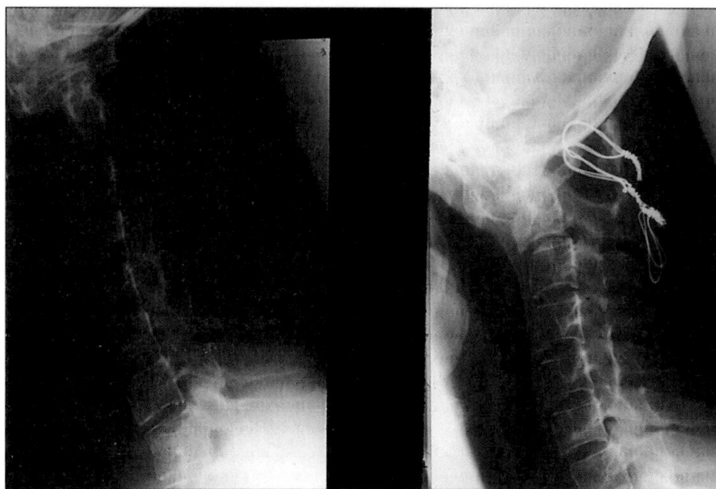

Fig 20.4 Pre- and postcervical fusion. The atlanto-axial subluxation seen preoperatively was accompanied by severe pain and numbness over the occiput. The symptoms were completely relieved by cervical fusion.

REFERENCES

1. Pal B. Use of simple analgesics in the treatment of ankylosing spondylitis. Br J Rheumatol. 1987;**26**: 207–9.
2. O'Brien BJ, Elswood J, Calin A. Perception of prescription drug risks: A survey of patients with ankylosing spondylitis. J Rheumatol. 1990;**17**:503–7.
3. Boersma JW. Retardation of ossification of the lumbar vertebral column in ankylosing spondylitis by means of phenylbutazone. Scand J Rheumatol. 1976;**5:**60–4.
4. Calin A, Elswood J. A prospective nationwide crosssectional study of NSAID usage in 1331 patients with ankylosing spondylitis. J Rheumatol. 1990;**17**:801–3.
5. Lehtinen R. Clinical and radiological features of ankylosing spondylitis in the 1950s and 1976 in the same hospital. Scand J Rheumatol. 1979;**8**:57–61.
6. Cox NL, Doherty SM. Non-steroidal antiinflammatories: out-patient audit of patient preferences and side-effects in different diseases. In: Rainsford KD, Velo GP, eds. Side effects of anti-inflammatory drugs. Part I: Clinical and epidemiological aspects. Lancaster: MTP Press; 1987:137–50.
7. Capell HA, Rennie JAN, Rooney PJ, et al. Patient compliance: A novel method of testing non-steroidal anti-inflammatory analgesics in rheumatoid arthritis. J Rheumatol. 1979;**6**:584–93.
8. Luggen ME, Gartside PS, Hess EV. Nonsteroidal antiinflammatory drugs in rheumatoid arthritis: duration of use as a measure of relative Value. J Rheumatol. 1989;**16**:1565–9.
9. Rooney PJ, Bjarnason I. NSAID gastropathy - not just a pain in the gut! J Rheumatol. 1991;**18**:796–8.
10. Morris AJ, Madhok R, Sturrock RD, Capell HA, MacKenzie JF. Enteroscopic diagnosis of small bowel ulceration in patients receiving non-steroidal antiinflammatory drugs. Lancet. 1991;**337**:520.
11. Moll JMH, Haslock I, Macrae IF, Wright V. Associations between ankylosing spondylitis, psoriatic arthritis, Reiter's disease, the intestinal arthropathies and Behcet's syndrome. Medicine (Baltimore). 1974;**53**:343–64.
12. Mielants H, Veys EM, DeVos M, Cuvelier C. Gut inflammation in the pathogenesis of idiopathic forms of reactive arthritis and in the peripheral joint involvement of ankylosing spondylitis. In: Spondyloarthropathies: involvement of the gut. Mielants H, Veys EM, eds. Amsterdam: Excerpta Medica; 1989:11–12.
13. Ferraz MB, Tugwell P, Goldsmith CH, Atra E. Meta-analysis of sulfasalazine in ankylosing spondylitis. J Rheumatol. 1990;**17**:1482–6.
14. McConkey B. Sulphasalazine and ankylosing spondylitis. Br J Rheumatol. 1990;**29**:2–5.
15. Sadowska-Wroblewska M, Garwolinska H, Maczynska-Rusiniak B. A trial of cyclophosphamide in ankylosing spondylitis with involvement of peripheral joints and high disease activity. Scand J Rheumatol. 1986;**15**:259–64.
16. Wordsworth BP, Pearcy MJ, Mowat AG. In-patient regime for the treatment of ankylosing spondylitis: an appraisal of improvement in spinal mobility and the effects of corticotrophin. Br J Rheumatol. 1984;**23**:39–43.
17. Somerville RW, Hawkey CJ. Non-steroidal antiinflammatory drugs and the gastrointestinal tract. Postgrad Med J. 1986;**62**:23–28.
18. Wynn Parry CB. Physical measures of rehabilitation. In: Ankylosing spondylitis. Moll J M H, ed. Edinburgh: Churchill Livingstone; 1980:214–26.
19. Kraag G, Stokes B, Groh J, Helewa A, Goldsmith C. The effects of comprehensive home physiotherapy and supervision on patients with ankylosing spondylitis - a randomised controlled trial. J Rheumatol. 1990;**17**:228–33.
20. Ormos G, Domjan L, Balint G. A controlled trial for assessing the effect of manual therapy on cervical spine mobility. Hung Rheumatol. 1987:(suppl.)77–80.
21. Gemignani G, Olivieri I, Rujo G, Pasero G. Transcutaneous electrical nerve stimulation in ankylosing spondylitis: a double-blind study. Arthritis Rheum. 1991;**4**:788–9.
22. Fisher LR, Cawley MID, Holgate ST. Relation between chest expansion, pulmonary function, and exercise tolerance in patients with ankylosing spondylitis. Ann Rheum Dis. 1990;**49**:921–5.
23. Bulstrode SJ, Barefoot J, Harrison RA, Clarke A K. The role of passive stretching in the treatment of ankylosing spondylitis. Br J Rheumatol, 1987:**26**;40–2.
24. Rassmussen J0, Hansen TM. Physical training for patients with ankylosing spondylitis. Arthritis Care Res. 1989;**2**:25–7.
25. Roberts WN, Larson MG, Liang MH, Harrison RA, Barefoot J, Clarke AK. Sensitivity of anthropometric techniques for clinical trials in ankylosing spondylitis. Br J Rheumatol. 1989;**28**:40–5.
26. Buckelew SP, Parker JC. Coping with arthritis pain. Arthritis Care Res. 1989;**2:**136–45.
27. Wordsworth BP, Mowat AG. A review of 100 patients with ankylosing spondylitis with particular reference to socio-economic effects. Br J Rheumatol, 1986;**25**:175–80.
28. Dunn N, Preston B, Lloyd Jones K. Unexplained acute backache in longstanding ankylosing spondylitis. Br Med J, 1985;**291**:1632–4.
29. Calin A, Elswood J. The outcome of 138 total hip replacements and 12 revisions in ankylosing spondylitis: high success rate after a mean follow-up of 7.5 years. J Rheumatol. 1989;**16**:955–8.
30. Will RK, Amor B, Calin A. The changing epidemiology of rheumatic diseases: should ankylosing spondylitis now be included? Br J Rheumatol. 1990;**29**:299–300.

ANKYLOSING SPONDYLITIS

21

PRACTICAL PROBLEMS

LOW BACK PAIN IN A YOUNG ADULT: IS IT INFLAMMATORY?

Kuntal Chakravarty

Definition of the Problem

Back pain is one of the commonest causes of primary care medical consultations (see Chapter 6). Most episodes are mechanical in origin and self-limiting. Detection of inflammatory causes, such as ankylosing spondylitis (AS) is often delayed.

The Typical Case

ER, a 22-year-old secretary, presented with a 5-month history of recurrent low back pain and stiffness. She had lately become tired, listless and depressed. She gave a history of a road traffic accident 5 years ago, when she was hit from the back by a speeding vehicle. She had been admitted to hospital, then treated by bed rest and traction for 3 months. Various investigations including CT scan of the lumbosacral spine were normal. Her pain increased in severity and she had recently taken long periods of time off work.

Further enquiry revealed that she had an attack of iritis in her right eye about 9 months ago, associated with recurrent low back pain and stiffness. The latter had become the major symptom and it was often severe after resting or periods of inactivity. Sometimes she noticed severe stiffness in her back very early in the morning. Clinical examination revealed severe restriction of forward and lateral flexions of her lumbosacral spine and localized tenderness over the sacroiliac joints. Investigations revealed a normochromic and normocytic anemia (hemoglobin 10.2g/dl) and elevated erythrocyte sedimentation rate (ESR) of 40mm in the first hour.

The biochemical, serologic and microbiologic tests were normal. A radiograph showed early sclerosis of the sacroiliac joints, although the possibility of osteitis condensansilii was also raised.

She was HLA B27-positive and further CT scan of her sacroiliac joints confirmed the presence of erosions, suggesting sacroiliitis.

She was treated with indomethacin and regular physiotherapy, which produced a significant clinical improvement. She has remained well, with occasional pain, and she has been able to resume her work.

Diagnostic Problems

Low back pain due to inflammatory causes such as AS is often misdiagnosed early in the disease, particularly in women. Moreover, certain features of the disease in women make definition of AS difficult. The previously held view of its rarity in women is no longer valid and it is now recognized that it is not uncommen in women. The association of low back pain and stiffness after rest or period of inactivity should alert the physician to an inflammatory cause. When these symptoms are associated with extra-articular features, such as uveitis, then the diagnosis of AS should be considered.

A detailed history and clinical examination is mandatory, not only to document the site of pain and limitation of spinal mobility, but also to look for any other extraspinal medical cause (Fig. 21.1).

The presence of radiologic sacroiliitis (Fig. 21.2) in a typical patient is sufficient for the diagnosis of AS, although tissue typing may be of particular help in early diagnosis when patients present atypically. A negative test for HLA B27 is 95% reliable in suggesting that AS is not present in the absence of sacroiliitis. Tissue typing is not indicated in an established disease. However, it is also important to consider other causes of similar presentation, such as psoriatic spondylitis and enteropathic and reactive arthritis, in which sacroiliitis may also be found.

MEDICAL CAUSES OF LOW BACK PAIN IN YOUNG ADULTS
Mechanical
Ligamentous Muscle sprain and prolapsed intervertebral disc Spondylosis and spondylolisthesis Spinal stenosis
Infectious
Pyogenic osteomyelitis Tubercular osteomyelitis
Inflammatory
Ankylosing spondylitis Reiter's syndrome Reactive arthritis Enteropathic arthritis
Neoplastic
Osteoid osteoma Extradural tumors
Visceral
Referred pain from kidney, duodenal ulcer or ovary

Fig. 21.1 Medical causes of low back pain in young adults.

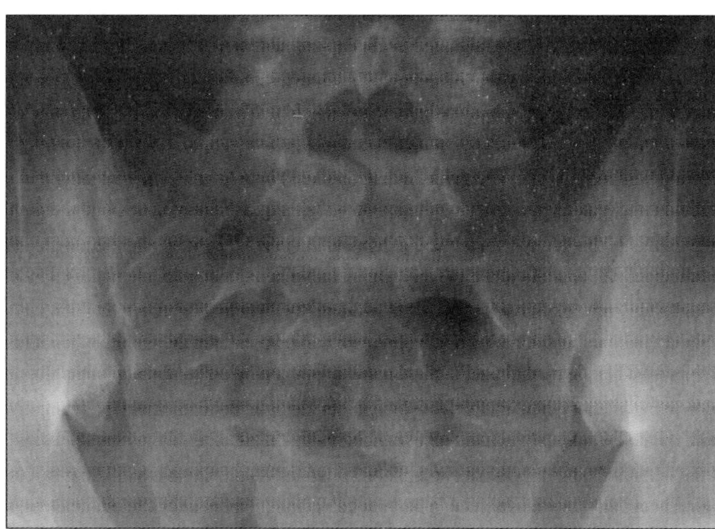

Fig. 21.2 The sacroiliac joints are somewhat widened and irregular, with ill-defined subchondral sclerosis on the iliac aspects.

In rare circumstances, as in the case cited, a radiologic suggestion of osteitis condensans-ilii can confuse the diagnosis; CT scanning is believed to be more helpful in the diagnosis of early changes in the sacroiliac joint than is bone scintigraphy.

In women, AS usually runs a benign mild course but a delay in diagnosis of up to 10 years has been reported.

REFERENCES

Back pain. London: Office of Health Economics; 1985.

Calin A. Ankylosing spondylitis. In: Kelly WN, Harris ED Jr, Ruddy S, Sledge CB. Textbook of rheumatology. 3E. Philadelphia: WB Saunders; 1989:1021–34.

Frymoyer JW. Back pain and sciatica. N Engl J Med. 1988;**318**: 291–300.

SPONDYLODISCITIS AND SPINAL FRACTURES IN ANKYLOSING SPONDYLITIS

Anthony Russell

Definition of the Problem

In AS, both spondylodiscitis and spinal fracture cause a relatively sudden onset of pain in a previously burned-out, rigid spine. It may be difficult clinically to distinguish between these conditions; indeed, it is likely that in a proportion of patients the two may be causally associated.

The Typical Case

A 50-year-old man with a 25-year history of AS presented with 6 weeks of increasing pain at the dorsolumbar junction. The pain was aggravated by standing, coughing and turning in bed and was poorly responsive to NSAIDs. Prior to this he had been only occasionally taking NSAIDs. The dorsolumbar spine had been virtually immobile (1cm flexion using Schober's method, and chest expansion of 0.5cm) and his occiput wall distance, which had been 4cm, was now 9cm, but spinal extension was markedly limited by pain and could not be fully assessed on this occasion. A radiograph showed classic changes of spondylitis with spinal fusion but no crush fractures nor other abnormalities. A bone scan, however, showed a focal area of increased uptake at T11. Single photon emission CT (SPECT) was not then available and no specific localization of the abnormal uptake within the vertebra could be made, i.e. anteriorly to suggest a discitis, or, if more posteriorly, a fracture. Tomograms were normal and it was assumed that no fracture was present. The patient was put in a brace. This helped, but over the next 4 months his pain persisted and further flexion deformity developed. Radiographs at that time showed a clear-cut discitis and he was subjected to an extension osteotomy with a resection at L3/L4 under local anesthetic. After recovery his position had improved, with an occiput wall distance of less than 1cm.

Diagnostic Problems and Therapeutic Options

The spine of AS patients, if rigid, is also osteoporotic and thus may fracture with even modest trauma. The most common site is at the C5/C6 interspace, and if there is instability paraplegia may result. C6/C7 and C7/T1 fractures are very difficult to see on normal views because of the overlap of other structures. The spectrum of injury ranges from a minor 'crack' to gross displacement, but what may seem at one moment to be a crack may be subject to major displacement. Undisplaced fractures heal well with external protection. Unstable cervical fractures must be reduced with halo traction, a hyperextension injury will usually fuse without external fixation, but a flexion injury may need a more radical correction and surgical stabilization. Fractures in the lower dorsal and dorsolumbar spine are uncommon and, as indicated above, it may be that, when undisplaced, these lead to a discitis. Crush fractures have been noted as a result of the osteoporosis but these can generally be managed in a conservative manner.

Spondylodiscitis, i.e. discitis seen in patients with ankylosing spondylitis, is radiologically similar to the rare spontaneous discitis (Fig. 21.3). The disc space is initially widened with erosion and breaking down of the vertebral endplates. The surrounding bone on both sides of the disc becomes sclerotic and this may happen very gradually. Generally, these lesions present with an increase in pain, most frequently located in the lower dorsal spine as in the case described, who had previously had relatively late asymptomatic disease with associated fusion of that region. They may, however, be entirely asymptomatic. If the discitis is in the dorsal spine and marked, an increasing kyphosis may be noted. Whether the discitis represents an inflammatory process directly related to the AS or is a reflection of trauma to a fused osteoporotic spine leading to a fracture and mild instability, is controversial. It is clear that a posterior fracture is often seen, but this could occur secondarily to the anterior erosions. These would lead to an increased kyphosis and thus to posterior fracture. Neurologic complications rarely ensue. The onset of symptoms is often sudden, more consistent with a fracture, and yet histologically there is usually granulation tissue at the bone ends. This is despite the fact that the AS has frequently been inactive at that site, bony ankylosis having developed some years earlier.

Some patients are asymptomatic. Earlier studies have suggested a discitis prevalence of 5% of AS patients, but there is reason to believe that it is now much less frequent, perhaps because of a more intense, aggressive approach to early disease management. Diagnosis is based on the characteristic radiologic features. A bone scan is especially helpful in confirming a focal cause for the increased pain prior to changes on conventional films but, unless SPECT scans are used, it cannot help distinguish between a fracture or discitis and, of course, as indicated above, some argue that the fracture may lead to discitis.

Conclusions

If there is a fracture and it is unstable, urgent immobilization and surgical fusion is required. If the lesion, fracture or discitis is stable, and

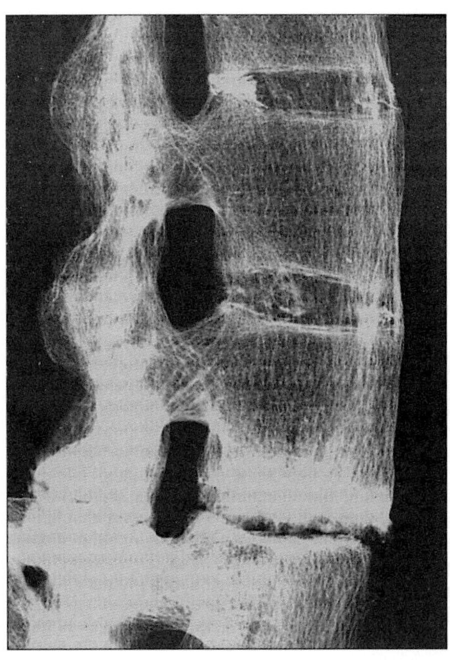

Fig. 21.3 Discitis in ankylosing spondylitis. The radiograph (taken postmortem) also shows pseudoarthrosis at a fracture site and vertebral fusion.

especially if it is in the dorsolumbar region, bracing may suffice. If there is a significant pre-existing kyphosis, surgery is likely to be required, either local fixation and grafting or, more particularly for kyphosis, a resection osteotomy below the level of the cord, making it a relatively safe procedure. This will alter the mechanical stress aggravating the discitis and tendency to kyphosis. The presence of a discitis lesion in the absence of symptoms does not warrant intervention.

REFERENCES

Cawley MID, Chalmers TM, Kellgren JH, Ball J. Destructive lesions of vertebral bodies in ankylosing spondylitis. Ann Rheum Dis. 1972;**31**:345–58.

Little H, Urowitz MB, Smythe HA. Asymptomatic spondylodiscitis: An unusual feature of ankylosing spondylitis. Arthritis Rheum. 1974;**17**:487–93.

Ralston SH, Urquhart GDK, Brzeski M, Sturrock RD. Prevalence of vertebral compression fractures due to osteoporosis in ankylosing spondylitis. Br Med J. 1990;**300**:563–5.

Simmons EH. Surgery of the spine in ankylosing spondylitis and rheumatoid arthritis. In: Chapman MW, ed. Operative orthopedics, Vol 3. New York: JB Lippincott; 1988:2077–114.

Will R, Palmer R, Bhalla AK, et al Osteoporosis in early ankylosing spondylitis: a primary pathological event. Lancet. 1989;**2**:1483–5(note).

CAUDA EQUINA SYNDROME IN ANKYLOSING SPONDYLITIS

Anthony S Russell

Definition of the Problem

Cauda equina lesions are a rare complication of late AS. The onset is usually insidious and early diagnosis requires a high index of clinical suspicion. Management can be a formidable problem.

The Typical Case

A 67-year-old man with a 40-year history of ankylosing spondylitis, a fused spine and a mildly kyphotic posture (occiput to wall distance 3cm) developed progressive pain in the right buttock, with a sciatic radiation, over a 6-year period. More recently he had also been complaining of pain in the left leg, and had developed some urinary incontinence with loss of bladder sensation. On examination, in addition to his ankylosing spondylitis he was found to have some abnormal neurologic signs. There was diminished sensation bilaterally from L4 to S2, some weakness of the right ankle plantar and dorsiflexion and bilateral loss of ankle jerks. Plantar responses were flexor. The anal reflex was absent.

The plain radiographs showed a fused lumbar spine with no vertebral damage. A lumbar myelogram was carried out through the suboccipital approach, and showed saccular diverticulae characteristic of the cauda equina syndrome (Fig. 21.4).

The Diagnostic Problem

Although rare and only first described in 196l, there have now been a large number of case reports of the cauda equina syndrome in late AS. The onset is generally very slow and insidious, and the condition usually takes many years to progress to an advanced state. The late, complete syndrome is very characteristic, and relatively easy to diagnose as long as one is aware of it. Neurologic signs and symptoms are fairly symmetric, all patients developing sensory loss in the L5 and sacral dermatomes. Lower motor neuron type sphincter disturbances are often present, and many patients experience pain in the rectum and lower limbs. The condition is confined to patients with a long history and relatively severe AS, but it is not related to previous radiotherapy. The pathology includes the development of arachnoiditis with an enlarged caudal sac and multiple diverticulae that may erode bone as well as causing the neurologic problems.

Early diagnosis is difficult. Any patient with AS who develops atypical lower limb pain or any neurologic signs should be fully investigated with this syndrome in mind. The differential diagnosis may include sciatica, a spinal fracture complicated by a hematoma, or an unrelated neurologic disorder. Disc prolapse is very rare in late AS.

Myelography may be very difficult to perform, because of the spinal fusion, and may not show the lesions early on. Alternative imaging techniques include CT scans (see Fig. 21.5) and MRI (see Fig. 21.6). In the case described, the late features were typical, leading to a confident diagnosis on clinical grounds; the investigation merely confirmed this suspicion, as well as ruling out any other neurologic disorder. Access to MRI should now obviate the need for myelography, which, in addition to being a difficult procedure, has been reported to make the condition worse.

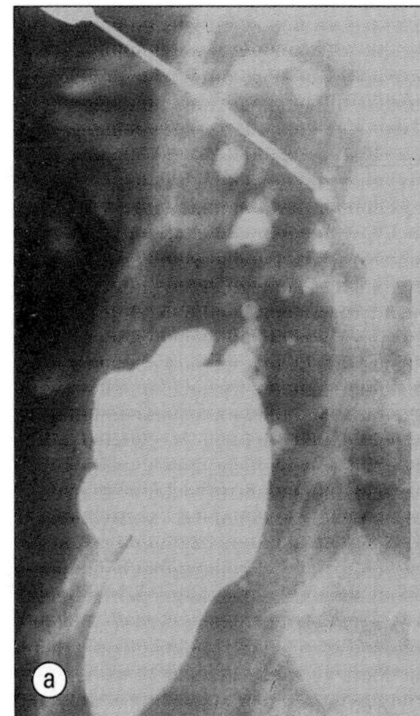

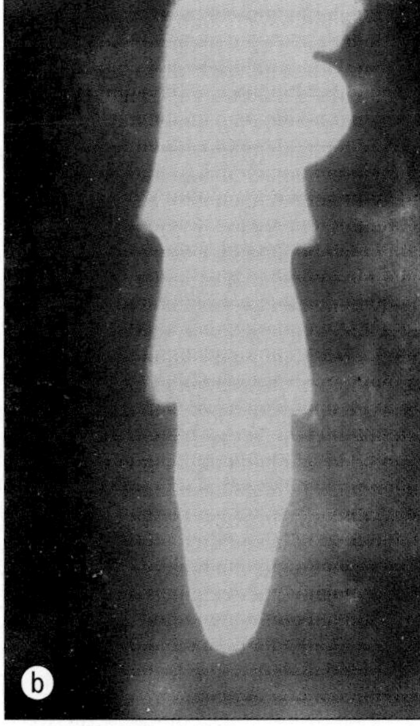

Fig. 21.4 Myelograms of the cauda equina syndrome in ankylosing spondylitis: voluminous lumbar sac (a) and posterior diverticulae (b). Courtesy of Duncan Gordon, Toronto Western Hospital.

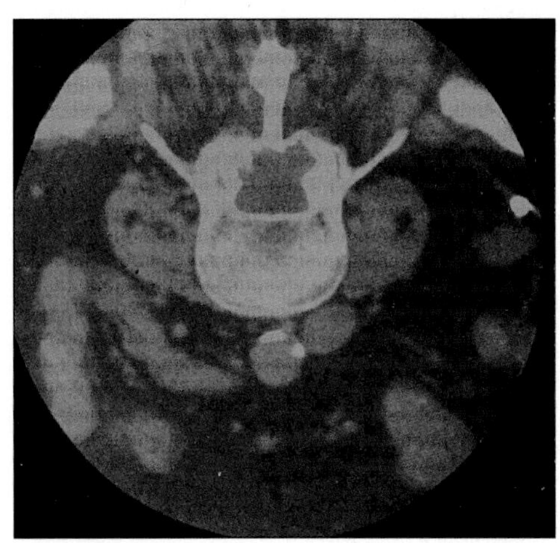

Fig. 21.5 CT scan in a patient with ankylosing spondylitis and the cauda equina syndrome, showing posterior diverticulae. Courtesy of Drs W Ginsberg and JD Barteson, Mayo Clinic.

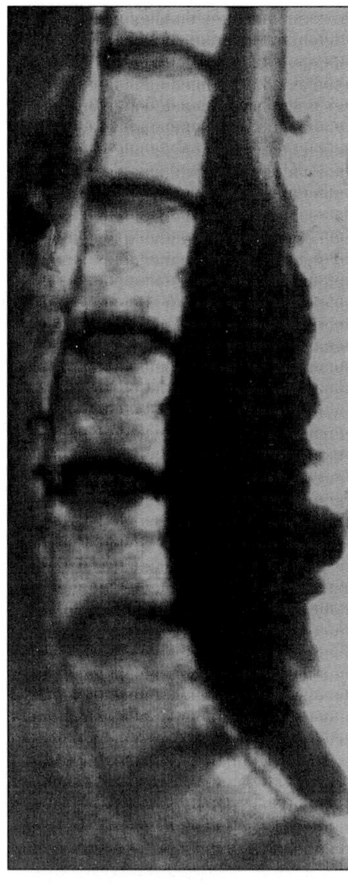

Fig. 21.6 MRI scan in a patient with ankylosing spondylitis and the cauda equina syndrome, showing posterior bulging of the arachnoid sac. Courtesy of Drs W Ginsberg and JD Barteson, Mayo Clinic.

The Management Problem

In this syndrome, diagnosis is the main management. It is obviously crucial to exclude any other, treatable cause of neurologic problems in AS patients. The cauda equina syndrome is not treatable, and it is important not to attempt surgery. Of the small number of cases reported, some have become much worse with spinal surgery, and one has died as a result of the procedure. Progression is very slow if there is no intervention, and the only thing that can be offered is supportive treatment, including standard methods of managing chronic incontinence.

Conclusions

- Cauda equina syndrome is a rare but characteristic complication of AS.
- Early diagnosis requires a high index of suspicion. Patients with atypical lower limb symptoms or any neurologic signs should be fully investigated to make the diagnosis and to rule out other, treatable causes.
- Myelography is difficult and may cause further damage. The investigations of choice are CT or, preferably, spinal MRI.
- There is no specific treatment, and attempts to treat the patients surgically must be resisted.

REFERENCES

Bowie J. Cauda equina lesions associated with ankylosing spondylitis. Br Med J. 1961;**2**:24–7.

Hunter T. The spinal complications of ankylosing spondylitis. Semin Arthritis Rheum. 1989;**19**:172–82.

Russell ML, Gordon DA, Ogryzlo MA, McPhedron RS. The cauda equina syndrome of ankylosing spondylitis. Ann Intern Med. 1973;**78**:551–4

Sparling MJ, Bartleson JD, McLeod PA, Cohen MD, Ginsberg WW. Magnetic resonance imaging of the arachnoid diverticulae associated with cauda equina syndrome in ankylosing spondylitis J Rheumatol. 1989;**16**:1335–7.

PULMONARY FIBROSIS IN ANKYLOSING SPONDYLITIS

Anthony S Russell

Definition of the Problem

Pulmonary problems in AS used to be frequent in patients with severe deforming disease. They are now less so. However, apical lung fibrosis remains as a specific rare complication of the disease, that may be difficult to differentiate from tuberculosis (TB), and can cause extensive problems of management.

The Typical Case

A 40-year-old White male with moderately severe AS and peripheral arthritis of 22 years' duration was receiving nonsteroidal anti-inflammatory drugs (NSAIDs) and sulfasalazine to control his joint disease. He developed a mild cough and lost 10kg in weight over a period of only 2 months. A chest radiograph initially showed right apical shadowing (Fig. 21.7), and a diagnosis of spondylotic lung disease was considered. Sputum cultures were taken for fungal and other organisms, and grew *Mycobacterium tuberculosis*. He was therefore treated with multiple drug therapy for TB for 1 year and made a complete recovery.

The Diagnostic Problem

Ankylosing spondylitis, when associated with severe kyphoscoliosis, can result in a significant ventilation–perfusion imbalance. However, deformities of that extent are rarely seen today, and symptomatic involvement of the lungs in AS is now uncommon. Patients with long-standing disease have a reduction of total lung capacity as well as vital capacity, but rarely complain of dyspnea or other respiratory problems, and their VO_2 max is usually not below expected normal values. Other lung function tests, such as residual volume and diffusion capacity, are

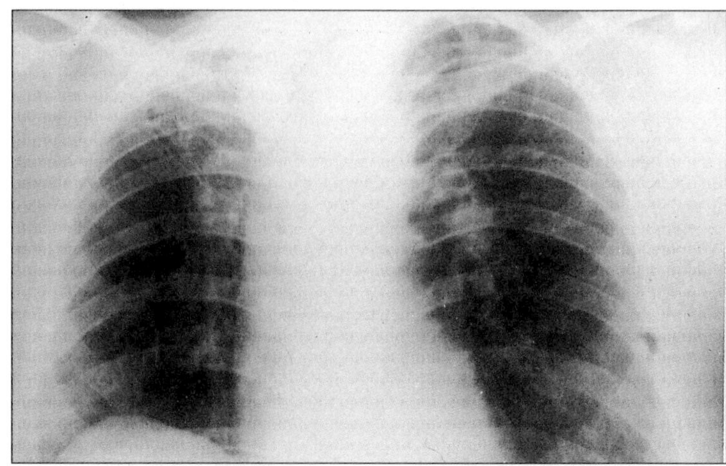

Fig. 21.7 Bilateral shadowing and fibrosis. No cause other than ankylosing spondylitis was found until sputum culture revealed TB.

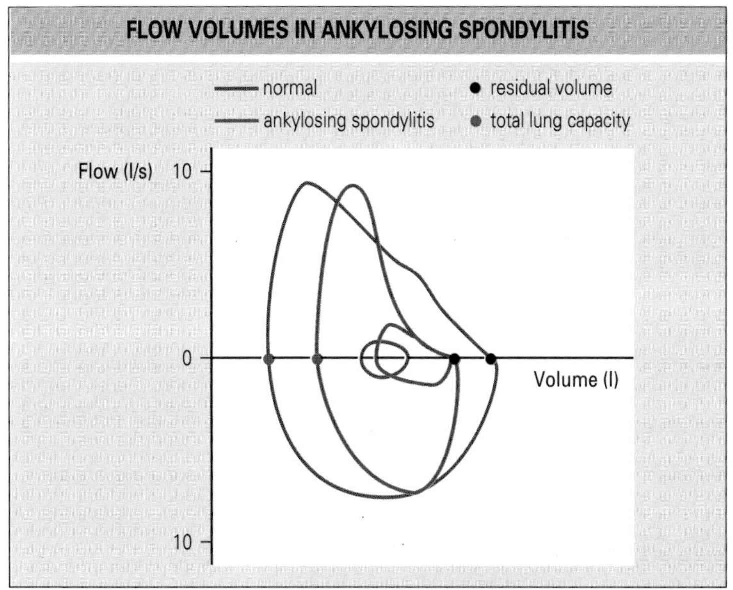

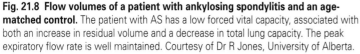

Fig. 21.8 Flow volumes of a patient with ankylosing spondylitis and an age-matched control. The patient with AS has a low forced vital capacity, associated with both an increase in residual volume and a decrease in total lung capacity. The peak expiratory flow rate is well maintained. Courtesy of Dr R Jones, University of Alberta.

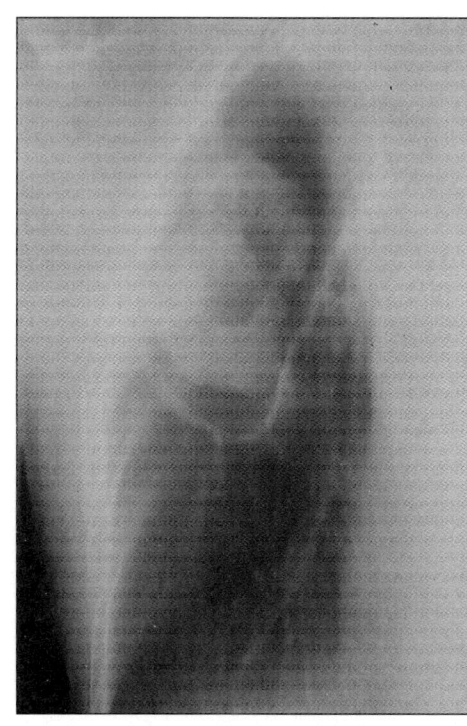

Fig. 21.9 Anteroposterior radiograph of the chest showing a large fungal ball in a cystic lesion within the right upper lobe of an ankylosing spondylitis patient. The position of the aspergilloma moved within the lung when the patient's position was changed.

generally normal as well, suggesting that the reduced lung volumes are directly related to the decreased costovertebral and costotransverse excursion. An increase in diaphragmatic movement is often a visible compensation that gradually develops as the movement of the rib cage becomes reduced. Typical flow loops from a patient with AS, and decreased thoracic excursion, are shown in Figure 21.8.

The one specific form of lung disease described in patients with AS is apical fibrosis. This is rare and must be differentiated from TB and other conditions, as outlined in the case illustration.

Apical fibrosis: is it AS, TB or another lung disorder?

The prevalence of apical fibrosis in AS has been quoted as 1%, but other experience, of only one patient out of over 500 cases, would suggest that it is much less common. It only occurs in patients with severe disease, and may be unilateral or bilateral at onset. The first signs on the radiograph are spotty and linear shadows confined to the apices; these subsequently develop into coarser coalescing shadows, cavities appearing in most cases, and finally a dense area of upper lobe consolidation. Bilateral involvement is usual in the later stages of the condition. It occasionally extends into the midzones of the lung, but has never been reported in the lower lobe. The symptoms that develop include a persistent cough with sputum and gradually increasing effort-related dyspnea.

The differential diagnosis of any case of apical fibrosis must include TB as well as other conditions, such as a pneumoconiosis, and any previous cause of lung damage, including other infections and radiotherapy. In most instances, TB will be the main differential in patients with AS, and in many parts of the world TB will be the more likely diagnosis. In the case illustration the extent of the systemic symptoms (e.g. weight loss), and relatively mild AS suggested that it was unlikely to be AS-related, prompting further investigation. Calcified lung foci or mediastinal nodes might indicate old TB, and in some countries skin testing may be of value, but full bacteriologic investigations should always be carried out to exclude active infection.

AS-Related fibrosis: is there secondary infection?

If TB and other conditions can be ruled out, a diagnosis of AS-related apical fibrosis is made by exclusion. Cavities usually form, and secondary infection is common. The formation of aspergillomas is particularly likely. Increasing general ill health, weight loss, dyspnea and fevers may suggest infection, and hemoptysis commonly occurs with aspergillomas. The hemoptysis is usually mild and recurrent, but extensive bleeding can occur, and the condition can cause massive, fatal hemorrhages. The radiograph will sometimes show the fungus ball (Fig. 21.9), but CT is often required to be sure of its presence or absence. Sputum cultures are often negative and, although all patients will develop IgG antibodies to the aspergillosis antigen, the many different types of the fungus may make it difficult to confirm the diagnosis serologically.

The Therapeutic Problem

There is no known preventative strategy and, once it has developed, there is no known therapy for the apical fibrosis. The main therapeutic dilemmas arise with the management of patients who develop secondary aspergillomas. It may be the wisest to do nothing.

The fungus ball can be removed surgically, but this is a high-risk procedure, usually made unwise by the general condition and lack of respiratory reserve in the AS patients. Intravenous amphotericin has been used, but it does not seem to work. More recently, attempts have been made to treat aspergillomas by local instillation of a cocktail of antifungal agents through an endobronchial tube, or by embolization of a bronchial artery.

Conclusions

- Reduced lung volumes, due to thoracic-wall immobility, are common in patients with advanced AS, but respiratory problems are rare.
- Apical fibrosis is a rare, specific complication of severe AS. It must be differentiated from other causes of apical fibrosis, especially TB.
- Patients with AS-related apical fibrosis commonly develop secondary aspergillomas in the lung cavities. These fungus balls may be diagnosed late, are difficult to treat, and can be fatal.

REFERENCES

Boshuea DK, Sundstrom WR. The pleuropulmonary manifestations of ankylosing spondylitis Semin Arthritis Rheum. 1989;**18**:277–81

Davies D. Ankylosing spondylitis and lung fibrosis. Q J Med.1972;**41**:395–417.

Feletius N, Hedenstrom H, Hillerdal G, Hallgren R. Pulmonary involvement in ankylosing spondylitis. Ann Rheum Dis. 1986;**45**:736–40.

Fisher LR, Cawley MID, Holgate ST. Relation between chest expansion, pulmonary function and exercise tolerance in patients with ankylosing spondylitis. Ann Rheum Dis. 1990;**49**:921–5.

Rosenow EC, Strimlan CV, Muhm JR, Ferguson RH. Pleuropulmonary manifestations of ankylosing spondylitis. Mayo Clin Proc. 1977;**52**:641–9.

UVEITIS IN ANKYLOSING SPONDYLITIS

Anthony S Russell

Definition of the Problem

Acute, unilateral anterior uveitis in the early stages may be ignored by AS patients if they have not been explicitly warned to expect it. Prompt management is critical to an uncomplicated outcome.

The Typical Case

A 25-year-old male with previously diagnosed AS and taking no medication developed some blurring of vision and redness of the left eye. Some over-the-counter drops were instilled and no medical advice sought as it was thought to be a minor problem. Over the next 4 days vision deteriorated and pain increased. He attended an emergency clinic; the eye was reddened, especially around the cornea. The pupil was small and vision poor. The right eye was normal. Ophthalmologic examination confirmed an acute uveitis with synechiae. Dilation of the pupil with atropine was only partially successful. The condition responded well to local steroid treatment. The patient had not been warned of this possible complication when the diagnosis of AS was initially made.

Prevalence

About 25–40% of AS patients may develop one or more attacks of nongranulomatous, acute anterior uveitis (AAU). There is little correlation between the activity of the AS and the development of AAU. It is nevertheless clear that the AAU is related to AS itself and does not occur merely because both are associated with HLA B27. Thus, it is 11 times more prevalent in AS patients than in HLA B27- positive relatives without AS. It is rare for both eyes to be clinically involved during the same attack, and such bilateral involvement, even in an individual with AS, would stimulate a search either for an alternative cause or for an initiating Reiter's syndrome. While synechiae are frequent if the problem is not treated promptly, severe progressive unresponsive disease is rare in comparison with, for example, patients with Behçet's disease; when seen, it is more likely to be found in those patients who have chronic Reiter's syndrome. Of 37 patients recently reported with AAU not due to known causes, e.g. herpes or sarcoidosis, at least 27/33 were HLA B27-positive and 25 had a spondyloarthropathy. Previous studies have shown a high prevalence of HLA B27 spondyloarthropathy in this group.

Like AS itself, the uveitis is seen more frequently in men, but there is some indication that it may be increased during pregnancy: in one study, it was seen in 10/50 pregnant women with AS. Control incidences are difficult to obtain, but one recent study of AS subjects found 4.4% developing it during a 6-month period.

Diagnosis and Therapeutic Options

The patient complains of a painful eye with photophobia, injection, lacrimation and impaired vision (Fig. 21.10). The pupil is initially small and may become irregular if posterior synechiae form. The therapy is directed toward urgent pupillary dilatation with atropine, and local steroids to reduce inflammation. Occasionally, subconjunctival injection of steroid is required. Because of the importance of prompt treatment, it is useful to warn all AS patients at the time of diagnosis of this possible complication and advise them to act promptly. Some individuals have multiple recurrences and can self-medicate successfully at the first sign of any such development. If it is not recognized and dealt with appropriately, synechiae, cataract and secondary glaucoma may ensue.

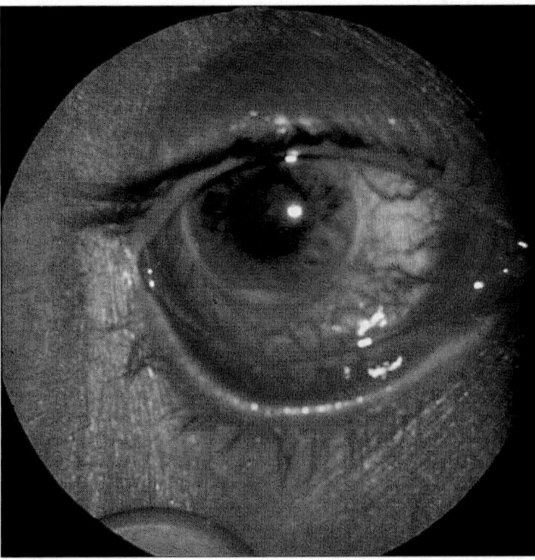

Fig. 21.10 Iritis in a patient with ankylosing spondylitis. In this severe case there is also considerable conjunctival injection and a hypopyon is also present.

REFERENCES

Beckingsale AB, Davies J, Gibson JM, Rosenthal AR. Acute anterior uveitis, ankylosing spondylitis, back pain and HLA-B27. Br J Ophthalmol. 1984;**68**:741–5.

Feltkamp TEW. HLA-B27, acute anterior uveitis, and ankylosing sponylitis. Adv Inflam Res. 1985;**9**:211–16.

Moller P, Vinje O, Kass E. How does Bechterew's syndrome start? Scand J Rheumatol. 1983;**12**:289–98.

Ostensen M, Romberg O, Husby G. Ankylosing spondylitis and motherhood. Arthritis Rheum. 1982;**25**:140–2.

Rosenbaum JT. Characteristics of uveitis associated with spondyloarthritis. J Rheumatol. 1989;**16**:792–6.

Van der Linden S, Rentsch HU, Gerber N, Cats A, Valkenburg HA. The association between ankylosing spondylitis, acute anterior uveitis and HLA B27: The results of a Swiss family study. Br J Rheum. 1988;**27**(suppl 2):39–41.

22

CLINICAL FEATURES OF PSORIATIC ARTHRITIS

Philip S Helliwell & Verna Wright

Definition
- An inflammatory arthritis associated with psoriasis.
- Rheumatoid factor negative.
- Rheumatoid nodules absent.

Clinical features
- Any form of psoriasis or a history compatible with psoriasis.
- Peripheral polyarthritis, frequently symmetrical.
- Typical inflammatory involvement of distal interphalangeal joints.
- Asymmetrical spondylitis and sacroiliitis.
- Uncommon but characteristic mutilating arthritis associated with telescoping of fingers.
- Dactylitis (sausage digits).

CLINICAL FEATURES

Onset of Skin and Joint Lesions

In the majority of cases (75%), psoriasis precedes joint disease but in a few cases (15%) the onset is synchronous and in 10% arthritis precedes psoriasis. It is worth repeating that in cases where there is asymmetrical seronegative oligoarthritis (especially with the presence of dactylitis or DIP joint involvement), previously unrecognized psoriasis may be found in a flexural region, scalp or nails (Fig. 22.1). Alternatively, there may be a history of widespread guttate psoriasis in childhood or a strong family history of psoriasis.

Oligoarthritis

A common presentation is of an oligoarthritis consisting of a large joint, such as a knee, together with one or two interphalangeal joints and a dactylitic digit or toe. On occasion, the arthritis appears to follow an episode of trauma so that initially the condition is misdiagnosed as 'mechanical'. The psoriasis may consist of one or two small patches of chronic stable psoriasis vulgaris with or without nail involvement (Fig. 22.2)

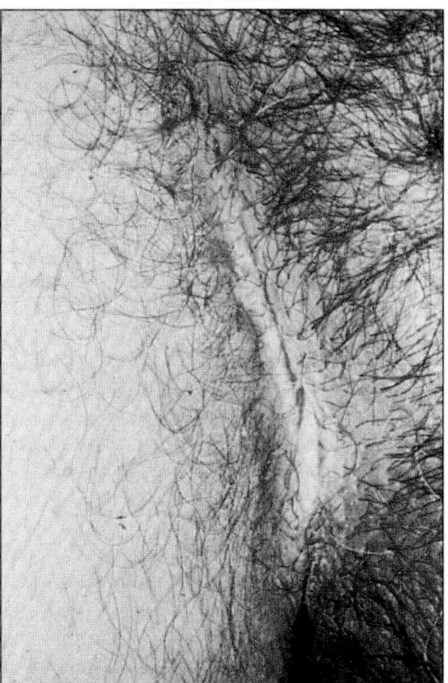

Fig. 22.1 Flexural psoriasis in the natal cleft.

Symmetrical Polyarthritis

Psoriatic arthritis may present with a symmetrical polyarthritis indistinguishable from RA involving small joints of the hands and feet, wrists, ankles, knees and elbows (Fig. 22.3). Indeed, cases of seronegative RA must occur coincidentally with psoriasis but, in the majority of cases, other features suggest that the symmetrical polyarthritis associated with psoriasis is a distinct clinical entity.

Distal Interphalangeal Joint Involvement

Inflammatory swelling of the DIP joint is a characteristic feature of psoriatic arthritis (Fig. 22.4). Involvement of the DIP joint is almost always associated with psoriatic changes in the associated nail (Fig. 22.5). Although DIP involvement may be the only clinical feature of psoriatic arthritis, these joints are more commonly part of a generalized arthropathy.

Spinal Involvement

Asymptomatic sacroiliitis occurs in up to one third of cases with psoriasis. The sacroiliitis is frequently asymmetrical and may be associated with spondylitis, sometimes clinically indistinguishable from AS. Radiologically, however, the spondylitis differs in certain respects from that of classical AS. Cervical spine involvement may occur more frequently where there is severe scalp involvement with psoriasis [1]. Inflammatory synovial tissue in cervical joints can cause atlantoaxial and subaxial subluxations, although, as in AS, the more common outcome is fusion of the cervical spine.

Clinical Subgroups

In order to provide a framework with which the distinctive features of psoriatic arthropathy could be assessed, a classification was provided by Moll and Wright [2]. Five groups were identified which are listed in Figure 22.6. The commonest manifestation, accounting for over 70% of the cases, was asymmetrical oligoarthritis involving scattered DIP, PIP, and metatarsophalangeal (MTP) joints. While this classification has proved robust and of use in studies of outcome, treatment and etiology, the precise frequency of patients in each subgroup has been challenged. Recent surveys suggest that the commonest manifestation is of a symmetrical polyarthritis

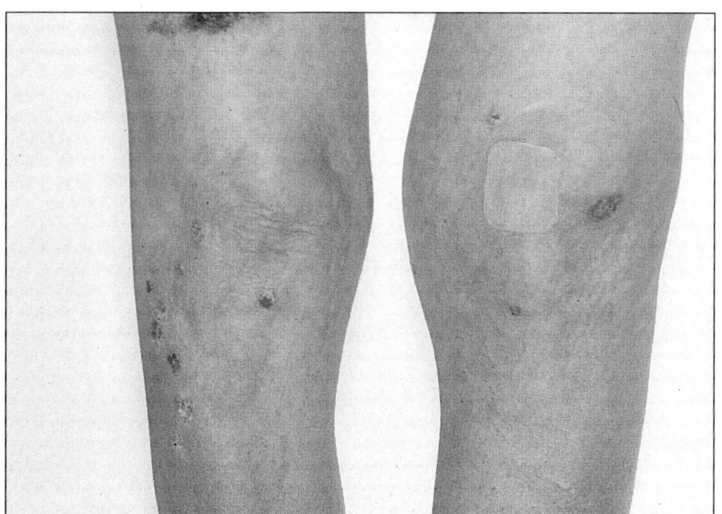

Fig. 22.2 Monoarthropathy associated with psoriasis vulgaris.

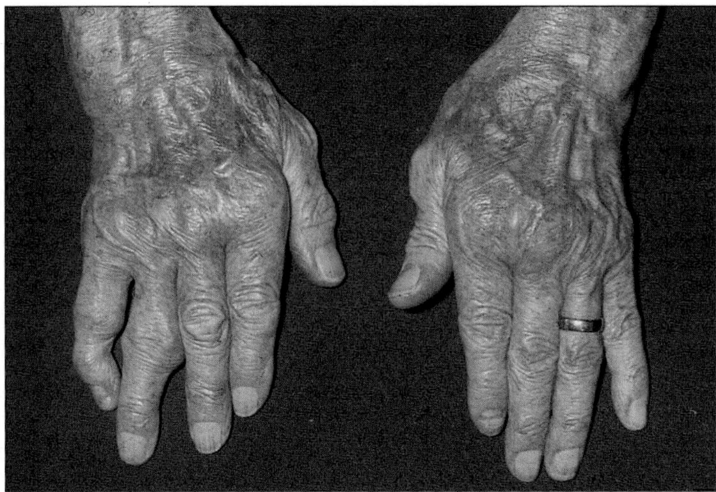

Fig. 22.3 Symmetrical psoriatic polyarthritis resembling rheumatoid arthritis.

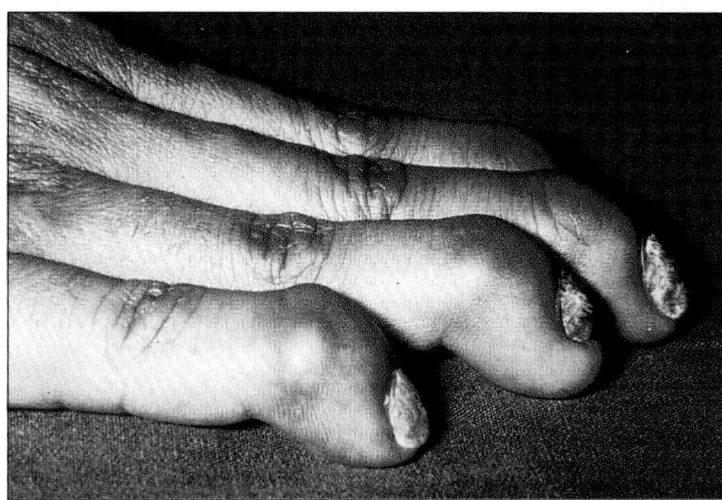

Fig. 22.4 Distal interphalangeal joint involvement.

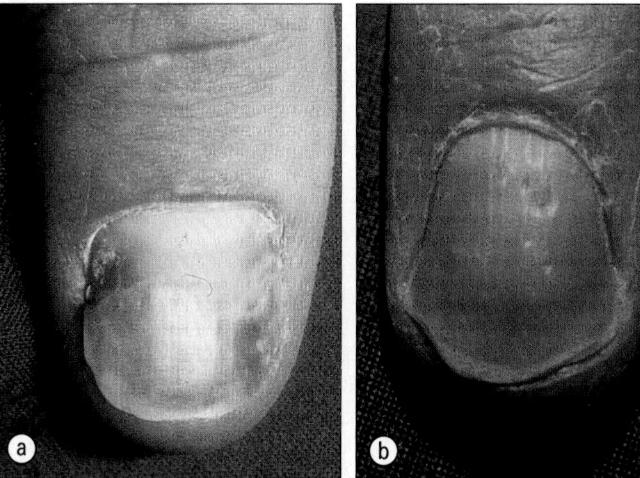

Fig. 22.5 Nail involvement with psoriasis. Note pitting, onycholysis (a) and hyperkeratosis (b).

CLASSIFICATION OF PSORIATIC ARTHRITIS
Classical psoriatic arthritis confined to distal interphalangeal joints of hands and feet
Arthritis mutilans with sacroiliitis
Symmetrical polyarthritis indistinguishable from rheumatoid arthritis but with negative serology
Asymmetrical, pauciarticular, small joint involvement, with 'sausage' digits
Ankylosing spondylitis with or without peripheral arthritis

Fig. 22.6 Clinical subgroups of psoriatic arthritis.

resembling RA [3,4] and a recent survey by Helliwell *et al.* using tighter definitions would support this [5]. Indeed, for the group as a whole the frequency of individual joint involvement, excluding DIP joints, resembles that of RA (Fig. 22.7).

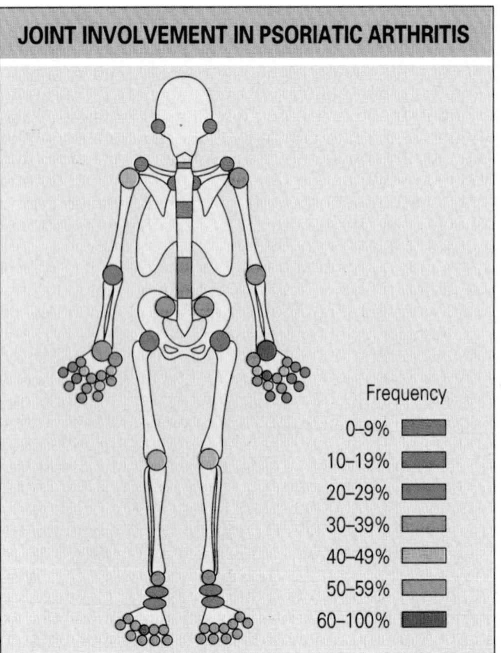

Fig. 22.7 Frequency of joint involvement in psoriatic arthritis.

Arthritis mutilans, while uncommon, provides an almost characteristic picture of this condition (Fig. 22.8). The clinical appearance is of a severely deformed, flail hand with shortening of one or two digits, the resulting redundant folds of skin enabling the examiner to extend the digit to its former length (telescoping) (Fig. 22.9). Similar destructive changes may appear in the feet, thus severely limiting function in the extremities.

Dactylitis or 'sausage digit' is a distinctive feature of psoriatic arthritis (Fig. 22.10). In appearance the whole digit (either toe or finger) is swollen as a result of inflammation in the digital joints and associated tendon sheaths. Dactylitic digits may also be seen in reactive arthritis.

A number of cases of unilateral limb edema associated with psoriasis have been seen and have also been reported by other authors [1]. Although it has been suggested that this may be the 'whole limb' version of dactylitis, in the authors' experience of such cases, individual limb joints are not particularly inflamed and the mechanism may be similar to that observed in limb edema in RA [6].

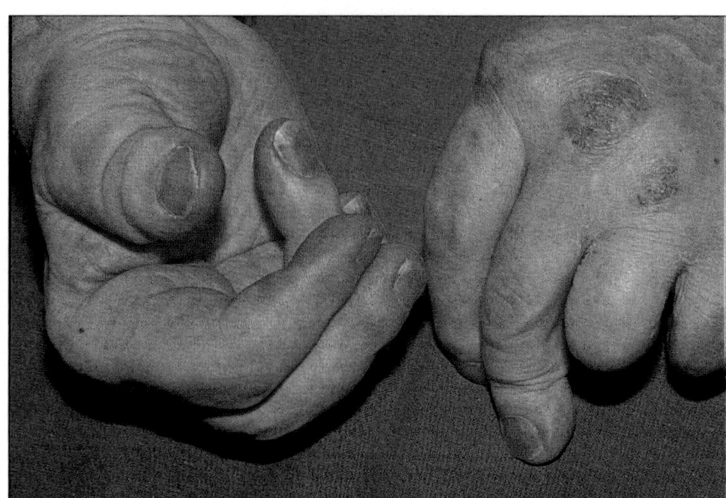

Fig. 22.8 Arthritis mutilans.

Enthesitis

A characteristic feature of the seronegative spondyloarthropathies is inflammation at the attachment of tendon and ligament to bone. In psoriatic arthritis, particularly common sites include the insertion of the Achilles tendon into the calcaneum (Fig. 22.11), plantar fasciitis and at musculotendinous insertions around the pelvis. Spondylitis may be regarded as an example of multiple enthesitic sites.

Ocular Involvement

In a survey of 112 patients with psoriatic arthritis, ocular inflammation was found in almost one third [7]. The commonest problem was conjunctivitis in 20%. However, as expected, iritis was found in a significant number (7%). These figures were confirmed in a more recent survey by Helliwell *et al.* [5].

Relationship Between Type of Psoriasis and Arthritis

There is no association between type of psoriasis and clinical subgroup of psoriatic arthritis. However, involvement of the DIP joints is virtually never found unless there is associated psoriatic involvement of the nails.

Histologically, palmoplantar pustulosis (pustular psoriasis of the palms and soles, PPP) is distinct from classical psoriasis and it has been suggested that the osteoarticular manifestations associated with PPP differ from classical psoriatic arthritis. Earlier reports of an inflammatory condition affecting particularly the anterior chest wall associated with PPP came from Japan [8], although this association has been found in Europe and North America [9]. The syndrome has now been widened to include PPP, acne conglobata, acne fulminans and hidrosadenitis suppurativa. The osteoarticular associations include sternoclavicular hyperostosis, chronic sterile recurrent multifocal osteomyelitis, hyperostosis of the spine and occasionally a peripheral arthritis – grouped with the acronym SAPHO (synovitis, acne, pustulosis, hyperostosis, osteomyelitis) [9]. Anterior chest wall involvement may be identified by isotope bone scan, although a definite diagnosis must be based on conventional X-ray changes [10]. Recent studies have demonstrated

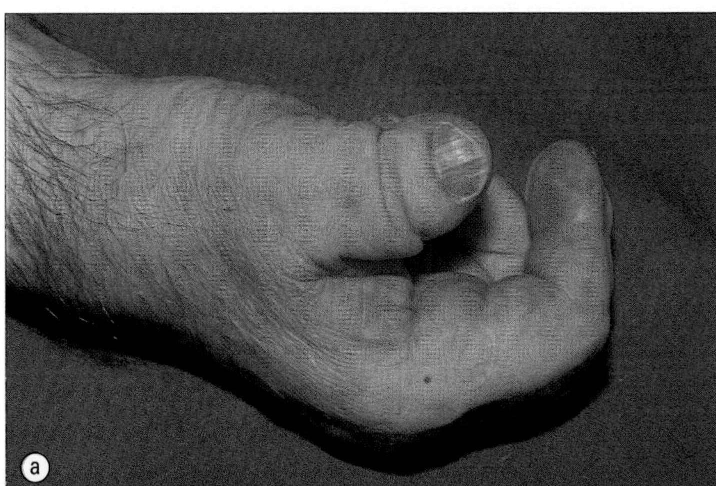
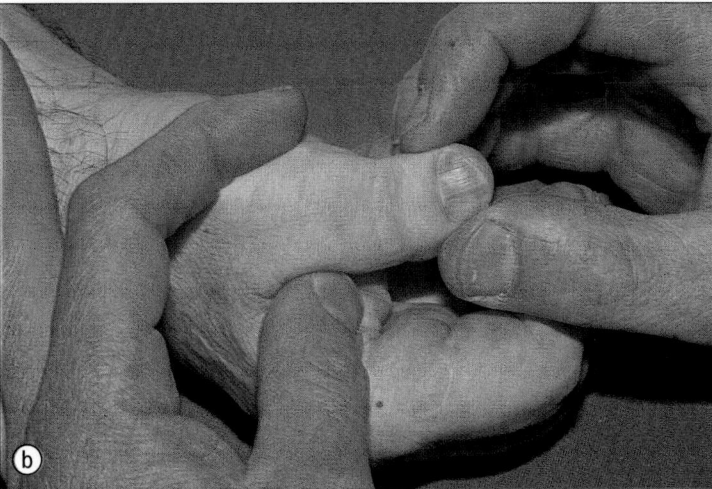

Fig. 22.9 Telescoping in psoriatic arthritis (a,b).

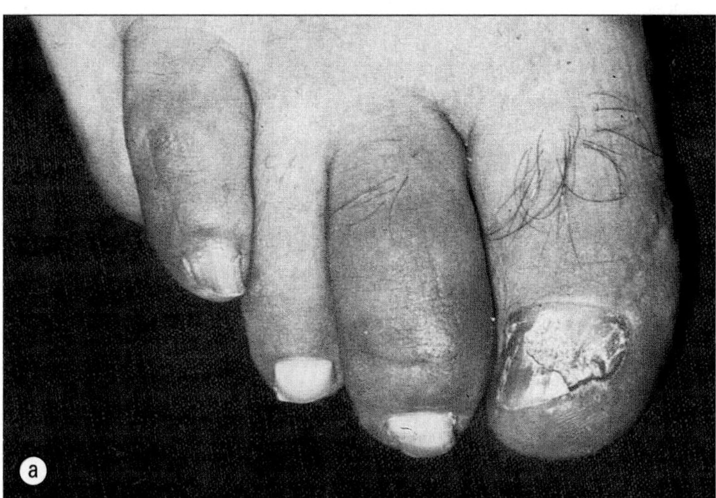
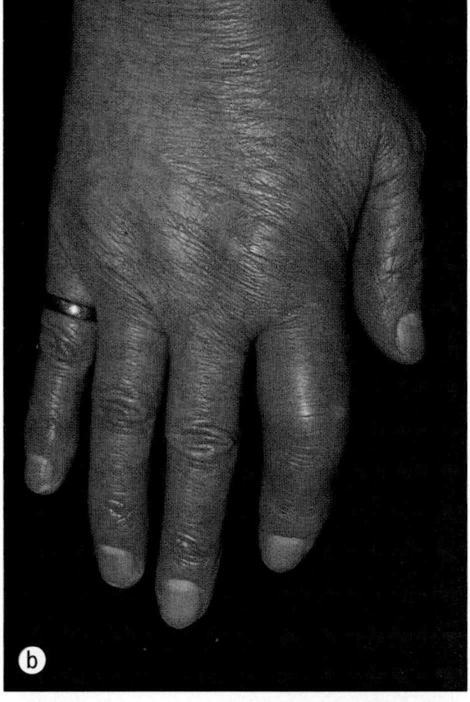

Fig. 22.10 Dactylitis of the toe (a) and finger (b).

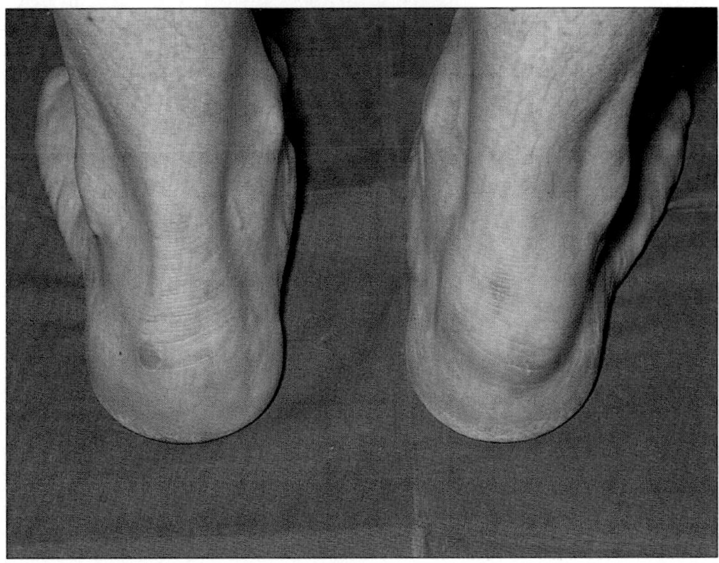

Fig. 22.11 Achilles insertional tendinitis.

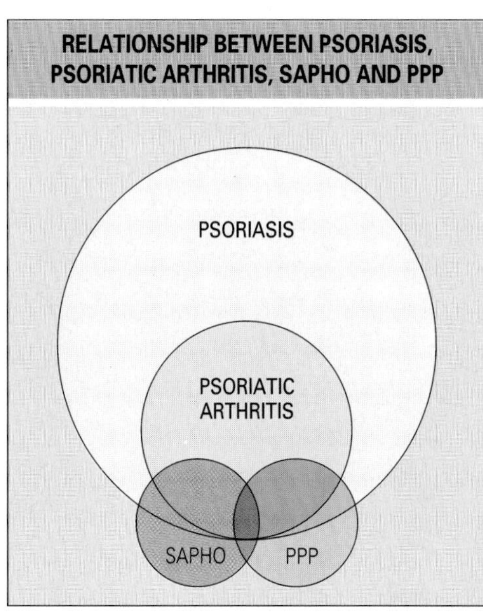

Fig. 22.12 Venn diagram to illustrate the relationship between psoriasis, psoriatic arthritis, SAPHO and PPP.

sternoclavicular and manubriosternal inflammation occurring in association with psoriasis vulgaris [5], thus suggesting SAPHO should be included within the clinical spectrum of psoriatic arthritis (Fig. 22.12).

HIV and Psoriatic Arthritis

An association between AIDS and psoriasis was first reported in 1985 in three cases; two of these patients already had chronic stable localized psoriasis and in one patient the psoriasis developed *de novo* [11]. Of interest was the extensive psoriasis which developed as a result of AIDS, including widespread confluent patches and severe onychodystrophy.

Subsequent reports have confirmed that an explosive and severe form of psoriasis may occur in association with HIV and that often this is a poor prognostic factor. There is, however, some dispute about the increased occurrence of psoriasis in association with HIV infection, reported prevalence rates ranging from 5% [12] to no more than the general population [13]. The only prospective study undertaken by a dermatologist reported no increase in the prevalence of psoriasis, although a severe form of seborrheic dermatitis did occur at a frequency of 12% [14]. It is possible therefore that severe seborrheic dermatitis has been mistaken by nondermatologists for psoriasis. It is clear, however, that existing psoriasis can deteriorate markedly in the presence of HIV and that a rapidly progressive psoriatic arthritis may supervene.

The prevalence of reactive arthritis is probably higher in HIV positive populations and immunogenetic factors such as HLA-B27 are important in susceptibility [15]. Furthermore, sexually acquired HIV infection is associated with a higher prevalence of reactive arthritis compared to the HIV infection acquired from blood products, suggesting co-infection with other arthritogenic agents (such as *Chlamydia* or *Neisseria gonorrhea*). In a prospective study of patients infected with HIV, the cumulative prevalence of reactive arthritis and psoriatic arthritis (over 2 years) was 1.7% in both cases but unclassified oligo- and polyarthritis occurred in a further 11.1% of patients [16]. In some cases reactive arthritis and psoriatic arthritis may be indistinguishable clinically. Although this field is still evolving, it is clear that the association of HIV with these conditions supports the distinctiveness of the arthropathy associated with psoriasis and that $CD4^+$ T-helper (TH) cells are not necessary for the expression of psoriasis or Reiter's syndrome (unlike RA). Many unusual infections occur in AIDS including fungal, bacterial and viral infections: the case for suggesting psoriatic arthritis is a reactive arthritis is therefore strengthened [17].

Juvenile Psoriatic Arthritis

The peak age of onset of psoriasis is between the ages of 5 and 15. However, psoriatic arthritis peaks at a much later age, possibly reflecting a necessary incubation period for this condition. Juvenile psoriatic arthritis, however, does exist and, unlike adult psoriatic arthritis, precedes psoriasis in the majority of cases (arthritis before psoriasis, 52%; psoriasis before arthritis, 41%; simultaneous, 7%). The commonest clinical manifestations in children are an asymmetrical polyarthritis, often involving the digits, pauciarticular arthritis involving mainly the knee, and spondylitis, each occurring with equal frequency [18,19]. Both dactylitis and eye involvement may occur. However, as in other juvenile chronic arthritides, chronic iridocyclitis is associated with a positive antinuclear factor.

Retinoids, Psoriasis and Hyperostosis

With the development of synthetic analogs of vitamin A as treatment for both psoriasis and severe acne has come the intriguing association between retinoid use and musculoskeletal abnormalities [20,21]. Hyperostosis may occur and is similar in site and extent to that seen in psoriatic arthritis, particularly in the spine; this may cause diagnostic confusion. In fact, the skeletal manifestations of retinoid therapy more closely resemble the condition known as diffuse idiopathic skeletal hyperostosis (DISH). Patients with DISH also have a higher blood level of vitamin A according to one report [21]. The mechanism by which retinoids cause hyperostosis is not understood but may be entirely different from the inflammatory reaction (with repair and ossification) seen in psoriatic arthritis.

PROGNOSIS

Intuitively it might be expected that patients with psoriatic arthritis would present with an oligoarthritis which, with the addition of further episodes of inflammation in other joints, would evolve into a symmetrical polyarthritis. There is some evidence to support this notion [3,22]. However, a retrospective series found only a 6% changing pattern after presentation [5]. An earlier study from Leeds in the United Kingdom suggested that psoriatic arthritis followed a mild course when measured in terms of admission to hospital and time off work [23]. Experience from other centers is different. In Toronto one in ten of a series of 220 patients were classified as ARA functional class IV [3]. Further studies from Toronto have shown that in terms of number of affected joints there is an inexorable and gradual progression with time although this may not necessarily be reflected in major changes in functional status [24]. Similar increments in syndesmophyte frequency have been observed in the thoracolumbar spine over an observation period of several years [25]. Functional outcome in juvenile psoriatic arthritis is generally good, although a small proportion of cases progress into adult life and some of these are confined to a wheelchair [18]. Currently, no predictive features for future outcome have been defined, although several prospective studies are underway (see also Chapter 23). Unlike RA, the presence of HLA-DR4 does not appear to predict a more severe course and worse functional outcome [3].

Patients with psoriatic arthritis have a dual disability in terms of employment since certain industries have self-imposed limitations on patients with any form of skin disease. In the study of Roberts *et al.* [23], the employment record was not adversely affected in the majority of patients with psoriatic arthritis. However, a more recent study from Canada found that patients with psoriatic arthritis were twice as likely to be unemployed compared to a group with psoriasis and other joint complaints [26]. This difference is almost certainly due to selection factors since the latter study included patients requiring PUVA treatment and presumably more severe psoriasis.

Unlike RA, psoriatic arthritis is not a multisystem disorder and therefore a large increase in mortality would not be expected. In the Leeds study there were 18 deaths in a total of 168 patients followed for more than 10 years [23]. Two of these were with pulmonary infection, possibly related to immobility as a result of the arthritis. One other death was related to hemorrhage associated with immunosuppressive treatment for psoriasis. Amyloid has been reported in juvenile psoriatic arthritis, occurring in 2 out of 43 cases reviewed retrospectively [18].

INVESTIGATIONS

Immunology

Although in the classical definition of psoriatic arthritis by Wright and Moll absence of rheumatoid factor was mandatory, subsequent authors have suggested that seropositivity does not necessarily exclude the diagnosis [3]. It has been argued that a proportion of the normal population will have rheumatoid factor in the serum (particularly in chronic inflammatory conditions) so that providing classical nodular RA is not present, rheumatoid factor positivity is allowed. Thus, in a series from Toronto, 9% were found to be seropositive [3]. While accepting that some cases of seronegative symmetrical polyarthritis classified as psoriatic arthritis are probably in fact cases of seronegative RA, one should have grave reservations about diagnosing psoriatic arthritis in the presence of a positive rheumatoid factor.

Histocompatibility typing has little place in the diagnosis of psoriatic arthritis or any of the group of the seronegative spondarthritides. The presence of HLA-B27 or other indicative antigens is helpful in cases of diagnostic doubt, but can rarely be of great predictive value in the clinical setting [27].

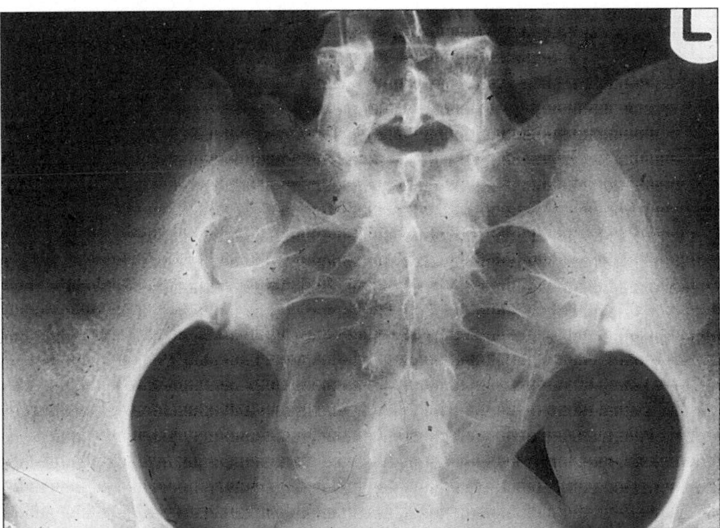

Fig. 22.13 Asymmetrical sacroiliitis.

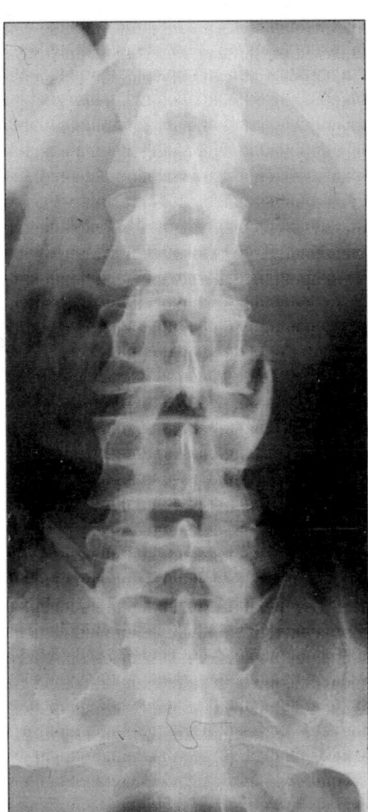

Fig. 22.14 Asymmetrical syndesmophytes and large other-than-marginal syndesmophytes.

Hematology and Biochemistry

Generally speaking, indices of inflammation such as acute phase reactants are elevated in proportion to the total body burden of inflamed synovium. In this respect, psoriatic arthritis is no different from RA and indeed is indistinguishable biochemically [28]. If spondylitis alone is present in association with psoriasis then, as in classical AS, there is little relationship between plasma viscosity, ESR and other acute phase reactants and clinical activity of disease.

A number of inflammatory indices in different subsets of psoriatic arthritis have recently been investigated [29]. As expected, symmetrical polyarthritis produced the greatest changes in ESR and C-reactive protein: overall, ESR was found to be the best laboratory guide to clinical disease activity. Cytidine deaminase was found to be unhelpful in monitoring synovial inflammation in psoriatic arthritis, in contrast to RA where this enzyme has proved a useful marker [30]. This explanation is not surprising since cytidine deaminase is derived from neutrophils, which are abundant in psoriatic skin.

Radiologic Features

Spinal disease

McEwen *et al.* found the radiologic features of spondylitis associated with psoriasis and reactive arthritis (Reiter's disease) were different from classical AS and the spondylitis accompanying ulcerative colitis and regional enteritis [31]. It was felt that the following features distinguished spondylitis associated with psoriasis and reactive arthritis:

- asymmetrical sacroiliitis (Fig. 22.13);
- less zygoapophyseal disease;
- fewer syndesmophytes;
- asymmetrical syndesmophytes (Fig. 22.14);
- syndesmophyte different in shape from those found in classical AS ('other-than-marginal' syndesmophytes first described by Bywaters and Dixon [32]) (Fig. 22.14).

A study of this type has not been repeated, although Helliwell *et al.* (unpublished data) recently carried out a survey similar to that of McEwen *et al.* and found the criteria for describing a syndesmophyte as 'other-than-marginal' or 'chunky' difficult to define. In some cases these bulky and slightly irregular syndesmophytes are indistinguishable from the hyperostotic lesions associated with DISH.

More recently Resnick has noted three other features associated with the spondylitis of psoriasis [33]:

- fluffy hyperostosis on the anterior surface of the vertebral bodies, particularly in the cervical spine (also described by Bywaters and Dixon [32]);
- severe cervical spine involvement and associated sacroiliitis with relative sparing of the thoracolumbar spine. Erosion of the odontoid peg and associated atlantoaxial subluxation may occur;
- paravertebral ossification.

Despite the above considerations, patients with psoriasis are seen who have developed the classical radiologic changes of AS.

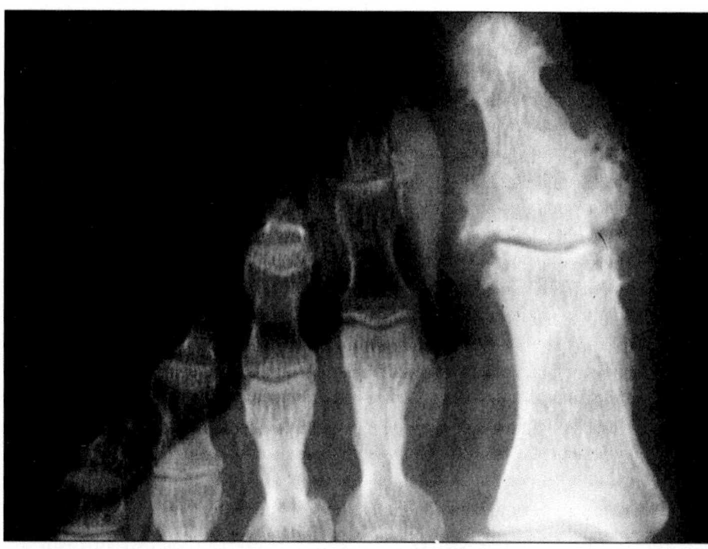

Fig. 22.15 Whiskering in the terminal interphalangeal joint of the great toe.

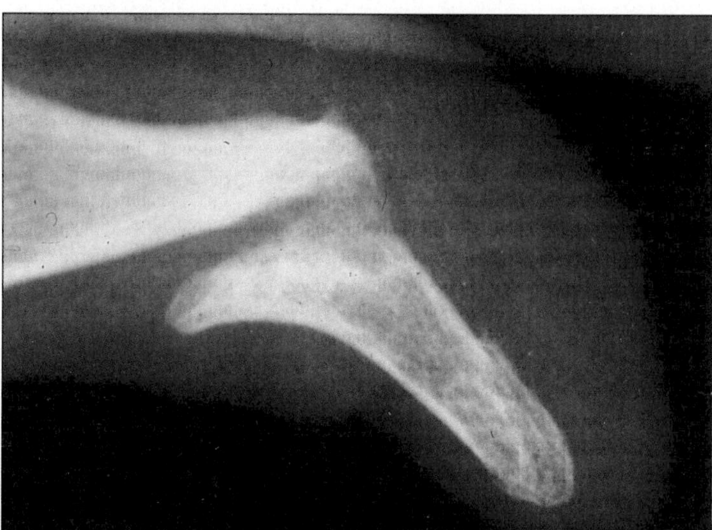

Fig. 22.16 Whittling.

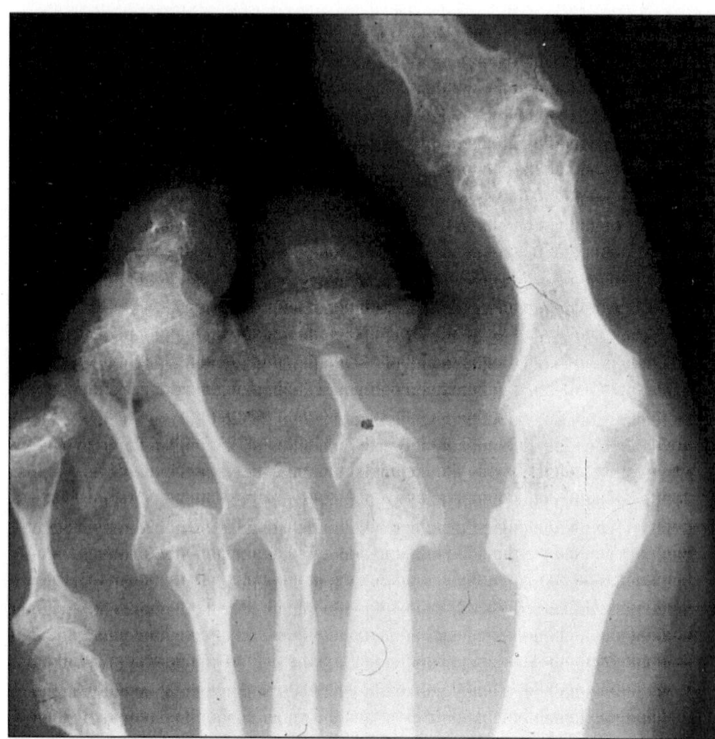

Fig. 22.17 Osteolysis.

Peripheral arthritis

The distinction between RA and psoriatic arthritis becomes more obvious when involved joints are examined radiologically. Characteristic features of psoriatic arthritis include:

- asymmetrical small joint involvement of the interphalangeal joints of the hands and feet;
- marginal erosion with adjacent proliferation of bone resulting in 'whiskering' (Fig. 22.15);
- a tendency to ankylosis of the joint;
- osteolysis involving phalangeal and metacarpal bone resulting in telescoping digits (Figs 22.16 & 22.17);
- characteristic pencil-in-cup deformity (Fig. 22.18);
- periostitis; and
- proliferative new bone formation at entheses, particularly around the pelvis and the calcaneum (Fig. 22.19).

Isotope Imaging

Scintigraphic imaging with bone seeking radioisotopes provides a sensitive indication of joint involvement in inflammatory arthropathies. As shown by Helliwell *et al.*, isotope imaging may also provide additional information on the pattern of joint involvement: over half of the isotope scans performed on 42 patients with psoriatic arthritis showed abnormal uptake in the region of the sterno-clavicular and manubriosternal joints, occasionally extending

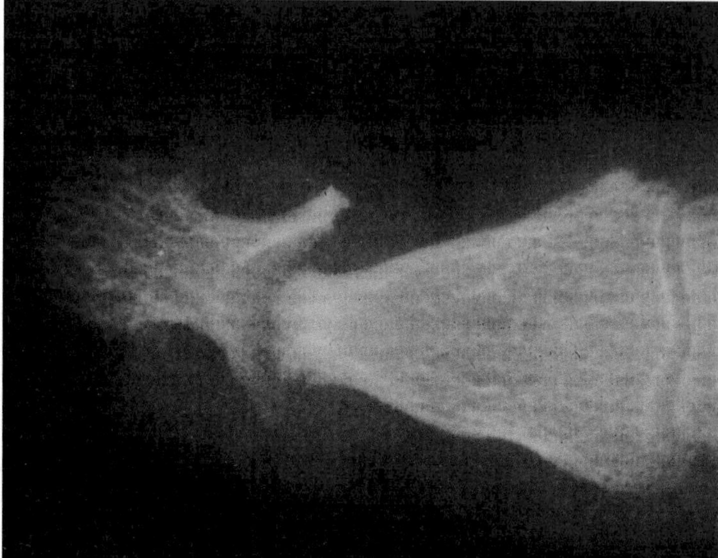

Fig. 22.18 Pencil-in-cup appearance.

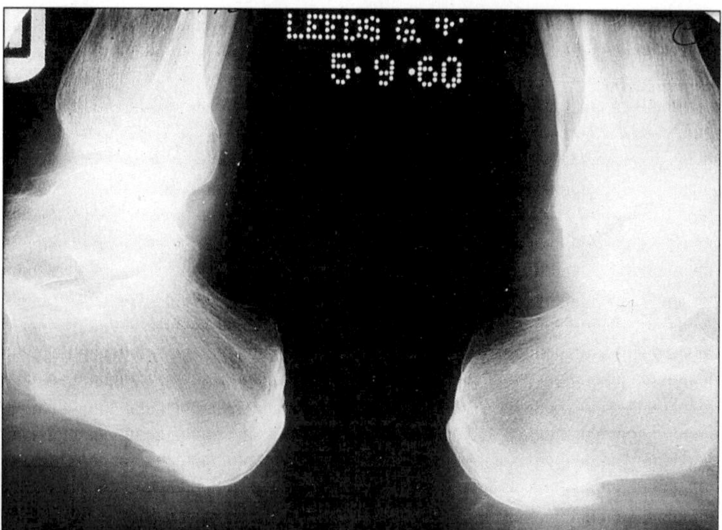

Fig. 22.19 Erosion and new bone formation on calcaneum.

into the clavicle [19]. In addition, unexplained abnormal uptake was seen at several sites in the long bones: this was unrelated to radiographic periostitis and possibly represents subclinical 'sterile' foci of osteomyelitis.

Namey and Rosenthal have demonstrated marked periarticular uptake using bone-seeking radioisotopes in 12 patients with psoriasis in the absence of an overt arthropathy and have suggested that this may occur as a result of deposition of immature collagen around the joints [34]. Interestingly, this abnormality improved with improvement in skin condition.

DIFFERENTIAL DIAGNOSIS

Since the majority of patients with peripheral arthritis associated with psoriasis have a rheumatoid-like pattern of arthritis, it must be accepted that some of these patients will have a seronegative RA and coincidental psoriasis. However, certain characteristics enable the two to be distinguished. Features in favor of psoriatic arthritis are:

- the pattern of joint involvement: in psoriatic arthritis DIP and anterior chest wall involvement commonly occur whereas hips and temporomandibular joints are infrequently involved [5];
- characteristic clinical features: these include dactylitis, iritis, unilateral limb edema, and enthesopathy, particularly around the heel;
- characteristic radiologic features: these include proliferative new bone formation at entheses, whiskering around the joints, acro-osteolysis, periostitis and pencil-incup deformities;
- associated spondylitis and sacroiliitis.

Clearly, the presence of nodules and rheumatoid factor in the serum favors the diagnosis of RA, as do systemic features of RA not seen in psoriasis. These include pulmonary and pleural involvement, systemic vasculitis, generalized lymphedanopathy, Felty's syndrome and renal involvement.

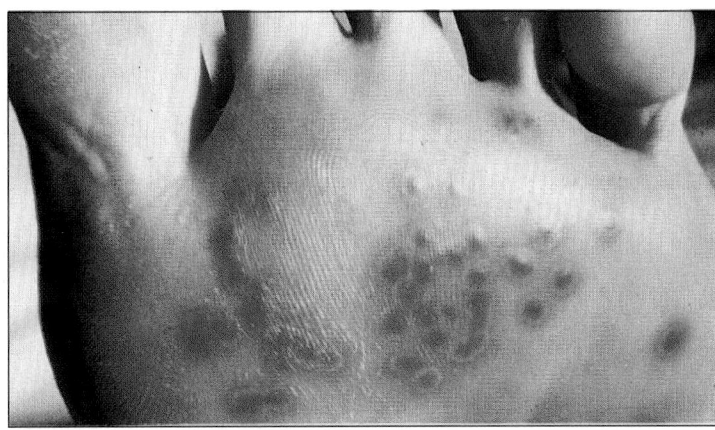

Fig. 22.20 Keratoderma blenorrhagicum.

The distinction between psoriatic arthritis and reactive arthritis, particularly where no infective trigger can be identified, is often impossible since these two diseases share common features within the group of seronegative spondarthritides. Indeed, it has been argued that psoriatic arthritis is a reactive arthritis, the trigger possibly being bacteria in psoriatic plaques [1]. However, where there has been a clear infective trigger, the appearance of keratoderma blenorrhagicum (Fig. 22.20) arising *de novo* in association with an asymmetrical oligoarthritis provides little problem in diagnosis.

REFERENCES

1. Vasey FB, Espinoza LR. Psoriatic arthropathy. In: Calin A, ed. Spondylarthropathies. New York: Grune and Stratton; 1984:151–85.
2. Moll JMH, Wright V. Psoriatic arthritis. Semin Arthritis Rheum. 1973;**3**:55–78.
3. Gladman DD, Shuckett R, Russell ML, Thorne JC, Schachter RK. Psoriatic arthritis: an analysis of 220 patients. Quart J Med. 1987;**62**:127–41.
4. Oriente CB, Scarpa R, Puccino A, Oriente P. Psoriasis and psoriatic arthritis. Dermatological and rheumatological co-operative clinical report. Acta Dermatol Venereol (Stockholm). 1989:**146**(Suppl.):69–71.
5. Helliwell PS, Marchessoni A, Peters M, Barker M, Wright V. A revaluation of the osteoarticular manifestations of psoriasis. Br J Rheumatol. 1991;**30**:339–45
6. De Silva RTD, Grennan DM, Palmer DG. Lymphatic obstruction in rheumatoid arthritis: a cause for upper limb oedema. Ann Rheum Dis. 1980;**39**:260–65.
7. Lambert JR, Wright V. Eye inflammation in psoriatic arthritis. Ann Rheum Dis. 1976;**35**:354–6.
8. Sonozaki H, Mitsui H, Miyanaga Y, et al. Clinical features of 53 cases with pustulotic arthro-osteitis. Ann Rheum Dis. 1981;**40**:547–53.
9. Benhamou CL, Shamot AM, Kahn MF. Synovitis acne pustulosis hyperostosis osteomyelitis syndrome (SAPHO). A new syndrome among the spondylo-arthropathies? Clin Exp Rheumatol. 1988;**6**:109–12.
10. Edlund E, Johnsson V, Lidgren L, et al. Palmoplantar pustulosis and sterno-costo-clavicular arthro-osteitis. Ann Rheum Dis. 1988;**47**:809–15.
11. Johnson TM, Duvik M, Rapini RP, Rios A. AIDS exacerbates psoriasis. N Engl J Med. 1985;**313**:1415.
12. Espinoza LR, Berman A, Vasez FB, Cahalin C, Nelson R, Germain B. Psoriatic arthritis and acquired immunodeficiency syndrome. Arthritis Rheum. 1988;**31**:1034–40.
13. Duvik N, Johnson TM, Rapini RP, Freeze T, Brewton G, Rios A. Acquired immuno-deficiency syndrome, associated psoriasis and Reiter's syndrome. Arch Dermatol. 1987;**123**:1622–32.
14. Valle SL. Dermatologic findings related to immuno-deficiency virus infection in high risk individuals. J Am Acad Dermatol. 1987;**17**:951–61.
15. Keat A, Rowe I. Reiter's syndrome and associated arthritides. Rheum Dis Clin North Am. 1991;**17**:25–42.
16. Calabrese LH, Kelley DM, Myers A, O'Connell M, Easley K. Rheumatic symptoms and human immunodeficiency virus infection. Arthritis Rheum. 1991;**34**:257–63.
17. Vasey FB, Seleznick MJ, Fenske NA, Espinoza LR. New signposts on the road to understanding psoriatic arthritis. J Rheumatol. 1989;**16**:1405–6.
18. Lambert JR, Ansell BM, Stevenson BE, Wright V. Psoriatic arthritis in childhood. Clin Rheum Dis. 1976;**2**:339–52.
19. Hamilton ML, Gladman DD, Shore A, Laxer RM, Silverman ED. Juvenile psoriatic arthritis and HLA antigens. Ann Rheum Dis. 1990;**49**:694–7.
20. Wendling D, Lamarque V, Portha P, Guidet M. Hyperostose induite par l'etretinate. Rheumatologie. 1991;**43**:41–8.
21. Kaplan G, Haettich B. Rheumatological symptoms due to retinoids. Bailliere's Clin Rheumatol. 1991;**5**:77–97.
22. Daunt SO'N, Robertson JC, Cox ML, Cawley MID. The natural history of psoriatic arthritis. A retrospective analysis of joint involvement. Br J Rheumatol. 1986;**25**:abstract 75.
23. Roberts MET, Wright V, Hill AGS, Mehra AC. Psoriatic arthritis. A follow-up study. Ann Rheum Dis. 1976;**35**:206–12.

24. Gladman DD, Stafford-Brady F, Chang CH, Lewandowski K, Russell ML. Longitudinal study of clinical and radiological progression in psoriatic arthritis. J Rheumatol. 1990;**17**:809–12.
25. Hanly JG, Russell ML, Gladman DD. Psoriatic spondyloarthropathy: a long-term prospective study. Ann Rheum Dis. 1988;**47**:386–93.
26. Stern RS. The epidemiology of joint complaints in patients with psoriasis. J Rheumatol. 1985;**12**:315–20.
27. Khan AK, Khan MK. HLA-B27 as an aid to diagnosis of ankylosing spondylitis. Spine: State of the Art Reviews. 1990;**4**:617–25.
28. Sitton NG, Dixon JS, Bird HA, Wright V. Serum of biochemistry in rheumatoid arthritis, seronegative arthropathies, osteoarthritis, SLE and normal subjects. Br J Rheumatol. 1987;**26**:131–5.
29. Helliwell PS, Marchessoni A, Peters M, Platt R, Wright V. Cytidine deaminase activity, C-reactive protein, histidine, and erythrocyte sedimentation rate as measures of disease activity in psoriatic arthritis. Ann Rheum Dis. 1991;**50**:362–5.
30. Thompson PW, Jones DD, Curry HLF. Cytidine deaminase activity as a measure of acute inflammation in rheumatoid arthritis. Ann Rheum Dis. 1986;**45**:9–14.
31. McEwen C, DiTata D, Lingg C, Porini A, Good A, Rankin T. Ankylosing spondylitis and spondylitis accompanying ulcerative colitis, regional enteritis, psoriasis and Reiter's disease. Arthritis Rheum. 1971;**14**:291–318.
32. Bywaters EGL, St J Dixon A. Paravertebral ossification in psoriatic arthritis. Ann Rheum Dis. 1965;**24**:313–31.
33. Resnick D, Niwayama G. Psoriatic arthritis. In: Resnick D, Niwayama G, eds. Diagnosis of Bone and Joint Disorders, Vol. 2. Philadelphia: WB Saunders; 1981:1103–29.
34. Namey TC, Rosenthal L. Periarticular uptake of ^{99m}technetium diphosphonate in psoriasis. Arthritis Rheum. 1976: **19**: 607–12.

23

MANAGEMENT OF PSORIATIC ARTHRITIS

Luis R Espinoza & Marta Lucia Cuellar

- Basic principles of management similar to those used in rheumatoid arthritis.
- Early, aggressive therapy may be important in subsets of psoriatic arthritis thought to have a poor prognosis, particularly polyarticular disease, and arthritis with extensive skin involvement.
- Disease-modifying drugs, particularly methotrexate and sulfasalazine, have an important role in drug management.
- Cyclosporin A and synthetic vitamin A derivatives are promising investigational drug therapies.

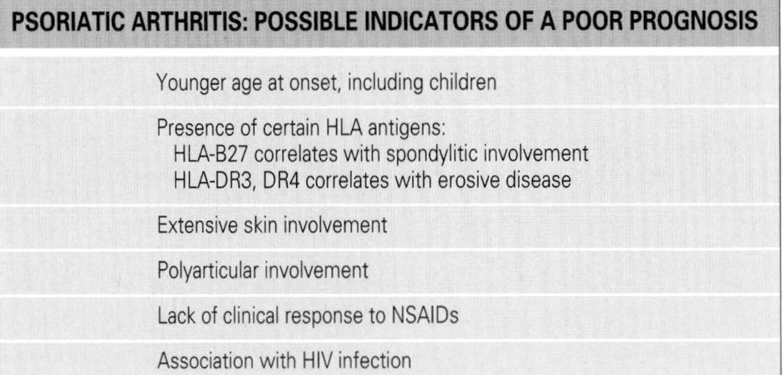

PSORIATIC ARTHRITIS: POSSIBLE INDICATORS OF A POOR PROGNOSIS
Younger age at onset, including children
Presence of certain HLA antigens: HLA-B27 correlates with spondylitic involvement HLA-DR3, DR4 correlates with erosive disease
Extensive skin involvement
Polyarticular involvement
Lack of clinical response to NSAIDs
Association with HIV infection

Fig. 23.1 Psoriatic arthritis: Possible indicators of a poor prognosis. Recognition of these indicators associated with disease severity is important in the planning of an early and aggressive therapeutic program.

INTRODUCTION

The medical management of patients with psoriatic arthritis includes suppression of joint inflammation, maintenance and improvement of musculoskeletal function, prevention of joint deformity and disability, and support in the emotional adjustment to the presence of arthritis and skin rash. The most important notion in the comprehensive medical management of patients with psoriatic arthritis is the need for a multidisciplinary approach, involving different health providers and supporting personnel regardless of the predominant manifestations of the disease. In this regard, the close cooperation among rheumatologists, dermatologists, orthopedists, psychiatrists, and rehabilitative team is essential.

The treatment of psoriatic arthritis remains essentially symptomatic and will depend on the clinical subset present. In general, patients with psoriatic arthritis suffer from less pain and disability than those with rheumatoid arthritis (RA). Most patients presenting with oligoarticular or distal interphalangeal (DIP) forms have mild disease that shows an episodic course. Recent reports, however, suggest a more aggressive behavior of psoriatic arthritis with a high frequency of deforming destructive arthropathy than previously believed [1]. Extensive skin involvement and younger age at onset appear to increase the severity of the prognosis. The presence of HLA-DR3 and DR4 may correlate with a greater frequency of erosive changes and more severe disease (Fig. 23.1) [1].

Patients presenting with polyarticular involvement and those with arthritis mutilans have a poor prognosis and will require aggressive therapeutic intervention including the early use of second-line agents (Fig. 23.2) [2]. It must be emphasized, however, that studies of second-line agents have been limited and to date only a few, long-term, uncontrolled studies have shown evidence that any treatment favorably influences the eventual outcome of psoriatic arthritis.

NONSTEROIDAL ANTI-INFLAMMATORY THERAPY

Initial therapeutic management includes the use of nonsteroidal anti-inflammatory drugs (NSAIDs). In contrast to RA, aspirin seems less effective in psoriatic arthritis than other, more recent agents, although there are few prospective controlled studies evaluating the efficacy of NSAID therapy. Available studies, however, do demonstrate the effectiveness of NSAIDs in the management of psoriatic arthritis [3–5].

Early studies claimed a better response to indomethacin [4], but more recent studies found no significant differences among the newer NSAIDs [6]. Scarpa *et al.* [6] studied the clinical response of 138 psoriatic arthritis patients to several NSAIDs, classified according to the criteria of Wright and Moll [7], and entered into a therapeutic program which also included rehabilitation. Eighty-five percent of their patients received NSAIDs which always proved adequate to relieve pain and articular inflammation. Several different NSAIDs were used including piroxicam, diclofenac, meclofenamate, nimesulide, naproxen and tiaprofenic, and proved to be equally effective. Side effects were not different from those observed in the treatment of RA.

Of particular concern about the use of NSAIDs in psoriatic arthritis is the potential harmful effect they may have on the psoriatic rash. Leukotrienes influence the evolution of the psoriatic skin rash through an effect on epidermal proliferation and inflammation [8]. NSAID-induced cyclooxygenase inhibition in the skin with diversion of arachidonate into the lipooxygenase pathway may result in worsening of the psoriatic cutaneous activity. Indeed, uncontrolled observations have shown worsening of the psoriatic rash with several NSAIDs including indomethacin, phenylbutazone, oxyphenbutazone and meclofenamate [9–11]. Other studies, however, have not

THERAPEUTIC MEASURES IN THE TREATMENT OF PSORIATIC ARTHRITIS
Pharmacologic measures
Nonsteroidal anti-inflammatory drugs Disease-modifying drugs Photochemotherapy with methoxypsoralen Miscellaneous
Surgical measures
Synovectomy Joint arthroplasty
Rehabilitative measures
Aggressive active and passive physical therapy Dynamic strengthening exercises Contact sports and heavy physical activity should be discouraged

Fig. 23.2 Therapeutic measures in the treatment of psoriatic arthritis. Initiation of an early aggressive comprehensive medical management program may prevent the development of joint deformity and disability.

been able to confirm this complication [7]. More important, perhaps, is the beneficial effect of certain NSAIDs on the psoriatic skin rash. This was first recognized with benoxaprofen, a purported cyclo- and lipo-oxygenase inhibitor [12]. This agent has since been withdrawn from the market because of serious liver toxicity. Another NSAID reported to benefit psoriatic skin rash is meclofenamate, although some conflicting reports about its efficacy exist [7–13]. Most patients with mildly active peripheral arthritis, as well as those with spondylitis, respond to NSAIDs. Usually, full doses of a given NSAID should be tried for 3–4 weeks before concluding that the drug has not been effective. There is no data about the influence of NSAIDs on the clinical and/or radiologic course of the disease.

DISEASE-MODIFYING AGENTS

Lack of clinical response to NSAID therapy, or the presence of progressive, severe and deforming arthritis, demand the use of 'disease-modifying' agents. Extrapolating from experience with RA, the use of second-line agents in psoriatic arthritis has proved to be a success.

A large variety of so-called 'disease-modifying' agents such as methotrexate, parenteral and oral gold preparations, antimalarials, and D-penicillamine have been used with varying success (Fig. 23.3). Better results are claimed with newer preparations including sulfasalazine, retinoic acid derivatives, azathioprine, cyclosporin A, vitamin D derivatives, somatostatin, psoralen and PUVA, and fumaric acid. Efficacy, however, is hampered by the high frequency of side effects.

Methotrexate Therapy

Gubner *et al.* were the first to describe the use of methotrexate in psoriatic arthritis in 1951 [14]. Their report was followed by others whose results have been largely encouraging. In a prospective placebo-controlled double-blind study of 21 patients, Black *et al.* showed that parenteral methotrexate was effective in suppressing skin and joint manifestations with relatively low toxicity [15]. A retrospective study in 1982 noted that 22 of 59 psoriatic arthritis patients were virtually asymptomatic after 1–11 years of methotrexate. Responses correlated directly with early treatment [16]. More recently, the same group reported the results of a prospective 12-month study of 28 patients with psoriatic arthritis treated with low-dose oral methotrexate. Most patients improved dramatically in pain and function, erythrocyte sedimentation rate (ESR), and intake of analgesics [17]. Conversely, a randomized, double-blind, placebo-controlled 12-week prospective study found that only the physician assessment of arthritis activity and the skin involvement improved [18].

Espinoza *et al.* [19] have recently reported their experience with this drug in psoriatic arthritis. The study group included 24 males and 16 females with a mean age of 47 years, with oligo- (13) or polyarticular (27) involvement, and a mean disease duration of 12 years. Patients received a mean dose of 11.2mg of methotrexate orally per week during a mean period of 34 months. Thirty-eight patients had an excellent or good clinical response and improvement in ESR. Only two patients had a rather poor response. Two patients discontinued the medication because of side effects (leukopenia in one and stomatitis in the other). Liver test abnormalities were seen in 11 patients, but cirrhosis and/or inflammation was not found in any. No changes in liver histology were found in seven patients who had repeated liver biopsies. The finding of mildly abnormal liver histology in 6–64% of patients with psoriatic arthritis who have not taken methotrexate or have other risk factors such as obesity and excessive alcohol intake is presumably attributable to the disease *per se* [20,21]. Other potentially hepatotoxic agents, e.g. NSAIDs, may be implicated in the genesis of liver abnormalities found in patients who had not taken methotrexate. Methotrexate-induced cirrhosis in psoriatic arthritis does occur, but with exceptions, and is not of an aggressive nature [22–25]. In fact, in most patients continuing methotrexate in spite of underlying cirrhosis, a cumulative index of grading for fibrosis, status of the limiting membrane, and regeneration shows a tendency to decrease [25]. This suggests that methotrexate can be tolerated despite an abnormal liver architecture. It has been shown that methotrexate does not seem to increase collagen production, but rather affects other factors involved in its turnover [26].

Furthermore, methotrexate has also been used preliminarily to treat hepatopathies such as primary biliary cirrhosis and primary sclerosing cholangitis [27,28]. The beneficial effect observed on these disorders suggests that methotrexate may be far less hepatotoxic than previously suspected. From available evidence it appears that liver biopsy is not necessary in the routine evaluation of patients with psoriatic arthritis, but should be considered in those patients with persistently elevated liver enzyme abnormalities despite discontinuation or reduction of methotrexate therapy. A recent report serves to illustrate this point. Gilbert *et al.* [29] described three psoriasis patients receiving high doses of methotrexate, in excess of 30–35mg/week for several years, who developed cirrhosis requiring liver transplantation. The first two patients had elevated liver enzymes and abnormal liver–spleen scan respectively. However, methotrexate dosage was not adjusted. The third patient took it for several years under no supervision.

The usual dosage of methotrexate is 7.5–15mg/week, given orally as a single dose or divided into two doses taken 12 hours apart on the same day. The amount can be increased to 25–30mg/week until improvement occurs, and then it can be tapered down to a maintenance dose that varies from patient to patient, but tends to be around 5–15mg/week. Most frequent side effects are abdominal pain and stomatitis. The major advantage of using this agent is the lack of evidence of oncogenesis, and also its effectiveness in suppressing both the psoriatic skin disease as well as arthritis.

DISEASE-MODIFYING AGENTS

Drug treatment	Main target cell	Possible mode of action
Methotrexate	Multiple cells	Cytokine release, antimetabolite
Gold compounds	Macrophage Endothelial cell	Inhibition of cytokine release IL-1 release inhibition Antigen presentation inhibition Inhibition of macrophage differentiation
Antimalarials	B cell Macrophage	PGE_2 inhibition Decrease antigen presentation Inhibition of cytokine release Inhibition of macrophage differentiation
D-Penicillamine	Macrophage T-helper cell	Enhance phagocytosis Decrease immune complex formation
Retinoids	Multiple cells	Inhibition of DNA replication
Cyclosporin A	T-helper cell	Inhibition of IL-2 release Inhibition of T-cell proliferation
Azathioprine	Macrophage	Inhibition of macrophage differentiation Powerful anti-inflammatory
Vitamin D derivatives	T cells	Inhibition of T-lymphocyte proliferation Inhibition of cytokine release
Corticosteroids	Multiple cells	Inhibition of PGE_2 formation Inhibition of cytokine release Increases IL-1 receptor Decreases antigen-presenting cells

Fig. 23.3 Disease-modifying agents. Drugs affect various aspects of the pathogenic process of psoriatic arthritis. Therapy directed at one process may be beneficial in modifying this disorder.

Gold Compounds

Gold has been shown to be beneficial in psoriatic arthritis, resulting in a significant clinical improvement in 50–75% of the patients [5,6,30–33]. Both intramuscular and oral preparations are effective, although there is a suggestion that parenteral gold may be more effective. Palit *et al.* [34] studied the efficacy and safety of the oral compound auranofin and intramuscular gold thiomalate in a placebo-controlled, double-blind, four-center trial in 82 patients with psoriatic arthritis requiring drug therapy. Significant falls were seen in Ritchie articular index, visual analog pain score, and ESR at 12 and 24 weeks following parenteral gold; no significant changes were observed in the auranofin-treated group. They concluded that intramuscular gold was safe and more effective than auranofin as a second-line, suppressive antirheumatic agent for patients with psoriatic arthritis when followed for 6 months.

A double-blind placebo-controlled study of auranofin in 238 patients with psoriatic arthritis found auranofin treatment superior to placebo treatment, according to physician's global assessment and functional scores. However, the therapeutic advantage over treatment with NSAIDs alone was modest [35].

Most studies have shown that the polyarticular subtype of psoriatic arthritis, and not the spondylitic and/or oligoarticular forms, is the one which responds best to gold compounds. Children with the juvenile form of psoriatic arthritis also respond well to gold. In general, chrysotherapy in psoriatic arthritis is accompanied by similar side effects to those seen in RA patients, except that photosensitivity and exacerbation of underlying psoriatic skin disease seem to be unique side effects [36].

Antimalarial Therapy

The use of antimalarial agents in psoriatic arthritis remains controversial. Earlier studies with quinacrine and chloroquine reported a high incidence of side effects, including flare-ups of psoriasis [37–39]. Other reports, however, suggest less frequent side effects and good control of arthritis with the use of hydroxychloroquine [5,40]. Given the availability of newer agents it is prudent to use antimalarial compounds in psoriatic arthritis with great caution.

D-Penicillamine Therapy

Evidence suggesting effectiveness of D-penicillamine in the therapy of psoriatic arthritis is available, but is based on a few small, uncontrolled studies. Side effects, including myasthenia gravis and pemphigus, are similar to those seen in RA patients [41,42].

Sulfasalazine Therapy

Psoriatic arthritis appears to respond to sulfasalazine [43,44]. A recently published double-blind, placebo-controlled trial of 30 patients showed greater improvement in those patients on active treatment than on placebo, with greater benefit observed in patients with a seronegative symmetrical polyarthritis associated with a high acute-phase response [45]. Overall, in the sulfasalazine group, five patients were good responders, seven were partial and two were poor or no responders. In the placebo group there were no good responders. Analysis of individual variables of clinical and laboratory parameters of disease activity showed the greatest improvement in some of the clinical indices, but no change in the laboratory parameters. Sulfasalazine was well tolerated and side effects were mild. The maintenance dose of sulfasalazine was 2g daily and the treatment period was 24 weeks.

Treatment with sulfasalazine represents a good alternative to other therapeutic modalities, especially if consideration is given to its effectiveness in controlling the psoriatic skin involvement. Gupta *et al.* [46] recently showed that sulfasalazine improves psoriasis. In an 8-week double-blind trial, they found that 7 of 17 patients (41%) receiving sulfasalazine experienced moderate improvement, and 3 (18%) demonstrated minimal change. A low incidence of severe side effects (skin rash, gastrointestinal distress) was observed.

Retinoid Therapy

Synthetic vitamin A derivatives (retinoids) have been shown to be effective in the treatment of psoriasis and psoriatic arthritis [47–49]. Retinoids may improve skin disorders, including psoriasis, by blockade of the cell cycle in G_1 and inhibition of collagenase synthesis [50]. Disorders of keratinization and also recalcitrant cystic acne appear to respond best [51].

Etretinate is the most studied retinoid in the treatment of psoriatic arthritis [47–49]. Klinkhoff *et al.* [52] recently reported their experience with this compound in 40 patients with psoriatic arthritis before and after treatment for 8–24 weeks. The number of tender joints fell from 22.0 ± 8.75 before treatment to 11.44 ± 8.50 after treatment. The duration of morning stiffness was 101.95 ± 62.45 minutes before therapy and 44.53 ± 82.10 minutes after treatment. Similar highly clinically and statistically significant improvement was seen in all the clinical outcome measures and in the ESR. A relatively major drawback with this compound, however, was the high incidence of side effects. Mucocutaneous side effects were seen in 39/40 patients and resulted in discontinuation of therapy before 24 weeks in nine patients. Relapse of arthritis usually occurs within 6 weeks of discontinuation of the drug.

Vitamin A derivatives are likely to be of great clinical benefit in the medical management of psoriatic arthritis. At present, however, they are limited by their high incidence of side effects, including hair loss, palmar dermatitis, dry lips, pruritus and bone pain secondary to periostitis. New compounds (e.g. acitretin, an active compound of etretinate) are potentially of great importance for their superior effectiveness and lesser incidence of side effects [53]. The teratogenic potential of the retinoids, however, remains a serious limitation in women of child-bearing age.

Cyclosporin Therapy

The effectiveness of cyclosporin in the treatment of psoriasis and psoriatic arthritis is clearly documented [54–56]. Improvement within 2–4 weeks of both skin and joint involvement is seen in most patients. Control studies show that cyclosporin leads to a rapid and thorough clearing of psoriasis, and an initial dose of 5mg/kg/day seems to be adequate. Concern exists, however, about significant neurologic and renal side effects even at this dose. Control studies in psoriatic arthritis are not available.

The short-term efficacy of cyclosporin in the treatment of six patients with moderately severe to severe psoriatic arthritis was evaluated in an open study [56]. Patients received oral cyclosporin (6mg/kg/day) for eight weeks. A significant clinical improvement was seen in all patients within 2–4 weeks. At the completion of the treatment, rheumatologic assessment revealed a decrease in the number of tender joints, joint tenderness index, duration of morning stiffness, and an increase in grip strength. There was a decrease in the number of swollen joints, joint swelling index, and the time taken to walk 50 feet. Overall disease activity significantly improved as assessed independently by the patient and physician. Discontinuation of cyclosporin was followed within 4 weeks by exacerbation of both psoriatic skin and joint involvement. The need for long-term studies is underscored by the high incidence of serious side effects, including the potential for the development of lymphoid malignancies.

Immunosuppressive or Cytotoxic Therapy

The purine analogs, azaribine, azathioprine and 6-mercaptopurine, and cytotoxic drugs such as nitrogen mustard and cyclophosphamide, have all been used in the treatment of psoriatic arthritis [57]. Several uncontrolled studies have shown the effectiveness of 6-mercaptopurine and azathioprine [58,59]. Efficacy for both psoriatic skin and joint involvement is reported, as well as low incidence of side effects. However, a potential for serious side effects, including lymphoid proliferative malignancy, limits their long-term use.

Vitamin D Derivatives

Recently, several groups have reported on the use of oral 1,25-dihydroxyvitamin D_3 [1,25$(OH)_2D_3$] in patients with psoriasis [60]. Up to 70% of the patients experienced significant improvement in their skin lesions. Vitamin D may have immunoregulatory effects that could ameliorate inflammatory articular disease. For instance, 1,25$(OH)_2D_3$ potentiates the inhibitory effect of cyclosporin A on T-helper cells from patients with RA, inhibits T-lymphocyte mitogenesis and also has varying effects on lymphokine production. In a 6-month open-label pilot study of 10 patients with active psoriatic arthritis receiving 2μg of oral 1,25$(OH)_2D_3$ daily, significant improvement in the tender joint count and physician global impression was measured [61]. Of the 10 patients, four had substantial (≥50%) improvement, and three had moderate (≥25%) improvement in the tender joint count. Two patients were unable to receive therapeutic doses because of hypercalciuria. Further studies with this compound appear to be indicated.

Somatostatin Therapy

Somatostatin, an inhibitor of human growth hormone, has been shown to be effective in ameliorating the skin lesions of psoriasis [62]. It has also been used with success in psoriatic arthritis. Eighteen patients with psoriatic arthritis were treated for 48 hours with an infusion of somatostatin, 250μg/hr diluted in a 5% glucose solution [63]. This therapy resulted in an immediate reduction of joint pain and satisfactory clearing of cutaneous lesions in eight patients, less marked results in four, and no response in four. Two patients were dropped from the study because of significant side effects during administration of the drug. Fifteen days after treatment the clearing of skin lesions and joint pain reduction were even more pronounced. Patients with erythrodermic and large plaque psoriasis and polyarticular inflammatory involvement responded better.

Zinc Therapy

The use of oral zinc sulfate has been reported to be of benefit to patients with psoriatic arthritis [64]. A double-blind cross-over trial in 24 psoriatic arthritis patients showed that most tolerated the medication well and nine demonstrated improvement in joint count while receiving zinc as compared with when they were treated with placebo. In this study, patients were maintained on steady doses of immunosuppressive agents throughout.

However, two other studies offer a conflicting view [65,66]. In an open uncontrolled trial 20 psoriatic arthritis patients received 200mg of zinc sulfate three times daily for 6 months. The 18 patients who completed the trial showed a significant decrease in the number of swollen and tender joints, Ritchie articular index, need for NSAIDs, ESR, and plasma copper level [65]. The other study investigated the effect of zinc sulfate (50mg elementary three times daily) on neutrophil chemotaxis and clinical course in patients with psoriasis vulgaris and psoriatic arthritis. They found no effect on the clinical course, although it restored both the random migration and directed neutrophil chemotaxis to normal in patients with psoriasis vulgaris [66]. Further studies are needed to confirm the value of zinc in psoriatic patients.

Photochemotherapy with Methoxypsoralen (Psoralen Ultraviolet A, PUVA)

PUVA treatment is of benefit for some psoriatic arthritis patients. Perlman *et al.* [67] prospectively studied 27 patients receiving photochemotherapy for treatment of psoriasis. Patients were classified as having either spondylitic or nonspondylitic joint involvement. A good response to PUVA, with a 49% improvement in peripheral joint activity, was observed in the nonspondylitic group. Skin improvement was also noted. Spondylitic patients did not experience improvement of either psoriasis or arthritis. These results support the notion that skin activity influences articular response in a subset of psoriatic arthritis patients.

DRUGS COMMONLY USED IN PSORIATIC ARTHRITIS

Drugs treatment	Main target cell	Mode of action
NSAIDs	Macrophage	Inhibits cyclooxygenase Decrease PGE_2 formation Increase leukotriene B_4 formation
Sulfasalazine	Undefined	Alters bowel flora Inhibits folate metabolism Inhibits and stimulates PGE_2 Inhibits leukotriene B_4 formation
Somatostatin	Not well defined	Inhibits human growth hormone
Zinc	Undefined	Stimulates cell-mediated immune responses
Colchicine	Multiple cells	Antimitotic Inhibits cytokine release
Bromocriptine	Lymphocytes	Inhibits prolactin release Immunomodulator

Fig. 23.4 Anti-inflammatory and other drugs commonly used in psoriatic arthritis. The use of some of these agents is gaining increasing popularity and may be useful to prevent long-term joint deterioration and disability.

Glucocorticosteroid Treatment

The use of steroids in psoriatic arthritis merits special consideration although they can only be recommended in special circumstances. Systemic steroids are often needed in high doses to control psoriatic arthritis, but unfortunately the disease usually relapses despite continued treatment. Generally, the adverse effects outweigh the benefits. The topical use of corticosteroids is effective in controlling skin disease and their intra-articular use in patients with monoarticular or oligoarticular involvement can be helpful. Special care should be taken to prepare the skin in order to minimize the likelihood of introducing infection into the joint. Children with psoriatic arthritis do not respond well to corticosteroids and the incidence of side effects is very high [68].

Colchicine Therapy

Colchicine has been found efficacious in the treatment of psoriasis [69]. A small number (n=15) of patients with psoriatic skin lesions and arthritis were given colchicine in a placebo-controlled, double-blind cross-over study of 16 weeks' duration. A significant improvement was observed in grip strength, Ritchie index, joint swelling and pain, and overall therapeutic assessment [70]. In this study, psoriatic rash was not improved by colchicine. The few side effects, mostly gastrointestinal intolerance, were easily controlled by temporary reduction of the dose. The results indicated that 1.5mg colchicine is effective in the treatment of psoriatic arthritis. Further studies are needed to confirm and expand this observation. A summary of some of the drugs commonly used in the management of psoriatic arthritis listing target sites and mode of action is given in Figure 23.4.

Miscellaneous Forms of Treatment

A variety of therapeutic modalities including gamma interferon (IFN-γ), razoxane, H_2-receptor antagonists, bromocriptine, total lymphoid irradiation, plasmapheresis, extracorporeal photochemotherapy, splenopentin, antibiotics, peptide-T, anti-CD4 monoclonal antibodies, monokine release inhibitor, allogenic bone marrow transplantation and radioactive synovectomy have all been reported to be potentially effective in the management of psoriatic arthritis (Fig. 23.5) [71–85]. However, prospective, controlled studies are needed to confirm their usefulness.

SURGICAL MANAGEMENT

Generally, the indications for surgical intervention in psoriatic arthritis patients are identical to those of patients with RA. Synovectomy may be used in selected cases, particularly in those patients with only few

AGENTS TRIED IN THE TREATMENT OF JOINT AND SKIN INVOLVEMENT	
Anti-CD4 monoclonal antibodies	Peptide-T
Gamma interferon	Total lymphoid irradiation
Razoxane	Plasmapheresis
H_2-receptor antagonists	Extra-corporeal photochemotherapy
Splenopentin	Radioactive synovectomy
Antibiotics	

Fig. 23.5 Treatment of joint and skin involvement. At times, treatment of both skin and joint involvement can be very complex and a multitude of agents have been sporadically used in an attempt to arrest the progress of the disease.

joints affected. Major reconstructive surgery, including joint arthroplasty, is reserved for severe forms of arthritis. Patients with psoriatic arthritis tolerate surgery well and standard presurgical skin preparation minimizes the risk for postoperative infection. However, they are at increased risk of up to six times the expected frequency in normal subjects [86]. In this regard, special attention should be given to the use of topical corticosteroid or other treatment when total joint arthroplasty is considered [87]. Methotrexate or any of the other immunosuppressive agents should be stopped at least 2 weeks preoperatively, and restarted about 1–2 weeks postoperatively.

REHABILITATIVE TREATMENT

Rehabilitative measures should be considered in every psoriatic arthritis patient, according to an individualized evaluation. Ideally, the goals to be achieved should also be identified on an individual basis and should be directed to maximize the patient's potential for normal physical and emotional activities.

In the presence of active synovitis, a combination of exercise, rest and relative immobilization is advisable. The type and intensity of exercise will depend on the degree of inflammation and the size, number and location of the affected joints. Generally, minimal passive or active-assisted stretching exercises should be instituted for inflamed large joints, such as the knees, ankles, hips and shoulders; this will help to avoid flexion contractures or even joint fusion, which can otherwise occur early in the course of psoriatic arthritis. Immediately after the acute synovitis subsides, isometric strengthening exercises may be implemented (to further avoid contractures and disease atrophy). As strength improves, dynamic strengthening exercises (isotonic and isokinetic) will gradually increase the range of motion. Resistant exercises should be gradually introduced to boost the effect of the strengthening exercises [88,89].

Hydrotherapy or local heat (diathermy) can render exercise therapy more feasible in the recovery phase. Cryotherapy in the form of cold (ice) packs, ethyl chloride or fluoromethane sprays, hydrotherapy, or ice massage is more helpful when joint inflammation is present. Any patient with acutely inflamed joints must rest intermittently. Rest does not imply physical inactivity, or this would lead to deleterious effects such as muscular wasting and atrophy as well as osteoporosis and articular ankylosis. The term 'rest' in this context refers to selective immobilization of the affected joints, avoiding injurious postures and placing joints in functional positions that may permit relaxation (often with the aid of orthotic devices such as braces, splints, etc.), but always alternating with increasingly longer and more intense periods of joint motion [88,89]. For example, many patients keep their knees in slight semiflexion to relieve the pain, a posture that is highly inconvenient for the further restoration of walking.

Foot and ankle synovitis is common in psoriatic arthritis, and renders the patient unable to bear weight or walk. In bed, the presence of the bed clothes on the feet will position the ankles in an extensor posture. This may rapidly lead to shortening of the Achilles tendon (which is frequently also inflamed), thus complicating the subsequent course. Sausage toes usually are swollen, painful, and unable to fit comfortably into standard shoes. Prescription of a shoe with a high toe box, or an extra-depth shoe, should alleviate this complication.

Small joints of the hand and wrist are frequently affected in psoriatic arthritis. Use of a functional wrist splint at the onset of synovitis may help preserve wrist function and alignment. Dactylitis (sausage deformity) of the entire finger or of just the DIP joint frequently occurs and may lead to flexion deformities and bony ankylosis. Passive stretching and ring splints may help avoid this.

If axial involvement is present, physical measures such as exercises designed to stretch the paravertebral musculature and correct the tendency toward a kyphotic posture should be advised, especially when the cervical segment of the spine is affected. The most important intervention is to preserve normal upright posture. All of the therapeutic modalities discussed can also be applied to the axial skeleton, and orthotic devices such as corsets or neck supports can be employed in accordance with each patient's needs.

The spine in psoriatic spondylitis is often osteoporotic and susceptible to fracturing with minimal trauma. Therapy to prevent osteoporosis should form part of the medical management and prolonged bed rest should be avoided. Contact sports and heavy physical activity should be discouraged and swimming encouraged.

The use of orthoses can be helpful for some other conditions in these patients. Wrist splints may relieve the pain in the presence of carpal tunnel syndrome. In addition, splints may provide support for hand movement. Likewise, the use of canes, crutches, and walkers must be advised in order to improve ambulation and the working capacity of a given joint. Disability in psoriatic arthritis patients is generally less severe than in patients with RA. However, significant limitation occurs in approximately 11% of cases, and up to 20% of the patients may have a more severe form of the disease most often with damage to five or more joints [1,90]. To prevent this from happening, it is imperative to initiate an early comprehensive medical management program such as outlined here.

REFERENCES

1. Gladman DD, Shuckett, R, Russell ML, Thorne JC, Schachter RK. Psoriatic arthritis (PSA) – an analysis of 220 patients. Quart J Med. 1987;**238**:127–41.
2. Wright V. What is the best treatment approach for a patient with the mutilating pattern of psoriatic peripheral arthritis? Br J Rheumatol. 1989;**28**:382.
3. Rothermich NO. An extended study of indomethacin. JAMA. 1966;**195**:1102–6.
4. Zbojanova M, Trnavsky K, Ulcek F. Indocid in the treatment of psoriatic arthritis. Cesk Dermatol. 1974;**49**:129–32.
5. Kammer GM, Soter MA, Gibson DJ, Schur PH. A clinical, immunologic and HLA study of 100 patients. Semin Arthritis Rheum. 1979;**9**:75–95.
6. Scarpa R, Pucino A, Iocco M, Sollazo M, Biondi-Oriente C, Oriente P. The management of 138 psoriatic arthritis patients. Acta Derm Venereol. 1989;**146**:199–200.
7. Wright V, Moll JMH. Seronegative polyarthritis. Amsterdam: Elsevier North Holland; 1976.
8. Voorhees JJ. Leukotrienes and other lipoxygenase products in the pathogenesis and therapy of psoriasis and other dermatoses. Arch Dermatol. 1983;**119**:541–6.
9. Katayama H, Kawada A. Exacerbation of psoriasis induced by indomethacin. J Dermatol. 1981;**8**:323–5.
10. Reshad H, Hargreaves GK, Vickers CFH. Generalized pustular psoriasis precipitated by phenylbutazone and oxyphenbutazone. Br J Dermatol. 1983;**108**:111–13.
11. Meyerhoff JO. Exacerbation of psoriasis with meclofenamate. N Engl J Med. 1983;**309**:496.
12. Kragbell K, Herlin T. Benoxaprofen improves psoriasis. Arch Dermatol. 1983;**119**:548.
13. Kuliev NA. Use of mefenamic acid as a connective tissue stabilizer in treating arthropathic psoriasis. Vestnik Dermatol Venerol. 1989:**4**:54–9.
14. Gubner R, August S, Ginsberg V. Therapeutic suppression of tissue reactivity. II. Effect of aminopterin in rheumatoid arthritis and psoriasis. Am J Med Sci. 1951;**221**:176–82.
15. Black RL, O'Brien WM, Van Scott EJ, Auerbach R, Eisen AZ, Bunin JJ. Methotrexate therapy in psoriatic arthritis. JAMA. 1964;**189**:743–7.

16. Kragballe K, Zachariae E, Zachariae H. Methotrexate in psoriatic arthritis. A retrospective study. Acta Derm Venereol. 1982;**63**:165–7.
17. Zachariae E, Zachariae H. Methotrexate treatment of psoriatic arthritis. Acta Derm Venereol. 1987;**67**:270–3.
18. Wilkens RF, Williams HJ, Ward JR, et al. Randomized, double-blind, placebo-controlled trial of low-dose pulse methotrexate in psoriatic arthritis. Arthritis Rheum. 1984;**27**:376–81.
19. Espinoza LR, Zakraoui L, Espinoza CG, et al. Psoriatic arthritis: clinical response and side effects to methotrexate therapy. J Rheumatol. 1992;**12**:872–77.
20. Almeyda J, Barnardo D, Baker H, Levene GM, Landells JW. Structural and function abnormalities of the liver in psoriasis before and during methotrexate therapy. Br J Dermatol. 1972;**72**:623–31.
21. Zachariae H, Søgaard H. Liver biopsy in psoriasis. A controlled study. Dermatologica. 1973;**146**:149–55.
22. Nyfors A, Poulsen H. Liver biopsies from psoriatics related to methotrexate therapy. I. Findings in 123 consecutive non-methotrexate treated patients. Acta Path Microbiol Scand. 1976; **84**:253–61.
23. Zachariae H, Kragballe K, Søgaard H. Methotrexate-induced liver cirrhosis. Studies including serial liver biopsies during continued treatment. Br J Dermatol. 1980;**102**:407–12.
24. Zachariae H, Søgaard H. Methotrexate-induced liver cirrhosis, A follow-up. Dermatologica. 1987;**175**:178–82.
25. Newman M, Auerbach A, Feiner H, et al. The role of liver biopsies in psoriatic patients receiving long term methotrexate treatment. Improvement in liver abnormalities after cessation of treatment. Arch Dermatol. 1989;**125**:1218–24.
26. Bjorkman D, Tolman K, Clegg D, Ward J. Hepatic fibrosis and serum procollagen-III peptide levels in methotrexate therapy for rheumatoid arthritis. Clin Res. 1991;**39**:34A.
27. Kaplan MM, Knox TA, Arora J. Primary biliary cirrhosis treated with low-dose oral pulse methotrexate. Ann Intern Med. 1988;**109**:249–51.
28. Kaplin MM, Arora J, Pincus SH. Primary sclerosing cholangitis and low dose oral pulse methotrexate therapy. Clinical and histological response. Ann Intern Med. 1987;**105**:231–5.
29. Gilbert SC, Klintmaln G, Menter A, Silverman A. Methotrexate-induced cirrhosis requiring liver transplantation in three patients with psoriasis. A word of caution in light of the expanding use of this 'steroid-sparing' agent. Arch Intern Med. 1990;**150**:889–91.
30. Dorwart B, Gall EP, Schumacher HR, Krauser RE. Chrysotherapy in psoriatic arthropathy. Arthritis Rheum. 1978;**21**:513–5.
31. Richter MB, Kinsella P, Corbett M. Gold in psoriatic arthropathy. Ann Rheum Dis 1980;**39**:279–80.
32. Koo E, Sesztak M. Gold salts in the treatment of psoriatic arthritis. Orv Hetil. 1990;**131**:179–81.
33. Salvarani C, Zizzi F, Macchioni P, et al. Clinical response to auranofin in patients with psoriatic arthritis. Clin Rheumatol. 1989;**8**:54–7.
34. Palit J, Hill J, Capell HA, et al. A multicenter double-blind comparison of auranofin, intramuscular gold thiomalate and placebo in patients with psoriatic arthritis. Br J Rheumatol. 1990;**29**:280–3.
35. Carette S, Calin A, McCafferty JP, Wallin BA. A double-blind placebo-controlled study of auranofin in patients with psoriatic arthritis. Arthritis Rheum. 1989;**32**:158–65.
36. Smith DL, Wernick R. Exacerbation of psoriasis by chrysotherapy. Arch Dermatol. 1991;**127**:268–70.
37. Cornbelt T. Action of synthetic malarial drugs on psoriasis. J Invest Dermatol. 1956;**26**:435–8.
38. Mackenzie A, Scherbel A. Chloroquine and hydroxychloroquine. Clin Rheum Dis. 1980;**15**:545–7.
39. Trnavsky K, Zbojanova M, Vlcek F. Antimalarials in psoriatic arthritis. J Rheumatol. 1983;**10**:883–5.
40. Slagel GA, James WD. Plaquenil-induced erythroderma. J Am Acad Dermatol. 1985:**12**:857–9.
41. Price R, Gibson T. D-Penicillamine and psoriatic arthropathy. Br J Rheumatol. 1986;**25**:228.
42. Ferbert A. D-penicillamine-induced ocular myasthenia in psoriatic arthritis. Nervenarzt. 1989;**60**:576–9.
43. Seideman P. Sulphasalazine treatment of psoriatic arthritis. Br J Rheumatol. 1990;**29**:491–2.
44. Farr M, Kitas GD, Waterhouse L, Jubb R, Felix-Davies DD, Bacon PA. Treatment of psoriatic arthritis and sulphasalazine. Clin Rheumatol. 1988;**7**:372–7.
45. Farr M, Kitas GD, Waterhouse L, Jubb R, Felix-Davies DD, Bacon PA. Sulphasalazine in psoriatic arthritis. A double-blind placebo-controlled study. Br J Rheumatol. 1990;**29**:46–9.
46. Gupta AK, Ellis CN, Siegel MT, et al. Sulfasalazine improves psoriasis: a double-blind analysis. Arch Dermatol. 1990;**126**:487–93.
47. Chieregato GC, Leoni A. Treatment of psoriatic arthropathy with etretinate. A two-year follow-up. Acta Dermatol Venereol. 1986;**66**:321–4.
48. Seppala J, Laulainen M, Reunala T. Comparison of etretinate (Tigason) and parenteral gold in the treatment of psoriatic arthropathy. Clin Rheumatol. 1988;**7**:498–503.
49. Giompi ML, Bazzichi L, Marotta G, Pasero G. Tigason (etretinate) treatment in psoriatic arthritis. Int J Tissue Reactions. 1988;**10**:25–7.
50. Brinckerhoff CE, McMillan RM, Dayer JM, Harris ED. Inhibition by retinoid acid of collagenase production in rheumatoid synovial cells. N Engl J Med. 1980;**303**:432–6.
51. Peck GL, Olsen TG, Yoder FW, et al. Prolonged remissions of cystic and conglobate acne with 13 cis retinoid acid. N Engl J Med. 1979;**300**:329–33.
52. Klinkhoff AV, Gertner E, Chalmers A, et al. Pilot study of etretinate in psoriatic arthritis. J Rheumatol. 1989;**16**:789–91.
53. Ruzicka T, Somnerburg C, Braun-Falco O, et al. Efficiency of acitretin in combination with UV-B in the treatment of severe psoriasis. Arch Dermatol. 1990;**126**:482–6.
54. Fradin MS, Ellis CN, Voorhees JJ. Management of patients and side effects during cyclosporin therapy for cutaneous disorders. J Am Acad Dermatol. 1990;**23**:1265–73.
55. Steinsson K, Jonsdottir I, Valdimarsson H. Cyclosporin A in psoriatic arthritis. An open study. Ann Rheum Dis. 1990;**49**:603–6.
56. Gupta AK, Matteson EL, Ellis CN, et al. Cyclosporin in the treatment of psoriatic arthritis. Arch Dermatol. 1990;**125**:507–10.
57. Wilke WS, Sexton C, Steck W. Parenteral nitrogen mustard for inflammatory arthritis. Cleve Clin J Med. 1990;**57**:643–6.
58. Baum J, Hurd E, Lewis D, Ferguson JL, Ziff M. Treatment of psoriatic arthritis with 6-mercaptopurine. Arthritis Rheum. 1973:**16**:139–47.
59. Levy J, Paulus HE, Barnett EV, Sokoloff M, Bangert R, Pearson CM. A double-blind controlled evaluation of azathioprine treatment in rheumatoid arthritis and psoriatic arthritis. Arthritis Rheum. 1972;**15**:116.
60. Smith EL, Pincus SH, Donovan L, Holick MF. A novel approach for the evaluation and treatment of psoriasis. J Am Acad Dermatol. 1988;**19**:516–28.
61. Hukins D, Felson DT, Holick M. Treatment of psoriatic arthritis with oral 1,25-dihydroxyvitamin D_3. A pilot study. Arthritis Rheum. 1990;**33**:1723–7.
62. Weber G, Klughardt G, Neidhardt M, Galle K, Frey H, Geiger A. Treatment of psoriasis with somatostatin. Arch Derm Res. 1982;**272**:31–6.
63. Matucci-Cerinic M, Lotti T, Cappugi P, Boddi V, Fattorini L, Panconesi E. Somatostatin treatment of psoriatic arthritis. Intern J Dermatol. 1988;**27**:56–8.
64. Clemmensen OJ, Siggaard-Andersen J, Worm AM, Stahl D, Frost F, Bloch I. Psoriatic arthritis treated with oral zinc sulphate. Br J Dermatol. 1980;**103**:411–5.
65. Frigo A, Tambalo C, Bambara LM, et al. Zinc sulfate in the treatment of psoriatic arthritis. Rec Prog Med. 1988;**80**:577–81.
66. Leibovici V, Statter M, Weinrauch L, Tzfoni E, Matzner Y. Effect of zinc therapy on neutrophil chemotaxis in psoriasis. Isr J Med Sci. 1988;**26**:306–9.
67. Perlman SG, Gerber LH, Roberts RM, Nigra TP, Barth WF. Photochemotherapy and psoriatic arthritis. Ann Intern Med. 1979;**91**:717–22.
68. Grishko TN. The unsuitability of using corticosteroid preparations in the treatment of psoriasis in children. Vestnik Dermatol Venerol. 1989;**9**:69–71 .
69. Wahba A, Cohen AS. Therapeutic trials with oral colchicine in psoriasis. Acta Dermatol Venereol. 1980;**60**:515–20.
70. Seideman P, Fjellner B, Johannesson A. Psoriatic arthritis treated with oral colchicine. J Rheumatol. 1987;**14**:777–9.
71. Fierlbeck G, Rassner G. Treatment of psoriasis and psoriatic arthritis with interferon gamma. J Invest Dermatol. 1990;**95**:138s–141s.
72. Atherton DJ, Wells RS, Laurent MR, Williams YF. Razoxane (ICRF 159) in the treatment of psoriasis. Br J Dermatol. 1980;**102**:307–17.
73. Nielsen HJ, Neilsen H, Georgsen J. Ranitidine for improvement of treatment-resistant psoriasis. Arch Dermatol. 1991;**127**:270.
74. Buskila D, Sukenik S, Holcberg G, Horowitz J. Improvement of psoriatic arthritis in a patient treated with bromocriptine for hyperprolactinemia. J Rheumatol. 1991;**18**:611–2.
75. Yazici H, Bilge N, Kinay M. Total lymphoid irradiation for psoriatic arthritis. Arthritis Rheum. 1983;**26**:1052–4.
76. Grivet V, Carli M, MacDonald F, Cancelli M, Pristera G. Plasmapheresis. An additional treatment of psoriatic arthritis. Acta Dermatol Venereol. 1989;**146**:130–1.
77. Wilfert H, Honigsmann H, Steiner G, Smolen J, Wolff K. Treatment of psoriatic arthritis by extra-corporeal photochemotherapy. Br J Dermatol. 1990;**122**:225–32.
78. Greiner J, Miehe M, Weber H, Stoimenov A, Sonnichsen N, Diezel W. Therapeutic use of splenopentin (DA SP-5) in patients with psoriasis arthropathica. Dermatol Monatsschr. 1990;**176**:157–62.
79. Caperton EM, Heim-Duthoy KL, Matzke GR, Peterson PK, Johnson RC. Ceftriaxone therapy of chronic inflammatory arthritis. A double-blind placebo controlled trial. Arch Intern Med. 1990;**150**:1677–82.
80. Kaplan MH, Sadick NS, Wieder J, Farber BF, Neidt GW. Antipsoriatic effects of zidovudine in human immunodeficiency virus-associated psoriasis. J Am Acad Dermatol. 1989;**20**:76–82.
81. Marcusson JA, Wetterberg L. Peptide-T in the treatment of psoriasis and psoriatic arthritis. A case report. Acta Dermatol Venereol. 1989;**69**:86–8.
82. Herzog C, Walker C, Muller W, et al. Anti-CD4 antibody treatment of patients with rheumatoid arthritis. I. Effect on clinical course and circulating T cells. J Autoimmun. 1989;**2**:627–42.
83. Seibel MJ, Bruckle W, Respondek M, Beveridge T, Schnyder J, Muller W. Initial clinical experience in the treatment of chronic polyarthritis with a new monokine release inhibitor. Z Rheumatol. 1989;**48**:147–51.
84. Eedy DJ, Burrows D, Bridges JM, Jones FGC. Clearance of severe psoriasis after allogenic bone marrow transplantation. Br Med J. 1990;**300**:908.
85. Szanto E. Long-term follow-up of yttrium treated knee joint arthritis. Scand J Rheum. 1977;**6**:209–12.
86. Lambert JR, Wright V. Surgery in patients with psoriasis and arthritis. Rheumatol Rehab. 1979;**18**:35–40.
87. Stern SH, Insall JN, Windsor RE, Inglis AE, Dines DM. Total knee arthroplasty in patients with psoriasis. Clin Orthop Rel Res. 1989;**248**:108–10.
88. Gerber LH. Psoriatic arthritis. Pharmacologic, surgical, and rehabilitative management. In: Gerber LH, Espinoza LR, eds. Psoriatic Arthritis. New York: Grune & Stratton; 1985:147–66.
89. Gutierrez FJ, Martinez-Osuna P, Seleznick M, Espinoza LR. Rheumatologic rehabilitation for patients with HIV. In: Mukand J, ed. Rehabilitation for patients with HIV disease. New York: McGraw-Hill; 1991:77–94.
90. Gladman DD, Stafford-Brady F, Chang CH, Lewandowski K, Russell ML. Longitudinal study of clinical and radiological progression in psoriatic arthritis. J Rheumatol. 1990;**17**:809–12.

PSORIATIC ARTHRITIS

24

PRACTICAL PROBLEMS

PSORIATIC ARTHRITIS *SINE* PSORIASIS

Werner F Barth

Definition of the Problem
In most patients with psoriatic arthritis, psoriasis is present many years before or appears concomitantly with the onset of arthritis. In a small percentage of adults, and more often in children, the arthritis appears before the classical skin or nail changes. The recognition of psoriatic arthritis *sine* psoriasis may thus pose a diagnostic problem.

Typical Case
A 37-year-old White male presented with a painful right knee and swollen calf of 3 weeks' duration. He worked with the Corps of Engineers and spent a good part of every day walking. His history and physical examination were unremarkable except for synovitis in the knee and swelling in the calf and lower thigh. A diagnosis of pseudophlebitis was suspected. The venogram was negative, but the right knee arthrogram confirmed dissection of a popliteal cyst into the calf. The knee fluid contained white blood cells at 7098/mm^3, 72% being polymorphonuclear leukocytes and the remainder mononuclear cells. No crystals were seen. His rheumatoid factor was negative and the erythrocyte sedimentation rate (ESR) only mildly elevated. Following a steroid injection into the knee, symptoms totally resolved.

He was not seen again until 6 years later when he presented with a painful left knee and swollen calf. The joint fluid again showed a low-grade inflammatory reaction similar to the first one and he again responded to an intra-articular steroid injection.

He returned again, 11 years after his initial presentation, with recurrent joint symptoms, now involving the left knee, left ankle and right great toe. This time, and for the first time, he had lesions of psoriasis on the knees and elbow. The great toe had a characteristic 'sausage' appearance. The diagnosis of psoriatic arthritis was finally established and nonsteroidal anti-inflammatory drug (NSAID) therapy instituted.

Diagnostic Problems
This case illustrates the development of psoriasis more than 10 years after the onset of an inflammatory polyarthritis and the lengthy follow up that may be necessary before the diagnosis is established. In some patients, an inflammatory polyarthritis may be present for several years and the diagnosis remain unclear until the classical skin or nail changes finally appear. In other patients, psoriasis may be present in so-called hidden areas and even unbeknown to the patient. It is important to examine the scalp, navel and the intergluteal cleft where the classical changes of psoriasis may be present. The diagnosis of psoriatic arthritis is based on the clinical presentation without specific laboratory tests and is made only after other possibilities have been excluded.

Major clues to the diagnosis (Fig. 24.1) include sausage digits, asymmetry, oligoarticular presentation and distal interphalangeal (DIP) joint involvement in a patient who is serologically negative and lacks subcutaneous nodules. The clinical course is characterized by remissions and exacerbations with long intervals between them. Radiographic clues (Fig. 24.2) include fluffy periostitis, new bone formation (see Fig. 24.3), lack of para-articular osteoporosis, widening of the joint space and asymmetric sacroiliitis. Asymmetry is sometimes seen in the syndesmophytes in patients with psoriatic spondylitis.

CLINICAL CLUES TO THE DIAGNOSIS OF PSORIATIC ARTHRITIS *SINE* PSORIASIS
Positive family history for psoriasis
Sausage digits
Asymmetric, oligoarticular involvement
Distal interphalangeal joint involvement
Waxing and waning course with frequent remissions
Absent serum rheumatoid factor
Lack of subcutaneous nodules

Fig. 24.1 Clinical clues to the diagnosis of psoriatic arthritis *sine* psoriasis.

RADIOLOGIC CLUES TO THE DIAGNOSIS OF PSORIATIC ARTHRITIS *SINE* PSORIASIS
Lack of para-articular osteoporosis
Widening of joint space
Fluffy periostitis
Arthritis mutilans
Asymmetry
Peripheral joints
Sacroiliitis
Syndesmophytes

Fig. 24.2 Radiologic clues to the diagnosis of psoriatic arthritis *sine* psoriasis.

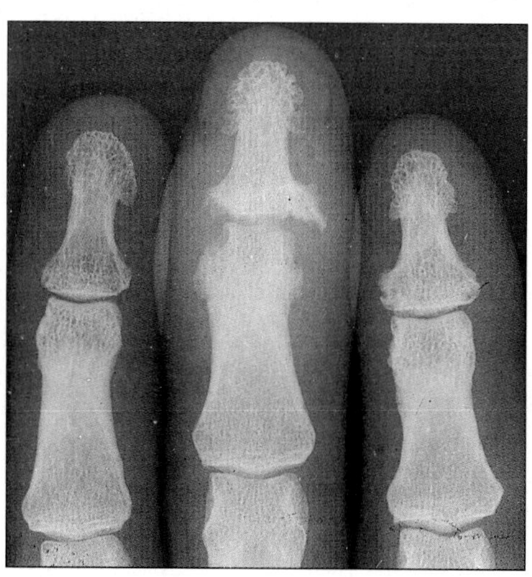

Fig. 24.3 Typical erosive arthritis due to psoriasis. Note the new bone growth around the erosions of the distal interphalangeal joint which distinguish this from rheumatoid erosive changes.

A positive family history is often a helpful clue. The clinical picture most closely resembles reactive arthritis but differs in the lack of urethritis and in the low incidence of ocular involvement.

REFERENCES

Avila R, Pugh DG, Slocumb CH, Winkelmann RK. Psoriatic arthritis: a roentgenographic study. Radiology. 1960;**75**:691–701.

Brower AC. The radiologic features of psoriatic arthritis. In: Gerber LH, Espinoza, LR, eds. Psoriatic arthritis. Orlando: Grune & Stratton; 1985;125–46.

Kammer GM, Soter NA, Gibson DJ, Schur PH. Psoriatic arthritis: a clinical, immunologic and HLA study of 100 patients. Semin Arthritis Rheum. 1979;**9**:75–9.

DOES THE PRESENCE OF EXTENSIVE SKIN INVOLVEMENT INFLUENCE THE THERAPY OF PSORIATIC ARTHRITIS?

Verna Wright

Definition of the Problem

In the majority of cases of psoriatic arthritis, both arthritis and skin lesions require only first-line treatment: NSAIDs and analgesics for arthritis, dithranol and coal tar for psoriasis. However, exceptionally, the severity of either or both components necessitate second-line therapy, the choice of which may be influenced by the associated pathology.

The Typical Case

AC is a 52-year-old man who developed patches of psoriasis vulgaris at the age of 33. This was controlled successfully by topical therapy. At the age of 43, he was referred to hospital with mild arthralgia in the hands but no obvious inflammatory synovitis. At the age of 50, both skin and joints deteriorated markedly: he presented with more than 50% of body surface involved with psoriatic plaques (Fig. 24.4), together with pain and stiffness in his neck, shoulders, and hips and he had an obvious arthropathy of the small joints of the hands. Radiographs showed his cervical spine was fused from C5 to C7; he had bilateral grade 3 sacroiliitis, occasional syndesmophytes in the lumbar spine, and an erosive arthritis particularly involving scattered DIP joints of the fingers. He was treated with ultraviolet B radiation (UVB), which caused erythema. Shortly after this, he was started on methotrexate for what amounted to generalized erythrodermic psoriasis and, within 3 weeks, both skin and joints had improved markedly. He subsequently developed nausea from methotrexate and his skin treatment was changed to psoralen and ultraviolet A (PUVA) and, again, as the skin improved so did his joint symptoms. At a later time he was started on etretinate therapy together with PUVA (REPUVA), which cleared his psoriasis completely and at the same time improved his joint symptoms. He has recently started hyroxychloroquine for persistent synovitis in peripheral joints.

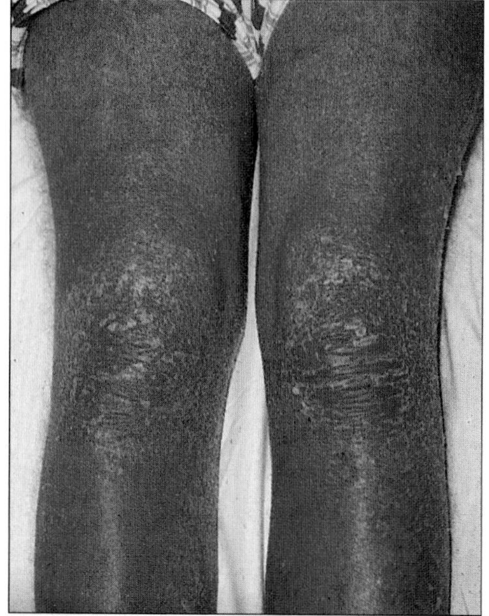

Fig. 24.4 Severe psoriasis with arthritis of the right knee. There is also a small joint effusion.

Diagnostic Problems

In cases of severe involvement of both skin and joints a combined dermatologic–rheumatologic approach is required (Fig. 24.5). The decision to start second-line treatment must be based primarily on the severity of involvement of each particular system, but the choice of which second-line agent to use would depend on the extent and severity of involvement of the other system (Fig. 24.6). Thus, if the peripheral arthropathy is particularly severe, requiring second-line treatment, but the skin involvement is only mild, then a choice of therapy with either sulfasalazine or intramuscular gold salts would be appropriate (Fig. 24.6). If, however, severe concomitant involvement of skin is present then an agent with therapeutic effect on both skin and joints, such as methotrexate, azathioprine or etretinate, would be indicated. In some patients, the severity of both skin and joint involvement vary together, and in these cases successful treatment of skin may also improve the arthropathy (although the converse does not occur). Generally speaking, the outcome of successful dermato-

AN APPROACH TO THE MANAGEMENT OF SKIN AND JOINT LESIONS IN PSORIATIC ARTHRITIS

- Base decision to start second-line therapy on severity of each particular system
- Skin and joint symptoms may fluctuate together so that specific dermatologic therapies may help the joints indirectly
- A number of preparations may help both skin and joint problems, including methotrexate, azathioprine, cyclosporin A and etretinate
- Selection of appropriate drug depends on several factors, including medical and social factors, and severity of joint and skin lesions

Fig. 24.5 An approach to the management of skin and joint lesions in psoriatic arthritis.

SECOND-LINE DRUGS USED IN PSORIASIS AND PSORIATIC ARTHRITIS		
Arthropathy alone		Dose
Antimalarials	Chloroquine, hydroxychloroquine	5mg/kg/day
Sulfasalazine	Benefits axial and peripheral arthropathy	40mg/kg/day
Gold compounds	Oral gold, auranofin Gold sodium thiomalate	6mg/day 50mg weekly
Arthropathy and skin		
Methotrexate		Oral or intramuscular 15–30mg weekly
Azathioprine		1–3mg/kg/day orally
Etretinate		0.5–1.0mg/kg/day orally
Cyclosporin A		3–5mg/kg/day orally

Fig. 24.6 Second-line drugs used in psoriasis and psoriatic arthritis.

logic treatment is 'normal' skin but the outcome of successful rheumatologic treatment will depend on the amount of joint damage incurred before remission is achieved. For this reason, dermatologists can employ short-duration treatments without fear of long-term skin damage but the rheumatologist may have to use long-duration treatment to ensure maintained improvement.

Therapeutic Options

Drugs may be divided into three groups: agents with favorable action on the course of the arthropathy but with no effect on the skin, agents that affect the skin but not the arthropathy directly, and agents that affect both skin and joints favorably.

Drugs with a favorable effect on course of arthritis but no effect on the skin

Although antimalarials have been shown to have a beneficial effect on the course of the arthritis associated with psoriasis, traditionally these drugs have been avoided because of early reports of severe dermatologic reactions and worsening of psoriatic skin lesions. Recent experience in my unit with hydroxychloroquine and chloroquine phosphate at doses less than 5mg/kg/day (Fig. 24.6) has been favorable without any adverse skin reactions. Gold, both injectable and oral, improve the arthropathy associated with psoriasis and appear to have little adverse effect on the course of the skin condition. Sulfasalazine (40mg/kg/day) provides useful antirheumatic activity and may, unlike the other second-line antiarthritic drugs, have a beneficial effect on the course of the spondylitis. Colchicine (1.5mg/day in divided doses) may be particularly helpful in arthro-osteitis and the inflammatory lesions associated with SAPHO (synovitis acne pustulosis hyperostosis osteitis).

Therapy for skin without specific benefit for joints

As far as can be discerned traditional treatments for psoriasis, such as dithranol and coal tar, have no direct effect on the arthropathy. Both UVB and PUVA are effective therapies for moderately severe involvement of skin by psoriasis. As the skin improves so may the peripheral, but not the axial, arthropathy.

Drugs with a favorable effect on both arthritis and skin lesions

Methotrexate either orally or intramuscular at a dose of 15–30mg weekly, azathioprine at a dose of 1–3mg/kg/day orally and cyclosporin A at a dose of 3–5mg/kg/day are all effective treatments for both skin and joint lesions in psoriatic arthritis. More recently, retinoids such as etretinate (at a dose of 50–150mg daily) have been shown to be effective for the arthritis associated with psoriasis.

Which drug to start would depend on a number of factors, including severity of psoriasis and type of psoriasis (etretinate is particularly good for generalized pustular psoriasis), social circumstances (methotrexate therapy requires weekly blood tests), alcohol intake and previous drug therapy. Particular precautions must be taken with etretinate in young females, who are liable to become pregnant, and close surveillance of serum lipids must be made while on this drug. It must be emphasized that there is no hierarchical arrangement of these drugs and that a decision to start one particular drug in favor of another is based on a number of factors, as indicated above. Currently, in combined therapy for skin and joint disease, the most popular drug is methotrexate.

Conclusions

Where extensive skin involvement is present, treatment of psoriatic arthritis requires a combined rheumatologic–dermatologic approach, using powerful drugs which may benefit both conditions. Rational drug selection requires familiarity with drug side-effect profiles, treatment schedules and monitoring protocols, and is governed by both medical and social factors.

REFERENCES

Farr M, Kitas GD, Waterhouse L, Jubb R, Felix-Davies D, Bacon PA. Sulphasalazine in psoriatic arthritis: a double-blind placebo controlled study. Br J Rheumatol. 1990;**29**:46–9.

Gupta AK, Matteson EL, Ellis CN, et al. Cyclosporin in the treatment of psoriatic arthritis. Archiv Dermatol. 1989;**125**:507–10.

Hopkins R, Bird HA, Jones H, et al. A double-blind controlled trial of etretinate (Tigason) and ibuprofen in psoriatic arthritis. Ann Rheum Dis. 1985;**44**:189–93.

Palit J, Hill J, Capell HA, et al. A multicentre double-blind comparison of auranofin, intra-muscular gold thiomalate and placebo in patients with psoriatic arthritis. Br J Rheumatol. 1990;**29**:280–2.

Perlman SG, Gerber LH, Roberts RM, Nigra TP, Barth WF. Photochemotherapy and psoriatic arthritis. Ann Intern Med. 1979;**91**:717–22.

PSORIATIC ARTHRITIS IN AN INDIVIDUAL WITH HIV INFECTION

Andrew CS Keat

Definition of the Problem

Amongst the plethora of pathologic lesions occurring in association with HIV infection, both inflammatory arthritis and psoriasis are well described. In addition, arthralgia and myalgia without objective signs of inflammatory disease are common, and septic musculoskeletal lesions in those with profound immunodeficiency require particular care in diagnosis. In this population inflammatory arthritis is most often oligoarticular and seronegative, although polyarticular disease and low-grade monoarthritis may occur. The prevalence of joint and skin disorders in HIV-infected populations varies widely from one study to another, but with the exception of septic arthritis there is no clear evidence that in either case HIV itself is either a causal or predisposing factor. Nevertheless, there remains a strong clinical suspicion that both psoriasis and arthritis may be unusually severe in the presence of HIV infection, and either may be the presenting feature in an individual with undiagnosed HIV infection.

In consequence, both the dermatologist and the rheumatologist are likely to come into contact with both known HIV-infected individuals and other, apparently generally healthy, patients in whom HIV infection is present but asymptomatic. It is therefore important to be aware of risk factors for HIV infection and clinical features of this condition and fully to consider the diagnostic procedures,

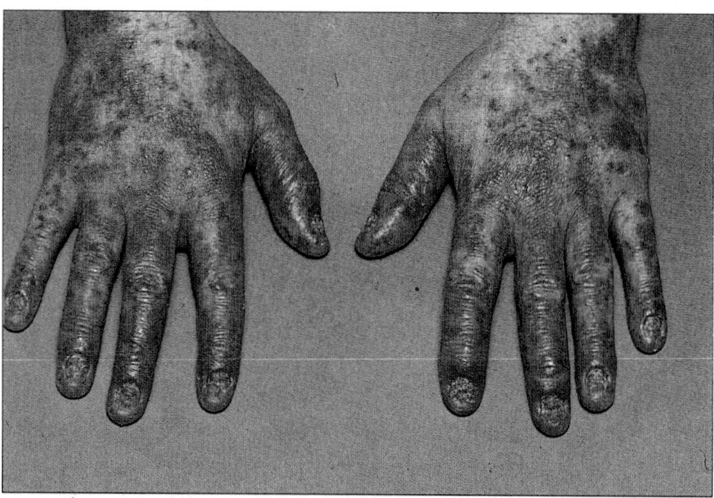

Fig. 24.7 Psoriatic lesions on the hands with cutaneous edema and nail dystrophy.

including HIV antibody testing. Moreover, although in the main the treatment of joint and skin disorders in the presence of HIV infection reflects practice in HIV-negative patients, some forms of therapy may carry special risks, and experience is now growing on which to base clinical practice in this group of patients.

Case Report

A 49-year-old male civil servant with a 4-month history of psoriasiform skin rash affecting the legs, trunk, scalp and genitals, with pustular lesions on the skin and palms, was referred to a dermatologist . For the previous 2 months he had also noticed increasingly severe thoracolumbar back pain and stiffness and pain at the right buttock, left knee, right ankle and both feet. He had become grossly disabled and was unable to work. He was therefore admitted to hospital immediately.

Clinically, he had widespread psoriasis affecting the trunk, scalp, hands (Fig. 24.7) and feet (Fig. 24.8), with an active polyarthritis with spinal pain, stiffness and restriction suggestive of spondylitis. Investigation at this time revealed an elevated ESR (Westergren) at 84mm in the first hour, negative tests for rheumatoid factor and antinuclear antibody, normal blood count, urea, alkaline phosphatase and urate, and no evidence of infection in the urogenital tract, gut or respiratory tract. Radiographs of the affected joints, including the sacroiliac joints and spine, were normal. A skin biopsy confirmed the diagnosis of psoriasis and an isotope bone scan showed increased uptake of technetium at the clinically affected peripheral joints but not in the spine or sacroiliac joints. An arthroscopic synovial biopsy taken from the left knee showed evidence of nonspecific synovitis and tissue typing for HLA B27 was positive.

A diagnosis of psoriatic arthritis was made and he was treated with topical dithranol, NSAIDs and physiotherapy, but both joint and skin lesions remained disabling and resistant to therapy. More aggressive therapy, including cytotoxic drugs, was therefore considered and the history and findings were reviewed. The patient was single and until 5 years before had worked in a 'white collar' capacity in South Africa. Apart from an episode of gonorrhea 13 years earlier he had been quite well until this episode, and the family history was unremarkable except for the development of a mild scaly rash over the knees of one sister. Because of the unusually aggressive, unremitting nature of the disease and the need to consider potentially toxic therapy, it was considered necessary to exclude HIV infection. Enquiry revealed that the patient was bisexual with numerous sexual contacts both in Africa and the UK, though not with prostitutes. He remained sexually active and did not usually use condoms. He had never used intravenous drugs nor had he received any blood products. He considered that exposure to HIV infection was possible but was reluctant to be tested for this condition. However, he did agree to discuss the issues, especially those relating to confidentiality, prognosis if positive, and such financial matters as personal insurance policies, with an experienced counselor. After due consideration he consented to testing and both enzyme-linked immunosorbant assay (ELISA) and Western blot tests for HIV antibody were positive. In spite of the normal routine blood count the $CD4^+$ lymphocyte count was reduced, $0.33 \times 10^9/mm^3$, with inversion of the T-helper/T-suppressor ratio. In view of his good general health and the absence of any opportunistic infections or lesions, the diagnosis of HIV infection CDC grade II was made.

No specific treatment for the HIV infection was indicated, nor was prophylaxis for pulmonary infection with *Pneumocystis aeruginosa,*

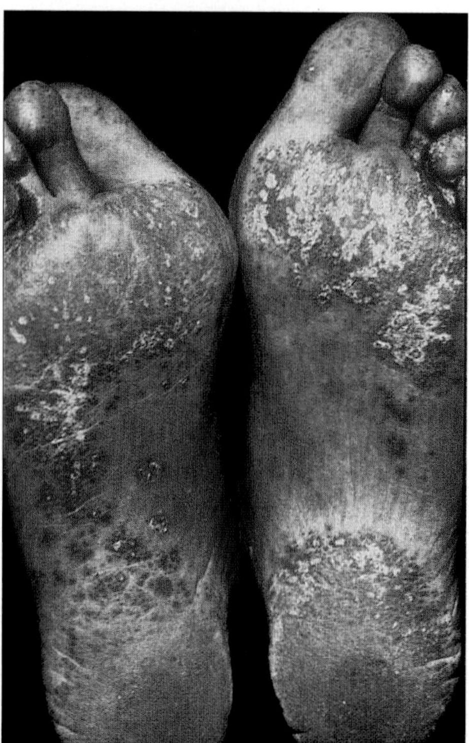

Fig. 24.8 Pustular psoriasis on the soles of the feet.

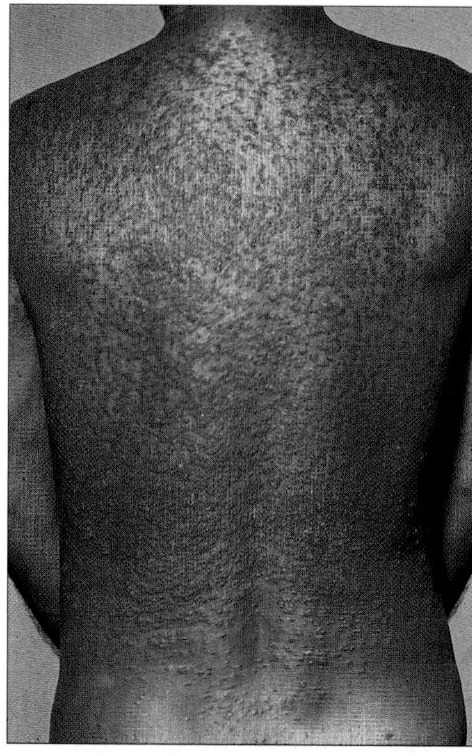

Fig. 24.9 Extensive lesions of guttate psoriasis after exposure to bright sunlight.

but follow-up was arranged. Methotrexate was considered inappropriate therapy and he was treated conservatively for the psoriasis and arthritis, but with the addition of etretinate and local steroid injections. On this regimen he gradually improved. After nearly 6 months he was able to return to work with only residual pain related to plantar fasciitis which was resistant to local steroid injections. A year later the patient, now generally feeling well, visited the Canary Islands for a sunny holiday. Within a few days of sunbathing he developed widespread guttate psoriasiform lesions (Fig. 24.9) with recurrence of pains at the left knee, ankles and heels. He required further admission to hospital for topical treatment of the skin, light exclusion with local steroid injections and NSAID therapy, on this occasion with a good response.

Three years after his initial presentation he developed a febrile illness attributed to septicemia secondary to a *Pseudomonas aeruginosa* urinary tract infection. He had had troublesome oral candidiasis and had lost 11kg in weight over the previous 12 months. By this time the $CD4^{+}$ lymphocyte count had fallen further and treatment with zidovudine was introduced, along with co-trimoxazole as prophylaxis against *P. carinii* infection, and intermittent antifungal treatment with fluconazole. Antibiotic treatment for the septicemia was rapidly successful and, in spite of the evident immunodeficiency and episodes of bacterial and fungal infection, he has remained reasonably well with only intermittent exacerbations of joint pain and enthesopathy, mainly at the heels.

Radiographs of the spine and peripheral joints have not revealed erosive damage, only the development of plantar spurs at both calcaneii. Good control of the skin disease has been maintained since the introduction of zidovudine

Diagnosis

Diagnosis of arthritis

The diagnosis of psoriatic arthritis is clinically apparent and readily confirmed by routine investigations. Arthroscopic examination and synovial biopsy is commonly useful in refining the diagnosis but in instances of HIV exposes the operator and other staff to significant risk. In retrospect, it was unwise to use this procedure in the case described above, and exclusion of HIV and hepatitis B infection by appropriate measures prior to such procedures should now be mandatory.

Diagnosis of HIV infection

In the case illustrated there were virtually no grounds to suspect the diagnosis, and no clinical features were related directly to it, the issue being raised by the severity of the psoriatic arthritis and the need to consider treatment with methotrexate. In practice, severity of arthritis or psoriasis should not be especially linked with HIV infection, although in some HIV-infected individuals particularly severe lesions are seen. However, the history can give clear clues as to the risk of HIV infection. The past history of sexually transmitted disease can provide a ready entry to enquiry about sexual orientation and exposure. A high number of sexual partners, including homosexual men outside of a stable relationship, and the lack of 'safe sex' practices indicates a clear high risk of HIV infection. Indeed, the patient may be aware of the possibility and freely discuss it. Consideration of other sexually transmitted diseases, including hepatitis B and syphilis, is also important, as is enquiry regarding other risk factors, including transfusion of blood products and intravenous drug abuse.

Testing for HIV antibody and lymphocyte subsets should be discussed with the patient, with expert counseling, before consent is obtained. In this way, the impact of the positive result can be anticipated and managed. Establishment of the diagnosis is vital in guiding the management of the clinical condition, principally by avoiding cytotoxic therapy and also in allowing regular surveillance of the immunodeficiency, allowing appropriate and timely introduction of zidovudine and PCP prophylaxis.

Safety

Handling of clinical samples in the laboratory should always involve adequate precautions against transmissible agents and should not therefore pose special problems. However, procedures such as arthroscopy, in which both the operator and others close by may be splashed by joint fluid or blood or may be exposed to an aerosol, clearly carry higher risk. Ideally, a remote viewing system should be used to increase the distance between the patient and the operator's face, and the diagnostic or therapeutic value of the procedure should be assessed in the light of the likelihood of HIV or other transmissible infection. Formal HIV testing before such procedures should not be essential, although the likelihood of infection must be considered and appropriate precautions taken at all times.

Therapy

Current experience indicates that most modalities of treatment for both arthritis and psoriasis may be used safely in HIV-infected individuals. This includes oral and injected steroids, though scrupulous care must be taken to exclude joint infection, as the classical signs of bacterial sepsis may be diminished or absent. Anecdotal evidence and basic principles indicate that cytotoxic therapy may carry special risks in this population of progression of HIV disease; drugs such as methotrexate and azathioprine should therefore be avoided in general, and decisions to use them in a patient with psoriatic arthritis should be met with the question 'has HIV infection been satisfactorily excluded?'

REFERENCES

Rowe IF. Arthritis in the aquired immunodeficiency syndrome and other viral infections. Curr Opin Rheumatol. 1991;**3**:621–7.

Arnett FC, Reveille JD, Duvic M. Psoriasis and psoriatic arthritis asscociated with human immunodeficiency virus infection. Rheum Dis Clin N Am. 1991;**17**:59–78.

Calabrese LH, Kelley DM, Myers A, O'Connell M, Easley K. Rheumatic symptoms and human immunodeficiency virus infection. Arthritis Rheum. 1991;**34**:257–63.

GOUT AND PSEUDOGOUT

25

GOUT

Michael G Cohen & Bryan T Emmerson

Definition
- Gout is a syndrome caused by an inflammatory response to the formation of monosodium urate monohydrate (MSUM) crystals which develop secondary to hyperuricemia.
- Acute and chronic forms are recognized. Hyperuricemia may be due to environmental and/or genetic factors.

Clinical features
- Most commonly affects middle-aged males.
- Acute and usually relapsing self-limiting arthropathy.
- Chronic form associated with tophus formation and bone and joint destruction.
- Commonly associated with obesity, heavy alcohol intake, hypertension, renal impairment and diuretic use.
- Target areas – first metatarsophalangeal joints (insteps, heels, ankles and knees).

EPIDEMIOLOGY

The urate concentrations in various populations have been studied extensively [1–15]. Furthermore, the risk of developing gout at a particular urate concentration has been the subject of several studies. However, the epidemiology of gout is different from that of hyperuricemia.

Hyperuricemia

Mean urate concentrations are age and sex dependent [2,3]. Prepubertally, the mean concentration is approximately 3.5mg/dl (0.21mmol/l), although there is probably a slow increase with increasing age. In males, there is a steep rise in urate concentrations at puberty to a mean of approximately 5.2mg/dl (0.31mmol/l) but, thereafter, there is no consistent rise with increasing age. In females, there is probably a very small rise at puberty with concentrations either remaining stable or slowly increasing until there is a more definite increment associated with the menopause. Premenopausally, the mean urate concentration in females is about 4.0mg/dl (0.24mmol/l) whereas it increases to 4.7mg/dl (0.28 mmol/l) after the menopause [2].

Hyperuricemia has been defined as a serum or plasma urate concentration greater than 7.0mg/dl (0.42mmol/l) in males and 6.0mg/dl (0.36 mmol/l) in females. It is important to note that these figures have not been calculated to be the mean plus two standard deviations of the serum urate concentrations of the population but rather represent a 'desirable' upper limit in a manner analogous with the current recommendations with regard to cholesterol concentrations. Despite the definition of hyperuricemia initially being determined somewhat arbitrarily, the choice of the particular values has been justified over time by the clinical applicability with respect to diagnosis as well as by defining a subgroup of the population at risk for the subsequent development of gout. In different populations there is considerable variation in the percentage of people with hyperuricemia.

INCIDENCE OF GOUT IN RELATION TO SERUM URATE CONCENTRATIONS		
Incidence (per 1000)		Serum urate concentration (mg/dl)
Per year	5 year cumulative	
0.8	5.0	<7.0 (0.42mmol/l)
0.9	6.0	7.0–7.9 (0.42–0.47mmol/l)
4.1	9.8	8.0–8.9 (0.48–0.53mmol/l)
49	220	>9.0 (0.54mmol/l)

Fig. 25.1 Incidence of gout in males in relation to serum urate concentrations [15].

Gout

Difficulty in determining the precise incidence rate and prevalence of gout relates to the remitting and relapsing nature of the disease, as well as the propensity to misdiagnosis by patients and, to a lesser extent, by clinicians. The difficulty is highlighted by the higher prevalence noted with patient-reported gout compared with physician-diagnosed gout, a disparity which is even greater in females than males. In addition, the epidemiology of gout is changing (e.g. the ratio of males to females afflicted with gout was formerly 20:1 but is now 2–7:1) [13,14]. This is probably related to changes in lifestyle, drugs and increasing longevity. Even so, gout is still recognized as the most common inflammatory arthropathy in males over 40 years of age.

Gout is rare in children and premenopausal females and is uncommon in males under 30 years of age. The peak age of onset in males is between 40 and 50 years whereas it is somewhat later in females. It will then often be associated with identifiable causes of hyperuricemia such as concomitant thiazide diuretic therapy.

The plasma urate concentration is the single most important determinant of the risk of developing gout (Fig. 25.1) [15]. Significantly, it appears that the risk of developing gouty arthritis is similar in males and females for a particular urate concentration. This suggests that the lower prevalence of gout in females is likely a reflection of their lower urate concentrations.

Figure 25.2 summarizes the epidemiology of gout. Some of the variability between the several studies arises as a consequence of the

EPIDEMIOLOGY OF GOUT	
Peak age (years)	Males: 40–50; females: >60
Sex distribution (M:F)	2–7:1
Prevalence rate (/1000)	Males: 5–28; females: 1–6
Annual incidence (/1000)	Males: 1–3; females: 0.2
Geography	Worldwide; regional differences may reflect environmental factors as well as racial predisposition
Genetic associations	Inherited enzyme abnormalities Inherited urate underexcretion
Environmental associations	Diet, drugs, toxins (e.g. lead)

Fig. 25.2 Epidemiology of gout. The serum or plasma urate concentration is the major determinant of risk for the development of gout.

different age ranges studied. Clearly, studies including children will give lower incidence rates and prevalence figures than those examining only adults. Although studies do show racial differences in the prevalence of hyperuricemia and gout, the relative importance of genetic and environmental factors (particularly with respect to diet) is difficult to determine. Gout was previously uncommon in ethnic Chinese as well as several groups of Polynesians but the prevalence has increased in recent years in these races. Moreover, ethnic Chinese, Polynesians, and Filipinos in different countries exhibit prevalences of hyperuricemia and gout that vary from those in their native countries [4,8,10–12]. These studies suggest that the increased prevalence of hyperuricemia and gout in these races is due to environmental factors (predominantly diet) superimposed upon a basic underexcretion of urate. On the other hand, a study of New Guineans demonstrated hyperuricemia in two population groups in absence of obesity or a Westernized diet [10].

The prevalence of tophi has decreased over the period 1948 to 1973 related to improved therapy. Yu *et al.* reported that 53% of patients in the period 1948 to 1953 had tophi in comparison with 17% in the period 1969 to 1973 [16]. Even now, however, tophaceous gout remains common in patients with untreated or inadequately treated gout.

CLINICAL FEATURES

Asymptomatic Hyperuricemia

It is important to recognize the clear distinction between hyperuricemia and gout. Hyperuricemia is clearly a risk factor for the development of gout, the risk increasing with a higher urate concentration. However, many years of hyperuricemia have usually elapsed before the development of acute gouty arthritis, and in some hyperuricemic people gout may never develop. Nonetheless, acute severe overproduction of urate, as may occur with cytotoxic chemotherapy, is associated with a high risk of acute renal failure from uric acid crystal deposition in the renal tubules.

The risk of damage beyond the musculoskeletal system from protracted hyperuricemia or recurrent attacks of gout is small. Calculi are uncommon with the annual incidence being approximately 1% in gout and 0.3% in otherwise asymptomatic hyperuricemia [17]. These may consist of either uric acid or calcium oxalate. Such calculi may cause an obstructive nephropathy and renal impairment. However, the calculi are usually passed or surgically removed with resolution of any transient renal impairment. In addition, microtophi may be deposited in the renal parenchyma and interstitial renal damage is likely to be found after 10 years of inadequately treated gout.

Acute Gout

Several sets of criteria for the diagnosis and classification of gout have been devised [18–20]. However, although these were developed principally for epidemiologic studies rather than for application to individual patients, they do highlight some of the distinctive clinical features.

Often quoted, Sydenham's classic description [21] still demonstrates the important clinical characteristics used to diagnose a typical attack of acute gout:

'The victim goes to bed and sleeps in good health. About two o'clock in the morning he is awakened by pain in the great toe; more rarely in the heel, ankle or instep. This pain is like that of a dislocation, and yet the parts feel as if cold water were poured over them. Then follows chills and shivers and a little fever. The pain, which was at first moderate, becomes more intense. With its intensity the chills and shivers increase. After a time this comes to its full height, accommodating itself to the bones and ligaments of the tarsus and metatarsus. Now it is a violent stretching and tearing of the ligaments – now it is a gnawing pain and now a pressure and tightness. So exquisite and lively meanwhile is the feeling of the part affected, that it cannot bear the weight of bedclothes nor the jar of a person walking in the room. The night is passed in torture, sleeplessness, turning of the part affected, and perpetual change of posture; the tossing about of the body being as incessant as the pain of the tortured joint, and being worse as the fit comes on. Hence the vain effort by change of posture, both in the body and the limb affected, to obtain an abatement of the pain.'

Acute gout is characterized by the rapidity of onset and build-up of pain, the exquisite nature of the pain and the swelling with associated redness of the affected joint [21,22]. In over half of the initial attacks, this occurs in the first metatarsophalangeal joint, and in time, this joint is affected in some 90% of patients with gout. Almost any joint can be affected. However, the lower limbs are involved more often than upper limbs. Symptomatic involvement of the axial joints is rare. After the first metatarsophalangeal joints, the order of frequency of involvement is the instep, heel, ankle and knee. Gout does not always need to be articular, with involvement of several sites including the olecranon bursa and the Achilles tendon being well recognized. Redness overlying the affected part is a feature that sets gout apart from most other noninfective arthropathies. Swelling can be marked and involve an entire region (Fig. 25.3). The natural history of the acute attack is variable and dependent in part on its severity. Mild attacks may resolve within one to two days. More severe attacks exhibit rapidly increasing pain reaching its peak usually within a few hours, remaining at this level for some one to three days, then slowly remitting such that the attack has often subsided within seven to ten days. It may take several weeks before very severe attacks settle completely.

Some 90% of initial attacks are monoarticular [23] and concurrent systemic features are mild or absent. Even so, occasional patients with just a single joint affected may have marked systemic features with high fever and leukocytosis suggestive of sepsis. Subsequent attacks may affect the same joint or progress to involve other joints. Later in the disease process, the incidence of polyarticular attacks increases, sometimes with a concomitant increase in the severity of systemic features. Nonetheless, these attacks still resolve completely with symptom free-intervals until finally chronic gout, in which symptoms resolve incompletely between exacerbations, becomes established. Occasionally, gout may present early in its course with polyarticular involvement and is then easily confused with other arthropathies.

In the elderly, gouty arthritis is often more indolent than that arising in younger patients and may be mistaken for osteoarthritis (OA) with a resultant delay in accurate diagnosis [24,25]. This is further complicated in some patients by the coexistence of both gout and OA, at times in the same joints (particularly Heberden's nodes) [26]. Moreover, more than one joint is involved in the initial attack in approximately 50% of patients. Antecedent and intercurrent medical disorders are common in this group.

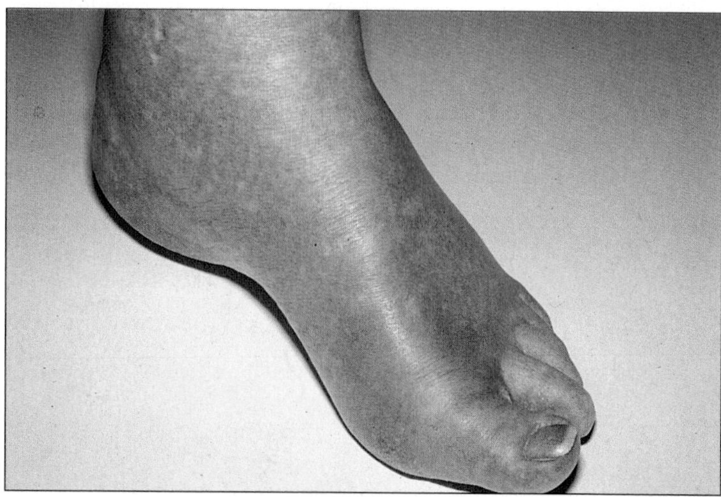

Fig. 25.3 Acute gout. There is redness of the skin of the dorsum of the foot with marked swelling of the entire foot and ankle.

Pauci- or polyarticular onset of gouty arthritis is more common in females than in males. This may largely reflect the age of onset because gout is predominantly found in women over the age of 60. In addition, tophi and concurrent diuretic use are all more common in females than males [27–30].

There are usually no obvious sequelae of an acute attack of gout apart from some desquamation overlying the affected joint. However, residual microtophi may remain in and around the joint. On rare occasions, a patient may present with a ruptured Baker's cyst which may be slow to resolve. It is likely that the resolution is slower than with noncrystal-related ruptured Baker's cysts because of the intense inflammatory response that may be associated with urate crystals.

Several factors have been recognized as precipitants of acute attacks of gout. These include acute illness, trauma, surgery, alcohol (especially beer and wines) and drugs that either increase or decrease the plasma urate concentration.

The periods between attacks when the patient is asymptomatic has sometimes been termed 'intercritical gout'. Since many patients with a single attack of gout are either not diagnosed or are overlooked in epidemiologic studies, it is not possible to determine the proportion of patients who have subsequent attacks. Nonetheless, it would appear that a significant majority of patients will have more than one attack, with the second attack usually occurring within one or two years. In a small minority of patients, many years may elapse between attacks.

Chronic Gout

Incomplete resolution of attacks early in the course of gout most often indicates a concurrent arthropathy, usually OA. Rarely, symptom free periods, characteristic of the early phase of gout, may not be seen and the disease may become chronic from an early stage. The proportion of patients who develop chronic gout is uncertain but this depends upon the number whose hyperuricemia is not controlled.

Tophi appearing within the first two years of gout are extremely rare and patients have usually suffered from gout for at least 10 years before tophi develop. Exceptions exist, particularly (i) some juvenile forms with severe hyperuricemia when tophi occasionally appear concurrently with an early, or even the first, attack of gout and (ii) secondary gout associated with myeloproliferative disorders.

Tophi appear as firm nodular or fusiform swellings (see Fig. 25.4). If there is associated significant local inflammation, the overlying skin may be erythematous. When they are indolent and when the tophi are close to the skin surface, they may appear yellowish in color. In ulcerated tophi, white chalky material may easily exude. Tophi may occur at virtually any site with the most common locations being the digits of the hands and feet. The olecranon bursa is also frequently involved. Tophi of the helix or the antihelix of the ear are classical albeit less common locations for gouty tophi.

The inflammatory process in chronic gout is often mild except when acute attacks supervene. Much of the disability in chronic gout is due to the presence of tophi. These may be associated with a destructive, deforming arthritis and may ulcerate, in which case secondary infection may be a problem.

Tophi may give rise to diagnostic difficulties when they arise in an unusual site, particularly when there is no good history of recurrent attacks of acute gout. Some of the reported locations for gouty tophi include different parts of the eye, several other structures within the head and neck, the heart (especially cardiac valves), the carpal tunnel and spine causing back pain and quadriparesis [31–37]. In these situations, the diagnosis is most often unsuspected until surgery.

Associated Disorders

Some conditions are associated with gout by causing hyperuricemia, whereas in others an etiologic role has not been fully defined.

- The strong association of obesity with hyperuricemia and gout [38], in so far as it reflects dietary excesses, is linked causally with hyperuricemia and gout. Weight loss will also facilitate renal elimination of urate [39,40].
- Hypertension may be associated with hyperuricemia in three ways apart from that due to concurrent diuretic therapy: (i) hypertension reduces renal excretion of urate [41,42]; (ii) renal damage from interstitial microtophi may lead to secondary renal hypertesion; (iii) excessive alcohol consumption may cause both hyperuricemia and hypertension.
- Hyperlipidemia is to be observed frequently in gouty patients, the common associated disorder being hypertriglyceridemia (Type IV lipoproteinemia) [21,41]. Whether this association has a genetic basis or occurs because both are secondary to other factors

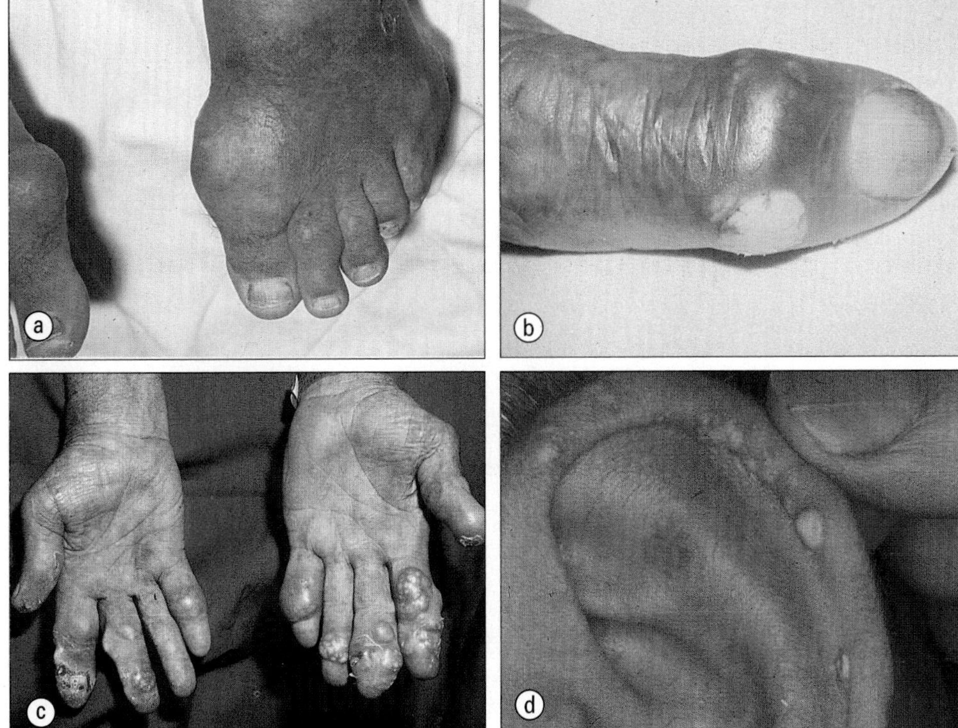

Fig. 25.4 Gouty tophi. Tophi involving the first, second and fifth metatarsophalangeal joints with little involvement of overlying skin (a). An ulcerating tophus of a distal interphalangeal joint with associated redness of the overlying skin (b). Extensive tophi of all digits (c). Auricular tophi. Courtesy of Dr J Webb (d).

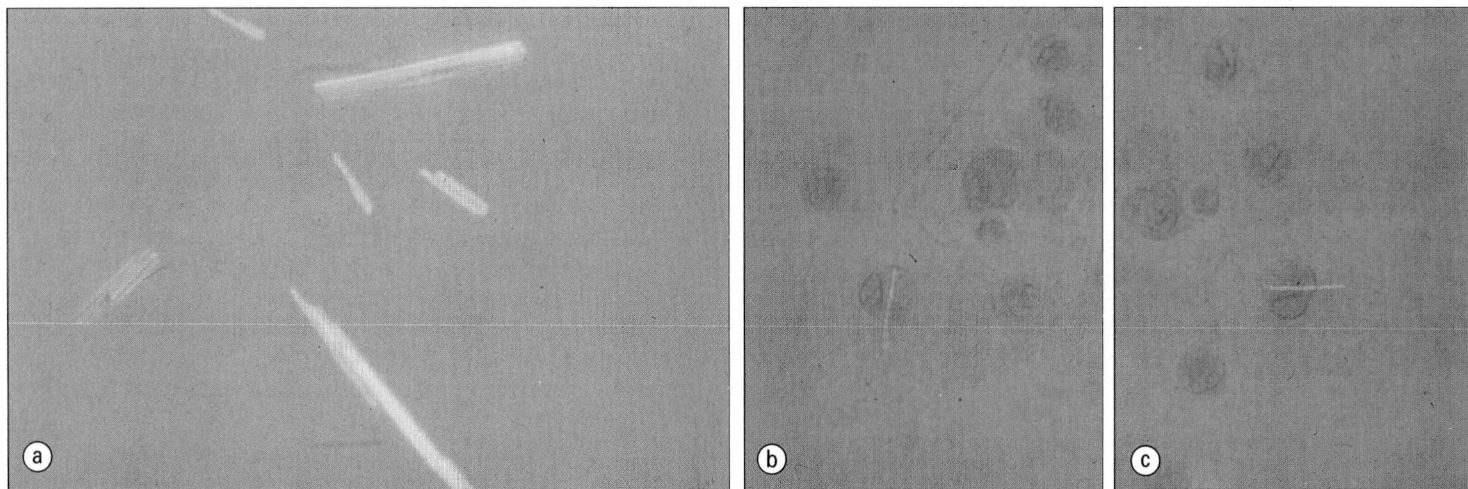

Fig. 25.5 Polarized light microscopy of urate crystals. Illustrated are extracellular (a) and intracellular birefringent needle-shaped urate crystals (b and c). Courtesy of Dr J Webb.

remains to be determined, but there is evidence for both of these alternatives [43,44].

- The association between gout and vascular disease is most likely dependent upon several factors other than hyperuricemia, particularly hypertension, obesity, platelet adhesiveness and possibly hyperlipidemia [45].

Some, although not all, studies have suggested an association between gout and diabetes mellitus or abnormal glucose tolerance [21,46]. However, plasma urate concentrations are lower in diabetic subjects than normal subjects in the absence of renal impairment. This may be due to the uricosuric effect of glycosuria or to the glomerular hyperfiltration that occurs in early diabetic nephropathy. It is probable, therefore, that any association is largely dependent on other factors such as the presence of obesity or renal impairment due to diabetic nephropathy.

In the absence of coexistent renal impairment, there is a negative association between gout and rheumatoid arthritis (RA) [47,48] and probably also between gout and systemic lupus erythematosus [49,50]. In most cases of gout and RA in the same patient, gouty arthritis preceded RA. These negative associations may be due to alterations in the protein constituents of the synovial fluid which may inhibit crystal formation. Changes in immunoglobulin and complement concentrations within the joint may also affect the inflammatory response to crystals but does not explain the rarity with which urate crystals are found in RA and systemic lupus erythematosus.

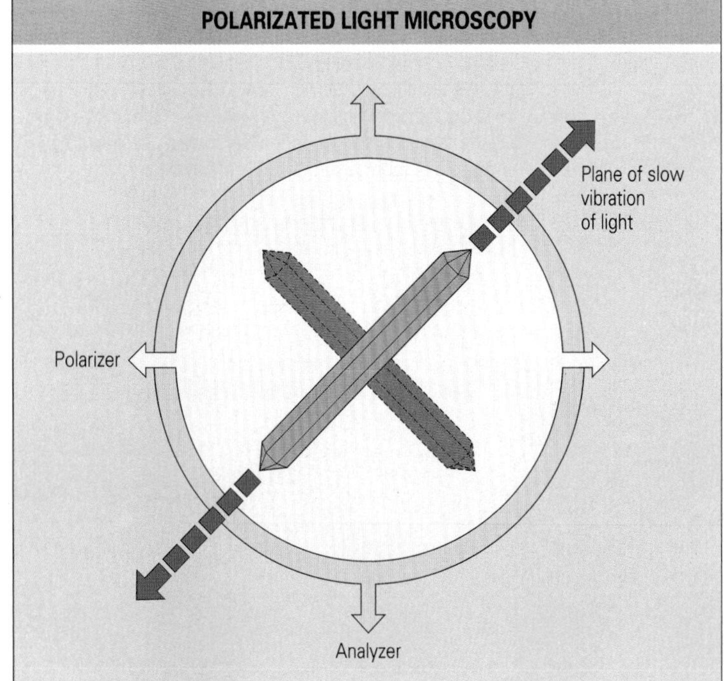

Fig. 25.6 Polarized light microscopy. Schematic representation of the effect of the orientation of a urate crystal with respect to the direction of the plane of slow vibration of light when using a red-plate compensator (retardation plate).

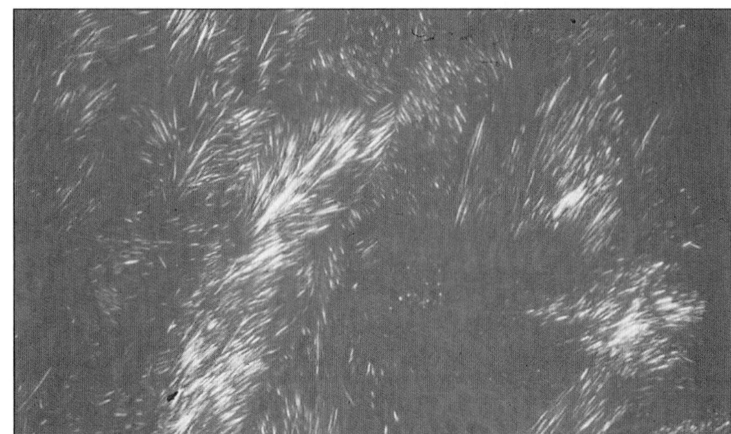

Fig. 25.7 Polarized light microscopy of a gouty tophus. There is a mass of urate crystals from a gouty tophus.

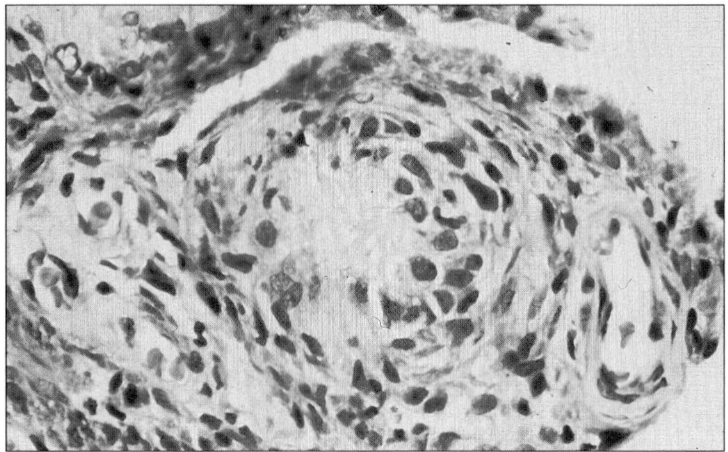

Fig. 25.8 Synovial gouty tophus. Synovium from a patient with gout where the urate crystals from the microtophus have been dissolved by formalin.

INVESTIGATIONS

Synovial Fluid Analysis and Crystal Identification

Joint fluid is examined in order to confirm the presence of urate crystals (in the form of monosodium urate monohydrate [MSUM]) and identify their intra- or extracellular location. If sufficient fluid is available, the cell count should also be determined. In order to identify crystals, only one or two drops of synovial fluid may be required. In small joints, the diagnosis has often been made by examination of the tiny quantity of fluid in the hub or shaft of the needle: this should not be discarded! If septic arthritis is considered to be a significant risk, fluid should be sent for culture. It is important to note that the identification of urate crystals does not exclude septic arthritis.

Crystals are identified by examination under polarized light (Fig. 25.5) [51]; initially, low power and a dark field are used to find crystals. High power is then employed to identify the crystals. In order to demonstrate the characteristic birefringence with certainty, the microscope needs to be equipped with a red-plate compensator and a rotating stage.

Joint fluid is best examined while fresh, although urate (and calcium pyrophosphate dihydrate) crystals can usually be demonstrated after many weeks if the synovial fluid has been kept in a sterile capped tube at 4°C [52,53]. Should urate crystals not be identified and there is sufficient synovial fluid, the remaining fluid can be centrifuged and the pellet examined. Although this is usually not necessary, this technique can increase the yield if only a few crystals are present.

Urate crystals are needle shaped, generally 5 to 25μm in length [54] and show strong negative birefringence under polarized light; thus crystals parallel to the line of slow vibration appear as brilliant yellow whereas those at right angles to the line of slow vibration are brilliant blue (Fig. 25.6). When the stage is rotated through 90°, the color of each crystal changes to the opposite of that which they were initially. These features are pathognomonic for urate crystals. In acute gout, most crystals will be seen to be within neutrophil leukocytes, with many of the longer crystals apparently extending beyond the leukocyte membrane. In contrast, between attacks and in chronic gout, many crystals are extracellular and free within the synovial fluid.

Gouty tophi may be examined in a similar manner. A small amount of the tophaceous material is smeared onto a slide and examined as before. There will rarely be any doubt as to the diagnosis in this situation as the entire smear is a mass of brilliantly birefringent needle-shaped crystals (Fig. 25.7). When tophi present atypically, the possibility that a mass may be a tophus may not initially be anticipated but operative inspection reveals chalky white material. Once a tophus is considered, it is important that at least some of the material is delivered fresh to the laboratory. The routine placement of a specimen in formalin will dissolve the urate crystals leaving 'ghosts' that may suggest a diagnosis of gouty tophus but may preclude a definitive diagnosis (Fig. 25.8).

Other features of synovial fluid in acute gout include its low viscosity and very high leukocyte count, usually more than 70% of which are neutrophils. The leukocyte count may exceed 50,000/mm^3 which is higher than usually observed in noncrystal-related and nonseptic inflammatory arthritides.

MANAGEMENT

Therapy in gout [16,21,22,56,57] is directed towards: (i) the management of acute attacks; and (ii) the prevention of further attacks and the complications of chronic gout. With regard to the complications of gout, treatment should also aim to reverse any of these that may have arisen. Attention should be given to any concomitant or etiologically related conditions such as renal impairment. Since hyperuricemia may be contributed to by an unhealthy lifestyle, identification of correctable factors such as obesity, hypertension, excessive alcohol consumption and hyperlipidemia may indicate the need to correct these with corresponding benefit to both the hyperuricemia and the patients general health. Unfortunately, significant lifestyle changes, which would often be the optimum therapy, are infrequently maintained. In the current era of health and diet consciousness, this may perhaps be changing.

It is important when considering therapy for gout to distinguish between therapy for reducing inflammation and that for managing hyperuricemia. Rarely does any agent offer clinically useful control of both factors [58]. Indeed, the inappropriate use of antihyperuricemic agents during acute gout can cause a severe exacerbation. An outline for the management of gouty arthritis is given in Figure 25.9.

The management of an acute attack is similar whatever the underlying cause of the gout. In determining the best method to prevent further attacks by normalizing the serum urate, however, attention should first be given to possible etiologic factors. It may be possible to identify a number of reversible factors such as thiazide diuretic therapy which, if able to be withdrawn, may obviate the need to introduce urate-lowering drugs. The decision to introduce drugs to normalize hyperuricemia depends in part on the number of previous attacks of acute gout, the degree of hyperuricemia, the presence or otherwise of reversible factors, and the presence of tophi. Urate-lowering drugs will not normally be used after just a single attack of gout but should be considered after the second or third attacks. Furthermore, they should virtually always be used for tophaceous gout. The patient needs to be informed that the decision to commence antihyperuricemic therapy usually implies life-long treatment and the patient, as well as the physician, needs to be committed to this policy.

Dietary restriction of purines rarely causes a fall in the plasma urate concentration of more than 1.0mg/dl (0.06mmol/l). Moreover, such dietary restriction can rarely be sustained for long and is only occasionally clinically useful. In contrast, alcohol restriction can have a much greater effect on the plasma urate concentration, depending upon the amount previously consumed. Consequently, permanent modification of excessive alcohol consumption should contribute significantly to lowering the plasma urate concentration. Maintaining a urine volume of at least 1400ml/day will also facilitate urate excretion, although this will usually only have a small impact on plasma urate concentrations.

Where gout and hyperuricemia are considered to be secondary to chronic lead nephropathy it is important to ensure that management of the renal failure takes first priority. The use of chelating therapy to reduce body stores of lead has no impact on the hyperuricemia and may be hazardous.

The familial nature of gout, whether genetic or environmental, has been recognized for almost two millennia. Since there is no indication to treat asymptomatic hyperuricemia, there is little reason to screen families unless one of the rarer enzyme abnormalities causing urate overproduction is demonstrated in the index case, or a familial reduction in the urate clearance can be demonstrated.

GENERAL PRINCIPLES IN THE MANAGEMENT OF GOUT	
Acute gout	Nonsteroidal anti-inflammatory drugs Colchicine Do not attempt to modify plasma urate concentrations
Recurrent gout or chronic gout	Reverse factors promoting hyperuricemia Maintain urine output > 1400ml/day When asymptomatic, add agent to lower plasma urate concentration (e.g. probenecid or allopurinol) Continue prophylactic doses of colchicine for at least 9 months after normalization of the plasma urate concentration

Fig. 25.9 General principles in the management of gout.

Management Techniques

The pharmacology of the drugs used in the treatment of gout has been described elsewhere [57]. Consequently, the discussion here will focus on specific details with respect to their use in gout.

Asymptomatic Hyperuricemia

Whereas the treatment of hyperuricemia is certainly of value in patients with recurrent attacks of gout, there is currently no evidence of benefit to be obtained from treating asymptomatic hyperuricemia except for severe hyperuricemia [>11.8mg/dl (> 0.7mmol/l)] or in situations where there may be acute urate overproduction as with tumor lysis. Although, as documented earlier, hyperuricemia is associated with a significant risk for the development of gout and a smaller risk of nephrolithiasis and possible renal impairment, it is usually many years between the detection of hyperuricemia and the presentation of any of these problems, if they arise at all. Only when acute severe overproduction of urate can be anticipated should prophylactic therapy with a xanthine oxidase inhibitor be considered. In patients with asymptomatic hyperuricemia, long-term urate-lowering drug therapy cannot be justified either in terms of the risks of drug complications or cost effectiveness.

Acute Gout

Colchicine and nonsteroidal anti-inflammatory drugs (NSAIDs) are effective in the treatment of acute gout and are much superior to paracetamol or aspirin. In addition, NSAIDs are superior to colchicine in terms of speed of onset of action. Thus, despite having been used for centuries, colchicine is usually reserved for patients in whom NSAIDs are contraindicated. Occasionally, a response to colchicine therapy may be of diagnostic value in patients in whom the diagnosis of gout has not been firmly established (though an apparent response to colchicine does not preclude other arthropathies). Whichever drug is chosen in acute gout, the earlier the therapy is instituted the quicker the resolution of the attack. Patients who have had previous attacks of gout learn and should be advised to have therapy readily available and to take it at the first indication of an attack. Taken so early, only one or two doses may be sufficient to abort an attack of gout. Amongst the various NSAIDs, indomethacin has been the most widely used. Phenylbutazone is now not used because of potential hematologic toxicity. Most other NSAIDs have been shown to be effective and provided they are used in appropriate doses, are probably effective in the treatment of an acute attack.

Numerous regimens exist for the use of these drugs in the acute attack and these recommendations provide a guide which may be altered depending upon the severity of the attack and the response to therapy. Nonetheless, it must be noted that the commonest cause of difficulty in controlling an attack is the simultaneous administration or withdrawal of drugs that alter the plasma urate concentration. Both increases and decreases in plasma urate concentrations may precipitate or prolong an attack of gout. Therefore, therapy aimed at reducing urate concentrations should be delayed until after the complete resolution of all signs of inflammation.

Indomethacin: Patients will often notice that the pain has begun to ease within two hours of taking the first dose. Generally, 50mg four times a day is an average and effective dose schedule although mild attacks may respond to lower doses. This dose may be doubled with benefit in particularly severe cases. The dose should be maintained for two days and then reduced to three times a day. Providing the attack continues to settle, the dose is further reduced to 25mg three times a day and continued for one to two days after the acute inflammation has settled completely.

Other NSAIDs: The doses of the several other NSAIDs used to treat gout tend to be towards the upper limit or above the usual therapeutic range. In most cases, a higher initial dose has been advocated and, as with indomethacin, the dose is generally reduced as the attack resolves. Some of the dose schedules are as follows: ibuprofen 800mg every 8 hours reducing to 400mg every six hours; diclofenac 50mg every 8 hours reducing to 25mg every 8 hours; naproxen 750mg initially then by 250mg every 8 hours; piroxicam 40mg daily for five days; and sulindac 200mg initially then 100mg every 6 hours.

Several of the NSAIDs available in suppository or injectable form may be useful in patients unable to take oral medications. In a severe attack of gout, an effective dose may be difficult to achieve with suppositories in which case parenteral therapy may be indicated.

Colchicine: The therapeutic and the toxic dose of colchicine are very similar and it is usually toxicity in the form of nausea, vomiting or diarrhea that limit the dose of colchicine that can be used in a particular patient. A dose of 1mg is given initially followed by 0.5mg at second hourly intervals until the attack begins to settle or diarrhea or vomiting occur. When used within the first few hours of an attack, there is most often a good response to colchicine. However, when the therapy is delayed, the response rate declines and there is frequently a delay of 24 hours before a response is demonstrated. Total effective dose rarely exceeds 8mg, although a larger dose may be administered to a large patient who is not responding.

Colchicine may also be given intravenously, although a suitable preparation is available only in some countries. Whereas gastrointestinal toxicity is largely absent when colchicine is administered this way, there is risk of other complications. Local tissue necrosis may occur if there is extravasation of the colchicine outside the vein. If it is to be used at all, intravenous colchicine should be reserved for patients in whom other forms of therapy are contraindicated.

Corticosteroids: Intra-articular administration of corticosteroids is a particularly effective means of terminating an attack of gout. Resolution is typically complete within 12–24 hours. This form of treatment is of particular value in some patients with renal impairment and other conditions where the use of full doses of other drugs may be relatively contraindicated. Prophylactic doses of colchicine or an NSAID should be instituted to decrease the likelihood of a recurrence. In contrast, the response to oral corticosteroids is variable and rebound attacks frequently occur on the withdrawal of this therapy.

Prophylactic Therapy

Clearly, the best prophylactic therapy would be correction of the hyperuricemia and this can be achieved by several means. Colchicine, used to treat acute attacks of gout, is also effective in preventing attacks whatever the plasma urate concentration. Prophylactic colchicine is usually required when drugs are introduced to correct hyperuricemia; it may still be needed even when urate concentrations have been normalized.

Colchicine in a dose of 0.5 to 2.0mg/day, usually 0.5mg twice or three times daily, has been shown by numerous investigators to be highly effective in reducing the frequency of attacks. It is also useful in reducing the likelihood of attacks when antihyperuricemic therapy is begun. Indomethacin 25mg twice daily is also widely used for prophylaxis although its value is less well documented and its potential complications are greater than those of colchicine. Prophylaxis should normally be continued for 9 to 12 months after normouricemia has been achieved and the patient has remained free of attacks. Even then, some patients will experience further attacks and may choose to continue prophylaxis.

Correction of Hyperuricemia

Despite the use of effective prophylaxis, only correction of the hyperuricemia can alter the underlying tendency to gout. Drugs to correct hyperuricemia act either by promoting the renal excretion of urate (uricosuric agents) or by decreasing urate production by inhibiting xanthine oxidase (allopurinol). Although it would be logical to use a uricosuric agent when there is primary urate underexcretion and a xanthine oxidase inhibitor when there is overproduction, many patients show features of both overproduction and underexcretion of urate. Xanthine oxidase inhibitors are effective in correcting hyperuricemia (Fig. 25.10). They may be used in most situations even when there is urate underexcretion and in the presence of modest renal impairment (provided the dose is suitably reduced). Uricosuric agents should be avoided if there is an inadequate urine volume or a history of renal colic or if there is significant renal failure (clearance less than half normal). Figure 25.11 lists the indications for the use of allopurinol (the only widely available xanthine oxidase inhibitor). Hypersensitivity to allopurinol sometimes necessitates its withdrawal. Should this occur, and a xanthine oxidase inhibitor is required, then a regimen of desensitization, as outlined by Meyrier [59], may be attempted. In some patients in whom the hypersensitivity has had mild manifestations, this is successful, whereas in others, adverse symptoms recur before an adequate therapeutic dose is achieved. The best solution usually is to change to a uricosuric agent and often the potent sulfinpyrazone is needed. A further uncommon situation is the patient in whom there is a history of renal calculi but the patient has also been intolerant to allopurinol. In such a patient, if urate lowering therapy is required, a uricosuric agent may be cautiously begun with strict attention to maintaining an alkaline urine and a high urine volume.

In the occasional patient, a full dosage of allopurinol (300–400 mg/day) will not cause the urate concentration to return to normal, and in such a case, another factor (e.g. regular alcohol consumption) is usually operating. This needs to be identified and corrected. Rare patients may need to be treated with the combination of a uricosuric drug and xanthine oxidase inhibitor but this should be avoided if at all possible because the uricosuric agents alter the pharmacokinetics of oxipurinol (the major active metabolite of allopurinol).

It cannot be stressed too much that antihyperuricemic drugs should not be commenced until an attack of gout has settled completely. In addition, prophylactic doses of colchicine should be administered concomitantly to minimize the risk of inducing an attack of acute gout.

Tophaceous Gout

The principle of treatment of tophi is to lower the plasma urate concentration to such a degree as to allow urate to be resorbed from the surface of the tophi. In effect, this implies maintaining the urate concentration within the middle of the optimal range. This requires the long-term use of urate-lowering drugs over many years. It is obvious that drugs such as colchicine and most NSAIDs, while controlling acute attacks, will not prevent the formation of tophi and may, by preventing the inflammatory response, actually increase the development of tophi unless hyperuricemia is controlled at the same time. Whether uricosuric NSAIDs such as azapropazone and diflunisal will have a role in the management of tophaceous gout remains to be demonstrated.

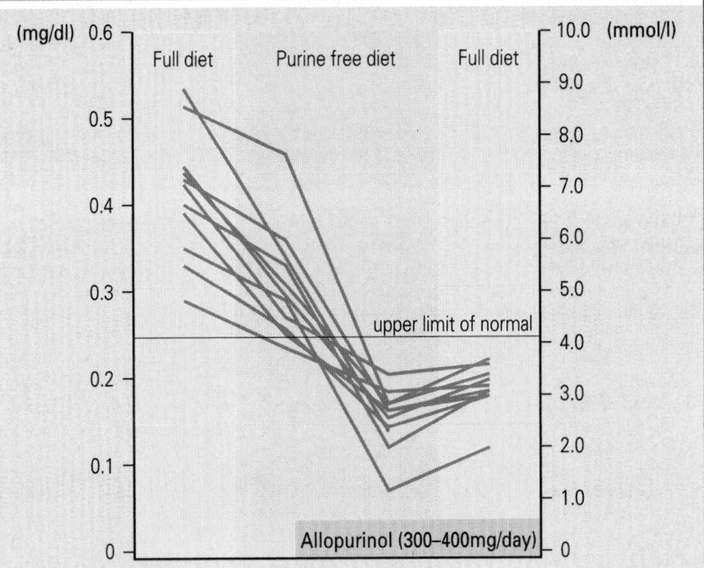

Fig. 25.10 The effect of a low purine diet and allopurinol on serum urate concentrations. There is a consistent but usually small fall in serum urate concentrations with low purine diet alone. The addition of allopurinol reliably normalizes the serum urate concentrations an effect which is largely maintained when the patients return to a full diet. Adapted from Emmerson BT. Aust Ann Med. 1969;**16**:205–14).

Surgery is rarely indicated for tophi except in the unusual presentations where tophi exert pressure on an important structure (e.g. spinal cord). In other less vital situations, control of the hyperuricemia will cause resorption of the tophi provided there is no urgency to have them removed. Infected tophi can usually be managed with antibiotics and local measures, but debridement may be needed particularly when there is associated vascular disease.

INDICATIONS FOR ALLOPURINOL WHEN AN ANTIHYPERURICEMIC AGENT IS REQUIRED
Urate overproduction, primary or secondary
Acute uric acid nephropathy, tumor lysis syndrome
Nephrolithiasis of any type
Renal impairment (dose 100mg/day per 30ml/min glomerular filtration rate)
Low urine volume
24 hour urinary uric acid > 0.42g (2.5mmol) (an arbitrary value on a low purine diet)
Intolerance or allergy to uricosuric agents

Fig. 25.11 Indications for allopurinol when an antihyperuricemic agent is required.

REFERENCES

1. Popert AJ, Venise Hewett J. Gout and hyperuricemia in rural and urban populations. Ann Rheum Dis. 1962;**21**:154–63.
2. Mikkelsen WM, Dodge HJ, Valkenburg H, Himes S. The distribution of serum uric acid values in a population unselected as to gout or hyperuricemia. Am J Med. 1965;**39**:242–51.
3. Hall AP, Barry PE, Dawber TR, McNamara PM. Epidemiology of gout and hyperuricemia. Am J Med. 1967;**42**:27–37.
4. Duff IF, Mikkelsen WM, Dodge HJ, Himes DS. Comparison of uric acid levels in some Oriental and Caucasian groups unselected as to gout or hyperuricemia. Arthritis Rheum. 1968;**11**:184–90.
5. O'Sullivan JB. Gout in a New England town. Ann Rheum Dis. 1972;**31**:166–9.
6. Yano K, Rhoads GG, Kagan A. Epidemiology of serum uric acid among 8000 Japanese–American men in Hawaii. J Chron Dis. 1977;**30**:171–84.
7. Munan L, Kelly A, Petitclerc C. Population serum uric acid levels and their correlates. Am J Epidemiol. 1976;**103**:369–82.

8. Zimmet PZ, Whitehouse S, Jackson L, Thoma K. High prevalence of hyperuricemia and gout in an urbanized Micronesian population. Br Med J. 1978;**1**:1237–9.
9. Badley EM, Meyrick JS, Wood PHN. Gout and serum uric acid levels in the Cotswolds. Rheumatol Rehab. 1978;**17**:33–42.
10. Prior I. Epidemiology of rheumatic disorders in the Pacific with particular emphasis on hyperuricemia and gout. Semin Arthritis Rheum. 1981;**11**:213–29.
11. Gibson T, Waterworth R, Hatfield P, Robinson G, Bremner K. Hyperuricaemia, gout and kidney function in New Zealand Maori men. Br J Rheumatol. 1984;**23**:276-82.
12. Prior IAM, Welby TJ, Ostbye T, Salmond CE, Stokes YM. Migration and gout: the Tokelau Island migrant study. Br Med J. 1987;**295**:457–61.
13. Roubenoff R. Gout and hyperuricemia. Rheum Dis Clin North Am. 1990;**16**:539–50.
14. Yu T-F. Some unusual features of gouty arthritis in females. Semin Arthritis Rheum. 1977;**6**:247–55.
15. Campion EW, Glynn RJ, DeLabry LO. Asymptomatic hyperuricemia. Am J Med. 1987;**82**:421–6.
16. Yu T-F. Milestones in the treatment of gout. Am J Med. 1974;**56**:676–85.
17. Fessel WJ. Renal outcomes of gout and hyperuricemia. Am J Med. 1979;**67**:74–82.
18. Wallace SL, Robinson H, Masi AT, Decker JL, McCarty DJ, Yu T-F. Preliminary criteria for the classification of the acute arthritis of primary gout. Arthritis Rheum. 1977;**20**:895–900.
19. C.I.O.M.S. Criteria, Rome. In: Kellgren JH, Jeffrey MR, Ball S, eds. The epidemiology of chronic rheumatism. Oxford: Blackwell; 1963:327.
20. C.I.O.M.S. Criteria, New York. In: Bennett PH, Wood PHN, eds. Population studies of the rheumatic diseases, 1966 (International Congress Series No. 168). Amsterdam: Excerpta Medica Foundation; 1968:457.
21. Wyngaarden JB, Kelley WN. Gout and hyperuricemia. New York: Grune and Stratton; 1976.
22. Emmerson BT. Hyperuricaemia and gout in clinical practice. Sydney: ADIS Health Science Press; 1983.
23. Lawry GV, Fan PT, Bluestone R. Polyarticular versus monoarticular gout: a prospective, comparative analysis of clinical features. Medicine (Baltimore). 1988;**67**:335–43.
24. Ter Borg EJ, Rasker JJ. Gout in the elderly, a separate entity? Ann Rheum Dis. 1987;**46**:72–6.
24. Campbell SM. Gout: How presentation, diagnosis, and treatment differ in the elderly. Geriatrics. 1988;**43**:71–7.
26. Lally EV, Zimmerman B, Ho G, Kaplan SR. Urate-mediated inflammation in nodal osteoarthritis: clinical and roentgenographic correlations. Arthritis Rheum. 1989;**32**:86–90
27. Macfarlane DG, Dieppe PA. Diuretic-induced gout in elderly women. Br J Rheumatol. 1985;**24**:155–7.
28. Meyers OL, Monteagudo FSE. Gout in females: an analysis of 92 patients. Clin Exp Rheumatol. 1985;**3**:105–9.
29. Meyers OL, Monteagudo FSE. A comparison of gout in men and women. S Afr Med J. 1986;**70**:721–3.
30. Lally EV, Ho G, Kaplan SR. The clinical spectrum of gouty arthritis in women. Arch Intern Med. 1986;**146**:2221–5.
31. Landau A, Reese DJ, Blumenthal DR, Chin NW. Tophaceous neck mass presenting as a thyroglossal duct cyst. Arthritis Rheum. 1990;**33**: 910–11.
32. Stark TW, Hirokawa RH. Gout and its manifestations in the head and neck. Otolaryngol Clin North Am. 1982;**15**:659–64.
33. Scalapino JN, Edwards WD, Steckelberg JM, Wooton RS, Callahan JA, Ginsberg WW. Mitral stenosis associated with valvular tophi. Mayo Clin Proc. 1984;**59**:509–12.
34. Martinez-Cordero E, Barriera-Mercado E, Katona G. Eye tophi deposition in gout. J Rheumatol. 1986;**11**:471–3.
35. Sequeira W, Bouffard A, Salgia K, Skosey J. Quadriparesis in tophaceous gout. Arthritis Rheum. 1981;**24**:1428–30.
36. Champion D. Gouty tenosynovitis and the carpal tunnel syndrome. Med J Aust. 1969;**1**:1030–32.
37. Arnold MH, Brooks PM, Savvas P, Ruff S. Tophaceous gout of the axial skeleton. Aust NZ J Med. 1988;**18**:865–7.
38. Grahame R, Scott JT. Clinical survey of 354 patients with gout. Ann Rheum Dis. 1970;**29**:461–8.
39. Yamashita S, Matsuzawa Y, Tokunaga K, Fujioka S, Tarui S. Studies on the impaired metabolism of uric acid in obese subjects: marked reduction of renal urate excretion and its improvement by a low-calorie diet. Int J Obesity. 1986;**10**:255–64.
40. Emmerson BT. Alteration of urate metabolism by weight reduction. Aust NZ J Med. 1973;**3**:410–12.
41. Emmerson BT. Abnormal urate excretion associated with renal and systemic disorders, drugs, toxins. In: Kelley WN, Weiner IM, eds. Uric acid (Handbook Exp Pharm, Vol 51). Berlin: Springer Verlag; 1978:287–324.
42. Messerli FH, Frohlich ED, Dreslinski GR, Suarez DH, Aristimuno GG. Serum uric acid in essential hypertension: an indication of renal vascular involvement. Ann Intern Med. 1980;**93**:817–21.
43. Matsubara K, Matsuzawa Y, Jiao S, Takama T, Kubo M, Tarui S. Relationship between hypertriglyceridemia and uric acid-production in primary gout. Metabolism. 1989;**38**:698-701.
44. Yu T, Dorph DJ, Smith H. Hyperlipidemia in primary gout. Semin Arthritis Rheum. 1978;**7**:233–44.
45. Emmerson BT. Atherosclerosis and urate metabolism. Aust NZ J Med. 1979;**9**:451–4.
46. Herman JB, Goldbourt U. Uric acid and diabetes: observations in a population study. Lancet. 1982;**2**:240–41.
47. Rizzoli AJ, Trujeque L, Bankhurst AD. The coexistence of gout and rheumatoid arthritis. J Rheumatol. 1980;**7**:316–24.
48. Atdjian M, Fernandez-Madrid F. Coexistence of chronic tophaceous gout and rheumatoid arthritis. J Rheumatol. 1981;**8**:989–92.
49. Greenfield DI, Fong JS, Barth WF. Systemic lupus erythematosus and gout. Semin Arthritis Rheum. 1985;**14**:176–9.
50. Bradley JD, Pinals RS. Tophaceous gout in patients with systemic lupus erythematosus. Clin Exp Rheumatol. 1984;**2**:151–5.
51. Phelps P, Steele AD, McCarty DJ. Compensated polarized light microscopy: identification of crystals in synovial fluids from gout and pseudogout. JAMA. 1968;**203**:508–12.
52. McKnight KM, Agudelo C. Comment on article by Kerolus *et al.* (Arthritis Rheum. 1989;**32**:271–8). Arthritis Rheum. 1991;**34**:118.
53. Schumacher JR. Reply to McKnight and Agudelo (Arthritis Rheum. 1989;**34**:118). Arthritis Rheum. 1991;**34**:118–9.
54. McCarty DJ. Crystal identification in human synovial fluids.Rheum Dis Clin North Am. 1988;**14**:253–67.
56. Scott JT. Long-term management of gout and hyperuricemia. Br Med J. 1980;**281**:1164–6.
57. Wallace SL, Singer JZ. Therapy in gout. Rheum Dis Clin North Am. 1988;**14**:441–7.
58. Emmerson BT, Hazelton RA, Whyte IMacG. Comparison of the urate lowering effects of allopurinol and diflunisal. J Rheumatol. 1987;**14**:335–7.
59. Meyrier A. Desensitisation in a patient with chronic renal disease and severe allergy to allopurinol. Br Med J. 1976;**2**:458.
60. Emmerson BT, Nagel SL. Duffy DL, Martin NG. Genetic control of the renal clearance of urate: a study of twins. Ann Rheum Dis. 1992;**51**:375–7.

26

CALCIUM PYROPHOSPHATE DIHYDRATE

Michael Doherty

Definition
- Arthropathy and other locomotor disease associated with calcium pyrophosphate dihydrate (CPPD) crystal deposition.
- Sporadic, familial, and metabolic disease-associated forms recognized.

Clinical features
- Predominantly a disease of the elderly.
- Acute self-limiting synovitis ('pseudogout').
- Chronic arthropathy showing strong association/overlap with osteoarthritis.
- Target joints – knees, wrists, shoulders, hips.

EPIDEMIOLOGY

Data on chondrocalcinosis (CC), derived from radiographic and pathologic surveys, is sparse and largely confined to the knee [1–4]. All studies, however, suggest female preponderance and striking association with aging, the prevalence for radiographic CC being rare under age 50, but rising from 10–15% in those aged 65–75, to 30–60% in those over 85 years [1,2]. The only large population-based radiographic survey is the Framingham study [4] which in the age range 63–93 showed an overall prevalence rate of 8%, ranging from 3% in those aged <70, to 27% in those >85 years. This study also confirmed female preponderance (age-adjusted relative risk 1.33), though less pronounced than that derived from patient series [1,2] (Fig. 26.1).

CC is reported from most countries and racial groups, but there is insufficient data to confirm racial predisposition. Familial predisposition, however, is well reported from several countries and different ethnic groups including Czechoslovakia, Chile, Holland, France, Canada, Germany, Sweden, United States, Spain, Japan, Israel and the United Kingdom [1,2,5–9]. Two different clinical phenotypes have been emphasized, the first characterized by early onset (3rd–4th decade), florid polyarticular CC with variable severity of arthropathy (ranging from mild to severe destructive [5,6,9]), the second by late-onset (6th–7th decade) oligoarticular CC (mainly knee) with arthritis resembling sporadic pyrophosphate arthropathy [7–9]. This latter form may be more common than generally recognized, the late onset of disease expression and geographic dispersal of families posing difficulties in this respect. An association with benign childhood fits has been reported in one UK family with early onset polyarticular CC [9]. The pattern of inheritance varies, though autosomal dominance occurs in most. Genetic associations have not been identified.

EPIDEMIOLOGY OF PYROPHOSPHATE ARTHROPATHY	
Peak age (years)	65–75
Sex distribution (F:M)	2–7:1
Prevalence rate (/100,000)	8100 (CC only, age range 63–93)
Annual incidence (/1000)	Unknown
Geography	Appears ubiquitous
Genetic associations	Nil identified

Fig. 26.1 Epidemiology of pyrophosphate arthropathy.

No epidemiologic data exists for pyrophosphate arthropathy. Most patient series concur in reporting a mean age at presentation of circa 65–75 years [1,2], with female predominance (2–3:1) particularly in older patients. Associated metabolic disease (Fig. 26.2) and familial predisposition are rarely identified in patient series, though each may associate with a younger age of presentation (<55 years) and tendency to florid, polyarticular CC. Though numerous metabolic associations have been suggested [10], many reflect chance concurrence of common age-related conditions as controlled studies have shown for diabetes, uremia, Paget's disease, and hypothyroidism. The strongest evidence undoubtedly relates to hyperparathyroidism and hemochromatosis [10–12], in which the independent effect of aging has also been demonstrated. With rare conditions, convincing evidence is provided by occurrence of premature CC in just a few cases, as reported for hypophosphatasia, hypomagnesemia and Wilson's disease [10–14].

CLINICAL FEATURES

Three common presentations are acute synovitis, chronic arthritis, and incidental finding [1,2,15,16]. Other presentations are rare.

Acute Synovitis ('Pseudogout')

This classic presentation is the commonest cause of acute monoarthritis in the elderly. Acute attacks may be the only manifestation of otherwise asymptomatic CC or pyrophosphate arthropathy; in older, predominantly female patients, however, they commonly superimpose upon a background of chronic symptomatic arthropathy. Although any joint may be involved (including 1st metatarsophalangeal joint 'pseudopodagra') the knee is by far the commonest site (Fig. 26.3), followed by the wrist, shoulder, ankle, and elbow. Concurrent attacks in more than one joint are uncommon (<10% of cases), and polyarticular attacks rare.

The typical attack develops rapidly with severe pain, stiffness and swelling, maximal within 6–24 hours of onset. As with gout, the patient may describe pain as the 'worst ever experienced', and be unable to tolerate even light pressure from clothing or bedding. Overlying erythema is common and examination reveals a tender

METABOLIC DISEASES PREDISPOSING TO CPPD CRYSTAL DEPOSITION	
Definite associations	Possible associations
Hyperparathyroidism Hemochromatosis Hypophosphatasia Hypomagnesemia Wilson's disease	Gout Ochronosis

Fig. 26.2 Metabolic diseases predisposing to CPPD.

joint, held in the loose-packed position, with signs of marked synovitis (increased warmth, large/tense effusion, joint line tenderness, and restricted movement with stress pain). Fever is common and occasionally marked. Elderly patients particularly may appear unwell and mildly confused, especially with knee or multiple joint involvement.

Acute attacks are self-limiting and usually resolve within 1–3 weeks. Transient, less severe 'petite' attacks are probably common but difficult to confirm. Although most pseudogout episodes develop spontaneously, several provoking factors are recognized which may precede the attack by 1–3 days (Fig. 26.4), the commonest being stress response of intercurrent illness or surgery.

Chronic Pyrophosphate Arthropathy

Symptomatic patients with this common condition are mainly elderly and female. The distribution of involvement is similar to that of pseudogout and principally involves large and medium-sized joints, the knees being the most common and severely affected sites followed by wrists, shoulders, elbows, hips and midtarsal joints (Figs 26.5 & 26.6). In the hand, metacarpophalangeal joints (particularly 2nd and 3rd) are the commonest, most severely affected sites. Presentation is with chronic pain, early morning and inactivity stiffness, limitation of movement, and functional impairment: acute attacks may be superimposed upon this chronic history. Symptoms are often restricted to just a few joints, though single or multiple joint involvement also occurs.

Affected joints usually reveal signs of OA (bony swelling, crepitus, restricted movement) with varying degrees of synovitis. Synovitis, represented by increased warmth, joint line/capsular tenderness, stress pain, effusion and soft tissue thickening, may be marked, and is usually most evident clinically at the knee, radiocarpal or glenohumeral joint. Knees typically show bi- or tricompartmental disease, with marked or predominant patello-femoral involvement. In severe cases fixed flexion with either valgus or varus deformity may occur (other deformities, e.g. recurvatum, posterior tibial subluxation, are less common).

Examination, particularly of elderly women, often reveals more widespread but asymptomatic joint abnormality. Generalized OA with Heberden's nodes, for example, is a common accompaniment, but pyrophosphate arthropathy is often clinically distinguished from uncomplicated, noncrystal associated OA by: (i) the pattern of affected joints (wrists, shoulders, ankles, elbows are uncommonly affected in OA; knee involvement usually predominates in the medial compartment), and; (ii) the often marked inflammatory component; and (iii) superimposition of acute attacks.

Inflammatory features may indeed be sufficiently severe to cause confusion with rheumatoid ('pseudorheumatoid arthritis') [1], though the infrequency of tenosynovitis and absence of extra-articular features usually permit ready distinction from rheumatoid arthritis (RA).

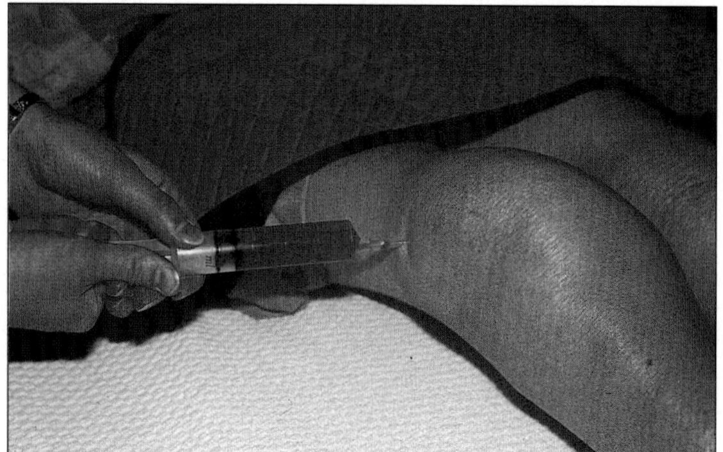

Fig. 26.3 Pseudogout affecting the knee. Seen here in an elderly lady with background chronic pyrophosphate arthropathy. Blood-staining of synovial fluid is common in this situation.

The natural history of chronic pyrophosphate arthropathy is poorly documented. However, despite often severe symptoms and structural change at presentation, one 5-year hospital-based prospective study [16] suggests that most patients run a benign course, particularly in respect of small and medium-sized joint involvement (Fig. 26.7). As expected, most symptom progression in this study occurred in large lower limb joints, but even in severely affected knees (the usual site of presentation) 60% showed stabilization or improvement of symptoms.

Nevertheless, it is recognized that progressive, severely destructive arthropathy may occasionally develop, particularly at the knee, shoulder or hip. Such destructive pyrophosphate arthropathy is virtually confined to elderly women, usually accompanied by severe night and rest pain, and associates with a poor outcome [17]. Some such patients have problematic recurrent hemarthrosis, particularly of the shoulder and knee; joint leakage may cause extensive bleeding, swelling and bruising of adjacent tissues. Because of radiographic similarity to hypertrophic Charcot joints in some cases, the term 'pseudoneuropathic joint' is sometimes used [1]. Interestingly, occurrence of rapidly destructive apatite-associated arthritis at the hip (without local CPPD deposition), showing radiographic similarity to atrophic Charcot joints, is reported particularly in patients with CC and pyrophosphate arthropathy at other sites, though the mechanism for this is obscure [2]. Again, such rapidly progressive arthropathy is virtually confined to elderly women.

Incidental Finding

Because isolated CC is a common age-associated phenomenon it is often observed as an incidental radiographic finding in elderly subjects. Though less well documented, it is likely that asymptomatic pyrophosphate arthropathy is also common in the 8th and 9th decades [3,4]. Therefore, as with OA, clinical or radiographic evidence of pyrophosphate arthropathy or CC may be a confounding factor, and only a thorough history and examination can elucidate the importance of such a finding in terms of symptom causation.

Uncommon Presentations

Atypical arthropathic and axial presentations

Marked proximal stiffness accompanying glenohumeral and polyarticular involvement may rarely lead to consideration of polymyalgia rheumatica. Severe spinal stiffness (particularly in Czech, Chilean and other familial forms) may cause 'pseudo-ankylosing spondylitis', and indeed true spinal ankylosis may occur in Chilean families [6]. The putative association with DISH [18] may further complicate this issue. Acute attacks in axial joints are difficult to confirm, and some self-limiting spinal syndromes, described in relation to the periodontoid ('crowned dens' syndrome), cervical

SITUATIONS WHICH MAY TRIGGER ACUTE PSEUDOGOUT
Direct trauma to joint
Intercurrent medical illness (e.g. chest infection, myocardial infarction)
Surgery (especially parathyroidectomy)
Blood transfusion, parenteral fluid administration
Institution of thyroxine replacement therapy
Joint lavage
Most cases of pseudogout develop spontaneously

Fig. 26.4 Situations which may trigger acute pseudogout.

and lumbar regions, may reflect pseudogout attacks. Certainly in elderly subjects acute self-limiting meningitic episodes may relate to CPPD deposition in degenerative ligamenta flava and cervical discs, and such deposits rarely associate with chronic myeloradiculopathy. Preferential deposition of CPPD in ligamenta flava at C3–C6 remains unexplained but corresponds to the level of greatest mobility.

Tendinitis and tenosynovitis

Acute inflammatory episodes relating to CPPD deposition in tendons are described for triceps, flexor digitorum, and Achilles tendons, and tenosynovitis is reported for hand flexors and extensors [19]. Tendinitis and tenosynovitis usually, but not inevitably, occur in patients with accompanying CC or pyrophosphate arthropathy. Flexor tendon involvement may associate with carpal tunnel syndrome, and less frequently combined median and ulnar nerve entrapment at the wrist [19,20], the entrapment appearing to relate more to soft tissue factors than structural arthropathy. Tendon rupture (hand extensors, Achilles) is a rare complication.

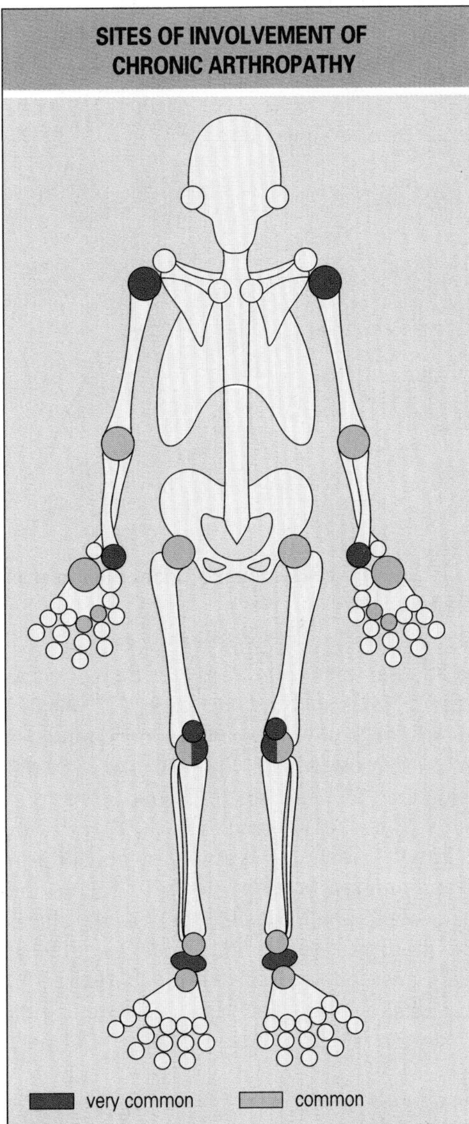

Fig. 26.5 Chronic arthropathy. Common sites of involvement of chronic pyrophosphate arthropathy.

Bursitis

Olecranon, infra-patellar and retrocalcaneal bursitis are rare clinical manifestations, again predominating in patients with widespread pyrophosphate arthropathy. It is thought most likely that CPPD crystals migrate to bursal tissues from adjacent sites (cartilage, capsule, tendon), rather than deposit *de novo* in soft tissues.

Tophaceous CPPD deposition

Tophaceous ('tumoral') CPPD deposition is rare, but reported in intra- or periarticular sites that include the elbow, finger, jaw, acromioclavicular joint, and hip [21]. Lesions are solitary and usually develop in areas of chondroid metaplasia without predisposing metabolic abnormality or evidence of CPPD deposition elsewhere. Malignancy is often suspected and the diagnosis follows examination of excised material.

INVESTIGATIONS

Central investigations for diagnosis are (i) fluid and tissue analysis (primarily synovial fluid, rarely bursal or tenosynovial aspirate, biopsy material) for presence of CPPD crystals, and (ii) plain radiographs. Other investigations may be undertaken to exclude alternative or coexisting arthropathy, and once the diagnosis is confirmed further investigation for predisposing metabolic disease may be indicated.

CPPD Crystal Identification

In pseudogout, aspirated fluid is often turbid or blood-stained, with diminished viscosity and greatly elevated cell count (usually > 90% neutrophils). Macroscopic appearance, viscosity and cell counts in chronic arthropathy are more variable and range across the 'inflammatory' – 'non-inflammatory' spectrum. CPPD crystals are poorly visualized by plain light microscopy, but compensated polarized light

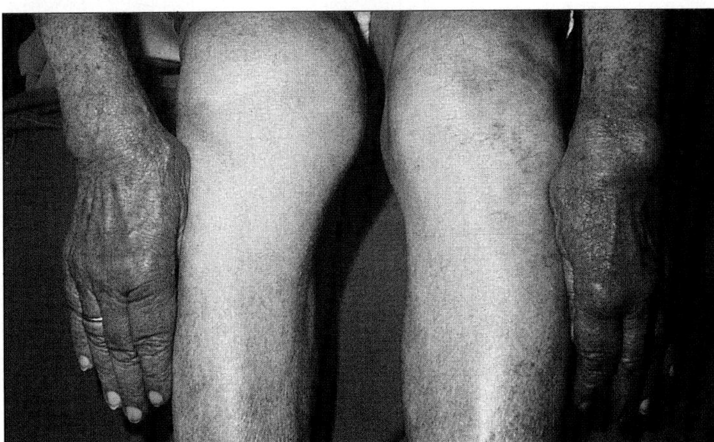

Fig. 26.6 Characteristic elderly female patient with marked knee, wrist, and metacarpophalangeal pyrophosphate arthropathy.

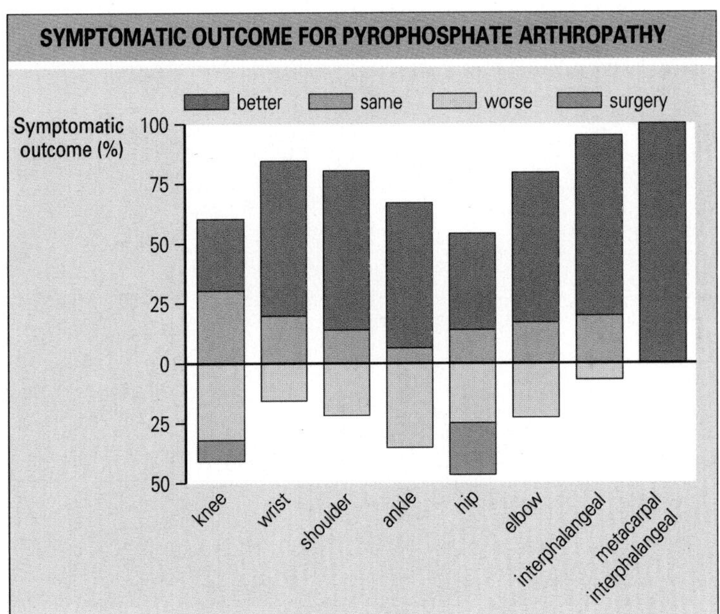

Fig. 26.7 Symptomatic outcome for pyrophosphate arthropathy at different joint sites in 64 patients followed over 5 years.

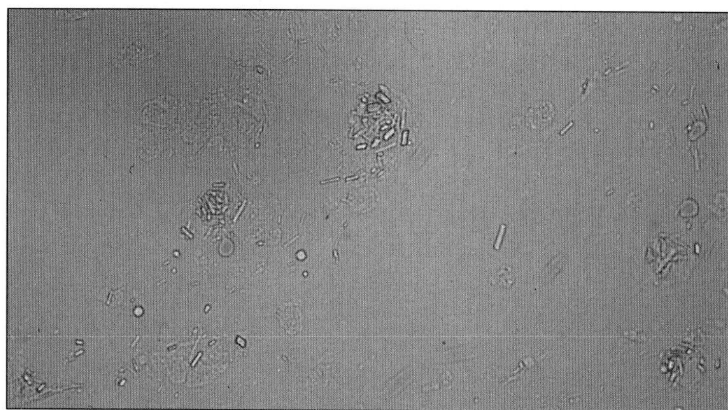

Fig. 26.8 Synovial fluid CPPD crystals.

microscopy (×400) will reveal predominantly intracellular CPPD crystals (Fig. 26.8), recognized by their morphology (usually rhomboids or rods, occasionally acicular, ~2–10μm long), weak positive birefringence, and inclined extinction (15–20°): 'twinning' of crystals, leaving a chip at one corner, is occasionally seen. CPPD are less readily identified and often less numerous than urate crystals, and may often be missed: careful search in areas of cellular debris and fibrin, and examination of a spun deposit may both increase detection. Although robust crystals, early examination of fresh fluid avoids problems of dissolution and postaspiration artefact. For histologic samples, tissue preparation in neutral buffers and stains should be used to avoid dissolution: crystals may readily be lost during decalcification (often done for tissue submitted with bone).

As with other synovial fluid particles, identification by polarized light microscopy associates with false positives (and negatives) and identification using more definitive analytical means (e.g. infra-red spectrophotometry, electron microscopic methods, X-ray diffraction) is ideal. However, such methods often require a high crystal load for analysis, are expensive, and take time. Therefore, for routine clinical purposes polarized microscopy of fresh fluid represents a convenient, rapid and adequate compromise.

Plain Radiographic Features

Radiographic aspects relate both to the calcification and arthropathy associated with CPPD deposition [22,23].

Calcification

This may affect several joint tissues (Fig. 26.9). CC most commonly affects fibrocartilage (particularly knee menisci, wrist triangular cartilage, symphysis pubis), but also occurs in hyaline cartilage (particularly knee, glenohumeral joint, hip) as thick linear deposits, parallel

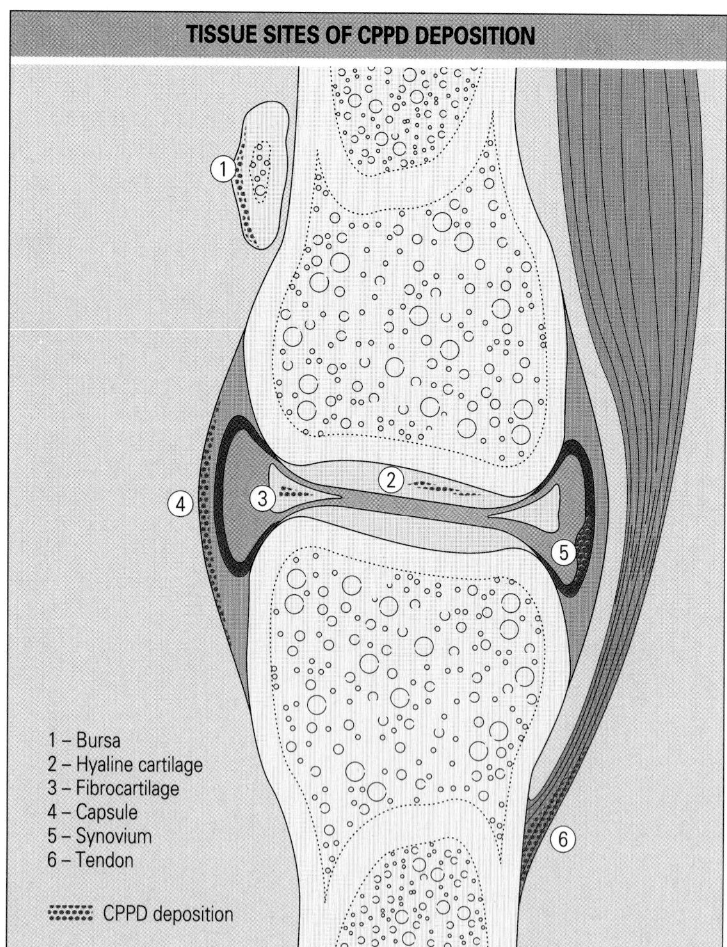

Fig. 26.9 Tissue sites of CPPD deposition.

to and separate from subchondral bone (Fig. 26.10). Although occasionally localized to a single joint such as one knee, CC usually affects several joints: if absent from knees, wrists or symphysis pubis it is unlikely to be present elsewhere. Capsular and synovial calcification is less common than CC, and usually is most obvious at metacarpophalangeal joints (Fig. 26.11) and the knee. Florid synovial calcification occasionally simulates synovial osteochondromatosis. Deposition in tendon insertions particularly favors the Achilles (Fig. 26.12), triceps, and obturators, and is typically linear and extensive compared to discrete, nummular calcification of apatite. Diffuse calcification of bursae (subacromial, olecranon, retrocalcaneal) is an occasional finding. Both CC and calcification are dynamic and may increase, or decrease with time. CC may

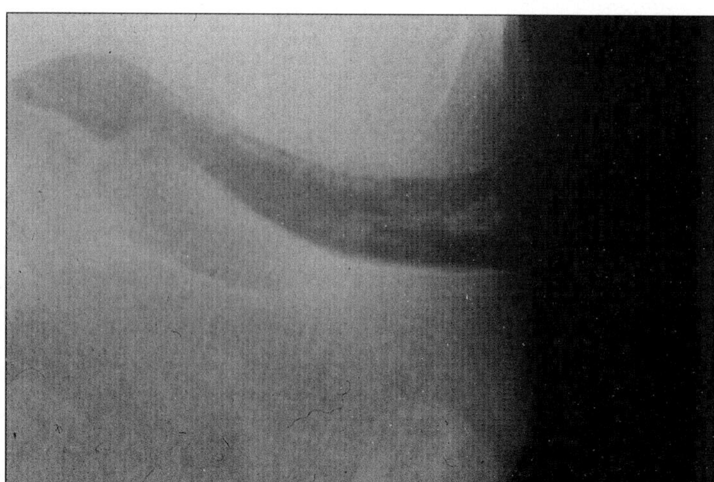

Fig. 26.10 Knee radiograph showing chondrocalcinosis of both fibrocartilage (meniscus) and hyaline cartilage.

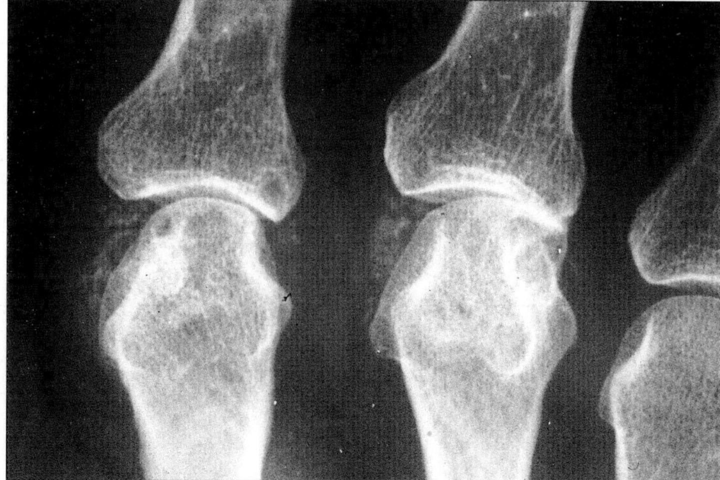

Fig. 26.11 Calcification affecting metacarpophalangeal joints.

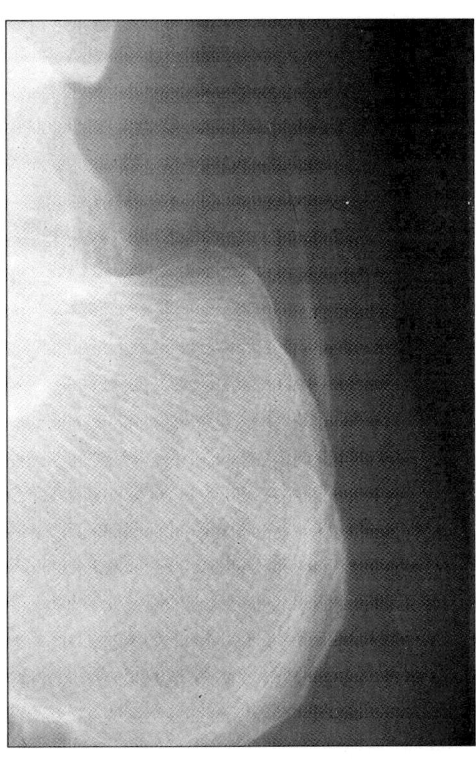

Fig. 26.12 Achilles tendon calcification.

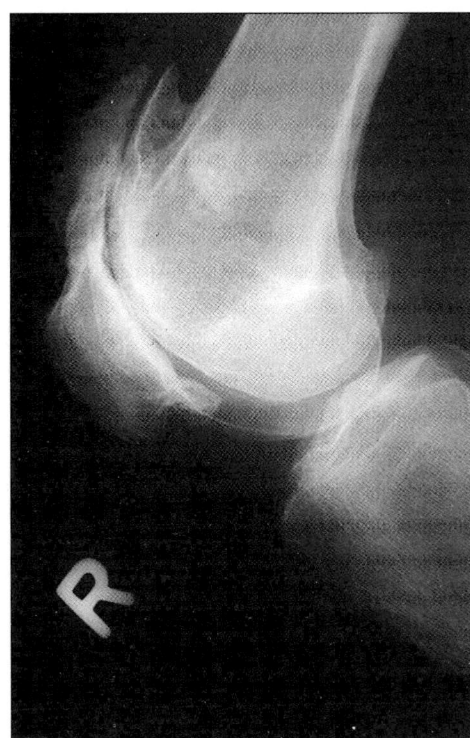

Fig. 26.13 Knee radiograph showing hypertrophic OA features. Note prominent patello-femoral involvement, typical of pyrophosphate arthropathy.

become less evident particularly if cartilage thickness is lost, or if crystals are 'shed' from cartilage during acute or recurrent inflammatory episodes [16,24].

CC and calcification may be readily visible on standard radiographs, though meticulous technique using optimal resolution undoubtedly enhances detection. Plain radiographs, tomography and CT imaging are relatively insensitive and detect only sizeable CPPD deposits. Presence of detectable calcification is not a prerequisite for diagnosis of CPPD associated syndromes.

Structural changes

Changes of pyrophosphate arthropathy are those of OA – namely cartilage loss, sclerosis, cysts, and osteophytes. Characteristics which may permit distinction, however, include:

- joint distribution and involvement within articulations that is atypical of OA. For example, glenohumeral, metacarpophalangeal, ankle or elbow disease; isolated or predominant involvement of patello-femoral compartment, radiocarpal joint (sometimes with characteristic scapho-lunate dissociation), or talocalcaneonavicular articulation; and
- often prominant, exuberant osteophyte and cyst formation (particularly at knee and wrist).

Such combined features may present a distinctive 'hypertrophic' appearance and distribution that suggest CPPD even in the absence of CC (see Figs 26.13 & 26.14). Many cases of pyrophosphate arthropathy, however, appear not dissimilar to 'uncomplicated' OA as regards structural change (and vice versa); furthermore, since nodal generalized OA often coexists in such patients it is common to find otherwise typical OA changes in some joints, with more distinctive changes of pyrophosphate arthropathy at others.

Sequential radiographic changes are variable, though in the 5-year study reporting a generally benign outcome [16], the commonest change was increase in osteophyte with bone remodeling, rather than progressive cartilage or bone attrition (Fig. 26.15). The few patients with destructive arthropathy show marked attrition of cartilage and bone, with occasional fragmentation and loose osseous bodies that may resemble 'disorganization' of a Charcot joint; such cases may show rapid, progessive change.

Marginal erosions (nonproliferative or proliferative) are not a feature of pyrophosphate arthropathy, though smooth 'pressure' erosions (reflecting chronic effusions or bone 'wear') are not infrequent, particularly on the anterior distal femur and around distal inferior radio-ulnar and radiocarpal joints. In patients with coexistant RA and CPPD (c.f. 'pseudorheumatoid arthritis') a modified

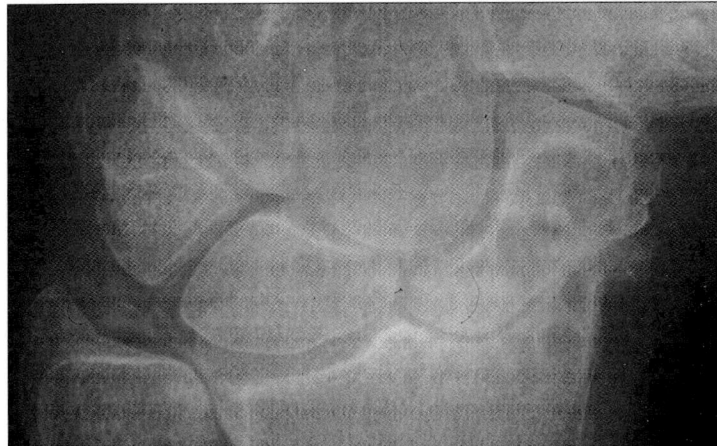

Fig. 26.14 Hand radiograph showing typical radiocarpal involvement. Note prominant cyst formation, and CC.

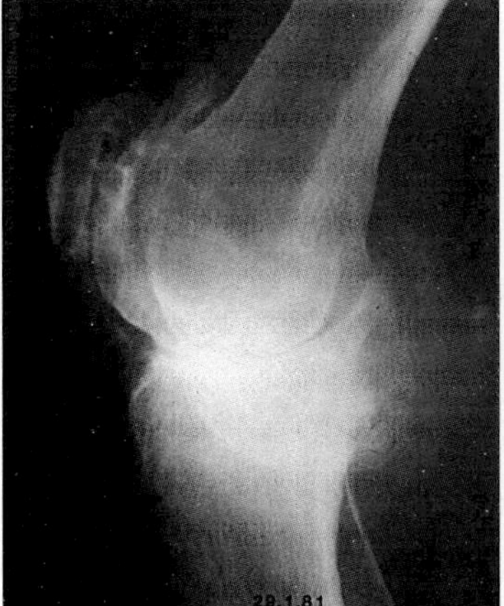

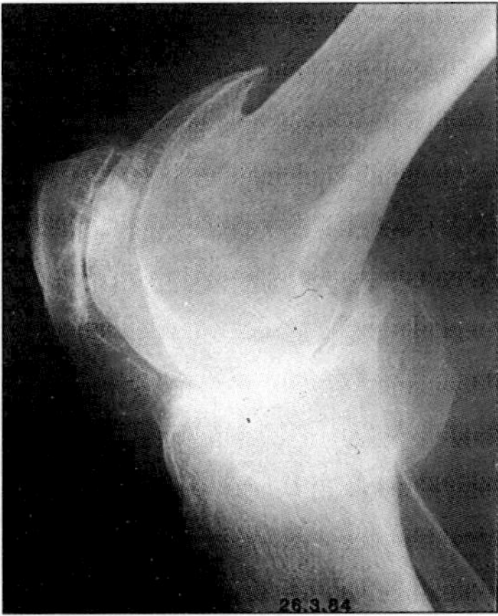

Fig. 26.15 Radiographic progression in the knee of a 67-year-old woman showing predominant bone remodeling. During this 3-year interval her symptoms and function improved (knee radiograph).

radiographic appearance may occur (Fig. 26.16) characterized by retained bone density, prominent osteophyte, prominent well-corticated cysts, and paucity of erosion [25].

Additional Investigations

In pseudogout, Gram stain and culture should always be performed on aspirated fluid: sepsis will be on the differential diagnosis, and concurrence with pseudogout occasionally occurs. Other synovial fluid investigations are of little diagnostic value in this situation: lactate levels, for example, are often in the range seen in sepsis. Pseudogout commonly triggers a moderate acute phase response with elevation of plasma viscosity, ESR, acute phase reactants (e.g. C reactive protein) and peripheral white cell count (predominantly neutrophils): such changes are occasionally impressive, particularly with pseudogout affecting multiple large joints and in patients with triggering intercurrent illness.

In chronic arthropathy, mild anemia with modest elevation of plasma viscosity and acute phase reactants (including ferritin) are not uncommon. The frequency of other biochemical and serologic abnormalities, however, is no different from other subjects of the same age.

Screening for Predisposing Metabolic Disease

Metabolic predisposition is rare and routine screening of all CPPD patients is unrewarding. Nevertheless, CC and arthritis may be the presenting feature of metabolic disease (Fig. 26.2), and a search is warranted in the following circumstances: (i) early onset arthritis (<55 yrs); (ii) florid polyarticular, as opposed to pauciarticular, CC; (iii) recurrent acute attacks > chronic arthropathy; and (iv) presence of additional clinical or radiographic clues that suggest the diagnosis.

A 'blanket screen' for young-onset, polyarticular CC includes serum calcium, alkaline phosphatase, magnesium, ferritin and liver function, but investigation may be more focused if additional clues suggest specific conditions. Hemochromatosis may present radiographic changes similar to sporadic pyrophosphate arthropathy, though possible differentiating features include more widespread metacarpophalangeal involvement, absence of scapho-lunate dissociation, multiple 'ring cysts' in large joints, and subchondral bone fragmentation at the hip [23,26]. In older patients with typical pauciarticular disease and no added features further tests other than calcium studies (performed for additional reasons in this age group) are probably unwarranted.

DIFFERENTIAL DIAGNOSIS

Acute Pseudogout

Occurrence of acute synovitis in one or a few joints, overlying erythema, pyrexia, systemic upset, and purulent joint fluid (particularly in the setting of preceding surgery, trauma, or infective illness) should always lead to consideration and exclusion of sepsis. Because sepsis may coexist with crystal synovitis, Gram stain and culture of joint fluid should always be undertaken (culture of blood and other body fluids may also be appropriate), even once CPPD crystals are identified or radiographic CC demonstrated.

Gout is the other principal condition to consider, diagnosis again resting on synovial fluid analysis. Occasionally heavy blood staining of joint fluid may lead to consideration of other causes of hemarthrosis, especially bleeding disorder or subchondral fracture (particularly with preceding, provoking trauma). However, if CPPD crystals are identified, the clotting screen is normal, there is no lipid in the aspirated fluid, and no radiographic fracture, the diagnosis of pseudogout alone can be accepted. If localized tenderness and pain on weight-bearing persist following resolution of synovitis, repeat radiographs (± subsequent bone scan) may be justified to detect missed fracture.

Chronic Pyrophosphate Arthropathy

In most cases the characteristic distribution, radiographic features, and joint fluid findings permit a ready diagnosis. Polyarticular involvement in elderly patients with modest elevation of ESR, however, may lead to consideration of RA, particularly since predominant large joint involvement may occur in elderly patients with RA. Nevertheless, with pyrophosphate arthropathy the following considerations usually permit distinction: infrequency of tenosynovitis; infrequency of severe systemic upset; absence of extra-articular features; lack of juxta-articular osteopenia and erosions; lack of strong seropositivity for rheumatoid factors; and positive joint fluid and radiographic findings for pyrophosphate arthropathy.

Patients with marked proximal stiffness and elevated ESR are differentiated from polymyalgia rheumatica mainly by careful locomotor examination, and positive joint fluid and radiographic findings. Oral steroids often improve symptoms in such patients but rarely give the rapid 'cure' of polymyalgia: response to local intra-articular steroid may be more impressive.

Differentiation from uncomplicated OA is often by: the different pattern of distribution between and within articulations; the more

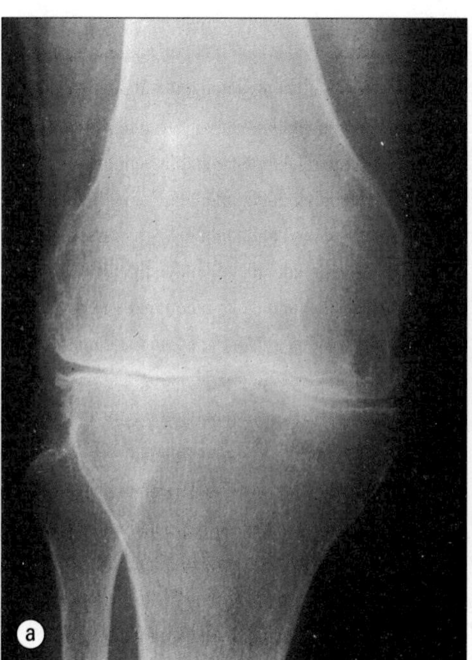

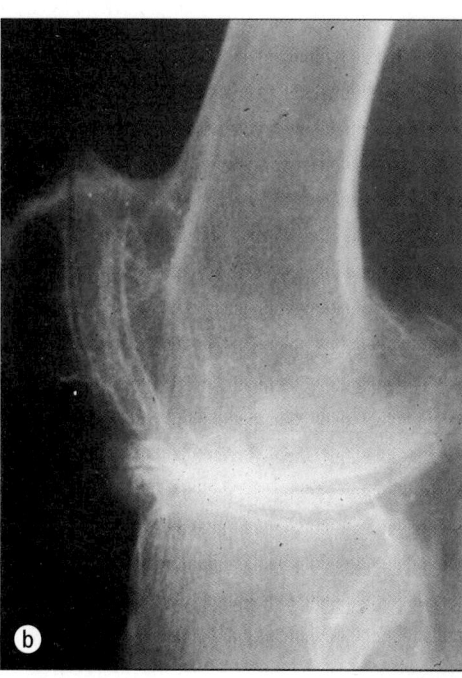

Fig. 26.16 Knee radiograph of patient with coexistant rheumatoid arthritis and CPPD deposition. On the AP view (a) there is widespread cartilage loss, but the lateral view (b) shows marked new bone formation atypical of RA.

florid inflammatory component; presence of superimposed acute attacks; radiographic findings of atypical distribution for OA, CC, calcification, prominant osteophyte and cyst; and synovial fluid CPPD crystals.

Although destructive pyrophosphate arthropathy may radiographically resemble a neuropathic joint (shoulder involvement suggesting syringomyelia, knee involvement tabes) such joints are severely symptomatic and arise in the absence of overt neurologic or serologic abnormality.

Although description of clinical presentations by addition of 'pseudo-' to other diagnostic labels suggests close mimicry of other joint disease, the diagnosis is usually suspected on clinical grounds alone, and confirmed by the synovial fluid and radiographic findings. However, CPPD deposition commonly coexists or is superimposed upon other recognizable joint disease, making the prefix 'pseudo-' clearly inappropriate [2]. The commonest associated condition is OA (generalized, pauciarticular, or post-traumatic) affecting the same or distant joints, though coexistent gout, sepsis, rheumatoid, apatite-associated destructive arthropathy, or true Charcot arthropathy may all occur. In such cases the diagnostic label should reflect both conditions, though the relative contribution of each may vary at different sites in the same individual.

Although rare, tophaceous CPPD should be considered with malignancy, tophaceous gout, and tumoral calcinosis in the differential diagnosis of calcified lesions involving periarticular soft tissues. Examination of biopsy material is inevitably required for correct diagnosis [21].

MANAGEMENT

Acute Synovitis

The aims of management for pseudogout are to: reduce symptoms; identify and treat triggering illness; and rapidly mobilize as inflammation settles.

Rapid mobilization is particularly important since many patients are elderly and especially prone to complications from prolonged immobility. Many also have coexisting medical problems and are especially at risk from drug side-effects and interactions. In general, therefore, local rather than systemic therapy is preferred, particularly since pseudogout affects usually only one or a few joints.

Aspiration and injection

In most cases aspiration alone greatly relieves symptoms and may be the only treatment required. Fluid reaccumulation, however, is common (particularly early in the attack), and for florid pseudogout intra-articular steroid injection is appropriate, either at the time of initial aspiration or as a second procedure following reaccumulation (some prefer the reassurance of a negative Gram stain and/or culture before injecting). Joint lavage (normal saline, room temperature) can help settle attacks but is reserved for troublesome relapsing or prolonged episodes unresponsive to steroid injection.

Oral drugs

Simple analgesic and nonsteroidal drugs may give additional benefit, but these must be used with caution in elderly or medically unfit patients. Colchicine (oral or intravenous) is effective but rarely warranted. For severe polyarticular attacks, unresponsive to aspiration and injection of the largest affected joints, oral steroid may be considered though its efficacy is anecdotal.

Additional measures

Identification of triggering illness that requires specific treatment (e.g. chest infection) is by appropriate patient enquiry and examination. Once the synovitis is settling, increasing mobilization with attention to muscle training exercises should be undertaken.

Chronic Pyrophosphate Arthropathy

Unlike gout there is no specific therapy and treatment of underlying metabolic disease does not influence outcome. The aims of management are to reduce symptoms and retain or improve function. A variety of strategies may be beneficial.

General principles

Reduction in obesity, use of a stick or other walking aid, education in appropriate joint usage, and improvement in muscle tone/strength may all reduce adverse mechanical stress and optimize chances of stabilization or improvement. Recognition and management of depression and use of coping strategies are as applicable to elderly patients with pyrophosphate arthropathy as young patients with RA.

Control of chronic synovitis

Despite presence of often marked mechanical abnormality, intra-articular steroid injection often greatly improves symptoms. Though often temporary, this may improve the patients optimism, encourage involvement in other aspects of treatment, and provide a useful interval for effective physiotherapy or enjoyment of an important life event (e.g. holiday).

Intra-articular radiocolloid (yttrium-90) should be considered in patients with troublesome knee (or shoulder) synovitis who show definite, but temporary, improvement following steroid injection. Prolonged symptomatic benefit may be obtained with such treatment, even in cases with gross structural change [2]. If synovitis recurs (again steroid responsive) single repeat treatment may be considered. Radiosynovectomy is also useful for recurrent hemarthrosis, presumably by induction of synovial fibrosis.

Symptomatic drugs

As for pseudogout, symptomatic drugs are used with caution in older patients. In general, simple analgesics are preferable to NSAIDs; the patient should be instructed on appropriate usage, the requirement for NSAIDs regularly reviewed, and 'repeat' prescribing avoided.

One 6-month placebo-controlled study of oral magnesium supplementation, given to enhance solubility and inhibit formation of CPPD, showed limited symptomatic benefit without alteration in radiographic CC [2]. Such treatment was well tolerated and further long-term studies seem warranted.

Surgery

Patients with progressive or destructive large joint arthropathy who require replacement appear to derive benefit equal to patients with uncomplicated OA, without increased risk of prosthetic failure.

REFERENCES

1. McCarty DJ. Calcium pyrophosphate dihydrate crystal deposition disease – 1975. Arthritis Rheum. 1976;**19**(suppl): 275–86.
2. Doherty M, Dieppe PA. Clinical aspects of calcium pyrophosphate dihydrate crystal deposition. Rheum Dis Clin North Am. 1988;**14**:395–414.
3. Mitrovic DR, Stankovic A, Iriarte-Borda O, et al. The prevalence of chondrocalcinosis in the human knee joint. An autopsy survey. J Rheumatol. 1988;**15**:633–41.
4. Felson DT, Anderson JJ, Naimark A, Kannel W, Meenan RF. The prevalence of chondrocalcinosis in the elderly and its association with knee osteoarthritis: the Framingham study. J Rheumatol. 1989;**16**:1241–5.
5. Bjelle AO. Morphological study of articular cartilage in pyrophosphate arthropathy. (Chondrocalcinosis articularis or calcium pyrophosphate dihydrate crystal deposition disease). Ann Rheum Dis. 1972;**31**:449–56.
6. Reginato AJ. Articular chondrocalcinosis in the Chiloe Islanders. Arthritis Rheum. 1976;**19**:395–404.
7. Rodriguez-Valverde V, Tinture T, Zuniga M, Pena J, Gonzalez A. Familial chondrocalcinosis. Prevalence in northern Spain and clinical features in 5 pedigrees. Arthritis Rheum. 1980;**23**:471–8.
8. Riestra JL, Sanchez A, Rodriguez-Valverde V, Alonson JL. Radiographic features of hereditary articular chondrocalcinosis. A comparative study with the sporadic type. Clin Exp Rheumatol. 1988;**6**:369–72.
9. Doherty M, Hamilton E, Henderson J, Misra H, Dixey H. Familial chondrocalcinosis due to calcium pyrophosphate dihydrate crystal deposition in English families. Br J Rheumatol. 1991;**30**:10–15.
10. Hamilton EBD. Diseases associated with CPPD deposition disease. Arthritis Rheum. 1976;**19**:353–7.
11. Dodds WJ, Steinbach HL. Primary hyperparathyroidism and articular cartilage calcification. Am J Roentgenol Rad Ther Nucl Med. 1968;**104**:884–92.
12. Hamilton EBD, Bomford AB, Laws JW, Williams R. The natural history of arthritis and idiopathic haemochromatosis: progression of the clinical and radiological features over ten years. Quart J Med. 1981;**199**:321–9.
13 Chuck AJ, Pattrick MG, Hamilton E, Wilson R, Doherty M. Crystal deposition in hypophosphatasia: a reappraisal. Ann Rheum Dis. 1989;**48**:57–6.
14. Milazzo SC, Ahern MJ, Cleland LG, Henderson DRF. Calcium pyrophosphate dihydrate deposition disease and familial hypomagnesemia. J Rheumatol. 1981;**8**:767–71.
15. Dieppe PA, Alexander GM, Jones H, Doherty M, Scott DG. Pyrophosphate arthropathy: a clinical and radiological study of 105 cases. Ann Rheum Dis. 1982;**41**:371–6.
16. Doherty M. Pyrophosphate arthropathy – a clinical study. MD thesis, Cambridge University; 1987.
17. Menkes CJ, Simon F, Delrieu F, Forest M, Delbarre F. Destructive arthropathy in chondrocalcinosis articularis. Arthritis Rheum. 1976;**19**:329–48.
18. Okazaki T, Saito T, Mitommo Y, Sicta Y. Pseudogout: clinical observations and chemical analyses of deposits. Arthritis Rheum. 1976;**19**:293–305.
19. Gerster JC, Lagier R. Upper limb pyrophosphate tenosynovitis outside the carpal tunnel. Ann Rheum Dis. 1989;**48**:689–91.
20. Pattrick M, Watt I, Dieppe PA, Doherty M.Peripheral nerve entrapment at the wrist in pyrophosphate arthropathy. J Rheumatol. 1988;**15**:1254–7.
21. Sissons HA, Steiner GC, Bonar F, et al. Tumoral calcium pyrophosphate deposition disease. Skeletal Radiol. 1989;**18**:79–87.
22. Resnick D, Niwayama G, Goergen TG, et al. Clinical, radiographic and pathologic abnormalities in calcium pyrophosphate dihydrate deposition disease (CPPD): pseudogout. Radiology. 1977;**122**:1–15.
23. Resnick D, Niwayama G. Calcium pyrophosphate dihydrate (CPPD) crystal deposition disease. In: Diagnosis of bone and joint disorders. Philadelphia: WB Saunders; 1981:1520–74.
24. Doherty M, Dieppe PA. Acute pseudogout: 'Crystal shedding' or acute crystallisation? Arthritis Rheum. 1981;**24**:954–7.
25. Doherty M, Dieppe PA, Watt I. Low incidence of calcium pyrophosphate dihydrate crystal deposition in rheumatoid arthritis with modification of radiographic features in coexistent disease. Arthritis Rheum. 1984;**27**:1002–9.
26. Adamson TC, Resnik CS, Guerra J, Vint VC, Weisman MH, Resnick D. Hand and wrist arthropathies of haemochromatosis and calcium pyrophosphate deposition disease: distinct radiographic features. Radiology. 1983;**147**:377–81.

GOUT AND PSEUDOGOUT

27

PRACTICAL PROBLEMS

ATYPICAL GOUT

Bryan T Emmerson

Description of the Problem

When gout presents with classical podagra, the diagnosis is usually simple. However, gout can affect virtually any joint, is sometimes polyarticular, may present with systemic features such as fever, and can mimic many other arthropathies. Atypical presentations can present difficult diagnostic and management problems.

Typical Case

A man of 52 years presented with a subacute onset of polyarthritis. The onset, some 10 weeks before presentation, was characterized by the development of pain and swelling of both forefeet. The problem subsequently spread to involve the metacarpophalangeal (MCP) joints, proximal interphalangeal (PIP) joints, wrists, elbows and knees. He had no significant past or family history and had been on no drug prior to the onset of arthritis. He was a heavy beer drinker and a smoker.

On examination he had a symmetrical polyarthritis affecting the symptomatic joints (Fig. 27.1). In addition, he had bilateral swellings over the elbows, clinically thought to be bursitis with firm nodules within their walls. Nodular swellings were also observed over the right ulna and the dorsum of both feet. He was mildly obese and hypertensive with a blood pressure of 150/95.

Initial investigations showed an elevated acute-phase response (erythrocyte sedimentation rate, ESR: 87mm/hour), a weakly positive rheumatoid factor (titer 1:40), and some erosions on radiographs of the hands. A diagnosis of rheumatoid arthritis (RA) was made, and the patient was prescribed a nonsteroidal anti-inflammatory agent (NSAID).

Subsequently, clinical suspicion was raised by acute exacerbations of the arthritis in selected joints, and the atypical nature of swellings. Further investigations showed that the plasma urate concentration was markedly elevated (10.5mg/dl; 0.63mmol/l), as were plasma lipid concentrations. Synovial fluid was aspirated from knee and elbow joints and contained numerous urate crystals. Excision of a 'nodule' revealed a gouty tophus.

Diagnostic Problems

Tophaceous gout or nodular rheumatoid arthritis?

Tophacous gout can mimic RA, as in the case described. Gout is polyarticular in onset in about 10% of cases, and may produce a symmetric polyarthritis. Tophi may have a similar distribution to rheumatoid nodules. A raised acute-phase response is usual, and the radiographs may show erosions. Screening tests for rheumatoid factor are sometimes positive, but the titers are rarely high.

Suspicion should always be raised by the presence of the associations of gout – obese middle aged men with hypertension are at risk. Other features of gout that should lead to the correct diagnosis being made at the onset include the characteristic erosions, which are quite

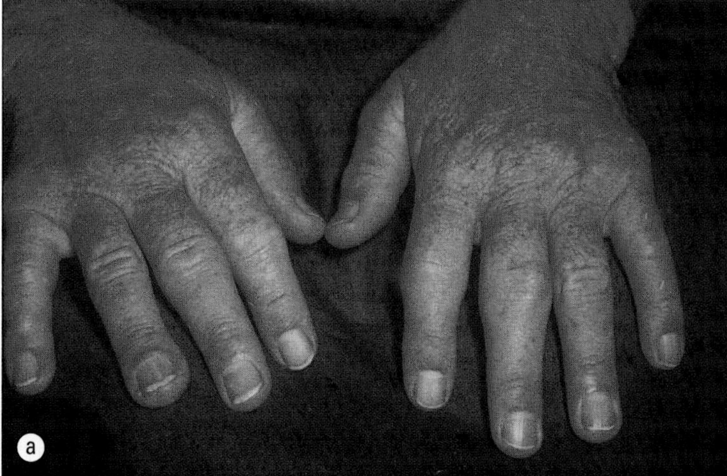

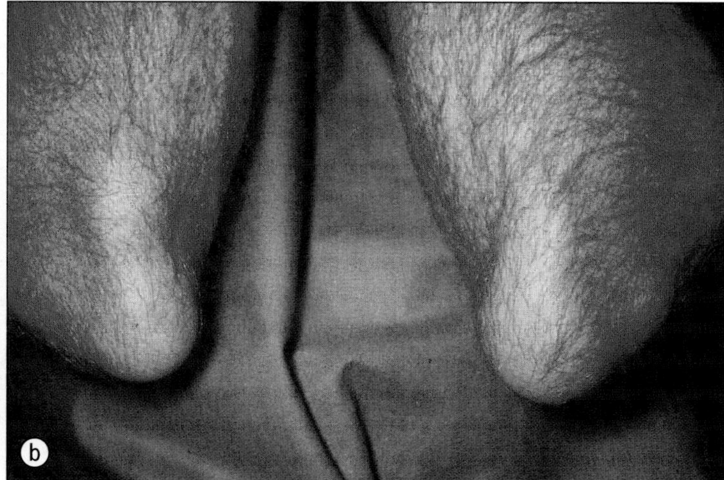

Fig. 27.1 Symmetrical polyarthritis in atypical gout. In this patient there is obvious bilateral swelling of the 2nd to 5th MCP joints and some of the PIP joints (a), as well as both olecranon bursae and the right proximal ulna border (b). Courtesy of Dr J Webb.

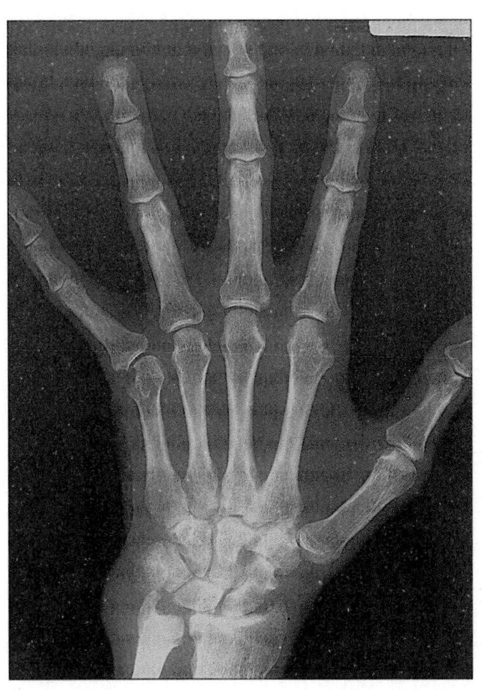

Fig. 27.2 Hand radiograph of the patient with gout masquerading as RA. Note the large tophaceous swelling over the ulnar border of the wrist. The erosions do not have the regular distribution (MCPs and PIPs) that is usual in RA. The large marginal erosion at the distal end of the 5th metacarpal has a 'punched out' appearance with a sclerotic margin and 'hook' at the edge – this is typical of gout. The ill-defined erosion of the 2nd metacarpal is less characteristic.

different from those of RA (Fig. 27.2) and the absence of a high titer of rheumatoid factor – nodular RA is always associated with high titers. These cases also emphasize the need for careful examination of the synovial fluid in any case of undiagnosed arthritis. Fluid samples should always be examined under polarized light microscopy and by culture, as well as for their cell content.

The negative association between rheumatoid arthritis and gout

There is a strong negative association between these two diseases, with only a handful of case descriptions of their coexistence in spite of the fact that both are common. The reasons for this are unknown, but physicians should always be wary of making the diagnosis of gout with RA, or of the development of one disease in patients known to have the other.

Management Problems

Hypertension and arthritis

Patients often need treatment for their hypertension, as well as for their arthritis. Patients of this sort often have problems with drug treatment, because NSAIDs can make the hypertension worse, and diuretics used for hypertension can counteract the effect of the NSAIDs as well as contributing to hyperuricemia. Diuretics should be avoided, and the hypertension treated with other agents such as β-blockers or angiotensin-converting enzyme (ACE) inhibitors if drug treatment is necessary. There are some theoretical advantages to an NSAID that is least likely to affect the kidney, such as sulindac, but the use of any NSAID should be cautious, with attention being paid to both the blood pressure and renal function. Colchicine is a valuable alternative in the treatment of gouty inflammation.

The patient described earlier is at risk of cardiovascular disease, and every attempt should be made to reduce this risk. He should be advised to lose weight and to give up smoking. Dietary advice, and possibly drug therapy, should be used to control the hyperlipidemia, and exercise, within the limits of the arthritis, should be recommended.

Long-term control of the hyperuricemia and gout

The patient's hyperuricemia should be fully investigated to differentiate between the rare overproducers of uric acid and the more common underexcretors. In the case described, 24-hour urine samples were collected after taking the patient off all drugs except for colchicine, and while on a low purine diet, and they showed that he was an underexcretor. Renal function was normal. In such a case this allows for the option to use a drug that increases excretion, such as probenecid, or one of the NSAIDs with more powerful uricosuric effects, such as azapropazone. In these circumstances care must be taken to keep urine volumes high, particularly when the treatment is first started. In practice, if drug therapy is needed allopurinol may still be the best hypouricemic agent, but it should be introduced slowly with coexistent use of prophylactic colchicine to reduce the problem of exacerbating the gout.

However, in many instances hypouricemic drug therapy may be less important than the patient's lifestyle. Obesity and a high alcohol intake, associated with a low urine volume, make a great contribution to the hyperuricemia. Advice to lose weight, reduce alcohol intake, increase fluid intake and reduce dietary fats may result in a marked weight loss and a fall in the uric acid levels. Such achievements depend on high motivation and are aided by careful, sustained educational input.

Conclusions

- The diagnosis of gout of atypical onset requires a high degree of clinical suspicion.
- If there is any uncertainty about the diagnosis of a polyarthritis, synovial fluid examination should be carried out, including a search for urate crystals.
- RA and gout rarely coexist, but gout is associated with other crystal arthropathies.
- Drug therapy of gouty patients with hypertension is difficult; diuretics as well as NSAIDs should be either avoided or used with great caution.
- Hyperuricemia and gout can often be controlled by alterations in lifestyle, rather than drug therapy provided that patients are well motivated.

REFERENCES

Diamond HS. Control of crystal-induced arthropathies. Rheum Dis Clin North Am. 1989;**15**:557–67.

Dieppe PA. Investigation and management of gout in the young and the elderly. Ann Rheum Dis. 1991;**50**:263–6.

Fessel WJ. High uric acid content as an indicator of cardiovascular disease; independence from obesity. Am J Med. 1980;**68**:401–4.

Lawry GV, Fan PT, Bluestone R. Polyarticular versus monoarticular gout; a prospective comparative analysis of clinical features. Medicine (Balt). 1988;**67**:335–43.

Wallace DJ, Klinenberg JR, Morhain D, Berlanstein B, Biren PC, Callis G. Coexistent gout and rheumatoid arthritis: case report and review of the literature. Arthritis Rheum. 1979;**22**:81–6.

THE MANAGEMENT OF TOPHACEOUS GOUT IN THE ELDERLY

Paul A Dieppe

Definition of the Problem

Tophaceous gout may develop in elderly people, especially women, with poor renal function. Such patients are frequently suffering from other conditions as well and may be taking several drugs, including diuretics. Several problems can arise in these patients, including the relatively rapid growth of painful, destructive, peripheral tophi, ulceration of the lesions and secondary infections. Drug treatment is made particularly difficult because of the high incidence of severe side effects. Anti-inflammatory drugs are particularly dangerous in this group, and allopurinol can cause fatal drug reactions.

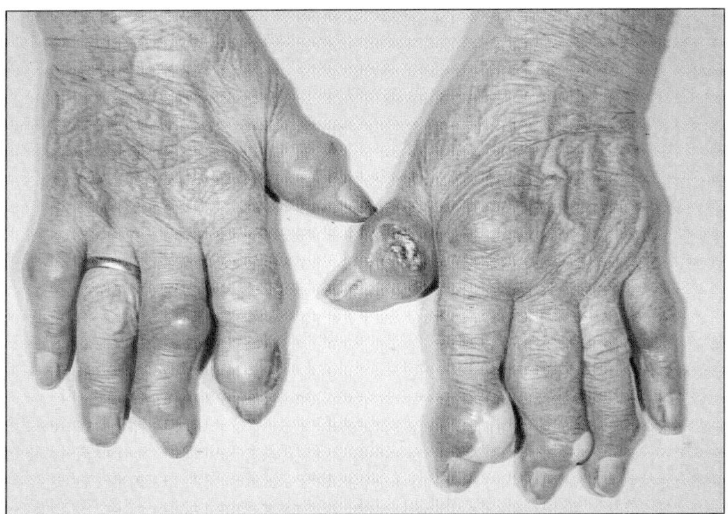

Fig. 27.3 Gouty tophi around the osteoarthritic interphalangeal joints of patient JG. Note the characteristic shiny, white deposits, many of which remain painless. One lesion on the thumb has ulcerated and is prone to secondary infection.

The Typical Case

JG is a 79-year-old woman who developed tophaceous gout at the age of 78. She has rheumatic heart disease and has required high-dose diuretic therapy for a number of years to control congestive cardiac failure. A year ago she noticed the development of painful lumps on her already 'knobbly' fingers (Fig. 27.3); she subsequently developed lumps over the toes, with ulceration over the left first metatarsophalangeal joint. Her primary-care physician initially diagnosed infection and prescribed antibiotics which had no effect. The diagnosis of gout was confirmed by obtaining a smear of material from the ulcerated lesion and examining it for urate crystals in a polarizing light microscope. Her serum uric acid was 11.8mg/dl (0.71mmol/l), with a urea of 35mg/dl (12.5mmol/l) and a much reduced creatinine clearance (43ml/min); radiographs showed evidence of extensive bony destruction. She was initially treated with NSAIDs. Several were tried, but all caused severe gastrointestinal side effects. Colchicine was prescribed but, even in low doses, resulted in diarrhea. Finally JG was treated with low-dose allopurinol (starting at 50mg on alternate days); after several months there was a gradual improvement in her condition.

Diagnostic Problems

Gout often presents atypically in the elderly. Acute attacks are less frequent and the formation of tophi more common. Tophi are particularly likely to occur in and around Heberden's nodes. The white ulcerating lesions cause confusion with sepsis. Other diagnoses that may have to be considered include other crystal arthropathies and other causes of tophi such as hyperlipidemia. However, the appearance of the deposits is usually highly characteristic (see Fig. 27.3), and the diagnosis is easily confirmed by polarizing light microscopy of material from one of the lesions. Secondary infections can occur, particularly in and around ulcerated lesions, and gout and joint sepsis can coexist. If there is any doubt, material should be sent for culture as well as crystal examination. Extensive investigations are unnecessary, but the extent of the hyperuricemia should be documented and renal function assessed.

AN APPROACH TO THE MANAGEMENT OF TOPHACEOUS GOUT IN THE ELDERLY

- Confirm diagnosis by crystal identification
  Beware coexistent infection
- Check serum uric acid, renal function and blood count
  Further investigations usually unnecessary
- Remove any avoidable factors contributing to hyperuricemia, such as unnecessary diuretics
- Consider the need for specific therapy
  (this is often unecessary)
- Use low-dose colchicine as the drug of first choice for painful inflammatory problems
- Beware of NSAIDs
  Consider renal disease, diuretics and high risk of gastrointestinal problems
- Beware of allopurinol
  If it has to be used, start with very low doses and look out for serious toxicity
  Avoid uricosuric drugs

Fig. 27.4 The management of tophaceous gout in the elderly.

Therapeutic Options

These patients are difficult to treat. They are often frail, may have multiple pathologies, and be on many drugs. Life expectancy may be short. Severe drug reactions are common.

The first decision is whether any treatment is necessary. The lesions are often relatively trouble free, and severe acute attacks of gout are uncommon. However, the tophi may be painful and/or destructive, and the hyperuricemia may be contributing to further renal damage, in which case treatment may be required.

Where possible, any factors contributing to the hyperuricemia should be removed. Diuretics may be unnecessary and are often the main culprit. Other drugs, obesity and alcohol may be contributing. Painful inflammatory reactions are probably best treated with low-dose colchicine in this age group. Doses of around 0.5mg twice daily often prevent attacks without causing side effects. Anti-inflammatory drugs are hazardous because of the age and sex of the patients, and the frequent coexistence of renal disease and diuretic therapy. Lack of efficacy and a high incidence of side effects, both gastrointestinal and neurologic, are frequent problems.

Hypouricemic therapy should be approached with extreme caution. Uricosuric agents are unlikely to be efficacious. Allopurinol produces a high incidence of rashes, sensitivity reactions and vasculitis, probably because of the concurrent renal problems. Several fatal reactions have been reported, and doses must be kept low. A starting dose of 100mg on alternate days, or less, is reasonable if it is deemed necessary to use the drug, and cover with low-dose colchicine to prevent worsening inflammation is advisable. Around 100mg daily is often sufficient to control the hyperuricemia. Local aspiration or surgery are hazardous because of the risk of secondary infection, although it is sometimes helpful to drain or remove a particularly troublesome lesion.

The management of these patients is quite different from that of the typical middle-aged gouty male. Priority must be given to the quality of life and avoiding serious toxicity from drugs. The emphasis given to long-term renal and cardiovascular issues in typical gout is often inappropriate in the elderly (Fig 27.4).

Conclusions

Elderly patients with tophaceous gout must be treated quite differently from the typical gouty patient (see Fig. 27.4). Drugs are dangerous in this group.

REFERENCES

Borg EGG, Rasker JJ. Gout in the elderly; a separate entity? Ann Rheum Dis. 1987;**46:**72–5.

Lally EV, Zimmerman B, Ho G, Kaplan SR. Urate-mediated inflammation in nodal osteoarthritis; clinical and roentgenographic correlations. Arthritis Rheum. 1989;**32:**86–90.

Macfarlane DG, Dieppe PA. Diuretic-induced gout in elderly women. Br J Rheumatol. 1985;**24:**155–7.

O'Connell PG, Milburn BM, Nashel DJ. Coexistent gout and septic arthritis; a report of two cases and literature review. Clin Exp Rheumatol. 1985;**3**:265–9.

Wordsworth BP, Mowat AG. Rapid development of gouty tophi after diuretic therapy. J Rheumatol. 1985;**12:**376–9.

Definition of the Problem

Pseudogout is the commonest cause of acute inflammatory monoarthritis in the elderly. Provocation by intercurrent illness, trauma or surgery, together with the physical signs, often suggest sepsis as the likely cause. This may cause delay in appropriate treatment, and cause side effects from inappropriate interventions.

The Typical Case

RS is a fit 76-year-old woman with no previous joint symptoms, admitted with acute appendicitis. On the third day following laparotomy she developed a painful, swollen right knee, pyrexia of 38.5°C, and mild confusion. A diagnosis of septic arthritis was made by the duty orthopedic staff after 70ml of blood-stained turbid fluid (white cell count 75,000/mm^3; polymorphs 98%) was aspirated from her knee. Her leg was splinted and she was commenced on parenteral antibiotics (flucloxacillin, fusidic acid, gentamicin). Gram staining and culture of the aspirate was negative, and the microbiology staff detected no crystals; the knee radiograph was considered normal. Because of persistent synovitis and pyrexia on day 6, the knee was again aspirated and arthrotomy considered. However, on day 7 she developed persistent bloody diarrhea, necessitating intravenous fluid replacement and deferral of arthrotomy. Her general state was poor and on day 9 the medical team were consulted.

Previous joint aspirates were re-examined and calcium pyrophosphate dihydrate (CPPD) crystals identified in all samples: faint lateral meniscal chondrocalcinosis (CC) was noted on her radiograph using bright light illumination. Sigmoidoscopy showed an inflamed mucosa but no pseudomembrane; clostridial toxin was not detected and stool culture grew no pathogens. Her parenteral antibiotics were stopped, her knee re-aspirated and injected with corticosteroid, the splinting was removed and physiotherapy (passive followed by increasing active) was instituted. Her synovitis quickly settled and her diarrhea subsided over the next 2 days. After slow mobilization (due mainly to the weakened left quadriceps muscle) she was discharged 4 weeks after admission.

Diagnostic Problems

Pseudogout may be difficult to distinguish from septic arthritis. Both may cause marked synovitis, overlying erythema, purulent synovial fluid, and a florid acute-phase response manifested by fever, malaise, and elevated ESR and C-reactive protein (CRP). Furthermore, triggering of pseudogout may occur in circumstances that particularly suggest sepsis (Fig.27.5), and pseudogout and sepsis may coexist. Nevertheless, certain features may make pseudogout the most likely diagnosis:

- In terms of frequency alone, pseudogout is more common than sepsis and should be considered first.
- Marked blood-staining of synovial fluid is rare in the early stages of septic arthritis but common in pseudogout (Fig. 27.6).
- Pseudogout may be the presentation of CPPD deposition, whereas sepsis is rare in a previously normal joint in adults with no systemic predisposition to infection.

Even when the possibility of pseudogout is considered, two factors (illustrated in the case above) commonly mitigate against ready diagnosis:

- CPPD crystals are easily missed unless carefully sought by experienced staff using appropriate equipment.
- Radiographic CC need not be florid, or even present, for the diagnosis of pseudogout.

The other principal condition to consider is gout. However, *de novo* presentation in the elderly, particularly women, is rare in the absence of preceding chronic diuretic therapy or a long-standing history of arthropathy.

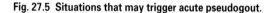

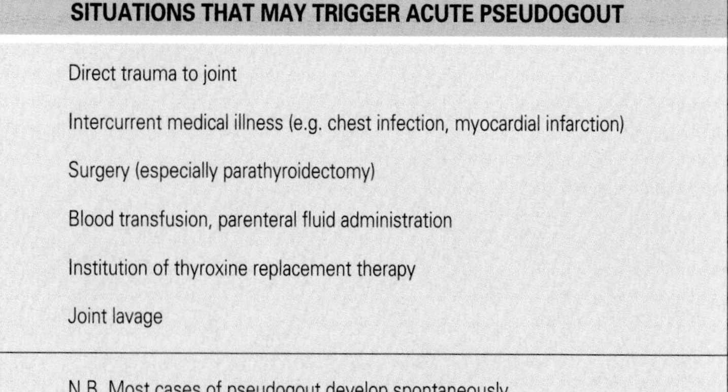

SITUATIONS THAT MAY TRIGGER ACUTE PSEUDOGOUT

Direct trauma to joint

Intercurrent medical illness (e.g. chest infection, myocardial infarction)

Surgery (especially parathyroidectomy)

Blood transfusion, parenteral fluid administration

Institution of thyroxine replacement therapy

Joint lavage

N.B. Most cases of pseudogout develop spontaneously

Fig. 27.5 Situations that may trigger acute pseudogout.

Correct diagnosis pivots around appropriate joint-fluid analysis – i.e. Gram stain and culture and compensated polarized microscopy. Both analyses must be undertaken. If pseudogout is misdiagnosed joint recovery may be unduly delayed and inappropriate, potentially harmful interventions employed. Conversely, missed sepsis carries serious consequences in terms of joint damage and mortality.

Therapeutic Options

If CPPD crystals are identified and the Gram stain is negative, the diagnosis will usually be pseudogout alone (Fig.27.7). Intra-articular corticosteroid may be used for brisk synovitis; antibiotics should not be given (unless for precipitating infective illness); and other aspects of management are along the lines already discussed. The 48-hour culture result should always be checked to avoid missing coexistent sepsis.

The uncommon exception to this strategy is if the patient is severely ill (unusual in pseudogout), or immunocompromised by disease or drugs. In such high-risk circumstances it seems reasonable to commence parenteral antibiotics pending the results of synovial fluid culture. If the culture is negative, however, antibiotics should be stopped, the diagnosis of uncomplicated pseudogout accepted and treatment of the joint adapted for this alone. This approach avoids complications resulting from inappropriate antibiotics or surgical drainage.

If it transpires that the patient receives corticosteroid into a joint subsequently proven to have sepsis, this is unlikely to be detrimental

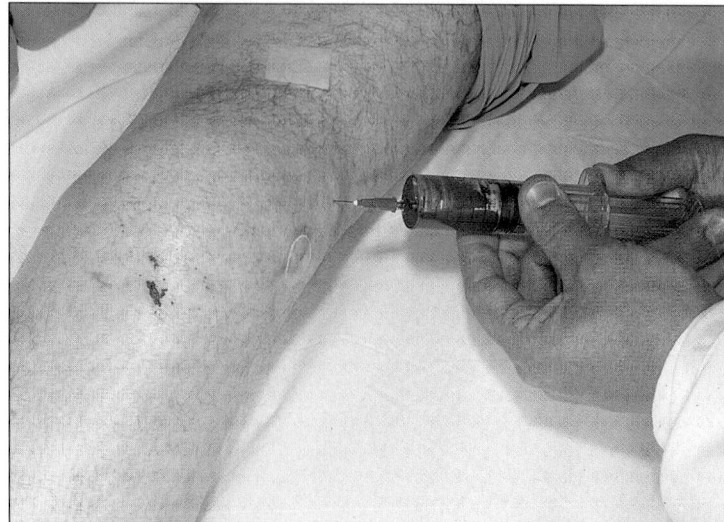

Fig. 27.6 Blood-stained synovial fluid in pseudogout. In this case pseudogout was exacerbated by minor trauma, resulting in an acutely inflamed knee joint.

providing antibiotics are commenced within 48–72 hours of the initial aspiration/injection. Corticosteroids are potent inhibitors of damaging host cell-derived enzymes in septic arthritis, and their use in this situation is arguably beneficial.

AN APPROACH TO THE MANAGEMENT OF PSEUDOGOUT IN THE ELDERLY

- Confirm diagnosis by crystal identification
- Always undertake Gram stain and culture, and check culture result at 48–72 hours
- If Gram stain is negative, treat as pseudogout alone
- Only consider i.v. antibiotics in the first 48 hours if the patient is severely ill or immunocompromised, or if indicated for triggering sepsis elsewhere
- Stop antibiotics if culture negative at 48–72 hours
- If appropriate, use intra-articular corticosteroids early

Fig. 27.7 An approach to the management of pseudogout in the elderly.

Conclusion

In acute mono- or oligoarthritis in the elderly, crystals and sepsis should both be sought. Apart from a few exceptional situations, pseudogout is most likely, and management for this should be instituted early. Misdiagnosis and treatment as sepsis is not without complications in the elderly.

REFERENCES

Doherty M, Dieppe P. Crystal deposition in the elderly. Clin Rheum Dis. 1986;**12**:97–116.

Haslock I. Arthritis in old age: drug treatment. In: Wright V, ed. Bone and joint disease in the elderly. Edinburgh: Churchill Livingstone; 1983:181–96.

Radcliffe K, Pattrick M, Doherty M. Complications resulting from misdiagnosing pseudogout as sepsis. Br Med J. 1986;**293**:440–1

CHRONIC PYROPHOSPHATE ARTHROPATHY OR RHEUMATOID ARTHRITIS?

Michael Doherty

Definition of the Problem

In polyarticular chronic pyrophosphate arthropathy (CPA) the diagnosis of RA, rather than a subset of osteoarthritis (OA), may be suggested by the combination of overt synovitis, atypical joint distribution and periarticular complications. The problem is compounded by occasional concurrence of RA and CPPD crystal deposition. Differentiation between CPA, RA or coexistent disease is by accurate clinical assessment and basic investigations (synovial fluid analysis, plain radiographs). Accurate diagnosis may have relevence to prognosis and selection of appropriate interventions.

The Typical Case

BS is a 72-year-old woman referred as a case of RA for consideration of second-line therapy. She gave a 3-year history of inflammatory arthropathy affecting the wrists, MCPs, shoulders, knees and left ankle. She had suffered prolonged early morning stiffness, particularly of the wrists and knees, and progressive difficulty with dressing and other activities of daily living. In the preceding year she had undergone right and then left carpal tunnel decompression. Investigations by her family doctor had revealed an elevated ESR (34mm in the first hour) and weakly positive Rose Waaler test (1:64). She had been prescribed sulfasalazine for 4 months with no benefit, and 4 months prior to referral had been commenced on prednisolone 7.5mg daily.

Examination revealed joint-line tenderness, restricted movement and crepitus affecting both wrists, glenohumeral joints and knees, with less marked changes in both 2nd to 4th MCPs, left ankle and right elbow. Synovitis (soft tissue swelling, effusion, warmth) was particularly evident in both wrists and knees. She had moderate muscle wasting and weakness around both shoulders and knees. Additional locomotor findings included several nontender Heberden's nodes; there were no extra-articular abnormalities of note. Examination of synovial fluid from both knees revealed CPPD crystals. Radiographs showed changes of pyrophosphate arthropathy in both wrists (Fig. 27.8), shoulders (Fig. 27.9) and knees; chondrocalcinosis was evident in both wrists and the right knee. She was

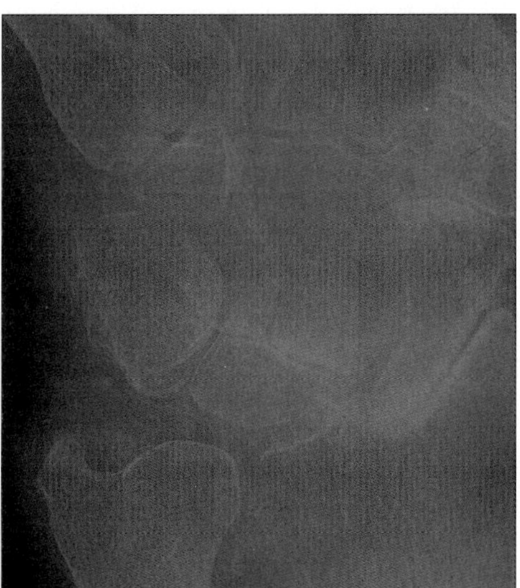

Fig. 27.8 Wrist radiograph in CPA. There is narrowing and sclerosis of radiocarpal and midcarpal joints, pressure erosion of scaphoid onto the radius (with mild scapholunate dissociation), and chondrocalcinosis.

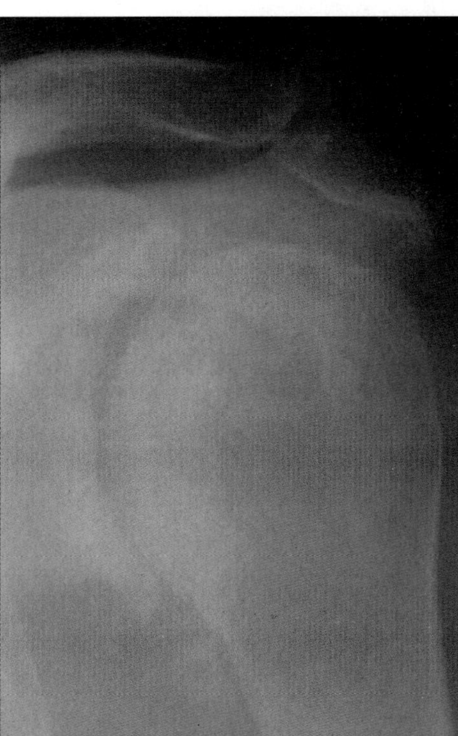

Fig. 27.9 Shoulder radiograph in CPA. The glenohumeral joint shows joint space narrowing, subchondral sclerosis and osteophytosis – the features of OA. Note the large inferior osteophyte. Features which suggest possible pyrophosphate-associated OA include the extensive subchondral cyst formation, as well as the amount of sclerosis and osteophytosis indicative of the 'hypertrophic' end of the spectrum of OA.

weaned off corticosteroid and made good progress from a combined approach employing local physical treatments, advice on muscle use, simple analgesics, and intra-articular corticosteroid injections and subsequently yttrium-90 to both knees.

Diagnostic Problems

Marked inflammatory symptoms, clinically evident synovitis, and predominant involvement of wrists, MCPs, shoulders and knees readily suggest late-onset RA as the diagnosis. Carpal tunnel syndrome may occur as an early, even presenting feature of RA, and elevated ESR and weakly positive rheumatoid factor may be interpreted as confirmatory of this diagnosis. Many elderly women have a few Heberden's nodes, and their presence, together with the absence of nodules or other extra-articular features, does not necessarily mitigate against the diagnosis of RA.

However, though the family doctor was correct to consider RA within the differential diagnosis of the inflammatory arthropathy of the case described, CPA was equally likely on her history and physical findings alone, and perhaps even more likely considering the age of the patient and evident structural damage, particularly in the shoulders and knees (these are usually late features of RA, but frequently present at presentation in CPA).

Carpal tunnel syndrome may accompany any inflammatory arthropathy or tenosynovitis at the wrist and is well associated with CPA. Although uncommon, even clinically evident wrist extensor or flexor tenosynovitis (with or without tendon rupture) would not rule out CPA. Initial investigations can be unhelpful in distinguishing RA from CPA: CPA may cause modest elevation of ESR, and low titer (particularly IgM) rheumatoid factors are of little significance in the elderly.

The more useful investigations are:

- Synovial fluid analysis (confirming CPPD), and
- Plain radiographs (showing features only of CPA).

The history, signs and investigations were thus all consistent with CPA alone in this case. She suffered no superimposed acute attacks – such a history may have more readily prompted consideration of an alternative diagnosis to RA. Absence of extra-articular features or radiographic evidence of RA (marginal erosions, widespread chondropathy) argue against coexistent RA. In coexistent disease, radiographic features of RA may be modified (retained bone density, paucity of erosions, prominent osteophyte and remodeling; Fig. 27.10).

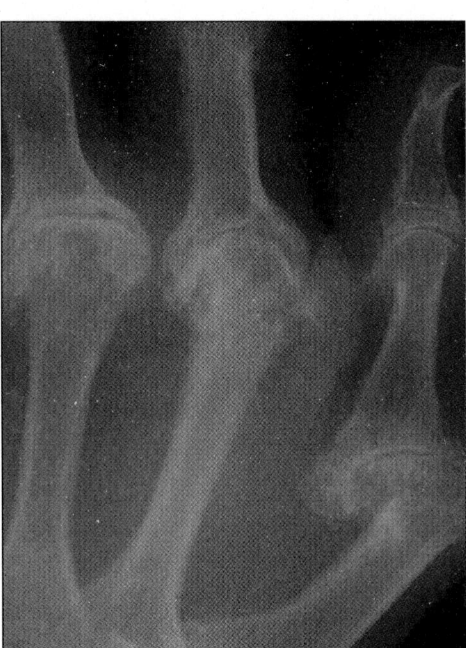

Fig. 27.10 Radiograph of MCPs of a 65-year-old woman with coexistent RA and CPPD deposition. Note the florid remodeling, sclerosis, retained bone density and paucity of marginal erosive change (more typical marginal erosions were evident in two metatarsophalangeal joints).

Therapeutic Options

Absence of coexistent RA makes 'second-line' and low-dose oral corticosteroid therapy inappropriate. Local approaches to synovitis and mechanical problems, with simple analgesics for symptom amelioration, are often most helpful. In those with coexistent RA and CPPD, second-line drugs may be added to control persistent synovitis or extra-articular disease.

Conclusions

In late middle-aged and elderly patients, CPA and RA may be difficult to distinguish on clinical grounds alone. Both should therefore be considered in the differential diagnosis of inflammatory arthritis in these age groups. Plain radiographs and synovial fluid analysis usually permit distinction and allow appropriate management strategies to be designed. Coexistent RA and CPA are uncommon and may associate with a modified radiographic appearance.

REFERENCES

Doherty M, Dieppe P, Watt I. Low incidence of calcium pyrophosphate dihydrate crystal deposition in rheumatoid arthritis with modification of radiographic features in coexistent disease. Arthritis Rheum. 1984;**27**:1002–9.

Hollingworth P, Williams PL, Scott JT. Frequency of chondrocalcinosis of the knees in asymptomatic hyperuricaemia and rheumatoid arthritis: a controlled study. Ann Rheum Dis. 1982;**41**:344–6.

Resnick D, Williams G, Weisman MH, Slaughter L. Rheumatoid arthritis and pseudo-rheumatoid arthritis in calcium pyrophosphate deposition disease. Radiology. 1980;**140**:615–21.

28

SEPTIC BONE AND JOINT LESIONS

Sven Åke Hedström & Lars Lidgren

Definitions

- Septic arthritis: inflammation of a joint caused by the presence of a microorganism.
- Prosthetic joint infection: a deep infection in a prosthetic joint.
- Septic bursitis: acute infection restricted to a bursa.
- Acute osteomyelitis: acute infection of bone, usually in the metaphysis of a long bone.
- Pelvic osteomyelitis: infection usually affecting the pubic symphysis, sacroiliac joint, os ileum or acetabulum.
- Chronic osteomyelitis: sustained or relapsing infection of bone, principally the long, tubular bones.
- Osteitis: a contiguous subacute or chronic infection of the cortical and/or cancellous bone, mainly in the short and flat bones.
- Spondylitis: infection of a vertebra.

HISTORY

Laudable pus was pointed out by Galen as helpful in open fractures and was the treatment of choice in most centers in Europe until the last century [1].

Hippocrates understood the importance of the reduction of fractures and the appliance of wound dressings, but it was not until Lister as a surgeon accepted Pasteur's findings that both antisepsis and asepsis slowly became standard practice. Bone infection in osteomyelitis is described in Greek, Roman and Arab texts from AD500–1200, and limited sequestrectomy was an accepted treatment. Chemotherapy in osteomyelitis was first used in 1936 [2] and rapidly gained popularity as penicillin was introduced.

For some orthopedic infections, such as septic arthritis and acute hematogenous ostemyelitis, there is still some dispute as to whether chemotherapy alone can control and cure the infection without surgical intervention. Randomized controlled studies in this area are lacking for obvious reasons.

EPIDEMIOLOGY

The annual incidence of acute osteomyelitis in Sweden is 10 per 100,000 children, the same as that of bacterial arthritis [3,4]. The incidence is higher in warm and humid geographic areas and is probably also related to socioeconomic conditions. In Western Australia, among European children, there are twice as many cases of acute osteomyelitis as in, for example, Scotland or Sweden.

In New Zealand the Maori have four times, and in Australia the Aborigines 12 times, as many hospital admissions for acute osteomyelitis compared with Europeans in both Australia and Europe [5]. The number of acute bone infections developing into chronic ones has been drastically reduced, by early antibiotic treatment and surgical decompression, from 10–20% to less than 2% [7].

The number of new cases of chronic osteomyelitis of post-traumatic, postoperative and hematogenous origin during the last decade has been estimated to be 15–30 per 100,000 population [3,5,8]. The annual incidence of vertebral osteomyelitis has been estimated to be 0.5–1.0 per 100,000 population [9,10].

Postoperative discitis has been reported to occur in about 1% [11,12] and only rarely is hematogenous discitis seen, especially in the cervical spine in children. Today at least 400,000 joint prosthetic implants and 1.5 million devices for hip fractures per year are implanted all over the world. In the 1970s, before any preventive measures were taken, about 10% of all major surgical hip procedures involving an implant resulted in infection.

Sterile enclosures, body exhaust systems, antibiotic prophylaxis, and, last but not least, improved surgical technique have led to a reduction of the infection rate, to less than 1% in hip surgery and 2% in knee prosthetic surgery [13].

CLINICAL FEATURES

Septic Arthritis

The presentation varies with age. Adults and elderly patients with arthrosis or rheumatoid arthritis (RA) more often have an acute septic arthritis. The lower extremities are most often affected, particularly the hip and knee joints.

In the neonatal period, up to about 1 year of age, the symptoms are usually systemic rather than local [14,15]. Small children develop high, septic fever (Fig. 28.1) and are usually rather ill. The clinical features are more those of sepsis than of local arthritis. Older children are also febrile and unwell, but the local signs are more prominent. Distension of the joint capsule and increased intra-articular pressure contribute to pain. If the hip joint is involved it is usually held in flexion, as this position gives maximum compliance. Adults often have severe pain and are febrile, but malaise is generally moderate [16]. Patients are reluctant to move and put weight on the joint.

The joint capsule is distended, warm and often reddened and edematous (Fig. 28.2). If detected and treated during the first 2–3 days

CLINICAL FEATURES OF SEPTIC BONE AND JOINT LESIONS

	Fever	Local pain	Inflammatory signs	Discharging purulence	Reduced function
Septic arthritis	+	+	+	–	(+) to +
Prosthetic joint infection	(+) to +	(+) to +	(–) to (+)	– to (+)	(–) to +
Septic bursitis	(+) to +	(+)	(+) to +	–	(–) to (+)
Acute osteomyelitis	+	+	(+) to +	–	– to (+)
Pelvic osteomyelitis	+	+	(–) to (+)	–	(+) to +
Chronic osteomyelitis	– to (+)	– to (+)	(–) to (+)	– to +	– to (+)
Osteitis	– to (+)	(+)	(–) to (+)	– to (+)	– to (+)
Spondylitis	(–) to +	(–) to (+)	(–)	–	– to +

– = absent (–) = low-grade (+) = moderate + = high-grade

Fig. 28.1 Clinical features of septic bone and joint lesions.

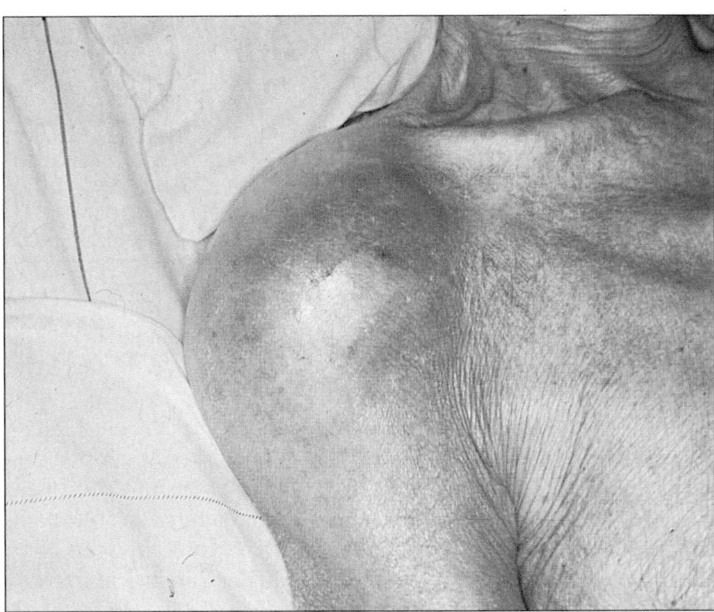

Fig. 28.2 Septic arthritis in an elderly patient, here recognized by distension, increased skin temperature and tenderness. The septic arthritis does not always differ from other kinds of arthritis.

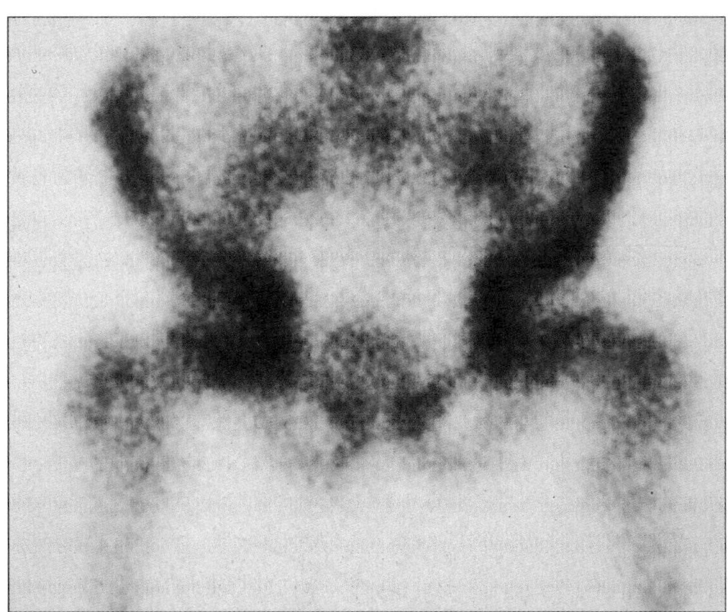

Fig. 28.3 Segmental femoral head necrosis in a left septic coxitis.

the outcome is favorable and there is no mortality. A delay in diagnosis, particularly in septic coxitis in children, often results in joint destruction [17] (Fig. 28.3).

Gonococcal Arthritis

In the main, septic arthritis is a disease of small children, the elderly and people who are immunosuppressed or have damaged joints. However, gonococcal arthritis affects young adults primarily, especially where access to free, high-quality treatment of sexually transmitted diseases is restricted. It occurs as a result of dissemination of infection in the genitourinary tract or rectum. Arthralgia is a common feature of disseminated gonococcal infection (DGI); arthritis occurs in 30–40% of cases [18]. In many instances arthritis following gonorrhoea is reactive and it is important to distinguish such reactive arthritis from septic gonococcal arthritis.

Presentation is most commonly with diffuse or migratory arthralgias and low grade fever, but there may be isolated mono- or oligoarthritis in an apparently well individual. Gonococcal arthritis is most common in women between the ages of 15 and 30 years but has also been recorded in children and is increasingly seen in homosexual men. In menstruating women, onset of gonococcal arthritis is particularly likely to occur within one week of a menstrual period or during pregnancy. In a high proportion of cases urogenital symptoms are absent despite positive urethral cultures, and it is essential to search for evidence of pharyngeal and rectal infection. Gonococcal arthritis has been reported in association with HIV infection, although it remains unclear whether homosexual men are especially susceptible to DGI.

During the early bacteremic phase of DGI painless skin lesions that may be macular, papular, vesicular, pustular or necrotic may be found, especially on the distal parts of the limbs. Tenosynovitis is also common at this stage. At this stage around 40% of patients will have positive blood cultures [19], but within 2–3 days skin lesions settle and isolation from blood is less likely. Mono- or oligoarthritis then follows over a few days as the bacteremic phase settles, mainly affecting large joints especially the knee, wrist and ankle. Uncommonly persistent low-grade monoarthritis has been reported and localized bone pain should suggest the possibility of osteomyelitis [20].

Isolation of the organism from the genital tract is successful in 50–80% of cases. In contrast only 30% of joint fluid samples yield isolates. The reason for this is not clear; in some instances a synovial membrane biopsy may yield an isolate when synovial fluid does not and in others microorganisms may be seen on light or electron

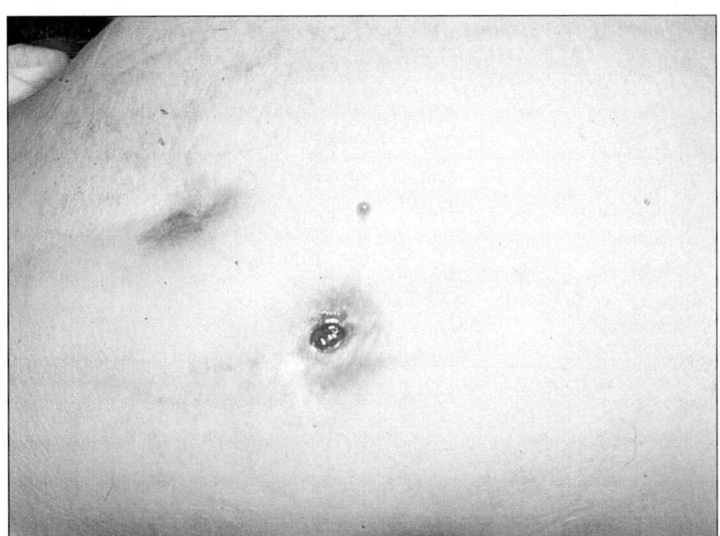

Fig. 28.4 In spite of a severe deep infection around a prosthesis, the only external signs may be a fistula and edema.

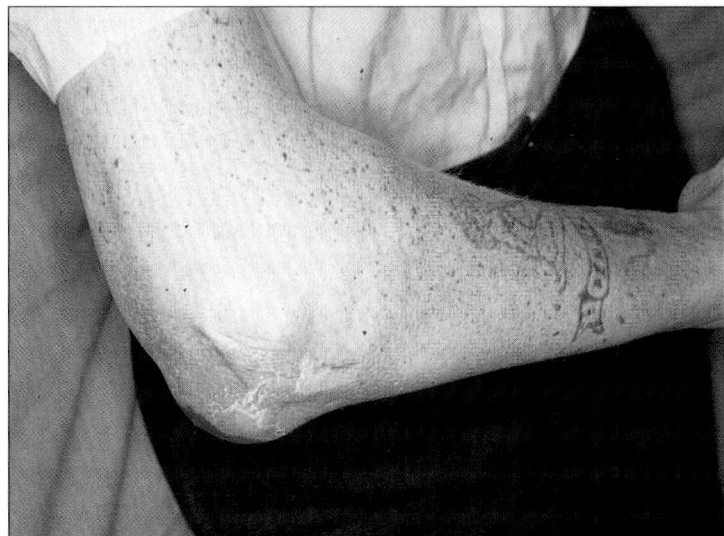

Fig. 28.5 Bursitis symptoms are similar to arthritis but a diagnostic puncture of the bursa containing purulent material in septic bursitis is easy to do.

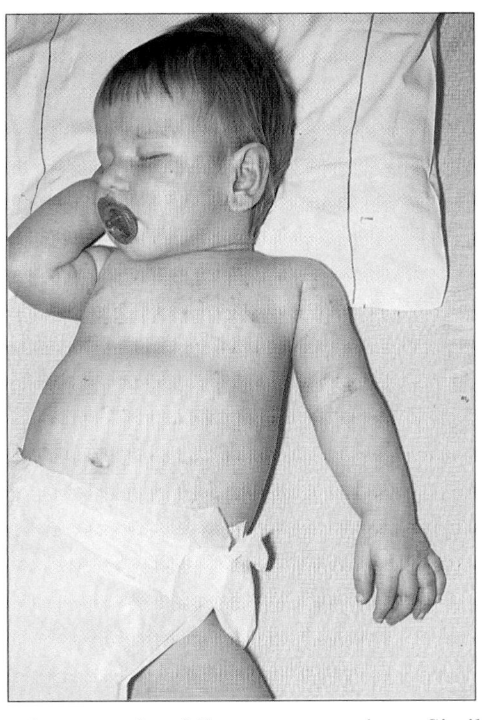

Fig. 28.6 An acute osteomyelitis in the proximal metaphysis of the left humerus. The child is not willing to move the affected limb. The roseola is consistent with a *Salmonella* infection, which was confirmed by fecal cultures.

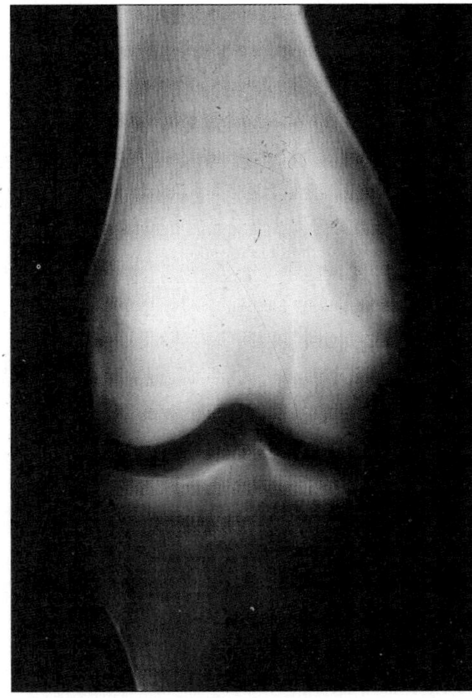

Fig. 28.7 Hematogenous chronic osteomyelitis (of the Brodie type) in the distal femur.

microscopy but fail to grow on culture. Similarly, attempts to isolate bacteria from skin lesions are usually but not always negative, though gonococci may be identified by immunofluoresence staining [19].

Pathogenesis

No evidence of specific genetic susceptibility to DGI or gonococcal arthritis has been detected. The association with arthritis of dissemination of microorganisms and a prompt response to antibiotic therapy suggests that viability of the microorganisms is an essential factor for the development of arthritis. However, both the difficulty in isolating from the joint and animal studies in which killed gonococci and purified gonococcal lipopolysaccharide have been shown to induce synovitis [21] suggest that arthritis may represent a combination of abscess formation in response to replicating bacteria and an aseptic inflammatory reaction to bacterial lipopolysaccharide.

Immune-complex-mediated mechanisms have been proposed on the basis of the finding of high levels of C1q-binding immune complexes in synovial fluid from patients with gonococcal arthritis, but this may be a nonspecific finding.

Prosthetic Joint Infection

The symptoms can differ in the early and late postoperative period. If an infection presents soon after surgery, staphylococci and streptococci are more common and the symptoms are more intensive, with high fever, general malaise and a wound discharging pus [22]. Later on, when the wound has healed or a sinus has developed, the patient may still have pain with soft tissue swelling (Fig. 28.4). In infections presenting late the general symptoms are usually not impressive and the local signs can be rather discrete, with slight tenderness and pain. In some cases of hip joint infection the joint effusion and the pressure can be so high that dislocation occurs [13]. In hematogenous infections the onset is usually acute, with high, septic fever and increasing pain even at rest. A prosthetic joint infection is always serious, with high morbidity and mortality. Patients with RA with *Staphylococcus aureus* infection around a hip or knee prosthesis have a mortality rate of about 10% [23].

Septic Bursitis

Acute bacterial bursitis is most common at the elbow and knee. Adults are mostly affected. The onset is rapid, often after repeated trauma. High fever, sometimes with chills, and a swelling of the bursa with increased warmth, redness, and pain are characteristic (Fig. 28.5). Joint function is generally not affected. In cases with olecranon bursitis without trauma, diabetes mellitus is a frequent underlying disease. The prognosis is good, with few sequelae [24].

Acute Osteomyelitis

This type of infection principally affects children and young adults [16]. In children below 1 year of age acute osteomyelitis presents with arthritis in about 75% of cases and septicemia in almost all [15]. The epiphysis is sometimes involved [25]. Older children will not move or put weight on the affected limb (Fig. 28.6). The metaphysis, mostly in the lower extremities around the knee joint, in the trochanter region or in the humerus, is tender to the touch and can be swollen and warm. In the proximal humerus and femur the joint may be involved due to the insertion of the joint capsule below the metaphysis. If the infection is diagnosed and treated during the first 2–3 days after onset the prognosis is good and chronic complications are rare. The mortality in acute osteomyelitis is almost nil.

Pelvic Osteomyelitis

This disease is seen in athletic youngsters in the form of an acute, hematogenous infection around the symphysis or the sacroiliac joints; it is caused by *S. aureus* [26]. In women with obstetric or gynecologic

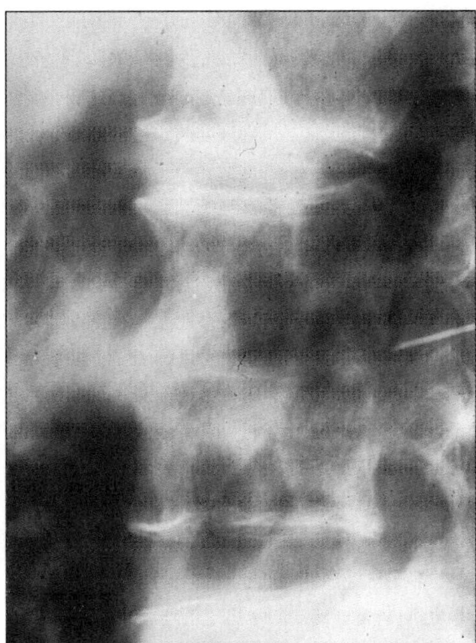

Fig. 28.8 Vertebral spondylitis of L3 and L4 with destruction of the disc and the adjacent end plates. The aspiration needle for culture and histology is seen. The position of the needle should always be documented with a radiogram.

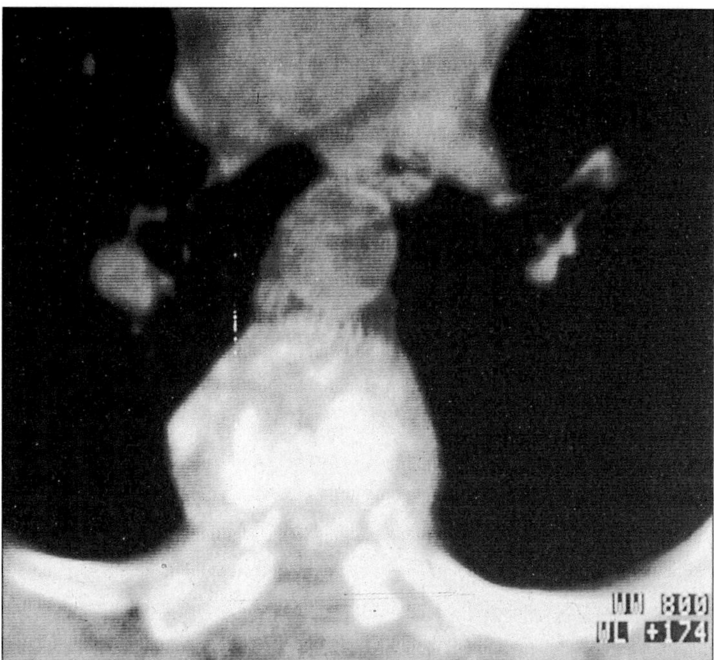

Fig. 28.9 CT showing osteomyelitic destruction of the fourth vertebral body with soft tissue swelling.

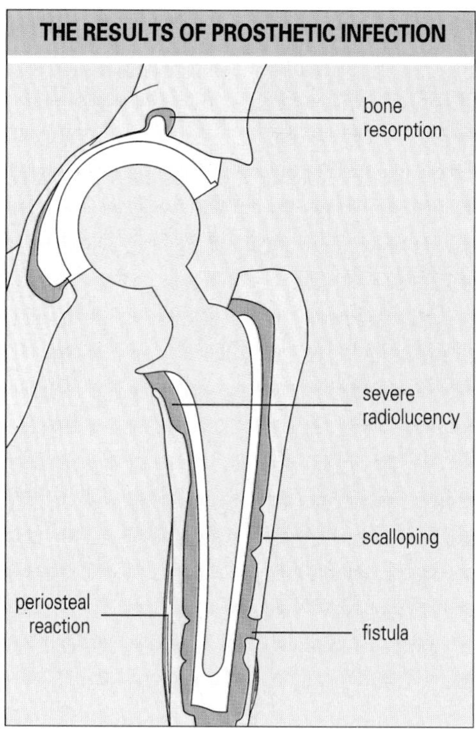

Fig. 28.10 The results of prosthetic infection. Periosteal reaction, scalloping, severe radiolucency at the interface, fistula through the bone, and severe bone resorption are illustrated. All these changes can also be seen in severe prosthetic mechanical loosening but do not progress as rapidly as in infection.

pelvic infections another clinical picture is seen, with a subacute onset and a contiguous dissemination from the pelvis. Gram-negative bacteria or anaerobes are usually the causative agents [13].

The symptoms can be diffuse and difficult to attribute to a skeletal infection; pain and fever are the most prominent symptoms. The condition may be difficult to detect and the diagnosis is often delayed. However, the prognosis is good and sequelae are rare.

Chronic and Subacute Osteomyelitis

Chronic osteomyelitis can be intermittent or continuous. The hematogenous form caused by *S. aureus* is now only present in elderly people who became infected before the antibiotic era [27], and chronic osteomyelitis in adults is usually post-traumatic or postoperative. The long tubular bones in the lower extremities are most often affected in both forms. The intermittent type presents symptoms either in the form of pain, swelling and increased skin temperature around the affected area, and possibly a moderate rise in body temperature, or as a sinus continuously discharging pus without swelling and often with only slight pain. Another type of osteomyelitis, the subacute Brodie abscess, presents with pain often without inflammatory signs (see Fig. 28.7).

There is almost no mortality in chronic osteomyelitis, but the relapse frequency is high (10–20%) and definitive healing is rare even after adequate treatment.

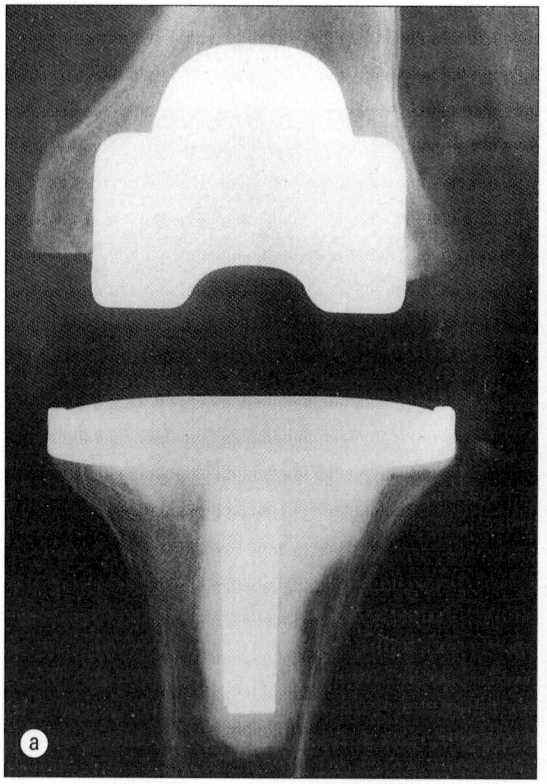

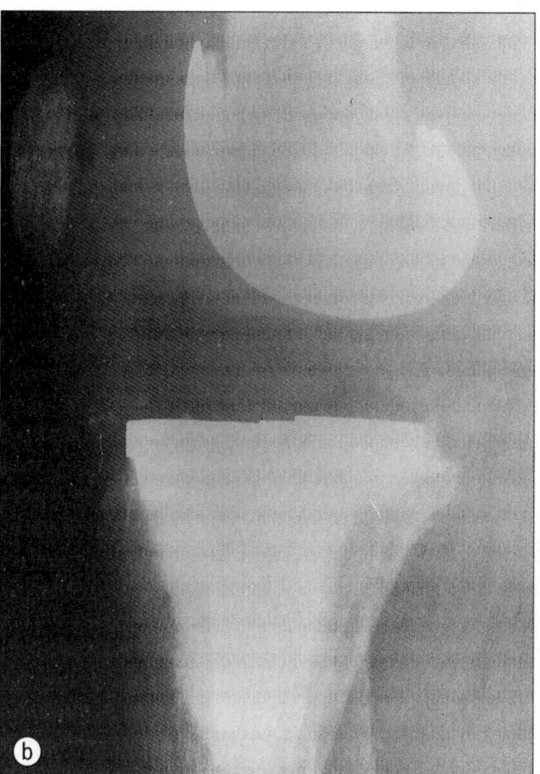

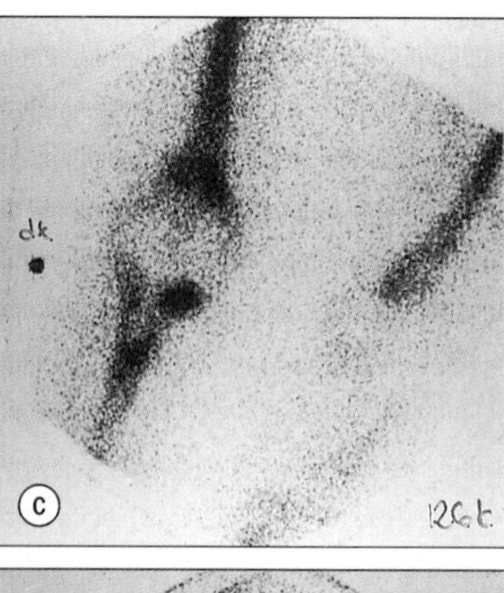

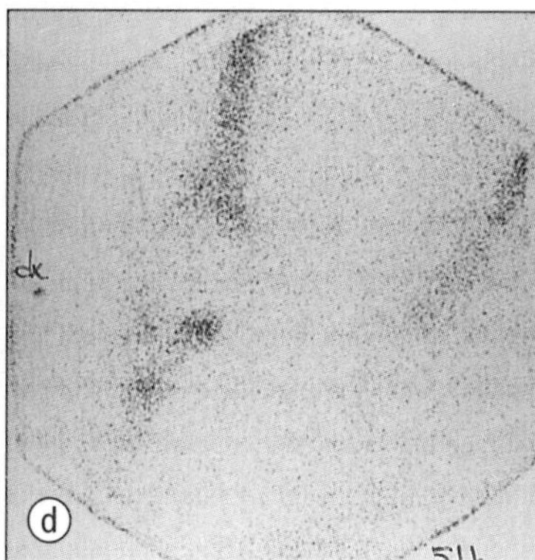

Fig. 28.11 A knee prosthesis 1 year after surgery in a patient with RA and severe pain at rest and on weightbearing. The radiograms (a and b) show no abnormalities and no radiolucency. 99Tc-NSCS (c) shows obviously increased uptake corresponding to the distal femur and proximal medial tibia. The uptake with ^{111}In-LS (d) was classified as slightly increased.

Osteitis

Infections of short and flat bones, particularly common in the feet but also occurring in the hands, and usually discrete, give rise to symptoms and are initiated by infections in the skin and/or soft tissue. The patients often have underlying diseases such as diabetes mellitus or arteriosclerosis. Due to the limited bone infection fever is not common, and pain and other symptoms commonly seen in osteomyelitis are not severe. Sometimes a thin fistula or an abrasion down to the bone surface can be the result of a penetrating infectious process. The chances of retaining the affected region intact are low as the condition most often requires various degrees of resection or amputation [13].

Spondylitis

The symptoms of septic spondylitis are often not distinct and may be misunderstood. However, there is often tenderness over the affected vertebrae. With the exception of postoperative discitis [28], which rarely proceeds to spondylitis, the route of infection is hematogenous. Spondylitis is most common in the elderly (50–70 years) and located in the lumbar spine. The onset can be insidious, with increasing fever and uncharacteristic back pain or radiating pain to the thorax or abdomen. In such cases the condition is often misinterpreted as myocardial infarction, pleuropneumonia, cholecystitis, or appendicitis [29]. Sometimes the onset is acute, with high body temperature, chills and severe back pain.

The process often starts as a discitis, with the vertebrae affected later (see Fig. 28.8) with abscess formation; the nerve roots can be involved, resulting in paresis. The purulent infection can also spread to the surrounding soft tissue, and an epidural abscess concomitant to the spondylitis is also possible (Fig. 28.9). Neurological or disabling sequelae occur in a small percentage of cases, but the prospects for complete healing of the infection are good. More sequelae are seen after tuberculous infection.

DIAGNOSTIC PROCEDURES AND INVESTIGATIONS

The definite diagnosis of deep, late, especially hematogenous, infection may sometimes be difficult. Erythrocyte sedimentation rate (ESR) together with C-reactive protein is usually quite sensitive in nonrheumatoid patients, especially in joint prosthetic infections. The presence of radiographic changes indicates that an infection has been present for 2–3 weeks or more. Plain radiographs, although not specific, often show a rapidly developing irregular resorption zone around implants, sometimes with an extensive periosteal reaction (Fig. 28.10).

Scintimetry employing sequential ^{99m}Technetium phosphate (three-phase bone scan) is an excellent diagnostic aid before radiographic changes appear. In acute hematogenous osteomyelitis with cold lesions caused by a deficient blood supply in a tubular bone, the scan can be repeated after 2–3 days. Computerized tomography (CT) and magnetic resonance imaging (MRI) are helpful for the diagnosis, but ideal diagnostic tests are still lacking. ^{111}Indium-labeled leukocytes have been used in a few studies and have shown high specificity and sensitivity (80%) [13]. Promising new isotopes, such as ^{99m}Tc nanocolloid, have recently been introduced. In a recent study at our department, where ^{111}indium was compared with ^{99m}Tc nanocolloid in 35 patients with suspected infections, nanocolloid showed a sensitivity of 90% and a specificity of 80%, which is comparable to indium. In clinical practice, however, ^{99m}Tc nanocolloid scanning has the advantage of being completed in 1 day, whereas indium requires the use of autologous granulocytes and a 2-day procedure (Fig. 28.11).

In acute septic arthritis the microbes are generally localized to the synovia, particularly in the initial stage. Bacteria can be killed by phagocytes and thus there is a risk of getting negative cultures from the aspirated joint fluid. It is advisable to dilute the aspirated material in a blood-culture bottle in a proportion of about 1:10 to inhibit the bactericidal components of the joint fluid [13].

In addition to cultures it is advisable to make smears for direct microscopy. If it is possible to perform an arthroscopy, or when a synovectomy is indicated, tissue samples should be used for culture [30]. The same procedures are recommended in prosthetic joint infections. Quantification of cultures, with positive tissue biopsies, is important for a clinical diagnosis of infection [13].

In suspected acute osteomyelitis, pelvic osteomyelitis, sacroiliitis and spondylitis, samples for culture and direct microscopy can often be obtained by needle aspiration or open biopsy [31]. In all these acute infections cultures from blood and suspected infectious foci can facilitate the etiologic diagnosis.

In chronic osteomyelitis and osteitis with fistulae it is not adequate to take cultures from the superficial orifice. This area is usually colonized by irrelevant bacteria [13]. In the surgical exploration of the infectious focus, tissue biopsies are suitable for culture. Blood cultures and cultures from other foci in the body are not indicated since the chronic infection is restricted to the bone.

In spondylitis, puncture and aspiration of the intervertebral space (see Fig. 28.8) or of a vertebra under fluoroscopy, for a smear and culture, is a rapid diagnostic method for determining the causative agent [13]. If the patient has septic fever or a focus of origin, blood cultures and a sample from the lesional area should be taken.

BACTERIOLOGICAL FINDINGS IN BONE AND JOINT INFECTIONS

	Acute septic arthritis	Prosthetic joint infection	Bursitis	Acute hematogenous osteomyelitis	Chronic osteomyelitis	Pelvic osteomyelitis	Spondylitis	Diabetes osteitis
Staphylococcus aureus	+++	+++	+++	+++	+++	+++	+++	++
Coagulase-negative staphylococci		+++			+			
Hemolytic streptococcus	++	++	++	++			++	++
Other streptococci	+	+		+			+	+
Skin anaerobes	+	+++		+	+			++
Gram-negative cocci	+			+				
Hemophilus influenzae	+	+		+				
Gram-negative aerobes	+	++	+	+	+	++	++	++
Pseudomonas aeruginosa	+	+		+	+		+	
Salmonella	+	+		+	+		+	
Intestinal anaerobes		+			+	++		++
Mycobacteria	+	+			+		+	

+++ = very common (30% or more) ++ = common (5–30%) + = occurs in some circumstances (age, underlying disease, foreign material)

Fig. 28.12 Bacteriological findings in bone and joint infections.

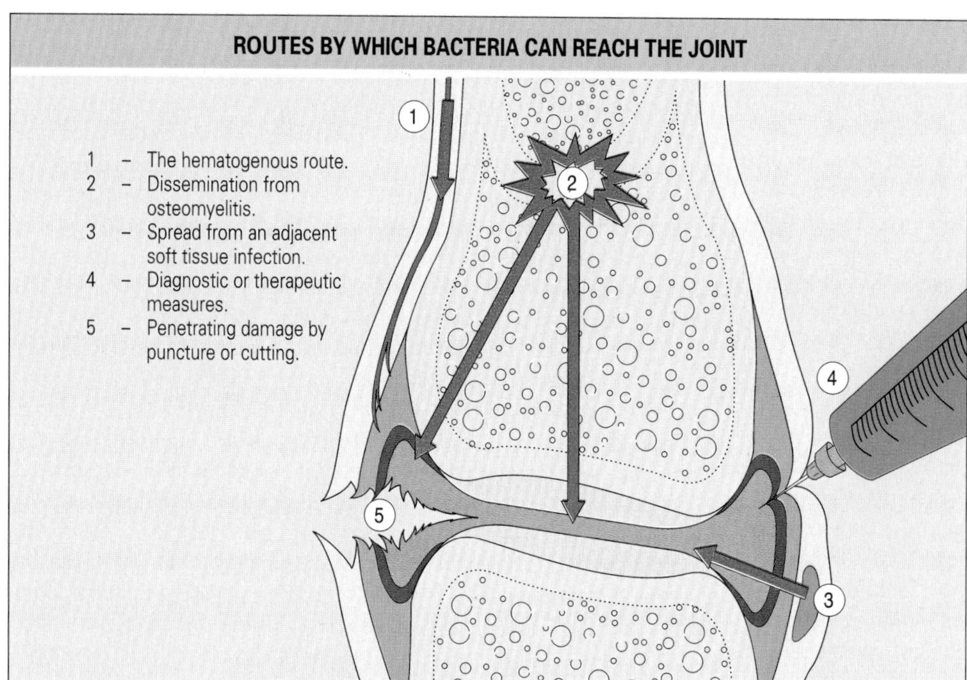

Fig. 28.13 Routes by which bacteria can reach the joint.

Recommended bacteriological investigations for acute febrile conditions and chronic conditions, respectively, are:

- Blood culture, culture from primary foci, smear and culture from the local infectious focus.
- Representative samples from the deep infectious focus: aspirate or biopsy.

ETIOLOGY

The bacterial etiology in bone and joint infections depends on the type and route of infection. Significant factors are: the course of the infection (acute or chronic), pathogenesis (hematogenous or contiguous), the localization of the infection (see Fig. 28.12), the age of the patient, and underlying disease. Of great importance for the findings are also the conditions for sampling and culturing: type and amount of material, media used, accessibility to the laboratory and the quality of the laboratory [13].

With regard to the different bacteria it is difficult to compare various patient materials and to state the relative frequency of microorganisms. *S. aureus* is always common in all entities. It is the most common bacteria found in osteomyelitis in all ages and is almost the sole cause of chronic hematogenous osteomyelitis [27]. Coagulase-negative staphylococci and skin anaerobes are opportunistic bacteria but are common in the presence of foreign material.

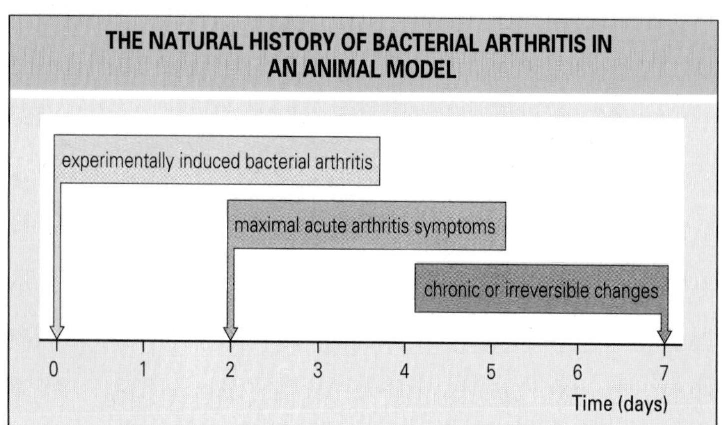

Fig. 28.14 The natural history of bacterial arthritis in an animal model is similar to the development in the clinical case. Data from Goldenberg and Reed 1985 [40].

Hemolytic *Streptococcus* group B is more often seen in neonatal osteomyelitis [32].

Hemophilus influenzae is most common in hematogenous arthritis in children of 1 month to 5 years of age [32]. *Escherichia coli* was common some years ago in neonatal arthritis and osteomyelitis, but as a result of better hygiene it is now less common and mostly seen in neonatal arthritis [32]. Gram-negative intestinal bacteria are more frequent in the elderly in conditions such as diabetes osteitis, spondylitis, and prosthetic joint infections. *Pseudomonas aeruginosa* is found in drug addicts with arthritis and spondylitis, and after trauma. In post-traumatic osteomyelitis Gram-negative aerobes are increasingly common when compared to the Gram-positive bacteria. *Salmonella* is more common in developing countries in osteomyelitis, particularly in sickle cell anemia, and in arthritis in children [33]. Anaerobes are found almost exclusively in diabetes osteitis and prosthetic joint infections.

Many types of microorganisms are found in orthopedic infections, but most of them occur only sporadically. Mycoplasma and ureaplasma are rare and can cause infections in immunocompromised patients [34]. Mycobacteria, including atypical varieties, can cause arthritis, spondylitis and osteomyelitis. In prosthetic joint infections some unusual bacteria spread by the hematogenous route are sometimes found [35].

Clavicular osteomyelitis can be caused by *S. aureus*, but *Propionibacterium acnes* is also reported as a putative agent [36] (Fig. 28.12).

PATHOGENESIS

Septic Arthritis

A prerequisite for the development of septic arthritis is that bacteria can reach the synovial membrane. This can take place in five different ways (Fig. 28.13). Firstly, bacteria may reach the joint from a remote infectious focus via the hematogenous route. Such foci are usually abscesses or infected wounds in the skin, infections in the teeth, upper or lower respiratory tract infections, urinary or intestinal tract infections, or endocarditis. In some cases no obvious primary focus is noted – a common experience in septicemia. The bacteria reach the deep vascular plexus terminating in the looped capillary anastomosis (circulus articularis vasculosus) [17,37].

A second route, particularly common in small children, is a dissemination of bacteria from an acute osteomyelitic focus in the metaphysis or epiphysis. The vessels through the physis and epiphysis are not

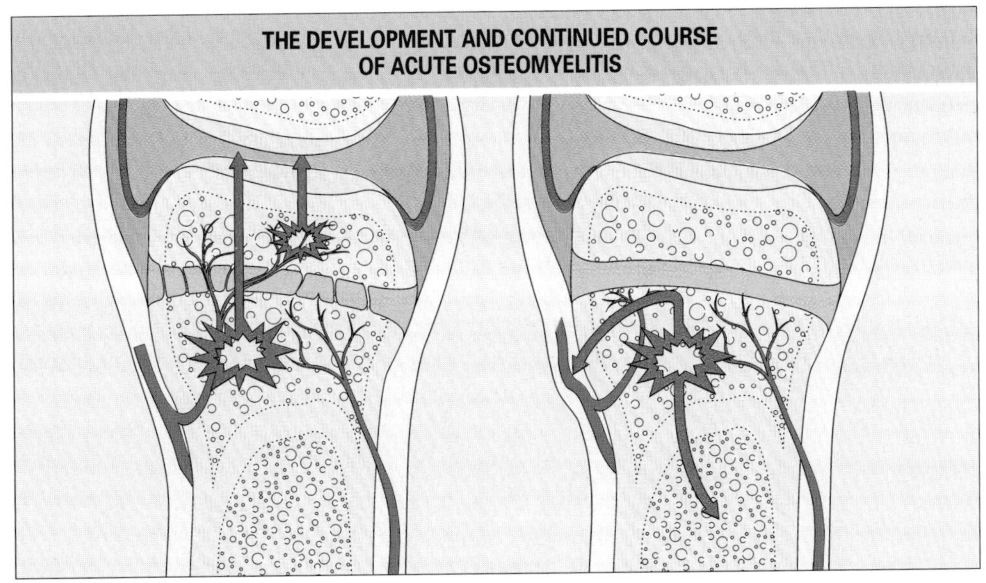

Fig. 28.15 The development and continued course of acute osteomyelitis differs with age. In infants below 1 year of age the epiphysis is nourished by penetrating arteries through the physis, allowing development of the condition within epiphysis. In children up to 15 years of age the infection is restricted to below the physis due to interruption of the vessels.

occluded as is usually the case above 1 year of age [38]. Above this age spread of bacteria can occur from the humerus and femur metaphysis or in the elbow where the joint capsule covers parts of the metaphysis, allowing bacteria to penetrate through the cortical bone and the periosteum to the joint cavity. In adults with closed growth plates there is a re-established connection between the metaphysis and the epiphysis, and spread of the infection to the synovial plexus is possible.

Thirdly, an infection in the vicinity of the joint can progress to the joint or spread via the lymphogenic route. This is most often seen in nonpenetrating traumatic and postoperative wound infections and in skin and soft tissue infections around the joint, particularly the knee joint.

A fourth possibility is iatrogenic infection caused by joint puncture for a diagnostic or therapeutic purpose. Although extremely rare it has not been completely eradicated.

Lastly, a penetrating trauma, often caused by dirty objects or by animal or human bites, often gives rise to a severe infection due to the high inoculate of bacteria and lacerated tissue. After joint surgery peroperatively implanted bacteria can cause a postoperative infection.

In the hematogenous infection, once the bacteria have reached the synovial membrane an inflammatory reaction starts. Leukocytes migrate to the focus and inflammatory proteins exude to the infectious focus. The synovial membrane proliferates and becomes tender, and the blood flow increases. There is an exudation of bacteria, cells and proteins to the joint cavity. The bacteria in the joint fluid can be killed by phagocytes. The joint becomes swollen and the joint pressure rises and can cause cartilage damage. Enzymes (i.e. elastase and collagenase) liberated from polymorphonuclear leukocytes and synovial cells degrade the cartilage. The infection and inflammation can spread in the subchondral bone [39]. Joint cartilage loses its resilience, tolerating only about a third of the normal pressure. The tissue changes become irreversible, often in a few days (Fig. 28.14) [40]. A proliferating pannus tissue will often result from persistent infection.

Acute Osteomyelitis

The metaphysis has a rich blood supply and a slow circulation time. On the other hand the perfusion is slow through the venous sinusoids. The endothelial cells of the sinusoids have a reduced phagocytic activity [41,42]. These factors are favorable for bacterial adherence and multiplication in the metaphysis (Fig. 28.15). The ensuing inflammatory reaction increases the intraosseous pressure, and microthrombi of the small vessels obstruct the blood flow. The result is an intraosseous inflammatory focus with abscess formation under high pressure, and a reduced blood supply resulting in the destruction of osseous trabeculae by osteoclasts followed by osteoblastic activity forming new bone tissue [43]. In chickens it has been shown that bacteria deposit in the growth plate and bacterial proliferation occludes the blood vessels within 24 hours [44]. Abscess formation usually occurs within 2–3 days. When the purulent infection has penetrated laterally through Haversian channels to the subperiosteal area and/or down to the medullary cavity, the lesion becomes chronic.

Chronic Osteomyelitis

Chronic osteomyelitis can develop from an untreated acute osteomyelitis or, more commonly, as a complication of an infected fracture or postoperative infection. Often the vessels are lacerated. The massive bacterial invasion to a vast area promotes a propagation of the infection, often in the whole diaphysis. Destruction of the bone tissue is prominent and sequestra and circumscribed abscesses arise. Lysis is followed by new bone deposition. This can grow centrifugally or encroach on the medullary cavity [13].

Sinus formation originating from intraosseous cavities is common, with discharge of pus, infected material and small bone pieces to the skin surface. Defective healing and skeletal malformation are common.

Pelvic Osteomyelitis

In young people, mostly men, *S. aureus* can usually reach the pelvic bones via the blood. The sacroiliac joints, the symphysis and the acetabulum are commonly affected. Osteomyelitis has been noted in

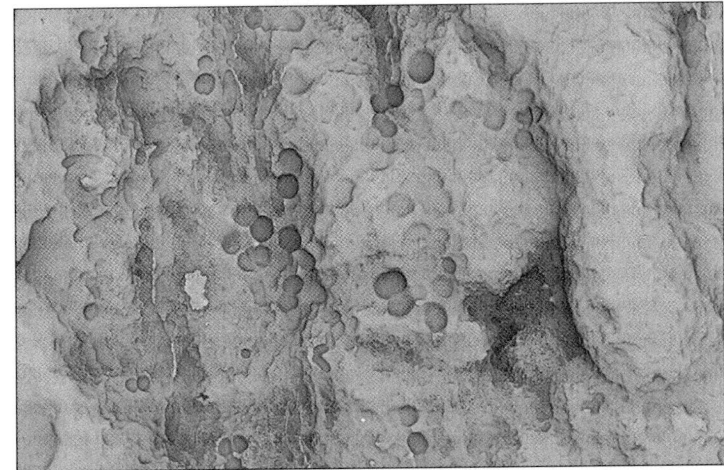

Fig. 28.16 Bone sequesters found in chronic osteomyelitis have no blood supply and function as a foreign body with a rough, irregular surface. In this scanning electron microscopy picture adherent cocci (*S. aureus* and *E. coli* were found in a culture) and a few rods are displayed. Also in this case the body defense system and antibiotics cannot reach the bacteria.

athletes, and it is possible that skin lesions with colonizing *S. aureus* are the source of bacteria [26].

In women, during the child-bearing period, bacteria, usually Gram-negative intestinal organisms and/or anaerobes, may spread contiguously from an infectious focus in the pelvic region as a complication of pregnancy or gynecological disease.

Spondylitis

Bacteria reach the vertebrae almost exclusively after a hematogenous dissemination from a known infectious or cryptogenic focus, as in the case of acute osteomyelitis. The intervertebral space is commonly infected first, with subsequent spread to the adjacent vertebrae. Destruction of the end plate follows and the disc and the vertebrae become compressed. Later this is often followed by spontaneous interbody vertebral fusion. Local spread of infection is common, with the formation of abscess masses localized in the epidural space or in the soft tissues.

Osteitis

If bacteria disseminate from a contiguous focus in the skin or soft tissues the cortical bone can be affected. Most often such infections occur in the feet. The short, cancellous bones are the site of a low-virulent infection. Destruction is seen but new bone formation is not as pronounced as in osteomyelitis of the long tubular bones.

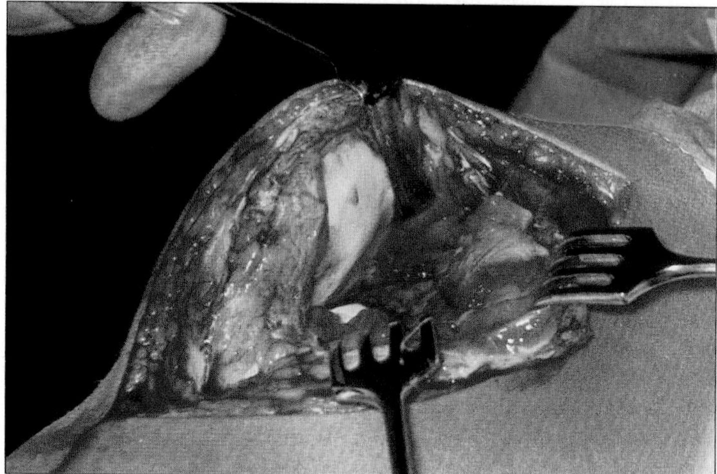

Fig. 28.17 Particularly in postoperative and post-traumatic arthritis with no response to antibiotic treatment a pannus formation, as seen here on the femoral condyle, may develop.

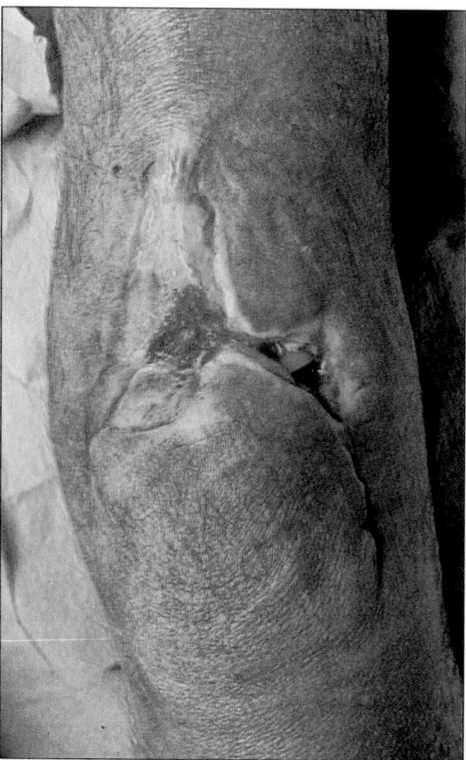

Fig. 28.18 Wound tissue breakdown in a rheumatoid knee caused by a faulty skin incision with sensitive atrophic skin.

MANAGEMENT OF BACTERIAL INFECTIONS IN BONE AND JOINTS

Treatment of infections in bone tissue is hampered by the impeded blood supply. Thus, penetration of antibiotics is impaired due to an elevated intraosseous pressure, occluded blood vessels, and edema [45].

Prerequisites for successful antibiotic therapy in acute hematogenous osteomyelitis are: susceptible causative bacteria, sufficient penetration of drugs to the bone tissue and the affected area, and the availability of appropriate forms of administration, i.e. parenteral and well-absorbed oral formulations [13].

In acute hematogenous osteomyelitis, the penetration of antibiotic therapy is impaired as the intraosseous pressure rises and the blood vessels become occluded by edema and microthrombi. At the time when an abscess has developed, the access of antibiotics to the infectious focus is very limited. Therefore, the antibiotics should be instituted within 2 or 3 days of the onset of the clinical symptoms [46].

Factors contributing to decreased efficacy of antibiotics in chronic osteomyelitis are diminished blood flow secondary to deranged bone structure, trauma and sclerosis, the presence of abscesses, sequestra and foreign material, and the development of glycocalyx [47] (Fig. 28.16). *S. aureus* can bind to blood and tissue components such as fibrinogen, immunoglobulin G, complement, fibronectin, collagen, vitronectin, laminin, and sialoprotein II [48].

Certain strains of *S. aureus*, such as phage-group I strains, are difficult to eradicate and there is an increase of penicillinase-producing or methicillin-resistant staphylococci [27]. The antimicrobial therapy recommendations made below are relevant for countries in which both the frequency of methicillin-resistant staphylococci and the bacterial resistance against antibiotics are low (i.e., the Nordic countries). In countries where methicillin-resistance is common, drugs such as vancomycin, teicoplanin, aminoglycosides, rifampicin, fusidic acid and quinolones must be used, either in single therapy or, preferably, in combination.

Septic Arthritis, Bursitis and Prosthetic Joint Infections

Early and aggressive therapy is imperative to prevent destruction – not least in childhood [49] – and mortality – particularly in elderly patients with RA or diabetes. The history, age and underlying diseases are valuable guides in the choice of antibiotic treatment. In all these entities *S. aureus* and other Gram-positive cocci are common, and *H. influenzae* dominates in children below 3 years of age with acute arthritis. The occurrence of Gram-negative organisms in the elderly with predisposing diseases, as well as *S. aureus* in RA, must be taken into account [27].

Isoxazolylpenicillins in suspected Gram-positive infection and a cephalosporin in suspected Gram-negative infection are effective in the ordinary acute case. We recommend parenteral cloxacillin 2g t.i.d. or 100mg/kg/day in Gram-positive infections, and cefuroxime 1.5g t.i.d. or 75–80mg/kg/day in Gram-negative infections. The duration of parenteral therapy should be 7–10 days, and thereafter oral drugs, flucloxacillin 1.5g t.i.d. or 75–80mg/kg/day or a cephalosporin, should be administered for up to a total of 6 weeks [13].

In prosthetic joint infections oral clindamycin and ciprofloxacin are alternatives, depending on the bacteriological findings. In these cases, which are often treated operatively, local treatment with antibiotic-containing bone cement or other vehicles is used [13]. Bursitis can be treated with drainage and a short course of parenteral cloxacillin or benzylpenicillin, depending on findings, and the oral treatment period can be short [24].

In bacterial coxitis surgical drainage of the joint is effective and necessary. In case of infection in other joints, repeated aspiration should be performed if no pus is found initially. However, if aspiration is unsuccessful or if the symptoms increase within the first 24–48 hours, an arthrotomy is necessary. Arthroscopy has been used as an alternative to repeated aspiration and for more effective irrigation of the joint. The early use of devices for passive motion has reduced the need for surgical mobilization after bacterial arthritis. The joint is protected from weightbearing for an average of 6 weeks. However, the patient is normally mobilized as soon as the pain has subsided. Late synovectomy has been performed in the knee joint to prevent cartilage destruction and subsequent arthrosis [30] (Fig. 28.17).

The treatment of infected joint implants is complicated. Factors influencing the choice of treatment include the condition of the patient and the adjacent joint soft tissue, the quality of the bone stock, the type of primary revision implants, type and sensitivity of the infected organism, the patient's daily requirements for activities, and finally the rarity of the problem. The treatment of these patients should be centralized, especially when deciding on definitive treatment from amongst long-term antibiotics, revision arthroplasty, arthrodesis, and amputation.

The surgical procedure in itself, involving meticulous removal of all foreign material in a staged procedure before the insertion of a new prosthesis, also calls for centralized treatment (Fig. 28.18). The fusion rate in arthrodesis and the healing rate of an infected knee prosthesis is improved if the patient is treated at experienced centers [50]. The septic complication in a joint implant carries an overall mortality from 5% in knee prostheses up to 15% for hip prostheses [50].

Acute Hematogenous Osteomyelitis

Streptococci and *S. aureus* dominate in juveniles and adults [51]. In addition to these *H. influenzae* and *E. coli* can also occur in neonatal osteomyelitis, and *E. coli* and other intestinal bacteria in the elderly.

Betalactam antibiotics, clindamycin, fusidic acid, certain quinolones, such as ciprofloxacin, and rifampicin are known to penetrate bone tissue in sufficient amounts. Erythromycin and aminoglycosides have inadequate penetration properties [13].

Administration of parenteral antibiotics is indicated initially in acute hematogenous osteomyelitis, followed by an oral regime. Penicillins with a spectrum against Gram-positive bacteria, or cephalosporins against Gram-positive and Gram-negative bacteria

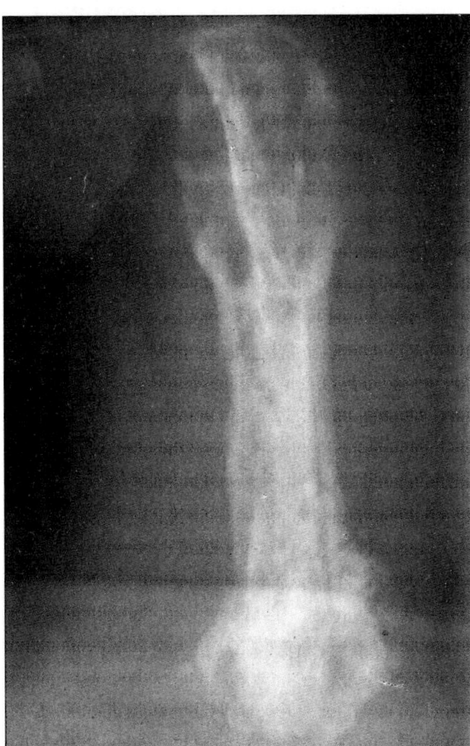

Fig. 28.19 Chronic osteomyelitis with sequestrum and involucrum in an 18-month-old boy.

are the drugs of choice for acute hematogenous osteomyelitis. Clindamycin, fusidic acid, and ciprofloxacin are alternatives in specified situations, based on bacteriological findings and/or penicillin hypersensitivity. Combinations containing erythromycin, aminoglycosides and rifampicin have been used but are second choices.

S. aureus must be covered in all age groups. We favor a combination of benzylpenicillin and isoxazolylpenicillin, or a corresponding drug. The former is more effective against penicillin-sensitive *S. aureus* and streptococci and the latter against penicillinase-producing staphylococci. High doses should be used, preferably 150mg/kg/day and 100mg/kg/day, respectively, in three divided doses [13].

In acute hematogenous osteomyelitis, abscesses should be drained since decompression prevents further obstruction of blood vessels and resulting bone necrosis. Drainage also results in dramatic improvement in the patient's general condition. If antibiotic treatment has not been started early and decompression has not been carried out, the trabecular bone may be sequestrated and eventually embedded in new bone (Fig. 28.19). Weight bearing on the extremity should be avoided until radiographic signs of bone restoration are present because there is a high risk for pathological fractures [13].

When culture results become available, one of the two antibiotics can be withdrawn. The duration of therapy has been discussed in several papers and is proposed to be 3 weeks [44]. However, there are great difficulties in keeping children in hospital on an intravenous catheter for such a long time. We have limited the parenteral treatment to 1 week followed by oral treatment up to a total of about 2 months [13].

In age groups in which *H. influenzae* or Gram-negative intestinal bacteria may be suspected as being the cause of acute hematogenous osteomyelitis, cloxacillin should be combined with ampicillin or, preferably, a cephalosporin effective on this flora, i.e. cefuroxime, should be chosen. This drug has also sustained good effect against Gram-positive bacteria. In cases of unknown etiology and in which either Gram-positive or Gram-negative bacteria are possible, cefuroxime is furthermore the more suitable choice [13].

In elderly patients, in whom Gram-negative bacteria are common as a consequence of urinary, biliary, intestinal and lower respiratory infections or invasive diagnostic measures in the named localizations, the treatment with broad spectrum antibiotics, for instance broad spectrum penicillins, cefuroxime, cefotaxime or trimethoprim-sulpha, is indicated.

Parenteral treatment should be given until fever and the local signs of infection have disappeared, which usually takes 7–10 days. Laboratory variables such as ESR or CRP should be monitored, and normalization of these variables may be interpreted as evidence of the effectiveness of the antibiotic treatment. If chronic osteomyelitis with radiographic changes develops, treatment should be continued for up to 6 months, particularly in cases of staphylococcal etiology [27]. By instituting early systemic antibiotic treatment, it is possible to prevent the development of radiographic changes. The prognosis is directly related to the time at which antibiotic therapy was instituted [46]. Only when an abscess is demonstrable is operative drainage superior to antibiotic treatment [52].

Spondylitis and Pelvic Osteomyelitis

The evolution of spondylitis is often slow and the prognosis mostly good. There is therefore no need for haste in instituting antibiotic therapy. It is better to first attain a confirmed diagnosis and establish the etiology as far as possible. Usually acute spondylitis with intensive symptoms such as fever, pain and disability is treated in the same way as acute hematogenous osteomyelitis, depending on disease history and bacterial findings. In hematogenous pelvic osteomyelitis *S. aureus* is the most common agent, particularly in patients below 50 years of age, and the onset is often more acute.

In cases of Gram-positive and *E. coli* infection, antibiotic therapy for 2–3 months is often sufficient if the radiographic findings are discrete. Salmonella-induced and tuberculous spondylitis are more difficult to heal, and longer treatment, 6–12 months, is often needed [13].

Chronic Osteomyelitis

The treatment of chronic osteomyelitis is more difficult and less well standardized than that of acute infections. Recurrences of infection are common in chronic osteomyelitis, and extensive surgery and debridement is an important part of successful therapy.

Bacteriologic and pharmacologic data make isoxazolylpenicillins the drugs of choice in chronic hematogenous osteomyelitis. They are tolerated well even in high doses, with a low rate of toxic side effects; rash and diarrhea are seen only in a few cases. There is a low risk of developing chromosomal resistance and this has not been a problem despite general long-term treatment. We have generally used oral drugs, such as flucloxacillin at a dose of 1.5g t.i.d. [13]. Probenecid, 1g b.i.d., enhances the serum concentration and lowers the protein binding of isoxazolylpenicillins. Clindamycin, fusidic acid and cephalosporins with effect against Gram-positive bacteria are alternatives for treatment of patients with penicillin allergy. If the treatment fails, rifampicin 0.6–0.9g daily, which penetrates into the granulocytes, may be added in combination with isoxazolylpenicillin. We have used parenteral antibiotics for only 1–3 days perioperatively in connection with the surgery, giving oral drugs for the rest of the long-term treatment period. Prolonged parenteral antibiotic therapy is not necessary but the total period of treatment should be extended. The duplication time and the metabolism of the bacteria are very slow in osteomyelitis, which necessitates prolonged treatment [53].

The long-term results are very good, and high dose oral antibiotics for at least 6 months are tolerable and sufficient in combination with surgery. In some cases when surgery is contraindicated or not accepted by the patient, antibiotics alone are usually sufficient.

Radiographic changes are already present, and careful planning is required in order to decide whether or not a sequestrum is present, and whether surgical intervention is necessary. This could include procedures from a simple sequestrectomy and removal of granulation tissue up to removal of an entire part of tubular bone followed by subsequent bone transplantation. Intramedullary reaming has been used for chronic hematogenous osteomyelitis with severe pain at rest, in order to re-establish a new medullary cavity and improve endosteal circulation [54].

REFERENCES

1. Bick E M. Source book of orthopaedics. Hafner: New York; 1968.
2. Le Cocq J F, le Cocq E. Use of neoarsphenamine in treatment of acute *S. aureus* septicaemia and osteomyelitis. J Bone Joint Surg. 1941;**23**:596–7.
3. Lidgren L, Lindberg L. Orthopedic infections during a 5-year period. Acta Orthop Scand. 1972;**43**:325–34.
4. Danielsson L, Uden A. Diagnostik och behandling av akut hematogen osteit hos barn. Lakartidningen. 1981;**4**:241–4.
5. Gillespie W J, Nade S. Musculoskeletal Infections. Blackwell Scientific Publications: Oxford; 1987.
6. Gillespie WJ, Mayo K M. The management of acute hematogenous osteomyelitis in the antibiotic area. J Bone Joint Surg. 1981;**63**-B:126–31.
7. Smith I. Staphylococcus aureus. In: Mandell G L, Douglas R, Bennett J E, eds. Principles and practice of infectious diseases. John Wiley & Sons: New York;1979:1530–2.
8. Boda A. The problem of osteomyelitis in Hungary. In: Meeting of the European study group on bone and joint infections. Vienna; August 27,1983.
9. Digby J M, Kersley J B. Pyogenic non-tuberculous spinal infection: an analysis of thirty cases. J Bone Joint Surg. 1979;**61-B**:47–55.
10. Silverthorn K M, Gillespie WJ. Pyogenic vertebrae osteomyelitis. NZ Med J. 1986;**99**:62–5.
11. El-Gindi S, Aref S, Salama M, Andrew J. Infection of intervertebral discs after operation. J Bone Joint Surg. 1976;**57**-A:1104–6.
12. Lindholm T S, Pylkkanen P. Discitis following removal of intervertebral disc: A report on 120 patients. Spine. 1982;**7**:618–22.
13. Hedström S Å, Lidgren L. Orthopedic infections, Studentlitteratur. Lund: 1988.
14. Fox L, Sprunt K. Neonatal osteomyelitis. Pediatrics. 1978; **62**:535–42.
15. Welkon CJ, Long S S, Fischer M C, Alburger P D. Pyogenic arthritis in infants and children: a review of 95 cases. Infect Dis. 1986;**5**:669–76.
16. Mitchell M, Howard B, Haller J, Sartoris DJ, Resnick D. Septic arthritis. Radiol Clin North Am. 1988;**26**:1295–1313.
17. Griffin PP. Acute septic arthritis of the hip in childhood: its pathogenesis and treatment. Hip. 1979;**4**:89–104.
18. O'Brien JP, Goldenberg DL, Rice PA. Disseminated gonococcal infection: a prospective analysis of 49 patients and a review of pathophysiology and immunological mechanisms. Medicine. 1983;**62**:395–406.
19. Barr J, Danielson D. Septic gonococcal dermatitis. Br Med J. 1971;**1**:482–5.
20. Black JR, Cohen MS. Gonococcal osteomyelitis: a case report and review of the literature. Sex Transm Dis. 1984;**11**:96–9.
21. Goldenberg DL, Reed JI, Rice PA. Arthritis in rabbits induced by killed *Neisseria gonorrhoeae* and gonococcal lipopolysaccharide. J Rheumatol; 1984;**11**:3–8.
22. Powers KA, Terpenning MS, Voice RA, Kauffman CA. Prosthetic joint infections in the elderly. Am J Med. 1990;**88**:9N–13N.
23. Vincent GM, Amirault JD. Septic arthritis in the elderly. Clin Orthop. 1990;**251**:241–5.
24. Söderqvist B, Hedström S Å. Predisposing factors, bacteriology and antibiotic therapy in 35 cases of septic bursitis. Scand J Infect Dis. 1986;**18**:305–11.
25. Sandberg-Sørensen T, Hedeboe J, Rostgaard-Christensen E. Primary epiphyseal osteomyelitis in children. J Bone Joint Surg. 1988;**70**-B:818–20.
26. Hedström S Å, Lidgren L. Acute hematogenous pelvic osteomyelitis in athletes. Am J Sports Med. 1982;**1**:44–6.
27. Hedström S Å. Staphylococcal problems in orthopedic infections. In: Hedström S Å, ed. Advances of staphylococcal infections. Astra Alab AB: Södertälje; 1987:87–99.
28. Dall BE, Rowe DE, Odette WG, Batts DH. Postoperative discitis. Diagnosis and management. Clin Orthop. 1987;**224**:138–146.
29. Musher DM, Thorsteinsson SB, Minuth JN, Luchi RJ. Vertebral osteomyelitis: still a diagnostic pitfall. Arch Intern Med. 1976;**136**:105–10.
30. Törholm C, Hedström S Å, Sundèn G, Lidgren L. Synovectomy in bacterial arthritis. Acta Orthop Scand. 1983;**54**:748–53.
31. Kasser JR. Hematogenous osteomyelitis. Untangling the diagnostic confusion. Postgrad Med. 1984;**76**:79–86.
32. Jackson MA, Nelson JD. Etiology and management of acute suppurative bone and joint infections in pediatric patients. J Pediatr Orthop. 1982;**2**:315–19.
33. Cavell B, Hedström S Å. Septic Salmonella bone and joint infections in 2 infants. Opuscula Medica. 1989;**34**:53–4.
34. Jorup-Rönström C, Ahl T, Hammarström L, Smith CIE, Rylander M, Hallander H. Septic osteomyelitis and polyarthritis with ureaplasma in hypogammaglobulinemia. Infection. 1989;**17**:301–3.
35. Hedström S ÅLidgren L. Les infections hèmatogènes sur prothèses articulaires et leur prèvention. In: L'infection en chirurgie ortopèdique GEEIOA, ed. Expansion Scientifique Franaise (SOFCOT) no. 37: Paris; 1990:102–5.
36. Alessi DM, Sercarz JA, Calcaterra TC. Osteomyelitis of the clavicle. Arch Otolaryngol Head Neck Surg. 1988;**114**:1000–2.
37. Freeland AE, Senter BS. Septic arthritis and osteomyelitis. Hand Clin. 1989;**5**:533–52.
38. Alderson M, Speers D, Emslie KR, Nade S. Acute hematogenous osteomyelitis and septic arthritis – a single disease. A hypothesis based upon the presence of transphyseal blood vessels. J Bone Joint Surg. 1986;**68**-B:268–74.
39. Lane Smith R, Schurman DJ, Kajiyama G, Mell M, Gilkerson E. The effect of antibiotics on the destruction of cartilage in experimental infectious arthritis. J Bone Joint Surg. 1987;**69-A**:1063–8.
40. Goldenberg DL, Reed JI. Bacterial arthritis. N Engl J Med. 1985;**312**:764–71.
41. Fitzgerald RH. Pathogenesis of musculoskeletal sepsis. In: Musculoskeletal infections. Hughes SPF, Fitzgerald RH, eds. Year Book Medical Publishers. Chicago:1986; 14–33.
42. Wald ER. Risk factors for osteomyelitis. Am J Med. 1985; **78**:206–12.
43. Peterson HA. Hematogenous osteomyelitis in children. Instr Course Lect. 1983;**32**:33–7.
44. Emslie KR, Nade S. Acute hematogenous staphylococcal osteomyelitis. A description of the natural history in an avian model. Am J Pathol. 1983;**110**:333–45.
45. Emslie KR, Nade S. Acute hematogenous staphylococcal osteomyelitis: evaluation of cloxacillin therapy in an animal model. Pathology. 1984;**16**:441–6.
46. Vaughan PA, Newman NM, Rosman MA. Acute hematogenous osteomyelitis in children. J Pediatr Orthop. 1987;**7**:652–5.
47. Gristina AG, Costerton JW. Bacterial adherence and the glycocalyx and their role in musculoskeletal infection. In: The Orthopedic Clinics of North America. Symposium on musculoskeletal sepsis. WB Saunders: Philadelphia; 1984:517–35.
48. Rydén C. Studies on interactions between staphylococcal cells and some connective tissue components. Thesis. Uppsala: 1987.
49. Shaw BA, Kasser JR. Acute septic arthritis in infancy and childhood. Clin Orthop. 1990;**257**:212–25.
50. Knutson K, Lindstrand A, Lidgren L. Arthrodesis for failed knee arthroplasty. A report of 20 cases. J Bone Joint Surg. 1985;**67**:47–52.
51. Armstrong EP, Rush DR. Treatment of osteomyelitis. Clin Pharmacy.1983;**2**:213–24.
52. LaMont RL, Anderson PA, Dajani AS, Thirumoorthi MC. Acute hematogenous osteomyelitis in children. J Pediatr Orthop. 1987;**7**:579–83.
53. Zak O, Reilly TO. Animal models as predictors of the safety and efficacy of antibiotics. Eur J Clin Microbiol Inf Dis. 1990;**9**:472–8.
54 Lidgren L, Törholm, C. Intramedullary reaming in chronic diaphyseal osteomyelitis. Clin Orthop. 1980;**151**:215–21.

29

REACTIVE ARTHRITIS

Auli Toivanen

Definition
- A sterile joint inflammation that develops after a distant infection.
- The disease is systemic and not limited to the joints, in spite of its name.
- Triggering infections most commonly originate in the throat, urogenital organs or gastrointestinal tract.
- The disease also occurs without obvious preceding infection, e.g. in association with inflammatory bowel disease.

Clinical features
- Arthritis.
- Enthesopathy, tendinitis, tenosynovitis, osteitis and muscle pains.
- Skin and mucous membrane lesions are frequent.
- Eye inflammations, e.g. uveitis and conjunctivitis.
- Visceral involvement, such as nephritis or carditis, is relatively rare.
- Severity ranges from mild arthralgia to disabling disease.
- Spontaneous recovery is common and the prognosis is, in general, good.
- Later, many patients suffer arthralgias and recurrences.
- Susceptibility to the disease is strongly linked to possession of the HLA-B27 antigen.

HISTORY

Reactive arthritis is often named Reiter's disease after Hans Reiter (1881–1969), who in 1916 described in an officer a dysenteric illness with arthritis, urethritis and conjunctivitis [1]. Reiter did not actually recognize that the arthritis and conjunctivitis were related to the dysentery, but called the disease 'spirochaetosis syphilitica'. As early as the 16th century Pierre van Forest, and in the 17th century Martinière, had recognized arthritis as a complication of urethritis.

The first description of the disease is attributed to Sir Benjamin Brodie (1783–1862) [2]. Ilmari Paronen described 344 cases of arthritis in connection to a *Shigella* outbreak that occurred on the Karelian isthmus at the end of the Second World War [3]. In 1969, Paronen and his coworkers published a follow-up study of 100 of these patients, illustrating the prognosis of the disorder [4]. The term 'reactive arthritis' was introduced by Aho *et al.* [5], and it has gained wide use even though it does not indicate the systemic character of the disease. The term 'Reiter's disease' is still in general use and refers to the triad of arthritis, urethritis and conjunctivitis; often the term 'incomplete Reiter's disease' is used. Both complete and incomplete Reiter's disease can be considered identical with reactive arthritis.

Observations of family clustering were soon confirmed by the finding that reactive arthritis is strongly associated with HLA–B27. In recent years, great research interest has been focused on reactive arthritis, partly because information gained regarding it may elucidate the pathogenetic processes involved in the development of other rheumatic diseases, such as rheumatoid arthritis and ankylosing spondylitis.

EPIDEMIOLOGY

Because the clinical severity varies greatly and milder cases apparently go unnoticed, the true incidence of reactive arthritis is hard to assess. Certainly, increasing awareness of reactive arthritis as a diagnostic possibility will increase the number of cases recognized. According to a Finnish estimation [6,7], the incidence of enteroarthritis or uroarthritis per 100,000 adults per year is 30, and that of seronegative oligoarthritis (probably often reactive arthritis) 40 per 100,000 (Fig. 29.1). Reactive arthritis has been described from several countries, and it can be assumed to affect people all around the world. The disease is considered to be more frequent in Scandinavia, but this is probably due to greater awareness and hence more frequent diagnosis. Rheumatic fever, also a type of reactive arthritis, occurs often in developing countries but has practically disappeared elsewhere.

Reactive arthritis affects males and females with the same frequency. Typically it is a disorder of young adults, rare in small children and in old people. Most patients are aged between 20 and 40 years [2,8].

Genetic factors play a role in susceptibility to the disease. Most patients report of relatives who have had a similar disease. Patients with reactive arthritis are positive for HLA-B27 in 65–96% of cases. Conversely, persons with the HLA-B27 antigen have a strongly increased risk of developing reactive arthritis [9–13]; Aho *et al.* [5] calculated the increase in risk to be fifty-fold. However, the association is not absolute; HLA-B27-positive individuals do not always get reactive arthritis even after a suitable triggering infection, and it can occur even in HLA-B27-negative individuals. This is illustrated by observations by van Bohemen *et al.* in connection with an outbreak of bacillary dysentery in The Netherlands: in three families, some but not all HLA-B27-positive members developed reactive arthritis after verified infection [14]. The clinical experience is that the disease is more severe and the tendency to chronic development is greater in HLA-B27-positive individuals [13,15–18].

The frequency of reactive arthritis following enteric infections due to *Salmonella, Shigella* and *Campylobacter* has been reported to be 1–4% in unselected populations [19–21]. In some yersiniosis outbreaks the frequency of this complication has been quite high and in others negligible [22,23]. The fact that bacteria of the same genus, or

EPIDEMIOLOGY OF REACTIVE ARTHRITIS

Most commonly affects young adults
Equally frequent in males and females
Annual incidence 30–40/100,000
Probably worldwide
Genetic associations
  Family clustering
  Strongly associated with HLA-B27
Frequency in connection with infection
  (e.g. enteric) varies

Fig. 29.1 Epidemiology of reactive arthritis.

species even, vary in their capacity to trigger reactive arthritis is of considerable theoretical interest.

CLINICAL FEATURES

History

Typically the patient seeks medical help because of joint discomfort. When a careful history is taken it may indicate symptoms of enteric or urogenital infection in the preceeding few days or a couple of weeks, and often the patient reports of such symptoms in other family members. Sometimes, for a few days before the appearance of joint symptoms, patients have suffered abdominal pains suspected to be due to acute appendicitis or salpingo-oophoritis; this is especially the case in young adults. They may even have been laparotomized, in which case usually only mesenteric lymphadenitis has been found. Yet it is remarkable that patients requiring hospital care for severe enteritis due to, for example, *Yersinia* have rarely developed reactive arthritis. A common clinical experience is that the symptoms of the triggering infection have often been mild and, in about 10% of cases, the infection has passed unnoticed [24–26].

Infections most commonly preceding reactive arthritis include *Salmonella, Shigella, Yersinia, Campylobacter, Borrelia, Chlamydia, Neisseria* and streptococci. In Whipple's disease, joint symptoms that can be considered reactive arthritis are seen. Several viruses have been implicated; those most often mentioned in connection with joint inflammation are rubella, hepatitis and parvovirus. Regarding *Salmonella, Borrelia* and *Neisseria,* it is worth keeping in mind that they can cause true septic arthritis as well as reactive arthritis. It is not unusual that a triggering infection cannot be identified, and in these cases the diagnosis remains uncertain. A preceding infection is not always necessary; it is well known that various inflammatory bowel diseases may be associated with reactive arthritis. Of some theoretical interest is that the disease is occasionally seen after an intestinal bypass operation, for example for morbid obesity [26]. It is obvious, however, that in these conditions the intestinal microbial flora and/or the mucosal defense mechanisms are altered.

General Symptoms

Reactive arthritis is a systemic disease (Fig. 29.2). Its severity varies greatly. Frequently, general symptoms such as malaise, fatigue and fever are seen.

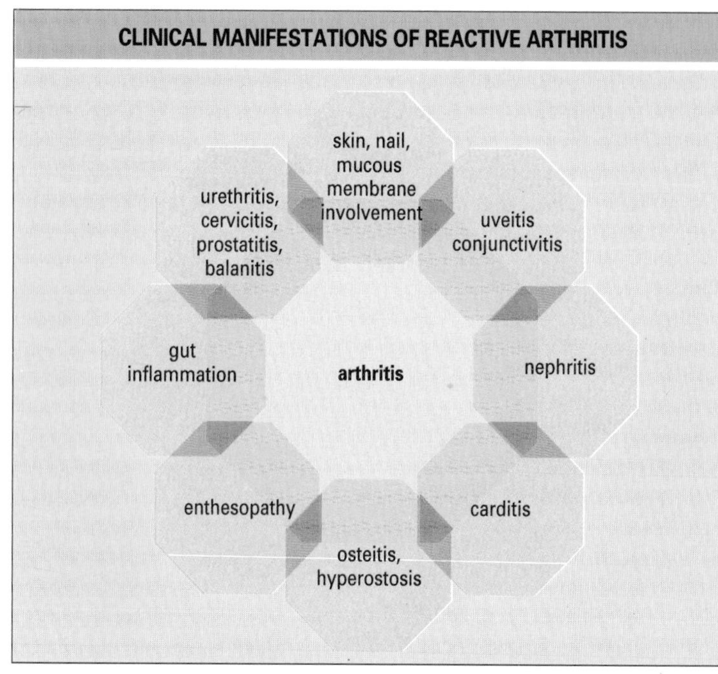

Fig. 29.2 Clinical manifestations of reactive arthritis.

Joint and Musculoskeletal Symptoms

The most prominent symptoms are usually those in the joints. They vary from mild arthralgias to severely disabling polyarthritis [2,13,18,24,25,27]. Typically there is asymmetric monoarthritis or oligoarthritis. Most often affected are the weightbearing joints (Figs 29.3 & 29.4) – knees, ankles and hips – but quite commonly other large joints such as the shoulders, elbows and wrists are also involved. The inflammation may vary from day to day and shift from one joint to another. Occasionally, reactive arthritis affects the small joints of hands and feet. Dactylitis is not an uncommon sign, and sometimes the condition may mimic rheumatoid arthritis. Especially in the later stages, patients often complain of pains in the sacroiliac joints. Other common symptoms are morning stiffness, clumsiness and back pain upon prolonged rest. The joints involved may be red and warm, and occasionally there is also erythema nodosum.

A diagnosis cannot be made on the basis of physical examination, since the findings vary greatly and may mimic any other diseases involving joint inflammation, including gout, rheumatoid arthritis or true purulent arthritis.

Reactive arthritis is not limited to the joints; various tendinitides, tenosynovitises and peritendinitides are present in most cases. Plantar fasciitis and tenosynovitis of the ankle region often results in difficulties in walking. Pain on palpation is frequent at the sites where tendons attach to bones, and this enthesopathy may also limit movement. In severe cases, muscle wasting may be quite prominent. Unusually severe cases may become bedridden. Rarely, the disease renders the patient quite helpless and disabled. Yet it should be emphasized that the outcome is not related to the severity of the disease in its initial phase.

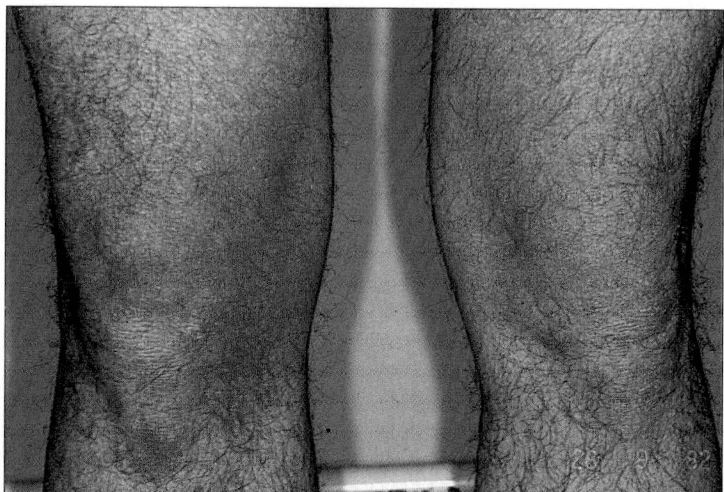

Fig. 29.3 Reactive arthritis of the knee.

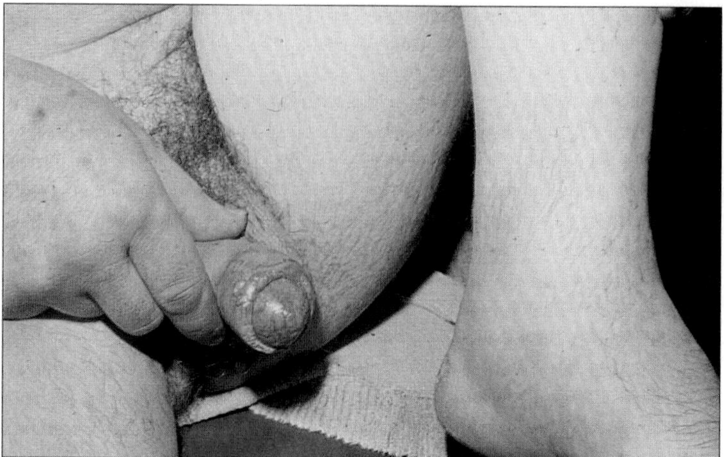

Fig. 29.4 Reactive arthritis of the ankle and non-typical circinate balanitis. (Courtesy of Professor VK Havu, Department of Dermatology, University of Turku.)

Skin and Mucous Membrane Symptoms

The skin lesion most commonly attributed to reactive arthritis is keratoderma blenorrhagicum (Fig. 29.5); another term frequently used is 'pustulosis palmoplantaris'. The lesions closely resemble psoriasis, and both clinically and histologically appear quite similar to it. The same holds for the nail lesions seen in both reactive arthritis and psoriasis. This similarity has not gained wide attention but may be of some theoretical interest when the pathogenesis of reactive arthritis and psoriatic arthropathy are considered. Erythema nodosum, which is often seen after *Yersinia* infection, is not common in connection with reactive arthritis and is not associated with HLA-B27.

When reactive arthritis is triggered by urogenital infection such as gonorrhea or *Chlamydia*, it is a uroarthritis. Sterile urogenital inflammation can also be part of the reactive disease. Thus, sterile urethritis has classically been considered part of the triad of Reiter's disease. Circinate balanitis (Fig. 29.6) that resembles the keratodermia elsewhere, cystitis and prostatitis may be present and can sometimes lead to complications such as shrinking of the bladder. Further, it seems that pelvic inflammatory disease, including salpingitis, may arise in women with reactive arthritis [28,29]. Inflammation of the urogenital tract has a tendency to relapse.

Various lesions are seen in the mouth. Wright and Moll [2] describe them as painless shiny patches, occurring on the palate, tongue and mucosa of the cheeks and lips. Erythema of the soft palate, uvula and tonsillar region has been described occasionally.

Gastrointestinal Symptoms

Enteric infections or inflammatory diseases can, like urogenital infections, be the etiologic triggering event. It has become apparent that, as in the urogenital system, the epithelium of the intestine may form part of the reactive disease itself. Patients may complain of occasional abdominal pains and diarrhea, but at this stage no pathogens can be isolated from stool cultures. When ileocolonoscopy has been carried out in patients with established reactive arthritis, either macroscopically or microscopically detectable lesions resembling ulcerative colitis or Crohn's disease have been seen [30,31].

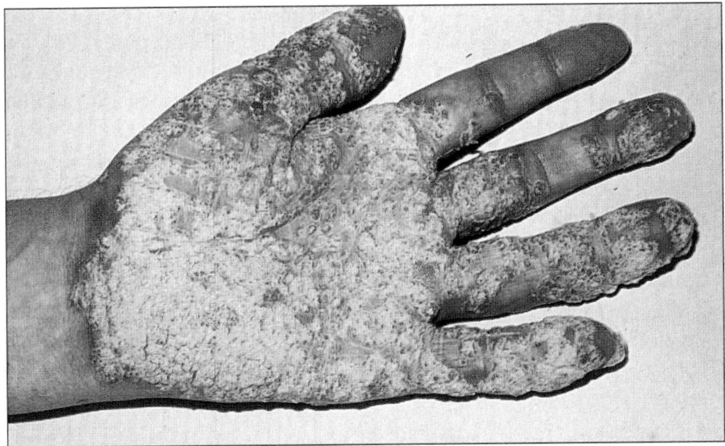

Fig. 29.5 Keratoderma blenorrhagicum of the palm in a patient with reactive arthritis. (Courtesy of Professor VK Havu, Department of Dermatology, University of

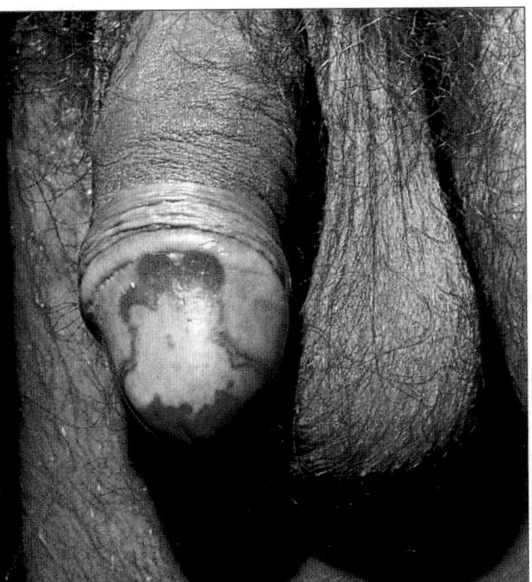

Fig. 29.6 Circinate balanitis in a man with reactive arthritis. (Courtesy of Professor VK Havu, Department of Dermatology, University of Turku.)

Ocular Lesions

Various eye inflammations form a classical part of the clinical picture. They may be either unilateral or bilateral. Conjunctivitis with sterile discharge is frequently seen. It usually subsides but may progress to produce episcleritis, keratitis or even corneal ulcerations [2]. Acute uveitis, especially anterior uveitis (iritis) is also common. The ocular lesions may be the only or the first manifestation of reactive arthritis. They have a strong tendency to recur. Patients with reactive iritis most commonly complain of redness, photophobia and pain, and some of them have diminution of vision and increased lacrimation [32]. In cases with ocular complaints, it is advisable to undertake careful ophthalmologic examination, since if left undiagnosed and untreated, permanent damage of vision may follow.

Visceral Manifestations

Carditis is classically connected to rheumatic fever, and in developing countries valvular disease as a late sequela is a major problem. In reactive arthritides seen after enteric or urogenital infections, cardiac involvement is not as prominent. With increasing awareness it has become apparent, however, that involvement may give rise to conduction disturbances that may even require a cardiac pacemaker [2,13,33].

Mild renal and urinary pathology, such as proteinuria, microhematuria and aseptic pyuria are seen in about 50% of reactive arthritis patients. Severe glomerulonephritis and IgA nephropathy are rare and hardly ever lead to permanently impaired renal function.

INVESTIGATIONS

In most cases, the patient seeks medical help for joint symptoms or for eye inflammation. The history and findings at the physical examination may immediately suggest the diagnosis, but confirmation requires laboratory and radiologic investigations (Fig. 29.7).

INVESTIGATION OF REACTIVE ARTHRITIS

- ESR
- C-Reactive protein
- Blood cell count
- Liver function tests, e.g. ALAT, GT
- Kidney function tests, e.g. serum creatinine or blood urea nitrogen
- Rheumatoid factor tests
- Urinalysis
- ECG
- Joint fluid sample with analysis of:
  - Cell count
  - Exclusion of crystals
  - Gram stain
  - Bacterial culture
- Bacterial culture of:
  - Feces
  - Urine or urethral swab
  - Cervical sample
  - Throat
- Blood culture (not always necessary)
- Antibody determination at admission
- HLA-B27 antigen (or HLA typing) after 2–4 weeks
- X-Ray of affected joints
- Ophthalmological examination if eye symptoms present

Fig. 29.7 Investigation of reactive arthritis.

Laboratory Investigations

The erythrocyte sedimentation rate (ESR) is markedly elevated in most cases of acute reactive arthritis, and values exceeding 60mm/hour are commonly seen. Also, C-reactive protein (CRP) is elevated at the onset of the disease. At a later stage, patients with chronic symptoms nevertheless have quite normal ESR and CRP values. The blood cell count may reveal moderate leukocytosis and mild anemia.

Urinalysis should be carried out at diagnosis and should be repeated during follow up, in order to detect possible aseptic pyuria due to urethritis. It is advisable to check renal function, for example by serum creatinine or blood urea nitrogen tests, and liver function by serum alaninea minotransferase (ALAT) or serum glutamyltransferase (GT). Tests for rheumatoid factor are usually negative.

An electrocardiogram should be performed and repeated in cases having a prolonged course, to exclude possible conduction disturbances. When endocarditis is suspected, especially in cases of rheumatic fever, it is essential to also follow cardiac function by echocardiography.

Joint fluid should always be aspirated when possible. Gram-stain and bacterial culture should be performed for a differential diagnosis. In reactive arthritis, bacteria are not demonstrable either by staining or even extensive culturing. Observation of microbial components in the synovial membrane or in the synovial fluid have been obtained with special techniques not suitable for routine clinical work; these include immunofluorescence, immunoelectronmicroscopy, immunoblotting and polymerase chain reaction (PCR) techniques [34]. As yet unpublished observations by several clinicians (P Kortekangas, HT Aro, J Tuominen, A Toivanen) and a recent comparative study [35] demonstrate that, at an early stage of reactive arthritis, the cell count in the synovial fluid can be quite high and polymorphonuclear leukocytes can dominate the picture. Later, lymphocytosis can develop. Demonstrations of specific antibodies and of T-cells specifically responding to an infectious agent are carried out in some laboratories and may be of diagnostic significance. However, these methods require elaborate techniques not available in most hospitals. Microscopy under polarized light should be performed to exclude gout or pseudogout. Blood culture is not routinely advisable but should be undertaken if septic infection is suspected.

Microbiologic and serologic studies form a cornerstone of diagnosis. Every effort should be taken to isolate the causative microorganism from the throat, feces or urogenital tract. Isolation of *Yersinia* requires special methods, and it is easily missed in routine fecal culture. In most cases, however, results are negative, which emphasizes the role of serology. The serological tests to be considered include antibodies against *Salmonella*, *Yersinia*, *Campylobacter*, *Chlamydia, Borrelia burgdorferi* and β-hemolytic streptococci. Depending on the infection history of the patient, antibodies against various viruses may yield a specific diagnosis.

It should be stressed that not all microorganisms triggering reactive arthritis have been identified, but the list is steadily rising. Thus, negative serology does not rule out a diagnosis of reactive arthritis; furthermore, in some patients the antibodies rise slowly and yield a positive result only a few weeks after the onset of disease.

Detection of the HLA-B27 antigen is helpful in the diagnosis and in considering the treatment and follow up of the patient. As noted before, however, the disease may occur also in HLA-B27-negative individuals.

Radiography and Other Imaging Procedures

Radiographic studies of symptomatic joints should be made not so much to confirm the diagnosis of reactive arthritis as to rule out erosive disease, for example rheumatoid arthritis. The findings in reactive arthritis are usually rather scanty, such as osteoporosis and soft tissue swelling. In recurrent and chronic cases they increase and may include erosions. More often, periosteal reaction and proliferation, especially at the insertion sites of tendons, are seen. Thus, plantar spurs are a common sign in chronic cases.

Chronic or recurring reactive arthritis also often leads to sacroiliitis and spondylitis that may be radiographically indistinguishable from ankylosing spondylitis. However, the changes remain limited, and severe ankylosing spondylitis as a late sequela of reactive arthritis is very rare.

Radionuclide scintigraphy is a sensitive technique for demonstrating inflammation and is superior to radiography, especially in cases of enthesopathy, periostitis or incipient sacroiliitis [2,36].

Other Investigations

It has been demonstrated that, in patients with reactive arthritis, inflammatory bowel disease (ulcerative colitis or Crohn's disease) may be a background factor. Ileocolonoscopy has revealed that in many patients either macroscopic or microscopic lesions of these conditions are present, in the absence of subjective symptoms. However, endoscopy or radiographic investigation of the colon is not recommended routinely. The same holds true for scintigraphy using radiolabelled leukocytes to search for inflammatory sites in the bowel area, especially in the terminal ileum.

In cases with eye symptoms, it is advisable to refer the patient to an ophthalmologist, since uveitis requires rapid diagnosis for prompt and proper treatment. Without a split-lamp examination, the uveitis may remain undiagnosed and result in serious damage.

DIFFERENTIAL DIAGNOSIS

The most important question at admission is whether the patient has reactive arthritis or true septic infection of the joint. Especially in children, a purulent arthritis may rapidly lead to destruction of the joint. As discussed above, the question may be difficult to solve rapidly. Therefore it is advisable to proceed with therapy on the assumption of purulent arthritis in uncertain causes. In case of intensive inflammation, the redness may lead to a suspicion of erysipelas.

Gout or pseudogout may present with symptoms and findings similar to reactive arthritis, but careful history taking, analysis of crystals in the joint fluid and serum urate determination clarify the situation in most instances.

Patients express much concern on the question of whether the disease is rheumatoid arthritis or ankylosing spondylitis. Demonstration of rheumatoid factor and radiographic observations are helpful. Sometimes the diagnosis can be established only after some follow up. Especially in chronic cases, it is of great value for the patient if rheumatoid arthritis or ankylosing spondylitis can be excluded.

Psoriatic arthropathy may resemble reactive arthritis, but radiography, history and observation over a period of time yield the correct diagnosis.

ETIOLOGY

There is no disagreement regarding the etiology of reactive arthritis: it is infection. With increasing awareness of this condition, the list of the causative agents is still growing. Although effort has been made to characterize the microorganisms linked to reactive arthritis, no common or definite feature has so far emerged. Many of the bacteria implicated are Gram-negative, have cell membranes that contain lipopolysaccharide and peptidoglycan, and are intracellularly invasive, i.e. able to enter cells and to survive (and even multiply) intracellularly. Many are quite common in the environment, and infection does not necessarily lead to reactive arthritis. In most instances, the triggering infection affects the throat, the intestine or the urogenital tract. Therefore it appears that mucosal immune defense mechanisms must be of importance – but how and why are not known. The frequency of reactive arthritis in connection with outbreaks of *Yersinia*, *Salmonella* and *Shigella* varies quite considerably. The evidence implies that some features of a microbe are important for its arthritogenicity [13,37].

PATHOGENESIS

The pathogenesis of reactive arthritis is interesting not only in itself but also as a putative model of other inflammatory diseases of the joints and connective tissue. Rheumatoid arthritis and ankylosing spondylitis develop slowly, and when the diagnosis can be established with the accuracy necessary for research work, several months and even years have lapsed. At such a late stage it is quite difficult to gain information on the early triggering or pathogenetic events. Reactive arthritis has a sudden onset, within days or a few weeks of the triggering infection, which often can be identified, and thus studies on its pathogenesis are possible. Much new information has been gained recently, and several groups are working on the pathogenesis.

The term reactive arthritis acknowledges the facts that the joint inflammation develops some time after the actual triggering infection and that the causative agent cannot be isolated from the site of inflammation. This strongly suggests that a breakdown of immunologic defense mechanisms plays a central role [37].

Role of HLA-B27

The role of HLA-B27 is of interest. Although not all HLA-B27-positive individuals develop reactive arthritis after a suitable triggering infection, while some negative individuals may do so, this tissue antigen undisputably plays an important role. It has been suggested that the granulocytes of HLA-B27-positive individuals would be especially active metabolically, perhaps thus enhancing an inflammatory response [38]. Another very plausible possibility is that HLA-B27 would lead to an aberrant immune response by presenting the HLA-B27-specific (microbe-derived?) peptides to helper T cells, leading to recognition of autoantigens by cytotoxic T cells. However, the picture is far from clear; for instance synovial T cell clones derived from patients with reactive arthritis have been almost exclusively helper T cells [39,40].

A hypothesis much studied and discussed has been that HLA-B27 could act as a receptor for a microbial antigen, which would modify the HLA-B27 antigen to be a target for harmful immune response [41,42]. However, studies concerning this receptor theory have revealed contradictory results.

Another theory that has gained wide attention is that of molecular mimicry, i.e. that the microorganisms share a structure with the HLA-B27 molecule [43]. The first examples were based on use of polyclonal antisera reacting with HLA-B27 and *Klebsiella pneumoniae* [44,45]. Since then, crossreactive structures have been identified with monoclonal antibodies. Sequencing of genes for HLA-B27 and microbial antigens has further made it possible to carry out comparisons at the nucleotide and amino acid level. Indeed, molecular mimicry in the form of amino acid homology has been observed between HLA-B27 and microbial antigens [46], but this apparently is not restricted to disease-associated HLA-B27. Work using synthetic peptides and their capacity to generate a response by either B or T cells has, however, raised suspicions about the biologic importance of this homology. Therefore the role of molecular mimicry in the pathogenesis of reactive arthritis or ankylosing spondylitis needs critical re-evaluation [39,47].

Recently, mouse and rat strains carrying a transgene for HLA-B27 have been developed. These may help to elucidate the role of HLA-B27 in the pathogenesis of reactive arthritis and ankylosing spondylitis.

IMMUNE RESPONSE IN YERSINIA-TRIGGERED REACTIVE ARTHRITIS
Initially, weak IgM-class antibody production
Later, strong and persisting IgG and especially IgA antibody production
IgA antibodies increase in avidity with time
Antibodies are directed against several antigenic epitopes of *Yersinia*
Nonspecific immune complexes are always found in serum
Specific immune complexes containing *Yersinia* and anti-*Yersinia* antibody may be found in serum and in synovial fluid
Peripheral blood T cells show weak response to *Yersinia*
T cells in the synovial fluid show vigorous but somewhat nonspecific response to *Yersinia* (or other arthritis-triggering microorganism)

Fig. 29.8 Immune response in *Yersinia*-triggered reactive arthritis.

Immune Response

In studies on the immune reaction against the triggering microorganism, several interesting findings have been obtained. As an example, the results for *Yersinia*-triggered reactive arthritis are presented in Figure 29.8.

The immune responses of patients developing reactive arthritis or recovering without postinfection complications have been compared in follow-up studies [13,37,48]. The most characteristic feature of patients with reactive arthritis is a strong and persisting IgA antibody formation. With time, the antibodies increase in avidity, indicating a maturation of the response. Considering the short half-life of IgA this indicates prolonged antigenic stimulation. The observation that the antibodies recognize a multitude of antigenic epitopes of *Yersinia* suggests that the driving force might be either whole microbes or large components of them.

The T-cell responses against *Yersinia* antigens are weak in peripheral blood samples of patients with reactive arthritis, compared with those of persons who do not develop postinfection complications. However, at the synovial level, a strong but relatively nonspecific response of T cells is seen [49]. It seems that T cells with slightly different specificities can be cloned from the synovial fluid, indicating that local stimulation may play a role [40].

Yersinia infection always causes formation of immune complexes. Such complexes composed of *Yersinia* antigen and specific antibody have been demonstrated in the blood, and even in the synovial fluid of a few patients with reactive arthritis [50].

All these observations suggest that, in patients with reactive arthritis, the microorganism may persist somewhere in the body, for example in the intestinal mucosa or in the mesenteric lymph nodes. Furthermore, microbial components might actually enter the site of inflammation itself, i.e. the synovium or the synovial fluid. Using immunofluorescence (see Fig. 29.9) and immunoblotting techniques as well as immunoelectronmicroscopy, positive reactions have been obtained in reactive arthritis triggered by *Chlamydia*, *Salmonella*, *Yersinia* and *Shigella* [51–57] It must be stressed, however, that viable organisms have not been isolated, in spite of extensive efforts.

Currently it seems, therefore, that reactive arthritis involves persistence of the triggering microorganisms in the host, and the spread of its components either as parts of immune complexes or within phagocytosing cells into the joints, where they activate the inflammatory cascade [58–60]. This would explain the inflammation of many different sites. However, many questions still remain unanswered.

MANAGEMENT

Acute Reactive Arthritis

The severity of reactive arthritis varies from mild arthralgias to a severe arthritis. The therapy has to be adjusted accordingly.

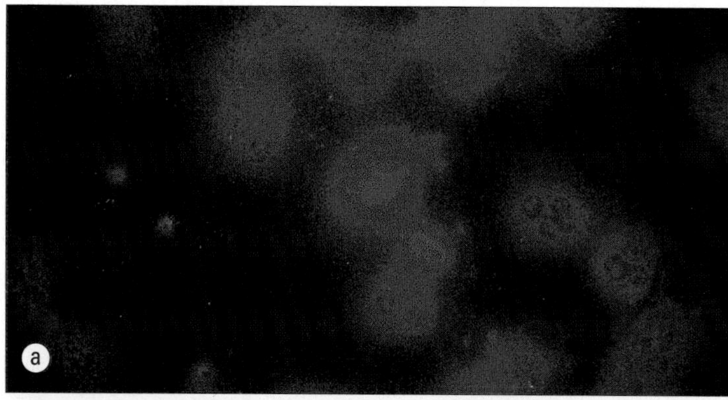

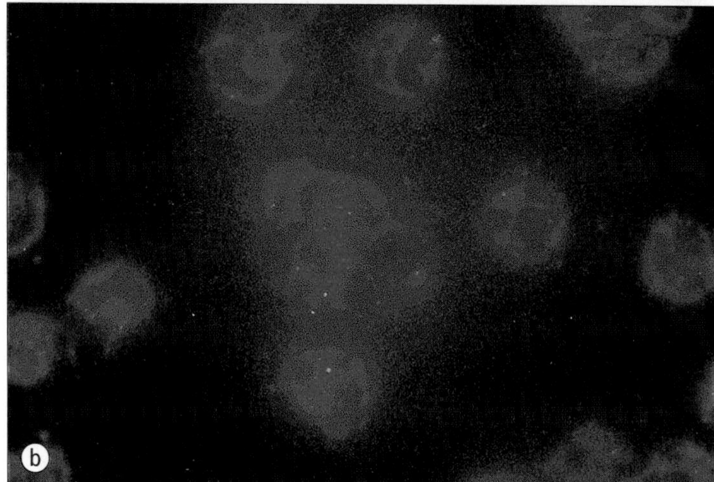

Fig. 29.9 Microbial material in synovial fluid cells of a patient with *Yersinia*-triggered reactive arthritis (a) and a patient with chronic *Yersinia*-triggered reactive arthritis (b). There is positive immunofluorescence staining by an antiserum obtained by immunizing a rabbit with live *Yersinia*. Most of the cells are polymorphonuclear granulocytes and, in the chronic case, nearly all are strongly positive. (From Granfors *et al.* [51], with permission.)

Nonsteroidal anti-inflammatory drugs (NSAIDs) form the basis of therapy (Fig. 29.10). They should be used regularly over some time in order to achieve maximum anti-inflammatory effect, and patients should be informed of this, otherwise they consider the drug as an analgesic. There is no definite drug of choice, since patients' responses differ.

Corticosteroids are a valuable asset in the treatment of reactive arthritis. In many cases, intra-articular administration gives prompt relief. However, purulent arthritis must be excluded before the injection. Systemic treatment with corticosteroids has also proved effective. They should be used in cases in which NSAIDs have not had a sufficient effect and when many joints are affected. The treatment can be started with a relatively high dose, 30–50mg daily of prednisolone or its equivalent, tapering down according to the improvement. Oral corticosteroids should be withdrawn slowly, while continuing NSAIDs. Corticosteroids should not be used more than for 2–4 months.

Antibiotic treatment should be given if a microbe is isolated. However, this is more to diminish spread of the infection than to influence the ongoing course of the disease. All the available information indicates that at the time of the first joint symptoms – when the patient usually comes to the physician – the pathogenic process cannot be reverted. The new quinolones offer a good alternative to the trimethoprim–sulfamethoxazole or tetracyclines often used. For streptococcal throat infection, penicillin or erythromycin are the drugs of choice. Recently lymecycline, administered for 3 months, has been studied [61] and found to have some beneficial effect in patients with *Chlamydia*-triggered disease. Currently, further studies on the value of long-term antibiotic therapy in reactive arthritis are underway.

TREATMENT OF ACUTE REACTIVE ARTHRITIS
Antibiotics if infection is still present
Rest
Nonsteroidal anti-inflammatory drugs
Intra-articular corticosteroid
Systemic corticosteroids
Rarely, second-line antirheumatic drugs

Fig. 29.10 Treatment of reactive arthritis.

Physical therapy using cold pads may alleviate the pain and edema of an inflamed joint. Rest is advisable, and splinting may be used to alleviate pain at night. However, immobilization should not be too complete. In severe cases, muscle wasting may be a problem and systematic rehabilitation may be required. During convalescence many patients tend to stop the analgesics too early; it is better to use them until pain no longer inhibits full use of muscles and joints, in order ensure a good end-result.

Cases with Chronic Symptoms

Recurrences of reactive arthritis are treated as the acute disease. The chronic arthralgias are a difficult therapeutic problem. With time, the patients often derive less and less benefit from the various NSAIDs, and side effects become more common with prolonged use. Nevertheless, these drugs are the best of the alternatives. Physiotherapy may give some patients relief but does not have a long-term effect. In chronic cases, corticosteroids are not advisable, since their therapeutic effect in this situation is not very good, and the prognosis is good in almost all cases.

Sulfasalazine is of interest because of the observations that patients with reactive arthritis often have more or less asymptomatic inflammation of the bowel. In some instances, it may give good results. The drug should be started at low dose, increasing to 2g, or even 3g if tolerated by the patient. Unfortunately, some patients cannot continue with the drug because of gastrointestinal intolerance.

When the symptoms resemble rheumatoid arthritis, classical antirheumatic treatment, for example gold salts (injected or by mouth), may prove quite useful and lead to rapid improvement. In these cases the treatment can be stopped after some months without the disease relapsing. There have been some reports regarding the use of methotrexate or azathioprine, but controlled trials with a large number of patients are not yet available.

The possibility of microbial persistence has opened the question of whether long-term antibiotic treatment should be used in chronic reactive arthritis. For rheumatic fever, permanent penicillin prophylaxis is commonly used to prevent relapses. In a recent double-blind prospective trial, the quinolone ciprofloxacin administered by mouth in a dose of 500mg twice daily has been evaluated. Although the drug did not have any dramatic effect, a decrease of symptoms in the active treatment group was observed (A Toivanen, T Yli-Kerttula, R Luukkainen *et al.*, unpublished observations). Further studies are needed to assess the value of long-term antibiotic treatment.

Many patients with chronic reactive arthritis suffer uncertainty and fear that they have a disease which leads to permanent disability. Because the findings are minimal, the diagnosis is often missed. Information on diagnosis and explanation of the disease, especially of its good prognosis, may be enough. With understanding and knowledge of the disorder, the patient is better able to tolerate its discomforts.

Extra-articular Disease

Ocular inflammations must be diagnosed and treated promptly, otherwise irreversible damage to the eyesight may occur. If possible, the patient should be referred to an ophthalmologist, since the diagnosis of uveitis requires use of a split lamp. Therapy consists of corticosteroids in the form of eye drops or even systemically, and of mydriatics. The patient should be informed about the strong possibility of recurrence. Excluding the endocarditis of rheumatic fever, the most common cardiac complications are conduction disturbance. In these instances a cardiac pacemaker is often indicated.

The nephritis that can be associated with reactive arthritis is usually mild, subsides spontaneously and does not require any treatment. The skin lesions, which by many dermatologists are considered identical to psoriasis, are treated accordingly. In mild cases keratinolytic agents, such as salicylic acid ointment or topical corticosteroid, may be used. In more severe cases, the patient is best referred to a dermatologist; retinoids or methotrexate are most commonly used.

Prognosis

The prognosis of reactive arthritis is generally good. The duration of the disease varies from a few days to several weeks. Even patients who are severely incapacitated and bedridden can look forward to full recovery. However, recurrences are frequent, and they can be triggered not only by new infections but also by nonspecific stress factors. Urogenital and eye inflammations, particularly, have a tendency to recur. Many patients complain of abdominal discomfort and occasional diarrhea for months and even years after the initial attack of the disease. Back pain and arthralgia are common, and also frank synovitis may be seen. Tendinitis and enthesopathy may lead to erosion or proliferation of bone at the tendon insertions. These joint symptoms may be precipitated by rather nonspecific factors, such as changes in the weather, and many patients report discomfort during the fall and winter seasons. Conversely, a new infection by bacteria known to trigger the disease may pass without any sequela. The nonsymptomatic period between recurrences may last for several years.

Follow-up studies of reactive arthritis suggest that 20–70% of patients later suffer some joint discomfort or other symptoms [2,4,16,18,62]. For the individual patient it is important to know that, in spite of unpleasant symptoms, severe destructive disease as a sequel of reactive arthritis is extremely rare. Of 100 patients who were studied 20 years after a *Shigella*-triggered reactive arthritis, none had rheumatoid arthritis [4]; and in another follow-up study of 60 patients, only one definite rheumatoid arthritis case was found [62]. Observations of sacroiliitis and radiologic findings suggest that ankylosing spondylitis can occur, but even in these cases the disease usually remains mild. Whether degenerative changes, such as osteoarthritis, develop more readily in a joint that has been affected by reactive arthritis remains an open question.

REFERENCES

1. Reiter H. Uber eine bisher unerkannte Spirochäteninfektion (Spirochaetosis arthritica). Dtsch Med Wochenschr. 1916;**42**:1535–6.
2. Wright V, Moll JMH, eds. Seronegative polyarthritis. Amsterdam: North-Holland Publishing Company; 1976.
3. Paronen I. Reiter's disease. A study of 344 cases observed in Finland. Acta Med Scand. 1948;suppl **212**:1–112.
4. Sairanen E, Paronen I, Mähönen H. Reiter's syndrome: a follow-up study. Acta Med Scand. 1969;**185**:57–63.
5. Aho K, Ahvonen P, Lassus A, Sievers K, Tiilikainen A. Yersinia arthritis and related diseases: clinical and immunogenetic implications. In: Dumonde DC, ed. Infection and immunology in the rheumatic diseases. Oxford: Blackwell Scientific Publications; 1976:341–4.
6. Isomäki H, Raunio J, von Essen R, Hämeenkorpi R. Incidence of inflammatory rheumatic diseases in Finland. Scand J Rheumatol. 1978;**7**:188–92.
7. Aho K. Bowel infection predisposing to reactive arthritis. In: Rooney PJ, ed. Baillière's clinical rheumatology, vol 3. London: Baillière Tindall; 1989:303–19.
8. Leino R, Kalliomäki JL. Yersiniosis as an internal disease. Ann Intern Med. 1974;**81**:458–61.
9. Aho K, Ahvonen P, Lassus A, Sievers K, Tiilikainen A. HLA-B27 in reactive arthritis: a study of yersinia arthritis and Reiter's disease. Arthritis Rheum. 1974;**17**:521–6.
10. Nicholls A. Reiter's disease and HLA-B27. Ann Rheum Dis. 1975;**34** (suppl): 27–8.
11. Laitinen O, Leirisalo M, Skylv G. Relation between HLA-B27 and clinical features with yersinia arthritis. Arthritis Rheum. 1977;**20**:1121–4.
12. Keat A. HLA-linked disease susceptibility and reactive arthritis. J Infect. 1982;**5**:227–39.
13. Lahesmaa-Rantala R, Toivanen A. Clinical spectrum of reactive arthritis. In: Toivanen A, Toivanen P, eds. Reactive arthritis. Boca Raton: CRC Press; 1988:1–13.
14. van Bohemen CG, Lionarons RJ, van Bodegom P, et al. Susceptibility and HLA-B27 in post-dysenteric arthropathies. Immunology. 1985; **56**:377–9.
15. Schultz JS, Good AE, Sing CF, Kapur JJ. HLA profile and Reiter's syndrome. Clin Genet. 1981;**19**:159–67.
16. Calin A, Fries JF. An "experimental" epidemic of Reiter's syndrome revisited. Follow-up evidence on genetic and environmental factors. Ann Intern Med. 1976;**84**:564–6.
17. van Bohemen ChG, Dinant HJ, Grumet FC, Landheer JE, Zanen HC. Significance of HLA-B27-like enterobacterial epitopes in the etiology of reactive arthritis. In: Toivanen A, Toivanen P, eds. Reactive arthritis. Boca Raton: CRC Press; 1988:51–63.
18. Leirisalo M, Skylv G, Kousa M, et al. Followup study on patients with Reiter's disease and reactive arthritis with special reference to HLA-B27. Arthritis Rheum. 1982;**25**:249–59.
19. Håkansson U, Löw B, Eitrem R, Winblad S. HLA-27 and reactive arthritis in an outbreak of salmonellosis. Tissue Antigens. 1975;**6**:366–7.
20. Simon DG, Kaslow RA, Rosenbaum J, Kaye RL, Calin A. Reiter's syndrome following epidemic shigellosis. J Rheumatol. 1981;**8**:969–73.
21. Eastmond CJ, Rennie JAN, Reid TMS. An outbreak of *Campylobacter* enteritis – a rheumatological followup survey. J Rheumatol. 1983;**10**:107–8.
22. Tertti R, Granfors K, Lehtonen O-P, et al. An outbreak of *Yersinia* pseudotuberculosis infection. J Infect Dis. 1984;**149**:245–50.
23. Tertti R, Vuento R, Mikkola PGK, Mäkelä A-L, Toivanen A. Clinical manifestations of *Yersinia* pseudotuberculosis infection in children. Eur J Clin Microbiol Infect Dis. 1989;**8**:587–91.
24. Leino R. Human yersiniosis. A clinical study with special reference to lymphocyte transformation in yersinia arthritis [Thesis]. Turku: Turku University; 1982.
25. Ahvonen P. Human yersiniosis in Finland. II. Clinical features. Ann Clin Res. 1972;**4**:39–48.
26. Leino R, Toivanen A. Arthritis associated with gastrointestinal disorders. In: Toivanen A, Toivanen P, eds. Reactive arthritis. Boca Raton: CRC Press; 1988:77–86.
27. Ahvonen P, Sievers K, Aho K. Arthritis associated with *Yersinia enterocolitica* infection. Acta Rheum Scand. 1969;1**5**:232–53.
28. Yli-Kerttula U. Reiter's syndrome or uro-arthritis in females with special emphasis on chlamydial infections [Thesis]. Acta Univ Tamperensis ser A. 1984;177.
29. Yli-Kerttula UI, Vilppula AH. Reactive salpingitis. In: Toivanen A, Toivanen P, eds. Reactive arthritis. Boca Raton: CRC Press; 1988:125–31.
30. De Vos M, Cuvelier C, Mielants H, Veys E, Barbier F, Elewaut A. Ileocolonoscopy in seronegative spondylarthropathy. Gastroenterology. 1989;**96**:339–44.
31. Mielants H, Veys EM. Inflammation of the ileum in patients with B27-positive reactive arthritis. Lancet. 1984;**i**:288.
32. Saari KM. The eye and reactive arthritis. In: Toivanen A, Toivanen P, eds. Reactive arthritis. Boca Raton: CRC Press; 1988:113–24.
33. Kovanen S, Viander M, Granfors K, et al. Heart-reactive antibodies in yersiniosis. Int J Immunopathol Pharmacol. 1988;**1**:63–7.
34. Viitanen A-M, Arstila TP, Lahesmaa R, Granfors K, Skirnik M, Toivanen P. Application of the polymerase chain reaction and immunofluorescence techniques to the detection of bacteria in Yersinia-triggered reactive arthritis. Arthritis Rheum. 1991;**34**:89–96.
35. Shmerling RH, Delbanco TL, Tosteson ANA, Trentham DE. Synovial fluid tests. What should be ordered? JAMA. 1990;**264**:1009–14.
36. Isomäki H, Anttila P. Radiology of reactive arthritis. In: Toivanen A, Toivanen P, eds. Reactive arthritis. Boca Raton: CRC Press; 1988:133–8.
37. Granfors K, Vuento R, Toivanen A. Host–microbe interaction in reactive arthritis. In: Toivanen A, Toivanen P, eds. Reactive arthritis. Boca Raton: CRC Press; 1988:15–49.
38. Repo H, Leirisalo-Repo M, Koivuranta-Vaara P. Exaggerated inflammatory responsiveness plays a part in the pathogenesis of HLA-B27 linked diseases – hypothesis. Ann Clin Res. 1984;**16**:47–50.
39. Lahesmaa R, Skurnik M, Toivanen P. Molecular mimicry: any role in the pathogenesis of spondyloarthropathies? Contrib Microbiol Immunol. 1992; **31**:221–9.
40. Hermann E, Mayet W-J, Poralla T, Meyer zum Buschenfelde K-H, Fleischer B. *Salmonella*-reactive synovial fluid T-cell clones in a patient with post-infectious salmonella-arthritis. Scand J Rheum. 1990;**19**:350–5.
41. Geczy AF, McGuigan LE, Sullivan JS, Edmonds JP. Cytotoxic T lymphocytes against disease-associated determinant(s) in ankylosing spondylitis. J Exp Med. 1986;**164**:932–7.
42. Keat A. Is spondylitis caused by *Klebsiella*? Immunol Today. 1986;**7**:144–9.
43. Oldstone MBA. Molecular mimicry and autoimmune disease. Cell. 1987;**50**:819–20.
44. Avakian H, Welsh J, Ebringer A, Entwistle CC. Ankylosing spondylitis HLA-B27 and *Klebsiella*. II. Cross-reactivity studies with human tissue typing sera. Br J Exp Pathol. 1980;**61**:92–6.
45. Welsh J, Avakian H, Cowling P, et al. Ankylosing spondylitis, HLA-B27 and *Klebsiella*. I. Cross-reactivity with rabbit antisera. Br J Exp Pathol. 1980;**61**:85–91.

46. Schwimmbeck PL, Oldstone MBA. *Klebsiella pneumoniae* and HLA B27-associated diseases of Reiter's syndrome and ankylosing spondylitis. Curr Topics Microbiol Immunol. 1989;**145**:45–56.
47. Tertti R, Toivanen P. Immune functions and inflammatory reactions in HLA-B27 positive subjects. Ann Rheum Dis. 1991;**50**:731–4.
48. Toivanen A, Granfors K, Lahesmaa-Rantala R, Leino R, Ståhlberg T, Vuento R. Pathogenesis of yersinia-triggered reactive arthritis: Immunological, microbiological and clinical aspects. Immunol Rev. 1985;**86**:47–70.
49. Gaston JSH, Life PF, Granfors K, et al. Synovial T lymphocyte recognition of organisms that trigger reactive arthritis. Clin Exp Immunol. 1989;**76**:348–53.
50. Lahesmaa-Rantala R, Granfors K, Isomäki H, Toivanen A. *Yersinia* specific immune complexes in the synovial fluid of patients with yersinia-triggered reactive arthritis. Ann Rheum Dis. 1987;**46**:10–4.
51. Granfors K, Jalkanen S, von Essen R, et al. *Yersinia* antigens in synovial-fluid cells from patients with reactive arthritis. N Engl J Med. 1989;**320**:216–21.
52. Toivanen A, Lahesmaa-Rantala R, Ståhlberg T, Merilahti-Palo R. Do bacterial antigens persist in reactive arthritis? Clin Exp Rheum. 1987;**5**(suppl 1):25–7.
53. Keat A, Thomas B, Dixey J, Osborn M, Sonnex C, Taylor-Robinson D. *Chlamydia trachomatis* and reactive arthritis – the missing link. Lancet. 1987;**i**:72–4.
54. Schumacher HR, Jr, Magge S, Cherian PV, et al. Light and electron microscopic studies on the synovial membrane in Reiter's syndrome. Immunocytochemical identification of chlamydial antigen in patients with early disease. Arthritis Rheum. 1988;**31**:937–46.
55. Granfors K, Jalkanen S, Lindberg AA, et al. *Salmonella* lipopolysaccharide in synovial cells from patients with reactive arthritis. Lancet. 1990;**335**:685–8.
56. Hammer M, Zeidler H, Klimsa S, Heesemann J. *Yersinia enterocolitica* in the synovial membrane of patients with *Yersinia*-induced arthritis. Arthritis Rheum. 1990;**33**:1795–800.
57. Merilahti-Palo R, Söderström K-O, Lahesmaa-Rantala R, Granfors K, Toivanen A. Bacterial antigens in synovial biopsy specimens in Yersinia-triggered reactive arthritis. Ann Rheum Dis. 1991;**50**:87–90.
58. Lipsky PE, Davis LS, Cush JJ, Oppenheimer-Marks N. The role of cytokines in the pathogenesis of rheumatoid arthritis. Springer Semin Immunopathol. 1989;**11**:123–62.
59. Ziff M. Role of endothelium in chronic inflammation. Springer Semin Immunopathol. 1989;**11**:199–214.
60. Toivanen A, Toivanen P. Pathogenesis of reactive arthritis. In: Toivanen A, Toivanen P, eds. Reactive arthritis. Boca Raton: CRC Press; 1988:167–78.
61. Lauhio A, Leirisalo-Repo M, Lähdevirta J, Saikku P, Repo H. Double-blind, placebo controlled study of three-month treatment with lymecycline in reactive arthritis, with special reference to *Chlamydia* arthritis. Arthritis Rheum. 1991;**34**:6–14.
62. Kalliomäki JL, Leino R. Follow-up studies of joint complications in yersiniosis. Acta Med Scand. 1979;**205**:521–5.

INFECTION AND REACTIVE ARTHRITIS 30

PRACTICAL PROBLEMS

RHEUMATIC FEVER IN ADULTS

Alan G Tyndall

Definition of the Problem

Rheumatic fever is relatively rare in the developed world, particularly so in adults. Therefore, most physicians have little first-hand experience of this previously devastating illness, and must rely on the literature from the middle of this century or from developing countries. The situation is complex, however, because:

- The epidemiology and virulence of rheumatogenic streptococcae are changing.
- The clinical expression of a poststreptococcal syndrome may vary from sterile reactive arthritis alone to major cardiac involvements.
- Modern cardiologic diagnostic tools (e.g. two-dimensional echocardiography or atrial stimulation electrocardiography) may demonstrate major cardiac involvement which was unsuspected on conventional testing.
- Guidelines for prophylaxis lack extensive supportive data.

Typical Cases

Case 1

A 26-year-old woman was referred to the rheumatology department after two attacks of inflammatory right hip synovitis over 6 weeks. There was no preceding sore throat or other infective episode, and no symptoms to suggest an associated rheumatologic disorder. Aspiration of the hip on the first occasion demonstrated markedly inflammatory sterile fluid. Antibiotics were given on the first occasion only. Each episode lasted 2–3 weeks. Laboratory investigation showed elevated acute-phase reactants, ESR 85mm/hour, C-reactive protein (CRP) 6mg/dl (normal 0.0–0.5) and elevated DNAase B antibody of 2400IU (normal up to 610); these parameters returned to normal after 6 months. The antistreptolysin O titer (ASOT) remained normal throughout. She remained symptom free in the next 2 years of follow-up. At no stage was cardiac involvement present clinically or on ECG or echocardiographic examination. Throat cultures failed to demonstrate pathogenic streptococcae on both occasions.

Case 2

A 34-year-old woman had three separate episodes of fixed inflammatory oligoarthritis of large joints over 3 months. The first episode was associated with a mildly sore throat and proven group A beta-hemolytic streptococcal infection on culture. The third episode was associated with erythema nodosum (Fig. 30.1) and marked systemic malaise. She had an elevated ESR, CRP, ASOT and DNAase B antibody. A full immunologic and rheumatologic laboratory investigation showed negative antinuclear antibodies, rheumatoid factors and HLA B27 antigen, and negative antibody testing to arthritogenic viruses such as parvovirus, hepatitis, Epstein–Barr virus and rubella. No antibodies to *Yersinia, Chlamydia, Salmonella, Shigella* or *Borrelia burgdorferi* were detected. There were no cardiac symptoms or signs, and the chest radiograph and electrocardiograph were normal. However, a routine two-dimensional echocardiograph demonstrated a definitively hypokinetic left ventricle. The arthritis and painful erythema nodosum was managed successfully with indomethacin, initially 50mg three times a day tapering to 25mg three times a day over 4 weeks. In addition, prophylactic penicillin was commenced at 250mg oral penicillin V twice per day. At follow up 3 and 6 months later she was symptom free, but the echocardiographic hypokinesis of the left ventricle remained. At least 12 months of prophylactic penicillin was recommended, to be reviewed.

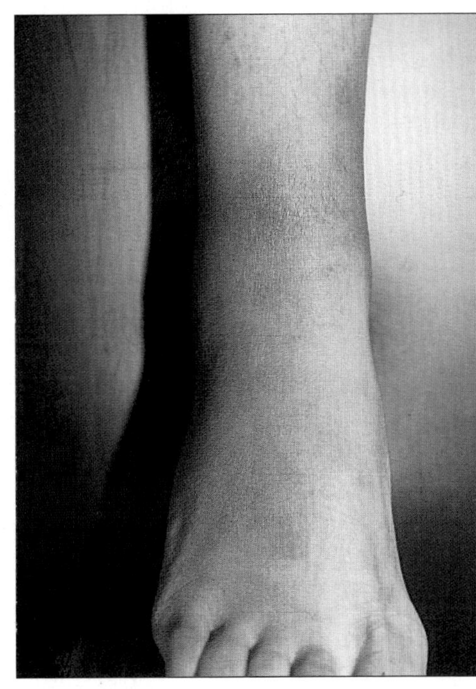

Fig. 30.1 Erythema nodosum associated with beta-hemolytic streptococcal infection and inflammatory oligoarthritis.

Diagnostic Problems

These two cases reflect the clinical and laboratory difficulties in diagnosing rheumatic fever. The first case probably represents a true poststreptococcal reactive arthritis. However, such apparently 'non-carditic cases' may progress later to cardiac involvement or have unsuspected cardiac involvement at the time of presentation, as seen in case 2. Neither case has the typical revised Jones criteria of 1965 with migratory oligoarthritis, and neither had cardiac involvement on simple ECG or clinical grounds.

Laboratory Data

The first case illustrates the absolute need for multiple streptococcal antigen testing.

Streptolysin O is produced by most group A streptococci and also by organisms of groups C and G. Antistreptolysin antibodies rise between 1 and 4 weeks after infection and fall after a period of 3–6 months. Laboratory reference ranges fluctuate according to the age of the patient and the time of the year. Normal values are generally quoted at less than 150IU for children under 5 years of age and less than 300IU in older children or young adults. However, some individuals have been documented with sustained levels between 400 and 800IU over a period as long as 12 months without obvious clinical correlation. Therefore, changing unequivocally raised titers should be demonstrated. Some beta-hemolytic streptococci induce no antistreptolysin antibodies, and other serologic parameters should be measured. Most group A streptococci produce significant amounts of the exoenzyme DNAase B, but apart from groups C and G no other streptococci produce this in significant amounts. Elevated levels are defined as being greater than 80IU in children less than 5 years of age, greater than 230IU in individuals 5–19 years old, and greater than 610IU in individuals over 20 years of age. Elevated DNAase B levels occur after both cutaneous and pharyngeal infection, whereas the ASOT is often not elevated after cutaneous infection. DNAase B antibodies do not show the false-positive result sometimes seen with ASOT after bacterial contamination of the specimen, liver diseases or oxidation of the ASO molecule. Throat culture is neither diagnostic nor exclusive.

Many patients do not recall a preceding pharyngitis before proven streptococcal infections with rheumatic fever sequelae (up to 40% in a series of young adults). In addition, asymptomatic, noninfective carriage of *Streptococcus* in the throat is well described. A serologic reaction should be demonstrated, since throat culture may be negative even without antibiotic therapy in definite clinically significant infections.

Great care must be taken to exclude streptococcal septic arthritis and bacteremia or septicemia, by appropriate blood and joint fluid cultures. *Streptococcus* A of different Lancefield groups may cause such infections of one or more joints; these infections are usually asymmetric with a poor response to antibiotics and are generally associated with an unfavorable outcome. This may be particularly difficult to distinguish from a true sterile reactive arthritis, particularly if partial antibiotic therapy has occurred prior to assessment.

The 'rheumatogenic' specificity resides mainly in the M-type protein seen in the outer coat of the three-layered cell wall of the *Streptococcus* and fimbriae. M-Typing is not routinely performed, but it is important as part of assessing a suspected epidemic. There are more than 80 subtypes of these M-types and, in general, the lower numbers are more associated with 'rheumatogenic' beta-hemolytic *Streptococcus* group A organisms. The recent outbreaks of rheumatic fever in the US have been associated with M-types 1, 3, 5, 6 and 18. These were mostly seen in clusters, either regional (e.g. Salt Lake City and surrounding areas of Utah, in 1985) or institutional (San Diego, California Naval Training Center, 1987, and Fort Leonard Wood Army Training Base in Missouri, 1987 and 1988). The latter involved adult army recruits.

Have there been changes in virulence?

Are these epidemics transient shifts in virulence or part of a generalized trend towards a world wide increase in beta-hemolytic streptococcal virulence? Certainly they have been associated with increased virulence in other ways, for example streptococcal toxic shock syndrome, invasive soft tissue infections, septicemia and septic arthritis. One study suggests that a gene encoding streptococcal pyrogenic toxin A (*spe-A*) is more common in invasive, clinically significant infections and was found in M 1 strains from eight states in the US, Norway, Canada and New Zealand. Such genes may be acquired by horizontal spread within bacterial species via bacteriophages.

This raises the possibility that a virulence gene, rather than a specific serotype, is important. More data are required.

The reason for an apparent worldwide trend is unclear, and exotoxins themselves are not directly or solely the cause of rheumatic fever. However, as a marker of generalized increased virulence the trend should be carefully followed (Fig. 30.2).

Therapeutic Options

Adequate (at least 10 days) treatment of a primary pharyngeal streptoccal infection should be given when diagnosed. Naturally, not every patient with an upper respiratory or throat infection should or could have bacteriologic culture, but particular attention should be paid during times of apparent epidemics. Whether such epidemics occur within households, institutions, suburbs or regions, culture should be performed and bacterial strain identification undertaken and notified to the appropriate authorities. Only in this way will we detect a worldwide or regional shift in virulence.

The question of secondary prophylaxis remains unanswered. Clearly those adults who have contracted rheumatic fever with cardiac sequelae should have up to 5 years secondary prevention with the appropriate antibiotic. Whether this is oral or monthly intramuscular depot treatment depends on local conditions, compliance, follow-up facilities, etc.

It would also seem prudent to treat similarly any adults contracting streptococcal infection in the presence of an epidemic – either institutional or regional – associated with a 'rheumatogenic' group A beta-hemolytic *Streptococcus* strain. Such a decision for prophylaxis would be strengthened if the patient had a documented brisk and marked serologic reaction, and if other patients had cardiac involvement. There are no data yet to support this 'common-sense', first-principles advice.

Conclusions

There appears to be a changing pattern of poststreptococcal sterile reactive arthritis in young adults different from that described in the middle of the century with classical rheumatic fever. Single

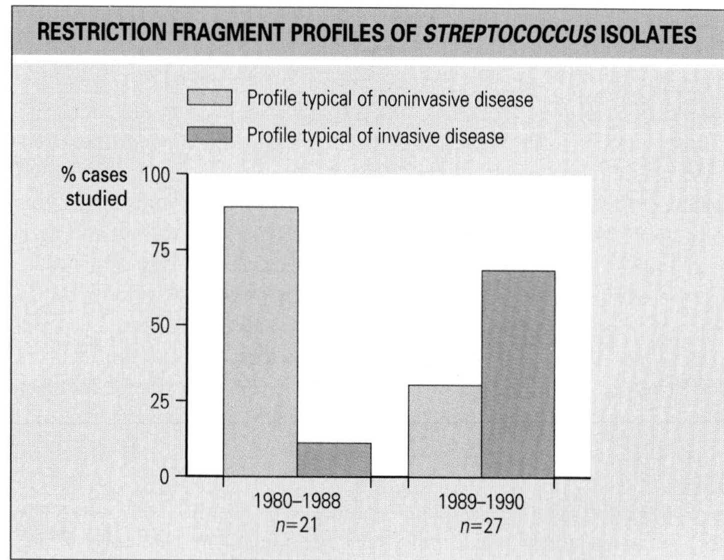

Fig. 30.2 Restriction profiles of *Streptococcus* isolates from cases of uncomplicated disease (pharyngitis). Over time, the DNA restriction fragment profile seen in invasive disease has become more common than that seen in noninvasive disease. Data from Clearly *et al.* (1992).

cases with no carditic involvement after modern assessment and unassociated with high antibody titers probably do not require years of antibiotic secondary prophylaxis. However, when occurring in epidemics, and associated with more virulent 'rheumatogenic' streptococcal A strains, secondary prophylaxis for up to 5 years would appear justified. Primary eradication of all proven cases of streptococcal throat infection should be attempted and careful, complete microbiologic data collected and reported on such cases. The apparent increase in 'rheumatogenic' virulent streptococcal infections in the western world in the 1980s has not been confined only to overcrowded, underprivileged urban areas or institutions, but also observed in so-called middle-class, well-to-do suburban and rural groups.

The possible re-emergence of this old adversary should be remembered and we should remain vigilant.

REFERENCES

Arnold MH, Tyndall AG. Poststreptococcal reactive arthritis. Ann Rheum Dis. 1989;**48**:686–8.

Bisno AL. Group A Streptococcal infections and acute rheumatic fever. N Engl J Med. 1991;**325**:738–93.

Cleary PP, Kaplan EL, Handly JP, et al. Clonal basis for resurgence of serious *Streptococcus pyogenes* disease in the 1980s. Lancet. 1992;**339**:518–21.

Fink CW. The role of the streptococcus in poststreptococcal reactive arthritis and childhood polyarteritis nodosa. J Rheumatol. 1991;**18**(suppl 29):14–20.

Wallace MR, Garst PD, Papadimos TJ, et al. The return of acute rheumatic fever in young adults. JAMA. 1989:**262**:2557–61.

POSITIVE LYME SEROLOGY WITH NONSPECIFIC SYMPTOMS

Daniel W Rahn

Definition of the Problem

Lyme disease is a relapsing and remitting illness with clinical manifestations that vary greatly among different patients and over time in individual patients. Because the possible vectors of Lyme disease, ticks of the *Ixodes ricinus* complex, are distributed widely around the world, large populations are conceivably at risk of contracting this illness. Individuals in both endemic and nonendemic areas seek medical attention with complaints that are within the possible clinical spectrum of Lyme disease. When there is no history of erythema chronicum migrans (ECM), Lyme disease may mimic or be mimicked by other disease processes. Even though there are often other more likely explanations for the individual's complaints, the physician may be faced with the need to 'rule out' Lyme disease. The usual approach chosen in this situation is to order a Lyme serology in the hope that a negative result will eliminate the unlikely but possible diagnosis of Lyme disease; but what happens if the serology is positive? Does this mean that the individual has Lyme disease? Statistically, the positive predictive value of a serology result varies according to the pretest probability of the disease being present. If this probability is low, a positive serology result may have very poor predictive value for the diagnosis of Lyme disease and, therefore, actually be misleading rather than helpful.

The Typical Case

LD is a 45-year-old woman who made an appointment for the evaluation of generalized musculoskeletal pain, fatigue and headache of 6 months' duration. She was concerned that she might have undiagnosed Lyme disease, although the area in which she lives is not known to be endemic for this illness. Her symptoms began a few weeks after a summer holiday in an area where Lyme disease is thought to occur. She did not recall any tick bites or expanding skin lesions but did have a red spot about a centimeter in diameter, located behind her knee, during this holiday. She saw a general practitioner on return from her vacation because of her concern about this skin lesion and was treated with penicillin for 7 days, during which time the lesion disappeared.

Her pains began shortly after the lesion resolved and became constant. They seemed to be located in bones, muscles, joints and periarticular areas. The discomfort was disturbing her sleep four to five times nightly. She would wake for the day with a feeling of exhaustion that worsened throughout the day. More recently she developed a generalized headache that was present more often than not. She also reported difficulty concentrating but could not identify specific intellectual deficits. She had seen three physicians prior to the consultation, none of whom found an explanation for her symptoms. She had had a series of laboratory tests including complete blood count, ESR, rheumatoid factor, antinuclear antibody, routine blood chemistries, thyroid function tests and urinalysis, all of which were normal, and she had had three Lyme serologies, two of which were negative and one weakly positive. She wanted her Lyme serology to be determined a fourth time and to be given antibiotic treatment for Lyme disease because of her concern about her decreased functional capacity and possible neurologic deterioration. She was particularly concerned because she had read that physicians often fail to recognize and correctly diagnose Lyme disease and that laboratory testing for this disease may be unreliable. She described herself as depressed but attributed this to the debilitating nature of her current symptoms.

On physical examination, she had a relatively flat affect but a generally healthy appearance. Her general examination was unremarkable. Examination of her musculoskeletal system revealed no evidence of joint inflammation. She was remarkably tender at many periarticular sites including subacromial bursae, the lateral epicondyles of both humeri, both greater trochanters and iliac crests. Her strength was normal and her neurologic examination, including bedside mental status testing, cranial nerves, peripheral nervous system and reflexes, was normal.

In reviewing the findings with her, she was told that she did not appear to have overt arthritis or neurologic deficits, and the clinical judgment was that it was very unlikely that she had Lyme disease. Because she was very concerned, however, it was decided to repeat her Lyme serology and to order an immunoblot to rule out the possibility that the previous weakly positive result could have been a false positive. The Lyme serology revealed an IgG titer in the 'borderline' range by enzyme-linked immunosorbant assay (ELISA); the immunoblot was reported to show faint bands of immunoreactivity at 41 and 60kDa. The interpretation accompanying these results stated that these were findings 'consistent with but not diagnostic of' Lyme disease.

Diagnostic Problems

The major dilemma posed when an individual has nonspecific symptoms and a positive serology is whether the patient has active Lyme disease. The data on which conclusions must be based are history, findings on physical examination and laboratory results.

It may be difficult to establish whether a patient has been exposed to an endemic area, since an area may only be suspected, or indeed not even suspected, but still harbor an occasional infected tick. To establish an area as endemic would ordinarily require the identification of *Borrelia burgdorferi* in ticks or animal reservoirs and in skin biopsy material of patients with lesions meeting the clinical description of ECM. If this information is unavailable, whether a patient has been at risk of acquiring Lyme disease cannot be known with certainty. The skin lesion of the patient discussed earlier was not ECM as classically described, but there was no opportunity to examine it and it may have responded to penicillin (alternatively it may have resolved spontaneously while the patient was taking penicillin).

Patients with positive serologies but no classic symptoms of Lyme disease have complaints that are within the general clinical spectrum of this disease: musculoskeletal pain and cognitive impairment. Such complaints must be explored thoroughly to determine the likelihood that they are due to Lyme disease. The arthritic manifestations of Lyme disease fall into three general categories (Fig. 30.3): intermittent, migratory musculoskeletal pain; intermittent, inflammatory mono- or oligoarticular, large joint arthritis; and chronic monoarthritis (particularly of the knee). It is worth remembering that, in 20% of individuals with Lyme disease, musculoskeletal complaints are generally transient and characterized by intermittent, migratory arthralgias and periarticular pain, rather than overt arthritis. On examination, one would expect little tenderness in such cases, since inflammation is minimal when Lyme disease causes only arthralgias. In contrast, the patient described earlier had constant pain and exquisite tenderness of periarticular sites; her rheumatic syndrome was not typical of Lyme disease but rather fits the clinical description of fibromyalgia, a syndrome characterized by the presence of widespread musculoskeletal pain and tender points.

It is also important to elicit any history of cognitive impairment. Lyme disease can cause a chronic mild encephalopathy, primarily affecting short-term memory. This deficit may be demonstrated with objective tests of higher cortical function. Although a patient may describe a deterioration from baseline intellectual function, if there is also a chronic sleep disturbance, daytime exhaustion and depression then these may be associated with blunting of higher intellectual function, and depression alone rather than encephalopathy may explain the cognitive complaints.

Finally, there is the issue of how to interpret Lyme serologies in clinical context. Lyme disease serologic test results vary considerably, in part due to problems associated with currently available test kits and clinical laboratory procedures. The immune response to *Borrelia burgdorferi* develops slowly, but almost all individuals with Lyme disease of 6 months' duration have significantly elevated IgG antibody levels (not a result in the indeterminate range between definite negative and definite positive). Antibiotic therapy given for ECM may blunt the immune response to *Borrelia burgdorferi* if initiated before dissemination and systemic immune challenge. Theoretically, if the organism had already spread silently to the nervous system, however, oral penicillin might eradicate it from the skin without eradicating it from the central nervous system. In this circumstance, chronic neurologic disease might occur with minimal immunoreactivity in serum, the immune response being restricted largely to the spinal fluid. A full evaluation for this possibility would require a lumbar puncture and examination of spinal fluid for anti-*Borrelia burgdorferi* antibodies. This is recommended only if a patient has a convincing history of Lyme disease and neurologic deficit unexplainable by other processes.

There are other possible explanations for weak seropositivity, including immunologic crossreactivity with other spirochetes (*Treponema pallidum*, oral and gut spirochetes, *Borrelia hermsii*) or other bacterial organisms (particularly at the 41kDa flagellar antigen), self-antigens (in the case of the 60kDa heat shock protein), or generalized B cell hyper-reactivity as has occured in systemic lupus erythematosus (SLE), subacute bacterial endocarditis, RA, and other diseases with immunologic components. When there is low likelihood of Lyme disease on clinical and epidemiologic grounds, positive serology is very likely falsely positive for one or more of these reasons (or even due to simple inconsistency in test performance). When individuals at low risk of Lyme disease are surveyed

MUSCULOSKELETAL MANIFESTATIONS OF LYME DISEASE		
Syndrome	Description	Prevalence (%)
Migratory musculoskeletal pain	Intermittent brief attacks of pain lasting hours to days and involving joints, tendons, bursae and entheses	20
Intermittent oligoarticular arthritis	Recurrent attacks of inflammatory arthritis lasting days to months and involving 1–3 large joints In 80% of cases, one or both knees are affected Effusions may be massive	50
Chronic arthritis	Persistent synovitis of 1–2 large joints lasting 1 year or longer without response to antibiotics	20
No musculoskeletal symptoms	In the US, approximately 10% of individuals with untreated erythema chronicum migrans have no subsequent musculoskeletal manifestations In Europe, musculoskeletal signs and symptoms may be less frequent	10

Fig. 30.3 Musculoskeletal manifestations of Lyme disease.

with current Lyme serology tests, some test in the indeterminate or low positive range due to antibody patterns, such as that of the patient described, even though there is no history to suggest Lyme disease. In clinical practice, one may well encounter more low-titer false-positive than low-titer true-positive results. As the titer increases, or if immunoblot analysis reveals reactivity against *B. burgdorferi*-specific epitopes (e.g. the 31, 34 or 39kDa antigens), it becomes more likely that the result reflects true immunoreactivity against *B. burgdorferi*, but even then there is not necessarily any relationship between symptoms under evaluation and immunoreactivity (Fig. 30.4). The bottom line is that serology results are not helpful in the evaluation of individuals who have a low likelihood of Lyme disease by clinical and epidemiologic criteria.

Conclusions

Lyme serologies are an adjunct to the diagnosis of Lyme disease. A positive serology increases the likelihood of Lyme disease if there is

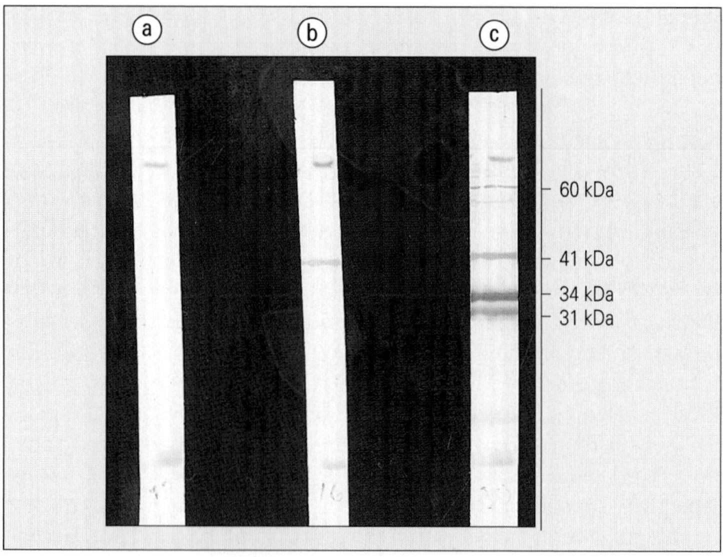

Fig. 30.4 Immunoblot analysis may be helpful in clarifying whether a positive ELISA assay for Lyme disease represents a true or false positive. Negative, equivocal and positive immunoblots are shown. An ELISA may be positive because of nonspecific immunoreactivity and be associated with a negative pattern on immunoblot (a). It may be positive due to reactivity at a commonly crossreactive epitope like the 41kDa flagellar antigen (b). Immunoblot analysis can confirm an ELISA result as a true positive only if immunoreactivity is seen against *B. burgdorferi*-specific antigens such as ospA (31kDa) or ospB (34kDa) (c). Courtesy of Ms Stella Cretella, Yale University School of Medicine.

a history of exposure and the clinical picture is consistent with this diagnosis. Both false positives and negatives occur with current techniques, however, so Lyme serologies cannot be used to screen individuals with nonspecific symptoms. Because of the relatively high incidence of low-titer false-positive results in particular, a weakly positive serology cannot be the basis of the diagnosis of Lyme disease when supporting data from history and physical examination are lacking. Even strongly positive immunoreactivity (high-titer antibody level accompanied by a definitely positive immunoblot) does not establish a causal link between symptoms and signs under evaluation and the serologic status for Lyme disease. In all cases, the diagnosis of Lyme disease must be based on clinical features; the certainty of the diagnosis may be increased by positive serologic results in the appropriate clinical setting.

REFERENCES

Barbour AG. The diagnosis of Lyme disease: rewards and perils. Ann Intern Med. 1989;**110**:501–2.

Halperin JJ, Krupp LB, Golightly MG, Volkman DJ. Lyme borreliosis-associated encephalopathy. Neurology. 1990;**40**:1340–3.

Logigian EL, Kaplan RF, Steere AC. Chronic neurologic manifestations of Lyme disease. N Engl J Med. 1990;**323**:1438–43.

Steere AC, Bartenhagen NH, Craft JE, et al. The early clinical manifestations of Lyme disease. Ann Intern Med. 1983;**99**76–82.

Steere AC, Schoen RT, Taylor E. The clinical evolution of Lyme arthritis. Ann Intern Med. 1987;**107**:725–31.

Sigal H. Summary of the first 100 patients seen at a Lyme disease referral center. Am J Med. 1990;**88**:577–81.

MANAGEMENT OF LATE LYME DISEASE

Daniel W Rahn

Definition of the Problem

It is believed that persistent infection with *Borrelia burgdorferi* drives the clinical manifestations of Lyme disease throughout its course. As the illness advances, however, it is progressively more difficult to recover organisms by culture and to demonstrate antibiotic responsiveness. The organism can be recovered readily from erythema chronicum migrans skin lesions if cultured in the appropriate medium but it is rarely possible to recover it from inflamed joints of individuals with chronic Lyme arthritis or from cerebrospinal fluid of individuals with chronic neurologic manifestations. Because of this problem, it is often difficult to prove definitively the diagnosis of late Lyme disease, to define the endpoint of antibiotic therapy or even to know for certain when antibiotic therapy is indicated. Finally, the response to therapy is usually delayed by weeks to months and may be incomplete, raising the question whether incomplete responses may be due to failure to eradicate the infection or alternatively to persistent reactive, parainfectious inflammation.

The Typical Case

ES, a 53-year-old construction company owner, in an area known to be endemic for Lyme disease, noted gradually progressive fatigue. He had a past medical history of diabetes mellitus and hypertension. He was diagnosed as having depression and was placed on an antidepressant agent. Six months prior to evaluation, his right knee suddenly swelled without trauma or injury. He was hospitalized and treated with a brief course of intravenous antibiotics until pyogenic bacterial infection was excluded by gram stain and culture. Antibiotics were then discontinued, he was discharged from the hospital, and the episode resolved within 7 days. Two weeks later his left knee swelled. At this juncture, because of his own suspicion that he had Lyme disease, he sought consultation with a rheumatologist. His left knee examination revealed a large effusion and synovial thickening; his right knee examination was normal. A left knee aspirate revealed inflammatory joint fluid with 20,000 cells/mm^3 and a serum sample contained an elevated level of IgG antibody against *B. burgdorferi*.

A diagnosis of Lyme arthritis was made and he was treated with doxycycline 100 mg twice daily for 1 month. His arthritis resolved slowly but he was completely well within 2 months of completion of his antibiotic therapy. Three months later, he and his wife noted a change in his cognitive function, with the development of new impairment of short-term memory. His neurologic examination was normal, as was an MRI scan of the head. A spinal fluid sample contained an elevated level of antibody against *B. burgdorferi* (the concentration of specific antibody relative to total immunoglobulin in spinal fluid was higher than a similar ratio in serum) but was otherwise normal. Neuropsychologic testing revealed a deficit in short-term recall. A diagnosis of neurologic Lyme disease was made and a decision was made to treat him with intravenous ceftriaxone at home, but he experienced throat tightening and tongue swelling during the infusion of the first dose. He was, therefore, hospitalized and treated with a 2-week course of aqueous penicillin, 20 million units daily. In subsequent follow-up his cognitive function improved but he did not completely recover to his previous baseline.

Diagnostic Problems

The primary diagnostic challenge posed by cases such as the one described is the recognition of Lyme disease in an individual who has had no identifiable symptoms to herald disease onset. Instead, there may be gradually progressive energy depletion and lack of interest, which may be misinterpreted as symptoms typical of depression. Erythema chronicum migrans (ECM), if present in such cases at disease onset, can escape recognition even in retrospect. Sudden swelling of a knee is the most common presentation of Lyme arthritis and by far the most common later manifestation of Lyme disease in the US (see Fig. 30.3). But knee swelling is obviously not diagnostic of Lyme disease and may be initially mistakenly diagnosed as septic arthritis, a diagnosis that can be dismissed only after cultures are negative. Spontaneous resolution of bouts of joint inflammation is, again, typical of Lyme arthritis, which also distinguishes it from pyogenic bacterial infection. If swelling of the other knee develops then the diagnosis of Lyme arthritis becomes even more likely. In individuals whose time of disease onset is marked by ECM, arthritis typically appears anywhere from a few weeks to as long as years later. If serologic testing confirms the diagnosis of Lyme disease by demonstrating IgG antibodies against *B. burgdorferi*, an expected finding in patients with untreated Lyme disease of more than 6 weeks' duration, a course of antibiotics should be administered, based on the clinical diagnosis of Lyme arthritis.

Complaints of difficulty concentating are common in clinical practice and are often not accompanied by a demonstrable cognitive deficit. However, Lyme disease has been demonstrated occasionally to cause both a chronic organic encephalopathy and peripheral neuropathy, so the emergence of the complaints could reflect persistent central nervous system Lyme disease (Fig. 30.5). This syndrome is uncommon and deficits are usually subtle, making precise diagnosis difficult. It is essential that complaints be formally evaluated prior to initiation of additional antibiotic therapy because of the difficulty in

CHRONIC NEUROLOGIC MANIFESTATIONS OF LYME DISEASE	
Syndrome	Description
Encephalopathy	Memory loss, depression, sleep disturbance, irritability, difficulty concentrating, word-finding difficulty Documented by objective tests of cognitive function
Polyneuropathy	Spinal or radicular pain, distal paresthesias, sensory loss Weakness and hyporeflexia are less common Typically associated with electrodiagnostic abnormalities
Focal demyelinating disease	Focal weakness, bulbar dysfunction, ataxia, spasticity

Fig. 30.5 Chronic neurologic manifestations of Lyme disease. Diagnosis is based on the occurrence of neurologic manifestations in an individual with evidence of current immunoreactivity against *B. burgdorferi* and, generally, a history of previous clinical features of Lyme disease. Alternative explanations for symptoms must have been ruled out. Immunoreactivity in spinal fluid, if present, is confirmatory of diganosis.

defining therapeutic endpoints when treatment is being administered for relief of symptoms without an objective deficit or lesion. The evaluation should include a search for structural, neoplastic or inflammatory brain disease, and formal evaluation of cognitive function to determine whether the symptoms are due to an organic encephalopathy, an affective disorder, or both. The only positive findings in the case described were a selective deficit in short-term recall (which is not explainable by depression alone) and selective concentration of specific anti-*Borrelia burgdorferi* antibody in the cerebrospinal fluid relative to serum concentration, a finding which is suggestive of local synthesis of antibody against *B. burgdorferi* in the central nervous system.

Therapeutic Options

Doxycycline 100mg twice daily for 1 month has been found to cure Lyme arthritis in 70% of patients. The advantage of oral antibiotic therapy over intravenous therapy for Lyme arthritis is its ease of administration and low cost. Not all patients are cured with oral antibiotics, however. Those who fail to respond, do so because of persistent arthritis or the subsequent development of neurologic disease. It is likely that the patient described earlier had clinically occult central nervous system spread of his disease before his initial antibiotic course. Perhaps his initial fatigue was in part due to a subtle encephalopathy which went undiagnosed. This occurrence simply highlights the importance of careful neurologic evaluation prior to administration of oral antibiotics for Lyme arthritis. Once the diagnosis of neurologic Lyme disease is made by the demonstration of a specific cognitive deficit and immunoreactivity in cerebrospinal fluid, a 2-week course of high-dose penicillin is administered intravenously. Ceftriaxone is often preferred to penicillin which, because of the once-daily dosage schedule of this drug, lends itself well to home administration. Optimal duration of therapy is still under debate; experience has taught that 2–4 weeks is usually sufficient. The response to therapy is typically gradual and may be incomplete. This does not necessarily indicate, however, that infection is persisting in the central nervous system; it may simply be that whatever lesion was present prior to institution of antibiotics was not fully reversible. If therapy has eradicated the infection, repeat neuropsychologic testing should reveal gradual improvement or absence of progression and serial cerebrospinal fluid examination over time should show resolution of the hyperconcentration of specific anti-*Borrelia burgdorferi* antibody.

Conclusions

The diagnosis of late Lyme disease with either arthritis or neurologic manifestations can usually be made to a high degree of accuracy with the combination of careful clinical evaluation and appropriate use of serologic tests. Test results only have meaning, however, when interpreted in clinical context. Information on the optimal therapy for manifestations of late Lyme disease is still emerging; guidelines must be re-examined as new data become available. Most patients with Lyme arthritis are cured with either a 4-week course of oral antibiotics or a 2- to 4-week course of intravenous antibiotics. Neurologic Lyme disease typically responds to properly chosen antibiotic therapy given intravenously for 2–4 weeks. In most cases, incomplete responders do not show progression after initial therapy. These individuals may have fixed lesions, persistent inflammation due to mechanisms other than continued infection, or partially treated infection. Careful clinical follow-up and further study should provide the means to differentiate among these possibilities.

REFERENCES

Halperin JJ, Luft BJ, Anand AK, et al. Lyme neuroborreliosis: Central nervous system manifestations. Neurology. 1989;**39**:753–9.

Liu NY, Dinerman H, Levin RE, et al. Randomized trial of doxycycline versus amoxicilin/probenecid for the treatment of Lyme arthritis: Treatment of non-responders with iv penicillin or ceftriaxone. Arthritis Rheum. 1989;**32**(suppl):s46(abstract).

Rahn DW, Malawista SE. Lyme disease: recommendations for diagnosis and treatment. Ann Intern Med. 1991;**114**:472–81.

Steere AC, Berardi VP, Weeks KE, Logigian EL, Ackermann R. Evaluation of the intrathecal antibody response to *Borrelia burgdorferi* as a diagnostic test for Lyme neuroborreliosis. Infect Dis. 1990;**161**:1203–9.

Steere AC, Schoen RT, Taylor E. The clinical evolution of Lyme arthritis. Ann Intern Med. 1987;**107**:725–31.

ARTHRALGIA/MYALGIA: IS IT DUE TO HIV?

Ian F Rowe

Definition of the Problem

The role of infectious agents in triggering inflammatory joint disease has been the source of much recent interest; the predisposition of HIV-positive individuals to infection, often with opportunistic microorganisms, combined with the often profound direct effects of the virus on the host's immune system, may affect the incidence and nature of rheumatologic conditions occurring in this population.

A wide variety of musculoskeletal conditions have now been reported in individuals infected with the HIV. Of particular importance is the occurrence of inflammatory joint disease, usually in the form of an oligoarthropathy, sometimes with features of Reiter's syndrome or associated with psoriasis. Other conditions described include polymyositis, Sjögren's syndrome, vasculitis, septic arthritis, and a range of soft tissue problems and myalgias. Not only is the pattern of rheumatic manifestations in HIV-positive individuals becoming clearer; in some patients presenting with musculoskeletal symptoms, it may be necessary to consider the possibility of previously undiagnosed HIV infection.

Clinical Example

NJ, a 48-year-old bisexual man, was admitted with a 3-month history of progressive low back pain associated with morning stiffness. For the previous month he had developed a psoriasiform rash on his legs, arms, trunk and scalp (Fig. 30.6). Over 2 weeks he developed acute pain and swelling in the left metatarsophalangeal joints, progressing to the right ankle, left knee and left elbow. Although he had contracted gonorrhea several years previously there had been no recent history of diarrhea or of sexually acquired or other infection. There was no previous history to suggest HIV infection and he had not been HIV tested.

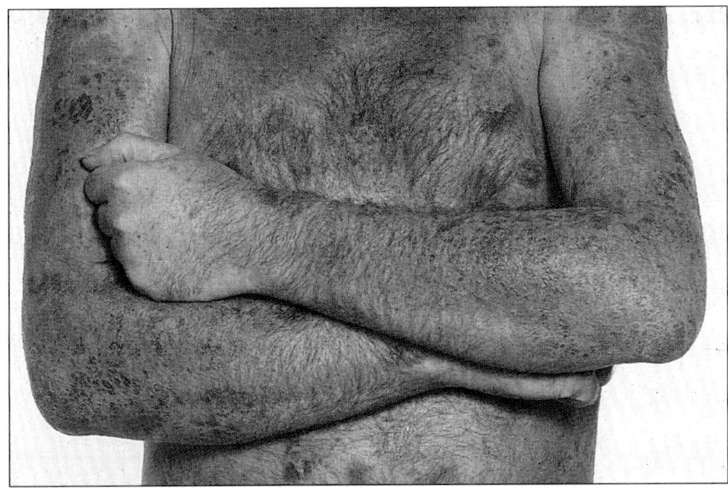

Fig. 30.6 Psoriasiform rash on the trunk and arms of a patient presenting with arthritis and myalgia, subsequently shown to be HIV-positive.

Examination confirmed acute arthritis in the affected joints as well as being highly suggestive of spondylitis. Investigations revealed hemoglobin 11.5g/dl, ESR 120mm/hour, CRP 115mg/l, white blood cell count 8×10^9/l (70% neutrophils, 17% lymphocytes, CD4 and CD8 lymphocyte subpopulations normal), HIV positivity, and HLA B27 positivity. Fluid aspirated from the left knee revealed white cells but no evidence of infection. Radiographs of spine, sacroiliac joints and peripheral joints were normal.

He was treated with bed rest, indomethacin and lavage with steroid injection into the left knee. He made considerable improvement and was eventually mobilized with physiotherapy support and discharged.

Diagnostic Problems

HIV positive or negative?

Rheumatologic conditions may present in individuals with HIV infection at any stage of illness, ranging from asymptomatic seropositivity to AIDS. However, symptoms may present in patients in whom HIV infection has not previously been diagnosed. If there is an appropriate history of risk factors, such as homosexuality or intravenous drug abuse, and features clinically suggestive of reactive arthritis or other conditions that are reported in HIV-positive patients, it may be necessary to counsel the patient and arrange for HIV testing. This may be especially important when considering therapeutic options.

Inflammatory joint disease or septic arthritis?

The occurrence in HIV-positive homosexual men of acute, peripheral, nonerosive oligoarthritis, generally affecting the lower limb joints, is now well recognized. Other features reported to develop concurrently with arthritis include keratoderma blennorrhagicum, plantar fasciitis, urethritis, conjunctivitis and anterior uveitis. This pattern of disease, associated with host HLA B27 positivity, and the demonstration in some patients of symptomatic bowel infection with *Yersinia*, *Campylobacter* or *Shigella* organisms in relation to the onset of rheumatic symptoms, suggests that they may be suffering from reactive arthritis. Other features, however, are atypical, such as the relative frequency of associated psoriasis and the apparent absence of chlamydial infection as a trigger in individuals from a sexually active population. In addition, many patients appear to suffer from more severe and persistent symptoms than is generally observed in reactive arthritis that is not associated with HIV.

Acute inflammation in joints occurring in individuals who may be severely immunosuppressed must always raise the possibility of septic arthritis. It is therefore necessary in many instances, especially if only one or two joints are affected without other features to suggest reactive or psoriatic arthritis, to obtain synovial fluid to exclude infection in the joint. This may be due to bacteria known to cause septic arthritis, such as staphylococci, or atypical microorganisms, such as *Histoplasma* or mycobacteria.

Joint, muscle or soft tissue pathology?

Much remains to be learned regarding the nature of rheumatic manifestation in HIV-positive individuals. An open mind must therefore be kept about symptoms in these patients, and attempts should not necessarily be made to classify conditions into pre-existing disease categories, although in the case described there was no doubt about the development of aseptic inflammatory joint disease associated with psoriasis. In addition to inflammatory joint disease, myositis has been reported in some individuals to be related to azidothymidine therapy and in others possibly as a direct consequence of viral infection. Others appear to present with severe myalgia of unknown cause. HIV-positive patients developing a form of Sjögren's syndrome, sometimes associated with diffuse lymphocyte infiltration and a variety of types of vasculitis, have also been described.

Are symptoms related to HIV infection?

Although the occurrence of aseptic oligoarthritis, with features suggestive of Reiter's syndrome and associated with HLA B27 positivity, is now well recognized in individuals with HIV infection, the necessary epidemiologic studies have not been performed to unequivocally establish that arthritis of this type occurs with increased frequency in this population. It is even less clear whether spondylitis or sacroiliitis, as suggested clinically in the case described, is associated with HIV infection. Although clearly rheumatic problems such as septic arthritis caused by opportunistic infection are almost certainly related to the underlying HIV infection, many conditions such as early degenerative change and soft tissue lesions (e.g. capsulitis) may be entirely coincidental to HIV infection.

Problems of handling biological material in HIV-positive individuals

In any person either infected with HIV or seriously suspected of having previously unconfirmed infection, extreme caution must be exercised with regard to handling of blood and tissue samples, including synovial fluid (which has been shown to contain the virus). Medical and paramedical staff must take care to ensure that no contact occurs with such specimens when they are being obtained, and wearing of appropriate clothing including gloves and goggles may be necessary. Similarly, clear marking of biologic material as potentially contaminated is important to alert laboratory staff to this possibility, as well as arranging for appropriate disposal of needles and other equipment.

Therapeutic Problems

Management of rheumatic lesions in HIV-positive patients may pose particular problems. Symptoms of inflammatory joint disease may be severe and, in many instances, may respond very poorly to NSAIDs. Although existing published data relate to very few cases, use of immunosuppressive drugs (given prior to the knowledge of HIV infection) may increase the risk of progression to AIDS. The possible therapeutic use of antirheumatic agents, such as sulfasalazine, or drugs acting against HIV, including azidothymidine, is not yet established. Moreover, use of some antirheumatic agents, in particular methotrexate, appears to accelerate AIDS progression and they are absolutely contraindicated in such patients. Appropriate analgesia and physiotherapy may be of great importance in many individuals. It appears that intraarticular steroid injection has not been associated with any significant adverse effect.

Treatment of any musculoskeletal pathology due to infection should ideally not be commenced at least until material has been sent for culture for a whole range of microorganisms, to ensure that appropriate antimicrobial agents may be administered.

Conclusions

Musculoskeletal symptoms are a source of considerable morbidity in patients with HIV infection and AIDS. In some circumstances they may indeed be a presenting feature. Of particular theoretical interest and practical significance may be the development of a generally asymmetric peripheral oligoarthropathy with features suggestive of reactive arthritis, Reiter's syndrome or psoriatic arthritis. Treatment may be difficult in view of the severity of symptoms, and the undesirability of administering immunosuppressive agents in these individuals. Consideration must always be given to infective causes of musculoskeletal symptoms, which may present atypically in these immunocompromised individuals. Extreme care must be exercised with regard to handling of potentially contaminated biologic material.

REFERENCES

Rowe IF, Forster SM, Seifert MH, et al. Rheumatological lesions in individuals with human immunodeficiency virus infection. Q J Med. 1989;**73**:1167–84.
Winchester R, Bernstein DH, Fischer HD, et al. The co-occurrence of Reiter's syndrome and acquired immunodeficiency. Ann Intern Med. 1987;**106**:19–26.
Winchester R, ed. AIDS and rheumatic disease. Rheum Dis Clin N Am. 1991;**17**(1).

VIRAL ARTHRITIS

Joachim R Kalden

Definition of the Problem

Viruses have long been implicated as a cause of acute self-limited forms of arthritis as well as in the pathogenesis of many autoimmune and chronic inflammatory joints diseases. The number of clearly defined viral arthritis syndromes, however, is limited.

The Typical Case

HC, a 26-year-old women presented with a 5-day history of fever, pain and stiffness of the hands, and a diffuse maculopapular rash confined to her trunk (Fig. 30.7). On careful history, it was learned that she had received a rubella vaccine (RA 27/3) 2 weeks prior to evaluation. On physical examination, no synovitis of the small joints of her hand or wrist was evident.

Diagnostic Problems

Among the recognized virus arthritis syndromes (Fig. 30.8), the arthridites associated with rubella virus, parvovirus, hepatitis virus, and recently the human immunodeficiency virus, are of most clinical interest.

Rubella Virus and Arthritis

Arthralgias and arthritis are reported to occur in up to 50% of infected women compared with up to 6% of adult men; they are uncommon in children. Rubella vaccine may cause joint symptoms in 15% or more of recipients. Joint symptoms usually start within 1 week of the skin rash in natural infection, or within 10–28 days after immunization. Fingers, wrist, elbow, knee, hip and toe joints are most frequently affected, usually asymmetrically. Sudden onset of symptoms is characteristic. Arthralgia and joint stiffness, as well as arthritis, may be accompanied by tenosynovitis and carpal tunnel syndrome. Usually, both the natural and the vaccine-induced arthritis resolve without residua within 30 days; however, some patients experience recurrent arthralgias and episodes of arthritis for up to 2 years, and sometimes longer. There are no specific laboratory findings, and reports of synovial fluid or synovial tissue analysis are limited.

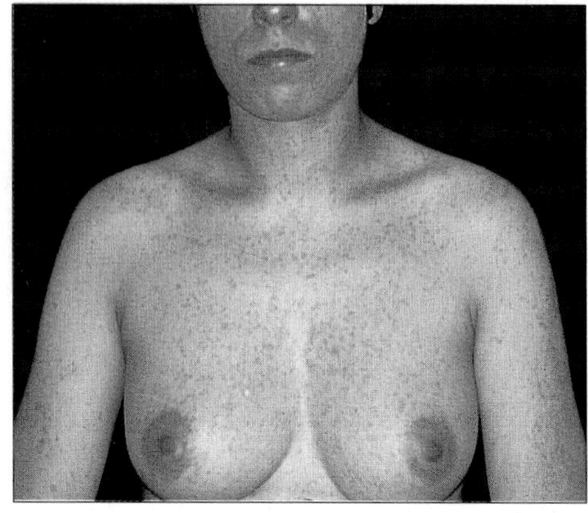

Fig. 30.7 The rash of rubella infection.

Parvoviruses and Arthritis

Parvoviruses are small, single-stranded DNA viruses; most of the interest in arthritis syndromes have focused on the human B19 parvovirus. In children, complications of infection can be severe with the development of chronic hemolytic anemia with aplastic crisis, hydrops fetalis, erythema infectiosum – the so-called fifth disease – and with rheumatoid-like polyarthritis in adults. Arthropathy occurs in up to 5% of children infected with the B19 virus, often with a characteristic skin rash which may produce a slapped cheek appearance

VIRUSES RELATED TO ARTHRITIS

Virus	Clinical features of associated arthritis
Togaviruses	
Rubella	15–30% of adult women affected, polyarticular (small and large joints), tendinitis common, self-limiting
Rubella vaccine	1–5% of children affected, polyarticular, recurrences possible, self-limiting
Hepadnaviruses	
Hepatitis B	Polyarticular (small joints), vasculitis with extra-articular manifestations, self-limiting
Arboviruses (alphaviruses)	
Ross river, sindbis	Polyarticular (small and large joints), epidemic in South East Asia, persistent for weeks to months
Ockelbo, Pogosta	Polyarticular (small and large joints), epidemic in Sweden, Finland
Chikungunya Mayaro, O'nyong-nyong	Polyarticular (small and large joints), epidemic in Africa, Asia, South America
Parvoviruses	
B19 RA-1	Polyarticular (small and large joints), erythema infectiosum (fifth disease), persistent for weeks to months
Enteroviruses	Probably involved in the postviral fatigue syndrome
Epstein–Barr	Transient arthritis of large joints. Postviral fatigue syndrome
Others	
Cytomegalovirus Varicella Zoster Herpes simplex	Mild, transient, arthralgia and arthritis, self-limiting
Paramyxoviruses	
Mumps	Oligoarthritis of large joints. Self-limiting
Retroviruses	
HTLV-1	Female preponderance, chronic oligoarthritis of large joints, extra-articular manifestations

Fig. 30.8 Viruses which have been related to arthritis. Of special interest are arthritides associated with rubella virus, parvoviruses and, more recently, retroviruses. In most cases of virus-related arthritis, joint inflammation is self-limiting and of short duration.

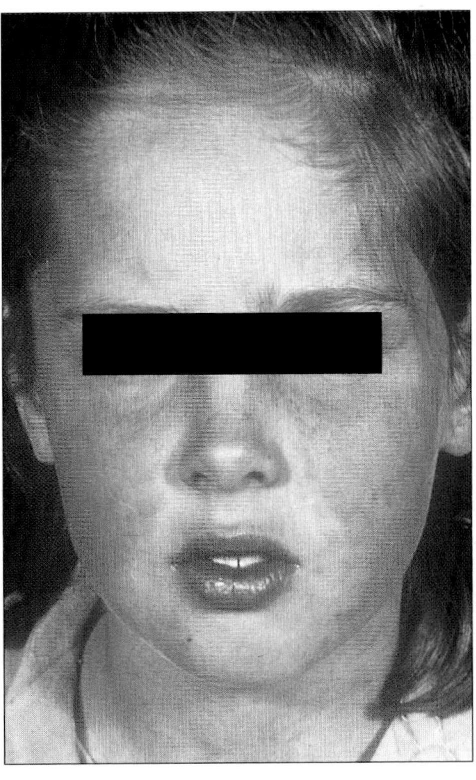

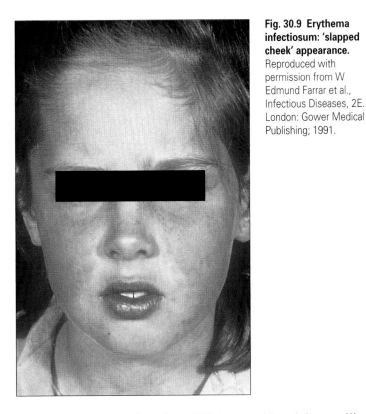

Fig. 30.9 Erythema infectiosum: 'slapped cheek' appearance. Reproduced with permission from W Edmund Farrar et al., Infectious Diseases, 2E. London: Gower Medical Publishing; 1991.

(Fig 30.9); however, less than 50% have evident joint swelling. Human parvovirus B19 can also cause an acute and occasionally persistent arthropathy in adults. The arthropathy is more common in women (60%) and is usually characterized by symmetrical polyarthropathy with pain, swelling and morning stiffness of affected joints. The finger joints, wrists and knees are occasionally painful. Acute costochondritis has been reported. Although the median duration of joint symptoms is about 10 days, pain and stiffness may persist for longer and may recur. Patients with acute parvovirus-induced arthritis exhibit significant levels of IgM and IgG antibodies to B19 parvovirus. Occasionally, the appearance of serum rheumatoid factor has been described.

Hepatitis B Virus and Arthritis

The hepatitis B virus (HBV) is for the most part transmitted sexually, but also partly parenterally and pre- or perinatally. Transient polyarthritis occurs during the prodromal stage of acute HBV infection in approximately one-third of patients and usually resolves with the onset of jaundice. Unlike rubella, vaccine-associated arthralgias or arthritis manifestations have been reported only rarely. Usually, small joints are affected symmetrically with arthralgias and/or arthritis. There is no predilection for either sex. Extrahepatic manifestations related to HBV infection, such as polyarthritis, glomerulonephritis, vasculodermatitis and vasculitic syndromes such as polyarteritis nodosa, mostly occur in patients with massive viremia. In patients with polyarteritis, significantly elevated serum titers of HBV, HBs-antigen (HBs-Ag) and HBe-antigen have been reported. Therefore, HBs-Ag-positive patients with arthritis or other extrahepatic disease manifestations must be considered as highly infectious at least until their serum HBV DNA is known.

Therapeutic Options

Virus-associated arthritis is usually self-limiting, and long-lasting clinical courses characterized by recurrent arthropathies have been reported only occasionally. In some cases of persisting arthritis it might be helpful to treat the underlying viral disease by drugs such as interferon-alpha, as in the case of HBV infection, or by antiviral drugs such as acyclovir as in rare cases of, for example, cytomegalovirus-associated arthritis. In most instances, the treatment of virus-associated arthritis is symptomatic: nonsteroidal anti-inflammatory drugs usually provide adequate relief.

The administration of immunoglobulin preparations has been reported to be successful in patients presenting with B19-parvovirus-induced pure red cell aplasia. The management of post-viral fatigue syndrome includes the application of drugs such as acyclovir and the use of non-steroidal anti-inflammatory drugs in cases of myalgia and arthralgia, as well as anti-anxiety and anti-depressive compounds.

REFERENCES

Nocton JJ, Miller LC, Tucker LB, Schaller JG. Human parvovirus B19-associated arthritis in children. J Pediatr. 1993;**32**:186–90.

Mitchell LA, Tingle AJ, Shukin R, Sangeorzan JA, McCune J, Braun DK. Chronic rubella vaccine-associated arthropathy. Arch Intern Med. 1993;**153**:2268–74.

Biasi D, De Sandre G, Bambara LM, Carletto A, Carmaschi P, Zanoni G, Tridente G. A new case of reactive arthritis after hepatitis B vaccination. Clin Exp Rheumatol. 1993;**11**:215.

Tai K-S, Whelan PI, Patel MS, Currie B. An outbreak of epidemic polyarthritis (Ross River virus disease) in the northern territories during the 1990–1991 west season. Med J Austral. 1993; **158**:522–5.

Kutzman G, Frickhofen N, Kimball J, Jenkins DW, Nienhuis AW, Young NS. Pure red-cell aplasia of 10 years' duration due to persistent parvovirus B19 infection and its cure with immunoglobulin therapy. N Engl J Med. 1989; **321**: 519–23.

GONOCOCCAL ARTHRITIS

John H Klippel

Definition of the Problem

Disseminated gonococcal infection (DGI) is the single most common type of bacterial arthritis. The clinical presentation is distinctive with fever, fleeting migratory polyarthritis and tenosynovitis and the development of diffuse vesiculopustular and hemorrhagic skin lesions. Immune complexes are thought to be involved in pathogenesis, although frank suppurative arthritis from *Neisseria gonorrhoeae* may occur in the late stages of the disease. Treatment with antibiotics is highly effective and residual joint damage from the infection very uncommon.

The Typical Case

A 22-year-old male student presented with a 7-day history of arthritis and fever. He had noted shaking chills with spiking fevers as high as 102°C. He described the arthritis as traveling from his finger joints, to his wrists and for the previous 2 days his right knee had been swollen and very painful. On physical examination, a large joint effusion was found in his right knee and red pustules were detected on his forearms and the dorsum of his left hand (Fig. 30.10). Aspiration of the knee yielded 35ml of yellow, cloudy fluid with a white blood cell count of 15,000/mm^3 with 90% polymorphonuclear cells on differential count; Gram stain of the fluid failed to show any organisms.

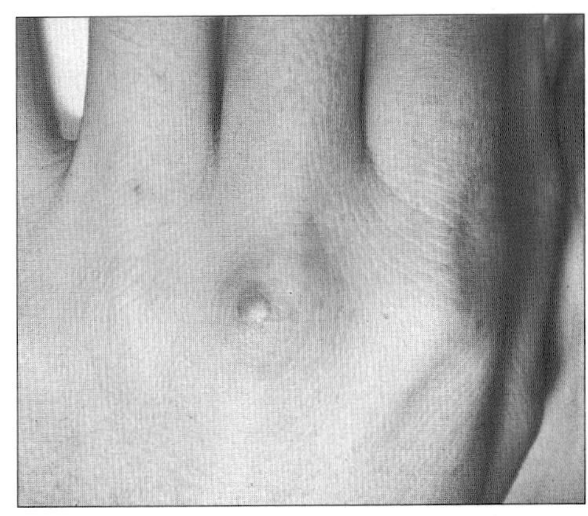

Fig. 30.10. Gonococcal skin lesion. A typical pustule on the back of the hand. Courtesy of Dr TF Sellers Jr.

Diagnostic Problems

The full clinical presentation of DGI with fever, arthritis and dermatitis in a sexually active person is generally promptly recognized. In females, infection often develops during menstruation or pregnancy; rare inherited deficiencies of late complement components are an added risk factor. Painful migratory tenosynovitis is a prominent feature early with the eventual development of mono- or oligoarthritis involving the small joints of the hands, wrists, elbows, knees or ankles. In the absence of antibiotic treatment, chronic osteomyelitis may develop. Skin lesions are found in about one-half of the patients, typically starting as an erythematous macule that progresses through stages of a pustular papule and eventual necrosis and ulceration. The lesions are diffusely located on the trunk and upper extremities; the lower extremities and oral mucosa are spared.

Patients seen early in the disease course with fever and polyarthralgias or tenosynovitis may be misdiagnosed with a viral syndrome, although the articular discomfort from DGI is major and patients are usually writhing in pain. A similar arthritis–dermatitis syndrome develops as a result of infection with *Neisseria meningitidis*. Patients typically present with a mild upper respiratory tract infection and may rapidly develop meningoencephalitis with shock. The finding of petechial lesions on mucosal surfaces, the trunk and lower extremities should suggest this diagnosis. In addition, the rheumatic manifestations of subacute bacterial endocarditis may mimic DGI.

Culture of *N. gonorrhoeae* is difficult since the organism is very sensitive to drying. Detection of the Gram-negative intracellular and extracellular diplococci on stains of synovial fluid, drainage from skin lesions or cervical swabs may help to confirm the diagnosis early. Cultures of all potential sites of infection, including synovial fluid, blood, cervix, urethral, rectal or pharyngeal swabs, and skin lesions should be taken at the bedside and immediately plated on chocolate agar or Thayer Martin medium. Blood and genitourinary cultures are often positive early on, but cultures from joints with tenosynovitis and skin lesions are generally negative. Recently, the polymerase chain reaction has been used to document the presence of organisms during this phase of the illness. The organism is easily cultured in instances of frank suppurative arthritis.

Therapeutic Options

Antibiotic treatment should be initiated promptly after appropriate cultures are obtained. Strains of penicillinase-producing *N. gonorrhoeae* are an increasing problem worldwide and current antibiotic recommendations are to begin treatment with intravenous ceftriaxone (Fig. 30.11). Daily needle aspirations of synovial fluid from the infected joint should be performed as long as it continues to accumulate; surgical fluid drainage is rarely, if ever, required.

RECOMMENDATIONS FOR THE TREATMENT OF DISSEMINATED GONOCOCCAL INFECTION

- Intravenous ceftriaxone, 1g daily for 7–10 days

or

- Intravenous ceftizoxime or cefotaxime 1g every 8 h for 2–3 days (or clinical improvement), then oral therapy with either cefixime 400mg twice daily or ciprofloxacin 500mg twice daily to complete 7–10 days of therapy

Fig. 30.11. Recommendations for the treatment of disseminated gonococcal infection.

REFERENCES

Hoosen AA, Mody GM, Goga IE, Kharsany AB, Van den Ende J. Prominence of penicillinase-producing strains of *Neisseria gonorrhoeae* in gonococcal arthritis – experience in Durban, South Africa. Br J Rheumatol. 1994;**33**;840-1.

Muralidhar B, Rumore PM, Steinman CR. Use of the polymerase chain reaction to study arthritis due to *Neisseria gonorrhoeae*. Arthritis Rheum. 1994;**37**:710-7.

O'Brien JP, Goldenberg DL, Rice PA. Disseminated gonococcal infection: a prospective analysis of 49 patients and a review of the pathophysiology and immune mechanisms. Medicine. 1983;**62**:395–406.

Center for Disease Control. 1989 sexually transmitted disease treatment guidelines. MMWR 1990;**38**:1–43.

Rompalo AM, Hook EW, Roberts PL, *et al*. The acute arthritis–dermatitis syndrome: the changing importance of *Neisseria gonorrhoeae* and *Neisseria meningitidis*. Arch Intern Med. 1987;**147**:281–3.

31

CLINICAL FEATURES OF SYSTEMIC LUPUS ERYTHEMATOSUS

Dafna D Gladman & Murray B Urowitz

Definition

- An inflammatory multisystem disease of unknown etiology with diverse clinical and laboratory manifestations and a variable course and prognosis.
- Immunologic aberrations give rise to excessive autoantibody production, some of which cause cytotoxic damage, while others participate in immune complex formation resulting in immune inflammation.

Clinical features

- Clinical manifestations may be constitutional or result from inflammation in various organ systems including skin and mucous membranes, joints, kidney, brain, serous membranes, lung, heart and occasionally gastrointestinal tract.
- Organ systems may be involved singly or in any combination.
- Involvement of vital organs, particularly the kidneys and central nervous system, accounts for significant morbidity and mortality.
- Morbidity and mortality result from tissue damage due to the disease process or its therapy.

HISTORY

The use of the term 'lupus', Latin for wolf, to describe various disfiguring cutaneous disorders dates to the medieval period. The first clinical description of rashes that continue to be recognized as lupus was by Biett, in 1833 [1]. Credit is generally given to Kaposi for describing the systemic nature of the disease, including fever, weight loss, lymphadenopathy and mental disturbances. Insights into the pathogenesis of systemic lupus erythematosus (SLE) were enhanced by the discovery of the LE cell phenomenon by Hargraves in 1948 [2] and the antinuclear factor by Friou [3]. Recognition of inflammatory and immunologic-mediated tissue injury of the disease has guided therapeutic approaches.

EPIDEMIOLOGY

SLE is recognized worldwide. Its prevalence in the US has been estimated to range between 15 and 50/100,000 population; elsewhere it has ranged from 12/100,000 in Britain, to 39/100,000 in Sweden.

SLE is more prevalent in women, particularly in their reproductive years. Ninety percent of patients in most studies of SLE are women. For the 14–64 age group, the ratios of age- and sex-specific incidence rates show a 6- to 10-fold female excess, which is not noted in patients below 14 or above 65 years. The effect of age and sex on the incidence and prevalence rates of SLE suggests a role for hormonal factors in its pathogenesis.

In the US it has been noted that SLE is three times more common among Blacks than Whites. Black patients with SLE have been shown to more often have Sm and RNP antibodies, discoid skin lesions, cellular casts and serositis [5]. These are not accounted for by age, gender or socioeconomic differences.

Genetic factors have long been considered to have a role in the etiopathogenesis of SLE. Support for this concept has come from the observation that there is a high prevalence of SLE among monozygotic twins [6]. Further evidence comes from family studies. It is estimated that 5–12% of relatives of patients with SLE develop SLE [7,8]. HLA studies have allowed for more detailed analysis of genetic epidemiology in SLE. The class II HLA antigens DR2 and DR3 occur more frequently among patients with SLE [9]. Several investigators have identified an association between SLE and the C4A null allele [10–12]. Genetic factors may also be important in select manifestations of the disease. For example, a recent study of with clinical evidence of lupus nephritis identified an increased frequency of DR2, DQw1, and especially DQβ1.AZH [13].

CLINICAL FEATURES

General

Constitutional complaints such as malaise, overwhelming fatigue, fever and weight loss are common presenting features of SLE. The presence of these features does not help the physician in the diagnosis of the disease, or in the identification of a flare, since they may just as likely represent the development of infection, or of fibromyalgia. Although some organ system involvements such as skin disease or arthritis are common in SLE, any system may be involved and present in variable combinations with other organ systems. Thus, SLE may have such diverse clinical presentations as rash and arthritis, or pleurisy and proteinuria, or Raynaud's phenomenon and seizures or pyrexia of unknown origin. It is only with a high index of suspicion, a careful history and physical examination, and obtaining appropriate laboratory confirmation that the diagnosis will become obvious. Figure 31.1 presents lupus manifestations at onset and at any time in the course of the disease in two of the largest reported SLE series in the English literature, the Toronto Clinic (602 patients) and the University of Southern California (USC) at Los Angeles Clinic (520 patients).

Skin Manifestations

The skin lesions seen in patients with lupus can be classified into those that are lupus-specific histologically, and those that are lupus-nonspecific [14,15]. The LE-specific lesions may be further divided into those that are acute, subacute cutaneous lupus, and chronic LE.

LE-Specific Lesions

Acute lesions

The most recognized skin manifestation of SLE is the 'butterfly' rash (Fig. 31.2), which usually presents acutely as an erythematous, elevated lesion, pruritic or painful, in a malar distribution, commonly precipitated by exposure to sunlight. The rash may last from days to weeks. Its presence facilitates the diagnosis of SLE and is commonly accompanied by other inflammatory manifestations of the disease. Pathologically, the lesions may show only nonspecific inflammation, although by immunofluorescence the classic immune deposits at the dermal–epidermal junction may be seen. The presence of immune

FREQUENCY OF LUPUS MANIFESTATIONS			
	At onset	Anytime	
Manifestations	(108)	(605)	(520)
Constitutional	73%	84%	86%
Arthritis	56%	63%	92%
Arthralgia	77%	85%	92%
Skin	57%	81%	72%
Mucous membranes	18%	54%	9%
Pleurisy	23%	37%	45%
Lung	9%	17%	–
Pericarditis	20%	29%	31%
Myocarditis	1%	4%	8%
Raynaud's phenomenon	33%	58%	18%
Thrombophlebitis	2%	8%	–
Vasculitis	10%	37%	21%
Renal	44%	77%	46%
Nephrotic syndrome	5%	11%	23%
Azotemia	3%	8%	–
CNS	24%	54%	26%
Cytoid bodies	5%	5%	10%
Gastrointestinal	22%	47%	49%
Pancreatitis	1%	4%	–
Lymphadenopathy	25%	32%	59%
Myositis	7%	5%	–

Fig. 31.1 Frequency of lupus manifestations. Frequency of lupus manifestations at onset based on 108 patients diagnosed at the University of Toronto Lupus Clinic and at anytime for 605 patients registered prior to December, 1990 and in 520 patients at the University of Southern California at Los Angeles.

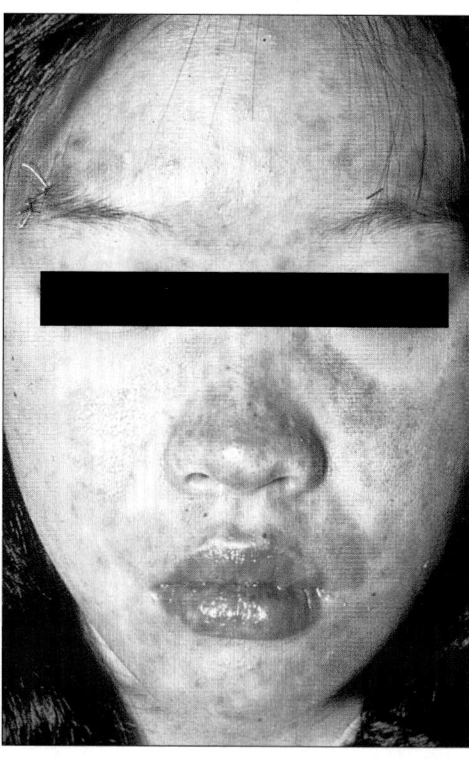

Fig. 31.2 Malar rash in a patient with SLE.

deposits in uninvolved skin in patients with SLE has been thought to be helpful in diagnosis, as well as of prognostic significance. Other acute lesions include generalized erythema, which may or may not be photosensitive, and bullous lesions. The latter lesions are uncommon cutaneous manifestations of SLE; their histology is characterized by acute inflammation, which may be immune-complex mediated, and which differentiates them from primary vesiculobullous disease [16].

Over 50% of patients with SLE demonstrate photosensitivity. In addition to the skin reaction, patients may develop exacerbations of their systemic disease. The mechanism for the photosensitivity is unknown, but it has been suggested that lymphocytes from patients with SLE are sensitive to 360–400nm light, related to a clastogenic factor in these cells [17]. The damaged chromatin may then provide a substrate for autoantibody production with the development of a local, or systemic, inflammatory response. Indeed, a recent study showed that UVB light increased the binding of antibody probes for Ro(SS-A) and La(SS-B) on keratinocytes in a dose-dependent manner [18].

Subacute cutaneous lupus erythematosus

Subacute cutaneous lupus erythematosus (SCLE) refers to a distinct cutaneous lesion which is nonfixed, nonscarring, exacerbating and remitting. This lesion is thus intermediate between the evanescent malar rash of active lupus, and the chronic lesions of the disease which usually cause scarring. SCLE lesions commonly occur in sun-exposed areas and may be generalized. The lesions originate as erythematous papules or small plaques with a slight scale and may evolve further into a plaque and scale, the papulosquamous variant, which mimics psoriasis or lichen planus, or merge and form polycyclic or annular lesions which may mimic erythema annular centrifugum (Fig. 31.3). SCLE may be accompanied by musculoskeletal complaints and serologic abnormalities, the most common of which is the antibody to Ro(SS-A), which has been demonstrated in the lesion. Many patients with ANA-negative lupus have demonstrated the annular lesions of SCLE. This subset of patients is also characterized by the increased frequency of HLA-DR3. The overall prognosis for

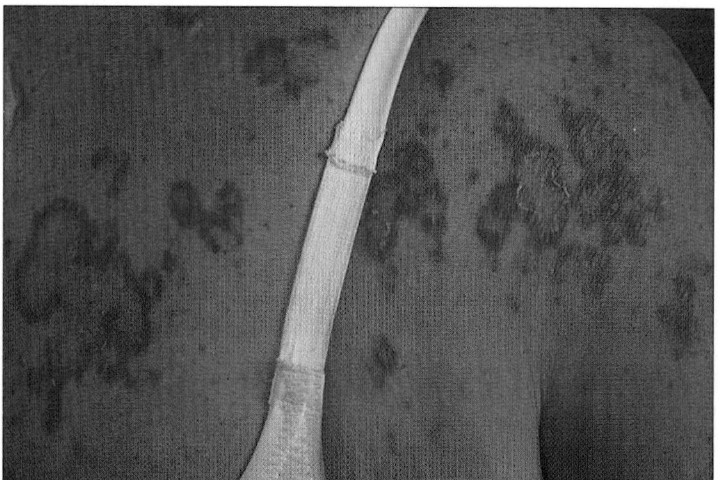

Fig. 31.3 Subacute cutaneous lupus lesions.

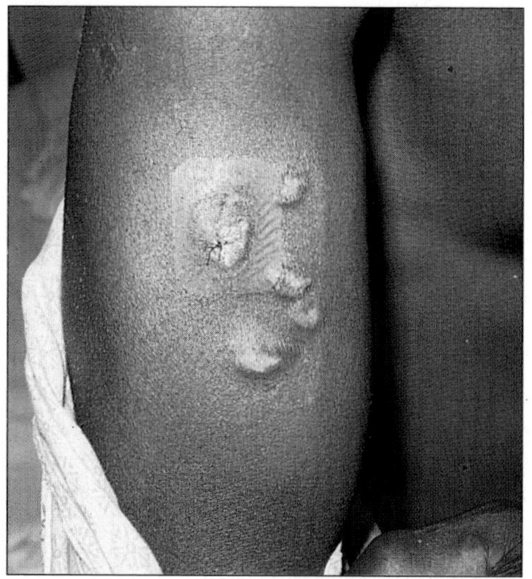

Fig. 31.4 Discoid lupus lesions.

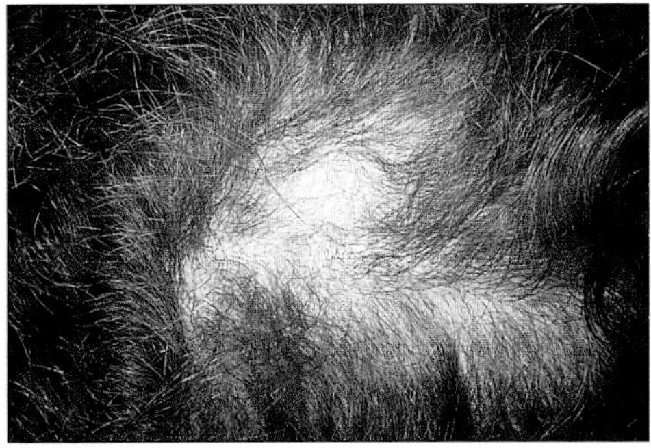

Fig. 31.5 Alopecia in a patient with SLE.

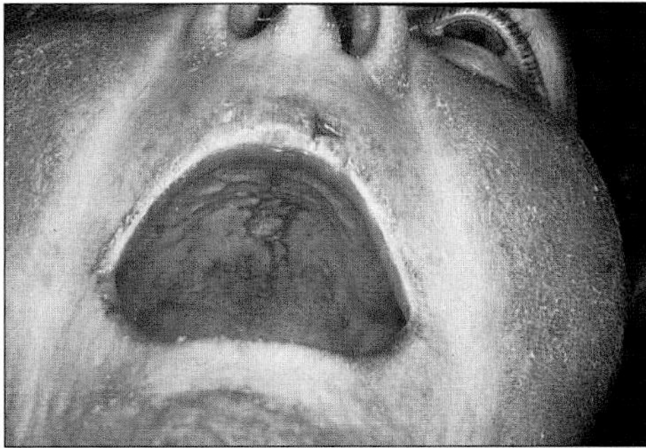

Fig. 31.6 Mouth ulcers in a patient with SLE.

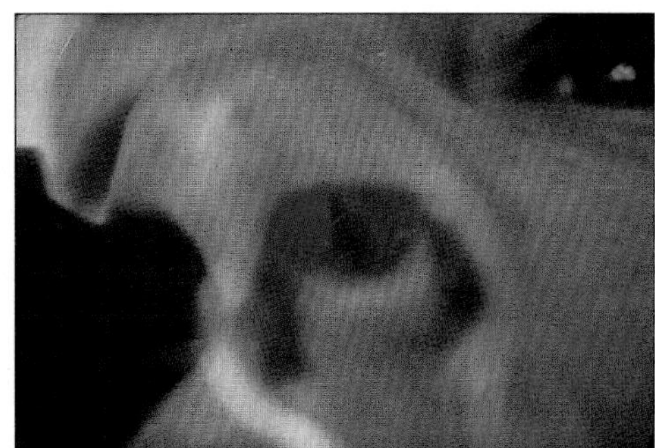

Fig. 31.7 Nasal septal perforation in a patient with SLE.

patients with SCLE is generally better than for patients with acute cutaneous lesions, although the skin lesions may be more refractory.

Chronic lupus

Discoid lesions are chronic cutaneous lesions which may occur in the absence of any systemic manifestations, as discoid lupus, or may be a manifestation of SLE. These lesions often begin as erythematous papules or plaques, with scaling which may become thick and adherent with a hypopigmented central area. As the lesion progresses follicular plugging occurs, with the development of scarring with central atrophy (Fig. 31.4). Discoid lesions may occur in the malar region, or in other sun-exposed areas. Lesions in the scalp lead to extensive and often permanent alopecia. Discoid lupus may be localized or generalized, the latter being more likely to be associated with systemic features and serologic abnormalities. Pathologically, the discoid lesion typically demonstrates hyperkeratosis, follicular plugging, edema and mononuclear cell infiltration at the dermal–epidermal junction.

LE-Nonspecific Lesions

Panniculitis is a rare cutaneous manifestation of SLE. The lesion presents as a deep, firm nodule, with or without a surface change. A biopsy may show perivascular infiltration of mononuclear cells and fat necrosis. There may be a skin lesion over the nodule which may demonstrate the perivascular infiltrate without fat necrosis, called lupus profundus.

Alopecia is a common feature of SLE. Hair loss may be diffuse or patchy. It may be associated with exacerbations of the disease, in which case it tends to regrow when the disease is under control. Alternatively, it may result from the extensive scarring of discoid lesions, in which case it may be permanent (Fig. 31.5). Alopecia may be drug-induced, for example by corticosteroids or cytotoxic drugs.

Mucous membrane lesions may result in ulcers of the mouth (Fig. 31.6) or vagina, or produce nasal septal erosions. The latter occasionally lead to nasal septal perforation (Fig. 31.7). Such lesions have been reported to result from vasculitis. Nail lesions (Fig. 31.8) are less well recognized, but may be associated with active lupus.

There are a number of dermatologic manifestations which occur in patients with SLE, but do not have the characteristic pathologic changes of cutaneous lupus. These include panniculitis, urticarial lesions, and vascular lesions. Urticarial lesions may occur in 5–10% of patients with SLE. These lesions are often chronic, and may represent vasculitis. Vasculitic lesions are among the LE-nonspecific lesions. They manifest as palpable purpura (Fig. 31.9), nail-fold or digital ulcerations, splinter hemorrhages, pulp-space and palmar vasculitic lesions simulating Osler's nodes and Janeway spots. Alternatively, these lesions may present as subcutaneous nodules. In addition, urticaria and livedo reticularis may represent a vasculitic process. Vasculitic lesions at the tip of a digit may result in gangrene (Fig. 31.10). Vasculitic skin lesions indicate active disease, and have been considered markers for systemic vasculitis in SLE. Other vascular lesions of lupus include periungual erythema or telangiectasia, and Raynaud's phenomenon. The latter may occur in more than 50% of patients. Unlike scleroderma, the Raynaud's phenomenon of lupus is not commonly associated with pulp-space pits or ulcerations.

Musculoskeletal Features

Arthritis

Arthralgias and/or arthritis constitute the most common presenting manifestation of SLE [19]. The acute arthritis may involve any joint but typically the small joints of the hands, wrists, and knees are involved. Most cases are symmetrical but a significant percentage may have an asymmetrical polyarthritis. Swelling is usually soft tissue with effusions tending to be minimal. The acute inflammation may be migratory in nature or persistent and become chronic. Nodules, formerly felt to be specific for rheumatoid arthritis (RA), are found in approximately 10% of patients with lupus. Synovial analysis reveals a mildly inflammatory fluid and if tested may reveal a positive ANA test and diminished complement levels.

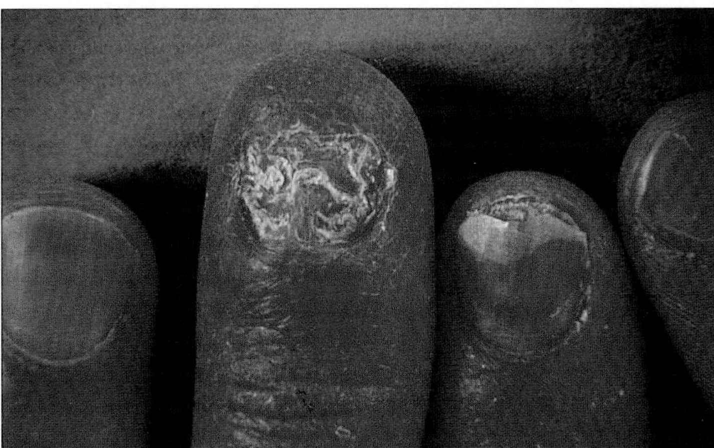

Fig. 31.8 Nail lesions demonstrating onycholysis in a patient with active SLE.

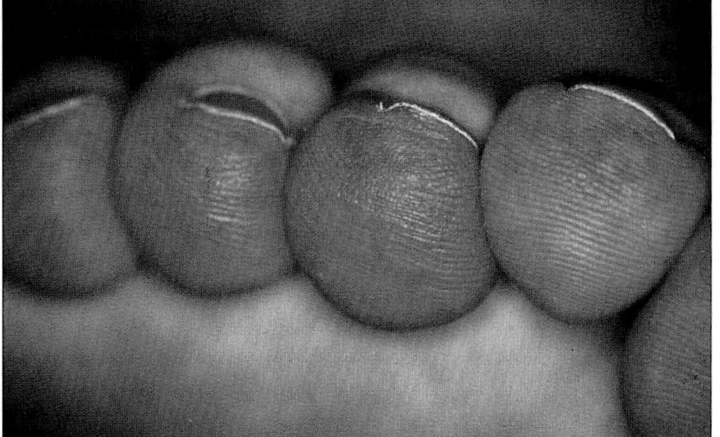

Fig. 31.9 Early vasculitic lesions over the tips of the toes in a patient with active SLE.

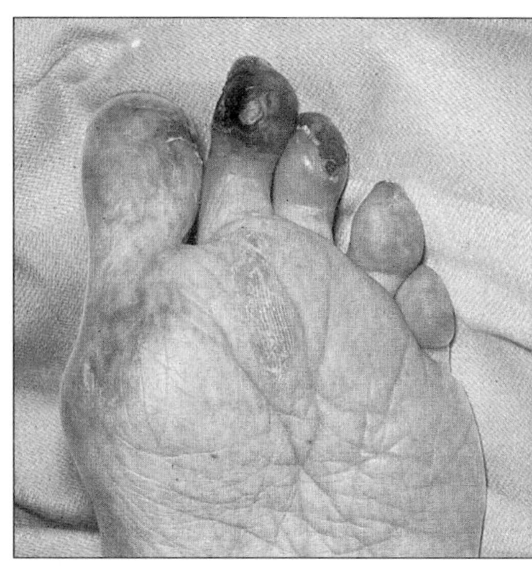

Fig. 31.10 Gangrene of the toe in a patient with SLE and vasculitis.

Unlike RA, the arthritis of systemic lupus is typically not erosive or destructive of bone. However, clinical deforming arthritis does occur and may take a number of different forms [20]. There may be mild synovial thickening about proximal interphalangeal joints or over tendon sheaths, ulnar deviation of the fingers and subluxations and contractures. When subluxations occur in the small joints of the hands, they are initially reversible (Figs 31.11 & 31.12) but can become fixed. This pattern of nonerosive but deforming disease has been called Jaccoud's arthritis [21]. Other authors have noted flexion contractures of the elbows [22], and deforming arthropathy of the feet [23]. Often patients who go on to develop deforming arthropathy have had continuous low-grade active arthritis, sometimes in the absence of other signs of SLE. Histologic examination of synovium in the acute stage reveals mild, usually perivascular inflammatory cell infiltrate, mild synovial cell proliferation and mild fibrinous deposition in synovial lining cells. In the more chronic stage, more synovial cell proliferation may be seen but not approaching the intensity seen in RA.

Radiographic findings in SLE arthritis are usually minimal but may be found in up to 50% of patients [20]. There may be periarticular or diffuse osteoporosis and soft tissue swelling, but unlike RA there are no erosions even when severe deformities from subluxations are present. Occasionally, one may see hook-like erosions of the metacarpal heads late in the disease, similar to the erosions described in postrheumatic fever Jaccoud's syndrome. These changes are more likely a result of bone trauma, due to misplaced tendon sheaths, rather than to erosions from a proliferative synovitis.

As tenosynovitis is an early manifestation of the synovitis of SLE, it is not surprising that tendon rupture syndromes have been reported in a number of different sites in the body, including the patellar tendons, the long head of the biceps, the triceps, and the extensor tendons of the hands. Patients who present with tendon ruptures may give a history of the sudden onset of pain, or disability in the joint or joints involved. Dramatic traumas are not often a part of the history; the rupture often occurs during the course of normal activity. In addition, patients have often been taking corticosteroids for long periods of time for their SLE. Histologic examination of the ruptured tendons has revealed inflammation in some instances but not invariably. Thus, one may incriminate either inflammation or corticosteroid-induced tendon degeneration as the mechanism for tendon damage.

Two complications of SLE or its treatment, septic arthritis and osteonecrosis, may confuse the diagnosis of acute synovitis in SLE. Although septic arthritis is not common in SLE, despite the immunosuppressed state, it should be suspected when one joint is inflamed out of proportion to all others. This state necessitates aspiration and culture of the synovial fluid.

Myositis

Patients with SLE may complain of muscle pain and weakness. The nature of the myalgia is not always clear. It may be secondary to joint inflammation, in which case the arthritis will be easily demonstrable on physical examination. Patients with SLE may develop a drug-related myopathy, secondary to corticosteroid use or as a complication of antimalarials. In addition, true muscle inflammation may be seen in patients with SLE, SLE being the second most frequent connective tissue disease to be associated with polymyositis. However, the histologic features of myositis in SLE may not be as striking as in idiopathic polymyositis [24].

Finol *et al.* [25] recently described the ultrastructural pathology in patients with SLE. Eleven of their 12 patients demonstrated myositis, with muscle atrophy, microtubular inclusions, and a mononuclear cell infiltrate, and in one patient with an elevated CPK, fiber necrosis. Vacuolar myopathy was found in one patient not treated with antimalarials.

Fibromyalgia

In the differential diagnosis of musculoskeletal complaints in patients with SLE one must consider the possibility of fibromyalgia [26]. Fibromyalgia may be distinguished from true arthritis or myositis by the presence of fibrositic tender points, and the absence of true inflammatory arthritis or evidence of muscle weakness. On the other hand, fibromyalgia may accompany true arthritis, and its presence needs to be taken into consideration when planning a treatment program for the patient.

Renal Disease

Specific symptoms referable to the kidney are not volunteered by the patient until there is advanced nephrotic syndrome or renal failure. The revised criteria for the classification of SLE recognizes proteinuria of more than 0.5g per 24 hours (or ⩾3+ if quantitative

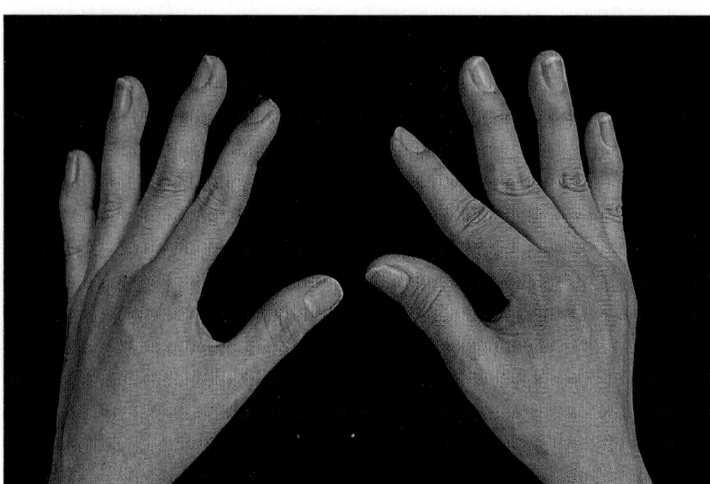

Fig. 31.11 Swan neck deformities in a patient with SLE.

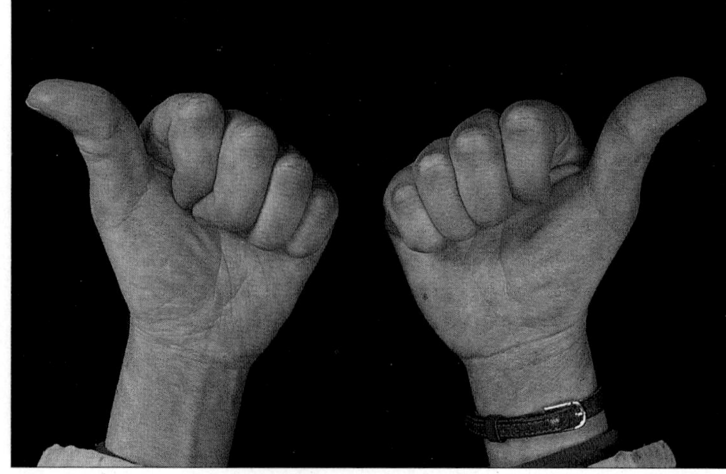

Fig. 31.12 Fists of the patient in Figure 2.13 showing the deformities reduced.

WHO CLASSIFICATION OF LUPUS NEPHRITIS IN 148 BIOPSIES	
I Normal glomeruli	12
a) Nil (by all techniques)	3
b) Normal by light but deposits on electron microscopy or immunofluorescence	9
II Pure mesangial alterations (mesangiopathy)	62
a) Mesangial widening and/or mild hypercellularity (+)	51
b) Moderate hypercellularity (++)	11
IIIA Focal segmental glomerulonephritis	19
a) 'Active' necrotizing lesions	14
b) 'Active' and sclerosing lesions	5
c) Sclerosing lesions	
IIIB Focal proliferative glomerulonephritis	3
a) 'Active' necrotizing lesions	1
b) 'Active' and sclerosing lesions	2
c) Sclerosing lesions	
IV Diffuse glomerulonephritis	37
a) Without segmental lesions	9
b) With 'active'necrotizing lesions	13
c) With 'active' and sclerosing lesions	14
d) With sclerosing lesions	1
V Diffuse membranous glomerulonephritis	11
a) Pure membranous glomerulonephritis	2
b) Associated with lesions of category II	7
c) Associated with lesions of category III	0
d) Associated with lesions of category IV	2
VI Advanced sclerosing glomerulonephritis	4

Fig. 31.13 WHO classification of lupus nephritis in 148 biopsies. Adapted from Gladman *et al.* [27].

evaluation is not done) or the presence of casts (including red blood cells (RBC), heme, granular, tubular, or mixed) as evidence of renal disease. In addition, the presence of hematuria (> 5 RBC/high power field), and/or pyuria (> 5 WBC/high power field), in the absence of infection, and the detection of an elevated serum creatinine, have been recognized as evidence for clinical renal disease. It is important to appreciate that in order to identify the presence of renal disease, a urinalysis, as well as a serum creatinine have to be performed regularly. A renal biopsy may provide a more accurate documentation of renal disease. Most lupus patients manifest some abnormality on renal biopsy, although in some cases it is only possible to document it with special techniques, such as immunofluorescence or electron microscopy.

The World Health Organization (WHO) has classified lupus nephritis according to the presence of changes on light, immunofluorescence and electron microscopy (Fig. 31.13). According to the WHO classification, patients with SLE may have normal biopsies (WHO class I), although this is rare. In a study of clinical–morphologic features in 148 patients with SLE, only three patients with truly normal biopsies were found [27] (Fig. 31.13). Mesangial alterations (WHO class II, Fig. 31.14) were most common, occurring in 62 biopsies (42.5%). These include mesangial widening or hypercellularity. Nineteen patients demonstrated focal segmental (class IIIA, Fig. 31.15), and three focal proliferative (class IIIB) glomerulonephritis, while 37 (25%) had diffuse proliferative glomerulonephritis (class IV, Fig. 31.16). In 11 patients, a predominantly membranous lesion was found (class V, Fig. 31.17), while four biopsies demonstrated advanced sclerosis (class VI, Fig. 31.18). Renal biopsies may demonstrate hematoxylin bodies, which are the tissue equivalent of

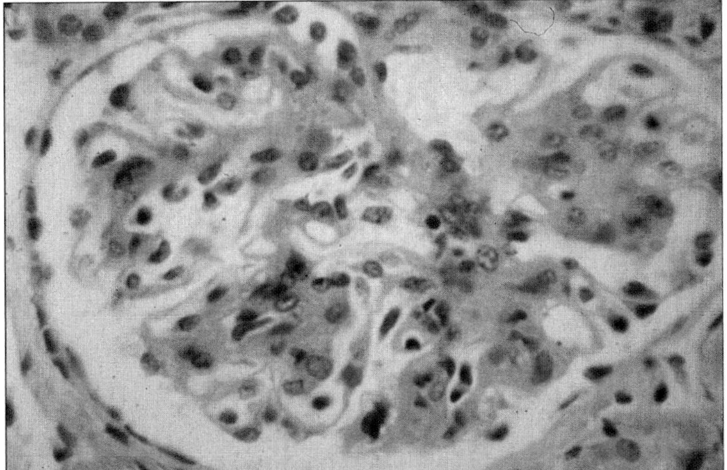

Fig. 31.14 Kidney biopsy specimen showing mesangial lesions.

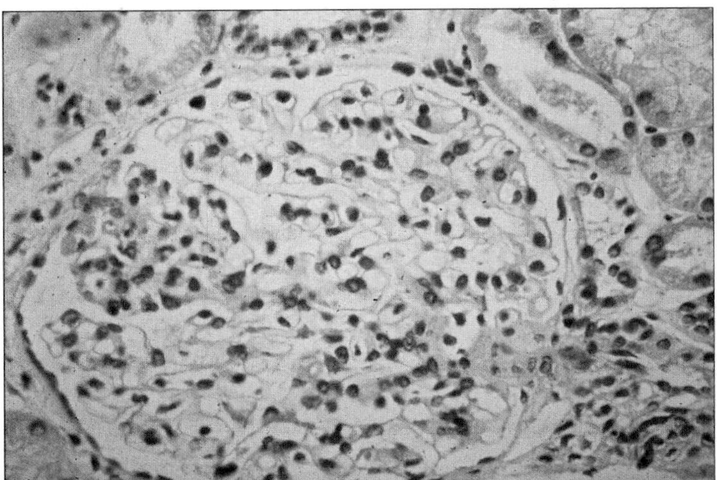

Fig. 31.15 Kidney biopsy showing focal proliferative glomerulonephritis (WHO class III).

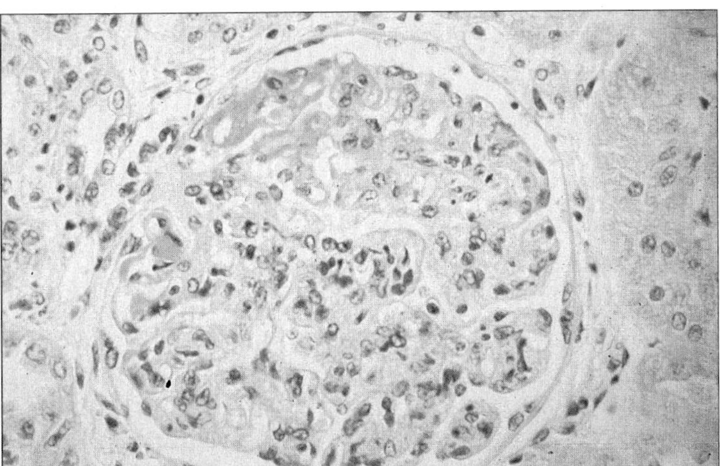

Fig. 31.16 Kidney biopsy showing diffuse proliferative glomerulonephritis (WHO class IV).

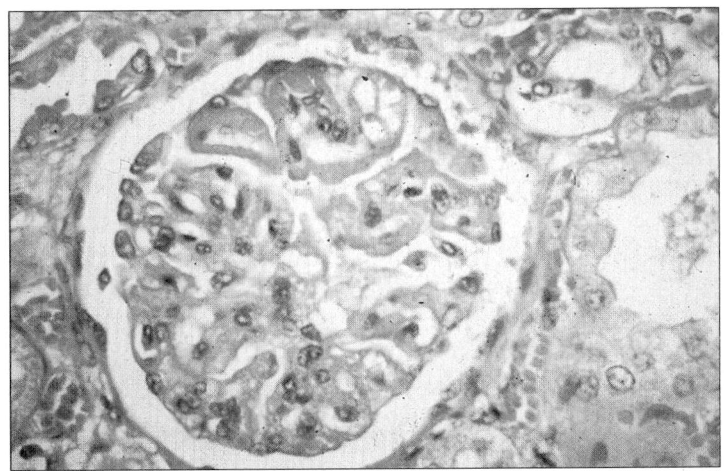

Fig. 31.17 Kidney biopsy showing membranous glomerulonephritis (WHO class V).

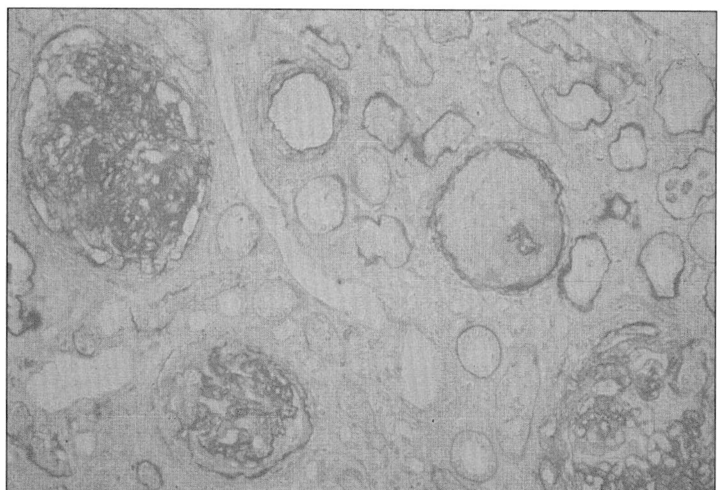

Fig. 31.18 Kidney biopsy showing advanced sclerosis (WHO class VI).

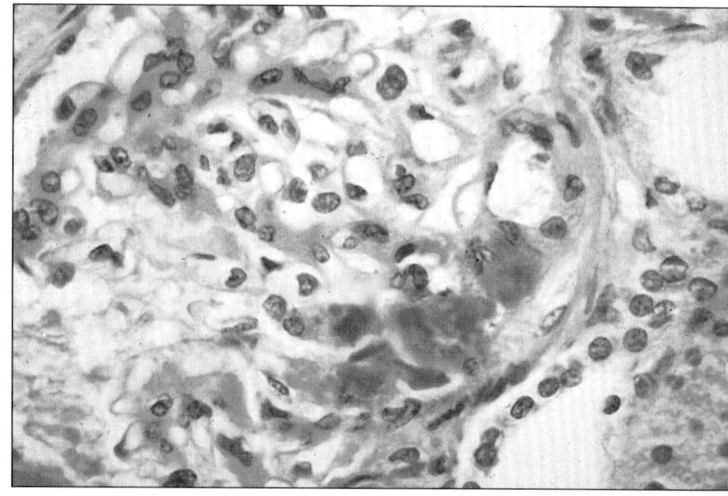

Fig. 31.19 Hematoxylin bodies in a glomerulus of a patient with lupus nephritis.

the LE cell phenomenon (Fig. 31.19). Most patients with mesangial lesions do not demonstrate clinical renal disease, as may be evidenced by the presence of an active sediment or elevated serum creatinine. However, patients with mesangial lesions may, on occasion, have prominent clinical evidence of renal involvement, and without a biopsy may be treated more aggressively than is perhaps indicated by the lesion itself [27]. Patients with class III and class IV disease tend to have evidence of clinical renal disease and impaired renal function; however, this is not universal. Other investigators have reported the finding of significant proliferative lesions on biopsy in the absence of clinical evidence of renal disease. Morel-Maroger *et al.* [28] have suggested that the various morphologic pictures may contribute to more appropriate choices of therapy. Further information may be derived from the renal biopsy with regards to the site of immune deposits, seen by either immunofluorescence (Figs 31.20 & 31.21), or by electron microscopy (Figs 31.22 & 31.23).

The role of kidney biopsy in the assessment of lupus nephritis has been controversial. Recent studies [29–32] have supported the concept that diffuse proliferative lupus nephritis is associated with poor prognosis, both in terms of renal function and in terms of patient survival. Other reports, however, have repudiated the usefulness of renal biopsy in predicting outcome, and claimed that the

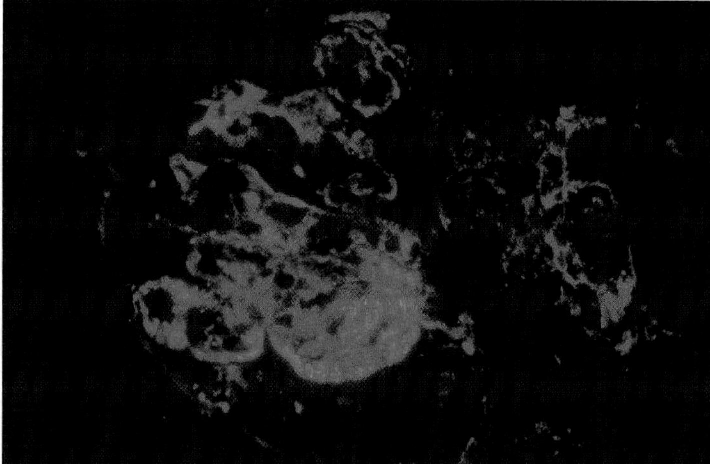

Fig. 31.20 Immunofluorescence showing IgG deposits in a mesangial distribution.

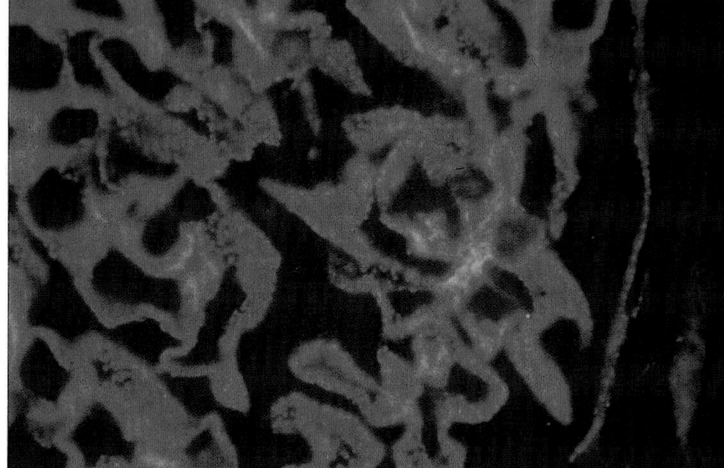

Fig. 31.21 Immunofluorescence showing C3 deposits in a capillary distribution.

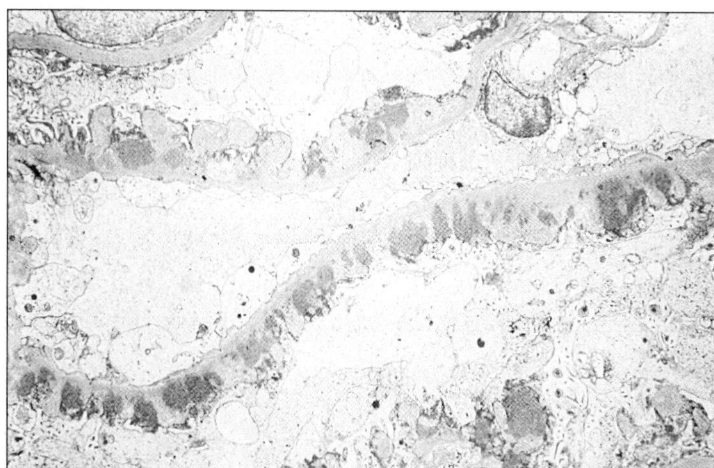

Fig. 31.22 Electron micrograph of a glomerulus showing intra-membranous immune deposits.

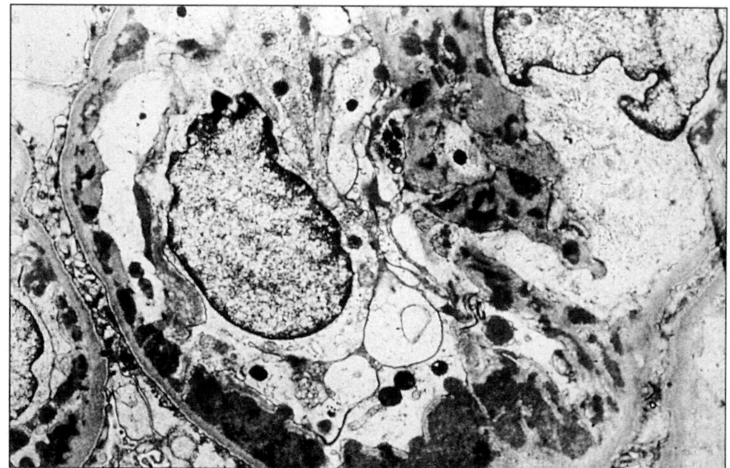

Fig. 31.23 Electron micrograph of a glomerulus showing subendothelial immune deposits.

ACTIVITY AND CHRONICITY INDICES FOR LUPUS NEPHRITIS		
	Activity	Chronicity
Glomerular lesions	1. Proliferation	1. Sclerotic glomeruli
	2. Necrosis/karyorrhexis	2. Fibrous crescents
	3. Hyaline thrombi	
	4. Cellular crescents	
	5. Leukocytic exudation	
Tubointerstitial lesions	1. Mononuclear cell infiltration	1. Tubular atrophy
		2. Interstitial fibrosis

Fig. 31.24 Activity and chronicity indices for lupus nephritis. Individual lesions are graded 0–3. Necrosis/karyorrhexis and cellular crescents are weighted by a factor of 2. Indices are composite scores of individual components, with activity index score ranging from 0–24, and chronicity index of 0–12.

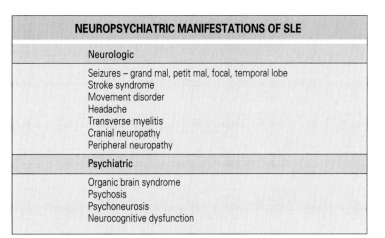

NEUROPSYCHIATRIC MANIFESTATIONS OF SLE
Neurologic
Seizures – grand mal, petit mal, focal, temporal lobe Stroke syndrome Movement disorder Headache Transverse myelitis Cranial neuropathy Peripheral neuropathy
Psychiatric
Organic brain syndrome Psychosis Psychoneurosis Neurocognitive dysfunction

Fig. 31.25 Neuropsychiatric manifestations of SLE.

renal morphology does not add to the clinical information obtained before biopsy [33]. Using a quantitative classification system (Fig. 31.24), it is clear that these morphologic features seen on kidney biopsies have both prognostic and therapeutic implications [34]. The presence of chronic lesions is clearly associated with lower survival, both for the patient and for the kidney. Moreover, the presence of active lesions would suggest that aggressive anti-inflammatory and/or immunosuppressive therapy should be considered.

Several studies have looked at the predictive value of clinical manifestations of renal disease using renal insufficiency as the outcome measure. Austin *et al.* [29] found increased risk of renal failure to be associated with younger age, male gender and an elevated serum creatinine level. This model was enhanced by including the renal chronicity index. Nossent *et al.* [32] further point out that a chronicity index greater than 3, especially in young patients, is the most important factor associated with decreased renal survival. Indeed, their findings suggest that renal function tests alone cannot distinguish between reversible and irreversible renal disease, as does a histologic evaluation. A recent study supports the importance of a renal biopsy, since it shows that for patients with evidence of diffuse proliferative glomerulonephritis with glomerular thrombosis, there may be improved prognosis through the use of ancrod [35].

Neuropsychiatric Manifestations

The diagnosis of neuropsychiatric involvement in SLE has been difficult. There are no widely accepted definitions for the clinical manifestations, and the relationship of neuropsychiatric features to the lupus disease process is not always clear [36]. There is a wide spectrum of clinical manifestations which may be grouped into neurologic, including the central nervous system (CNS), cranial and peripheral nerves, and psychiatric, including psychosis and severe depression. Many patients present with mixed neurologic and psychiatric manifestations [37]. Patients may have more than one manifestation at a time, a fact that makes their classification more difficult. Figure 31.25 lists the neuropsychiatric features reported to occur in SLE. These manifestations may be further divided on the basis of the presumed pathogenesis, into those that reflect diffuse involvement, such as seizures, organic brain syndrome or psychosis, and those that result from more focal disease, such as the neuropathies, cerebrovascular accidents, chorea, or transverse myelitis.

Neurologic features

Intractable headaches, unresponsive to narcotic analgesics, are the most common feature of neurologic disease in patients with lupus. The headaches may be migrainous in type, and may accompany other neuropsychiatric features. Seizure may be either focal or generalized. The occurrence of chorea in SLE has also been recognized [38]. Chorea occurs early in the course of the disease and resembles Sydenham's chorea. Its association with the anticardiolipin antibody has recently been suggested [39]. Cerebrovascular accidents, including paresis or subarachnoid hemorrhage, like chorea, have been related to the anticardiolipin syndrome as they may result from vessel occlusion, a feature of this syndrome. Cranial neuropathies may present with visual defects, blindness, papilledema, nystagmus or ptosis, tinnitus and vertigo, or facial palsy. By far the commonest are those related to the function of the eye. The retinopathy seen in patients with SLE is likely secondary to vasculitis [40]. The majority of patients have cotton-wool spots (cytoid bodies) (Fig. 31.26), hemorrhages, or areas of vasculitis (Fig. 31.27). Abnormalities of the optic nerve head manifested by papilledema or optic atrophy may also be seen.

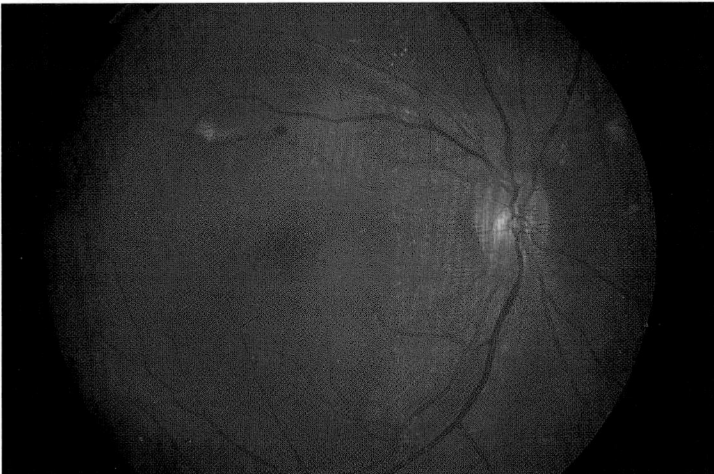

Fig. 31.26 Funduscopic examination in a patient with SLE demonstrating cytoid bodies.

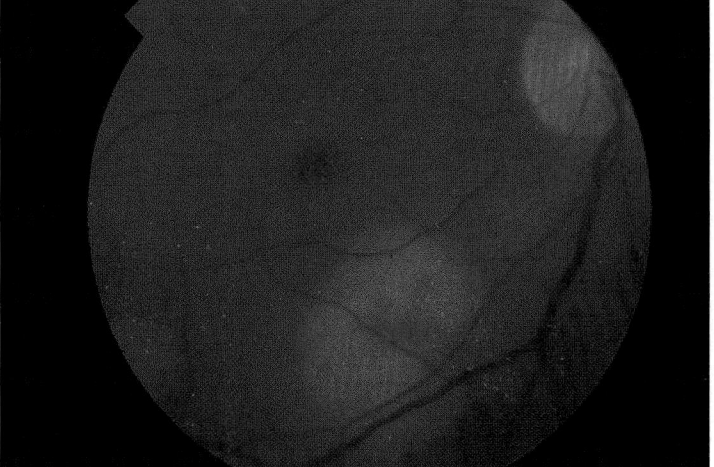

Fig. 31.27 Funduscopic examination in a patient with SLE demonstrating choroidal vasculitis.

Peripheral neuropathy is uncommon, but may include motor, sensory (stocking glove distribution), or mixed motor and sensory polyneuropathy or mononeuritis multiplex. An acute ascending motor paralysis indistinguishable from Guillain–Barré has been reported. Transverse myelitis, presenting with lower extremity paralysis, sensory deficits and loss of sphincter control, has rarely been reported in SLE patients [41].

Psychiatric features

Frank psychosis has long been recognized as a manifestation of SLE [42–45]. The use of steroids has been implicated in causing psychosis in some patients; however, stopping the drug in these patients and demonstrating that the psychosis gets worse confirms its relationship to the lupus process. Furthermore, the recently noted association between lupus psychosis and antiribosomal P protein antibodies supports the organic nature of this manifestation and its relationship to disease. Severe depression may also be part of the psychiatric manifestations of SLE and has resulted in a number of suicides. The presence of antiribosomal P proteins were found to be associated with severe depression in SLE, and may help distinguish true psychiatric features of SLE from drug-induced problems.

Organic brain syndrome in SLE is defined as a state of disturbed mental function with delirium, emotional inadequacy, impaired memory or concentration in the absence of drugs, infection or a metabolic cause. The prevalence of cognitive impairment in SLE is likely underestimated. Kremer attempted to systematically define the broader range of psychiatric symptoms in lupus patients using a combination of a standard psychiatric interview and several well validated measures, and reported a high prevalence of psychopathology [44]. There was a lack of correlation between the presence of nonorganic nonpsychotic psychopathology (NONPP) and underlying organic CNS disease or SLE disease activity. No correlation was found with NONPP and use of corticosteroids. In a similar study of neurocognitive function in SLE, it has been found that more than 80% of SLE patients with either active or inactive neuropsychiatric involvement, and 42% of patients who had never had neuropsychiatric manifestations, demonstrated significant cognitive impairment, as compared with 17% of patients with RA and 14% of the normal controls. However, a variety of cognitive deficits were present in patients with SLE, without a significant association with emotional disturbances [45].

Pathogenesis

The pathogenesis of CNS lupus is not well understood, but it is generally believed that more than one mechanism must be postulated to encompass the wide spectrum of clinical findings. The most common finding in autopsy series is the presence of multiple microinfarcts [46,47]. Noninflammatory thickening of small vessels by intimal proliferation is also seen, which may result from the reaction of antibodies with the phospholipids in the vascular endothelial cell membranes. Other pathologic findings include thrombotic occlusion of major vessels, which are the likely cause of some cerebrovascular accidents, while others may be related to the anticardiolipin antibody, intracerebral hemorrhage or embolism from mitral valve endocarditis. The pathologic findings do not always correlate with the clinical picture. A true vasculitis with inflammatory cell infiltrate and fibrinoid necrosis has rarely been demonstrated in brain pathology. However, it should be remembered that unlike skin and renal disease, where biopsies are readily available, most of the available pathology in the CNS comes from autopsy studies, and therefore vasculitis would be hard to demonstrate even if it existed. Support for vascular inflammation comes from studies showing enhanced cerebral blood flow during episodes of CNS activity [48,49]. Autoantibodies which cross-react with neuronal membrane antigens, and lymphocytotoxic antibodies have been found in both the serum and cerebrospinal fluid (CSF) of patients with SLE. These antibodies may be produced locally or pass through an immunologically damaged cerebral circulation or choroid plexus [50]. Changes in antineuronal antibodies frequently parallel concurrent changes in anti-DNA antibodies and overall disease activity, as well as cognitive dysfunction [51]. These antibodies may exert their effects by binding to molecules on neuronal membranes preventing signal responses or propagation. Potentially important target molecules on the cell surface include the very late activating (VLA) family of integrins and heat shock proteins [52]. An increased incidence of antineurofilament antibody has been found in SLE patients with 'diffuse' neuropsychiatric manifestations, and was frequently negative in 'focal' neuropsychiatric disease [53]. The association between antiribosomal P protein and psychiatric manifestations of SLE may have a similar mechanism [42,43].

Diagnosis

The diagnosis of neuropsychiatric lupus is primarily clinical. Exclusion of possible etiologies such as sepsis, uremia and severe hypertension is mandatory. Evidence of disease activity in other organs is helpful, but not always present. Nonspecific CSF abnormalities such as elevated cell count, elevated protein, or reduced glucose may be present in one third of the patients. Immune complexes have been detected in the CSF but have not been particularly helpful. Low levels of C4 and other complement components have also been detected in the CSF, but are difficult to measure in routine laboratories. Elevations of IgG, IgA and/or IgM indices have been described in patients with CNS lupus, and proposed as evidence of CNS disease activity [54]. Electroencephalogram (EEG) abnormalities are common in patients with neuropsychiatric lupus, but are nonspecific. The development of computerized quantitative EEG may be more sensitive to subtle electrophysiologic changes associated with lupus and requires evaluation. Evoked potentials have been proposed as a sensitive measure of CNS involvement in SLE [55]. Radionuclide scans (Fig. 31.28) have not uniformly been

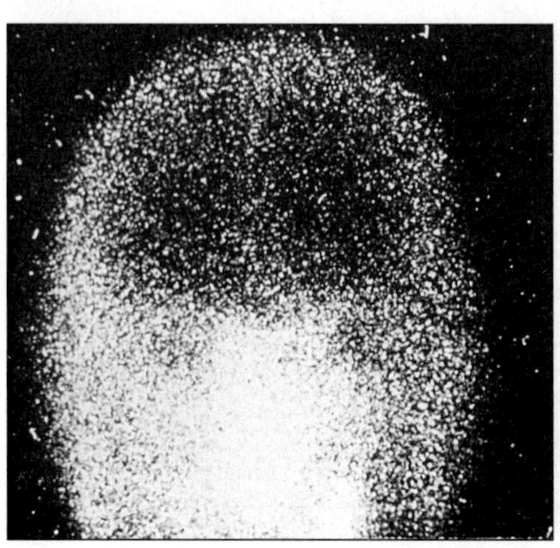

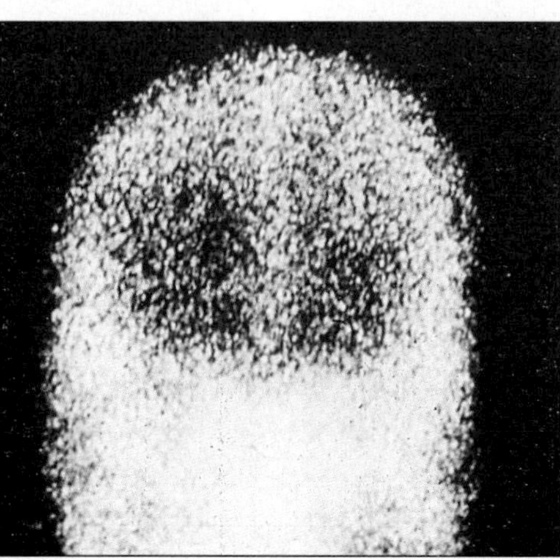

Fig. 31.28 Technetium brain scan demonstrating increased uptake in a 'draped curtain' pattern on the anterior view. A normal anterior view is shown on the left for comparison.

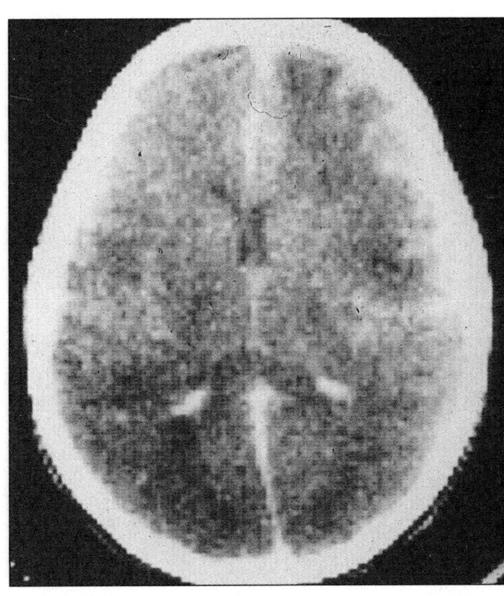

Fig. 31.29 CT scan of the brain demonstrating microinfarcts.

helpful. However, positron emission tomography (PET) showing areas of low attenuation which may represent areas of disturbed cerebral circulation and metabolism appear promising [56]. Computer tomography (CT) findings such as evidence of cerebral infarction (Fig. 31.29) and hemorrhage may reflect specific pathologic processes. Cortical atrophy (Fig. 31.30) may be found in SLE but does not necessarily reflect CNS disease [57].

Magnetic resonance imaging (MRI) appears to be superior to conventional CT, and particularly useful in the evaluation of patients with 'diffuse' presentations [58]. Some of the lesions seen on MRI, particularly the small focal areas of increased signal intensity in both the cerebral white matter and the cortical gray matter, tend to disappear after therapy with corticosteroids. These lesions may therefore represent either areas of local edema or inflammatory infiltrates which resolve with treatment. A more advanced technique, ^{31}P nuclear magnetic resonance (NMR) spectroscopy, may provide better demonstration of brain lesions in neuropsychiatric lupus [59].

Serositis

Serositis in SLE is common and may present as pleurisy, pericarditis, or peritonitis. Pleural manifestations have been variously reported in 30–60% of patients with SLE [60]. A clinical history of pleuritic pain is more common than radiographic change. Pleural rubs are found less frequently than either clinical pleurisy or radiographic abnormalities. However, autopsy findings of pleural involvement are more common than clinical diagnoses.

Pleural effusions may occur, are usually small, but can occasionally be massive. They are also frequently bilateral. Pleural effusions are seen more frequently in the aged and in drug-induced lupus. When pleural effusions are significant, other causes of effusion such as infection must be ruled out by thoracocentesis before initiating therapy. The fluid is usually an exudate and the glucose level is usually normal in contrast to RA where it is low. The white blood cell count is moderately elevated and the differential count commonly reveals polymorphs in the acute stage and lymphocytes in the later stages of the illness. LE cells have been described in the pleural fluid and immune complexes and reduced levels of complement are also found. Some investigators have suggested that a positive ANA in the pleural fluid is the most sensitive test for lupus pleuritis [61].

Pericarditis is the most common presentation of heart involvement in SLE but is less frequent than pleurisy as a feature of serositis. Clinical pericarditis has an incidence of 20–30% in most large series but may be found in over 60% of lupus patients at autopsy [62]. The clinical diagnosis is frequently difficult and depends on a constellation of clinical findings, including typical precordial chest pain and a pericardial rub. However, pericarditis may also be painless and clinically silent. On the other hand, posterior pericardial effusions may be found in patients on echocardiography who have no suspected history of pericarditis. Pericardial effusions (Fig. 31.31) are seen frequently as a feature of pericarditis in lupus, but cardiac tamponade is rare. However, this complication does occur and on rare occasions may be the presenting manifestation of SLE [63]. Pericardial fluid has been examined only in a small number of cases. Most samples demonstrated a leukocytosis with a high percentage of neutrophils. Glucose levels are significantly lower than the serum samples and several reports have documented reduced complement activity as well as elevated ANA levels and positive LE cells in the pericardial effusions.

Certain patients may be more predisposed to large pericardial effusions due to concomitant diseases such as uremia. In addition, infectious pericarditis in SLE has been reported both with bacteria and fungi [64,65]. Although early reports suggested some danger in performing pericardiocentesis in SLE because of the possibility of myocardial and coronary artery lacerations, this procedure should not be withheld in the presence of cardiac tamponade or in patients in whom superinfection is suspected. The use of fluoroscopy or echocardiographic guidance for the aspiration may decrease the risk. Constrictive pericarditis can occasionally develop in patients with pericardial involvement although this is very uncommon.

The gastrointestinal syndrome of acute SLE usually manifested by diffuse abdominal pain, anorexia, nausea and occasionally vomiting, has a number of possible etiologies including diffuse peritonitis, bowel vasculitis, pancreatitis, or inflammatory bowel disease. It is likely that in the majority of such cases, peritoneal inflammation is the cause of the symptoms. Ascites may be associated with peritonitis in about 11% of cases. However, at autopsy evidence of peritoneal inflammation may be found in up to 60% of cases [66]. When ascites presents in conjunction with abdominal pain and active lupus elsewhere, it generally follows the course and response to treatment of

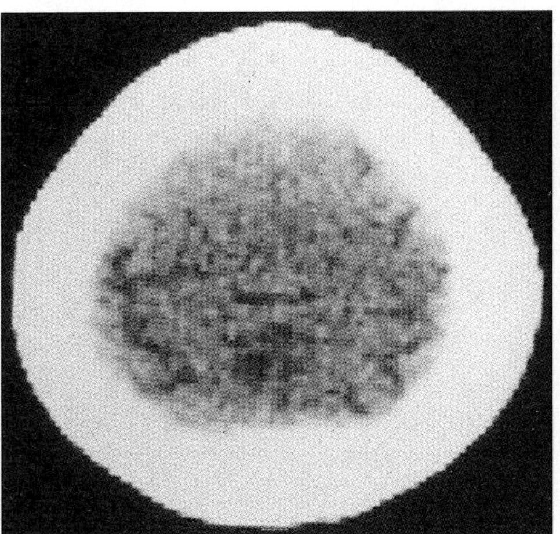

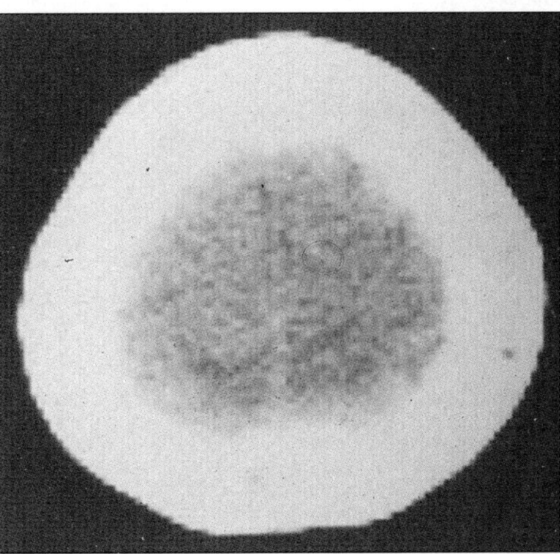

Fig. 31.30 CT scan of the brain demonstrating diffuse cerebral atrophy.

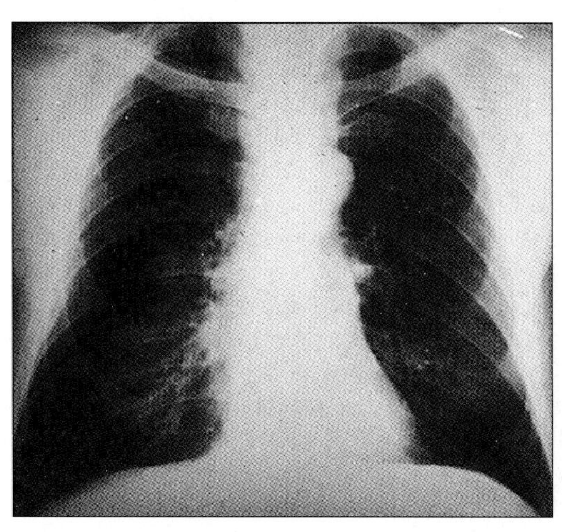
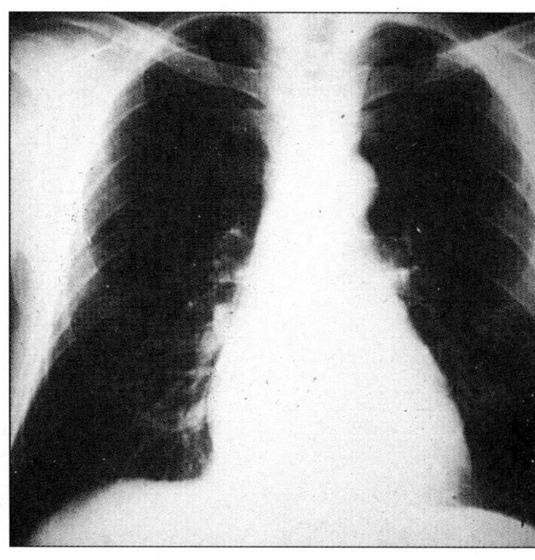

Fig. 31.31 Chest radiographs demonstrating the development of a pericardial effusion in a patient with SLE.

the other features of lupus. However, in a small number of patients ascites may become chronic. In those circumstances it may be painless and associated with only minimal or no other manifestations of active lupus. Autoantibodies such as antibodies to double-stranded DNA (dsDNA) may be found in ascitic fluid in these patients. The peritoneum may also be thickened with adhesions.

Acute lupus peritonitis must be differentiated from bowel infarction with perforation, acute pancreatitis, or bacterial peritonitis. Chronic lupus peritonitis must be differentiated from congestive heart failure, constrictive pericarditis, nephrotic syndrome, Budd–Chiari syndrome, intra-abdominal malignancy and intra-abdominal sepsis with a chronic infectious agent such as tuberculosis. When infection or malignancy is suspected, aspiration of ascitic fluid is required.

Pulmonary Involvement

Pulmonary involvement in SLE may consist of lupus pleuritis, lupus pneumonitis, pulmonary hemorrhage, pulmonary embolism, or pulmonary hypertension [67].

Pneumonitis

Lupus pneumonitis may present as both an acute and chronic illness. The acute illness simulates pneumonia and may present with classic symptoms of fever, dyspnea, cough and occasionally hemoptysis. The pulmonary infiltrates are usually associated with other signs of active SLE. The chronic form of lupus pneumonitis presents as a diffuse interstitial lung disease and is characterized by dyspnea on exertion, nonproductive cough and basilar rales. The pathophysiology of both of these forms of pulmonary involvement likely involve immune complex deposition in blood vessels and alveolar walls with or without associated vasculitis.

The acute pneumonitis syndrome must be differentiated from infection and when doubt persists, invasive investigation is indicated including bronchoalveolar lavage. In chronic lupus pneumonitis, the major clinical question revolves around whether the pulmonary fibrosis has an active component. There is a suggestion that gallium scanning of the lung may help differentiate active from inactive disease.

On occasions, the lupus pneumonitis may present as a lymphocytic interstitial pneumonia simulating a lymphangitic pulmonary malignancy. Usually this lesion is associated with active disease and will respond to the treatment of active lupus.

Pulmonary hemorrhage

Pulmonary hemorrhage presenting with cough and hemoptysis or as a pulmonary infiltrate is an uncommon but very serious feature of SLE [68,69]. It is presumed to be due to pulmonary vasculitis. Other causes of hemorrhagic pneumonia, such as some forms of viral pneumonia, must be considered in differential diagnoses.

Pulmonary hypertension

Lupus pulmonary involvement may also give rise to a syndrome of pulmonary hypertension which is similar to idiopathic pulmonary hypertension [70]. In this syndrome, patients present with dyspnea and a normal chest radiograph. They are found to be mildly hypoxic and to have a restrictive pattern on pulmonary function testing. Carbon dioxide diffusion capacity is reduced and Raynaud's phenomenon is frequently present. Doppler studies and cardiac catherization confirm pulmonary hypertension. Although patients are frequently treated with systemic vasodilators, the prognosis is generally grave. One must always rule out secondary pulmonary hypertension by searching for sites of deep venous thrombosis and for multiple pulmonary emboli. When there is any doubt, pulmonary angiography should be performed as a diagnosis of multiple pulmonary emboli might lead to potential life saving therapy. One must also rule out the antiphospholipid antibody syndrome with intrapulmonary clotting.

Cardiac Involvement

Cardiac involvement in SLE may consist of pericarditis, myocarditis, endocarditis, and coronary artery disease.

Myocarditis

Myocarditis may be suspected in patients who present with arrhythmias or conduction defects, unexplained cardiomegaly with or without congestive heart failure, or an unexplained tachycardia. Such patients usually have associated pericarditis and other features of active SLE. Peripheral myositis may be an associated feature. Congestive heart failure is a less common feature of SLE and is usually secondary to a combination of factors which may include myocarditis. However, associated hypertension and the use of corticosteroids are usually more important contributing factors.

The myocardial involvement may be more subtle in systemic lupus with abnormalities only being detected with a number of noninvasive investigations. Badui found 16 of 100 consecutive patients with SLE to have evidence of ischemic heart disease as judged by electrocardiography and/or echocardiography [71]. Hosenpud described abnormal thallium scans in 10 of 26 patients with SLE selected randomly [72]. These abnormalities included reversible defects suggesting ischemia, as well as persistent defects suggesting scarring. These findings may suggest either previous myocarditis or coronary artery disease. In patients with suspected myocarditis, endomyocardial biopsy may help confirm the diagnosis [73].

Endocarditis

The true incidence of endocarditis is very difficult to discern in lupus since the majority of murmurs heard clinically are not associated with any organic valvular disease on investigation or at postmortem. Nonbacterial verrucous vegetations described by Libman and Sacks are much less commonly found clinically at present than they were in the presteroid era. They are found, however, in 15–60% of patients at autopsy [62]. Vegetations may vary from mere valvular thickening detected by two-dimensional echocardiography, to very large lesions causing significant valvular dysfunction [74]. Valvular replacement has been required on occasion with significant mortality. Acute and subacute bacterial endocarditis may occur on previously involved valves. For this reason, prophylactic antibiotics for certain surgical procedures are advisable in patients with lupus endocarditis.

Coronary heart disease

Coronary artery disease in lupus is at the present time primarily a manifestation of generalized atherosclerosis which is discussed in greater detail in the section on late stage lupus. Coronary vasculitis on the other hand, is much less common in SLE [75], and when it occurs is usually associated with other features of active disease, in contradistinction to atherosclerotic coronary artery disease which is usually associated with inactive lupus. Coronary artery occlusion may also occur in association with a circulating anticoagulant.

Gastrointestinal Involvement

The gastrointestinal (GI) tract may be involved in many different ways in systemic lupus. Many patients complain of a nondescript dyspepsia and nausea associated with active disease without clear evidence of involvement of the GI tract. However, this may represent low-grade peritoneal inflammation, vascular disease of the bowel, or be related to medication. Gastrointestinal involvement may in addition present as esophageal disease, mesenteric vasculitis, inflammatory bowel disease, pancreatitis, and liver disease. Esophageal complaints, especially dysphagia, are uncommon in systemic lupus but may be associated with esophageal dysrhythmias seen in these patients who frequently also manifest Raynaud's phenomenon.

Mesenteric vasculitis

The presentation of greatest significance is that associated with mesenteric vasculitis [76]. Patients generally present with lower abdominal pain which may be insidious and may be intermittent over a period of weeks or months. Arteriography may reveal the presence of vasculitis. Bleeding per rectum may occur and both small bowel and colonic ulcerations may be seen on colonoscopy. Intestinal perforations from mesenteric vasculitis have been described. Although patients with mesenteric vasculitis often have evidence of vasculitis elsewhere, this is not always the case [77]. Thus, if mesenteric vasculitis is suspected, intensive investigation should be undertaken and treatment instituted to abort perforation. However, if perforation is suspected or does occur, surgical intervention is necessary.

Inflammatory bowel disease

Inflammatory bowel disease has been reported in SLE [78]. It may be difficult to distinguish the pathogenesis of this lesion between idiopathic inflammatory bowel disease and lupus enteritis. If due to SLE, other features of this illness are usually present.

Pancreatitis

Acute pancreatitis occurs in about 8% of patients with lupus. Presentation includes the typical symptoms of abdominal pain, nausea and vomiting and an elevated serum amylase. Although one may question whether the pancreatitis is due to lupus or corticosteroids, pancreatitis has been described in some patients not receiving corticosteroids [79].

Liver Disease

Although hepatomegaly occurs commonly in SLE, overt clinical liver disease is uncommon. The most common abnormality is elevated liver enzymes including SGOT, SGPT, LDH, and alkaline phosphatase. These abnormalities have been associated with active SLE and the administration of nonsteroidal anti-inflammatory medications, especially salicylates. So striking is this coincidence that if a young woman presents with a polyarthritis, is treated with aspirin and develops liver enzyme elevations, one should suspect SLE. Liver enzyme abnormalities return to normal when the lupus is under control and the anti-inflammatory medications are stopped.

Lupoid hepatitis is a subset of chronic active hepatitis, with an array of immunologic phenomena both serologically and clinically. However, in that condition the liver is the primary organ of involvement and this may result in liver damage and its consequences. An association between primary biliary cirrhosis and autoimmune disease has been suggested, and several patients with primary biliary cirrhosis who present with a multisystem disease consistent with SLE have been reported. Whether this is a chance coexistence of the two diseases or a direct relationship remains to be seen.

Reticuloendothelial System Involvement

Periarterial fibrosis, or 'onion-skin lesions' in the spleen, has been considered pathognomonic of SLE. It has been suggested that the saturation of the reticuloendothelial system contributes to the prolonged circulation of immune complexes and their subsequent tissue deposition [80]. Indeed, defective Fc receptor function in patients with SLE has been demonstrated and varies with disease activity. Splenic atrophy has been reported in patients with SLE [81] and the occurrence of splenic lymphoma has also been recognized [82].

Lymphadenopathy is a common nonspecific feature of SLE. The nodes are usually soft, nontender, and vary in size. In some patients, there may be fluctuation of the lymphadenopathy with disease exacerbations. Pathologically, the lymph nodes demonstrate reactive hyperplasia.

LABORATORY FEATURES

Hematologic Abnormalities

Cytopenias, including anemia, leukopenia or lymphopenia, and thrombocytopenia, are frequent manifestations of SLE and are included in the revised criteria for classification.

Anemia

Although anemia in SLE may have many different etiologies, including those secondary to chronic inflammatory disease, renal insufficiency, blood loss, or drugs, the most significant in acute SLE is the autoimmune hemolytic anemia due to autoantibodies directed against RBC antigens. Occasionally, the hemolytic anemia in lupus is Coombs' negative. Similarly, one may find a positive Coombs' test in the absence of any evidence of hemolyis.

Leukopenia/lymphopenia

Leukopenia generally ranges between 2500 and 4000/mm^3 and is often associated with active disease. One must always consider other causes for leukopenia such as drugs and infection. When the leukopenia is secondary to active lupus the bone marrow is usually normal. The white blood count rarely falls below 1500/mm^3 in active SLE unless there is an additional cause. In some instances, when the total white count does reach these levels, patients have been noted to have high spiking fevers requiring significant doses of corticosteroids to suppress the active disease. Lymphocytopenia is usually associated with antibodies to lymphocytes and is associated with active SLE.

Thrombocytopenia

As with anemia, other etiologies such as infection or drugs must be ruled out as a cause of thrombocytopenia in patients with lupus.

Although antiplatelet antibodies are a frequent finding in SLE, they are not always associated with thrombocytopenia. Two distinct subsets of patients with thrombocytopenia have been identified in SLE: a subset where the thrombocytopenia is one feature of a severely active patient with SLE and a second subset where the thrombocytopenia is an isolated finding. In the former, the thrombocytopenia tends to be refractory and follows the course of the acute lupus and its response to treatment. The latter subset of patients usually present with a platelet count of under 50,000/mm^3, without serious bleeding. In both groups, patients may present with mild petechiae or purpura.

Other findings

A variety of hemostatic abnormalities have been reported in lupus, the most common being the lupus anticoagulant. The most frequent laboratory accompaniments of this syndrome include a prolonged PTT, the presence of anticardiolipin antibody, and a false positive VDRL test for syphilis. The false positive VDRL test may precede the onset of the other symptoms of SLE by many years.

The ESR is frequently elevated during the course of active SLE, but it does not mirror the activity of the disease, and in lupus in remission may remain elevated for long periods of time. A positive CRP test, at one time purported to measure infection in lupus, has not been proven to be a constant indicator of a superimposed infection.

Serologic Abnormalities

Complement levels, measured as either total hemolytic complement or complement components C3 and C4, have been shown to be depressed in active SLE indicating consumption by immune complexes. Tests to directly measure the presence of immune complexes in the serum are less useful in routine clinical monitoring in systemic lupus.

Some of the antibodies seen in SLE are more specific for certain disease states and may therefore be useful in diagnosis. These include anti-Sm, which is seen primarily in systemic lupus, antihistone antibody, which is seen primarily in drug-induced lupus, and anti-Ro and La antibodies which are seen in Sjögren's syndrome as well as in systemic lupus. Antibodies to dsDNA are seen primarily in lupus.

Antibodies such as anti-DNA antibodies were initially felt to reflect disease activity in SLE and therefore to be monitors of therapy in this disease [83]. However, clinical experience indicates that DNA antibodies and depressed levels of serum complement are an imperfect predictor of clinical disease activity. Elevated levels do not appear to consistently correlate with any clinical feature except renal disease. In some patients, these abnormalities may persist for many years and on occasion return to normal without any intervening flare of disease.

Approximately 5% of patients with SLE do not demonstrate the classical antibody systems for SLE, namely antinuclear antibody and LE cells, and have been referred to as ANA-negative lupus. These patients have clinical evidence of SLE and tend to have more skin rash, photosensitivity, Raynaud's phenomenon and serositis. Some of these patients have subsequently been shown to have the anti-Ro(SS-A) antibody.

THE EVOLVING SPECTRUM OF SLE

Disease Patterns

The many different combinations of organ system involvement in SLE have long been known in medicine. Current concepts of pathogenesis implicate an immune complex inflammation in a variety of tissues, giving rise to clinical symptoms. However, patients may present with signs and symptoms loosely tied to SLE but with a different underlying pathogenesis and natural history, thus requiring different therapeutic approaches. One must be aware of these presentations so that not all patients will be painted with the same therapeutic brush. Some of these altered patterns include latent lupus, drug-induced lupus, antiphospholipid antibody syndrome, and late stage lupus (Fig. 31.32).

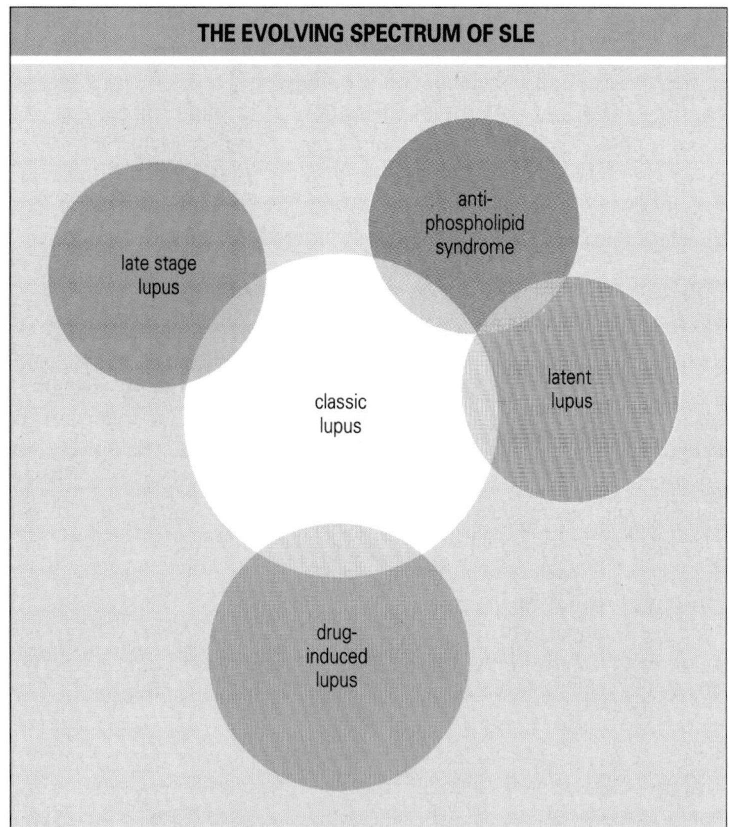

Fig. 31.32 The evolving spectrum of SLE.

Latent Lupus

Latent lupus describes a group of patients who present with a constellation of features suggestive of SLE but who do not qualify by 'criteria' or by a rheumatologist's intuition as having classic SLE [84,85]. These patients usually present with either one or two of the ACR classification criteria for SLE, and then a number of additional features suggestive of lupus. These criteria may include lymphadenopathy, fever, headache, nodules, Sjögren's syndrome, fatigue, neuropathy, less than two active joints, an elevation in PTT, hypergammaglobulinemia and an elevated ESR, depressed complement, positive rheumatoid factor, or aspirin-induced hepatotoxicity.

Many of these patients will persist with their constellation of signs and symptoms over many years without ever evolving into classic lupus. They generally do not respond well to therapy for lupus and are best followed with symptomatic treatment. A small number do evolve into classic lupus sometime after presentation. However, none of the presenting features of the illness are predictive for those patients who will eventually evolve into classic lupus. Patients with latent lupus tend to have a milder form of disease, not presenting with CNS involvement or renal disease.

Drug-Induced Lupus

Drug-induced lupus may be diagnosed in a patient in whom there is no prior history suggestive of SLE, in whom the clinical and serologic manifestations of lupus appear while on the drug, and in whom improvement in clinical symptoms occurs quickly on stopping the drug with a more gradual fall in the serologic abnormalities [86,87].

The drugs associated with drug-induced lupus can be classified into three categories: those where proof of the association is definite and appropriate controlled, prospective studies have been performed; those drugs that are only possibly associated; and finally, drugs where the association is still questionable. Examples of drugs in the first category include chlorpromazine, methyldopa, hydralazine, procainamide, and isoniazid. Examples of drugs in the second category include dilantin, penicillamine, and quinidine, and the third category is represented by a wide variety of drugs including gold salts, a number of antibiotics, and griseofulvin.

The clinical features of drug-related lupus are usually less severe than those of idiopathic SLE. The most commonly reported clinical features are constitutional symptoms, fever, arthritis and serositis. Central nervous system and renal involvement are distinctly uncommon. Laboratory tests reveal the presence of cytopenias, a positive LE prep, antinuclear antibody, and rheumatoid factor tests. Antibodies to ssDNA are commonly found but antibodies to dsDNA are not. Complement levels are generally not depressed. Antihistone antibodies occur in over 90% of cases. However, antihistone antibodies are not specific as they are also found in 20–30% of idiopathic SLE patients.

There is current interest in the association between acetylator phenotype and the predisposition to development of drug-induced lupus [88]. Patients receiving drugs which require acetylation by hepatic enzymes and who are slow acetylators develop antinuclear antibody sooner, and a symptom complex of drug-induced lupus more rapidly than patients who are fast acetylators. Thus, it is conceivable that at some time determination of acetylator status may help predict which patients may be susceptible to drug-induced lupus.

A number of possible pathogenic mechanisms for drug-induced lupus have been suggested including (i) molecular mimicry, which proposes that the drug or its metabolites may be cross-reactive with a nucleic acid, (ii) the drug or its metabolites may alter nucleic acid in such a way as to make it more immunogenic, (iii) the drug or its metabolites may have a direct effect on cells involved in immunoregulation, and (iv) the drug or its metabolites may interfere with the complement pathway [86]. There is not yet a universally accepted mechanism for the pathogenesis of this condition.

An interesting clinical question arises when patients with idiopathic SLE require drugs known to induce drug-induced lupus in other instances. The general practice is to use these drugs in such patients when they are necessary since generally they pose no increased problems in patients with idiopathic lupus.

Late Stage Lupus

Although short-term prognosis in lupus has improved dramatically over the past three decades, the mortality rates in patients surviving more than 5 years, and especially more than 10 years, have not shown similar dramatic improvement. Patients with disease duration of greater than 5 years tend to die of causes other than active SLE [89]. In such patients, mortality and morbidity are affected by long-term complications in SLE that result either from the previous SLE itself or as a consequence of its treatment (Fig. 31.33).

Atherosclerosis

Patients who have presented with atherosclerotic heart disease have usually demonstrated a significantly increased frequency of pericarditis, myocarditis, congestive heart failure and hypertension in their earlier active phase of systemic lupus. Furthermore, metabolic risk factors such as hyperlipidemia, hyperglycemia, and frank diabetes are more common among patients who develop atherosclerosis than in lupus patients in general. There has been no reported difference in the use of corticosteroids in patients with or without atherosclerosis although the average corticosteroid dose has generally been found to be higher. Vasculitis has not been shown to be increased in patients who later present with atherosclerosis, and cigarette smoking has also not been shown to be a clear predisposing factor.

LATE COMPLICATIONS OF SLE

Acute episodes	Chronic morbidity
Glomerulonephritis	End-stage renal disease, dialysis, transplantation
Vasculitis	Atherosclerosis, venous syndromes, pulmonary emboli
Arthritis	Osteonecrosis
Cerebritis	Neuropsychiatric dysfunction
Pneumonitis	Shrinking lung syndrome

Fig. 31.33 Late complications of SLE.

Thrombophlebitis/pulmonary emboli

Approximately 10% of patients with systemic lupus may demonstrate acute thrombophlebitis as a feature of their illness, either as a manifestation of lupus vasculitis or associated with a circulating anticoagulant [90]. In the former instance there will usually be other signs of active systemic lupus. However, either early or late in the course of the lupus patients may present with a bland phlebothrombosis with or without pulmonary emboli (Fig. 31.34). In some patients, multiple pulmonary emboli may be the first indication that there is a venous problem. In such instances, one may presume that previous venous inflammation gave rise to secondary thrombosis followed by multiple pulmonary emboli.

Osteonecrosis

Acute joint pain presenting in the later stages of systemic lupus, especially localized to a very few areas, most commonly the hips, may indicate the development of osteonecrosis. In most large series now, osteonecrosis is recognized as an important cause of disability in late lupus, occurring in about 10% of patients followed over a long period of time [91]. Patients with osteonecrosis are generally in the younger age group and have an interval between diagnosis of lupus and osteonecrosis of about 4 years. The hip is the most commonly involved joint, although most joints in the body have been reported to have been affected. One-half to two-thirds of patients with osteonecrosis will have multiple sites and typically will have been on high-dose corticosteroids at some time during the course of their illness.

There is no general agreement as to the predictive role of any specific manifestation of SLE, such as Raynaud's phenomenon or vasculitis in the subsequent development of osteonecrosis, and there is currently no general consensus on pathogenesis.

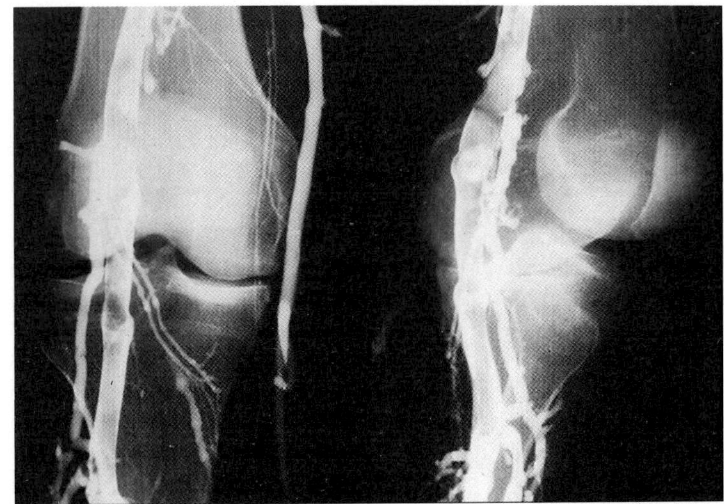

Fig. 31.34 A venogram showing venous thrombosis in a patient with SLE.

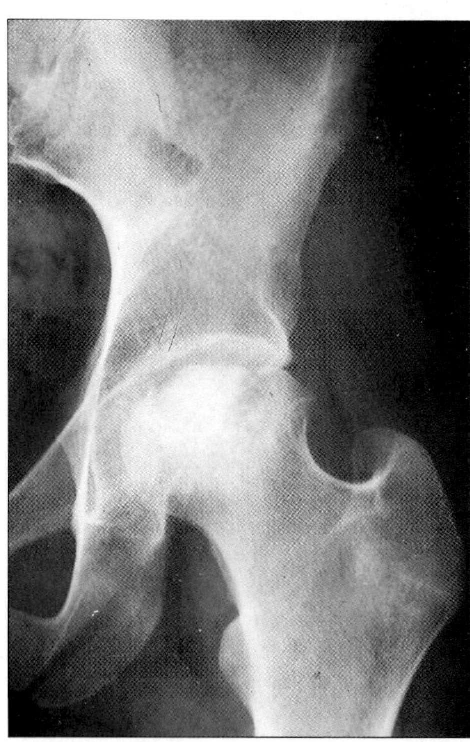
Fig. 31.35 A radiograph demonstrating advanced osteonecrosis of the hip.

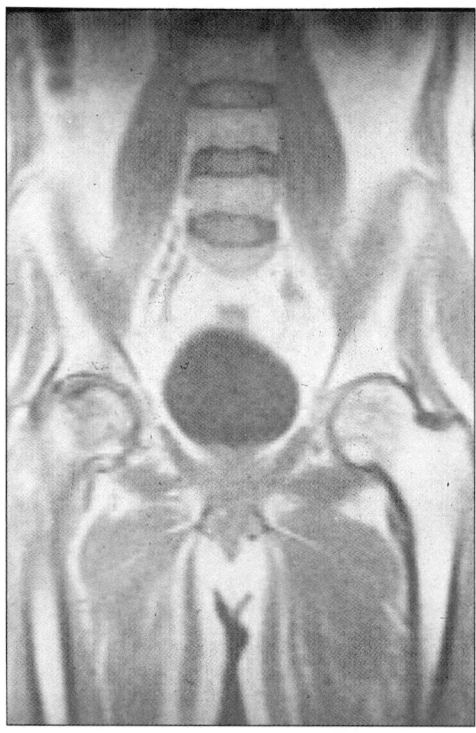
Fig. 31.36 Magnetic resonance imaging showing advanced changes of osteonecrosis of the right hip and early changes on the left.

Diagnosis of osteonecrosis in patients presenting with focal pain can be difficult. Changes in the routine radiographs (Fig. 31.35) are late findings. Earlier diagnosis can be made using radionuclide bone scans or MRI to demonstrate bone abnormality (Fig. 31.36). Although many patients with osteonecrosis have a poor outcome with respect to pain and disability, leading to joint replacement, some patients do respond to decreased weight-bearing and time. These patients may be left with some joint irregularity but adequate joint space, but do not require surgery. The size and exact location of the avascular area may determine the future necessity for joint replacement. Core decompression with or without bone grafting has not yet been demonstrated to be useful therapy [92–94].

Neurologic disorders

Assessments of cognitive function changes in SLE patients have demonstrated definite deterioration in mental function. In the acute illness, both active systemic lupus and corticosteroids have been implicated as causative factors in organic brain dysfunction, as discussed previously. However, in late stage lupus, when there is no longer any evidence of active disease and the patient is taking little or no corticosteroids, neurocognitive disabilities remain a frequent complaint. Patients often complain of decreased memory, decreased ability to do mathematical chores and increased speech disabilities. When such patients are submitted to a battery of neurocognitive tests, they are in fact shown to have significant impairment [45].

In addition, patients with systemic lupus undergoing neurologic investigation have been shown to demonstrate significant cortical atrophy on CT scanning. This has been shown both in patients who have had previous CNS disease due to lupus and in those who have not, as well as in those who have current neurocognitive symptoms and in those who do not. Thus, the exact pathogenesis of the neurocognitive disabilities that occur in latent lupus are not clear at this point. They may be a feature of SLE in general, CNS disease of SLE in particular, or related to the corticosteroids used to treat SLE, or a combination of these factors.

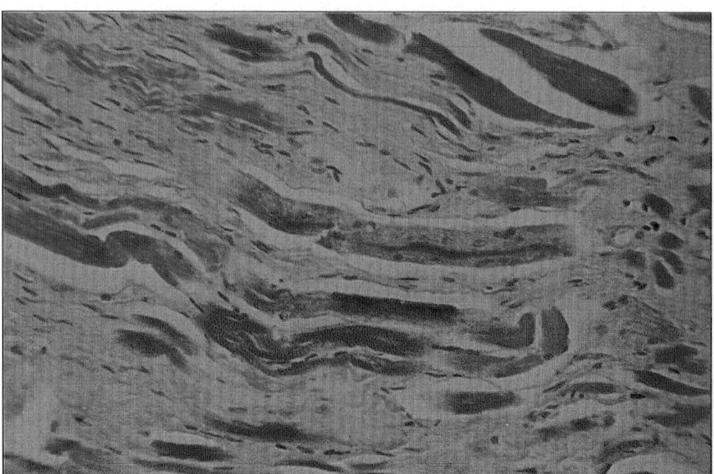
Fig. 31.37 Micrograph of the diaphragm in a patient with a shrinking lung syndrome demonstrating fibrosis.

Shrinking lung syndrome

Patients may present in the late stages of lupus with the symptom of increasing dyspnea in the face of a normal chest examination. Chest radiographs may reveal elevated diaphragms but normal lung fields. Pulmonary function tests will usually reveal small lung volumes and a restrictive pattern. This syndrome, usually referred to as shrinking lung syndrome, is a result of altered respiratory mechanics either on the basis of impaired respiratory muscle or diaphragmatic function, or problems in the respiratory skeletal apparatus. Some studies have demonstrated specific intercostal muscle weakness or diaphragmatic weakness [95]. One postmortem study revealed the diaphragm in a patient with shrinking lung syndrome in late lupus to be fibrotic and thinned [96] (Fig. 31.37). When shrinking lung syndrome occurs in the face of late stage lupus without other signs of active disease, the prognosis is grave.

REFERENCES

1. Smith CD, Cyr M. The history of lupus erythematosus. From Hippocrates to Osler. Rheum Dis Clin North Am. 1988;**14**:1–14.
2. Hargraves MM, Richmond H, Morton R. Presentation of two bone marrow elements. The 'tart' cell and the 'L.E.' cell. Proc Mayo Clin. 1948;**23**:25–8.
3. Friou GJ. Identification of the nuclear component of the interaction of lupus erythematosus globulin and nuclei. J Immunol. 1958;**80**:476–81.
4. Hochberg MC. Systemic lupus erythematosus. Rheum Dis Clin North Am. 1990;**16**:617–39.
5. Ward MM, Studenski S. Clinical manifestations of systemic lupus erythematosus. Identification of racial and socioeconomic influence. Arch Intern Med. 1990;**150**:849–953.
6. Block SK, Winfield JB, Lockshin MC, D'Angelo WA, Christian CL. Studies of twins with systemic lupus erythematosus. A review of the literature and presentation of 12 additional sets. Am J Med. 1975;**59**:533–52.
7. Lawrence JS, Martins L, Drake G. A family survey of lupus erythematosus. J Rheumatol. 1987;**14**:913–21.
8. Hochberg MC. The application of genetic epidemiology to systemic lupus erythematosus. J Rheumatol. 1987;**14**:867–9.
9. Reinersten JL, Klippel JH, Johnson AH, Steinberg AD, Decker JL, Mann DL. B-lymphocyte alloantigens associated with systemic lupus erythematosus. N Engl J Med. 1978;**299**:515–8.
10. Schur PH, Marcus-Bagley D, Awdeh Z, Yunis EJ, Alper CA. The effect of ethnicity on major histocompatibility complex complement allotypes and extended haplotypes in patients with systemic lupus erythematosus. Arthritis Rheum. 1990;**33**:985–92.
11. Hartung K, Fontana A, Klar M, et al. Association of class I, II, and III MHC gene products with systemic lupus erythematosus. Results of a central European multicenter study. Rheumatol Int. 1989;**9**:13–18.
12. Dunckley J, Gatenby PA, Hawkins B, Naito S, Serjeantson SW. Deficiency of C4A is a genetic determinant of systemic lupus erythematosus in three ethnic groups. J Immunogenet. 1987;**14**:209–18.
13. Fronek A, Timmerman LA, Alper CA, et al. Major histocompatibility complex genes and susceptibility to systemic lupus erythematosus. Arthritis Rheum. 1990;**33**:1542–53.
14. Gilliam JN. Systemic lupus erythematosus and the skin. In: Lahita RG, ed. Systemic lupus erythematosus. New York: Churchill Livingstone; 1987:615–42.
15. Callen JP. Mucocutaneous changes in patients with lupus erythematosus. The relationship of these lesions to systemic disease. Rheum Dis Clin North Am. 1988;**14**:79–97.
16. Gammon RW, Briggaman RA, Inman AO, Merritt CC, Wheller CE. Evidence supporting a role for immune complex-mediated inflammation in the pathogenesis of bullous lesions of systemic lupus erythematosus. J Invest Dermatol. 1983;**81**:320–25.
17. Emerit I, Michelson AM. Mechanism of photosensitivity in systemic lupus erythematosus patients. Proc Natl Acad Sci USA. 1984;**78**:2537–40.
18. Furukawa P, Kshihara-Sawami M, Lyons MB, Norris DA. Binding of antibodies to the extractable nuclear antigens SS-A/Ro and SS-B/La is induced on the surface of human keratinocytes by ultraviolet light (UVL): implications for the pathogenesis of photosensitive cutaneous lupus. J Invest Dermatol. 1990;**94**:77–85.
19. Cronin ME. Musculoskeletal manifestations of systemic lupus erythematosus. Rheum Dis Clin North Am. 1988;**14**:99–116.
20. Reilly PA, Evison G, McHugh NJ, Maddison PJ. Arthropathy of hands and feet in systemic lupus erythematosus. J Rheumatol. 1990;**17**:777–84.
21. Bywaters EGL. Jaccoud's syndrome: A sequel to the joint involvement of systemic lupus erythematosus. Clin Rheum Dis. 1975;**1**:125–48.
22. Esdaile JM, Danoff D, Rosenthal L, Gutowsko A. Deforming arthritis in systemic lupus erythematosus. Ann Rheum Dis. 1981;**40**:124–6.
23. Morley KD, Leung A, Rynes RI. Lupus foot. Br Med J. 1982; **284**:557–8.
24. Isenberg DA, Snaith ML. Muscle disease in systemic lupus erythematosus: a study of its nature, frequency and cause. J Rheumatol. 1981;**8**:917–24.
25. Finol HR, Montagnani S, Marquez A, Montes de Oca I, Müller B. Ultrastructural pathology of skeletal muscle in systemic lupus erythematosus. J Rheumatol. 1990;**17**:210–19.
26. Smythe H, Lee D, Rush P, Buskila D. Tender shins and steroid therapy. J Rheumatol. 1991;**18**:1568–72.
27. Gladman DD, Urowitz MB, Cole E, Ritchie S, Chang CH, Churg J. Kidney biopsy in SLE. I. A clinical–morphologic evaluation. Quart J Med. 1989;**73**:1125–53.
28. Morel-Maroger L, Méry J-Ph, Droz D, et al. The course of lupus nephritis: contribution of serial renal biopsies. Adv Nephrol. 1976;**6**:79–118.
29. Austin HA, Muenz LR, Joyce KM, et al. Prognostic factors in lupus nephritis. Contribution of renal histologic data. Am J Med. 1983;**75**:382–91.
30. McLaughlin J, Gladman DD, Urowitz MB, Bombardier CB, Farewell VT, Cole E. Renal biopsy in SLE. II: Survival analyses according to biopsy results. Arthritis Rheum. 1991;**34**:1268–73.
31. Esdaile JM, Levinton C, Federgreen W, Hayslett JP, Kashgarian M. The clinical and renal biopsy predictors of long-term outcome in lupus nephritis: a study of 87 patients and review of the literature. Quart J Med. 1989;**72**:779–833.
32. Nossent HC, Nenzen-Logmans SC, Vroom TM, Berden JHM, Swaak TJG. Contribution of renal biopsy data in predicting outcome in lupus nephritis. Arthritis Rheum. 1990;**33**:970-77.
33. Whiting-O'Keefe Q, Riccardi PJ, Henke JE, Shearn MA, Hopper J, Epstein WV. Recognition of information in renal biopsies of patients with lupus nephritis. Ann Intern Med. 1982;**96**(part 1):723-7.
34. Austin HA, Muenz LR, Joyce KM, Antonovych TT, Balow JE. Diffuse proliferative lupus nephritis: identification of specific pathologic features affecting renal outcome. Kidney Int. 1984;**25**:689–95.
35. Hariharan S, Pollak VE, Kant KS, Wess MA, Wadhwa NK. Diffuse proliferative lupus nephritis: long-term observations in patients treated with ancrod. Clin Nephrol. 1990;**34**:61-9.
36. Kaell AT, Shetty M, Lee BCP, Lochshin M. The diversity of neurologic events in systemic lupus erythematosus. Arch Neurol. 1988;**43**:273–6.
37. Abel T, Gladman DD, Urowitz MB. Neuropsychiatric lupus. J Rheumatol. 1980;**7**:325–33.
38. Bruyn GW, Padberg G. Chorea and systemic lupus erythematosus. A critical review. Eur Neurol. 1984;**28**:435–48.
39. Asherson RA, Derksen RHWM, Harris EN, et al. Chorea in systemic lupus erythematosus and 'lupus-like' disease: association with antiphospholipid antibodies. Semin Arthritis Rheum. 1987;**16**:253–359.
40. Stafford-Brady FJ, Urowitz MB, Gladman DD, Easterbrook M. Lupus retinopathy. Patterns, associations and prognosis. Arthritis Rheum. 1988;**31**:1105–10.
41. Warren RW, Kredich DW. Transverse myelitis and acute central nervous system manifestations of systemic lupus erythematosus. Arthritis Rheum. 1984;**27**:1058–60.
42. Bonfa E, Golombek SJ, Kaufman LD, et al. Association between lupus psychosis and anti-ribosomal P protein antibodies. N Engl J Med. 1987;**317**:265–71.
43. Schneebaum AB, Singleton JD, West SG, et al. Association of psychiatric manifestations with antibodies to ribosomal P proteins in systemic lupus erythematosus. Am J Med. 1991;**90**:54–62.
44. Kremer JM, Rynes RI, Bartholomew LE, et al. Non-organic non-psychotic psychopathology (NONPP) in patients with systemic lupus erythematosus. Semin Arthritis Rheum. 1981;**11**:182–9.
45. Denburg SD, Carbotte RM, Denburg JA. Cognitive impairment in systemic lupus erythematosus: a neuropsychological study of individual and group deficits. J Clin Exp Neuropsychol. 1987;**9**:323–9.
46. Johnson RT, Richardson EP. The neurological manifestations of systemic lupus erythematosus: a clinico-pathological study of 24 cases and review of the literature. Medicine. 1968;**47**:337–69.
47. Ellis SG, Verity MA. Central nervous system involvement in systemic lupus erythematosus: a review of neuropathological findings in 57 cases, 1955–1977. Semin Arthritis Rheum. 1979;**8**:212–21.
48. Tan RF, Gladman DD, Urowitz MB, Milne N. Brain scan diagnosis of central nervous system involvement in systemic lupus erythematosus. Ann Rheum Dis. 1978;**37**:357–62.
49. Pinching AJ, Travers RL, Hughes GRV. Oxygen-15 brain scanning for detection of cerebral involvement in systemic lupus erythematosus. Lancet. 1978;**1**:898–900.
50. Bluestein HG, Pischal KD, Woods JL Jr. Immunopathogenesis of the neuropsychiatric manifestations of systemic lupus erythematosus. Springer Semin Immunopathol. 1986;**9**:237–49.
51. Long AA, Denburg SD, Carbotte RM, Sinal DP, Denburg JA. Serum lymphocytotoxic antibodies and neurocognitive function in systemic lupus erythematosus. Ann Rheum Dis. 1990;**49**:249–53.
52. Minota S, Koyasu S, Yahara I, Winfield J. Autoantibodies to the heat shock protein hsp90 in systemic lupus erythematosus. J Clin Invest. 1988;**81**:106–109.
53. Robbins ML, Kornguth SE, Bell CL, et al. Antineurofilament antibody evaluation in neuropsychiatric systemic lupus erythematosus. Combination with anticardiolipin antibody assay and magnetic resonance imaging. Arthritis Rheum. 1988;**31**:623–31.
54. Hirohata S, Hirose S, Miyamoto T. Cerebrospinal fluid IgM, IgA, and IgG indexes in systemic lupus erythematosus. Their use as estimates of central nervous system disease activity. Arch Intern Med. 1985;**145**:1843–6.
55. Mongey AB, Glynn D, Hutchinson M, Bresnihan B. Clinical neurophysiology in the assessment of neurological symptoms in systemic lupus erythematosus. Rheumatol Int. 1987;**7**:49–52.
56. Hirawa M, Nonaka C, Abe T, Ilo M. Positron emission tomography in systemic lupus erythematosus: relation of cerebral vasculitis to PET findings. AJNR. 1983;**4**:541-3.
57. Carette S, Urowitz MB, Grossman H, St. Louis EL. Cranial computerized tomography in systemic lupus erythematosus. J Rheumatol. 1982;**9**:855–9.
58. Bell CL, Partington C, Robbins M, Graziano F, Turski P, Kornguth S. Magnetic resonance imaging of central nervous system lesions in patients with systemic lupus erythematosus. Correlation with clinical remission and antineurofilament and anticardiolipin antibody titers. Arthritis Rheum. 1991;**34**:432–41.
59. Griffey RH, Brown MS, Bankhurst AD, Sibbitt RR, Siggitt WL JR. Depletion of high-energy phosphates in the central nervous system of patients with systemic lupus erythematosus, as determined by phosphorus-31 nuclear magnetic resonance spectroscopy. Arthritis Rheum. 1990;**33**:827–33.
60. Segal AM, Calabrese LH, Ahmad M, Tubbs RT, White CS. The pulmonary manifestations of systemic lupus erythematosus. Semin Arthritis Rheum. 1985;**14**:202–24.
61. Good Jr JT, King TE, Antony VB, Sahn SA. Lupus pleuritis: Clinical features and pleural fluid characteristics with special reference to pleural fluid antinuclear antibodies. Chest. 1983;**84**:714–8.
62. Bulkley BH, Roberts WC. The heart in systemic lupus erythematosus and the changes induced in it by corticosteroid therapy. Am J Med. 1975;**58**:243–64.

63. Zashin SJ, Lipsky PE. Pericardial tamponade complicating systemic lupus erythematosus. J Rheumatol. 1989;**16**:374–7.
64. Kaufman LD, Seifert FC, Eilbott DJ, Zuna RE, Steigbigel RT, Kaplan AP. Candida pericarditis and tamponade in a patient with systemic lupus erythematosus. Arch Intern Med. 1988;**148**: 715–7.
65. Coe MD, Hamer DH, Levy CS, Milner MR, Nam MH, Barth WF. Gonococcal pericarditis with tamponade in a patient with systemic lupus erythematosus. Arthritis Rheum. 1990;**33**:1438–41.
66. Schoshoe JT, Koch AE, Chang RW. Chronic lupus peritonitis with ascites: Review of the literature with a case report. Semin Arthritis Rheum. 1988;**18**:121–6.
67. Carette S. Cardiopulmonary manifestations of systemic lupus erythematosus. Rheum Dis Clin North Am. 1988;**14**:135–47
68. Eagen JW, Mendi VA, Roberts JL, Lewis EJ. Pulmonary hemorrhage in systemic lupus erythematosus. Medicine. 1978;**57**:545–60.
69. Mintz G, Galindo LF, Fernandez-Diaz J, Jimenez FJ, Robles-Saavedra E, Enriquez-Casillas RD. Acute massive pulmonary hemorrhage in systemic lupus erythematosus. J Rheumatol. 1978;**5**:39–50.
70. Asherson RA, Oakley CM. Pulmonary hypertension and systemic lupus erythematosus. J Rheumatol. 1986;**13**:1–5.
71. Baduie E, Garcia-Rubi D, Robles E, et al. Cardiovascular manifestations in systemic lupus erythematosus. Angiology. 1985;**36**:431–41.
72. Hosenpud JD, Montanaro A, Hart MV, et al. Myocardial perfusion abnormalities in asymptomatic patients with systemic lupus erythematosus. Am J Med. 1984;**77**:286–92.
73. Tamburino C, Fiore C, Foti R, Salomone E, DiPacola R, Grimaldi GR. Endomyocardial biopsy in diagnosis and management of cardiovascular manifestations of systemic lupus erythematosus. Clin Rheumatol. 1989;**8**:108–12.
74. Klinkhoff AV, Thompson CR, Reid GD, Tomlison CW. M-mode and two-dimensional echocardiographic abnormalities in systemic lupus erythematosus. JAMA. 1985;**253**:3273–7.
75. Korbet SM, Schwartz MM, Lewis EJ. Immune complex deposition and coronary vasculitis in systemic lupus erythematosus. Am J Med. 1984;**77**:141–5.
76. Zizic TM, Classen JN, Stevens MB. Acute abdominal complications of systemic lupus erythematosus and polyarteritis nodosa. Am J Med. 1982;**73**:525–31.
77. Gladman DD, Ross T, Richardson B, Kulkarni S. Bowel involvement in systemic lupus erythematosus: Crohn's disease or lupus vasculitis. Arthritis Rheum. 1985;**28**:466–70.
78. Nagata M, Ogawa Y, Hisano S, Ueda K. Crohn's disease in systemic lupus erythematosus: A case report. Eur J Pediatr. 1989;**148**:525–6.
79. Reynolds JC, Inman RD, Kimberly RP, Chuong JH, Kovacs JE, Walsh M. Acute pancreatitis in systemic lupus erythematosus: Report of twenty cases and a review of the literature. Medicine. 1982;**61**:25.
80. Haakenstad AO, Mannik M. Saturation of the reticuloendothelial system with soluble immune complexes. J Immunol. 1974;**112**:1939–48.
81. Dillon AM, Stein HB, English RA. Splenic atrophy in SLE. Ann Intern Med. 1982;**96**:40–43.
82. Buskila D, Gladman DD, Hanna W, Kahn HJ. Primary malignant lymphoma of the spleen in systemic lupus erythematosus. J Rheumatol. 1989;**16**:993–6.
83. Lloyd W, Schur PH. Immune complexes, complement, and anti-DNA in exacerbations of systemic lupus erythematosus (SLE). Medicine. 1981;**60**:208–7.
84. Ganczarczyk L, Urowitz MB, Gladman DD. Latent lupus. J Rheumatol. 1989;**16**:475–8.
85. Lom-Orta H, Alarcon-Segovia D, Diaz-Jouanen E. Systemic lupus erythematosus – differences between patients who do and do not fulfil classification criteria at the time of diagnosis. J Rheumatol. 1980;**7**:831–7.
86. Hess EV. Drug-related lupus. N Engl J Med. 1988;**318**:1460–62.
87. Mongey AB, Hess EV. Drug-related lupus. Curr Opin Rheumatol. 1989;**1**:353–9.
88. Solinger AM. Drug-related lupus. Clinical etiologic considerations. Rheum Dis Clin North Am. 1988;**14**:187–202.
89. Rubin LA, Urowitz MB, Gladman DD. Mortality in systemic lupus erythematosus – the bimodal pattern revisited. Quart J Med. 1985;**55**:87–98.
90. Gladman DD, Urowitz MB. Venous syndromes and pulmonary embolism in systemic lupus erythematosus. Ann Rheum Dis. 1980;**39**:340–43.
91. Zizic TM, Marcoux C, Hungerford DS, Dansereau J-V, Stevens MB. Corticosteroid therapy associated with ischemic necrosis of bone in systemic lupus erythematosus. Am J Med. 1985;**79**:596–604.
92. Hungerford DS, Zizic TM. The treatment of ischemic necrosis of bone in systemic lupus erythematosus. Medicine. 1980;**59**:143.
93. Ganczarczyk ML, Lee P, Fornasier V. Early diagnosis of osteonecrosis in systemic lupus erythematosus with magnetic resonance imaging. Failure of core decompression. J Rheumatol. 1986;**13**:814.
94. Steinberg ME, Brighton CT, Steinberg DR, Tooze SE, Hayken GD. Treatment of avascular necrosis of the femoral head by a combination of bone grafting, decompression, and electrical stimulation. Clin Orthop Rel Res. 1984;**186**:137.
95. Jacobelli S, Moreno R, Massardo L, Rivero S, Lisboa C. Inspiratory muscle dysfunction and unexplained dyspnea in systemic lupus erythematosus. Arthritis Rheum. 1985;**28**:781–8.
96. Rubin LA, Urowitz MB. Shrinking lung syndrome in SLE – a clinical pathologic study. J Rheumatol. 1983;**10**:973.

32

MANAGEMENT OF SYSTEMIC LUPUS ERYTHEMATOSUS

John H Klippel

- Therapy for acute flares must be distinguished from long-term management strategies.
- Corticosteroids are important for serious, acute, active SLE; but NSAIDs are the first line of treatment for many manifestations.
- Antimalarials are effective for skin and other organ involvement.
- Renal function is preserved by intravenous cyclophosphamide in patients with nephritis.

Although systemic lupus erythematosus (SLE) is a chronic rheumatic syndrome, its clinical course is typically one of relapses and remissions. Disease management must include both interventions directed at acute flares of the disease, that on occasion may be life-threatening, and strategies directed at the progressive chronic disease course. Advances in lupus management, in particular the influences of corticosteroids and agents that suppress immune function, have contributed to improvements in survival and reduced disease morbidity over the past several decades (Fig. 32.1) [1].

MONITORING DISEASE ACTIVITY

Many of the decisions regarding lupus management, particularly those involving drug therapies, are guided by the concept of lupus disease activity. In simplest terms, this is a determination of the extent to which inflammation secondary to lupus is contributing to the clinical setting and, in addition, an assessment of the likelihood that the involvement will produce morbidity or mortality. Although in many patients it is a relatively easy and straightforward matter of knowing that lupus is active and deciding whether it is mild or severe and life-threatening, in others it is far more complicated. Typical examples of the latter include patients who have an elevated serum creatinine in whom active lupus nephritis, reversible effects of drug therapy, or irreversible scarring within the kidneys, become important considerations. Similarly, in patients who are grossly confused, active central nervous system lupus, drug side effects, metabolic imbalances and primary psychiatric disturbance must all be considered.

Identification of changes in lupus activity over time to decide whether lupus is improving, remaining the same, or worsening is essential in drug management. For manifestations such as anemia or thrombocytopenia, proteinuria, or nephritis, there are objective laboratory measures that may be followed to guide therapy. In the instance of lupus nephritis, a quantitative scoring system to determine the degrees of active and chronic changes on renal biopsy has been developed [2]. However, for most clinical manifestations, determinations of lupus activity are highly subjective and less well defined. Moreover, the patient who has an additive or migratory pattern of lupus involvement poses separate problems in the assessment of lupus activity. To provide a more reproducible and quantitative assessment of lupus activity, standardized scoring systems have been developed. The Systemic Lupus Erythematosus Disease Activity Index (SLE-DAI) is shown in Figure 32.2. These global measures of lupus activity are valuable for the conduct of clinical trials and in following the long-term course of individual lupus patients.

Immunologic studies, particularly antibodies to double-stranded DNA and serum complement levels, are often used as surrogate markers of lupus activity. Patients with clinically active lupus typically have increased levels of anti-DNA antibodies and depressed complement levels. Moreover, resolution in these abnormalities has been shown to correlate with improvements in the clinical course of lupus nephritis [3]. Based on these observations, immunologic studies are often used as early, preclinical markers of changing lupus activity (Fig. 32.3). Whether these immunologic studies predictably identify a window of preclinical flare in the broad population of lupus patients and, more importantly, whether therapeutic interventions

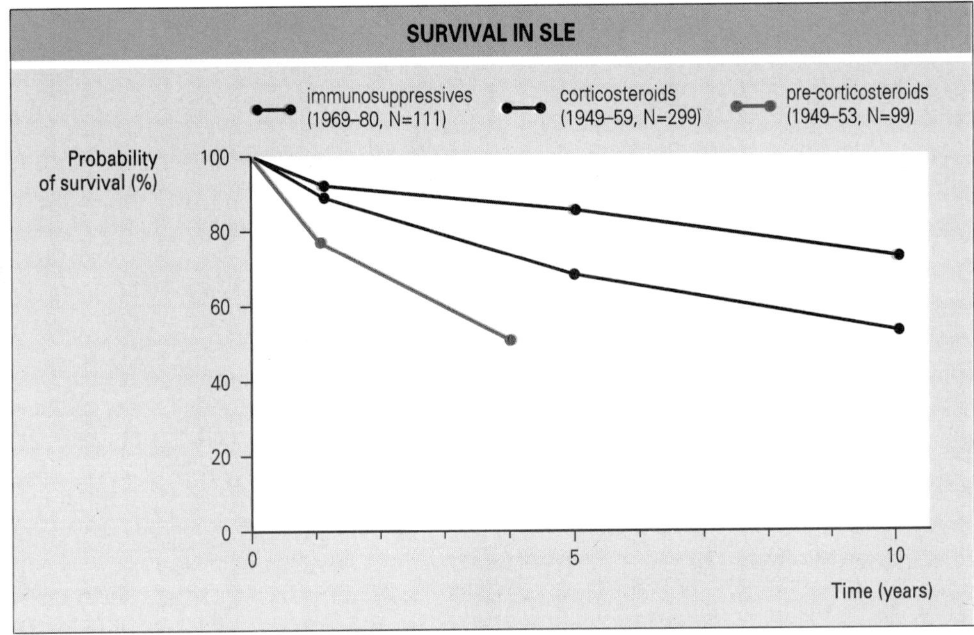

Fig. 32.1 Survival in SLE. With immunosuppressives (Ann Intern Med. 1987;**106**:79–94); corticosteroids (Arch Intern Med. 1964;**113**:200–207); and pre-corticosteroids (J Chronic Dis. 1955;**1**:12–32).

SYSTEMIC LUPUS ERYTHEMATOSUS DISEASE ACTIVITY INDEX (SLE-DAI)			
Weighted score	SLE-DAI score	Descriptor	Definition
8		Seizure	Recent onset. Exclude metabolic, infectious, or drug-related causes.
8		Psychosis	Altered ability to function in normal activity due to severe disturbance in the perception of reality. Includes hallucinations; incoherence; marked loose associations; impoverished thought content; marked illogical thinking; bizarre, disorganized, or catatonic behavior. Exclude the presence of uremia and offending drugs.
8		Organic brain syndrome	Altered mental function with impaired orientation or impaired memory or other intellectual function, with rapid onset and fluctuating clinical features. Includes a clouding of consciousness with a reduced capacity to focus and an inability to sustain attention on environment and at least two of the following: perceptual disturbance, incoherent speech, insomnia or daytime drowsiness, increased or decreased psychomotor activity. Exclude metabolic, infectious and drug-related causes.
8		Visual	Retinal changes from systemic lupus erythematosus: cytoid bodies, retinal hemorrhages, serous exudate or hemorrhages in the choroid, optic neuritis (not due to hypertension, drugs, or infection).
8		Cranial nerve	New onset of a sensory or motor neuropathy involving a cranial nerve.
8		Lupus headache	Severe, persistent headache; may be migrainous; nonresponsive to narcotic analgesia.
8		Cerebrovascular accident	New syndrome. Exclude arteriosclerosis.
8		Vasculitis	Ulceration, gangrene, tender finger nodules, periungual infarction, splinter hemorrhages. Vasculitis confirmed by biopsy or angiogram.
4		Arthritis	More than two joints with pain and signs of inflammation (such as tenderness, swelling, or effusion).
4		Myositis	Proximal muscle aching or weakness associated with elevated creatine phosphokinase/aldolase levels, electromyelographic changes, or a biopsy showing myositis.
4		Casts	Heme granule or erythrocyte.
4		Hematuria	More than 5 erythrocytes per high power field. Excluding other causes (stone, infection).
4		Proteinuria	More than 0.5g of urinary protein excreted per 24 hours. New onset or recent increase of more than 0.5g per 24 hours.
4		Pyuria	More than 5 leukocytes per high power field. Exclude infection.
2		New malar rash	New onset or recurrence of an inflammatory type of rash.
2		Alopecia	New or recurrent. A patch of abnormal, diffuse loss of hair.
2		Mucous membrane	New onset or recurrence of oral or nasal ulcerations.
2		Pleurisy	Pleuritic chest pain with pleural rub or effusion, or pleural thickening.
2		Pericarditis	Pericardial pain with at least one of the following; rub, effusion. Confirmation by electrocardiography or echocardiography.
2		Low complement	A decrease in CH_{50}, C3, or C4 level (to less than the lower limit of the laboratory-determined normal range).
2		Increased DNA binding	More than 25% binding by Farr assay (to more than the upper limit of the laboratory-determined normal range, for example 25%).
1		Fever	More than 38°C after the exclusion of infection.
1		Thrombocytopenia	More than 100,000 platelets.
1		Leukopenia	Leukocyte count of less than $3000/mm^3$ (not due to drugs).
Total SLE-DAI score		Enter the weighted score for each descriptor in the SLE-DAI score column if the descriptor was present at the time of the visit or in the preceding 10 days	

Fig. 32.2 Systemic lupus erythematosus disease activity index (SLE-DAI).

given during this period alter the clinical course, have never adequately been demonstrated in a prospective trial. Recent additional immunologic studies thought to be of potential use in following lupus activity include serum levels of complement split products (Bb, Ba, and Sc5b-9) and serum levels of the soluble interleukin-2 receptor.

PREVENTION

Preventive practices are aimed at the early detection of changing lupus activity and, where possible, efforts to reduce the likelihood of acute lupus flares or the development of confounding illnesses (Fig. 32.4). Regular physician evaluations for assessment of lupus activity and adjustments of drug therapies are essential. Several of the more serious aspects of lupus, such as renal disease or hematologic complications, can be detected only by laboratory studies. Routine screening of chemistries, blood counts, and a urinalysis need to be included as part of the regular evaluation. Whereas patients with worsening lupus may need to be seen as often as weekly, patients with stable, more established disease need to be seen less frequently. In addition, patients should be alerted to warning signs, such as unexplained weight loss, extreme fatigue, fluid retention, or fever, that might require an unscheduled visit. Finally, it is extremely important to recognize the role of general medicine skills in lupus management. Control of hypertension, correction of fluid and electrolyte disturbances, and treatment of seizure disorders, hyperlipidemia, and infections are common needs in lupus patients.

Many lupus patients are photosensitive and must be reminded of the importance of avoiding sun exposure. This includes practical advice about wearing long-sleeved clothing and big-brimmed hats, going outdoors only during early morning or evening hours, and the liberal use of sun screens. Changes in the work setting may be required; outdoor occupations may not be possible and office workers may need to avoid sunlight from a window or even overhead fluorescent lights. In addition, care must be taken in the use of various photosensitizing drugs, particularly antibiotics, in lupus patients.

Infections are common in lupus patients and require careful and prompt evaluation of all febrile individuals. This is particularly

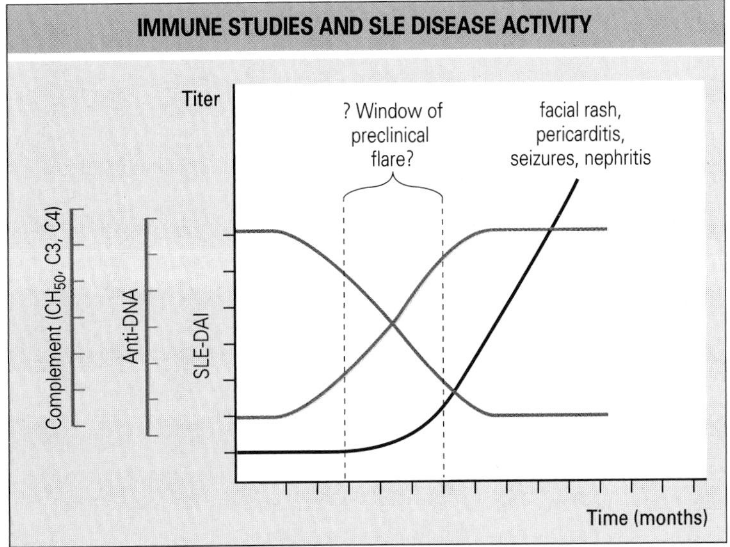

Fig. 32.3 Immune studies and SLE disease activity.

important in populations of lupus patients at heightened risk of infection, such as those with renal failure, complement deficiencies, ulcerative skin lesions, or cardiac valvular abnormalities. Patients treated with high doses of corticosteroids, or immunosuppressive drugs, and patients with splenectomy are at increased risk of infection. Antibiotic prophylaxis should be used for all dental and genitourinary procedures. Patients need to be immunized with influenza vaccine yearly, and pneumococcal vaccine should be given to lupus patients following splenectomy.

Birth control is important in female patients receiving drug therapies in which pregnancy would be contraindicated (i.e. cytotoxic or antimetabolite drugs). Birth control is also important in patients with very active lupus, particularly nephritis. Pregnancy in the lupus patient poses concerns of possible exacerbations of lupus in the mother and separate risks to the fetus. This requires more careful and frequent monitoring of lupus activity in the pregnant lupus patient and obstetric care provided by a specialist trained in the management of high risk pregnancies.

EDUCATION AND PSYCHOSOCIAL INTERVENTIONS

Education and psychosocial interventions are important and may easily be overlooked. The newly diagnosed patient with lupus generally has never heard of the disease and is understandably anxious. The physician must anticipate this response and be in a position to provide a clear explanation of what lupus is in language the patient can understand. Booklets specifically written for patients are often extremely helpful for this purpose and provide patients with basic information about the disease. In many hospitals and communities, lupus support groups have been organized. In addition to the educational function provided by these groups, many patients benefit enormously by having the opportunity to interact with other patients with the disease. In particular, this type of forum often provides patients with the coping skills needed for dealing with a chronic illness.

DRUG THERAPIES

Although an understanding of the exact mechanisms of action of many of the drugs used in lupus management is still incomplete, presumably direct effects on inflammatory pathways or immune events are important. The specific clinical manifestations of lupus to be treated serve as a reasonable guide to drug options (Fig. 32.5). In very few instances, however, have these therapies been subjected to testing by randomized controlled trials.

Nonsteroidal Drugs

Nonsteroidal anti-inflammatory drugs (NSAIDs), including salicylates, are widely prescribed for the symptomatic treatment of musculoskeletal manifestations and systemic features such as fever and mild serositis. Surprisingly, there are very few formal clinical studies of NSAIDs in lupus [4,5]. NSAIDs are often given for very mild lupus activity before low-dose corticosteroids or antimalarials. In addition, NSAIDs are often given in combination with corticosteroids in an effort to minimize corticosteroid dose or to suppress lupus activity when alternate day corticosteroids are used. There is no reason to believe that one NSAID is superior to another in lupus,

PREVENTIVE MEASURES IN LUPUS MANAGEMENT

Regular evaluation	Assess lupus activity. Routine chemistries, blood counts, urinalysis. Control of blood pressure, edema, and hyperlipidemia.
Photoprotection	Avoid intense sun exposure. Sun screens.
Infection control	Suspect infection in all febrile lupus patients. Antibiotic prophylaxis for dental and genitourinary procedures. Influenza and pneumococcal immunizations.
Pregnancy issues	Birth control with very active lupus (especially nephritis) and with cytotoxic or antimetabolite drugs. High-risk obstetrical care required.

Fig. 32.4 Preventive measures in lupus management.

DRUGS USED IN LUPUS MANAGEMENT

	Manifestations of SLE				
Approved	Constitutional	Musculoskeletal	Serositis	Cutaneous	Major Organ
Nonsteroidal drugs	+	+	+		
Corticosteroids					
Topical				+	
Low dose					
(i.e. prednisone ≤ 0.5mg/kg/day)	+	+	+	+	
High dose					
(i.e. prednisone 1.0mg/kg/day)					+
or 1g i.v. methylprednisolone					+
Antimalarials	+	+	+	+	
Investigational					
Azathioprine		+	+	+	+
Cyclophosphamide/chlorambucil					+
Methotrexate		+?	+?		
Dapsone	+?			+	
Immune globulin					+ (thrombocytopenia)
Danazol					+ (thrombocytopenia)
Cyclosporin A					??

Fig. 32.5 Drugs used in lupus management.

CORTICOSTEROIDS IN LUPUS	
Indication	**Corticosteroid regimen**
Rashes	Topical Short-acting Hydrocortisone (0.125–1.0%) Intermediate-acting Triamcinalone (0.025–0.5%) Long-acting Betamethasone (0.01–0.1%) Intralesional (discoid lupus) Triamcinolone acetonide
Minor disease activity	Oral prednisone (or equivalent) <0.5mg/kg in single or divided daily dose
Major disease activity	Oral prednisone (or equivalent) 1mg/kg in single or divided daily dose or Intravenous methylprednisolone (1g or 15mg/kg), often repeated for 3 consecutive days

Fig. 32.6 Corticosteroids in lupus.

and factors such as how well the patient tolerates the drug and cost often become considerations. As with other rheumatic diseases for which NSAIDs are used, there appears to be marked variability in patient responsiveness, and several different drugs may need to be tried before settling on the single best drug for an individual patient.

Several of the potential adverse reactions of NSAID therapy are important since they may be easily confused with active lupus, particularly renal and neurologic drug effects. In the kidney, NSAIDs inhibit renal prostaglandin synthesis and may lead to reversible impairments of renal blood flow, glomerular filtration, and tubular function. The patient with lupus nephritis may, if anything, be more susceptible to these influences due to a heightened dependency on prostaglandins for maintenance of renal function. Rarely, NSAIDs may produce membranous nephropathy, acute interstitial nephritis or acute tubular necrosis. Thus, it is very important in the lupus patient who presents with evidence of loss of renal function, edema, or hyperkalemia that consideration be given to the possibility of NSAID-induced effect. Nonsteroidal drugs should be discontinued in all patients with suspected lupus nephritis prior to baseline studies to assess renal function or when a renal biopsy is being considered.

Nonsteroidal drugs may cause a variety of neuropsychiatric complaints, including headache, dizziness, confusion, and depression, that might be confused with central nervous system lupus. Patients with lupus appear to be particularly susceptible to an aseptic meningitis syndrome induced by several of the NSAIDs, particularly ibuprofen [6]. The typical clinical presentation includes headache, meningism, and fever; pruritis, facial edema, and conjunctivitis may occur on occasion. Lymphocytosis, an elevated protein and a sterile culture are findings in the cerebrospinal fluid. The syndrome promptly resolves with discontinuation of the NSAID.

Corticosteroids

Corticosteroids are unquestionably the single most important class of drugs available for the management of acute, active manifestations of lupus [5]. The administration of corticosteroids typically results in prompt and complete resolution of most manifestations of lupus. In select patients with fulminate disease, corticosteroids can be life-saving. There are multiple uses for corticosteroids in lupus, including topical preparations for inflammatory rashes, intralesional injections for discoid lupus, low-dose oral therapy for active, mild disease, and high-dose oral or bolus, intravenous infusions for acute, severe manifestations (Fig. 32.6). There is little reason to suspect major clinical differences among the various oral corticosteroid preparations. For oral drug therapy, prednisone is most often used due to its shorter plasma half-life and the availability of multiple different tablet sizes which facilitate dose changes. It is usually preferable to avoid dexamethasone with its long half-life.

Corticosteroid toxicities limit long-term use, particularly when given in high doses or in multiple daily dose schedules. Oral therapy is generally begun as a single, daily morning dose. In patients who fail to show improvement, the dose of corticosteroids may either be increased or given in divided doses two or three times daily. The maximum daily dose of corticosteroids usually need not exceed 60mg prednisone (or equivalent), nor should the duration of high-dose corticosteroids exceed 6–8 weeks. Patients who fail to respond or relapse with these doses of corticosteroids, or who develop unacceptable toxicities from corticosteroids, are candidates for other forms of aggressive therapy.

Once lupus activity is judged to be under control, reductions of the corticosteroid dose should be undertaken. For patients on multiple daily dose regimens, the initial step should involve efforts to change the patient to a single morning dose regimen. With reductions of the corticosteroid dosage, patients need to be monitored carefully for signs of increasing lupus activity. Many patients appear to have a corticosteroid threshold below which disease activity predictably develops. In patients with prolonged periods of disease remission, reduction and eventual discontinuation of the corticosteroid should be a goal of patient management.

Antimalarials

Antimalarials are useful in the management of the cutaneous, musculoskeletal, and mild constitutional features of lupus, such as fever, fatigue, and malaise. The precise mechanism of action of these drugs is unknown. Both anti-inflammatory and immunosuppressive properties have been described. Antimalarials have a high affinity for DNA and intercalate between adjacent base pairs to inhibit cellular division as well as RNA transcription and translation. In addition, antimalarials are concentrated within mononuclear cells and inhibit phagocytosis, migratory properties, and metabolism of membrane phospholipids. Although inhibition of macrophage and B cell functions have been described *in vitro*, there are conflicting data in humans as to whether antibody responses are suppressed.

Both 4-aminoquinolone derivatives (hydroxychloroquine and chloroquine) and the 9-aminoacridine compound quinacrine are used (Fig. 32.7). The 8-aminoquinolone primaquine phosphate is specifically contraindicated in lupus. Therapy is often initiated at twice the recommended maintenance dose with reduction of the dose after 4–6 weeks once lupus activity has subsided. Antimalarials should be used with caution in lupus patients with glucose-6-phosphate dehydrogenase (G6PD) deficiency or in patients with liver disease.

Quinacrine and hydroxychloroquine are the best studied of the antimalarials; the clinical experience with chloroquine is substantially less [7,8]. Although some differences in onset of action and toxicities between quinacrine and hydroxychloroquine have been

ANTIMALARIALS USED IN LUPUS	
Drug	**Daily dose**
4-Aminoquinoline derivatives	
Hydroxychloroquine	200–400mg*
Chloroquine	250mg*
9-Aminoacridine derivative	
Quinacrine (mepacrine)	100mg*

* In patients weighing less than 45kg, dose reductions are necessary: 5–7mg/kg for hydroxychloroquine, 4mg/kg for chloroquine, 1–2mg/kg for quinacrine

Fig. 32.7 Antimalarials used in lupus.

noted, the choice between these agents is largely a matter of physician preference. Improvements in cutaneous manifestations, including both discoid and erythematous inflammatory lesions, can be remarkably rapid and often evident in a matter of days after starting therapy. In patients who fail to respond to a particular antimalarial, either substitution or addition of an alternative antimalarial drug is often beneficial.

In general, there is a reluctance to ever completely discontinue antimalarials in stable lupus patients on long-term therapy, particularly in those who have clearly benefitted from the drug. The discontinuation of antimalarials is clearly associated with an increased risk of clinical lupus flares, including major exacerbations of the disease such as vasculitis, transverse myelitis, and nephropathy [9]. Gradual reduction of the dose to one or two tablets a week in such patients is often worthwhile.

This poses a particular dilemma in the lupus patient on antimalarials who becomes pregnant. Antimalarials cross the placenta, and rare instances of congenital defects such as cleft palate, sensorineural hearing loss, and posterior column defects have been reported. The physician must decide whether the risk to the pregnancy of flaring lupus from discontinuing the antimalarials exceeds the risks of drug-induced fetal abnormalities. There is no ready answer to this question; however, the relative safety of antimalarials given during pregnancy has been noted in a small series of lupus patients[10].

In general, the low-doses of antimalarials used in patients with lupus are well tolerated and rarely need to be discontinued for an adverse reaction. Of the various toxicities associated with antimalarials, gastrointestinal intolerance, cutaneous eruptions, and nonspecific constitutional complaints are most frequent. Central nervous system toxicities including headaches, emotional changes, psychosis, ataxia, and seizures have been rarely reported such that antimalarials should be discontinued in patients with suspected neuropsychiatric manifestations of lupus. Long-term antimalarial therapy may cause a neuromyopathy, and assessment for muscle strength and reflexes should be done periodically. Although hematologic toxicities with antimalarials are distinctly uncommon, complete blood counts should be obtained regularly.

Much of the concern regarding antimalarial use in lupus has focused on potential ocular toxicities of which two forms are recognized. Deposition of the drug in the cornea may lead to complaints of blurred vision, photophobia, focusing difficulties, and visual halos. These are often noted within the first several weeks after starting therapy and generally resolve with continuation of the drug. In the retina, antimalarials bind to the melanin of the pigmented epithelial layer and may damage rods and cones. Retinal damage from antimalarials is thought to be related to daily drug dose and not cumulative drug dose. Moreover, there is some evidence that retinal toxicity may be less common with hydroxychloroquine than chloroquine [11]. Early retinal changes are typically first detected in the macula, with findings of macular edema, increased pigmentation and granularity, and loss of the foveal reflex. Although patients with early macular disease (so-called premaculopathy) generally have no visual complaints, on careful testing a paracentral scotomata to a red, but not white, test object may be detected. These early types of retinal changes are reversible upon discontinuation of the antimalarial drug. Advanced macular disease is characterized by a central area of patchy depigmentation of the macula surrounded by a concentric ring of pigmentation (the bull's eye lesion). Narrowing of the retinal vessels, optic atrophy, and diffuse depigmentation of the peripheral retina are very late changes.

It is important to emphasize that the risk of retinal toxicity in patients with lupus treated with low doses of antimalarials is extremely small. As a precaution, however, ophthalmologic examinations to include visual acuity, slit-lamp, funduscopic, and visual field testing should be performed prior to the start of therapy and at least yearly.

INVESTIGATIONAL THERAPIES

A number of therapies for lupus management, including both drug and nondrug interventions, have not received formal approval for use in lupus by drug regulatory agencies (in the USA the US Food and Drug Administration). Thus, although many of these therapies are used widely in clinical practice, they are all regarded as investigational.

Azathioprine

The purine analog azathioprine is an imidazolyl derivative of 6-mercaptopurine. The drug alters cellular purine biosynthesis through the formation of mono-, di-, and triphosphate nucleosides of methylthiopurines. Both anti-inflammatory and immunosuppressive properties have been described with azathioprine.

Clinically, azathioprine is regarded as an alternative to cyclophosphamide as an immunosuppressive agent in drug management of lupus. Although comparisons between the two drugs are difficult, azathioprine is generally considered to be less efficacious, but a far safer drug. Azathioprine (1–4mg/kg/day) is widely used in the management of nonrenal lupus manifestations as a corticosteroid-sparing agent. The drug has been extensively studied in lupus nephritis and may reduce proteinuria, improve or stabilize renal function, and reduce mortality in patients with diffuse proliferative glomerulonephritis [12].

The most common side effects of azathioprine that limit therapy involve various forms of gastrointestinal intolerance and bone marrow toxicity. Both erythroid and myeloid elements of the bone marrow are affected. The onset of anemia or leukopenia may be abrupt, and blood counts need to be monitored regularly during therapy [13]. Bone marrow toxicity is generally reversible with reduction of the dose or discontinuation of the drug.

It is generally recommended that azathioprine not be given during pregnancy and that birth control be used during therapy. Both congenital defects and evidence of severe immune deficiency have been described in infants born to mothers treated with azathioprine during pregnancy. Azathioprine is known to induce chromosome abnormalities as well as increases in sister chromatid exchanges. The relationship of chromosomal defects to teratogenicity is unknown.

Azathioprine can produce elevations of liver enzymes, particularly the glutamic pyruvic and glutamic oxaloacetic transaminases. On liver biopsy hepatocellular necrosis and mild biliary stasis have been seen. Hepatotoxicity is thought to result from drug hypersensitivity and may be accompanied by clinical features such as fever, diffuse abdominal pain, diarrhea, and a maculopapular skin rash [14]. Hepatic abnormalities are typically reversible upon stopping the drug.

There is concern that azathioprine may increase the risk of malignancy, particularly of hematopoietic or lymphoreticular origin. Case reports of the non-Hodgkin's lymphoma and leukemia [15,16] and a four-fold increase in cervical atypia [17] have been documented in lupus patients treated with azathioprine. An epidemiologic survey identified statistically increased frequencies of non-Hodgkin's lymphoma and reticulum cell sarcomas in patients treated with azathioprine for indications other than organ transplantation [18].

Cyclophosphamide/Chlorambucil

Several different nitrogen mustard alkylating agents have been used in lupus management. The nitrogen mustard alkylating drugs contain highly reactive radicals capable of forming cross-linkages. Drug effects on nucleic acids, particularly DNA, are thought to be of primary importance. Although alkylating agents act throughout the cell cycle including nonproliferating cells, cells in the S phase (the phase of DNA synthesis) are particularly vulnerable to drug actions. Alkylating agents may cause simple miscoding errors by substitution of incorrect base pairs, or produce internal cross-linkages leading to major alterations of the double-helical structure and cell death.

ORAL AND INTRAVENOUS CYCLOPHOSPHAMIDE IN LUPUS

	Oral	Intravenous
Pharmacology		
Dose	1–3mg/kg*	0.5–1.0g/m²*
Frequency	daily	monthly
Bladder Protection		
Fluids	2–3 liters daily	2–3 liters in 24-hour period post i.v. dose
Mesna	??	??
Monitoring Therapy		
CBC	q 4–6 wks	10–14 days post dose
Urinalysis	q 4–6 wks	q 4–6 wks
Urine cytology	to evaluate unexplained hematuria	to evaluate unexplained hematuria
* dose needs to be reduced in patients with impaired renal function		

Fig. 32.8 Oral and intravenous cyclophosphamide in lupus.

Nitrogen mustard alkylating agents have potent effects on the immune system, particularly cell-mediated functions, as well as anti-inflammatory properties.

Mechlorethamine is of historical interest since it was the first nitrogen mustard alkylating drug used in lupus during the early 1950s. In comparison to other agents, it is highly unstable, may be given only by an intravenous route, and is considered to have relatively weak effects on immune function.

Cyclophosphamide has been the best studied of the alkylating agents in systemic lupus. Cyclophosphamide must be metabolized within the liver before alkylating metabolites are generated, and both oral and intravenous schedules are used (Fig. 32.8). Since cyclophosphamide is excreted by the kidneys, the drug dose must be reduced in patients with impairments of renal function. The cytotoxic action of cyclophosphamide is commonly expressed on bone marrow function, particularly white blood cells. Thus, the drug must be given with caution in patients with leukopenia, and regular monitoring of white blood counts, hematocrit, and platelet counts are essential. As a general rule, the absolute white blood count should not be allowed to go below 2000 cells/mm^3 or the absolute neutrophil count below 1000 cells/mm^3. Finally, cyclophosphamide is a well established teratogen so tests to exclude pregnancy before starting therapy and effective birth control during therapy are essential [19].

In randomized controlled trials in lupus nephritis, cyclophosphamide has been shown to retard progressive scarring within the kidney [20] and reduce the risk of end-stage renal failure requiring dialysis or renal transplantation [21] (Fig. 32.9). The studies suggest that boluses of intravenous cyclophosphamide may be particularly beneficial.

Intravenous cyclophosphamide has also been reported to be effective in the management of several other serious forms of lupus, including hematologic, central nervous system, and vascular manifestations [22,23].

The potential toxicities of cyclophosphamide are substantial. Gastrointestinal complications with nausea and vomiting are common and many patients require antiemetic therapy, particularly for high-dose, intravenous therapy. Alopecia may on occasion be severe and require the use of a wig; however, patients need to be reassured that the hair will regrow even with continued therapy. Patients treated with cyclophosphamide are at heightened risk for infections and require careful evaluation for unexplained fever [24].

Long-term cyclophosphamide therapy may produce damage to gonadal tissue and lead to ovarian failure and azoospermia. In very young patients consideration should be given to the storage of ova or sperm prior to beginning therapy. In females, the risk of ovarian failure increases with patient age and is an almost universal complication in patients treated with cyclophosphamide after the age of 30 years. The recovery of ovarian function or spermatogenesis is unpredictable.

Cyclophosphamide may damage the bladder mucosa to cause hemorrhagic cystitis, bladder fibrosis, and transitional and squamous cell carcinoma [25,26]. A metabolite, acrolein, appears to be the irritant responsible for acute cystitis. Attention to generous fluid intake to reduce concentrations of acrolein in the bladder are helpful in minimizing these complications. In addition, mesna (2-mercaptoethane-sulfonate), a sulfonate that binds acrolein, should be considered in patients with known cyclophosphamide-induced bladder damage in whom continued drug administration is required. Patients treated with cyclophosphamide who develop evidence of reduced bladder capacity, such as frequency and small urinary volumes, should undergo cystometric evaluation. The findings of hematuria, particularly of new onset and after prolonged drug administration, should be assessed by urine cytology and cystoscopy for possible malignant changes of the bladder. Patients treated with prolonged courses of cyclophosphamide probably should be screened indefinitely for malignant changes in the bladder.

Malignancies of hematopoietic or lymphoreticular origin have been of particular concern in lupus patients treated with cyclophosphamide [27]. Although the actual risks have not been clearly defined, it is generally accepted that they exceed the risks associated with the use of azathioprine.

There are very few clinical studies of chlorambucil in systemic lupus [28]. A randomized trial concluded that chlorambucil (0.1–0.2mg/kg/day) was better than corticosteroids alone for extrarenal symptoms and roughly comparable to azathioprine and cyclophosphamide for the management of lupus nephritis [29]. Hematologic toxicity appears to be more severe and less predictable than with cyclophosphamide. In addition, the clear documentation of increased risks of leukemia with chlorambucil have greatly diminished enthusiasm for the drug [30].

Methotrexate

Studies of the folate antagonist methotrexate in lupus are very limited but suggest that it may be a reasonable alternative to antimalarials or low-dose corticosteroids in lupus patients with arthritis, skin rashes,

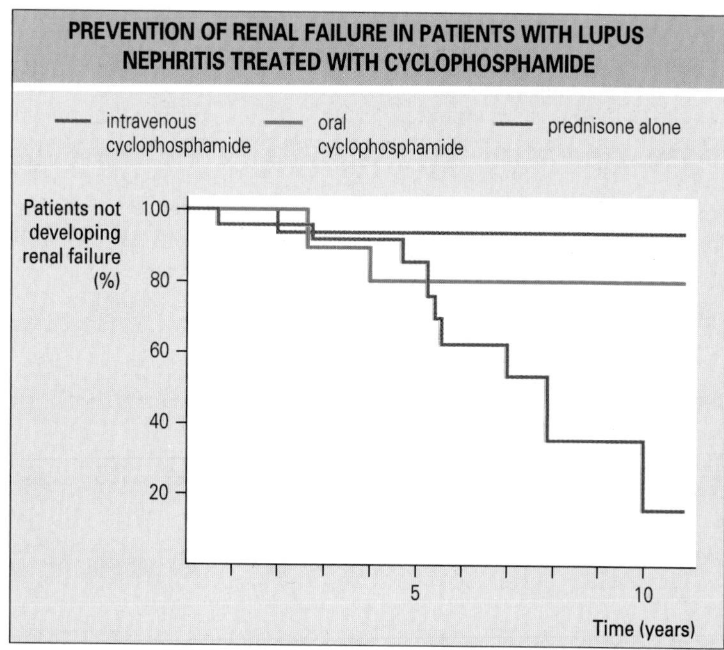

Fig. 32.9 Prevention of renal failure in patients with lupus nephritis treated with cyclophosphamide.

serositis, or fever [31]. The drug is given in weekly oral or, if needed, parenteral doses of 7.5–15mg; this is similar to drug schedules in rheumatoid arthritis. Since methotrexate is eliminated by both glomerular filtration and active tubular secretion, dose reductions are necessary in lupus patients with compromised renal function. The principal toxicities of low-dose methotrexate consist of mucositis, various forms of gastrointestinal intolerance and elevations of serum liver enzymes.

Cyclosporin A

Clinical studies of cyclosporin A in systemic lupus are limited, with no clear evidence of clinical efficacy [32,33]. Adverse drug reactions include nausea, anorexia, skin flushing and burning; a peculiar angioedema with reduction of C1 esterase inhibitor levels has been reported. The side effects of hypertension and direct renal toxicity from cyclosporin A, in particular, would appear to limit the usefulness of the drug in the management of lupus.

Dapsone

Dapsone (diaminodiphenylsulfone) is used in the management of various cutaneous features of lupus including discoid, subacute cutaneous, bullous, and lupus profundus lesions [35–37]. Therapy is typically begun with 50mg daily with gradual increases of the dose up to a maximum of 150mg/day. Hematologic side effects of dapsone are common and require careful monitoring. A dose-related hemolysis is evident in most patients. This is particularly severe in patients with G6PD deficiency, and routine screening for G6PD deficiency prior to therapy is recommended. In addition, methemoglobinemia with weakness, tachycardia, nausea, headache, and abdominal pain may develop.

Immune Globulin

Intravenous immune globulin has a number of effects on immune function including the suppression of antibody formation, suppression of T lymphocyte proliferation and reduction of natural killer cell activity. The mechanism of action is not entirely clear although it is thought to involve interference with Fc receptor function or interaction of anti-idiotype antibodies with antibody-producing cells or secreted antibody. A number of different immune globulin preparations are available. Typical dose schedules used in investigational studies in lupus have ranged from 300–400mg/kg/day given for 5 consecutive days, often followed by maintenance monthly therapy. The major contraindication is IgA deficiency, an occasional finding in lupus patients. Adverse reactions include fever, chills, myalgias, and abdominal or chest pain typically seen during or shortly after infusion; true anaphylactic reactions are very rare.

The principal indication for immune globulin in lupus is for the management of lupus thrombocytopenia [38]. Therapy is associated with a prompt rise in the platelet count in the majority of patients; however, the rate of relapse is high. This suggests that the primary role of immune globulin in lupus thrombocytopenia may be for control of acute bleeding or to rapidly increase the platelet count to permit splenectomy or other surgery. In addition, immune globulins are often used in combination with other forms of slow-acting drug therapy, such as immunosuppressives or danazol. Immune globulin has also been used in the investigational treatment of children with lupus nephritis [39] and cerebral vasculitis [40].

Danazol

The attenuated androgen, danazol, is useful in the management of lupus thrombocytopenia [41] and perhaps discoid lupus [42]. The mechanism of action of the drug has not been defined but may involve the influences of endocrine changes (suppression of pituitary follicle stimulating hormone and luteinizing hormone) on immune or reticuloendothelial functions. Pregnancy, breast feeding or unexplained genital bleeding are absolute contraindications to danazol therapy, and the drug must be used with caution in patients with liver or renal involvement. The principal adverse reactions relate to hormonal changes induced by the drug, such as vaginitis, irregular menses including amenorrhea, virilization, and emotional lability. Drug effects on the liver require monitoring of liver chemistries [43]; hepatic tumors have been reported with long-term danazol therapy [44,45].

Plasma Exchange

Since immune complexes or pathologic antibodies in the serum of lupus patients are thought to mediate tissue inflammation, theoretically their removal by plasma exchange (plasmapheresis) should be beneficial in lupus management. Although concentrations of serum immunoglobulins may be reduced by plasma exchange, the changes are only transient and rapidly return to normal levels once plasma exchange is stopped. Despite numerous clinical trials, however, it has been very difficult to actually prove that plasma exchange improves lupus activity or has a role in chronic management. Recent interest in plasma exchange in lupus has focused on its combination with intravenous cyclophosphamide (stimulation–depletion) [46] and the use of immunoabsorbent columns for the selective removal of autoantibodies [47].

Total Lymphoid Irradiation

Fractionated radiotherapy to central lymphoid structures (total lymphoid irradiation) has been used experimentally in the treatment of a small group of patients with lupus [48,49]. Total lymphoid irradiation produces a rather marked lymphopenia, with a preferential depletion of CD4 lymphocytes that may persist for several years or longer. This results in impairments of both cell-mediated immunity and T-cell-dependent antibody production. In patients with lupus nephritis, reductions in proteinuria, increases in serum albumin, and improvements in renal function have been noted following total lymphoid irradiation. Patients treated with total lymphoid irradiation appear to be at substantial risk for infectious complications and perhaps increases in the risks of acute leukemia and solid tumors and cardiovascular disease [50].

REFERENCES

1. Klippel JH. Systemic lupus erythematosus. Treatment-related complications superimposed on chronic disease. JAMA. 1990;**263**:1812–15.
2. Balow JE, Austin HA III. Renal disease in systemic lupus erythematosus. Rheum Dis Clin North Am. 1988;**14**:117–33.
3. Laitman RS, Glicklich D, Sablay LB, et al. Effect of long-term normalization of serum complement levels on the course of lupus nephritis. Am J Med. 1989;**87**:132–8.
4. Karsh J, Kimberly RP, Stahl NI, Plotz PH, Decker JL. Comparative effects of aspirin and ibuprofen in the management of systemic lupus erythematosus. Arthritis Rheum. 1980;**23**:1401–4.
5. Kimberly RP. Treatment. Corticosteroids and anti-inflammatory drugs. Rheum Dis Clin North Am. 1988;**14**:203–21.
6. Bouland DL, Specht NL, Hegstad DR. Ibuprofen and aseptic meningitis. Ann Intern Med. 1986;**104**:731.
7. Callen JP. Chronic cutaneous lupus erythematosus: Clinical, laboratory, therapeutic, and prognostic examination of 62 patients. Arch Dermatol. 1982;**118**:412–16.
8. Wallace DJ. The use of quinacrine (atabrine) in rheumatic diseases: a reexamination. Semin Arthritis Rheum. 1989;**18**:282–96.
9. The Canadian Hydroxychloroquine Study Group. A randomized study of the effect of withdrawing hydroxychloroquine sulfate in systemic lupus erythematosus. N Engl J Med. 1991;**324**:150–4.
10. Parke AL. Antimalarial drugs, systemic lupus erythematosus and pregnancy. J Rheumatol. 1988;**15**:607–10.
11. Finbloom DS, Silver K, Newsome DA, Gunkel R. Comparison of hydroxychloroquine and chloroquine use and the development of retinal toxicity. J Rheumatol. 1985;**12**:692–4.
12. Felson DT, Anderson J. Evidence for the superiority of immunosuppressive drugs and prednisone over prednisone alone in lupus nephritis. Results of a pooled analysis. N Engl J Med. 1984;**311**:1528–33.
13. Nossent JC, Swaak AJG. Pancytopenia in systemic lupus erythematosus related to azathioprine. J Intern Med. 1990;**227**:69–72.
14. Jeurissen MEC, Boerbooms AM Th, van de Putte LBA, Kruijsen MWM. Azathioprine induced fever, chills, rash, and hepatotoxicity in rheumatoid arthritis. Ann Rheum Dis 1990;**49**:25–7.
15. Vismans JJ, Briët E, Meijer K, den Ottolander GJ. Azathioprine and subacute myelomonocytic leukemia. Acta Med Scand. 1980;**207**:315–9.
16. Woolf AS, Conway G. Systemic lupus erythematosus and primary cerebral lymphoma. Postgrad Med J. 1987;**63**:569–72.
17. Nyberg G, Eriksson O, Westberg NG. Increased incidence of cervical atypia in women with systemic lupus erythematosus treated with chemotherapy. Arthritis Rheum. 1981;**24**:648–50.
18. Kinlen LJ, Peto J, Doll R, Sheil AGR. Cancer in patients treated with immunosuppressive drugs. Br Med J. 1981;**282**:474.
19. Kirshon B, Wasserstrum N, Willis R, Herman GE, McCabe ERB. Teratogenic effects of first-trimester cyclophosphamide therapy. Obstet Gynecol. 1988;**72**:462–4.
20. Balow JE, Austin HA III, Muenz LR, et al. Effect of treatment on the evolution of renal abnormalities in lupus nephritis. N Engl J Med. 1984;**311**:491–5.
21. Austin HA III, Klippel JH, Balow JE, et al. Therapy of lupus nephritis: Controlled trial of prednisone and cytotoxic drugs. N Engl J Med. 1986;**314**:614–9.
22. Winkler A, Jackson RW, Kay DS, et al. High-dose intravenous cyclophosphamide treatment of systemic lupus erythematosus-associated aplastic anemia. Arthritis Rheum. 1988;**31**:693–4.
23. McCune WJ, Golbus J, Zeldes W, Bohlke P, Dunne R, Fox DA. Clinical and immunologic effects of monthly administration of intravenous cyclophosphamide in severe systemic lupus erythematosus. N Engl J Med. 1988;**318**:1423–31.
24. Kattwinkel N, Cook L, Agnello V. Overwhelming fatal infection in a young woman after intravenous cyclophosphamide therapy for lupus nephritis. J Rheumatol. 1991;**18**:79–81.
25. Pedersen-Bjergaard J, Ersbll J, Hansen VL, et al. Carcinoma of the urinary bladder after treatment with cyclophosphamide for non-Hodgkin's lymphoma. N Engl J Med. 1988;**318**:1028–32.
26. Thrasher JB, Miller GJ, Wettlaufer JN. Bladder leiomyosarcoma following cyclophosphamide therapy for lupus nephritis. J Urol. 1990;**143**:119–21.
27. Gibbons RB, Westerman E. Acute nonlymphocytic leukemia following short-term, intermittent, intravenous cyclophosphamide treatment of lupus nephritis. Arthritis Rheum. 1988;**31**:1552–4.
28. Snaith MI, Holt JM, Oliver DO, et al. Treatment of patients with systemic lupus erythematosus including nephritis with chlorambucil. Br Med J. 1973;**2**:197–201.
29. Ivanova MM, Nassonova VA, Solovyo SK, et al. Controlled trial of cyclophosphamide, azathioprine, and chlorambucil in lupus nephritis (a double-blind trial). Vopr Revum. 1981;**2**:11–18.
30. Patapanian H, Graham S, Sambrook PN, et al. The oncogenicity of chlorambucil in rheumatoid arthritis. Br J Rheumatol. 1988;**27**:44–7.
31. Rothenberg RJ, Graziano FM, Grandone JT, et al. The use of methotrexate in steroid-resistant systemic lupus erythematosus. Arthritis Rheum. 1988;**31**:612–5.
32. Isenberg DA, Snaith ML, Morrow WJW, et al. Cyclosporin A for the treatment of systemic lupus erythematosus. Int J Immunopharmacol. 1981;**3**:163–9.
34. Favre H, Miescher PA, Huang YP, Chatelanat F, Mihatsch MJ. Cyclosporin in the treatment of lupus nephritis. Am J Nephrol. 1989; **9**(Suppl 1): 57–60.
35. Holtman JH, Neustadt DH, Klein J, Callen JP. Dapsone is an effective therapy for the skin lesions of subacute cutaneous lupus erythematosus and urticarial vasculitis in a patient with C2 deficiency. J Rheumatol. 1990;**17**:1222–5.
36. Fleming MG, Bergfeld WF, Tomecki KJ, et al. Bullous systemic lupus erythematosus. Int J Dermatol 1989;**28**:321–6.
37. Yamada Y, Dekio S, Jidoi J, Ozasa S. Lupus erythematosus profundus – report of a case treated with dapsone. J Dermatol. 1989;**16**:379–82.
38. Maier WP, Gordon DS, Howard RF, et al. Intravenous immunoglobulin therapy in systemic lupus erythematosus-associated thrombocytopenia. Arthritis Rheum. 1990;**33**:1233–9.
39. Lin CY, Hsu HC, Chiang H. Improvement of histological and immunological change in steroid and immunosuppressive drug-resistant nephritis by high-dose intravenous gamma globulin. Nephron. 1989;**53**:303–10.
40. Sturfelt G, Mousa F, Jonsson H, et al. Recurrent cerebral infarction and the antiphospholipid syndrome: effect of intravenous gammaglobulin in a patient with systemic lupus erythematosus. Ann Rheum Dis. 1990;**49**:939–41.
41. West SG, Johnson SC. Danazol for the treatment of refractory autoimmune thrombocytopenia in systemic lupus erythematosus. Ann Intern Med. 1988;**108**:703–6.
42. Englert HJ, Hughes GV. Danazol and discoid lupus. Br J Dermatol.1988;**119**:407–9.
43. Chevalier X, Awada H, Baetz A, Amor B. Danazol induced pancreatitis and hepatitis. Clin Rheumatol. 1990;**9**:239–41.
44. Weill BJ, Menkes CJ, Cormier C, et al. Hepatocellular carcinoma after danazol therapy. J Rheumatol. 1988;**15**:1447–9.
45. Hubscher O, Elsner B. Nodular transformation of the liver in a patient with systemic lupus erythematosus. J Rheumatol. 1989;**16**:410–12.
46. Schroeder JO, Euler HH, Löffler H. Synchronization of plasmapheresis and pulse cyclophosphamide in severe systemic lupus erythematosus. Ann Intern Med. 1987; **107**:344–6.
47. Schneider M, Berning T, Waldendorf, Glaser J, Gerlach U. Immunoadsorbent plasma perfusion in patients with systemic lupus erythematosus. J Rheumatol. 1990; **17**:900–7.
48. Strober S, Field E, Hoppe RT, et al. Treatment of intractable lupus nephritis with total lymphoid irradiation. Ann Intern Med. 1985;**102**:450–8.
49. Ben-Chetrit E, Gross DJ, Braverman A, et al. Total lymphoid irradiation in refractory systemic lupus erythematosus. Ann Intern Med. 1986;**105**:58–60.
50. Klippel JH. Radiation rheumatology. J Rheumatol. 1987;**14**:4–5.

33

CLINICAL FEATURES OF SYSTEMIC SCLEROSIS

James R Seibold

Definition
- A generalized disorder of connective tissue affecting skin and internal organs.
- Characterized by fibrotic arteriosclerosis of peripheral and visceral vasculature.
- Variable degrees of extracellular matrix accumulation (mainly collagen) occur in both skin and viscera.
- Associated with specific autoantibodies, most notably anticentromere and anti-Scl-70.

Clinical features
- Raynaud's phenomenon.
- Tightening and thickening of skin (scleroderma).
- Involvement of internal organs, including gastrointestinal tract, lungs, heart and kidneys, accounts for increased morbidity and mortality.
- Risk of internal organ involvement strongly linked to extent and progression of skin thickening.

EPIDEMIOLOGY OF SYSTEMIC SCLEROSIS	
Peak age (years)	30–50
Sex distribution (F:M)	4:1
Prevalence rate (/100,000)	10–20
Annual incidence (/100,000)	1–2
Geography	Unrestricted
Genetic associations	?? DR5, DRw52, DR4
Relative risk	Unknown

Fig. 33.1 Epidemiology of systemic sclerosis.

HISTORY

Although there are allusions to diseases of hardening of the skin in the writings of Galen and Hippocrates, the first convincing description of scleroderma was of a 17-year-old woman in Naples in 1753. Her attending physician, Carlo Curzio, successfully managed her case with bloodletting, warm milk and 'small doses of quicksilver' [1]. The relationship of scleroderma to Raynaud's phenomenon was first described by Maurice Raynaud himself in 1865 and was a well-accepted association by the turn of the century. Strangely, the systemic nature of scleroderma and its characteristic internal organ features were more slowly recognized. In 1945, Goetz proposed the term *progressive systemic sclerosis* based on his detailed review of the visceral lesions [2]. Acceptance of the syndrome of limited scleroderma followed Winterbauer's 1964 description [3] of what subsequently became termed 'CREST syndrome' (Calcinosis, Raynaud's phenomenon, Esophageal dysmotility, Sclerodactyly and Telangiectasia). A detailed case controlled autopsy study in 1969 directed attention to the ubiquitous nature of the vascular lesion [4]. The etiology and pathogenesis remain unknown and no effective therapies for the basic disorder have been developed. Breakthroughs in treatment of specific clinical features have derived from agents developed for other purposes and include angiotensin-converting enzyme (ACE) inhibitors for the hypertension associated with renal involvement and histamine-2 (H2) receptor antagonists for chronic acid reflux.

EPIDEMIOLOGY

Precise epidemiologic information regarding systemic sclerosis is lacking. Studies based on hospital records and death registries suggest occurrence in between 4 and 12 individuals per million population per year (Fig. 33.1) [5]. It is likely that many cases of systemic sclerosis are unrecognized, particularly in limited disease where skin manifestations are often clinically subtle. For example, directed examination by rheumatologists of clinical probands of 'primary' biliary cirrhosis, 'primary' pulmonary hypertension and isolated Raynaud's phenomenon have found surprisingly frequent cases of systemic sclerosis. A population based study in South Carolina identified subjects through a questionnaire for the presence of Raynaud's phenomenon. Subsequent validation of subjects with more detailed questioning and examination, nailfold capillaroscopy and serologic study found evidence of substantial numbers of previously undiagnosed connective tissue disease [6]. These data suggest that true prevalence may be more than four-fold higher than previously recognized and lead to estimates that there are perhaps 100,000–200,000 cases of systemic sclerosis in the United States.

Onset of systemic sclerosis is highest in the fourth and fifth decade of life and is 3–4 times more common in women than men [7]. Disease is not linked to race, season, geography, occupation or socioeconomic status in any consistent way [5,7]. Environmental etiologies are nonetheless possible and include silica dusts, silicone surgical implants [8,9], vinyl chloride, epoxy resins, and trichloroethylene as implicated vectors. Familial occurrence of systemic sclerosis is quite rare [10] and convincing genetic associations are lacking.

CLINICAL FEATURES

Systemic sclerosis is a remarkably heterogeneous disorder with diverse initial presentations and variable disease course including wide differences in pace, extent and severity of any of its clinical manifestations. Unlike rheumatoid arthritis (RA) or systemic lupus erythematosus (SLE), periodic waxing and waning of symptoms and laboratory features is unusual. Consideration of pathogenesis and clinical presentations must include attention to vascular features, the prominent abnormalities of extracellular matrix, the evidence of immunologic derangement and the characteristic visceral features.

Vascular Abnormalities

Raynaud's phenomenon

Raynaud's phenomenon is defined as episodic color changes (pallor, cyanosis, erythema) occurring in response to environmental cold

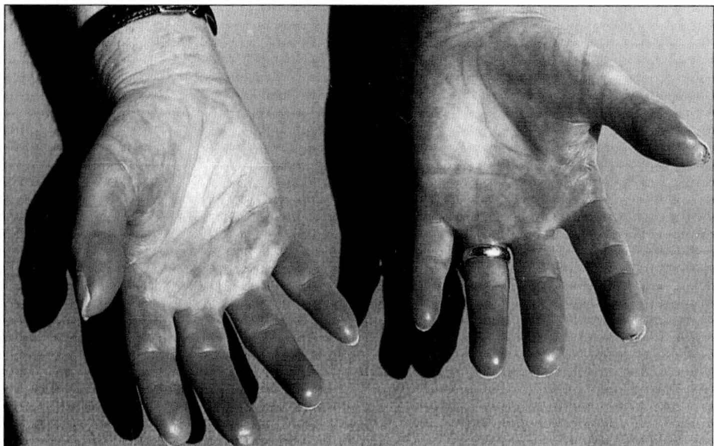

Fig. 33.2 The hands of a young woman with Raynaud's phenomenon. There is sharply demarcated cyanosis of the fingers with more proximal livedoid venular congestion.

and/or emotional stress. Although most typically noted in the fingers (Fig. 33.2), the circulation of the toes, ears, nose and tongue is also frequently affected. Individuals with Raynaud's phenomenon complain of symptoms of numbness and pain associated with the phases of pallor and cyanosis and of tingling and burning during the hyperemic recovery phase. The impact on hand function in cold environments can be substantial.

The prevalence of Raynaud's phenomenon in the general population is not precisely known but may be as high as 10–20% [11,12]. Reconciliation of these figures with the relative rarity of systemic sclerosis is difficult. In one population survey of nearly 7000 individuals, around 12% complained of subjective cold intolerance. Subsequent clinical review and examination suggested that only one quarter of these individuals could be accurately described as Raynaud's phenomenon but within this latter group, about 10% of these individuals had evidence of evolving systemic sclerosis [6].

Raynaud's phenomenon is the initial complaint in around three-quarters of patients with systemic sclerosis and in virtually all of those destined to evolve into systemic sclerosis with limited scleroderma (formerly CREST syndrome) (see below). The small subgroup (5%) of patients who never develop Raynaud's phenomenon are more frequently male and have poor survival principally due to their high risk for developing renal and myocardial involvement [13].

Perfusion to the skin normally exceeds that required for nutrition and oxygenation by 10–20-fold and reflects the role of skin blood flow as a principal mechanism of thermoregulation. Peripheral vasoconstriction in response to cold is physiologic and vasoconstriction sufficient to produce digital pallor or cyanosis may occur in normals, given a prolonged or severe enough cold exposure. Individuals with Raynaud's phenomenon have markedly reduced tolerance to environmental cold. This may occur in the absence of an underlying disease and in the absence of definable abnormalities of peripheral vascular structure and is termed primary or idiopathic Raynaud's phenomenon. Alternatively, there may be an underlying disease with one or more pathophysiologic abnormalities, so called secondary Raynaud's phenomenon, of which systemic sclerosis is an excellent example.

The potential importance of Raynaud's phenomenon in systemic sclerosis cannot be understated. It is an early and ubiquitous feature of disease and taken alone has considerable clinical impact. However, abnormalities similar to those of the peripheral circulation are widely distributed in the visceral vasculature as well and have major effects on morbidity and mortality.

In systemic sclerosis, structural narrowing of the digital arteries causes severe (>75%) attenuation of the arterial lumen [14] (Fig. 33.3). The principal lesion is one of intimal hyperplasia consisting of collagen and to a lesser degree of ground substance. While lesser degrees of fibrosis are noted in the adventitia, the media (smooth muscle) is little affected [14]. Normal peripheral vasoconstriction in response to cold superimposed on the structurally narrowed vessel would cause occlusion of the lumen [14]. Similarly, treatment of

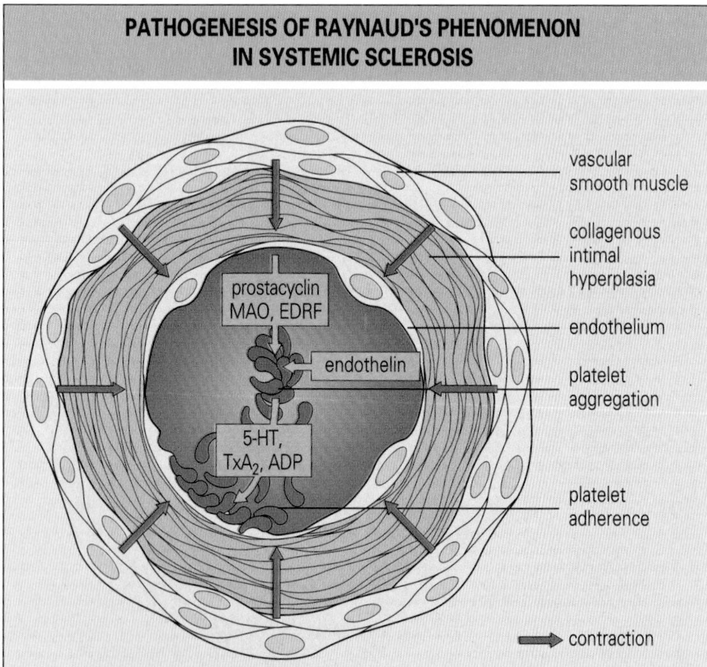

Fig. 33.3 Pathogenesis of Raynaud's phenomenon in systemic sclerosis. Endothelial injury results in secondary platelet activation. Platelets both adhere to subendothelium and aggregate locally leading to release of vasoconstrictive substances (5-HT, 5-hydroxytryptamine; TXA_2, thromboxane A_2; and ADP). Healthy endothelium opposes these effects with prostacyclin, monoamine oxidase (MAO), endothelium-dependent relaxation factor (EDRF) and by catabolism of 5-HT. Injured endothelium is less able to respond and also releases potent constrictive substances such as endothelin-I. In the setting of narrowed vessels from intimal hyperplasia, occlusive contraction is inevitable.

DIFFERENTIAL DIAGNOSIS OF RAYNAUD'S PHENOMENON
Structural vasculopathies
Large and medium arteries
Thoracic outlet syndrome
Brachiocephalic trunk disease (atherosclerosis, Takayasu's)
Crutch pressure
Small artery and arteriolar
Systemic lupus erythematosus
Dermatomyositis
Overlap syndromes
Cold injury
Vibration disease
Arteriosclerosis (thromboangiitis obliterans)
Chemotherapy (bleomycin, vinblastine)
Polyvinyl chloride disease
Normal vessels – abnormal blood elements
Cryoglobulinemia
Cryofibrinogenemia
Paraproteinemia
Cold agglutinin disease
Polycythemias
Normal blood vessels – abnormal vasomotion
Primary (idiopathic) Raynaud's phenomenon
Drug-induced (beta blockers, ergots, methysergide)
Pheochromocytoma
Carcinoid syndrome
Other vasospastic disorders (migraine, Prinzmetal)

Fig. 33.4 Differential diagnosis of Raynaud's phenomenon.

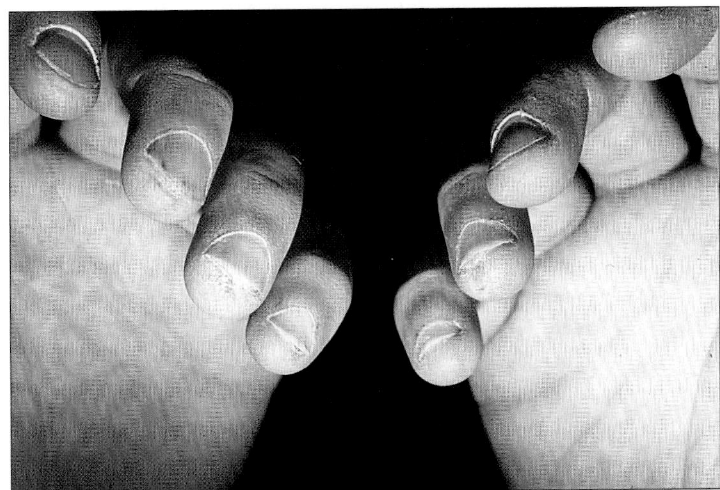

Fig. 33.5 Multiple digital ischemic ulcerations. Small areas of infarction at different stages of development and of variable severity of the fingertips of a young woman with several months of rapidly progressive scleroderma.

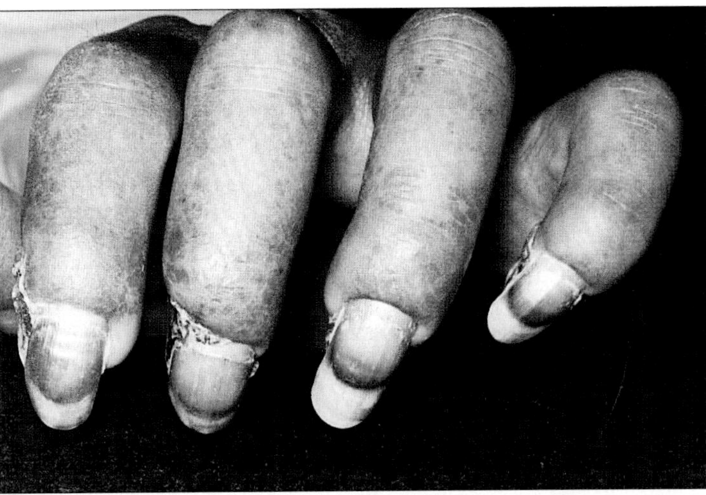

Fig. 33.6 Digital gangrene. Sharply demarcated gangrene of several weeks duration of multiple fingertips of a woman with recent onset of systemic sclerosis. Ultimately, these were managed with surgical debridement.

Raynaud's phenomenon with smooth muscle relaxants is less likely to work in the presence of a fixed obstructive lesion. Similar histopathologic changes are present in the small arteries and arterioles of internal organs [4,15]. Their presence serves to explain important clinical syndromes including scleroderma renal crisis and pulmonary hypertension.

Many factors other than structure are operative in the Raynaud's phenomenon of systemic sclerosis (Fig. 33.3). Platelet activation [16,17] causes local release of potent vasoconstrictors such as thromboxane A_2 and serotonin (5-hydroxytryptamine; 5-HT). Endothelial release of prostacyclin and endothelial monoamine oxidase (MAO) activity in the catabolism of serotonin represent the opposing vasodilatory influences and are reduced in the setting of endothelial injury [16]. Potent local vasoconstrictors may be released by injured endothelium, e.g. endothelin-I, while other local vasodilators may be lessened, e.g. nitric oxide or endothelium-dependent relaxation factor (EDRF) [18]. Hemorheologic abnormalities are well characterized in systemic sclerosis and may further reduce perfusion of the microvasculature. These include mild thrombocytosis, diminished red blood cell filtration and increased plasma viscosity.

The differential diagnosis of Raynaud's phenomenon is extensive and includes a variety of conditions which share pathophysiologic features of systemic sclerosis (Fig. 33.4).

Digital ischemic injury

The hallmark of severity of Raynaud's phenomenon in systemic sclerosis is the frequency of digital ischemic injury (Fig. 33.5). Around one third of patients experience at least one digital ulceration per year and patients are at risk of catastrophic peripheral digital gangrene (Fig. 33.6). Many of the factors thought to be involved in the pathogenesis of critical tissue ischemia are present in the microvasculature of scleroderma (Fig. 33.7). These include impaired vasomotion of afferent arterial circulation, enhanced neutrophil and platelet adherence to damaged endothelium, and impaired venous outflow possibly due to the altered hydrostatics of increased tissue pressure in affected digits.

Internal organ Raynaud's phenomenon

The fibrotic arteriosclerotic changes of the small artery and arteriole are omnipresent in the internal organs of patients with systemic sclerosis [4,15] and have great clinical significance. There is increased incidence of scleroderma renal crisis during cold weather months [19]. There are a variety of modern clinical studies suggesting that the internal organs sustain Raynaud-like intermittent ischemia during cold exposure. Heart involvement has been particularly well studied in this regard. The histopathologic finding of contraction band necrosis suggests intermittent myocardial ischemia [20]. Cold challenge in a laboratory setting has been shown to evoke both fixed and reversible thallium perfusion abnormalities [21] as well as transient regional wall motion abnormalities [22] and impaired left ventricular systolic function [23]. A study using ^{81}M krypton scanning demonstrated transient cold-induced perfusion decreases in the lungs of around one half of patients [24].

Microvascular abnormalities

There are characteristic architectural abnormalities of the microvasculature in systemic sclerosis which are easily appreciated by widefield microscopy of the nailfold capillary bed [25]. The changes of systemic sclerosis include enlargement and tortuosity of individual capillary loops interspersed with areas of capillary loop dropout. The mechanism of the capillary loop injury remains unresolved. At later stages of clinical disease, punctate telangiectasias develop (see Fig. 33.8) with typical locations including fingers, face, lips and oral mucosa.

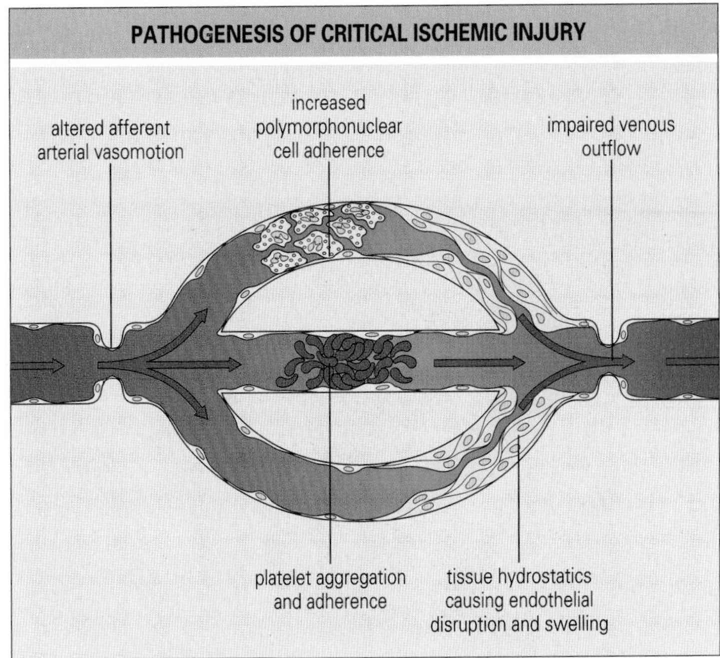

Fig. 33.7 Pathogenesis of critical tissue ischemia. Altered afferent vasomotion in scleroderma is but one factor in the pathogenesis of digital ulcers. Venous outflow is diminished and the microvasculature features endothelial swelling, local platelet plugging, leukocyte adherence and hydrostatic distortion of the capillary bed.

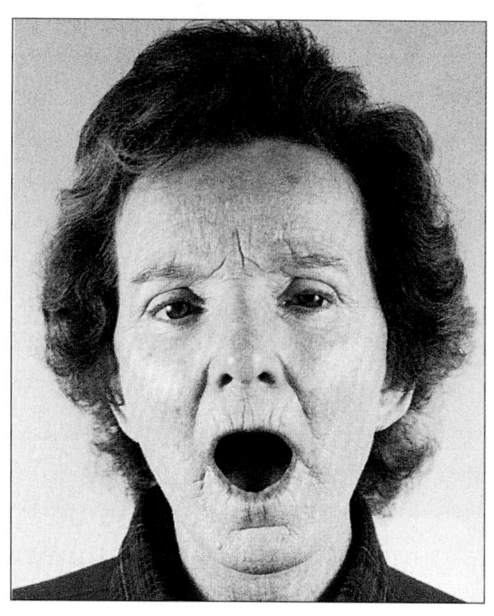

Fig. 33.8 Facial telangiectasias. Punctate telangiectasias are present on the lips and cheeks of this woman with long-standing limited scleroderma.

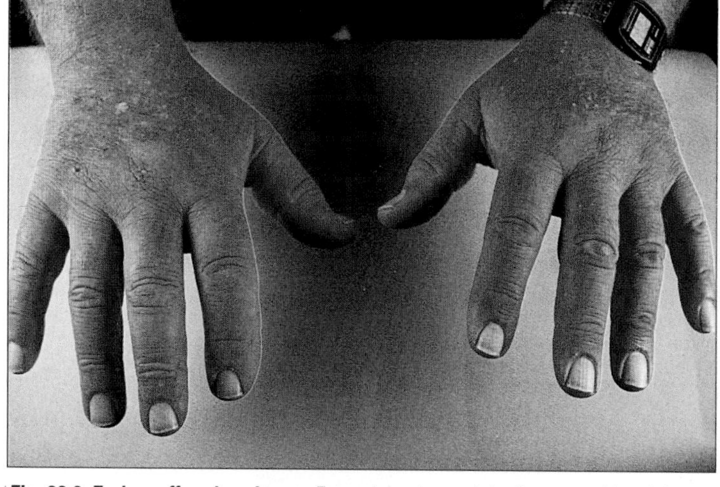

Fig. 33.9 Early, puffy scleroderma. Extensive edema of the fingers and hands in a man with several months of preceding Raynaud's phenomenon. Skin was not clinically thickened but became so on follow up.

Skin Involvement

The early tissue lesion of systemic sclerosis features ingress of immigrant inflammatory cell populations including helper-inducer lymphocytes, monocytes and mast cells. Autocrine effects of cytokine/growth factor from nonlesional cell populations such as circulating platelets, need to be considered as well. The net effect of this array of cells and signals is accumulation of extracellular matrix including collagen, glycosaminoglycan, fibronectin, adherence molecules and tissue water. The patient with scleroderma and the clinician recognize the result as the tightened and thickened skin (scleroderma) which is the clinical hallmark of disease.

Edematous change

An intrinsic feature of early systemic sclerosis is the painless swelling of the fingers and hands known as early 'puffy' or edematous scleroderma. Similar presentations are described in RA and SLE and is the most common early sign of overlap syndromes. Symptoms include morning stiffness and arthralgia. Carpal tunnel syndrome from median nerve compression is a frequent occurrence. Pitting edema of the fingers and dorsum of the hands is present on physical examination (Fig. 33.9) as well as in other locations including the upper arms, face and trunk. There are no differences in extent and severity of skin edema related to either duration or classification of disease. The edema is in part related to deposition of glycosaminoglycan in the dermis but may also reflect local inflammation, hydrostatic effects and microvascular disruption. Biopsy data suggest that edema does not regress with evolution of disease but rather becomes harder to detect clinically as superficial fibrosis develops.

Scleroderma

Scleroderma skin thickening begins on the fingers and hands in virtually all cases. The skin initially appears shiny and taut and may be erythematous at early stages (Fig. 33.10). Pruritus is common and may be intense. Digital skin creases are obscured and hair growth is reduced. The skin of the face and neck is usually involved next. Facial scleroderma causes an immobile and pinched facies (Fig. 33.11). The lips become thin and pursed and radial furrowing may develop about the mouth. The local skin thickening limits the ability to fully open the mouth impairing effective dental hygiene. Skin thickening may stay limited in extent to fingers, hands and face and may remain relatively mild. Extension to the forearms is frequently followed by spontaneous arrest of progression. In other patients, there is rapid centripetal spread to the upper arms, shoulders, anterior chest, back, abdomen and legs (Fig. 33.12). Prominent localized areas of hyperpigmentation and hypopigmentation may develop. Other patients experience generalized deepening of skin tone.

Skin thickening and disease classification

A multicenter study of the American College of Rheumatology proposed preliminary criteria for the classification of systemic sclerosis based on comparison of clinical and laboratory features of systemic

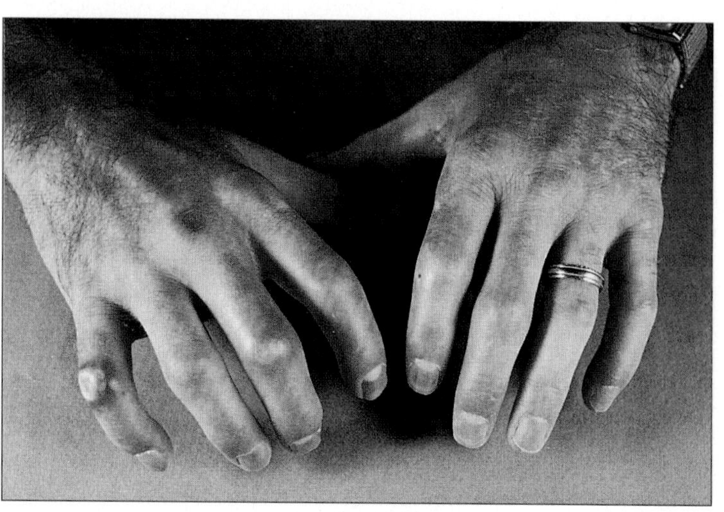

Fig. 33.10 Digital scleroderma. Advanced changes of scleroderma in the hand of a man with diffuse disease of several months duration. Fingers are held at maximum active extension.

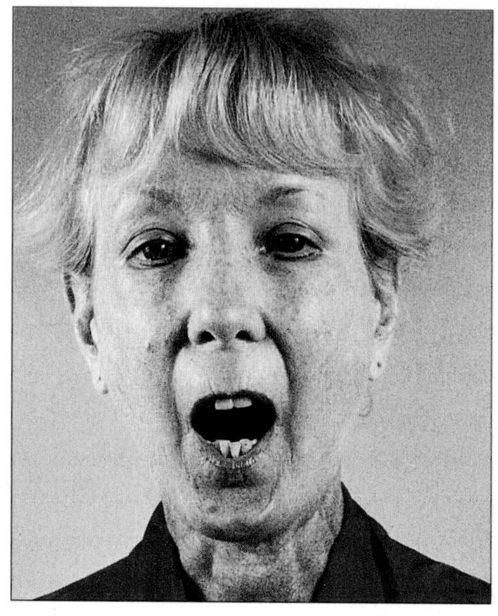

Fig. 33.11 Facial scleroderma. Taut smooth skin over the face of a woman with long-standing disease. Oral aperture is reduced and radial furrowing is present about the lips.

Gastrointestinal involvement

The third most common feature of systemic sclerosis, following Raynaud's phenomenon and scleroderma, is involvement of the gastrointestinal tract. There is no difference in prevalence or clinical severity of esophageal involvement between diffuse and limited scleroderma, and esophageal involvement is a principal feature of systemic sclerosis sine scleroderma.

Incompetence of the lower esophageal sphincter is suggested by symptoms of intermittent heartburn and associated bitter regurgitation. The pain is most commonly described as retrosternal burning. Impaired contractility of the smooth muscle portion (lower two-thirds) of the esophagus presents as dysphagia and odynophagia for solid foods. Complaints of a 'sticking' sensation of consistent location and variable severity are typical. Although thorough chewing of food can improve ability to swallow, many patients ultimately reduce their dietary intake to control symptoms. The lower esophageal dysmotility is an important cofactor in the symptoms of reflux by allowing pooling of acid in the esophagus [38].

The esophageal changes include smooth muscle atrophy; fibrosis of the muscularis, submucosa and lamina propria; and varying degrees of mucosal erosion [4,39]. Motility studies at early stages of involvement have shown disordered myoelectric function attributed to impaired cholinergic neural function [40]. Although Raynaud-like responsiveness has not been demonstrated, vascular injury including endothelial swelling and basement membrane lamination of esophageal capillaries has been demonstrated at early stages [39].

Esophageal function may be assessed by manometrics [40], thin-barium recumbent cine-esophagraphy (Fig. 33.16), radionuclide transit studies [41] and by endoscopy [38]. Choice of test should be guided by the clinical information sought for management decisions.

Complications include erosive esophagitis, stricture and bleeding [38]. The presence of lower esophageal dysmotility is the principal influence on the development of erosive esophagitis which may be present in surprising degree even in the asymptomatic patient [38]. Nocturnal aspiration contributes to pulmonary complaints and should be suspected in clinical presentations of productive cough, pulmonary infiltrates and evidence of reactive airway disease.

Involvement of the stomach is common in systemic sclerosis but is rarely a source of important clinical complaint. Symptoms include ease of satiety and, rarely, presentations of acute gastric dilatation or gastric outlet obstruction. Telangiectases of the gastrointestinal tract are frequently seen on endoscopy but are rarely a source of gastrointestinal bleeding.

Small intestine involvement is a major source of morbidity in systemic sclerosis and one of the most frustrating clinical syndromes for both the patient and the physician. Although most frequent and most severe in patients with long-standing limited scleroderma, subtle involvement occurs in the majority of patients. Symptoms include intermittent bloating with abdominal cramps, intermittent or chronic diarrhea and presentations of intestinal obstruction and pseudo-obstruction. Malabsorption is detected as impaired D-xylose absorption or as increased quantitative fecal fat elimination. The underlying mechanism is similar to that of the esophagus where fibrosis and smooth muscle atrophy are noted although interspersed with areas of minimal change [40]. Bacterial overgrowth in areas of intestinal stasis is well documented. Flares of diarrhea and bloating often respond to empiric courses of broad spectrum oral antibiotics such as tetracycline, vancomycin or metronidazole. Jejunal cultures and the bile acid breath test are useful in diagnosis [42]. Pneumatosis intestinalis cystoides is a rare but ominous clinical sign. Volvulus and intestinal perforation have been reported.

Colon involvement is present in the majority of patients with systemic sclerosis but uncommonly a source of clinical symptoms. Constipation and pseudo-obstruction are the principal presentations.

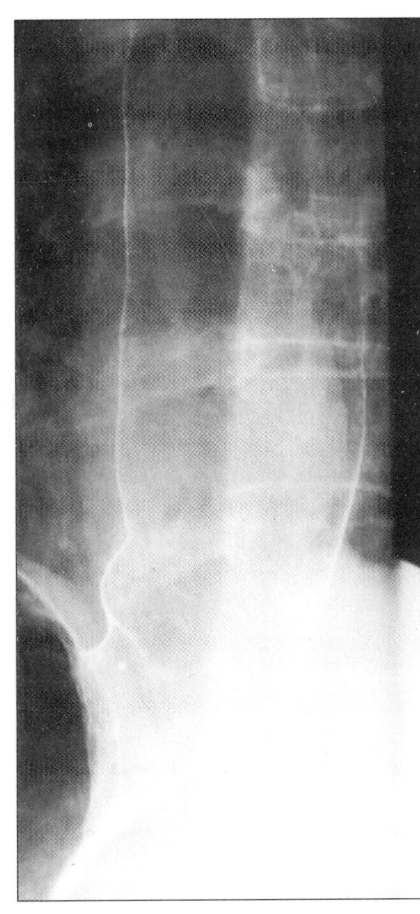

Wide-mouthed diverticula along the a
colon are characteristic but are neither
abscess. Rectal prolapse and fecal incon
ment of the anal sphincter.

Primary biliary cirrhosis occurs in ov
mainly as a late feature of limited diseas
fibrosis are distinctly uncommon.

Musculoskeletal features

The majority of patients with systemic
gia and morning stiffness. Joint line te
proliferation may be appreciated but o
Erosive arthropathy is demonstrable o
patients [44]. Loss of hand function is the
the tethering effects of skin thickening t
Inflammatory and fibrinous involvem
mimic arthritis. Tendon friction rubs can
passive motion of involved areas. The
over the wrists, ankles and knees. Inv
bursae may mimic the symptoms and au
friction rubs.

Muscle weakness, proximal greater t
disuse atrophy and from a disease-relat
drome is characterized by elevations
(typically 2–4-fold normal) including
phokinase [45]. Electromyographic abno
polyphasic potentials of normal and de
tion. The insertional irritability and fibr
polymyositis/dermatomyositis are unc
reveals interstitial fibrosis and fiber atro
tration and muscle fiber degeneration oc
that of polymyositis [46]. The clinical
waxing and waning of symptoms an
levels in a syndrome generally unrespon

Resorption of bone of the digital tuft
long-standing disease and is best ex

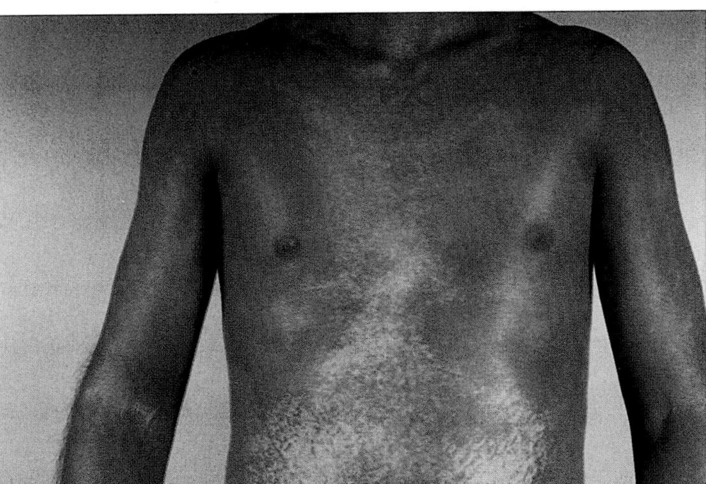

Fig. 33.12 Truncal scleroderma. Skin thickening of the chest and abdomen permit classification as diffuse scleroderma. There is both hyperpigmentation of the chest and hypopigmentation of the upper abdomen.

sclerosis with SLE, inflammatory muscle disease and isolated Raynaud's phenomenon [26]. Scleroderma skin thickening in any location proximal to the metacarpophalangeal joints was the single major criterion for classification of systemic sclerosis. The presence of two or more of the following features contributed further as minor criteria; sclerodactyly, digital pitting scars of fingertips or loss of digital finger pad substance, and bibasilar pulmonary fibrosis [26]. Many patients with confident diagnoses of systemic sclerosis do not fulfill these criteria and proximal skin thickening is a common clinical feature of many unrelated disorders (see Fig. 33.23).

Veteran clinical observers recognize subgroups of clinical and prognostic importance within the diagnosis of systemic sclerosis [27] which are not discriminated by the ACR classification criteria. A consensus proposal on nomenclature has been developed to permit separation of systemic sclerosis by clinical features alone with extent of skin involvement serving as a principal guide (Fig. 33.13) [27].

Clinical patterns of skin thickening

Study of systemic sclerosis is hampered by the absence of firm understanding about pathogenesis of disease. The absence of laboratory markers of disease progression and activity further impair study of the natural history of disease. Assessment of skin thickening as descriptive phenomenology is used as a clinical surrogate for monitoring disease progression and is the principal basis for classification of systemic sclerosis. Systemic sclerosis with *limited scleroderma* and systemic sclerosis with *diffuse scleroderma* are the two principal

CLASSIFICATION OF SYSTEMIC SCLEROSIS	
I	Diffuse scleroderma – skin thickening present on the trunk in addition to the face, proximal and distal extremities.
II	Limited scleroderma – skin thickening restricted to sites distal to the elbow and knee but also involving the face and neck. Synonym – CREST syndrome (C – subcutaneous Calcinosis, R – Raynaud's phenomenon, E – Esophageal dysmotility, S – Sclerodactyly, T – Telangiectasias).
III	Sine scleroderma – no clinically apparent skin thickening but with characteristic internal organ changes, vascular and serologic features.
IV	In overlap – criteria fulfilling systemic sclerosis occurring concomitantly with criteria fulfilling diagnoses of SLE, RA or inflammatory muscle disease.
V	Undifferentiated connective tissue disease – Raynaud's phenomenon with clinical and/or laboratory features of systemic sclerosis. These features include serum anticentromere antibody, abnormal nailfold capillaroscopy, finger edema and ischemic injury.

Fig. 33.13 Classification of systemic sclerosis.

clinical syndromes. These entities are of near equal prevalence and are so disparate in pace, severity and outcome as to warrant approach as two distinct conditions.

A typical natural history of limited scleroderma would begin with Raynaud's phenomenon as an isolated clinical finding to be followed by finger edema, although sometimes not for years. Clinically recognizable skin thickening follows edema after a time course ranging from months to years. Involvement remains limited in extent to fingers, hands, forearms, face and neck although the distal lower extremities may be involved as well. Change in extent of skin thickening and change in local severity of skin thickening are so slowly progressive as to remain undetectably different from year to year. Just as skin involvement is slowly progressive and limited, these patients enjoy a protracted disease course before the onset of visceral involvement.

At the other end of the scleroderma spectrum are individuals with rapidly progressive diffuse scleroderma. Finger edema and arthralgia are common first symptoms and have nearly contemporaneous onset (within months) with Raynaud's phenomenon. Skin thickening again begins on the fingers but with subsequent rapid worsening of extent and severity. In diffuse scleroderma, the pace of extension of skin change is somewhat variable ranging from development of total body skin thickening within a few months to more insidious progression over several years. Whereas some patients experience relapsing patterns with intermittent periods of rapidly progressive skin involvement interspersed with periods of clinical quiescence, the typical pattern is of unremitting progression. There appear to be important differences between early and late diffuse scleroderma. Limited data suggest that untreated diffuse scleroderma is uniphasic, with peaking of skin involvement in both extent and severity within 2–3 years of disease onset [28,29]. Following the plateau phase, many patients spontaneously lessen their skin thickening although the rate and ultimate extent of improvement are quite variable.

Clear and reliable information about the natural history of skin thickening is lacking. Even early in the development of diffuse scleroderma, clinical course is quite variable. In some patients, spontaneous arrest of disease progression occurs as early as a few months whereas others progress in unrelenting fashion over years.

At very late stages of disease and in both syndromes, atrophy develops leading to fragility and laxity of the dermis although tethering to deeper tissues may still be appreciated. The clinical observation of improving skin change in late diffuse scleroderma may reflect in part this atrophic phase.

The diagnosis of systemic sclerosis is clinically obvious once skin thickening has developed. Accurate and early classification is the paramount clinical issue because the relative risk of accruing new internal organ involvement closely parallels the pace, progression and extent of skin involvement (see below).

Assessment of skin thickening

The clinical ability to assess serial change in extent and severity of skin thickening is necessary for (i) accurate classification as diffuse vs limited disease, (ii) monitoring the stage and activity of disease and (iii) in assessing response to therapy. Clinical palpation of skin is the most widely employed system. The total skin score [30] uses a rating scale (0 – normal skin, 1 – mild, 2 – moderate, 3 – severe and 4 – extreme skin thickening) of findings on clinical palpation of multiple body areas (see Fig. 33.14). Other proposed systems estimate both skin thickening as well as tethering [31]. Skin thickness ratings of experienced clinical investigators by clinical palpation correlate closely with skin core biopsy weights as well as with total hydroxyproline content [30]. The usefulness of the total skin score and more simplified versions (fewer body areas and 0–3 rating scales: normal, mild, moderate and severe thickening) are increasingly used in clinical research studies. Interobserver variability is low (10–15%) and the techniques are easily taught and reproduced [32,33].

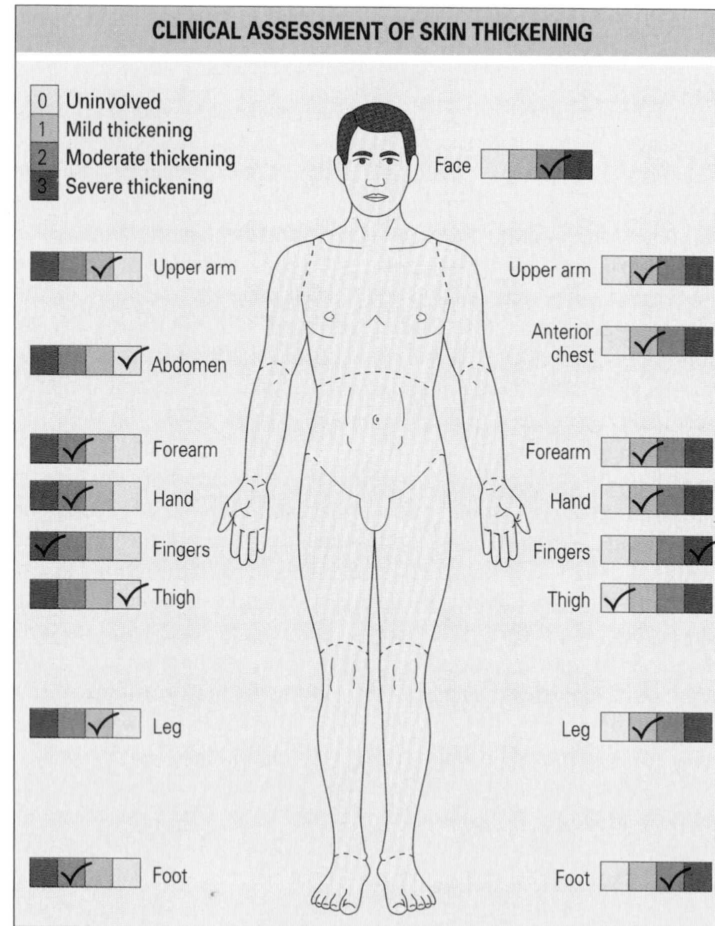

Fig. 33.14 Total skin score. Semiquantitative estimates by clinical palpation of the extent and severity of scleroderma skin change. In all cases, the initial areas involved are peripheral and are the most severely affected. The mild skin change on the chest permits classification of this subject as diffuse scleroderma.

Skin, visceral involvement and disease outcome

Skin involvement alone is symptomatic and by virtue of local tethering contributes to loss of motion, impaired hand function, cosmetic problems and lessened sense of well being [34]. It is thought unlikely that a treatment that worked for skin alone would gain approval for use in scleroderma. An individual patient who experienced lessening of skin thickening would likely be pleased with such an outcome. However, an individual with severe lung involvement, intractable intestinal dysmotility, recurrent digital ulcerations or severe loss of hand function should not be expected to accept softening of the skin as successful therapy.

The importance of skin involvement in systemic sclerosis stems from its linkage with visceral changes. Individuals at early stages of progressing diffuse scleroderma are at the highest risk of developing new internal organ involvement [29,31,35]. At later stages of diffuse disease, slowly improving skin change is typical. Skin involvement in late diffuse disease can improve to such an extent as to mimic clinical features of limited disease but complete remission is exceedingly rare [36]. In later disease, the risk of developing new visceral involvement is much reduced although still present. It should be emphasized that spontaneous improvement in established internal organ dysfunction is most uncommon.

Limited scleroderma is typified by insidious progression of skin involvement. Internal organ involvement other than renal occurs with frequencies close to that of diffuse disease but onset of involvement is delayed for years. Patients with long-standing diffuse and limited scleroderma, matched for sex, age and disease duration, differ only in terms of frequency of skeletal muscle involvement and extent of scleroderma [37]. Thus, systemic sclerosis incorporates two syndromes that are clinically divergent at early stages and clinically convergent late in the disease course (Fig. 33.15).

THE NATURAL H... CLA...

— diffus...
Total skin score
50
40
30 GI lung kidney heart
20
10
0
0 1

Fig. 33.15 Natural history of... rapid progression of skin invol... occurs most frequently during... Limited disease slowly increas... involvement is typically delaye... divergent in early years. In late... disease are nearly indistinguis...

Assuming that truly eff... of outcome and goals o... any given group. A drug... would be applicable (an... disease. In later years of... to speed spontaneous i... involvement would not l... derma at either early or l...

The same approach w... involvement. Early diff... which therapeutic benef... goal of therapy was pre... Therapy to improve pre... be directed at homogene... stall internal organ in... require trials of many ye...

These basic tenets of... bedside as well. Rational... with applicable measur... studies of systemic scler... trols matched for durat... inappropriate choices o... points; and lack of stand...

Systemic Features of Di...

General manifestations

The patient with system... symptoms ranging from... organ involvement to th... is uncommon in system... search for infection or o... the absence of gastrointe... frequently and is often a... unrelenting persistence c... impact of disease lead... sclerosis is uncommon. I... prior to their diagnosis.... chance to meet another p...

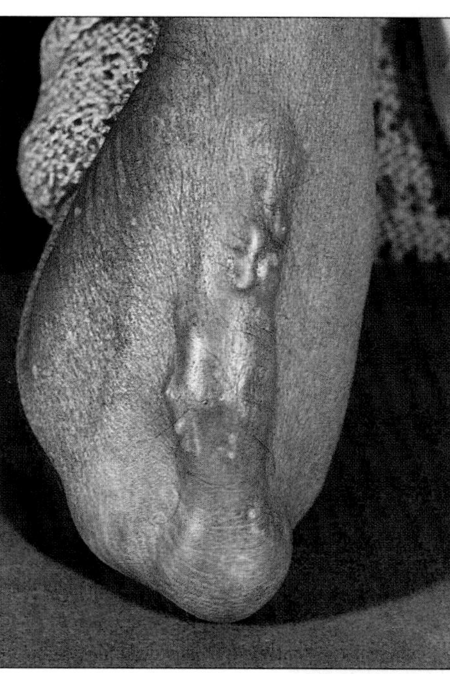

Fig. 33.17 Subcutaneous calcinosis. Extensive calcinosis is present in the preolecranon area of this woman with long-standing limited scleroderma.

ischemia. Resorption of the mandibular condyles and thickening of the periodontal membrane occurs as a sequelum of disordered mechanics of the temporomandibular joint secondary to facial skin thickening [47].

Subcutaneous calcinosis occurs in about one-half of patients with limited scleroderma and in about 10% of those with diffuse scleroderma (Fig. 33.17). Common locations include the fingers, preolecranon area, olecranon and prepatellar bursae. These areas become intermittently inflammed and a source of discomfort. Spontaneous extrusion through the skin is a frequent occurrence and a source of local infection. Protein rich in gamma-carboxyglutamic acid is increased locally [48] and has led to unsuccessful trials with warfarin.

Pulmonary involvement

Pulmonary involvement is the leading cause of mortality and morbidity in later stages of systemic sclerosis. Any combination of vascular obliteration, fibrosis and inflammation may be present. Clinical presentations are insidious and include exertional dyspnea, diminished effort tolerance and nonproductive cough. Chest pain, pleuritic or anginal, are uncommon. Physical examination reveals early inspiratory fine to crackling rales in patients with interstitial fibrotic disease. In the case of pulmonary hypertension, findings include an audibly increased and palpable pulmonic component of the second heart sound, right ventricular gallops, murmurs of pulmonic and tricuspid insufficiency, jugular venous distention, hepatojugular reflux and pedal edema [49].

Patients with diffuse scleroderma are at risk for progressive interstitial fibrotic lung disease. Diffuse fibrosis and variable degrees of inflammatory infiltrate affect the alveoli, interstitium and the peribronchiolar tissues.

Individuals with limited scleroderma are also at risk for interstitial disease but also develop progressive pulmonary hypertension in the relative absence of parenchymal fibrosis. Both presentations are more often seen in long-standing disease [50]. Intimal hyperplasia and medial myxomatous degeneration are present in the small-to-medium sized pulmonary arteries in nearly one-half of patients with limited scleroderma [39,51]. Pulmonary arterial hypertension was present by right heart catheterization in 33% of all patients and in 50% of those with limited scleroderma in one series [52].

Chest radiographs are insensitive screening tests but at advanced stages of disease reveal increased interstitial markings most prominently at the bases or the changes of pulmonary hypertension (Figs. 33.18 and 33.19). High resolution computerized tomography (CT) reveals extensive interstitial change at early stages of disease but is expensive, poorly standardized, of dubious quantitative value and does not discriminate fibrosis from inflammation. Pulmonary function testing is the mainstay of clinical diagnosis and serial assessment. Evidence of restriction including reduced vital capacity, diminished compliance and increased ratios of forced expiratory volume to vital capacity is typical in interstitial disease [53,54]. Isolated or disproportionately decreased diffusing capacity should suggest pulmonary vascular involvement [50,54].

Pulmonary involvement, once established, is continually progressive and prevalence increases in parallel with duration of systemic sclerosis [53]. Occasionally patients improve either their measures of volume or diffusing capacity. Isolated severe (<40%) reduction in diffusing capacity confers a poor prognosis. Obstructive disease is best attributed to cigarette smoking or chronic aspiration.

Bronchoalveolar lavage findings include elevated proportions of neutrophils, lymphocytes and, less frequently, eosinophils [55] as well

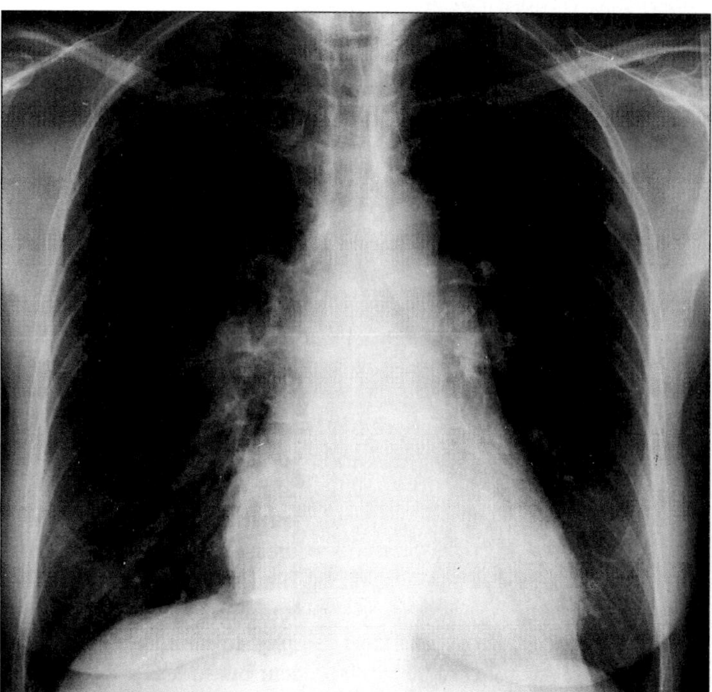

Fig. 33.18 Pulmonary hypertension. This patient had severe pulmonary hypertension documented on right heart catheterization. The lung fields are clear but the left heart border is straightened from elevation of the pulmonary conus and there is enlargement of the pulmonary arteries. This syndrome is most typical of later years of limited scleroderma.

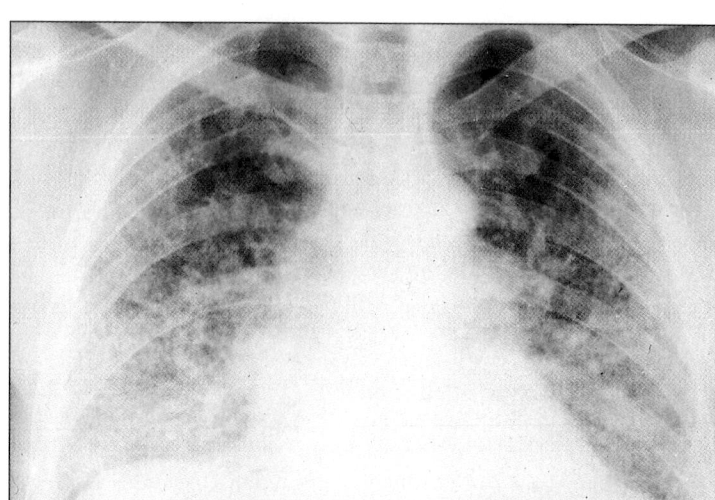

Fig. 33.19 Pulmonary interstitial fibrosis. Extensive parenchymal disease is apparent on this chest radiograph. Pulmonary functions confirmed severe restriction in this syndrome which occurs in both diffuse and limited scleroderma.

as increased concentration of immune complexes and fibronectin. It is unclear, based on current data, if the presence of inflammation should guide subsequent therapy. Pulmonary tissue has little capability to regenerate. Theoretically, a therapy which arrested pulmonary inflammation might slow the pace of fibrosis. Treatment of established fibrosis might improve measures of lung elasticity but would be unlikely to improve patient functional status.

Myocardial involvement

Patchy fibrosis of the myocardium is present at autopsy in as many as 81% of patients with systemic sclerosis [4,20]. Myocardial involvement is a principal determinant of survival in systemic sclerosis [56]. Presentations of chest pain and left ventricular failure are uncommon whereas many patients complain of diminished effort tolerance, palpitations and dyspnea. Separating myocardial from pulmonary involvement in clinical assessment is difficult.

Physical findings are nonspecific and include ventricular gallops, sinus tachycardia, signs of congestive heart failure and occasional pericardial friction rubs. Echocardiography is abnormal in 50% of patients and includes evidence of pericardial thickening or fluid but clinical presentations of pericarditis and of tamponade are infrequent [57].

Electrocardiographic abnormalities including atrial and ventricular arrhythmias and conduction disturbances. Ambulatory electrocardiographic study confirms a high prevalence of both supraventricular and ventricular tachyarrhythmias [58], the latter are strongly associated with both overall mortality and the syndrome of sudden death. Patients with limited systemic sclerosis are at only slightly decreased risk of myocardial involvement [59] although onset is typically delayed.

Renal involvement

Sudden onset of accelerated hypertension, rapidly progressive renal insufficiency, microangiopathic hemolysis, and consumptive thrombocytopenia in the setting of hyperreninemia constitutes the syndrome of 'scleroderma renal crisis' [19,60]. Peak risk is in early stages of diffuse scleroderma in association with rapid progression of skin involvement [35]. Renal involvement is distinctly uncommon in limited scleroderma.

Patients at risk for development of scleroderma renal disease cannot be identified by elevations of plasma renin activity [35]. Biopsy studies show pathologic evidence of renal vascular disease in many patients without clinical renal disease [4]. Elevations of plasma renin activity and diminished cortical perfusion are induced by cold challenge but do not predict impending renal disease. Markedly elevated plasma renin activity is encountered in virtually all patients at the onset of hypertension [35,60]. Functional vasospasm superimposed on pre-existing renal arteriolar fibrotic change is hypothesized to trigger release of renin. The subsequent vasoconstrictive effects of angiotensin II induce further renal cortical ischemia and the accelerated hypertension contributes as injury to the arteriolar media resulting in a fixed loss of cortical blood flow and necrosis. Extrarenal vascular injury is a hallmark of the syndrome and includes with intimal disruption, fibrin deposition and microangiopathic hemolysis. Normotensive renal failure related to arteriolar thrombosis is less common and has been linked to the use of corticosteroid therapy [61].

Profound anemia develops as well as thrombocytopenia with intravascular hemolysis as the dominant mechanism. Peripheral blood smears demonstrate fragmented red cells, serum fibrinogen levels decreased from previous values, and detection of fibrin degradation products. Urinalyses typically reveal protein and red cells although casts and nephrosis are unusual. Progression to anuric renal failure is the expected outcome if diagnosis is not promptly established and hypertension controlled.

Minor clinical features

Dryness of the eyes and mouth are prominent complaints in 20–30% of patients with systemic sclerosis (Fig. 33.20). Salivary gland enlargement is uncommon and relates to the presence of fibrotic gland replacement with minimal mononuclear cell infiltration noted on minor salivary gland biopsy [62]. Antibodies to the Sjögren's precipitins (Ro[SS-A] and La[SS-B]) are found in one-half of patients. Dryness of the mouth, in the setting of limited oral aperture and impaired hand function, renders adequate dental hygiene a difficult task.

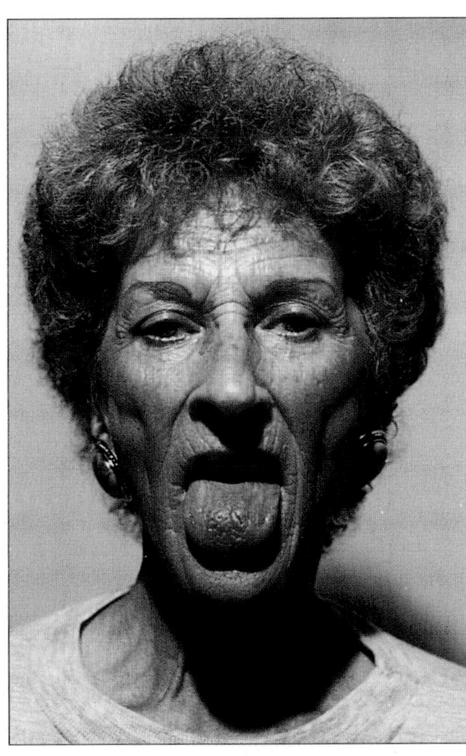

Fig. 33.20 Sicca syndrome in scleroderma. The tongue is parched and hypopapillated in this woman with sicca syndrome complicating long-standing diffuse scleroderma.

Thyroid gland fibrosis occurs in around one-fifth of patients and hypothyroidism is noted in as many as a quarter of patients [63]. Serum antithyroid antibodies, lymphocytic infiltration of the gland and clinical presentations of acute autoimmune thyroiditis are uncommon.

Impotence is an early clinical presentation of scleroderma [64] and is thought to represent an abnormality of penile vascular function.

Systemic sclerosis spares the central nervous system. Clinical neurologic presentations are principally those of entrapment neuropathy and include carpal tunnel syndrome, meralgia paresthethica, trigeminal neuropathy and facial nerve palsies. Autonomic dysfunction has been demonstrated [65] including disordered gastrointestinal cholinergic and peripheral adrenergic nervous function.

Pregnancy

Menstrual irregularities and amenorrhea occur in women with scleroderma in relation to the severity of illness. Difficulty with conception is frequent. Intrauterine growth retardation and low birth weights have been reported [66]. Pregnancy is not associated with worsening of scleroderma [66]. During the course of pregnancy, worsened symptoms of reflux esophagitis and cardiopulmonary decompensation may develop.

Scleroderma and malignancy

The coincidence of malignancy and scleroderma has been described although pathogenic interrelationships are unlikely. A syndrome of contemporaneous onset of systemic sclerosis with breast carcinoma has been suggested [67]. Surveys of malignancy in disease have revealed relative risks of lung carcinoma ranging from 1.8 to 16.5. There is no increased risk of esophageal cancers [68].

Immunologic Features

Systemic sclerosis occurs in overlap with other connective tissue disorders including SLE, polymyositis, RA and Sjögren's syndrome. Clinical associations with organ specific autoimmune disorders such as Hashimotos' thyroiditis and primary biliary cirrhosis are also well described. More frequently, patients with systemic sclerosis will present with clinical features and laboratory abnormalities insufficient to diagnose but reminiscent of a second specific overlapping condition.

Serologic abnormalities – nonspecific

Antinuclear antibodies are present in the sera of over 90% of patients with systemic sclerosis. These antibodies are not generally complement-fixing and are resistant to antigen-denaturation with ribonuclease and deoxyribonuclease. Antibody to native DNA is either lacking or present in extremely low titer. Patients with systemic sclerosis lack anti-Sm antibody and only about 20% have antibody directed against nuclear ribonucleoprotein (anti-nRNP) [69]. Serum rheumatoid factor and serum cryoglobulins are present in 30–50% of patients. Serum immune complexes have been found in systemic sclerosis [70] and have been correlated with cardiopulmonary involvement and overall severity of disease.

Serologic abnormalities – disease specific

Anticentromere antibodies give rise to coarse speckled patterns on interphase nuclei and appear as centromeric clustering on metaphase nuclei. Point prevalence surveys have suggested that between 50 and 96% of patients with limited systemic sclerosis had detectable serum anticentromere antibody [71,72]. In contrast, anticentromere antibody is found in less than 10% of individuals with diffuse scleroderma and is infrequent in other nonsystemic sclerosis connective tissue diseases. Patients with limited scleroderma and serum anticentromere antibody are more likely to have telangiectasias and calcinosis and less likely to have restrictive lung disease than those lacking anticentromere antibody [73]. The presence of serum anticentromere antibody is of great value in the differential diagnosis of Raynaud's phenomenon.

Between 20 and 40% of individuals with systemic sclerosis and diffuse scleroderma have serum antibody reactive with an extractable nuclear antigen of 70 kDa termed Scl-70 [74]. The antigen has been definitely characterized as DNA topoisomerase I, an intracellular enzyme involved in the initial uncoiling of supercoiled DNA prior to transcription, present at both centromeric and other intracellular locations [75]. Anti-Scl-70 (anti-topoisomerase I) antibodies inhibit function of the enzyme. Antigenicity to DNA topoisomerase I has been isolated to an 11 amino acid sequence which contains 6 sequential amino acids identical to a sequence present in the group-specific p30gag of mammalian retrovirus [76]. Serum antibody to retroviral p24gag is present in 25% of patients with diffuse scleroderma but unrelated to the presence of anti-Scl-70 [77]. Others have identified other antigenic epitopes of DNA topoisomerase I unrelated to the region of retroviral homology.

Abnormalities of cellular immunity

Total peripheral lymphocyte counts are typically normal in untreated systemic sclerosis. Subset analysis of T lymphocyte subpopulations demonstrates relative increased proportion of $CD4^+$ (T helper) cells with absolute reduction in $CD8^+$ (T suppressor) cells [78]. Plasma levels of the soluble CD8 molecule are elevated suggesting increased turnover or activation of the $CD8^+$ population [73]. Serum or plasma levels of soluble interleukin-2 (IL-2) receptors are increased in patients with systemic sclerosis [79] and correlate with disease severity, progression and mortality. The proportion of T lymphocytes expressing IL-2 receptors ($CD25^+$) is slightly increased in systemic sclerosis [78]. Prospective studies of both soluble IL-2 receptor and CD8 levels are in progress. A point prevalence survey of circulating cytokine levels found inconsistent results [80]. A reliable biologic marker of disease activity is much needed but lacking.

Clinically, patients with systemic sclerosis are not prone to opportunistic infection nor is there evidence overall of increased incidence of infection.

INVESTIGATIONS

Systemic sclerosis is a complex multisystem disorder which may present with many independent clinical problems requiring both accurate initial diagnosis and serial monitoring of progression. The potential for injudicious and cost-ineffective use of laboratory testing is substantial.

The diagnosis of systemic sclerosis should be made on clinical grounds and supported by confirmatory laboratory testing. The initial clinical problem involves differentiation from primary Raynaud's phenomenon (Fig. 33.21). Serologic studies of good specificity for systemic sclerosis (anticentromere and anti-Scl-70 antibodies) and performance of widefield nailfold capillaroscopy are established tests. Measures of in-vivo platelet activation and of endothelial integrity remain investigational.

Once systemic sclerosis is diagnosed, the clinical issue becomes one of accurate classification (Fig. 33.22). The above mentioned serologic studies support classification but are adjunctive to the clinical features. All patients deserve baseline assessments of the extent and severity of internal organ involvement. This would include, as a minimum, measures of pulmonary, esophageal, myocardial and renal status in addition to consideration of thyroid function. Choice of test to employ should be governed by the information sought and the expertise of the local laboratory.

As an example, consider the diverse assessments available for esophageal function. Radionuclide meals give quantitative information as to transit time and are sensitive screens for the presence of involvement. However, delayed transit could reflect either impaired motility or stricture. Endoscopy would permit measures of lower esophageal sphincter function, assessment of degree of erosive esophagitis and both assessment and treatment of stricture and ulceration. Cost and discomfort to the patient are considerable and use as a tool for serial assessment is impractical. Barium contrast studies describe both function and structure well but are limited again by discomfort, cost, and hazard to the patient. Their major limitation lies in lack of reliably standardized techniques of performance and interpretation. Manometry is sensitive and quantitative but produces little information of use for managing the individual patient.

As discussed above, there are no reliable laboratory tests of disease activity and progression. Nonspecific tests of immune activation including soluble IL-2 levels, soluble CD8, IL-2 and 4 levels [79,80]

CLINICAL AND LABORATORY FEATURES IN THE DIFFERENTIAL DIAGNOSIS OF RAYNAUD'S PHENOMENON

Feature	Primary Raynaud's	Systemic sclerosis
Sex	F:M 20:1	F:M 4:1
Age at onset	Puberty	25 years or older
Frequency	> 10 attacks per day	Usually < 5 per day
Precipitants	Cold, emotional stress	Cold
Ischemic injury	Absent	Present
Other vasomotor phenomena	Yes	No
Antinuclear antibodies	Absent	90–95%
Anticentromere antibody	Absent	50–60%
Anti-Scl-70 antibody	Absent	20–30%
Abnormal capillaroscopy	Absent	> 95%
In-vivo platelet activation	Absent	> 75%

Fig. 33.21 Clinical and laboratory features in the differential diagnosis of Raynaud's phenomenon.

COMPARISON OF CLINICAL AND LABORATORY FEATURES OF DIFFUSE SCLERODERMA AND LIMITED SCLERODERMA		
	Diffuse scleroderma	Limited scleroderma
Raynaud's phenomenon	90%	99%
Finger swelling	95%	90%
Tendon friction rubs	70%	5%
Arthralgia	98%	90%
Proximal weakness	80%	60%
Calcinosis	20%	40%
Telangiectasias	60%	90%
Esophageal dysmotility	80%	90%
Small bowel involvement	40%	60%
Interstitial lung disease	70%	35%
Pulmonary hypertension	5%	25%
Myocardiopathy	15%	10%
Renal 'crisis'	20%	1%
Sicca syndrome	15%	35%
Antinuclear antibody	90%	90%
Anticentromere antibody	5%	50–90%
Anti-Scl-70 antibody	20–30%	10–15%
Cumulative survival (5 year) (10 year)	70% 50%	90% 70%

Fig. 33.22 Comparison of clinical and laboratory features of diffuse scleroderma and limited scleroderma.

are under study and have promise. Additional tests need be developed to serially and quantitatively assess vascular status and matrix production.

There are sufficient data available to permit reasoned judgments as to which investigations warrant serial performance as measures of disease progression. These would include pulmonary function testing on a yearly basis in early diffuse scleroderma and on a biannual basis in all other circumstances. The insidious onset of hypothyroidism mandates performance of thyroid function testing on an annual basis.

The clinician should continually consider testing in light of reproducibility, accuracy, sensitivity to change, complexity and validity in addition to cost factors, discomfort and hazard to the individual patient. There is no defined panel of investigations that should be performed in all subjects with systemic sclerosis.

DIFFERENTIAL DIAGNOSIS

The differential diagnosis of systemic sclerosis is extensive (Fig. 33.23). In addition to the disorders that must be considered in the recognition of systemic sclerosis at the initial presentation of Raynaud's phenomenon (Fig. 33.4), early stages of disease often share clinical and laboratory features of other connective tissue diseases such as SLE and RA. Often the most prudent label would be one of undifferentiated connective tissue disease. Once skin thickening has developed, the differential diagnosis includes a wide array of other disorders in which tightening and thickening of the skin are prominent features. Finally, systemic sclerosis must be considered in the clinical approach to patients with specific disorders in which internal organ features are similar. For example, a young woman with pulmonary hypertension and Raynaud's phenomenon or an older patient with esophageal dysmotility would represent diverse clinical presentations in which underlying systemic sclerosis would warrant consideration.

DIFFERENTIAL DIAGNOSIS OF SCLERODERMA
Disorders characterized by Raynaud's phenomenon
Disorders characterized by similar presentations
Systemic lupus erythematosus Rheumatoid arthritis Inflammatory myopathy
Disorders characterized by similar visceral features
Primary pulmonary hypertension Primary biliary cirrhosis Idiopathic intestinal hypomotility Collagenous colitis Idiopathic interstitial pulmonary fibrosis
Disorders characterized by skin thickening
Affecting the fingers Diabetic digital sclerosis Vinyl chloride disease Vibration syndrome Bleomycin-induced scleroderma Chronic reflex sympathetic dystrophy Amyloidosis Acrodermatitis Sparing the fingers Scleredema/scleromyxedema Eosinophilic fasciitis Eosinophilia-myalgia syndrome Generalized subcutaneous morphea Fibrosis associated with augmentative mammoplasty Amyloidosis Carcinoid syndrome Pentazocine-induced scleroderma

Fig. 33.23 Differential diagnosis of scleroderma.

With the notable exception of the digital sclerosis complicating diabetes mellitus [81], the disorders characterized by tightening and thickening of the skin should be suspected when skin involvement spares the fingers.

Localized Scleroderma

Localized scleroderma includes several conditions of clinical and histopathologic similarity to the skin involvement of systemic sclerosis but in which systemic features are absent. Linear scleroderma is characterized by a band of sclerotic induration and hyperpigmentation of skin. Typically, linear scleroderma is restricted to a single extremity or the face. Disease begins with a localized band of erythema which evolves to thickening of skin with tethering to deeper tissues. Irregular atrophy of underlying subcutaneous fat is typical and extension to underlying muscle and bone may occur. Involvement of the face (coup de sabre) in children is associated with asymmetric growth and progressive facial disfigurement. Asymmetric growth of an affected extremity in childhood leads to leg length discrepancy (Fig. 33.24).

Morphea is a variety of localized scleroderma characterized by either small discrete spots (guttate morphea) or by larger patches (morphea en plaque) of scleroderma-like skin change. Lesions typically are 'target' with an erythematous or violaceous border and with central hypopigmentation. Disease may occur in many locations either simultaneously or serially over several years. Atrophy with persistent pigmentary change, spontaneous improvement and even total clinical resolution of morphea is typical after periods of

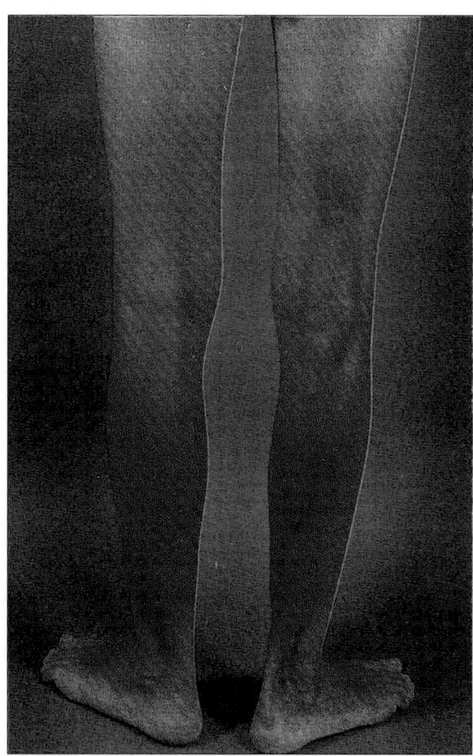

Fig. 33.24 Linear scleroderma. Present since age 5 in this 12-year-old girl, atrophy of the thigh and calf are apparent. As growth continues, leg length discrepancy would be anticipated.

several months to several years [82]. Morphea can be more generalized and occur with systemic symptoms including fatigue and weight loss. Generalized subcutaneous morphea is an exceedingly rare condition in which inflammation and fibrosis of the subcutaneum develops with extension to the dermis and to the underlying fascia [83].

Eosinophilic Fasciitis

Eosinophilic fasciitis is characterized by inflammation and thickening of the deep fascia. Extension superficially to the dermis is common. Onset frequently follows periods of unusual physical exertion and trauma, particularly in males [84]. A typical disease course would begin with precipitous onset of pain and swelling of the extremities soon followed by progressive induration of the skin and subcutaneous tissues. Areas of involvement include the forearms, legs and, on occasion, the hands, feet and trunk. The affected skin is shiny and erythematous with a coarse orange peel appearance. Carpal tunnel syndrome may occur and contractures develop early in the course of illness. Raynaud's phenomenon and internal organ features of systemic sclerosis do not occur. Laboratory abnormalities include peripheral eosinophilia and modestly elevated erythrocyte sedimentation rates. Diagnosis is made by full thickness (skin to skeletal muscle) wedge biopsy in which the deep fascia and subcutis are edematous and infiltrated with inflammatory cells including eosinophils. As the disease progresses, fibrosis of the fascia, subcutaneum and dermis develops which mimics the tissue features of scleroderma. The natural history of eosinophilic fasciitis remains unclear. Many patients improve spontaneously or while on glucocorticoids over periods of 2 to 5 years, although histopathologic evidence of fibrosis persists. Others have a disease course of recurrent relapse and remission. Later years of disease are typified by painful symmetric arthritis.

Eosinophilia-Myalgia Syndrome

An epidemic of now more than 1500 cases of abrupt onset of myalgia, fatigue and peripheral eosinophilia was recognized in 1989. Use of contaminated L-tryptophan dietary supplement traced to a single manufacturer was identified as the precipitating agent and attributed to both use of a new strain of *Bacillus amyloliquefaciens* in the fermentation process and reduced use of powdered carbon in a purification step [85]. The clinical features of eosinophilia-myalgia syndrome (EMS) are (i) dermal and fascial induration of the extremities (lower more than upper), (ii) dyspnea, dry cough and mild hypoxemia occasionally with a Löffler syndrome-like pneumonitis or with apparent pulmonary microvascular disruption, (iii) peripheral neuritis and (iv) hepatitis. Disabling muscle pain is frequent. Skin involvement typically evolves to mimic that of eosinophilic fasciitis [86].

Scleredema/Scleromyxedema

Scleredema (scleredema adultorum of Buschke) and scleromyxedema (papular mucinosis, lichen myxedematosus) are connective tissue disorders characterized by widespread induration and thickening of the skin resulting from accumulation of collagen and proteoglycan in the dermis. The distribution of skin involvement is typically face, neck, mantle and cape. The sparing of the fingers and hands, as well as the absence of Raynaud's phenomenon and of visceral involvement, permit clinical differentiation from systemic sclerosis. Histopathologically, both scleredema and scleromyxedema show minimal epidermal changes, whereas the dermis is markedly thickened with variable degrees of proteoglycan, hyaluronic acid and collagen deposits [87]. Scleredema and scleromyxedema have both been linked to underlying plasma cell dyscrasia and around one-half of adult scleredema patients have diabetes mellitus.

REFERENCES

1. Rodnan GP, Benedek TG. An historical account of the study of progressive systemic sclerosis (diffuse scleroderma). Ann Intern Med. 1962;**57**:305–19.
2. Goetz RH. Pathology of progressive systemic sclerosis (generalized scleroderma) with special reference to changes in the viscera. Clin Proc (S Africa). 1945;**4**:337–42.
3. Winterbauer RH. Multiple telangiectasia, Raynaud's phenomenon, sclerodactyly, and subcutaneous calcinosis: a syndrome mimicking hereditary hemorrhagic telangiectasia. Bull Johns Hopkins Hosp. 1964;**114**:361–83.
4. D'Angelo WA, Fries JF, Masi AT, Shulman LE. Pathologic observations in systemic sclerosis (scleroderma). A study of fifty-eight autopsy cases and fifty-eight matched controls. Am J Med. 1969;**46**:428–40.
5. Medsger TA. Epidemiology of progressive systemic sclerosis. In: Black CM, Myers AR, eds, 1E. Systemic sclerosis (scleroderma): New York: Gower Medical Publishing; 1985:53–60.
6. Maricq HR, Weinrich MC, Keil JE, et al. Prevalence of scleroderma spectrum disorders in the general population of South Carolina. Arthritis Rheum. 1989;**32**:998–1006.
7. Medsger TA, Masi AT. Epidemiology of systemic sclerosis (scleroderma). Ann Intern Med. 1971;**74**:714–21.
8. Varga J, Schumacher HR, Jimenez SA. Systemic sclerosis after augmentation mammoplasty with silicone implants. Ann Intern Med. 1989:**111**:377–83.
9. Spiera H. Scleroderma after silicone augmentation mammoplasty. JAMA. 1988;**260**:236–8.
10. Gray RG, Altman RD. Progressive systemic sclerosis in a family. Case report of a mother and son and review of the literature. Arthritis Rheum. 1977;**20**:35–41.
11. Heslop J, Coggon D, Acheson ED. The prevalence of intermittent digital ischaemia (Raynaud's phenomenon) in a general practice. J R Coll Gen Pract. 1983;**33**:85–8.
12. Olsen N, Nielson SL. Prevalence of primary Raynaud phenomenon in young females. Scand J Clin Lab Invest. 1978;**37**:761–6.
13. Young EA, Steen VD, Medsger TA. Systemic sclerosis without Raynaud's phenomenon. Arthritis Rheum. 1986;**29**(suppl 4): S51 (abstract).
14. Rodnan GP, Myerowitz RL, Justh GO. Morphologic changes in the digital arteries of patients with progressive systemic sclerosis (scleroderma) and Raynaud phenomenon. Medicine. 1980;**59**:393–408.
15. Norton WL, Nardo JM. Vascular disease in progressive systemic sclerosis (scleroderma). Ann Intern Med. 1970;**73**:317–24.
16. Seibold JR, Harris JN. Plasma beta-thromboglobulin in the differential diagnosis of Raynaud's phenomenon. J Rheumatol. 1985;**12**:99–103.
17. Kahaleh MB, Osborn I, LeRoy EC. Elevated levels of circulating platelet aggregates and beta-thromboglobulin in scleroderma. Ann Intern Med. 1982;**96**:610–13.
18. Yamane K, Kashiwagi H, Suzuki N, et al. Elevated plasma levels of endothelin-I in systemic sclerosis. Arthritis Rheum. 1991;**34**:243–4.
19. Traub YM, Shapiro AP, Rodnan GP, et al. Hypertension and renal failure (scleroderma renal crisis) in progressive systemic sclerosis. Review of a 25-year experience with 68 cases. Medicine. 1983;**62**:335–52.
20. Bulkley BH, Ridolfi RL, Salyer WR, Hutchins GM. Myocardial lesions of progressive systemic sclerosis. A cause of cardiac dysfunction. Circulation. 1976;**53**:483–90.
21. Follansbee WP, Curtiss EI, Medsger TA, et al. Physiologic abnormalities of cardiac function in progressive systemic sclerosis with diffuse scleroderma. N Engl J Med. 1984;**310**:142–8.
22. Alexander EL, Firestein GS, Weiss JL, et al. Reversible cold-induced abnormalities in myocardial perfusion and function in systemic sclerosis. Ann Intern Med.1986;**105**:661–8.
23. Ellis WW, Baer AN, Robertson RM, Pincus T, Kronenberg MW. Left ventricular dysfunction induced by cold exposure in patients with systemic sclerosis. Am J Med. 1986;**80**:385–92.
24. Furst DE, Davis JA, Clements PJ, Chpora SK, Theofilopoulos AN, Chia D. Abnormalities of pulmonary vascular dynamics and inflammation in early progressive systemic sclerosis. Arthritis Rheum. 1981;**24**:1403–8.
25. Maricq HR. Widefield capillary microscopy. Technique and rating scale for abnormalities seen in scleroderma and related disorders. Arthritis Rheum. 1981;**24**:1159–63.
26. Subcommittee for Scleroderma Criteria of the American Rheumatism Association Diagnostic and Therapeutic Criteria Committee. Preliminary criteria for the classification of systemic sclerosis (scleroderma). Arthritis Rheum. 1980;**23**:581–90.
27. LeRoy EC, Black C, Fleischmajer R, et al. Scleroderma (systemic sclerosis): classification, subsets and pathogenesis. J Rheumatol. 1988;**15**:202–5.
28. Medsger TA. Progressive systemic sclerosis. Clin Rheum Dis. 1983;**9**:9–16.
29. Steen VD, Medsger TA, Rodnan GP. D-Penicillamine therapy in progressive systemic sclerosis (scleroderma). A retrospective analysis. Ann Intern Med. 1982;**97**:652–8.
30. Rodnan GP, Lipinski E, Luksick J. Skin thickness and collagen content in progressive systemic sclerosis and localized scleroderma. Arthritis Rheum. 1979;**22**:130–40.
31. Clements PJ, Lachenbruch PA, Ng SC, Simmons M, Sterz M, Furst DE. Skin score. A semiquantitative measure of cutaneous involvement that improves prediction of prognosis in systemic sclerosis. Arthritis Rheum. 1990;**33**:1256–63.
32. Brennan P, Silman A, Black C, et al. Reliability of skin involvement measures in scleroderma. Br J Rheumatol. 1992; **31**:457–60.
33. Seibold JR, Furst DE, Clements PJ. Why everything (or nothing) seems to work in the treatment of scleroderma. J Rheumatol. 1992;**19**:673–6
34. McCloskey DA, Patella SJ, Seibold JR. Health assessment questionnaire in systemic sclerosis. Proc Allied Health Prof. 25th Mtg. 1990; 182.
35. Steen VD, Medsger TA, Osial TA. Factors predicting development of renal involvement in progressive systemic sclerosis. Am J Med. 1984;**76**:779–86.
36. Black C, Dieppe P, Huskisson T. Regressive systemic sclerosis. Ann Rheum Dis. 1986;**45**:384–7.
37. Furst DE, Clements PJ, Saab M, Sterz M, Paulus HE. Clinical and serological comparison of 17 chronic progressive systemic sclerosis (PSS) and 17 CREST syndrome patients matched for sex, age and disease duration. Ann Rheum Dis. 1984;**43**:794–801.
38. Zamost BJ, Hirschberg J, Ippoliti AF, Furst DE, Clements PJ, Ueinstein WM. Esophagitis in scleroderma. Prevalence and risk factors. Gastroenterology. 1987;**92**:421–8.
39. Russell ML, Friesen D, Henderson RD, Hanna WM. Ultrastructure of the esophagus in scleroderma. Arthritis Rheum. 1982;**25**:1117–23.
40. Cohen S, Laufer I, Snape UJ, Shiau Y-F, Levine GM, Jimenez S. The gastrointestinal manifestations of scleroderma: pathogenesis and management. Gastroenterology. 1980;**79**:155–66.
41. Davidson A, Russell C, Littlejohn GO. Assessment of esophageal abnormalities in progressive systemic sclerosis using radionuclide transit. J Rheumatol. 1985;**12**:472–7.
42. Isaacs PET, Kim YS. The contaminated small bowel syndrome. Am J Med. 1979;**67**:1049–57.
43. Miller F, Lane B, D'Angelo WA. Primary biliary cirrhosis and scleroderma. The possibility of a common pathogenetic mechanism. Arch Pathol Lab Med. 1979;**103**:505–14.
44. Blocka KLN, Bassett LW, Furst DE, Clements PJ, Paulus HE. The arthropathy of advanced progressive systemic sclerosis: a radiographic survey. Arthritis Rheum. 1981;**24**:874–84.
45. Clements PJ, Furst DE, Campion DS, et al. Muscle disease in progressive systemic sclerosis. Diagnostic and therapeutic considerations. Arthritis Rheum. 1978;**21**:62–71.
46. Medsger TA. Progressive systemic sclerosis skeletal muscle involvement. Clin Rheum Dis. 1979;**5**:103–22.
47. Osial TA, Avakian A, Sassouni V , Agarwal A, Medsger TA, Rodnan GP. Resorption of the mandibular condyles and coronoid processes in progressive systemic sclerosis (scleroderma). Arthritis Rheum. 1981;**24**: 729–33.
48. Lian JB, Pachman LM, Gundberg CM, Partridge REH, Maryjowski MC. Gamma-carboxyglutamate excretion and calcinosis in juvenile dermatomyositis. Arthritis Rheum. 1982;**25**:1094–110.
49. Seibold JR, Molony RR, Turkevich D, Ruddy MC, Kostis JB. Acute hemodynamic effects of ketanserin in pulmonary hypertension secondary to systemic sclerosis. J Rheumatol. 1987;**14**: 519–24.
50. Salerni R, Rodnan GP, Leon DF, Shavers J. Pulmonary hypertension in the CREST syndrome variant of progressive systemic sclerosis (scleroderma). Ann Intern Med. 1977;**86**:394–9.
51. Young RH, Mark GJ. Pulmonary vascular changes in scleroderma. Am J Med. 1978;**64**:998–1004.
52. Ungerer RG, Tashkin DP, Furst D, et al. Prevalence and clinical correlates of pulmonary arterial hypertension in progressive systemic sclerosis. Am J Med. 1983;**75**:65–74.
53. Schneider PD, Wise RA, Hochberg MC, Wigley FM. Serial pulmonary function in systemic sclerosis. Am J Med. 1982;**73**:385–94.
54. Owens GR, Fino GJ, Herbert DL, et al. Pulmonary function in progressive systemic sclerosis. Comparison of CREST syndrome variant with diffuse scleroderma. Chest. 1983;**84**:546–50.
55. Silver RM, Metcalf JF, Stanley JH, LeRoy EC. Interstitial lung disease in scleroderma. Analysis by bronchoalveolar lavage. Arthritis Rheum. 1984;**27**:1254–62.
56. Medsger TA, Masi AT, Rodnan GP. Survival with systemic sclerosis (scleroderma). A life-table analysis of clinical and demographic factors in 309 patients. Ann Intern Med. 1971;**75**:369–78.
57. McWhorter JE, LeRoy EC. Pericardial disease in scleroderma (systemic sclerosis). Am J Med. 1974;**57**:566–72.
58. Kostis JB, Seibold JR, Turkevich D, et al. Prognostic importance of cardiac arrhythmias in systemic sclerosis. Am J Med. 1988;**84**:1007–15.
59. Follansbee WP. The cardiovascular manifestations of systemic sclerosis (scleroderma). Curr Prob Cardiol. 1986;**11**:242–78.
60. Kovalchik MT, Guggenheim SJ, Silverman MH, Robertson JS, Steigerwald JC. The kidney in progressive systemic sclerosis. A prospective study. Ann Intern Med. 1978;**89**:881–7.
61. Helfrich DJ, Banner B, Steen VD, Medsger TA. Normotensive renal failure in systemic sclerosis. Arthritis Rheum. 1989;**32**:1128–34.
62. Cipoletti JF, Buckingham RB, Barnes EL, et al. Sjögren's syndrome in progressive systemic sclerosis. Ann Intern Med. 1977;**87**:535–41.
63. Gordon MB, Klein I, Dekker A, Rodnan GP, Medsger TA. Thyroid disease in progressive systemic sclerosis: increased frequency of glandular fibrosis and hypothyroidism. Ann Intern Med. 1981;**95**:431–5.
64. Nowlin NS, Brick JE, Weaver DJ, et al. Impotence in scleroderma. Ann Intern Med. 1986;**104**:794–8.
65. Sonnex C, Paice E, White AG. Autonomic neuropathy in systemic sclerosis: a case report and evaluation of six patients. Ann Rheum Dis. 1986;**45**:957–62.
66. Steen VD, Conte C, Day N, Ramsey-Goldman R, Medsger TA. Pregnancy in women with systemic sclerosis. Arthritis Rheum. 1989;**3**:151–7.
67. Roumm AD, Medsger TA. Cancer and systemic sclerosis. An epidemiologic study. Arthritis Rheum. 1985;**28**:1336–40.
68. Segel MC, Campbell WL, Medsger TA. Systemic sclerosis (scleroderma) and esophageal adenocarcinoma: is increased patient screening necessary? Gastroenterology. 1985;**89**:485–91.
69. Ginsburg WW, Conn DL, Bunch TW, McDuffie FC. Comparison of clinical and serologic markers in systemic lupus erythematosus and overlap

syndrome. A review of 247 patients. J Rheumatol. 1983;**10**:235–41.
70. Seibold JR, Medsger TA, Winkelstein A, Kelly RH, Rodnan GP. Immune complexes in progressive systemic sclerosis (scleroderma). Arthritis Rheum. 1982;**25**:1167–73.
71. Moroi Y, Peebles C, Fritzler MJ. Autoantibody to centromere (kinetochore) in scleroderma sera. Proc Natl Acad Sci USA. 1980;**77**:1627–33.
72. Fritzler MJ, Kinsella TD, Garbutt E. The CREST syndrome: a distinct serologic entity with anticentromere antibodies. Am J Med. 1980;**69**:520–7.
73. Steen VD, Ziegler GL, Rodnan GP, Medsger TA. Clinical and laboratory associations of anticentromere antibody in patients with progressive systemic sclerosis. Arthritis Rheum. 1984;**27**:125–31.
74. Tan EM, Rodnan GP, Garcia I, Moroi Y, Fritzler MJ, Peebles C. Diversity of antinuclear antibodies in progressive systemic sclerosis. Anti-centromere antibody and its relationship to CREST syndrome. Arthritis Rheum. 1980;**23**:617–5.
75. Maul GG, French BT, van VenrooiJ WJ, Love U, Moore ML. Topoisomerase I identified by scleroderma 70 antisera: enrichment of topoisomerase I at the centromere in mouse mitotic cells before anaphase. Proc Natl Acad Sci USA. 1986;**83**:5145–50.
76. Maul GG, Jimenez SA, Riggs E, Ziemnicki-Kotula D. Determination of an epitope of the diffuse systemic sclerosis marker antigen DNA topoisomerase-I: sequence similarity with retroviral p^{30} gag protein suggests a possible cause for autoimmunity in systemic sclerosis. Proc Natl Acad Sci USA. 1989;**86:**8492–96.
77. Dang H, Dauphinee MJ, Talal N, et al. Serum antibody to retroviral GAG proteins in systemic sclerosis. Arthritis Rheum. 1991;**34**:1336–7.
78. Degiannis D, Seibold JR, Czarnecki, Raskova J, Raska K. Soluble and cellular markers of immune activation in patients with systemic sclerosis. Clin Immunol Immunopath. 1990;**56**:259–70.
79. Degiannis D, Seibold JR, Czarnecki M, Raskova J, Raska K. Soluble interleukin-2 receptors in patients with systemic sclerosis. Clinical and laboratory correlations. Arthritis Rheum. 1990;**33**: 375–80.
80. Needleman BW, Wigley FM, Stair RW. Interleukin-I, interleukin-2, interleukin-4, interleukin-6, tumor necrosis factor alpha, and interferon-gamma levels in sera from patients with scleroderma. Arthritis Rheum. 1992;**35**:67–72.
81. Seibold JR. Digital sclerosis in children with insulin-dependent diabetes mellitus. Arthritis Rheum. 1982;**25**:1357–61.
82. Falanga V, Medsger TA, Reichlin M, Rodnan GP. Linear scleroderma. Clinical spectrum, prognosis, and laboratory abnormalities. Ann Intern Med. 1986;**104**:849–57.
83. Person JR, Su WPD. Subcutaneous morphea: a clinical study of sixteen cases. Br J Dermatol. 1979;**100**:371–83.
84. Moore TL, Zucker J. Eosinophilic fasciitis. Semin Arthritis Rheum. 1980;**9**:228–35.
85. Belongia EA, Hedberg CW, Gleich GJ, et al. An investigation of the cause of the eosinophilia-myalgia syndrome associated with tryptophan use. N Engl J Med. 1990;**323**:357–65.
86. Martin RW, Duffy J, Engel AG, et al. The clinical spectrum of the eosinophilia-myalgia syndrome associated with L-tryptophan ingestion. Clinical features in 20 patients and aspects of pathophysiology. Ann Intern Med. 1990;**113**:124–34.
87. Venencie PY, Powell FC, Su WPD. Scleredema: a review of thirty-three cases. J Am Acad Dermatol. 1984;**11**:128–43.

34

MANAGEMENT OF SYSTEMIC SCLEROSIS

Virginia D Steen

- Disease heterogeneity (stage, severity, pace and pattern) is an important factor in the therapeutic plan.
- Success with 'disease-modifying' therapy is modest.
- Organ-specific treatments can be dramatically successful (e.g. ACE inhibitors for renal crisis).

Systemic sclerosis is a connective tissue disease which is often extremely difficult to manage. Historically, much of the treatment has been ineffective, although progress on understanding the pathogenesis of the disease has resulted in new specific therapy. Angiotensin-converting enzyme (ACE) inhibitors and calcium channel blockers have brought dramatic changes in the treatment of renal crisis and Raynaud's phenomenon. Innovative surgery for hand contractures is now being performed by many hand surgeons and new drugs are available to treat symptoms of the gastrointestinal involvement. These advances in management, coupled with active research, have led to an optimistic view that scleroderma is not a hopeless disease [1].

EVALUATION OF THERAPY

The evaluation of therapy in systemic sclerosis has been a major challenge. However, new approaches to evaluation, in the context of both the individual patient and clinical trials, hold significant promise (Fig. 34.1).

Objective measures of organ involvement are essential to quantify disease changes and responses to therapy. The extent and severity of skin thickening can be assessed by skin thickness scores [2,3]. Changes in pulmonary function tests, cardiac ejection fraction (echocardiogram, MUGA scan) and creatinine clearance are useful to monitor progress in lung, heart or kidney involvement. The patient-derived Health Assessment Questionnaire results correlate with severity of disease [4] and may also reflect changes in disease over time. Promising laboratory tests include levels of soluble interleukin-2 receptors [5] and serum type III procollagen peptide [6] which have been shown to correlate with survival, disease severity and improving or worsening disease. All these factors may aid in determining the most effective therapy. There is a wide spectrum of disease manifestations and disease severity which must be considered in any therapeutic plan. Patients with long-standing, 'fixed' disease and patients with very mild, nonprogressive disease may not benefit from therapeutic intervention.

Similarly, patients with primary clinical features which historically do not respond to therapy may not benefit from agents in our current armamentarium. Additionally, there is great variability in the pace of disease. Some patients have such a slow-paced disease that they will never have severe disease. Spontaneous improvement may occur and can interfere with the interpretation of the response. Accordingly, it is often useful to consider disease subsets or variants in formulating a therapeutic approach.

The most frequently used classification divides patients into two groups; limited scleroderma and diffuse scleroderma [7]. Patients with limited scleroderma, previously called the CREST syndrome (see Fig. 34.2), generally have a slow-paced disease. These patients may have disabling disease with severe recurrent digital ulcers, reflux esophagitis, malabsorption and isolated pulmonary hypertension, the most deadly and untreatable of all scleroderma manifestations [8]. There has been little evidence that these patients would be helped by a potential disease-modifying agent.

Patients with diffuse scleroderma often have an acute onset of disease. Arthritis and tendon involvement along with extensive skin thickening commonly result in severe contractures. Tendon friction rubs, which are palpated in flexor and extensor tendons of fingers, wrist, elbows, knees and ankles, are seen almost exclusively in diffuse scleroderma and are very helpful in the early diagnosis of patients with diffuse disease. The rapid pace of progression in diffuse

EVALUATION OF THERAPY IN SYSTEMIC SCLEROSIS

Problem in evaluating therapy	Approaches to solving problem	Potential for overcoming problem
Lack of objective measures to quantify clinical changes	Health assessment questionnaire	Reliable measure of disease severity
	Organ system measures	
	Skin thickness scores	Validated method; evaluator needs training
	Pulmonary function tests	Quantitates function (medium to late changes)
	Cardiac ejection fraction	Quantitates function (medium to late changes)
	Creatinine clearance	Quantitates function (medium to late changes)
Lack of laboratory marker to measure disease status	Interleukin-2 receptor and type III procollagen peptide	Promising disease correlations
Need for long-term assessment	Follow-up long-term survival after completion of short-term studies	Tracking methods successful; statistical capabilities for complex analyses much improved
Wide spectrum of disease manifestations	Identify clinically significant subsets of patients	Natural history studies suggest meaningful disease subsets
Variable pace of progression	Blinded, controlled trials	Trials underway
Rare disease	Multicenter trials with vigorous patient and physician support	Trials underway

Fig. 34.1 Evaluation of therapy in systemic sclerosis is a major challenge. There has been an aggressive attempt to solve the many problems in order to adequately initiate and interpret therapeutic trials.

CLINICAL DIFFERENCES BETWEEN LIMITED AND DIFFUSE DISEASE	
Limited scleroderma	**Diffuse scleroderma**
Long duration of Raynaud's phenomenon	Short duration of Raynaud's with skin changes often occurring before Raynaud's
Puffy fingers intermittently for long time	Swollen hands and legs
Slow pace of progression	Rapid pace of progression
Mild constitutional symptoms, mild arthralgias, rare tendon rubs	Many constitutional symptoms, arthralgias/arthritis, carpal tunnel and tendon rubs
Most common problems – digital ulcers, esophageal, small bowel, pulmonary fibrosis	All organ systems involved – pulmonary fibrosis, cardiac and renal crisis most common causes of death
Pulmonary hypertension (10%) fatal	Rare pulmonary hypertension
Anticentromere antibody (50–90%)	Anticentromere antibody (5%)
Anti-Scl-70 antibody (10–15%)	Anti-Scl-70 antibody (20–30%)

Fig. 34.2 Clinical differences between limited and diffuse disease. These lists show the important differences in clinical features between limited scleroderma and diffuse scleroderma. The knowledge of these findings is needed to determine what subset the patient is in or is most likely to evolve to when some of the classic manifestations are not present. These features and the resultant understanding of the disease are helpful in determining the type of therapy that is needed.

scleroderma occurs primarily in the early stages of the disease, followed by a plateau and perhaps eventual modest improvement.

Systemic sclerosis has presented special challenges for clinical trials designed to evaluate therapy. The importance of objective outcome measures, the need to recognize patients with the potential to respond therapeutically; the need to stratify patients into clinically meaningful subsets, and the need for long-term follow-up data have all been significant issues in appropriate study design. Scleroderma is a rare disease with an incidence of 10–20 per million. Double-blind, randomized, controlled trials require the participation of many centers and prolonged time for patient accrual. Patients may be so eager to receive help that they will be unwilling to accept enrollment in a placebo-controlled trial. Nonetheless, the importance of such trials is now accepted, and the need for vigorous enrollment is clearly recognized; several trials are currently underway.

PREVENTION

Although disease-modifying agents capable of interrupting the disease process in the earliest stages are not yet identified, preventive measures can make significant contributions to the management of patients with systemic sclerosis. For patients with Raynaud's phenomenon, practical advice about dressing warmly, avoiding cold exposure and complete avoidance of smoking can help to decrease the frequency and severity of attacks. Good skin care and prompt attention to small wounds and bruises may prevent the development of more severe skin ulcerations. Patients with esophageal hypomotility and reflux can often prevent symptoms by eating frequent small meals and by elevating the head of their bed on blocks. Similarly, attention to proper diet can facilitate gastrointestinal motility and regular stool formation. The importance of general medical care – maintenance of adequate nutritional status, prompt correction of fluid and electrolyte abnormalities, control of hypertension – cannot be overemphasized in the management of patients with systemic sclerosis.

EDUCATION AND PSYCHOSOCIAL SUPPORT

Education about practical aspects of the disease and social support are essential for effective overall management of patients with systemic

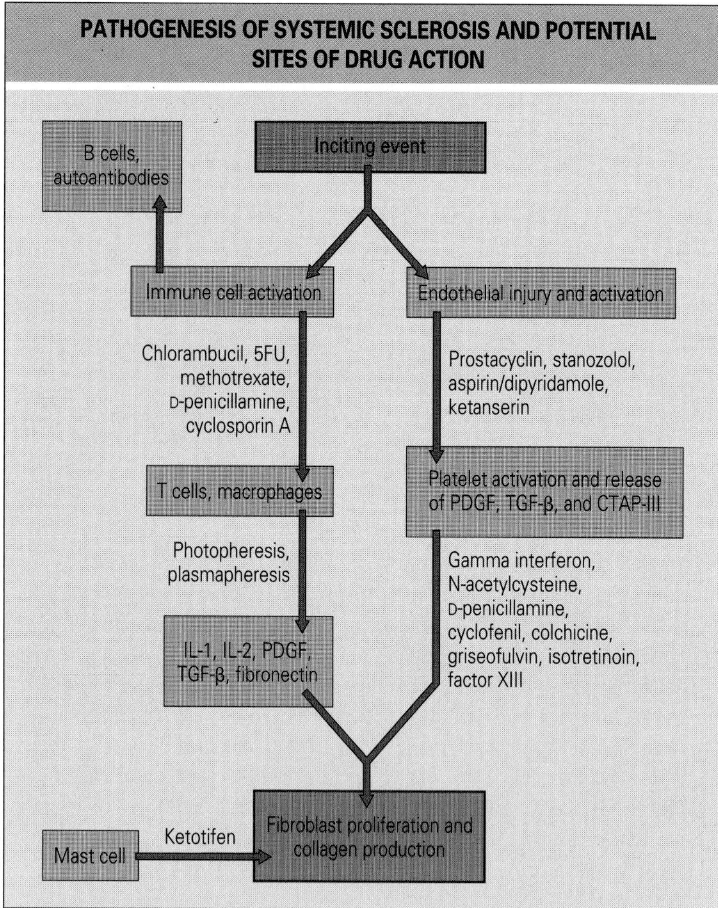

Fig. 34.3 Hypothetical pathogenesis of systemic sclerosis and the location of the possible sites where drugs might be useful for therapeutic intervention. Identification of inciting events, the alteration of T cell function, and endothelial cell activity may interfere with the stimulation of fibroblast production of collagen. There are a variety of ways in which drugs can interfere with collagen production directly. Further investigation will greatly influence the future treatment of systemic sclerosis.

sclerosis. Written material specifically oriented to patients is available through several foundations and provides a basic understanding of the disease. Local support groups often provide a forum for discussion and an opportunity to develop the skills necessary for dealing with a chronic disease which may be severely debilitating. Success in these initiatives can greatly facilitate the management of each patient.

DISEASE-MODIFYING AGENTS

Research over the last decade has led to a much better understanding of the pathogenesis of systemic sclerosis and to a more rational approach to therapy. Environmental factors, vascular biology, and cellular and humoral immunity interact in a complex fashion to cause increased collagen production and arterial narrowing.

Figure 34.3 summarizes one hypothetical scheme of the pathogenesis of systemic sclerosis and the potential sites of action of various drugs. These sites of action include modification of vascular, immunologic and fibroblast abnormalities (Fig. 34.4). Of course, therapy aimed at modifying the entire disease process is very important, but persuasive documentation of efficacy is difficult to gather.

Drugs Affecting Vascular Changes

Aspirin and dipyridamole affect platelet function and theoretically should be helpful. However, a controlled trial did not find any efficacy with these drugs [9]. Ketanserin, a serotonin antagonist, was studied in a double-blind controlled trial in 24 patients [10]. No objective changes were found in skin thickening or organ damage,

POTENTIAL DISEASE REMITTING DRUGS		
Drugs affecting vascular changes	**Drugs affecting immune abnormalities**	**Drugs affecting fibroblast changes**
Aspirin/dipyridamole	Chlorambucil	D-Penicillamine
Ketanserin	5-Fluorouracil	Gamma interferon
Stanozolol	Methotrexate	Cyclofenil
Iloprost (prostacylin)	Cyclosporin A	Factor XIII
Calcium channel blockers	Photopheresis	Colchicine
Tissue plasminogen activating factor	Antithymocyte globulin	N-acetylcysteine
	Thymopentin	Isotretinoin
	FK-506	Griseofulvin

Fig. 34.4 Potential disease remitting drugs used in the treatment of systemic sclerosis. Drugs affect various aspects of the pathogenetic process of systemic sclerosis. Although there are multiple interactions of these different events, therapy directed at one process may be successful in modifying this disease.

although it may be useful in Raynaud's and digital ulcers. Stanozolol, an anabolic steroid with fibrinolytic activity, has been studied in Raynaud's phenomenon [11]. A double-blind study showed improvement in objective measures of blood flow but little effect on clinical features. Iloprost, a vasodilatory prostacyclin analog, seems very promising in early studies [12], and additional controlled trials are underway.

Drugs Affecting Immunologic Changes

Chlorambucil, studied in an excellent double-blind controlled trial with a 3-year follow-up at a single center, was not any more effective than placebo [13]. Likewise 5-fluorouracil, which was very promising in open studies, has shown little efficacy in a controlled trial [14].

Many anecdotes and several small series studying the effectiveness of methotrexate and cyclosporin A in systemic sclerosis have been reported. Methotrexate has been used in scleroderma-myositis overlap patients, and although other immunosuppressive drugs have been ineffective in scleroderma, there is hope that methotrexate will be different. Randomized, double-blind, controlled studies are necessary. Cyclosporin A has been used in two series of closely monitored patients and promising results have been found. Unfortunately, cyclosporin has a high frequency of renal toxicity and there are reports of cyclosporin-induced renal crisis [15,16]. Again, careful, closely monitored, controlled studies are mandatory.

Photopheresis, a special procedure which seems to selectively interfere with T cell function, has been compared to D-penicillamine. Preliminary results suggest that both groups had significant improvement from baseline at 10 months, but there was no significant difference between groups [17]. Several other new therapeutic approaches have been tried in a few patients. Antithymocyte globulin, thymopentin and FK-506 (an investigational agent used for transplant rejection) may potentially be effective therapy [18]. Controlled trials are necessary before any judgment of their effectiveness as disease-modifying agents in systemic sclerosis can be made. Total lymphoid irradiation, studied in only 6 patients, was totally ineffective.

Drugs Affecting Fibroblast Changes

D-Penicillamine (DPA) has the longest history and widest support in the treatment of scleroderma. In the early 1970s, reports from several countries claimed improved outcomes in treated patients compared to historical controls. A large retrospective study showed a significant improvement in skin thickening at two years and an improved 5-year survival compared to similar historical controls [2]. An updated analysis of this cohort from the University of Pittsburgh now includes 152 patients treated with D-penicillamine and 80 patients in a comparison group from the same time period. The two groups initially had similar demographic and clinical features including sex, age, disease duration (2.5 years), total skin score, and presence of organ system involvement. Improvement in skin thickening as measured by the total skin score [3] was significantly greater

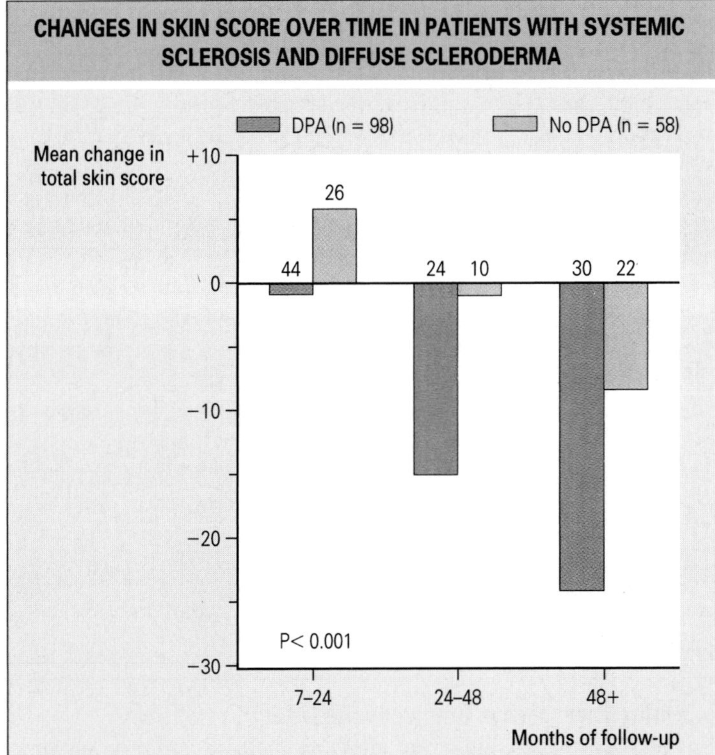

Fig. 34.5 Changes in skin scores over time in patients with systemic sclerosis and diffuse scleroderma. This shows the improvement in the total skin score seen in patients treated with D-penicillamine (DPA). Throughout the time period, treated patients had a significantly greater improvement in skin thickening than in a comparison untreated group of patients.

in DPA treated patients (Fig. 34.5). More importantly, the treated patients appear to have an improvement in survival (see Fig. 34.6). Although uncontrolled, there is another large cohort of early diffuse scleroderma patients who had a 75% improvement in skin involvement and an 80% 5-year cumulative survival rate [19].

Interferon-γ, which inhibits fibroblast proliferation and collagen production *in vitro*, resulted in significant improvement in total skin scores, joint mobility and grip strength but no change in Raynaud's phenomenon and carbon monoxide diffusing capacity in a small

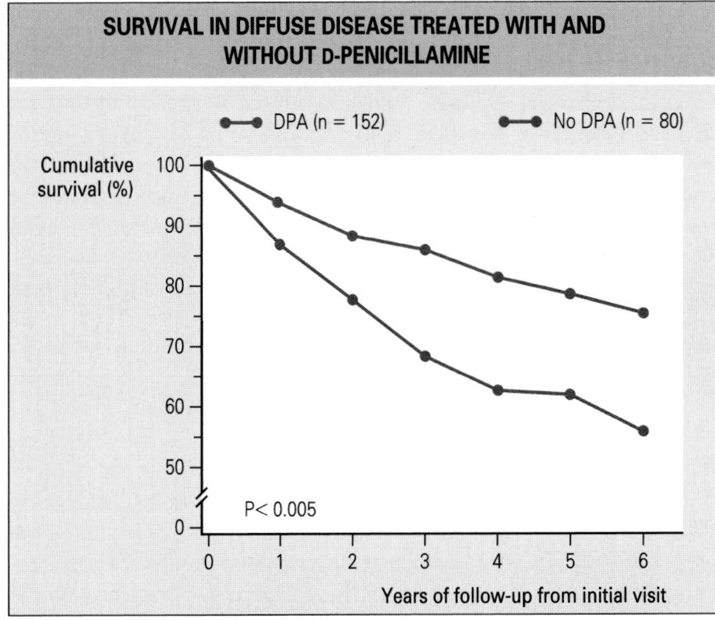

Fig. 34.6 Survival in diffuse disease treated with and without D-penicillamine. Survival of 152 patients with early diffuse scleroderma treated with D-penicillamine (DPA) is significantly better than the 80 untreated comparison patients. The 5-year survival from date of diagnosis of treated patients was 80%, which is one of the best outcomes in any survival study.

series of patients [20]. These findings need to be confirmed in a blinded, controlled setting. Colchicine, which affects collagen deposition, has been evaluated in two conflicting small studies but inadequate long-term follow-up does not support the use of colchicine in systemic sclerosis [18]. Similarly, ketotifen, a mast cell stabilizing agent, prevents skin fibrosis in the tight skin mouse [21] and had dramatic effects on two patients [22]. Unfortunately, a double-blind controlled study performed showed no significant improvement in any of the parameters studied except pruritus [23].

N-Acetylcysteine, which may be capable of promoting collagen breakdown, was studied in a small, but well designed double-blind, controlled trial [24] which showed no differences between groups. Cyclofenil, which inhibits production of proteoglycans, induced slight changes in skin softening and joint mobility in two small controlled trials but had a poor side-effect profile with allergic and hepatic reactions [25,26]. Factor XIII, which may participate in collagen clearance, had a favorable outcome in a very short (3 week) crossover study, but the study was too short to interpret for long-term therapy [27].

ORGAN-SPECIFIC THERAPIES

Vascular Tree: Spasm and Ischemic Injury

Raynaud's phenomenon is the most common symptom in systemic sclerosis patients and shows a wide spectrum of severity. The most important aspect in the management of Raynaud's phenomenon is total abstinence from smoking. Avoidance of the cold, keeping the entire body warm, and biofeedback may help control symptoms [28]. Patients with mild Raynaud's rarely need medication to control their symptoms. When Raynaud's becomes complicated by the presence of digital tip infarctions and ulcerations or when the frequency and severity of episodes interfere with daily life, calcium channel blockers such as nifedipine (10–30mg three times daily) have been effective in decreasing frequency and severity of Raynaud's episodes in double-blind studies [29,30]. Ketanserin, an investigational serotonin antagonist, has also been very effective in improving Raynaud's ulcers [31]. Prazosin [32] and topical nitroglycerine [33] have been used with variable effects. Dimethyl sulfoxide (DMSO) has been reported to have a therapeutic effect on ulcer healing [34] but a controlled, double-blind study failed to confirm these findings [35].

Local management of digital tip ulcers, as well as ulcers occurring over the proximal interphalangeal (PIP) joints (which are usually related to taut skin or trauma rather than vasospasm), is very problematic. The initial approach is to soak fingers in antiseptic fluid, air dry and then cover the ulcer with antibiotic ointment and a sterile bandage. This occlusive type of dressing promotes wound healing, and it also gives protection from trauma and infection. Duoderm, a bio-occlusive bandage, is particularly helpful on uninfected ulcers. Ulcers may become secondarily infected with evidence of swelling, erythema and a striking increase in pain. Oral antistaphylococcal antibiotics and extra soaking can often treat the infection, but at times surgical debridement and intravenous antibiotics covering pseudomonas and staphylococci species may be necessary. Severe ulcers, including those with impending gangrene, may require intermittent cervical sympathetic blocks, digital sympathectomy, hand surgery, intravenous prostaglandin E [36] or prostacyclin infusions [12], or intra-arterial phentolamine. Adequate pain control is necessary because of the cycle of pain and secondary vasospasm which exacerbates the ischemia and ulceration. Although surgical debridement may be necessary, amputation should be avoided except in the cases of extreme pain or nonresponsive infection.

Integument: Skin Thickening and Calcinosis

Skin thickening occurs in almost all patients but shows a marked variability in the extent, severity, and progression over time. Spontaneous improvement may occur, but only after several years. Dryness and pruritus may be relieved with decreased water contact or creams containing lanolin. Pruritus and the pain associated with rapidly progressive cutaneous thickening usually decrease in intensity over time.

Calcinosis occurs predominantly in limited scleroderma but may also appear in patients with long-standing diffuse scleroderma. Besides digital calcinosis, patients may also develop calcium deposits along the forearm, elbow, buttock, thigh, knee or shin. Attempts to dissolve or prevent development of additional calcinosis with probenecid, colchicine and warfarin [37] have been particularly unsuccessful. Fortunately, for about half of the patients, calcinosis is an asymptomatic, radiographic finding. For others, an acute intense, painful inflammation similar to other crystal-related problems may respond to colchicine [38] and nonsteroidal anti-inflammatory drugs (NSAIDs). Calcinosis causing chronic, ulcerating lesions requires vigorous local measures, antibiotics for infection and occasionally surgical debulking. Inadequate wound healing and recurrent calcinosis are concerns following surgical removal of these deposits.

Musculoskeletal System: Arthritis, Tendon and Muscle Involvement

Arthralgias and arthritis are common and may result from skin tightening with swollen, puffy fingers, or from synovial inflammation. Treatment with NSAIDs may be helpful, but adequate pain relief is often difficult to achieve. Later in the course of disease, symptoms may result from contractures, severe erosive arthritis or silent telescoping of digits. Surgical reconstruction of contracted fingers by straightening, shortening and fusing PIP joints improves appearance, decreases development of PIP ulcers and improves function of these hands [39]. The erosive arthritis and telescoping of digits are rare and are refractory to medication, including penicillamine and methotrexate.

Tendon rubs, unique to diffuse scleroderma, result from tendon inflammation and thickening and are found in characteristic anatomic regions. Although often asymptomatic, they may be extremely painful and may significantly limit joint function. Low dose oral corticosteroids (<10mg prednisone per day) may be necessary for tendon or joint involvement to keep a patient moving.

Early aggressive physical therapy is important in preventing contractures which may result from swollen fingers, arthritis, tenosynovitis and rapidly progressive skin thickening (Fig. 34.7). Clinical experience suggests that aggressive active and passive extension and flexion exercises are necessary to prevent further loss of motion as well as to regain function. Exercises may be quite painful, and the use of adequate analgesia is needed to optimize participation in the exercise program. Improvement occurs slowly, and steadfast encouragement by the physician and the therapist is essential. Resting wrist splints may be helpful for carpal tunnel symptoms which often

TREATMENT OF JOINT AND TENDON INVOLVEMENT

Pharmacologic measures:
- Nonsteroidal anti-inflammatory drugs
- Adequate analgesia
- Rarely, low dose steroids

Physical measures:
- Aggressive active and passive physical therapy
- Extension and flexion exercise to preserve and prevent loss of joint motion
- Dynamic splinting not well tolerated

Fig. 34.7 Treatment of joint and tendon involvement. The treatment of joint and tendon involvement plays a very important role in the management of systemic sclerosis. Skin thickening, arthritis, tendon inflammation or thickening all work towards development of contractures. Aggressive therapy may slow down the loss of function.

occur, even prior to the diagnosis of scleroderma. Local steroid injections are effective, and since symptoms often resolve as the disease progresses, surgery is not usually necessary. Dynamic splinting has been studied but has not been found to be effective in retarding progression of contractures [40].

An inflammatory myopathy, indistinguishable from polymyositis, can occur in scleroderma and, like polymyositis, is treated with high dose prednisone and/or methotrexate. In the absence of inflammation, patients may have a chronic proximal weakness resulting from a bland myopathy. Such patients have little or no increase in creatine kinase; the EMG shows few polyphasic potentials and no insertional irritability. Muscle biopsy typically shows interstitial fibrosis, non-specific fiber changes and occasional small foci of inflammatory cells. Management is primarily muscle strengthening exercises although a trial of oral prednisone (20–30 mg per day) may improve strength in severe cases.

Gastrointestinal Disturbances

Esophageal dysmotility is the most common gastrointestinal manifestation in systemic sclerosis and may lead to dyspepsia and dysphagia (Fig. 34.8). Dyspepsia usually results from both distal esophageal hypomotility and decreased lower esophageal pressure with esophageal reflux. Persistent reflux esophagitis requires several special, albeit simple, measures. These include small frequent meals eaten in upright position, avoidance of late evening meals, elevation of the head of the bed on 8in. blocks, and frequent nonabsorbable antacids. Histamine receptor (H2) blocking agents or a slurry of a cytoprotective agent such as sucralfate are usually helpful. Refractory cases may respond to short (1–2 month), intermittent courses of omeprazole, a potent inhibitor of acid production [41]. Nifedipine lowers esophageal sphincter pressure and may aggravate esophageal symptoms [42]. When esophageal symptoms are prominent and the treatment of Raynaud's phenomenon necessary, the use of a calcium channel blocker other than nifedipine may be helpful. Similarly, nonsteroidal anti-inflammatory drugs which may cause gastric irritation need to be used with discretion.

Dysphagia may result from severe esophageal dysmotility but may also be compounded by esophageal scarring and stricture formation. Barium swallow or endoscopy will differentiate symptoms due to esophageal dysmotility from those due to an esophageal stricture. Metoclopramide can be used to stimulate esophageal muscle function [43], but it is often marginally effective and poorly tolerated. Cisapride has fewer side effects and also improves esophageal function [44]. Periodic dilatation of strictures relieves the discomfort of dysphagia in this setting. Surgical intervention has not achieved general acceptance because of the high frequency of failure or recurrence.

Intestinal hypomotility underlies a spectrum of symptoms including nausea, vomiting, bloating and distension, diarrhea and constipation. Delayed gastric emptying may aggravate both esophageal and small bowel dysfunction; cisapride [45] is, and erythromycin [46] may be, effective in this situation. Small bowel hypomotility is often seen only as dilatation or delayed transit of contrast on small bowel radiographs. Symptoms from small bowel hypomotility include abdominal distension (or bloating) and malabsorption with diarrhea and weight loss due, in part, to bacterial overgrowth. Broad spectrum antibiotics, such as ampicillin, tetracycline, trimethoprim-sulfamethoxazole, metronidazole or ciprofloxacin given for intermittent 2-week courses, or in low continuous doses, can be dramatically effective. Refractory cases may require antibiotics chosen by specific identification of bacteria through duodenal or small intestinal aspiration. Careful attention to nutritional supplementation is essential to assist in stabilizing weight loss. At times parenteral hyperalimentation may be required [47].

Severe abdominal distension (pseudo-obstruction) may be confused with a mechanical obstruction. Patients with pseudo-obstruction do not usually have fevers or leukocytosis, and radiographs usually shows dilatation throughout the intestine. However, the differential diagnosis of these two entities can be difficult. In general, one should take a conservative approach to management with nasogastric suction, bowel rest, and patience, since these episodes usually spontaneously improve. Surgical intervention, which may aggravate the ileus and delay recovery even further, should be strongly discouraged. Pneumatosis cystoides intestinalis which results in dissection of luminal gas in the bowel wall is typically benign and does not require treatment.

Pulmonary Dysfunction

Pleural disease with pleural thickening, effusion or pleural rub is often asymptomatic. Acute, symptomatic pleuritis usually responds to an NSAID but occasionally steroids are necessary.

TREATMENT OF GASTROINTESTINAL INVOLVEMENT

Symptom	Gastrointestinal abnormality	Treatment
Heartburn	Esophageal reflux from decreased lower esophageal pressure	Mild – simple eating adjustments, antacids Moderate – H2 receptor blocking agents, cytoprotective agent (sucralfate), avoid calcium channel blockers and nonsteroidal anti-inflammatory drugs Severe – omeprazole
Dysphagia, vomiting	Esophageal dysmotility	Eat upright with liquids Prokinetic drugs (metaclopromide, cisapride)
	Esophageal stricture from chronic esophagitis	Esophageal dilatation Reflux treatment (above)
Nausea, vomiting, bloating	Gastric atony (infrequent)	Prokinetic drugs, ? erythromycin
Bloating, diarrhea	Small bowel hypomotility Bacterial growth	Prokinetic drugs Broad spectrum antibiotics Nutritional or parenteral supplement as needed
Bloating, pseudo-obstruction	Small and large intestinal hypomotility and dilatation	Conservative decompression with nasogastric suction and bowel rest Avoid surgery Prokinetic drugs Antibiotic trial
Constipation	Large intestinal hypomotility	Stool softeners Bulk to stimulate muscles

Fig. 34.8 Treatment of gastrointestinal involvement. Treatment of gastrointestinal scleroderma is very complex, but careful review of every option will optimize a patient's care. Only a small percentage of patients cannot be controlled with these regimens.

With improved survival in renal crisis over the last 20 years, pulmonary fibrosis is now the most frequent cause of death (11%) (Fig. 34.9). Since fixed fibrotic disease is not amenable to treatment, efforts have been directed toward identifying early stages of fibrosis. Bronchoalveolar lavage may frequently document increased neutrophils and lymphocytes in patients with early lung disease [48]. High resolution CT scanning is a very sensitive tool for early fibrosis and perhaps even alveolitis [49]. The course of pulmonary fibrosis and restrictive lung disease, reflected in pulmonary function tests, is extremely variable. Most of the decline in lung volume occurs in the first four years of disease [50], but many patients remain completely stable while others have a rapid deterioration. A few untreated patients even improve with time. Males are at increased risk for severe pulmonary disease. Anti-Scl-70 is seen more frequently in patients with pulmonary fibrosis, but this autoantibody does not predict severity of disease [51].

Steroids have had variable success in altering the downhill course of pulmonary fibrosis. When interstitial fibrosis has been present for many years, D-penicillamine has resulted in minimal improvement but stabilization of disease [52,53]. Several centers have had preliminary success with cyclophosphamide [54] (Fig. 34.10). Until therapy is more effective, prevention of pulmonary complications including aspiration and pneumonia is very important. Future treatment of severe fibrosis may include the cutting-edge technologies of single or double lung transplants.

Isolated pulmonary hypertension usually occurs in limited scleroderma patients with little or no interstitial fibrosis but with intimal proliferation of pulmonary arteries. Such patients may manifest only Raynaud's, telangiectasias or an anticentromere antibody, but they have a marked decrease in the diffusing capacity which is out of proportion to their normal or near normal forced vital capacity [55]. Attempts to lower pulmonary artery pressures with calcium channel blockers [56], prostaglandin E and prostacyclin [57] and other vasodilators are not very effective. The efficacy of early intervention, (e.g. with vasodilators and possibly disease-modifying drugs), in potentially high-risk limited scleroderma patients with a diffusing capacity less than 50% of predicted, is unknown. Patients with isolated pulmonary hypertension die from arrhythmias, pulmonary thrombosis, cardiac or respiratory failure 0.5 to 5 years after the diagnosis; supplemental oxygen, anticoagulation to prevent pulmonary thromboembolism, and control of heart failure, are the best supportive measures available. Two recent successful single lung transplants in patients with isolated pulmonary hypertension due to scleroderma at the University of Pittsburgh encourages optimism that this may be realistic therapy.

Patients with severe pulmonary fibrosis also develop pulmonary hypertension secondary to the severe fibrosis. These patients have a slightly better survival than patients with the vascular etiology of their pulmonary hypertension.

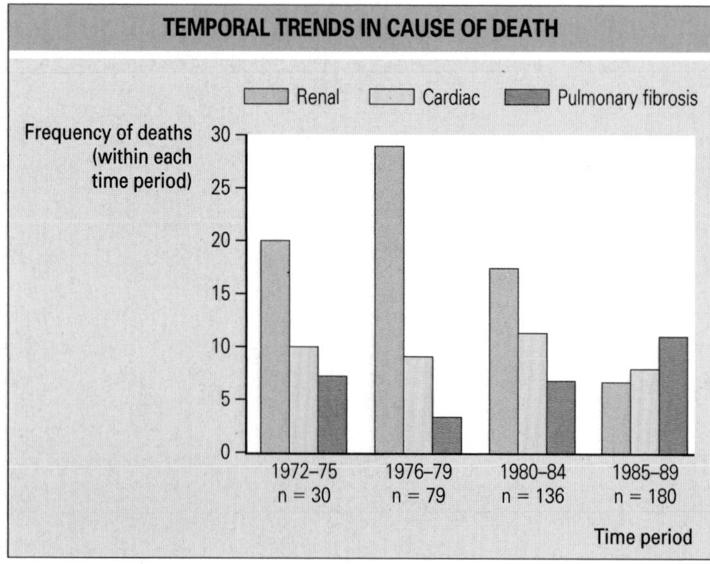

Fig. 34.9 Temporal trends in cause of death. This shows the change in the causes of deaths in 1068 systemic sclerosis patients over the last 20 years. In the 1970s, the unavailability of treatment for renal crisis resulted in large numbers of deaths. The introduction of ACE inhibitors has decreased death from renal crisis. In the last 15 years there is an increasing frequency of deaths from pulmonary fibrosis.

Cardiac Abnormalities

Pericarditis is uncommon but responds well to anti-inflammatory drugs. Steroids may be needed in more severe cases. Pericardial tamponade requiring pericardiocentesis or surgery is rare. Asymptomatic pericardial effusions are frequent – as high as 50% in some series – and while they may persist for prolonged periods of time, they rarely cause problems and do not need treatment. Large effusions are usually associated with a cardiomyopathy, pulmonary hypertension, severe pulmonary fibrosis, or renal crisis.

Myocardial fibrosis does not cause typical angina or myocardial infarction but may cause a cardiomyopathy with congestive heart failure. Defects in probable fibrotic areas found on thallium perfusion scans at rest, and reperfusion changes noted with exercise or a cold pressor test [58], suggest that repeated coronary vasospasm may contribute to the fibrosis. Perfusion statistically improved after short term use of calcium channel blockers or dipyridamole [59,60]. After one year of captopril, patients with these asymptomatic perfusion defects showed improved perfusion on repeat thallium scans [61]. An increased amount of thallium defects is strongly associated with decreased survival and new cardiac symptoms, but their alteration by drugs is not clear.

Conduction defects, arrhythmias and other electrocardiographic abnormalities are also very common. In general they correlate with a poor prognosis but most changes are asymptomatic and do not require intervention. There is no evidence that any of these cardiac abnormalities have been significantly altered by any disease modifying medication. Thus, therapy with cardiovascular medication is guided primarily by cardiovascular indications to optimize function.

Renal Dysfunction

Prior to the availability of ACE inhibitors, scleroderma renal crisis caused death in 90% of patients within 1 year. However, with the introduction of ACE inhibitors, the hypertension can now be controlled and end organ damage prevented (Fig. 34.11) [62]. Patients with early diffuse scleroderma and rapidly progressive skin thickening and those with anemia or new cardiac problems, are at greatest risk to develop renal crisis [65]. Mild hypertension does not predict the onset of malignant

TREATMENT OF PULMONARY INTERSTITIAL ALVEOLITIS WITH CYCLOPHOSPHAMIDE WITH OR WITHOUT CORTICOSTEROIDS

	Medical University of South Carolina (n = 7)	University of Pittsburgh (n = 15)	University of Pittsburgh untreated patients (n = 27)
Baseline FVC% of predicted	51.4%	53.5%	59.1%
Change in FVC	400ml/year	389ml/year	−14ml/year

Fig. 34.10 Treatment of pulmonary interstitial alveolitis with cyclophosphamide with or without corticosteroids. The effects of cyclophosphamide with or without steroids on pulmonary interstitial fibrosis in systemic sclerosis is shown from two centers, along with a comparison untreated group also with severe restrictive disease and similar disease duration. The University of Pittsburgh using intervenous monthly pulse cyclophosphamide and the Medical University of South Carolina using oral cyclophosphamide have both found improvement in small groups of patients with severe restrictive lung disease in the first 1–2 years after treatment. Early disease and inflammatory alveolitis may predict positive outcome with this treatment, but further controlled studies are definitely needed.

hypertension. Renal crisis occurs with the sudden onset of new malignant hypertension, microangiopathic hemolytic anemia, thrombocytopenia and azotemia; not all patients experience the entire complex of problems, and those with normotensive renal crisis (about 11% of renal crisis patients) are particularly difficult to diagnose and treat [63].

The cornerstone of successful management is early diagnosis and normalization of blood pressure. ACE inhibitors are the most effective agents and are started first at low doses and then with increasing amounts within the first few days in order to titrate the blood pressure to normal levels. When maximum doses of ACE inhibitors do not control the blood pressure, other antihypertensive agents, including calcium channel blockers or minoxidil can be used as needed. Some patients, especially those with severe renal dysfunction at presentation, fail to respond and progress to renal failure [64].

Figure 34.12 describes the University of Pittsburgh's experience using ACE inhibitors in renal crisis [63]. Thirty-one of 55 (56%) patients treated with ACE inhibitors had a good outcome with 20 patients never requiring dialysis and 11 patients (20% of the total) able to discontinue dialysis within 18 months. These latter patients were continued on ACE inhibitors throughout their course on dialysis. Of the 24 patients with a poor outcome, 9 patients required permanent dialysis and 15 died. Patients (especially older men) with congestive heart failure, a higher initial creatinine, or with inadequate control of blood pressure within 3 days of presentation, were more likely to have a poor outcome. Importantly, of the patients able to survive dialysis for 3 months, more than half were able to regain adequate independent renal function and discontinue dialysis. Renal transplantation can be done successfully.

Sjogren's Vasculitis

Keratoconjunctivitis sicca is common and may result from fibrosis of the glands [65]. Symptomatic treatment of the dryness includes artificial tears, sucking on sugarless candy, good dental care, and possibly electronic stimulation of salivary glands [66]. In some systemic sclerosis patients, most often those with limited scleroderma, Sjögren's syndrome and Ro(SS-A) and/or La(SS-B) antibody [67], a vasculitis may develop. Cutaneous and neurologic symptoms from the vasculitis usually respond to steroids.

SUMMARY

Although curative disease intervention is not presently possible, appropriate management of specific problems will improve both patient comfort and survival. The essential elements of effective management of systemic sclerosis are an understanding of the extent and pattern of organ involvement and the anticipation of the complications most likely to occur. The progress in basic pathophysiologic research and the potential for new and effective therapy clearly indicates that scleroderma is not a hopeless disease.

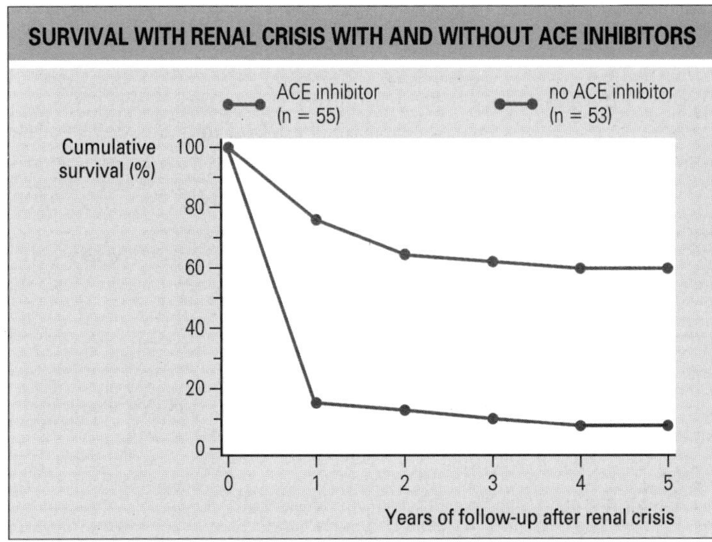

Fig. 34.11 Survival with renal crisis with and without ACE inhibitors. Scleroderma renal crisis had a very poor outcome prior to the availability of ACE inhibitors as demonstrated in this survival graph. The use of these drugs has helped to turn an almost uniformly fatal complication into a treatable problem.

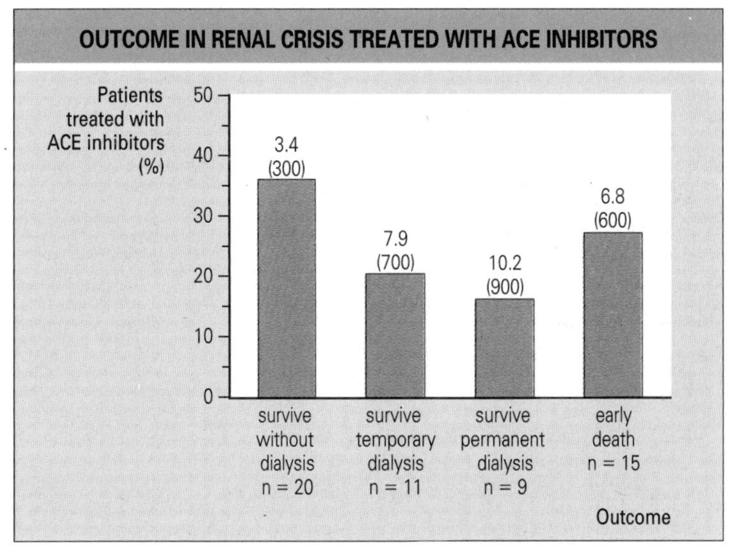

Fig. 34.12 Outcome in renal crisis treated with ACE inhibitors. ACE inhibitors are the drugs of choice in the management of scleroderma renal crisis. Unfortunately, there are still some patients who have an early death (27%) or require permanent dialysis (17%). Fortunately, a greater percentage (20%) were able to successfully discontinue dialysis after 3–18 months of treatment. Another 35% never required dialysis. The mean peak serum creatinine for each group in mg/dl is listed on top of bar with values for μmol/l in parentheses.

REFERENCES

1. Medsger TA Jr. Treatment of systemic sclerosis. Rheum Dis Clin North Am. 1989;**15**:513–31.
2. Steen VD, Medsger TA Jr, Rodnan GP. D-Penicillamine therapy in progressive systemic sclerosis (scleroderma). Ann Intern Med. 1984;**97**:652–9.
3. Kahaleh MB, Sultany GI, Smith EA, et al. A modified scleroderma skin scoring method. Clin Exp Rheumatol. 1986;**4**:367–9.
4. Poole J, Steen VD. The use of the Health Assessment Questionnaire (HAQ) to determine the physical disability in systemic sclerosis. Arthritis Care and Research. 1992;**4**:27–31.
5. Clements PJ, Peter JB, Agopian MS, et al. Elevated serum levels of soluble interleukin 2 receptor, interleukin 2 and neopterin in diffuse and limited scleroderma: effects of chlorambucil. J Rheumatol. 1990;**17**:908–10.
6. Black CM, McWhirter A, Harrison NK, et al. Serum type III procollagen peptide concentrations in systemic sclerosis and Raynaud's phenomenon: relationship to disease activity and duration. Br J Rheumatol.1989;**28**:98–103.
7. LeRoy EC, Black CM, Fleischmajer R, et al. Scleroderma (systemic sclerosis): classification, subsets and pathogenesis. J Rheumatol. 1988;**15**:202–5.
8. Steen VD, Medsger TA Jr, Rodnan GP, Ziegler GL. Clinical associations of anticentromere antibody (ACA) in patients with progressive systemic sclerosis. Arthritis Rheum. 1984;**27**:125–316.
9. Beckett VL, Conn DL, Fuster V, et al. Trial of platelet-inhibiting drug in scleroderma. Double-blind study with dipyridamole and aspirin. Arthritis Rheum. 1984;**27**:1137–43.
10. Ortonne JP, Torzuoli C, Dujardin P, et al. Ketanserin in the treatment of systemic sclerosis: a double-blind controlled trial. Br J Dermatol. 1989;**120**:261–6.

11. Jayson MIV, Holland CD, Keegan A, et al. A controlled study of stanozolol in primary Raynaud's phenomenon and systemic sclerosis. Ann Rheum Dis. 1991;**50**:41–7.
12. Constans T, Diot E, Lasfargues G, et al. Iloprost for scleroderma. Ann Intern Med. 1991;**114**:606.
13. Furst DE, Clements PJ, Hillis S, et al. Immunosuppression with chlorambucil, versus placebo, for scleroderma. Results of a three-year, parallel, randomized, double-blind study. Arthritis Rheum. 1989;**32**:584–93.
14. Alarcon GS, Casas JA, Saway PA, et al. 5-Fluorouracil in the treatment of scleroderma: a randomized, double-blind, placebo controlled international collaborative study. Ann Rheum Dis. 1990;**49**:926–8.
15. Clements PJ, Paulus HE, Sterz M, et al. A preliminary report on cyclosporin A (CSA) in systemic sclerosis (SSc). Arthritis Rheum. 1990;**33**:S66.
16. Zachariae H, Halkier-Sorensen L, Heickendorff L, Zachatiae E, Hansen HE. Cyclosporin A treatment of systemic sclerosis. Br J Dermatol. 1990;**122**:677–81.
17. Rook AH, Freundlich B, Jegasothy BV, et al. Treatment of systemic sclerosis with extracorporeal photochemotherapy: Results of a multicenter trial. Arch Dermatol. 1992;**128**:337–46.
18. Torres MA, Furst DE. Treatment of generalized systemic sclerosis. Rheum Dis Clin North Am. 1990;**16**:217–41.
19. Jimenez SA, Sigal SH. A 15-year prospective study of treatment of rapidly progresive systemic sclerosis with D-penicillamine. J Rheumatol. 1991;**18**(10):1496–1503.
20. Kahan A, Amor B, Menkes CJ, et al. Recombinant interferon-gamma in the treatment of systemic sclerosis. Am J Med. 1989;**87**:273–7.
21. Walker M, Harley R, LeRoy EC. Ketotifen prevents skin fibrosis in the tight skin mouse. J Rheumatol. 1990;**17**:57–9.
22. Gruber BL, Kaufman LD. Ketotifen-induced remission in progressive early diffuse scleroderma: evidence for the role of mast cells in disease pathogenesis. Am J Med. 1990;**89**:392–5.
23. Gruber BL, Kaufman LD. A double-blind randomized controlled trial of ketotifen versus placebo in early diffuse scleroderma. Arthritis Rheum. 1991;**34**:362–6.
24. Furst DE, Clements PJ, Harris R, Ross M, Levy J, Paulus HE. Measurement of clinical change in progressive systemic sclerosis: A 1 year double-blind placebo-controlled trial of N-acetylcysteine. Ann Rheum Dis. 1979;**38**:356–61.
25. Gibson T, Grahame R. Cyclofenil treatment of scleroderma: a controlled study. Br J Rheumatol. 1983;**22**:218–23.
26. Wollheim FA, Akesson A. Treatment of systemic sclerosis in 1988. Semin Arthritis Rheum. 1989;**18**:181–8.
27. Guillevin L, Chouvet B, Mery C. Treatment of progressive systemic sclerosis using factor XIII. Pharmatherapeutica. 1985;**4**:76–80.
28. Yocum DE, Hodes R, Sundstrom WR, et al. Use of biofeedback training in treatment of Raynaud's disease and phenomenon. J Rheumatol. 1985;**12**:90–3.
29. Smith CD, McKendry RJR. Controlled trial of nifedipine in the treatment of Raynaud's phenomenon. Lancet. 1982;**2**:1299–1301.
30. Finch MB, Dawson J, Johnston GD. The peripheral vascular effects of nifedipine in Raynaud's syndrome associated with scleroderma: a double-blind crossover study. Clin Rheumatol. 1986;**5**:493–8.
31. Seibold JR, Jageneau AHM. Treatment of Raynaud's phenomenon with ketanserin, a selective antagonist of the serotonin 2 (5-HT2) receptor. Arthritis Rheum. 1984;**27**:139–46.
32. Surwit RS, Gilgor RS, Allen LM, et al. A double-blind study of prazosin in the treatment of Raynaud's phenomenon in scleroderma. Arch Dermatol. 1984;**120**:329–31.
33. Franks AG Jr. Topical glyceryl trinitrate as adjunctive treatment in Raynaud's disease. Lancet. 1982;**1**:76–7.
34. Scherbel AL. The effect of percutaneous dimethyl sulfoxide on cutaneous manifestations of systemic sclerosis. Ann NY Acad Sci. 1983;**411**:120–30.
35. Williams HJ, Furst DE, Steen VD, et al. Double-blind multicenter controlled trial comparing dimethyl sulfoxide and normal saline in treatment of hand ulcers in patients with scleroderma. Arthritis Rheum. 1985;**28**:308–14.
36. Langevitz P, Buskila D, Lee P, et al. Treatment of refractory ischemic skin ulcers in patients with Raynaud's phenomenon with PGEI infusions. J Rheumatol. 1989;**16**:1433–5.
37. Berger RG, Featherstone GL, Raasch RH, et al. Treatment of calcinosis universalis with low-dose warfarin. Am J Med. 1987;**83**:72–6.
38. Fuchs D, Fruchter L, Fishel B, Holtzman M, Yaron M. Colchicine suppression of local inflammation due to calcinosis in dermatomyositis and progressive systemic sclerosis. Clin Rheumatol. 1986;**5**:527–30.
39. Jones NF, Imbriglia JE, Steen VD, et al. Surgery for scleroderma of the hand. J Hand Surg. 1987;**12A**:391–400.
40. Seeger MW, Furst DE. Effects of splinting in the treatment of hand contractures in progressive systemic sclerosis. Am J Occup Ther. 1987;**41**:118–21.
41. Olive A, Maddison PJ, Davis M. Treatment of oesophagitis in scleroderma with omeprazole. Br J Rheumatol. 1989; **28**:553.
42. Kahan A, Bour B, Couturier D, Amor B, Menkes CJ. Nifedipine and esophageal dysfunction in progressive systemic sclerosis. A controlled manometric study. Arthritis Rheum. 1985;**28**:490–95.
43. Johnson DA, Drane WE, Curran J, et al. Metoclopramide response in patients with progressive systemic sclerosis. Effect on esophageal and gastric motility abnormalities. Arch Intern Med. 1987;**147**:1597–1601.
44. Kahan A, Amor B, Menkes CJ, et al. Disapride in the treatment of esophageal abnormalities in systemic sclerosis. Arthritis Rheum. 1989;**32**:S-120.
45. Horowitz M, Maddern GJ, Maddoz A, et al. Effects of cisapride on gastric and esophageal emptying in progressive systemic sclerosis. Gastroenterology. 1987;**93**(2):311–5.
46. Dull JS, Raufman J-P, Zakai D, et al. Successful treatment of gastroparesis with erythromycin in a patient with progressive systemic sclerosis. Am J Med. 1990;**89**:528–30.
47. Levien DH, Kiallos F, Barone R, et al. The use of cyclic home hyperalimentation for malabsorption in patients with scleroderma involving the small arteries. J Paren Enter Nutrition. 1985;**9**:623–5.
48. Steen VD. Pulmonary involvement in systemic sclerosis. Chapter 10. In: Gannon GW, Zimmerman GA, eds. The lung in rheumatic disease. New York: Marcel Dekker Inc; 1990:279–302.
49. Schurawitzki H, Stiglbauer R, Graninger W, et al. Interstitial lung disease in progressive systemic sclerosis: high resolution CT versus radiography. Radiology. 1990;**176**:755–9.
50. Steen VD, Conte C, Owens G, et al. Natural history of severe pulmonary fibrosis in systemic sclerosis (SSc). Arthritis Rheum. 1990;**33**:S157.
51. Steen VD, Powell DL, Medsger TA Jr. Clinical correlations and prognosis based on serum autoantibodies in systemic sclerosis. Arthritis Rheum. 1988;**31**:196–203.
52. deClerck LS, Dequeker J, Francx L, Demedts M. D-Penicillamine therapy and interstitial lung disease in scleroderma. A long-term follow up study. Arthritis Rheum. 1987;**30**:643–50.
53. Steen VD, Owens GR, Redmond C, et al. The effect of D-penicillamine on pulmonary findings in systemic sclerosis. Arthritis Rheum. 1985;**28**:882–8.
54. Silver RM, Miller KS, Kinsella MB, et al. Evaluation and management of scleroderma lung disease using bronchoalveolar lavage. Am J Med. 1990;**88**:470–6.
55. Stupi AM, Steen VD, Owens GR, et al. Pulmonary hypertension in the CREST syndrome variant of systemic sclerosis. Arthritis Rheum. 1986;**29**:515–24.
56. Rich S, Brundage BH. High dose calcium channel-blocking therapy for primary pulmonary hypertension: evidence for long-term reduction in pulmonary arterial pressure and regression of right ventricular hypertrophy. Circulation. 1987;**76**:135–41.
57. Rubin LJ, Mendoza J, Hood M, et al. Treatment of primary pulmonary hypertension with continuous intravenous prostacyclin (epoprostenol). Results of a randomized trial. Ann Intern Med. 1990;**112**:485–91.
58. Follansbee WP. The cardiovascular manifestations of systemic sclerosis (scleroderma). Curr Prob Cardiol. 1986; **11**(5):245–98.
59. Kahan A, Devaux JY, Amor B, et al. Pharmacodynamic effect of nicardipine on left ventricular function in systemic sclerosis. J Cardiovasc Pharmacol. 1990;**15**(1):249–53.
60. Kahan A, Devaux JY, Amor B, et al. Pharmacodynamic effect of dipyridamole on thallium-201 myocardial perfusion in progressive systemic sclerosis with diffuse scleroderma. Ann Rheum Dis. 1986;**45**:718–25.
61. Kahan A, Devaux JY, Amor B, et al. The effect of captopril on thallium 201 myocardial perfusion in systemic sclerosis. Clin Pharmacol Ther. 1990;**47**:483–9.
62. Steen VD, Costantino JP, Shapiro AP, et al. Outcome of renal crisis in systemic sclerosis: relation to availability converting enzyme (ACE) inhibitors. Ann Intern Med. 1990;**113**:352–7.
63. Steen VD, Medsger TA Jr, Osial TA Jr, et al. Factors predicting the development of renal involvement in progressive systemic sclerosis. Am J Med. 1984;**76**:779–86.
64. Helfrich DJ, Banner B, Steen VD, Medsger TA Jr. Renal failure in normotensive patients with systemic sclerosis. Arthritis Rheum. 1989;**32**: 1128–1134.
65. Osial TA Jr, Whiteside TL, Buckingham RB. Clinical and serologic study of Sjögren's syndrome in patients with progressive systemic sclerosis. Arthritis Rheum. 1983;**26**:500–8.
66. Vivino FB, Sokol JN, Chapman EB, Hoffman BI, Katz WA. Treatment of xerostomia with salivary gland electrostimulation. Arthritis Rheum. 1990;**33**:S89.
67. Oddis CV, Eisenbeis CH Jr, Reidbord HE, et al. Vasculitis in systemic sclerosis: a subset of patients with the CREST variant, Sjögren's syndrome and neurologic complications. J Rheumatol. 1987;**14**:942–8.

35

CLINICAL FEATURES OF INFLAMMATORY MUSCLE DISEASE

Thomas A Medsger & Chester V Oddis

Definition

- A member of the connective tissue disease family as evidenced by autoimmune disease associations and other immunologic features.
- Characterized by chronic inflammation of striated muscle (polymyositis) and sometimes the skin (dermatomyositis).
- Autoantibody associations (e.g. anti-Jo-1, anti-Mi-2) define homogeneous clinical subsets of disease.

Clinical features

- Painless proximal muscle weakness with or without rash is the hallmark feature.
- Elevation of serum muscle enzymes, most notably creatine kinase.
- Other organ systems affected include joints, lungs (fibrosis), heart and gastrointestinal tract.
- Probable association with malignancy in elderly population.

HISTORY

Between 1886 and 1891 several German clinicians published accounts of patients with polymyositis/dermatomyositis although the first American case was not documented until 1888 [1]. Two thirds of the 19th century descriptions best fit polymyositis, which had been introduced by Wagner in 1886 [2], while one third described dermatomyositis, a term coined by Unverricht in 1891 [3]. The first reported case of unequivocal dermatomyositis associated with carcinoma was in 1916 [4], although a causal association between these two disease processes was not suggested until 1935 [5].

EPIDEMIOLOGY

Classification

The purposes of disease classification are to separate the disease of interest from others in order to determine incidence and prevalence, to describe the occurrence of disease in large populations, to compare one patient group with others and to identify clinically homogeneous subsets of patients. This will facilitate clinical studies of natural history and response to therapy as well as laboratory investigations of pathogenesis and etiology. It should be obvious that such attempts at classification, with no knowledge of cause and with inadequate understanding of pathogenesis, are necessarily preliminary and must ultimately be revised as appropriate.

In polymyositis/dermatomyositis, several different classification systems have been proposed (Fig. 35.1) [6–10]. Although all classifications identify these disorders as part of a single disease spectrum, certain important features are used to separate subsets, including the distinctions between childhood and adult onset, polymyositis versus dermatomyositis and the presence or absence of malignancy and other connective tissue diseases. The classification system of Bohan and Peter is relatively simple, but does not separate polymyositis from dermatomyositis in the categories of childhood, associated connective tissue disease or malignancy. The most complete classification is that of Banker and Engel [9], which distinguishes between all major forms of polymyositis and dermatomyositis with the exception that it does not include childhood polymyositis, admittedly the rarest of all subgroups. Inclusion body myositis is a morphologically distinct entity which may be part of the idiopathic polymyositis/dermatomyositis spectrum or, perhaps, a separate entity, which is discussed later.

In the future, it is likely that disease subsets will be identified according to serum autoantibodies and/or other immunologic characteristics. Such classifications are now in common use in systemic lupus erythematosus (SLE) and systemic sclerosis (scleroderma) where they now account for over 90% and over 80% of patients, respectively (see Chapters 31 and 33). In polymyositis/dermatomyositis, approximately 50% of patients can now be classified by myositis-specific autoantibody status, and for several of these autoantibodies, strong HLA associations have been described.

Incidence by Age, Race and Sex

The reported overall annual incidence of polymyositis/dermatomyositis ranges from 2 to 10 new cases per million persons at risk in various populations (Fig. 35.2) [11–15]. All published rates are most

PUBLISHED CLINICAL CLASSIFICATION SYSTEMS FOR POLYMYOSITIS/DERMATOMYOSITIS

	Author				
Disease subtype	Bohan and Peter [6]	Banker and Engel [9]	Walton and Adams [7]	Kagen [10]	Devere and Bradley [8]
Polymyositis					
Childhood	4		I/II	1	I
Adult	1	I	I/II	1	I
CTD	5	V	III	5	II/III
Malignancy	3	VII	IV	4	IV
Dermatomyositis					
Childhood	4	III	II	3	II/III
Adult	2	II	II	2	II/III
CTD	5	IV	III	5	II/III
Malignancy	3	VI	IV	4	IV

Fig. 35.1 Published clinical classification systems for polymyositis/dermatomyositis.

INCIDENCE RATES OF POLYMYOSITIS/DERMATOMYOSITIS FROM DIFFERENT POPULATIONS				
Author (year)	Geographic area	Inclusive dates of study	Incidence (per million)	Pertinent features
Rose and Walton (1966)	Northeast England	1954–1964	2.25	Patients included were classified using Walton and Adams criteria [7]
Kurland *et al.* (1969)	Rochester, MN, USA	1951–1967	6.0	Almost exclusively White population
Findlay *et al.* (1969)	Transvaal, South Africa	1960–1967	7.5	Includes incidence of dermatomyositis only
Medsger *et al.* (1970)	Memphis and Shelby County, TN, USA	1947–1968	5.0	40% population was Black
Benbassat *et al.* (1980)	Israel	1960–1976	2.2	Includes only hospital-diagnosed cases. Bohan and Peter criteria used for diagnosis
Oddis *et al.* (1990)	Allegheny County, PA, USA	1963–1982	5.5	Predominantly White population (91%). Incidence rate 8.9/million during 1973–1982

Fig. 35.2 Incidence rates of polymyositis/dermatomyositis from different populations.

likely underestimates since not all possible sources of ascertainment were examined. There is a trend toward increasing incidence in several communities over time [11–15], probably due to increased physician awareness rather than a true increase in disease occurrence.

In the northeast of England, Rose and Walton identified 89 new cases in a population of 3.2 million over an 11-year period, an annual incidence of 2.25 per million [14]. In the small, homogeneous, almost exclusively White population of Rochester and Olmstead County, Minnesota, Kurland and colleagues found an incidence of 6.0 new cases per million population per year [12]. Medsger and associates observed 5.0 new cases per million persons at risk annually in the large, racially mixed population of Memphis and Shelby County, Tennessee, which had a high proportion (40%) of Blacks [11]. The incidence during the last 6 years of the survey was 8.4 per million per year. Oddis and coworkers reported an overall annual incidence in Pittsburgh and Allegheny County, Pennsylvania, of 5.5 per million which was higher (8.9) during the last 10 years of the study [15]. In the same population, systemic sclerosis was twice as frequent and SLE approximately four times as frequent as polymyositis/dermatomyositis.

Although inflammatory myopathy can occur at any age, the observed pattern of incidence includes childhood and adult peaks and a paucity of patients with onset in the adolescent and young adult years [11,15]. This finding supports the concept of separating childhood from adult forms of the disease. The incidence sex ratio is 2.5:1 female to male. This ratio is lower (nearly 1:1) in childhood disease and with associated malignancy, but is very high (10:1) when there is an associated connective tissue disease. Polymyositis/ dermatomyositis has a 3–4:1 Black to White incidence ratio, with a Black young adult onset peak. The clinical–epidemiologic characteristics of each of the classification subsets of Rose and Walton are summarized in Figure 35.3.

Environmental Factors

No striking associations with environmental factors have been identified. Disease onset is more frequent in the winter and spring months, especially in childhood cases, consistent with precipitation by viral and bacterial infections [11]. Serum antibodies to coxsackie B viruses are more frequent in childhood dermatomyositis compared with juvenile RA controls [16]. In one study, polymyositis/dermatomyositis patients reported excessive physical exercise antedating illness significantly more frequently than controls [17], but this association has not been confirmed. D-penicillamine is a drug capable of inducing true myositis [18].

Genetic Factors

The occurrence of polymyositis/dermatomyositis in monozygotic twins [19] and first degree relatives of cases [20] supports a genetic predisposition, at least in some families. It is not uncommon to find that close relatives suffer from other autoimmune diseases [21].

The reported associations of certain HLA types with clinical subsets of disease are weak. White children with dermatomyositis and adults with polymyositis have an increased frequency of HLA-B8/DR3 [22–24], and HLA-B14 and B40 have been observed more commonly in adults with dermatomyositis coexisting with another connective tissue disease [25]. In polymyositis, Whites were noted to have HLA-B8/DR3, while Blacks more often had HLA-B7/ DRw6 [24]. HLA is considerably more closely linked to several recently identified

EPIDEMIOLOGIC CHARACTERISTICS OF POLYMYOSITIS/DERMATOMYOSITIS CLINICAL CLASSIFICATION SUBSETS						
	Adult poly-myositis	Adult dermato-myositis	Childhood	Connective tissue disease overlap	Malignancy overlap	All patients
Proportion of all patients	50%	20%	10%	10%	10%	
Age at diagnosis (mean)	45	40	10	35	60	45
Incidence sex ratio (F:M)	2:1	2:1	1:1	10:1	1:1	2.5:1
Incidence race ratio (B:W)	5:1	3:1	1:1	3:1	2:1	3:1

Fig. 35.3 Epidemiologic characteristics of polymyositis/dermatomyositis clinical classification subsets.

FREQUENCIES OF PRESENTING CLINICAL SYNDROMES IN POLYMYOSITIS/DERMATOMYOSITIS	
Syndrome	Estimated freqeuncy
1. Painless proximal weakness (over 3–6 months)	55%
2. Acute or subacute proximal pain and weakness (over weeks–2 months)	30%
3. Insidious proximal and distal weakness (over 1–10 years)	10%
4. Proximal myalgia alone	5%
5. Dermatomyositis rash alone	<1%

Fig. 35.4 Types and frequencies of presenting clinical syndromes in polymyositis/dermatomyositis.

GRADING OF MUSCLE WEAKNESS IN DERMATOMYOSITIS/POLYMYOSITIS	
1.	No abnormality on examination
2.	No abnormality on examination, but easy fatiguability and decreased exercise tolerance
3.	Minimal degree of atrophy of one or more muscle groups without functional impairment
4.	Waddling gait; unable to run but able to climb stairs without needing arm support
5.	Marked waddling gait; accentuated lordosis; unable to climb stairs or rise from a standard chair without arm support
6.	Unable to walk without assistance

Fig. 35.5 Grading of muscle weakness in dermatomyositis and polymyositis. Adapted with permission from Rose AL, Walton JN [14].

serum autoantibodies which have been found to define clinically homogeneous patient groups. Anti-Jo-1 antibody patients, who have predominantly polymyositis, have a significantly increased frequency of HLA-DRw52 compared with control persons [26], and those with anti-PM-Scl, who often have a polymyositis/ scleroderma overlap syndrome, nearly all possess HLA-DR3 or DRw52 [27].

Presentations

The clinical syndromes at presentation vary considerably from patient to patient (Fig. 35.4) [28–30]. The most frequent problem is insidious, progressive painless proximal muscle weakness over the course of 3–6 months prior to the first physician visit. Some patients, especially children and young adults with dermatomyositis, have a more acute onset with muscle pain and weakness developing rapidly over the course of several weeks. In the latter case, constitutional features such as fever and fatigue are more common. A few patients complain only about proximal myalgias. There is also a subset of patients with very slowly evolving weakness over the course of 5–10 years before diagnosis; they are typically men with pelvic girdle and distal extremity muscle weakness who have inclusion body myositis on muscle biopsy. Differentiation from muscular dystrophy may be difficult in this circumstance. The degree of muscle weakness at the time of first physician evaluation is highly variable. Several classifications for the severity of muscle weakness have been proposed [14,31]. One simple and useful scheme which combines physical examination and functional ability has been suggested by Rose and Walton [14] (Fig. 35.5). Using this system the mean disability grade in polymyositis/ dermatomyositis patients at presentation was 4.5 [8].

When the presenting musculoskeletal and cutaneous findings are listed according to disease classification, a somewhat different picture is found (Fig. 35.6). Of particular note are the rarity of Raynaud's

MUSCULOSKELETAL AND CUTANEOUS FINDINGS AT PRESENTATION IN 118 POLYMYOSITIS/DERMATOMYOSITIS PATIENTS

Signs	PM (%)	PM or DM; mild connective tissue disease (%)	PM or DM; severe connective tissue disease (%)	PM or DM; malignancy (%)	All cases (%)
Upper limb weakness	77	97	83	89	86
Lower limb weakness	88	97	93	89	92
Neck muscle weakness	37	50	54	71	47
Facial weakness	2	3	7	0	4
Respiratory muscle weakness	2	11	0	0	4
Bulbar weakness					
Palate and pharynx	0	17	10	0	6
Masseters	5	3	0	13	4
Muscle tenderness	34	47	46	57	43
Joint involvement	0	14	40	0	22
Contractures					
Upper limb	12	11	14	0	11
Lower limb	5	8	3	22	7
Skin rash	0	46	23	67	25
Skin tethering	0	8	33	0	11
Acrosclerosis	0	41	17	22	19
Distal ulceration or clinical calcinosis	0	0	13	0	3

Fig. 35.6 Musculoskeletal and cutaneous findings at presentation in 118 dermatomyositis/polymyositis patients. Adapted with permission from Bradley WG, Tandan R [28].

phenomenon and arthralgias in pure polymyositis (except anti-Jo-1 disease), the very similar features of dermatomyositis and myositis associated with connective tissue disease, and the absence of distal extremity and neck extensor weakness in patients with malignancy.

In addition to the shoulder and pelvic girdle, other striated muscles may be weak. On occasion, weakness in these muscle groups is the most prominent aspect of the illness. Examples of such findings, which each occur at presentation in approximately 5% of patients, are bulbar muscle weakness with dysphonia, pharyngeal dysphagia leading to aspiration pneumonia and respiratory muscle weakness, with or without interstitial lung disease causing dyspnea.

The rash of dermatomyositis can precede myositis [32,33]. Anti-Jo-1 antibody patients may first note Raynaud's phenomenon, polyarthralgias and/or polyarthritis, or dyspnea due to interstitial lung disease [34]. When an overlap syndrome is present, one may encounter early scleroderma symptoms and signs such as puffy fingers, sclerodactyly, and distal esophageal dysphagia or lupus findings including photosensitive and/or malar skin rash, alopecia, pleurisy or oral ulceration.

CLINICAL FEATURES

Constitutional

Fatigue in the sense of 'loss of well-being' is present in most patients with polymyositis/dermatomyositis. Fever occurs in a few individuals with dermatomyositis, especially children and young adults. Significant weight loss is uncommon.

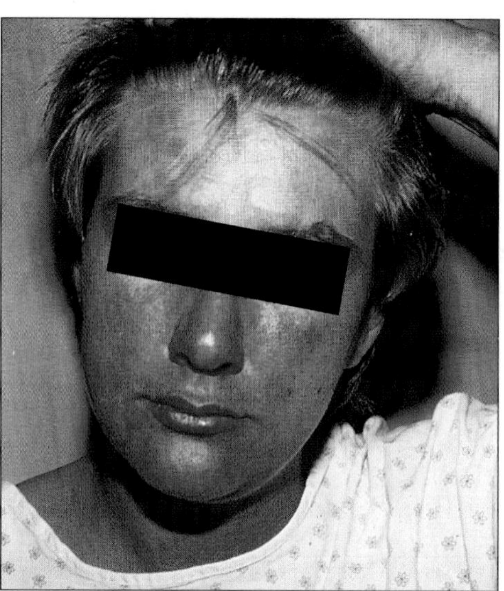

Fig. 35.7 The facial rash of dermatomyositis. Note the malar-like rash of dermatomyositis which involves the nasolabial area (an area often spared in SLE). Patchy involvement of the forehead and chin is also present in this patient.

Skeletal Muscle

Patients complain of difficulty in performing activities requiring normal upper and/or lower limb strength [28]. Pelvic girdle weakness leads to reduced strength in running, climbing stairs, and arising from a chair or toilet seat. Walking may become clumsy with a 'waddling' gait, and the patient may fall more frequently and if so, be unable to arise from the floor without assistance. Upper extremity weakness is manifested by difficulty raising an object overhead, inability to keep one's arms up while combing hair, or loss of grip strength. Neck flexor weakness is appreciated by difficulty raising the head from a pillow. Bulbar weakness results in hoarseness or dysphonia, difficulty in initiating swallowing with regurgitation of liquids through the nose and episodic coughing immediately after swallowing. Muscle pain is present in up to a half of patients but is seldom volunteered during history taking.

Physical examination is necessary to confirm weakness of individual muscles or groups of muscles. The severity of muscle weakness at each visit should be recorded. Serial quantitative assessment of muscle strength is an important measurement in these patients since laboratory tests do not always accurately reflect disease activity. In addition to the system noted earlier (Fig. 35.5), a rapid method for evaluation of lower extremity strength has been age and sex standardized [35]. A simple reproducible modified sphygmomanometer has been used to measure shoulder abductor muscle strength [36] and can be applied to other muscle groups.

The distribution of the muscle weakness is usually symmetric, affecting all proximal muscles. The shoulder and hip girdles are involved equally. The severity of weakness is almost always less in the distal muscles of the extremities, except in the circumstance of inclusion body myositis. Overall, distal muscles are weak in only 10–20% of patients. Ocular and facial muscles are rarely involved.

Muscle tenderness is present in half of patients but is not a prominent finding. Swelling of muscle is usual, and atrophy is a presenting feature only in long-standing previously undiagnosed myopathy, particularly inclusion body myositis. Firmness to touch and incomplete passive stretching suggest fibrous replacement of muscle and contracture, respectively. True muscle hypertrophy is not observed in polymyositis/dermatomyositis; this finding favors one or another of the forms of muscular dystrophy.

Skin

When typical, the skin lesions of dermatomyositis are often virtually pathognomonic of this disease (Figs 35.7, 35.8 & 35.9). The sites of predilection are the upper eyelids, malar areas, bridge of the nose and nasolabial folds, 'V' areas of the anterior chest and neck, upper

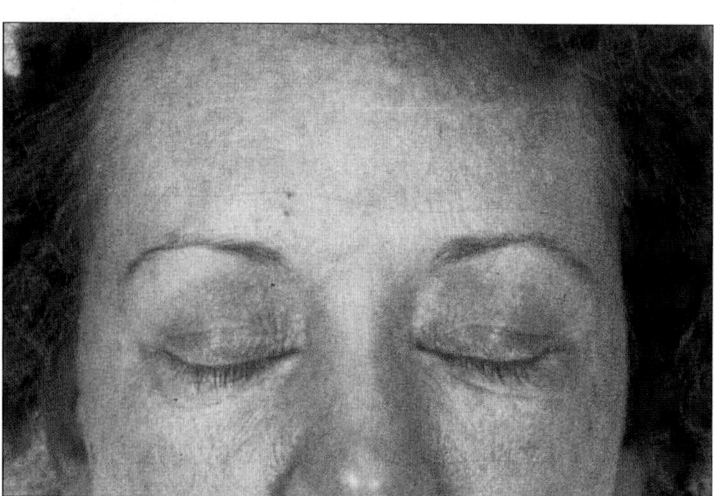

Fig. 35.8 Heliotrope rash of dermatomyositis. The erythematous/violaceous rash over the eyelids of this patient with dermatomyositis and breast cancer is a characteristic cutaneous feature.

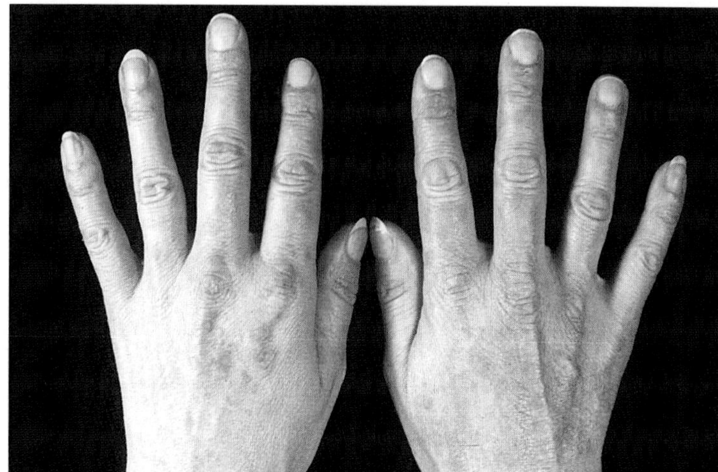

Fig. 35.9 Gottron sign. This erythematous, scaling rash over the knuckles and dorsum of the hand is a common early sign in dermatomyositis. It can be distinguished from the rash of SLE which usually affects the phalanges and spares the knuckles.

back, extensor surfaces of the elbows, knees, metacarpophalangeal and proximal interphalangeal joints and the periungual areas. Characteristic early lesions are erythematous or violaceous (heliotrope, lilac) and scaling is a prominent feature. Edema may be present, especially where the subcutaneous tissue is loose, such as the upper eyelids. Slightly raised or flat plaques over the finger joints are known as Gottron's papules. Cracking or fissuring of the distal digital pad skin has been termed 'machinist' or 'mechanic' hands (Fig. 35.10).

Later in their evolution, the affected skin lesions become shiny, atrophic and often hypopigmented. Cuticular hypertrophy and hemorrhage, as well as periungual erythema and telangiectasia are often visible to the naked eye, and nail-fold microscopy shows dilated capillary loops, as in other connective tissue diseases [37]. The skin may ulcerate and be difficult to heal because of motion at the site, trauma and hypovascularity. Photosensitivity and pruritus are observed but are not common. Other cutaneous findings reported to be associated with polymyositis/dermatomyositis include panniculitis, cutaneous mucinosis, vitiligo, and multifocal lipoatrophy [38–40].

Other Features

Joints

Polyarthralgias and/or polyarthritis, if they occur, are rheumatoid-like in distribution [41]. The wrists, knees and small joints of the hands are most frequently affected. Arthritis tends to occur early in the course of disease and to be mild and transient. Deforming arthritis is unusual but has been reported [42].

Calcinosis

Calcification can be a disabling late problem in polymyositis/dermatomyositis. It occurs most commonly in chronic dermatomyositis, especially with onset in childhood [43] and is rare in adult onset disease [44]. Myositis may be well-controlled or inactive at the time when calcinosis appears. Intracutaneous, subcutaneous, and fascial sites are affected, as well as the connective tissue surrounding muscle bundles. There is a predilection for sites of repeated microtrauma (elbows, knees, flexor surfaces of fingers, buttocks). When overlying or involved skin ulcerates with drainage of calcareous material, there may be complicating bacterial infection with chronic draining sinuses.

Respiratory

Dyspnea on exertion is a nonspecific but serious symptom in patients with polymyositis/dermatomyositis. It may be due to nonpulmonary problems such as inspiratory and expiratory respiratory muscle (diaphragm, intercostal) weakness [45,46], or congestive heart failure or cardiac arrhythmia from myocardial or conduction system involvement. Intrinsic causes of dyspnea include interstitial alveolitis or fibrosis, aspiration pneumonia from pharyngeal dysmotility, superimposed bacterial infection, and methotrexate pulmonary toxicity [47]. Cough is frequent, especially with advanced interstitial disease. Pleurisy and pleural effusion are rarely noted. Physical examination findings include decreased chest expansion with weakness of the muscles of respiration and bibasilar fine, crepitation 'velcro' rales in the case of alveolitis or interstitial fibrosis.

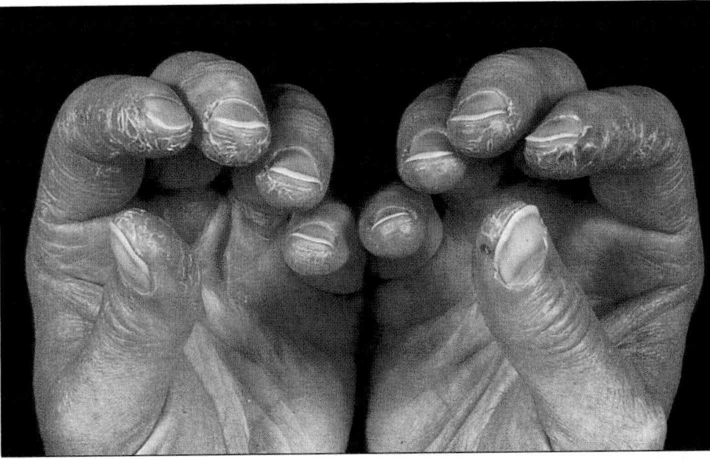

Fig. 35.10 'Machinist's hands'. Note the cracking and fissuring of the distal digital skin of the fingerpads in this patient with dermatomyositis. Courtesy of Dr. Frederick W. Miller.

There are three common presentations of lung disease in polymyositis/dermatomyositis. The most severe is an aggressive form of diffuse alveolitis with a nonproductive cough and rapid progression of dyspnea. In this situation pulmonary findings may be so prominent that the presence of myositis is overlooked. The opposite is the case in a more slowly progressive form of lung disease in which disability from myopathy may mask the severity of the pulmonary involvement. Finally, many asymptomatic persons have radiographic and/or physiologic manifestations of interstitial lung disease.

Cardiac involvement

Cardiac involvement is common but seldom symptomatic until it is very advanced [48]. Its true prevalence has been difficult to estimate because of conflicting results, biases of reported series, and probable under-ascertainment. The most frequent abnormality is a rhythm disturbance, and, thus, palpitations or symptomatic arrhythmias may occur [49]. Less common is congestive heart failure due to myocarditis or fibrous replacement of the myocardium. Dyspnea on exertion and orthopnea occur, and on physical examination one might detect tachycardia, neck vein distention, a left ventricular gallop sound, tender hepatomegaly and peripheral edema. Symptomatic pericarditis is rare.

Gastrointestinal tract

Cervical (pharyngeal) dysphagia in myositis is characterized by difficulty in initiating swallowing, nasal regurgitation of liquids and dysphonia. When severe, there may be aspiration into the tracheobronchial tree. The differential diagnosis includes cricopharyngeal muscle dysfunction [50].

Involvement of the smooth muscle of all portions of the intestinal tract from the thoracic esophagus through the colon is uncommon, except when there is overlap with systemic sclerosis. Such patients virtually always have associated Raynaud's phenomenon. Lower esophageal (thoracic) dysphagia results in the sensation that food, especially bread and meat, is 'sticking' in the retrosternal area during the act of swallowing. A weak lower esophageal sphincter leads to reflux of gastric acid into the lower esophagus with the symptom of heartburn, which is worse on reclining. Chronic distal esophagitis predisposes to stricture formation, the symptoms of which are progressive reduction in the caliber of food that can be swallowed until only liquids are tolerated, and vomiting of undigested food. Duodenal and small intestinal hypomotility are unusual; they may cause postprandial bloating, pain and distention as well as frequent diarrhea and weight loss. Constipation is the most common symptom of colonic hypomotility.

A unique type of gastrointestinal involvement in some patients with childhood dermatomyositis is ulceration and hemorrhage related to vasculopathy with ischemia [51].

Peripheral vasculature

Raynaud's phenomenon is a frequent accompanying complaint, particularly in individuals with dermatomyositis and/or features of systemic sclerosis or systemic lupus. Periungual infarction and fissuring of the digital pads without ulceration ('machinist's' hands) occur in some patients with Raynaud's phenomenon (Fig. 35.10). Digital tip ulceration due to ischemia is unusual but is claimed to be associated with underlying malignancy [52].

Renal involvement

Renal disease is rare in polymyositis/dermatomyositis. An occasional patient has proteinuria, and nephrotic syndrome has been described. Mild focal and mesangial proliferative glomerulonephritis without renal insufficiency may occur [53]. In the case of overlap syndrome the typical renal involvement of systemic sclerosis or lupus may be present. Myoglobinuria with acute renal insufficiency also has been observed [54].

Association with malignancy

The relationship between myositis and malignancy is controversial. Although one case-control study showed an increased risk of cancer prior to or concurrent with the diagnosis of inflammatory myopathy [55], another failed to detect any association [56]. Longitudinal observation of myositis patients after diagnosis has not identified a long-term increased frequency of malignancy [57]. A large retrospective literature review published in 1976 identified 258 cases of malignant neoplasm and concurrent myositis [58]. In over 80% of instances, the diagnosis of myositis and that of tumor were made within one year of each other. The most common relationship (50%) is myopathy preceding evidence of malignancy [59,60]. The frequency of malignancy in myositis derived from large medical center case series is regarded to be 10–15%, but community studies would suggest a lower figure, closer to 5% [11]. In cancer, dermatomyositis is three times as commonly found as polymyositis and the female to male ratio is approximately one. Although myositis in those under the age of 40 is distinctly unusual, and in children is rare [58], care must be taken to consider potential sites of malignancy appropriate for the patients' age in myositis cases over age 40 [61,62]. Interestingly, primary therapy of the tumor has been reported to result in regression of dermatomyositis manifestations [63], suggesting a close pathogenetic link between the two disorders.

Cancer in myositis patients is most frequently obvious rather than occult [55,56]. Thus, work-up for malignancy in myositis patients should consist of a careful history and physical examination and routine laboratory evaluation with directed individualized follow-up of any abnormalities found which cannot be explained by myositis, e.g. iron-deficient anemia or microscopic hematuria. An increased index of suspicion of malignancy is warranted if the patient has digital vasculitis [64] or a normal serum creatine kinase level [65].

DIFFERENTIAL DIAGNOSIS

History and Physical Examination

In patients with reduced muscle function, only half voluntarily complain about 'weakness'. Other frequent symptoms are 'tiredness' and 'fatigue'. Thus we must differentiate between difficulty in performing a certain motor task (weakness) or its repetitive performance (fatigue of muscle), from difficulty doing activities of daily living which require more endurance than muscle strength [66].

The two former problems imply primary disease of muscle or the neuromuscular unit, while the latter may include or be solely due to cardiovascular, metabolic, endocrine or psychiatric disorders. Fatigue describes a variety of patient complaints which have the common feature of loss of sense of well-being. Fatigue may include indifference to tasks at hand, preoccupation with unimportant activities or difficulty initiating or sustaining an activity. The patient often does not separate physical from mental activity. For example, disinclination to interact with one's family members and friends during leisure hours may be termed 'fatigue' by the patient but be interpreted as a symptom of depression by the discerning physician. Some of these non-neuromuscular causes of weakness are listed in Figure 35.11.

Noninflammatory Myopathies

The differential diagnosis of adult polymyositis is broad and includes numerous conditions capable of affecting skeletal muscle [28] (Fig. 35.12). History, physical examination and laboratory test result differences serve as the primary distinguishing features between these conditions. However, even the muscle biopsy may not be diagnostic in a number of patients with polymyositis/dermatomyositis.

NON-NEUROMUSCULAR CAUSES OF WEAKNESS
Episodic weakness (acute-attacks with recurrence)
Hypotension, cardiac arrhythmias
Hypoxia, hypercapnia
Hyperventilation
Hypoglycemia
Cerebrovascular insufficiency
Emotional states; anxiety attacks
Persistent weakness
Anemia
Chronic and acute infection
Malignancy
Malnutrition
Advanced organ system failure (lung, heart, liver, kidney)
Metabolic (hyperthyroidism, hyperparathyroidism, hypophosphatemia)

Fig. 35.11 Non-neuromuscular causes of weakness. Adapted with permission from Medsger TA Jr [66].

DIFFERENTIAL DIAGNOSIS OF MUSCLE WEAKNESS
Denervating conditions: spinal muscular atrophies*, amyotrophic lateral sclerosis*
Neuromuscular junction disorder: Eaton–Lambert syndrome*, myasthenia gravis*
The genetic muscular dystophies: Duchenne's facioscapulohumeral, limb girdle*, Becker's, Emery–Dreifuss type*, distal, ocular
Myotonic diseases: dystrophia myotonica*, myotonia congenita
Congenital myopathies: nemaline, mitochondrial, centronuclear, central core
Glycogen storage diseases: adult onset acid maltase deficiency*, McArdle's disease
Lipid storage myopathies: carnitine deficiency*, carnitine palmityltransferase deficiency*
The periodic paralyses
Myositis ossificans*: generalized and local
Endocrine myopathies*: hypothyroidism, hyperthyroidism, acromegaly, Cushing's disease, Addison's disease, hyperparathyroidism, hypoparathyroidism, vitamin D deficiency myopathy, hypokalemia, hypocalcemia
Metabolic myopathies*: uremia, hepatic failure
Toxic myopathies*: acute and chronic alcoholism, drugs including penicillamine*, clofibrate*, chloroquine, emetine
Nutritional myopathies: vitamin E deficiency*, malabsorption*
Carcinomatous neuromyopathy*: carcinomatous cachexia
Acute rhabdomyolysis*
Proximal neuropathies: Guillain–Barre syndrome*, acute intermittent porphyria*, diabetic lower limb chronic plexopathies*, chronic autoimmune polyneuropathy
Microembolization by atheroma or carcinoma
Polymyalgia rheumatica*
Other collagen vascular diseases: rheumatoid arthritis, scleroderma, systemic lupus erythematosus, polyarteritis nodosa
Infections: acute viral, including influenza, mononucleosis, rickettsia, coxsackie virus, rubella and rubella vaccination, acute bacterial including typhoid
Parasites: including toxoplasma, trichinella, schistosoma, cysticerci, sarcosporidia
Septic myositis: including staphylococcus, streptococcus, *clostridium welchii*, and leprosy
* Indicates the conditions that are most commonly confused with muscle weakness.

Fig. 35.12 Differential diagnosis of muscle weakness. The asterisk indicates the conditions that are most commonly confused with muscle weakness. Adapted with permission from Bradley WG, Tandan R [28].

Primary diseases of nerve include the spinal muscular atrophies, autosomal recessive disorders leading to slowly progressive degeneration of spinal anterior horn cells (weakness, wasting) and amyotrophic lateral sclerosis, which results in more rapid degeneration of both lower and upper motor neurons (bulbar or pseudobulbar palsy).

Myasthenia gravis is the prototypical disorder of the neuromuscular junction, in which weakness often affects the extraocular and bulbar muscles and becomes worse with repetitive contraction. A similar pattern of activity-increased weakness is found in Eaton–Lambert syndrome. Both of these diseases can cause proximal muscle weakness, but can be separated from polymyositis/dermatomyositis by their characteristic electromyographic patterns as well as absence of serum muscle enzyme elevation.

The muscular dystrophies are hereditary conditions with onset of symptoms either in childhood or adulthood and slow but steady progression. Their primary genetic and clinical features have been well described.

Glycogen storage diseases result from enzyme deficiencies involving the glycolytic pathway. McArdle's disease, or myophosphorylase deficiency, is caused by failure to degrade glycogen for energy under anaerobic conditions. It is characterized by acute episodes of pain, weakness, and swelling of muscles which are contracted frequently or for a prolonged period of time. On occasion, a late proximal myopathy occurs which can simulate polymyositis. Ischemic exercise testing results in failure to produce lactate and muscle biopsy shows glycogen accumulation and absence of myophosphorylase. Acid maltase deficiency results in excessive accumulation of glycogen in membrane-bound lysosomes. Progressive proximal weakness, myotonic changes on electromyogram and glycogen deposition on muscle biopsy are observed.

Disorders of muscle lipid metabolism may mimic polymyositis. Carnitine deficiency results in inability to transport long-chain fatty acids into mitochondria for oxidation, leading to lipid accumulation in muscle fibers and a chronic proximal myopathy. The enzyme carnitine palmityltransferase may also be lacking, resulting in a syndrome resembling McArdle's disease, with exertional pain and weakness due to inadequate ATP production from lipids. A similar symptom complex can occur with myoadenylate deaminase deficiency.

Other causes of proximal myopathy include vitamin D deficiency, adrenal insufficiency, hypophosphatemia, hyperthyroidism, carcinomatous neuromyopathy and exposures to various toxic substances. A variety of drugs are capable of producing inflammatory or noninflammatory myopathy (Fig. 35.13).

Other Inflammatory Myopathies

Inclusion body myositis is characterized by painless proximal and distal muscle weakness of insidious onset, typically in older men (Fig. 35.14). The serum creatine kinase level is normal or minimally elevated. Other connective tissue disease features are usually absent. Muscle biopsy shows vacuoles with basophilic granules and both intranuclear and intracytoplasmic tubulofilamentous inclusions. Although these inclusions resemble viral particles, the presence of large numbers of activated T cells in the endomysial infiltrate suggests immune-mediated muscle damage.

Infectious agents are capable of producing polymyositis [28]. Viruses reported to cause widespread, generally mild and self-limited myositis include influenza A and B, hepatitis B, coxsackie, rubella (both natural infection and following immunization with live attenuated virus), echo, and human immunodeficiency virus. Echovirus has been associated with myositis in patients with X-linked hypogammaglobulinemia.

Bacterial infection (pyomyositis) due to staphylococcal or streptococcal organisms results in acute focal suppuration with abscess formation, chiefly in children and young adults. Although initially reported to occur primarily in persons residing in tropical areas, pyomyositis recently has been more frequently diagnosed in temperate climates [67]. This disorder is potentially fatal if unrecognized and disabling if foci of osteomyelitis develop.

One parasitic infection capable of causing myositis is trichinosis, which is characterized by associated conjunctivitis, eosinophilia and elevated antibody titers. Toxoplasmosis may also cause a polymyositis-like illness in which the organisms are identified in muscle biopsies and an antibody response develops. Interestingly, antitoxoplasma antibody titers were significantly increased in a series of idiopathic polymyositis patients [68].

Focal nodular myositis, presenting with tumor-like masses and curiously limited to one or several extremities, has been noted. Giant cell myositis is rare but can be encountered in sarcoidosis. Regenerating muscle in other conditions may have a multinucleate appearance which must be distinguished from true giant cells in a typical granuloma.

Myositis with an eosinophilic inflammatory infiltrate has been reported; it may be part of the spectrum of the hypereosinophilic syndrome, may be focal or nodular, or be associated with eosinophilic fasciitis or the newly described eosinophilic myalgia syndrome due to the ingestion of contaminated L-tryptophan [69]. In the latter two disorders, the infiltrates occur in perimysial locations and true myofiber necrosis with weakness and creatine kinase elevation are unusual.

INVESTIGATIONS

General

Low-grade but rarely severe anemia is present in polymyositis; usually it is classified as the anemia of chronic disease. The erythrocyte

DRUGS ASSOCIATED WITH MYOPATHY	
Chloroquine	Ipecac
Cimetidine	Levadopa
Clofibrate	Lovastatin
Colchicine	Penicillamine
Corticosteroids	Penicillin
Cyclosporin	Phenylbutazone
Danazol	Phenytoin
Emetine	Procainamide
Epsilon amino-caproic acid	Nicotinic acid
Ethanol	Rifampicin
Gemfibrozil	Sulfonamides
Heroin	Vincristine
Hydralazine	Zidovudine (AZT)

Fig. 35.13 Drugs associated with myopathy.

CLINICAL FEATURES OF INCLUSION BODY MYOSITIS
1. Insidious yet progressive proximal and distal muscle atrophy and weakness
2. Affects predominantly elderly male population
3. Rare or no association with malignancy or other connective tissue diseases
4. Creatine kinase normal or only minimally elevated (usually <5–6 times normal)
5. Mixed myopathic and neuropathic electromyographic features
6. Resistance to corticosteroids and immuno-suppressive drugs

Fig. 35.14 Clinical features of inclusion body myositis.

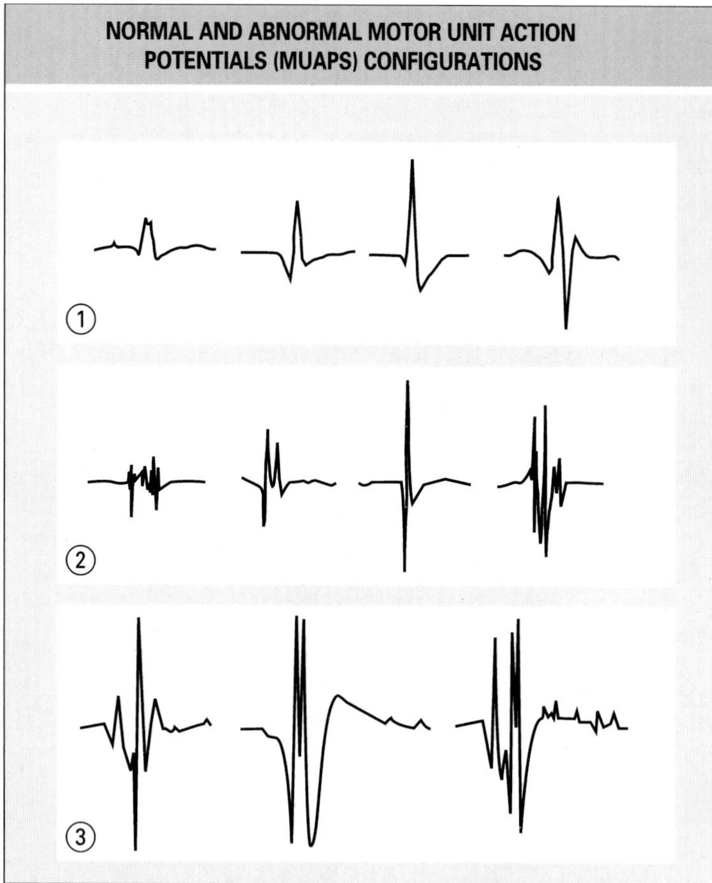

Fig. 35.15 Normal and abnormal motor unit action potentials (MUAPs) configurations. Normal MUAPs (1). Short duration, low amplitude, polyphasic MUAPs seen with myositis (2). Large amplitude, long duration polyphasic MUAPs as seen in neuropathic disorders (3). Adapted from Bromberg MB, Albers JW [73].

sedimentation rate (ESR) may be normal or mildly elevated (30–50mm/hour by the Westergren method) but seldom is increased to levels seen in RA or SLE.

Musculoskeletal

Enzymes

Elevated serum levels of enzymes which leak from injured skeletal muscle are valuable aids in detecting active muscle inflammation. In order of sensitivity, they are creatine kinase, aldolase, the transaminases (AST and ALT) and lactate dehydrogenase [70].

During disease exacerbations, creatine kinase levels rise several weeks or even months preceding clinical evidence of muscle weakness. Conversely, levels of this enzyme fall to normal or near normal weeks prior to objective improvement of muscle strength in a remission. For these reasons, and because of its specificity for muscle, creatine kinase is accepted as the most reliable enzyme test [71]. It is elevated at some time during the course of polymyositis/dermatomyositis in 95% of cases [63]. Three exceptions in which creatine kinase levels have been normal in biopsy-proven myositis are cases with a circulating inhibitor of creatine kinase activity [72], late-stage disease with severe atrophy and a few instances of early disease [65]. The latter situation should raise the suspicion of malignancy [65].

Electromyogram

Electrical testing is a sensitive but nonspecific method of evaluating inflammatory myopathy. Typical findings include irritability of myofibrils (fibrillation potentials) on needle insertion and at rest, and short duration, low amplitude, complex (polyphasic) potentials on contraction [73] (Fig. 35.15).

Over 90% of patients with polymyositis/dermatomyositis have these changes at first presentation in weak but not atrophic muscles, including paraspinal muscles. In addition, the electromyogram is a useful method for following disease activity, especially in the circumstance where serum enzyme levels and physical examination of muscle strength are difficult to interpret. However, there is little correlation between the amount of weakness or functional disability and the electromyographic findings. Many patients also have alterations which suggest involvement of terminal branches of intramuscular nerves, especially after several years of disease [74].

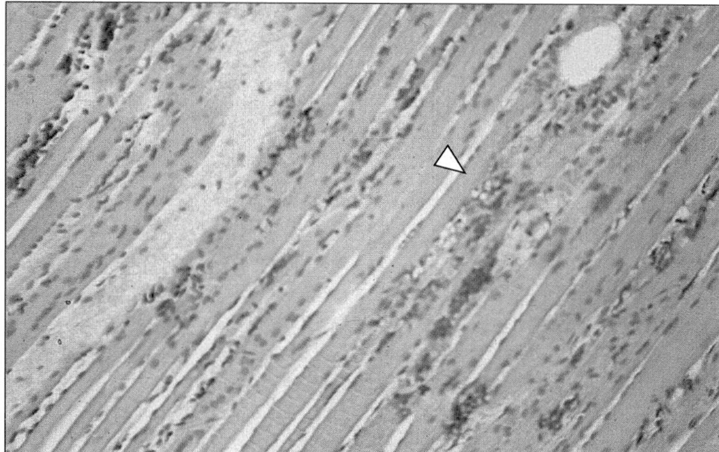

Fig. 35.16 Longitudinal section of fresh-frozen muscle from a patient with polymyositis. Multiple areas of interstitial involvement with myofiber destruction are seen. The arrow demonstrates an area of degeneration and necrosis of myofibers in association with interstitial lymphocytic and histiocytic cellular infiltration. (Hematoxylin and eosin, medium power.)

The electromyogram is helpful in the selection of a muscle for biopsy (see below). It should be performed unilaterally and an opposite side muscle chosen to avoid the interpretation problem presented by finding focal inflammation which could be an artifact secondary to needle insertion [10].

Biopsy

Muscle biopsy should be performed in all cases to confirm the diagnosis of inflammatory myopathy. The presence of chronic inflammatory cells in the perivascular and interstitial areas surrounding myofibrils, present in 80% of cases, is pathognomonic (Fig. 35.16). The infiltrate consists predominantly of lymphocytes, but other cells are often present, including histiocytes, plasma cells, eosinophils and polymorphonuclear leukocytes. Immunocytochemical studies have shown that a large number of activated T cells are present in the endomysial inflammation [75]. More common than inflammation are degeneration and necrosis of myofibrils, phagocytosis of necrotic cells, and myofibril regeneration (90% of cases). Damage to

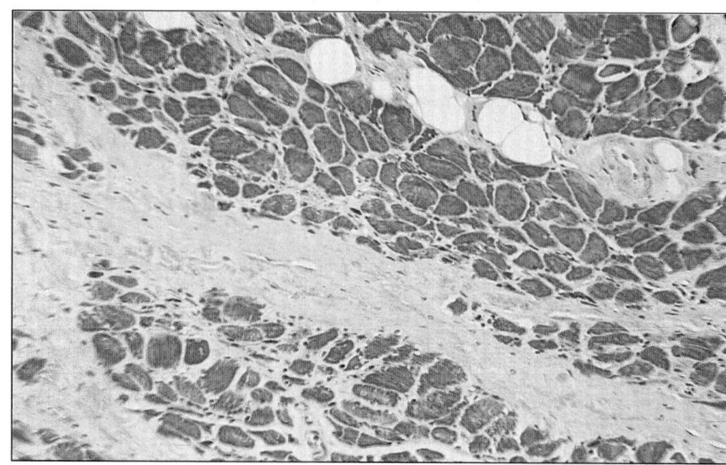

Fig. 35.17 Transverse fresh-frozen section of muscle from a patient with dermatomyositis. Note the atrophic, small fibers in the periphery of the fascicles (perifascicular atrophy) and the increase in fibrous tissue separating bundles of myofibers from a patient with chronic myositis. (Trichrome stain, low power.)

MUSCLE BIOPSY FINDINGS IN A GROUP OF 118 PATIENTS WITH MYOSITIS

Findings	Percentage of totals	
1. Fiber destruction, regeneration, perivascular and interstitial inflammation	46	65
2. Perivascular and interstitial inflammatory infiltrate with minimal fiber destruction	19	
3. Myofiber destruction and regeneration without inflammatory cell infiltrates	8	
4. Fiber atrophy and other nonspecific changes	11	
5. Normal tissue	17	

Fig. 35.18 Muscle biopsy findings in a group of 118 patients with myositis. Adapted with permission from DeVere R, Bradley WG [8].

muscle fibers, as well as atrophy, is concentrated at the periphery of fascicles, for unknown reasons. In long-standing myositis, fibrous connective tissue replaces necrotic myofibers and separates bundles of myofibers (Fig. 35.17). A summary of the histologic findings in a large series of patients is presented in Figure 35.18.

Overall, 15–20% of muscle biopsies in otherwise typical cases of polymyositis are not diagnostic of this disease [8]. This finding indicates the patchy nature of histologic changes and the rationale for basing diagnostic criteria on several clinical and laboratory abnormalities. Muscle histopathologic alterations in dermatomyositis and polymyositis are different in several important respects. Features more frequent in dermatomyositis include endothelial hyperplasia of blood vessels and deposition of immune complexes in the walls of intramuscular arteries [75–77].

Planning and proper technique can increase the yield of muscle biopsy [10]. A weak but not end-stage proximal muscle with electromyographic abnormalities on the opposite side is the best choice. It is preferable to choose a muscle not previously traumatized by injections. Open surgical biopsy is the current standard and has the advantage over needle biopsy of a larger specimen for review.

Serum myoglobin

Another substance which is released into the circulation from damaged skeletal muscle and cleared by the kidney is myoglobin. The majority of persons with active untreated myositis have increased serum myoglobin levels, but myoglobinuria is less frequent [78]. Myoglobinemia may be more sensitive than the serum creatine kinase level in some patients and can be used as an adjunct to serum muscle enzyme tests in diagnosis and follow-up [79].

Skin

Skin biopsy of early, active lesions reveals epidermal atrophy, liquefaction and degeneration of the basal cell layer, and perivascular infiltration of lymphocytes and histiocytes in the upper dermis [80]. In dermatomyositis, a striking vasculopathy of small vessels is found [81,82]. Immunofluorescence does not show immunoglobulin or complement at the dermal–epidermal junction as is found in systemic lupus.

Joints

In one form of polymyositis associated with serum anti-Jo-1 antibody, arthritis may become chronic and deforming with a characteristic radiographic feature of joint subluxation without erosions (Fig. 35.19) [83].

Lung

Reduced respiratory muscle strength is determined by measuring inspiratory pressures at the mouth. Affected individuals are unable to generate an adequate cough and thus are at increased risk of aspiration pneumonia [45–47]. The chest radiograph in interstitial lung disease shows bilateral basilar thickening (Fig. 35.20). In some patients with a normal chest film, thin section computerized axial

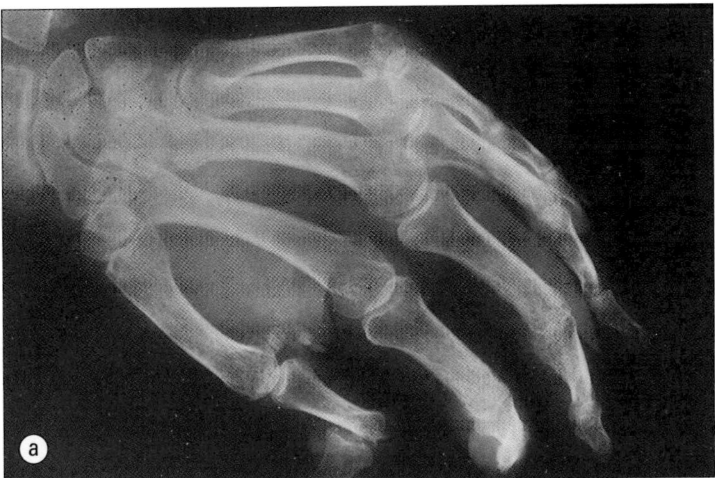

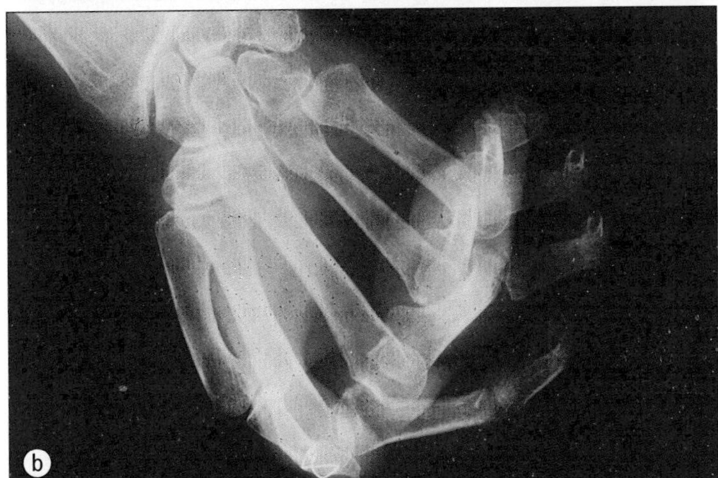

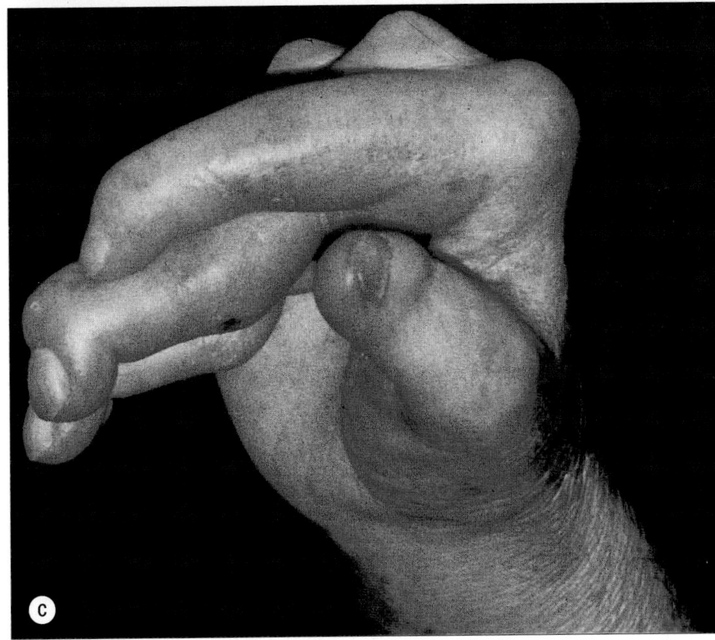

Fig. 35.19 Deforming arthropathy of polymyositis. Radiograph of the right hand of a patient with the anti-Jo-1 antibody taken in 1985 showing subluxation of the interphalangeal joint of the thumb (i.e. floppy thumb) [42]. No erosive changes were seen (a). Radiograph of the same patient's right hand taken in 1989, showing progressive deformity with numerous metacarpophalangeal, proximal interphalangeal, and distal interphalangeal joint subluxations, but no bony erosive changes (b). Photograph of the patient's right hand taken in 1989 showing significant deformity of multiple joints. The 'floppy thumb', present in the 1985 radiograph, was surgically fused at an earlier time (c).

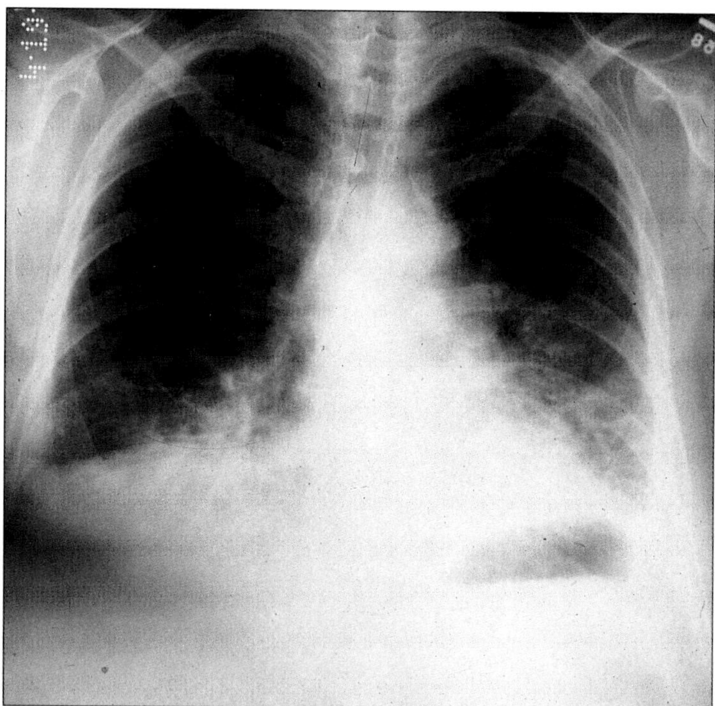

Fig. 35.20 Interstitial lung disease of polymyositis/dermatomyositis. Chest radiograph of a patient with interstitial lung disease and dermatomyositis demonstrating severe basilar fibrosis and mid-lung interstitial changes as well. Patients with myositis and interstitial lung disease often have antibodies to one of the amino-acyl-tRNA synthetase enzymes, as did this patient with anti-PL-12 (alanyl-tRNA synthetase).

tomography reveals evidence of interstitial fibrosis [84]. Advanced disease may result in the radiographic picture of 'honeycomb' lung. Ventilation–perfusion studies are abnormal, and pulmonary function tests show a restrictive physiologic pattern with reduced forced vital capacity and, often, reduced diffusing capacity for carbon monoxide. Vital capacity levels less than 55% of predicted normal are associated with carbon dioxide retention, especially in patients who also have respiratory muscle weakness [44].

In active alveolitis, the gallium scan is often abnormal [85], and bronchoalveolar lavage fluid contains increased numbers of macrophages, lymphocytes and neutrophils. Open lung biopsy typically shows excessive alveolar macrophages along with other chronic inflammatory cells, interstitial fibrosis and vascular thickening [47,86].

In late-stage disease, secondary pulmonary hypertension may ensue and progress slowly but with the ultimate development of clinical, radiographic and echocardiographic evidence of right ventricular dilatation and right heart failure.

Heart

There is disagreement about the frequency of cardiac disease. In one small prospective study, only 2 of 14 patients had abnormalities [87]. In contrast, in another report one-third of patients had electrocardiographic abnormalities (Fig. 35.21) [49], although none of these changes was specific for polymyositis/dermatomyositis. The most common alterations encountered are conduction defects and atrial and ventricular dysrhythmias, including complete heart block, which are due to involvement of working myocardium and/or the conducting system [48]. Left anterior hemiblock and right bundle branch block are the most frequently encountered conduction abnormalities. As in SLE and Sjögren's syndrome, the presence of maternal serum anti-Ro(SS-A) antibody is associated with an increased risk of infant cardiac conduction abnormalities [88].

Cardiomegaly and reduced left ventricular ejection fraction, along with congestive heart failure, are found in less than 5% of patients [63]. A series of endomyocardial biopsies has not been performed, but post-mortem examination shows myocardial fibrosis and, less commonly, myocarditis [48,89]. The latter and the extensive myocardial fibrosis are associated with congestive heart failure, as expected.

The MB fraction of creatine kinase is frequently elevated in patients with myositis, independent of clinical signs of cardiac involvement [90]. It appears most likely that this isoenzyme is produced by regenerating myofibrils in damaged skeletal muscle [91].

Intestine

In patients with pharyngeal dysphagia, the barium swallow shows cricopharyngeus muscle spasm, poorly coordinated motion of the pharyngeal musculature and vallecular pooling [92,93]. Distal esophageal hypomotility can be demonstrated by cine-esophagram or manometry in a high proportion of patients [94]. Such involvement of smooth muscle does not require the presence of associated connective tissue disease. Delayed gastric emptying and small bowel dilatation and hypomotility are infrequent; they are documented by barium studies [95]. A series of patients with both polymyositis and adult celiac disease has been reported [96]. The cause of the myopathy was not identified, although it was not considered to be secondary to osteomalacia.

Other Disorders

Miscellaneous conditions reported in association with polymyositis/dermatomyositis include autoimmune hypothyroidism [97,98], ophthalmologic abnormalities such as ophthalmoplegia, retinopathy (rare) and Evans syndrome or autoimmune hemolytic anemia with thrombocytopenia [99].

Serum Autoantibodies

An important new development in the connective tissue diseases is the identification of serum antibodies which are associated with clinically homogeneous patient subsets. In polymyositis/dermatomyositis, greater than 80% of patients have autoantibodies to nuclear and/or cytoplasmic antigens [100], and approximately half these patients have been shown to have myositis-specific antibodies [101] (Fig. 35.22). Autoantibodies typically associated with other connective tissue diseases may be found in myositis or overlap syndromes but are not myositis-specific. They include antiU1-RNP (15%), anti-PM-Scl (<10%), anti-Ro(SS-A) (<10%), anticentromere, antimitochondrial and others. Although a few patients have more than one autoantibody, multiple myositis-specific serum antibodies are rarely if ever detected in the same patient.

The most frequently identified antibody, anti-Jo-1, is found in only about 20% of all myositis patients tested [102]. Anti-Jo-1 is the most common of a group of anticytoplasmic aminoacyl-tRNA synthetase enzymes and is itself directed against histidyl-tRNA synthetase (Fig. 35.23). Due to the cytoplasmic location of the antigens

FREQUENCY OF ECG ABNORMALITIES IN 77 POLYMYOSITIS PATIENTS

	Number	(%)	Abnormalities (%)
Right bundle branch block	7	(9%)	28
Left bundle branch block	2	(3%)	8
Left anterior hemiblock	10	(13%)	40
Left ventricular hypertrophy	2	(3%)	8
Poor R wave progression	2	(3%)	8
Arrhythmia	2	(3%)	8
Total	25	(33%)	

Fig. 35.21 Frequency of ECG abnormalities in 77 polymyositis patients. Adapted from Stern R *et al.* [49].

SERUM AUTOANTIBODIES IN POLYMYOSITIS AND DERMATOMYOSITIS PATIENT SUBSETS					
Autoantibody	Polymyositis	Dermatomyositis	Childhood	Overlap	Malignancy
Jo-1	30% *	5%	0	15%	0
PM-Scl **	10%	<5%		10%	0
nRNP	10%	5%	<5%	30–40% ***	0
Others					
Ku				5%	
Mi-2		10%			
PL-7, PL-12, OJ, EJ	–<5%–				
SRP	<5%				

* Associated with interstitial lung disease
** Predominantly overlap with systemic sclerosis
*** Predominantly overlap with systemic lupus erythematosus

Fig. 35.22 Serum autoantibodies in polymyositis/dermatomyositis patient subsets. Adapted from Plotz PH [29].

to which they are directed, such autoantibodies are often found in patients who are antinuclear antibody (ANA) negative. Patients with these antisynthetase antibodies often have polymyositis, dermatomyositis or myositis in overlap rather than nonmyositis diagnoses. The 'antisynthetase syndrome' is characterized by fever, inflammatory and sometimes deforming polyarthritis, Raynaud's phenomenon, and interstitial lung disease [83].

Antibodies to signal recognition particle (anti-SRP) mark a separate subgroup of myositis patients with anticytoplasmic antibodies. These patients have the acute onset of severe muscle disease (polymyositis without rash) and respond poorly to therapy. They have no increase in interstitial lung disease, arthritis or Raynaud's phenomenon, but have greater than expected cardiac complications.

Anti-Mi-2 is an antinuclear antibody found in 5–10% of myositis patients overall and is strongly associated with the rash of dermatomyositis [104]. It is also identified in juvenile dermatomyositis. Anti-Mi-2 patients have none of the clinical associations seen with the antisynthetase antibodies. Anti-PM-Scl is an antinucleolar antibody that identifies a subset of myositis patients with features of systemic sclerosis [105]. This antibody may also be seen in persons with polymyositis, dermatomyositis or systemic sclerosis alone, i.e. without being called 'overlap'. Anti-U1 RNP antibodies are found in patients with so-called 'mixed connective tissue disease' [106].

Myositis-specific antibodies may be important in the pathogenesis of the inflammatory myopathies, as supported by their association with particular disease subsets, their selective response against particular antigens and the occasional reported variation of antibody titer with disease activity [107]. In addition, immunogenetic mechanisms appear to play a role, as the anti-Jo-1 antibody is associated with HLA-DR3 in Whites [108] and the other antibodies to translation-related antigens are associated with HLA-DRw52 [109]. Anti-PM-Scl has increased expression of HLA-DR3 compared with control populations [27]. Anti-SRP antibody positive patients have HLA-DR5 in a higher than expected proportion [101].

NATURAL HISTORY OF DISEASE

In some patients, dermatomyositis (but seldom polymyositis) is an illness of brief duration followed by remission which does not require continued therapy. The majority of patients, however, have multiple exacerbations and remissions or persistent disease activity necessitating chronic use of corticosteroids and/or immunosuppressive drugs. Milder, more easily controlled myositis is reported in community studies as compared with medical center-based series [111].

With each episode of myositis, there is the potential for absolute loss of muscle mass. The rate of progression and amount of muscle loss differ according to clinical classification and serum autoantibody subtype [112]. The best functional outcome occurs in dermatomyositis, while the worst is in inclusion body myositis and polymyositis with the anti-SRP antibody.

PROGNOSIS

Assessment of prognosis in polymyositis/dermatomyositis is difficult for several reasons. First, the disease is relatively rare, and some studies involve single referral centers reporting retrospectively on small numbers of patients followed for brief periods of time. Second, many reports are cross-sectional in design and combine patients with early and late stage disease. A classification system, with disease subsets based on meaningful pathophysiologic and serologic data, has not been developed. Finally, objective criteria for improvement (or deterioration) are not standardized. It is obvious that we need long-term prospective follow-up of well-defined incident cohorts of myositis patients utilizing validated outcome measures [113].

Survival

After reviewing the studies published before the availability of corticosteroids, one must conclude that a high proportion (up to 50%) of untreated polymyositis/dermatomyositis patients seen at major medical centers died of its complications [113]. Although nearly all studies during the past 30 years have confirmed the benefit of corticosteroids on muscle weakness, there is no double blind placebo-controlled documentation of their effect on survival. However, because of their nearly universal acceptance, corticosteroids cannot be withheld for ethical reasons in today's controlled prospective trials. Published uncontrolled studies during the corticosteroid era clearly support

ANTI-AMINOACYL-tRNA SYNTHETASE ANTIBODIES AND THEIR ASSOCIATED ANTIGENS IN POLYMYOSITIS/DERMATOMYOSITIS		
Antibody	Antigen	Polymyositis/ dermatomyositis patients with antibody (%)
Anti-Jo-1	Histidyl-tRNA synthetase	20
Anti-PL-7	Threonyl-tRNA synthetase	<3
Anti-PL-12	Alanyl-tRNA synthetase	<3
Anti-OJ	Isoleucyl-tRNA synthetase	<3
Anti-EJ	Glycyl-tRNA synthetase	<3

Fig. 35.23 Anti-aminoacyl-tRNA synthetase antibodies and their associated antigens in polymyositis/dermatomyositis.

improved survival (Fig. 35.24). During the 1960s, three large series described 265 patients followed for 1.8–5.0 years with mortality rates varying from 14 to 40% [63,114,115]. A similar 3-study composite of 288 patients reported during the 1970s had only 56 (19%) deaths [64,116,117]. At the present time, the expected survival in incident cases of polymyositis/dermatomyositis, excluding those associated with malignancy, is over 90% at 5 years after initial diagnosis.

Factors associated with poor survival in these reports include older age, malignancy, delayed initiation of corticosteroid therapy, pharyngeal dysphagia with aspiration pneumonia, myocardial involvement, and complications of corticosteroid and/or immunosuppressive drugs. Additional adverse risk factors for survival among childhood dermatomyositis patients are gastrointestinal vasculitis and sepsis.

Survival can also be determined according to clinical and autoantibody subsets. Pooling unpublished data from Miller [112] and Medsger, the 5-year cumulative survival rate from the time of first physician diagnosis is worst for cancer-associated myositis (55%) and dermatomyositis (80%) and best for inclusion body myositis (95%) and connective tissue disease related myositis (85%). Among the serum autoantibodies, anti-SRP is the worst prognostic marker (5-year survival 30%), followed by the antisynthetase group (65%). The best survival is among patients with anti-PM-Scl (95%) and anti-Mi-2 (95%).

Disability

The determinants of functional status in polymyositis/dermatomyositis are quite different from those of survival. For example, inclusion body myositis has the worst functional outlook but a good survival because of the lack of visceral involvement. Each major exacerbation of myositis likely results in a reduction in muscle strength, but therapy almost never returns the patient to the preceding level of total body muscle mass or strength [112]. Fortunately, a minor amount of atrophy and weakness in one or more muscle groups most often does not translate into functional impairment. In one 20-year follow-up study of 118 patients, two-thirds of the 82 survivors had no functional disability [8]. Other disease-related sequelae include calcinosis (especially in juvenile dermatomyositis), arthropathy, Raynaud's phenomenon, pulmonary interstitial fibrosis with respiratory insufficiency and myocardial involvement leading to congestive heart failure or ventricular arrhythmias.

The contribution of corticosteroid and immunosuppressive drug toxicity to long-term disability has not been adequately addressed, but the frequency of serious adverse reactions has been reported to be 20–40% [6,111,116,117,121,122]. The most commonly encountered disabling side effects include osteoporotic bone fractures, osteonecrosis of bone, serious bacterial and fungal infections, and cataracts. Problems which are inconvenient and require frequent physician visits, expense for medications and toxicity monitoring are diabetes mellitus, hypertension and peptic ulcer disease. Early cytopenias, with complications including septicemia, and late hematologic malignancies are serious concerns in patients treated with immunosuppressive drugs.

MORTALITY STATISTICS AND PROGNOSTIC FEATURES OF SEVERAL POLYMYOSITIS/DERMATOMYOSITIS SERIES STRATIFIED BY TREATMENT AND DECADE OF PATIENT ENTRY

Author (year)	Dates of patient entry	Number of patients	Mean follow-up from entry (years)	Mortality rate	
			Noncorticosteroid-treated patients		Comments
O'Leary (1940)	1926–1939	38	not stated	50%	36/38 with dermatomyositis
Sheard (1951)	1927–1950	25	5.0	52%	22/25 with dermatomyositis; 5/7 under age 20 died
Winkelmann (1968)	before 1959	122	3.0	29%	(see below)
			Corticosteroid-treated patients		Poor prognostic features
Rose (1966)	1954–64	89	6.1	30%	Malignancy, other connective tissue disease, acute course
Winkelmann (1968)	before 1959	157	3.0	35%	Malignancy, scleroderma, rapid progression
Medsger (1971)	1947–1968	124	2.5 (median)	36%	Pulmonary infiltrates, dysphagia, severe weakness, age >50, Black race
Carpenter (1977)	1947–1971	62	not stated	45%	Dysphagia, severe weakness
Bohan (1977)	1956–1971	153	4.3	14%	Malignancy, older age, delayed treatment
Benbassat (1985)	1956–1976	92	1.8	32%	Dysphagia, older age, leukocytosis, fever, failure to induce remission, shorter disease remission
Riddoch (1975)	1960–1970	20	5.0	40%	Study excluded children and patients with cancer and connective tissue disease
Henriksson (1982)	1967–1978	107	5.0	23%	Malignancy, older age, delayed treatment, cardiac involvement
Hochberg (1986)	1970–1981	76	not stated	17%	Age >45, cardiac involvement
Tymms (1985)	1970–1982	105	4.0	18%	Older age, delayed treatment

Fig. 35.24 Mortality statistics and prognostic features of several polymyositis/dermatomyositis series stratified by treatment and decade of patient entry. Adapted from Oddis CV, Medsger TA Jr [113].

REFERENCES

1. Jacoby GW. Subacute progressive polymyositis. J Nervous Mental Dis. 1888;**13**:697–726.
2. Wagner E. Ein Fall von akuter Polymyositis. Deutsch Arch klin Med. 1886;**40**:241–66.
3. Unverricht H. Dermatomyositis acuta. Deutsch Med Wchnscher. 1891;**17**:41–4.
4. Kankeleit. Uber primare nichteitrige Polymyositis. Deutsch Arch klin Med. 1916;**120**:335–49.
5. Bezecny R. Dermatomyositis. Arch f Dermat u Syph. 1935;**171**:242–51.
6. Bohan A, Peter JB. Polymyositis and dermatomyositis. N Engl J Med. 1975;**292**:344–7,403–7.
7. Walton JN, Adams RD, eds. Polymyositis. Baltimore: Williams & Wilkins; 1958.
8. DeVere R, Bradley WG. Polymyositis: its presentation, morbidity and mortality. Brain. 1975;**98**:637–66.
9. Banker BQ, Engel AG. The polymyositis and dermatomyositis syndromes. In: Engel AG, Banker BQ, eds. Myology, vol. 2. McGraw-Hill: New York; 1986:1385–422.
10. Kagen LJ. Polymyositis/dermatomyositis. In: McCarty DJ, ed. Arthritis and allied conditions, 11E. Philadelphia: Lea and Febiger; 1989:1092–117.
11. Medsger TA, Dawson WN, Masi AT. The epidemiology of polymyositis. Am J Med. 1970;**48**:715–23.
12. Kurland LT, Hauser WA, Ferguson RH, Holley KE. Epidemiologic features of diffuse connective tissue disorders in Rochester, Minnesota, 1951–1967, with special reference to systemic lupus erythematosus. Mayo Clin Proc. 1969;**44**:649–63.
13. Benbassat J, Geffel D, Zlotnick A. Epidemiology of polymyositis–dermatomyositis in Israel, 1960–76. Isr J Med Sci. 1980;**16**:197–200.
14. Rose AL, Walton JN. Polymyositis. A survey of 89 cases with particular reference to treatment and prognosis. Brain. 1966;**89**:747–68.
15. Oddis CV, Conte CG, Steen VD, Medsger TA Jr. Incidence of PM–DM: A 20-year study of hospital diagnosed cases in Allegheny County, PA 1963–1982. J Rheumatol. 1990;**17**:1329–34.
16. Christensen ML, Pachman LM, Schneiderman R, Patel DC, Friedman JM. Prevalence of Coxsackie B virus antibodies in patients with juvenile dermatomyositis. Arthritis Rheum. 1986;**29**:1365–70.
17. Lyon ME, Bloch DA, Hollak B, Fries JF. Predisposing factors in PM–DM: Results of a nationwide survey. J Rheumatol. 1989;**16**:1218–24.
18. Morgan GL, McGuire JL, Ochoa J. Penicillamine-induced myositis in rheumatoid arthritis. Muscle Nerve. 1981;**4**:137–40.
19. Harati Y, Niakan E, Bergman EW. Childhood dermatomyositis in monozygotic twins. Neurology. 1986;**36**:721–3.
20. Leonhardt T. Familial occurrence of collagen diseases. II. Progressive systemic sclerosis and dermatomyositis. Acta Med Scand. 1961;**169**:735–42.
21. Walker GL, Mastalgia FL, Roberts DF. A search for genetic influence in idiopathic inflammatory myopathy. Acta Neurol Scand. 1982;**66**:432–3.
22. Pachman LM, Cooke N. Juvenile dermatomyositis: A clinical and immunologic study. J Pediatr. 1980;**96**:226–34.
23. Behan WMH, Behan PO, Dick HA. HLA-B8 in polymyositis. N Engl J Med. 1978;**298**:1260–61.
24. Hirsch TJ, Enlow RW, Bias WB, Arnett FC. HLA-D related (DR) antigens in various kinds of myositis. Hum Immunol. 1981;**3**:181–6.
25. Wilcox CB. HLA and serum complement in polymyositis. Lancet. 1977;**2**:978–9.
26. Goldstein R, Duvic M, Targoff IN, et al. HLA-D region genes associated with autoantibody responses to histidyl-transfer RNA synthetase (Jo-1) and other translation related factors in myositis. Arthritis Rheum. 1990;**33**:1240–48.
27. Genth E, Mierau R, Genetzly P, et al. Immunogenetic associations of scleroderma-related antinuclear antibodies. Arthritis Rheum. 1990;**33**:657–65.
28. Bradley WG, Tandan R. Inflammatory diseases of muscle. In: Kelley WN, Harris Jr ED, Ruddy S, Sledge CB, eds. Textbook of rheumatology, 3E. Philadelphia: WB Saunders; 1989:1263–87.
29. Plotz PH (moderator). Current concepts in the idiopathic inflammatory myopathies: polymyositis, dermatomyositis and related disorders. NIH Conference. Ann Intern Med. 1989;**111**:143–57.
30. Callen JP. Dermatomyositis. Disease-a-Month. 1987;**5**:237-305.
31. Gardner-Medwin D, Walton JN. The clinical examination of the voluntary muscles. In: Walton JN, ed. Disorders of voluntary muscle. Edinburgh: Churchill Livingston; 1974:517–60.
32. Krain LS. Dermatomyositis in six patients without initial muscle involvement. Arch Dermatol. 1950;**111**:241–45.
33. Rockerbie NR, Woo TY, Callen JP, Giustina T. Cutaneous changes of dermatomyositis precede muscle weakness. J Am Acad Dermatol. 1989;**20**:629–32.
34. Bernstein RM, Morgan SH, Chapman J, Bunn CC, Mathews MB, Turner-Warwick M. Anti-Jo-1 antibody: A marker for myositis with interstitial lung disease. Br Med J. 1984;**289**:151–2.
35. Csuka ME, McCarty DJ. A rapid method for measurement of lower extremity muscle strength. Am J Med. 1985;**78**:77–81.
36. Helewa A, Goldsmith CH, Smythe HA. Patient, observer and instrument variation in the measurement of strength of shoulder abductor muscles in patients with rheumatoid arthritis using a modified sphygmomanometer. J Rheumatol. 1986;**6**:1044–9.
37. Maricq HR, LeRoy EC. Patterns of finger capillary abnormalities in connective tissue diseases by 'wide-field' microscopy. Arthritis Rheum. 1973;**16**:619–28.
38. Winkelman WJ, Billick RC, Srolovitz H. Dermatomyositis presenting as panniculitis. J Am Acad Dermatol. 1990;**23**:1278.
39. van Linthoudt D, Gabay C, Ott H. Vitiligo and polymyositis. Clin and Exp Rheumatol. 1989;**7**:334–5.
40. Commens C, O'Neill P, Walker G. Dermatomyositis associated with multifocal lipoatrophy. J Am Acad Dermatol. 1990;**22**:966–9.
41. Schumacher HR, Schimmer B, Gordon GV, et al. Articular manifestations of polymyositis and dermatomyositis. Am J Med. 1979;**67**:287–92.
42. Bunch TW, O'Duffy JD, McLeod RA. Deforming arthritis of the hands in polymyositis. Arthritis Rheum. 1976;**19**:243–8.
43. Blane CE, White SJ, Braunstein EM, Bowyer SL, Sullivan DB. Patterns of calcification in childhood dermatomyositis. Am J Radiol. 1984;**142**:397–400.
44. Cohen MG, Nash J, Webb J. Calcification is rare in adult-onset dermatopolymyositis. Clin Rheumatol. 1986;**5**:512–16.
45. Braun NMT, Arora NS, Rochester DF. Respiratory muscle and pulmonary function in polymyositis and other proximal myopathies. Thorax. 1983;**38**:616–23.
46. Martin L, Chalmers IM, Dhingra S, McCarthy D, Hunter T. Measurements of maximum respiratory pressures in polymyositis and dermatomyositis. J Rheumatol. 1985;**12**:104–7.
47. Dickey BF, Myers AR. Pulmonary disease in polymyositis/dermatomyositis. Semin Arthritis Rheum. 1984;**14**:60–76.
48. Haupt HM, Hutchins GM. The heart and cardiac conducting system in polymyositis–dermatomyositis. Am J Cardiol. 1982;**50**:998–1006.
49. Stern R, Goodbold JH, Chess Q, Kagen LJ. ECG abnormalities in polymyositis. Arch Intern Med. 1984;**44**:2185–9.
50. Dietz F, Logeman JA, Sahgal V, Schmidt FR. Cricopharyngeal muscle dysfunction in the differential diagnosis of dysphagia of polymyositis. Arthritis Rheum 1980;**23**:491–5.
51. Banker BQ, Victor M. Dermatomyositis (systemic angiopathy) of childhood. Medicine. 1966;**45**:261–89.
52. Feldman D, Hochberg MC, Zizic TM, Stevens MB. Cutaneous vasculitis in adult polymyositis/dermatomyositis. J Rheumatol. 1983;**10**:85–9.
53. Dyck RF, Katz A, Gordon DA, et al. Glomerulonephritis with polymyositis. J Rheumatol. 1979;**6**:336–44.
54. Kagan LJ. Myoglobinemia and myoglobinuria in patients with myositis. Arthritis Rheum.1971;**14**:457–64.
55. Manchul LA, Jim A, Pritchard KI, et al. The frequency of malignant neoplasms in patients with polymyositis–dermatomyositis. Arch Intern Med. 1985;**145**:1835–1939.
56. Lakhanpal S, Bunch TW, Ilstrup DM, Melton LJ. Polymyositis–dermatomyositis and malignant lesions: does an association exist? Mayo Clin Proc. 1986;**61**:645–53.
57. Bonnetblanc JM, Bernard P, Fayol J. Dermatomyositis and malignancy: a multicenter cooperative study. Dermatologica. 1990; **180**:212–16.
58. Barnes BE. Dermatomyositis and malignancy. Ann Intern Med. 1976;**84**:68–76.
59. Arundell FD, Wilkinson RD, Haserick JR. Dermatomyositis and malignant neoplasms in adults. Arch Dermatol. 1960;**82**:772–5.
60. Callen JP, Hyla JF, Bole GG Jr, Kay DR. The relationship of dermatomyositis and polymyositis to internal malignancy. Arch Dermatol. 1980;**116**:295–8.
61. Schulman P, Kerr LD. A reexamination of the relationship between myositis and malignancy. J Rheumatol. 1991;**18**:1689–92.
62. Callen JP, Hyla JF, Bole GG Jr, Kay DR. The relationship of dermatomyositis/polymyositis to malignancy. J Rheumatol. 1991;**18**:1645–6.
63. Bohan A, Peter JB, Bowman RI, Pearson CM. A computer-assisted analysis of 153 patients with polymyositis and dermatomyositis. Medicine. 1976;**55**:89–104.
64. Hochberg MC, Feldman D, Stevens MB. Adult onset polymyositis/dermatomyositis: an analysis of clinical and laboratory features and survival in 76 patients with a review of the literature. Semin Arthritis Rheum. 1986;**15**:168–78.
65. Fudman EJ, Schnitzer TJ. Dermatomyositis without creatine kinase elevation. A poor prognostic sign. Am J Med. 1986;**80**:329–32.
66. Medsger TA. Approach to the patient with weakness. In: Kelley WN, ed. Textbook of internal medicine, vol 1. Philadelphia: JB Lippincott; 1989:1068–71.
67. Gibson RK. Pyomyositis: increasing recognition in temperate climates. Am J Med. 1984;**77**:768–72.
68. Kagan LJ, Kimball AC, Christian CL. Serologic evidence of toxoplasmosis among patients with polymyositis. Am J Med. 1974;**56**:186–91.
69. Kaufman LD, Seidman RJ, Gruber BL. L-tryptophan-associated eosinophilic perimyositis, neuritis and fascitis. A clinico–pathologic and laboratory study of 25 patients. Medicine. 1990;**69**:187–99.
70. Pennington RT. In: Walton JN, ed. Biochemical aspects of muscle disease. New York: Churchill Livingstone; 1981:415–47.
71. Vignos PJ, Goldwin J. Evaluation of laboratory tests in diagnosis and management of polymyositis. Am J Med. 1972;**263**:291–308.
72. Kagen LJ, Aram S. Creatine kinase activity inhibitor in sera from patients with muscle disease. Arthritis Rheum. 1987;**30**:213–17.
73. Bromberg MB, Albers JW. Electromyography in idiopathic myositis. Mt Sinai J Med. 1988,**55**:459–64.
74. Henricksson KG, Stalberg E. The terminal innervation pattern in polymyositis; a histochemical and SFEMG study. Muscle Nerve. 1978;**1**:3–13.
75. Jerusalem F, Rakusa M, Engel AG, McDonald RD. Morphometric analysis of skeletal muscle capillary structure in inflammatory myopathies. J Neurol Sci. 1974;**23**:391–402.
76. Whitaker JN, Engel WK. Vascular deposits of immunoglobulin and complement in idiopathic inflammatory myopathy. N Engl J Med. 1972;**286**:333–8.

77. Heffner RR, Barron SA, Jenis EH, Valeski JE. Skeletal muscle in polymyositis. Arch Pathol Lab Med. 1979;**103**:310–13.
78. Nishikai M, Reichlin M. Radioimmunoassay of serum myoglobin in polymyositis and other conditions. Arthritis Rheum. 1977;**20**:1514–18.
79. Kagan LJ. Myoglobinemia in inflammatory myopathies. JAMA. 1977;**237**:1448–52.
80. Janis JF, Winkelmann RK. Histopathology of the skin in dermatomyositis. Arch Dermatol. 1968;**97**:640–50.
81. Banker BQ. Dermatomyositis of childhood. J Neuropathol Exp Neurol. 1975;**34**:46–75.
82. Crowe WE, Bove KE, Levinson JE, Hilton PK. Clinical and pathogenic implications of histopathology in childhood polydermatomyositis. Arthritis Rheum. 1982;**25**:126–39.
83. Oddis CV, Medsger TA Jr, Cooperstein LA. A subluxing arthropathy associated with the anti-Jo-l antibody in polymyositis/dermatomyositis. Arthritis Rheum. 1990;**33**:1640–45.
84. Warrick JH, Bhalla M, Schabel SI, Silver RM. High resolution computed tomography in early scleroderma lung disease. J Rheumatol. 1991;**18**:1520–28.
85. Crystal RG, Gadek JE, Ferrans UJ, et al. Interstitial lung disease. Current concepts of pathogenesis, staging and therapy. Am J Med. 1981;**70**:542–68.
86. Schwarz MI, Matthay RA, Sahn SA, Stanford RE, Marmorstein BL, Scheinhorn DJ. Interstitial lung disease in polymyositis and dermatomyositis: analysis of six cases and review of the literature. Medicine. 1976;**55**:89–104.
87. Agrawal CS, Behari M, Schrivastava S, et al. The heart in polymyositis–dermatomyositis. J Neurol. 1989;**236**:249–50.
88. Behan WM, Behan PO, Gairns J. Cardiac damage in polymyositis associated with antibodies to tissue ribonucleoproteins. Br Heart J. 1987;**57**:176–80.
89. Denbow CE, Lie JT, Tancredi RG, Bunch TW. Cardiac involvement in polymyositis. Arthritis Rheum. 1979;**22**:1088–92.
90. Brownlow K, Elevitch FR. Serum creatine phosphokinase isoenzyme (CPK2) in myositis. JAMA. 1974;**230**:1141–4.
91. Lough J, Bischoff R. Differentiation of creatine phosphokinase during myogenesis. Quantitative fractionation of isoenzymes. Devel Biol. 1977;**57**:330–34.
92. Kagen LJ, Hochman RB, Strong EW. Cricopharyngeal obstruction in inflammatory myopathy (polymyositis/dermatomyositis). Arthritis Rheum. 1985;**28**:630–36.
93. DeMerieux O, Verity MA, Clements PJ, Paulus HE. Esophageal abnormalities and dysphagia in polymyositis and dermatomyositis. Arthritis Rheum. 1983;**26**:961–8.
94. Jacob H, Berkowitz D, McDonald E, Bernstein LH, Beneventano T. The esophageal motility disorder of polymyositis. Arch Intern Med. 1983;**143**:2262–4.
95. Horowitz M, McNeil JD, Maddern GJ, Collins PJ, Shearman DJC. Abnormalities of gastric and esophageal emptying in polymyositis and dermatomyositis. Gastroenterology. 1986;**90**:434–9.
96. Henriksson KG, Hallert C, Norrby K, Walan A. Polymyositis and adult coeliac disease. Acta Neurol Scand. 1982;**65**:301–19.
97. Gamsky TE, Chan MK. Coexistent dermatomyositis and autoimmune thyroiditis. West J Med. 1988;**148**:213–14.
98. Miller FW, Cronin ME, Love LA. Increased prevalence of hypothyroidism and its association with pulmonary fibrosis in patients with idiopathic inflammatory myopathy. Arthritis Rheum. 1987;**30**(Suppl):S64.
99. Hay EM, Makris M, Winfield J, Winfield DA. Evans syndrome associated with dermatomyositis. Ann Rheum Dis. 1990;**49**:793–4.
100. Reichlin M, Arnett FC. Multiplicity of antibodies in myositis sera. Arthritis Rheum. 1984;**27**:1150–56.
101. Medsger TA Jr. Inflammatory diseases of muscle. In: Kelley WN, ed. Textbook of internal medicine, vol 1. Philadelphia: JB Lippincott; 1989:1007–9.
102. Arnett FC, Hirsch TJ. Bias WB, Nishekai M, Reichlin M. The Jo-1 antibody system in myositis: Relationships to clinical features and HLA. J Rheumatol. 1981;**8**:925–30.
103. Targoff IN, Johnson AE, Miller FW. Antibody to signal recognition particle in polymyositis. Arthritis Rheum. 1990;**33**:1361–70.
104. Targoff IN, Reichlin M. The association between Mi-2 antibodies and dermatomyositis. Arthritis Rheum. 1985;**28**:796–803.
105. Treadwell EL, Alspaugh MA, Wolfe JF, Sharp GC. Clinical relevance of PM-l antibody and physicochemical characterization of PM-l antigen, J Rheumatol. 1984;**11**:658–62.
106. Sharp GC, Irvin WS, Tan EM, Gould RG, Holman HR. Mixed connective tissue disease – an apparently distinct rheumatic disease associated with a specific antibody to an extractable nuclear antigen (ENA). Am J Med. 1972;**52**:148–59.
107. Love LA, Leff RL. Fraser DD, et al. A new approach to the classification of idiopathic inflammatory myopathy: Myositis-specific autoantibodies define useful homogeneous patient groups. Medicine. 1991;**70**:310–74.
108. Arnett FC, Hirsch RJ, Bias WB, Nishikai M. Reichlin M. The Jo-l antibody system in myositis. Relationships to clinical features and HLA. J Rheumatol. 1981;**8**:825–930.
109. Goldstein R, Duvic M, Targoff IN, et al. HLA-D region genes associated with autoantibody responses to histidyltransfer RNA synthetase (Jo-l) and other translation-related factors in myositis. Arthritis Rheum. 1990;**33**:1240–48.
110. Miller FW. Humoral immunity and immunogenetics in the idiopathic inflammatory myopathies. Curr Opin Rheumotol. 1991;**3**:902–10.
111. Hoffman GS, Franck WA, Raddatz DA, Stallones L. Presentation, treatment and prognosis of idiopathic inflammatory muscle disease in a rural hospital. Am J Med. 1983;**75**:433–8.
112. Miller FW. Treatment problems in idiopathic inflammatory myopathy. Presented at American College of Rheumatology Polymyositis Symposium, San Antonio, Texas: March 21; 1991.
113. Oddis CV, Medsger TA Jr. Polymyositis–dermatomyositis. In: Bellamy N, ed. Prognosis in the rheumatic diseases, Lancaster: Kluwer Academic Publishers; 1991:233–49.
114. Benbassat J, Gefel D, Larholt K, Sukenik S. Morgenstern V, Zlotnick A. Prognostic factors in PM–DM: A computer assisted analysis of 92 cases. Arthritis Rheum. 1985;**28**:249–55.
115. Riddoch D, Morgan-Hughes JA. Prognosis in adult polymyositis. J Neurol Sci. 1975;**26**:71–80.
116. Henriksson KG, Sandstedt P. Polymyositis – treatment and prognosis: a study of 107 patients. Acta Neurol Scand. 1982;**65**:280–300.
117. Tymms KE, Webb J. Dermatopolymyositis and other connective tissue diseases. A review of 105 cases. J Rheumatol. 1986;**12**:1140–48.
118. Spencer CH, Hanson V, Singsen BH, Bernstein BH, Kornreich JH, King KK. Course of treated juvenile dermatomyositis. J Pediatr. 1984;**105**:399–408.
119. Yoshioka M, Okuno T, Mikawa H. Prognosis and treatment of polymyositis with particular reference to steroid resistant patients. Arch Dis Child. 1985;**60**:231-44.
120. Miller LC, Michael AF, Kim Y. Childhood dermatomyositis: clinical course and long-term follow-up. Clin Pediatr. 1987;**26**:561–6.
121. Baron M, Small P. Polymyositis/dermatomyositis: clinical features and outcome in 22 patients. J Rheumatol. 1985;**12**:283–6.
122. Oddis CV, Medsger TA Jr. Relationship between serum creatine kinase level and corticosteroid therapy in polymyositis–dermatomyositis. J Rheumatol. 1988;**15**:807–11.

36

MANAGEMENT OF INFLAMMATORY MUSCLE DISEASE

Lawrence J Kagen

- Therapy should halt the inflammatory process *and* preserve muscle function and strength.
- Corticosteroids are the mainstay of treatment.
- Methotrexate and azathioprine may be important adjunctive agents.
- Therapeutic approaches to dermatomyositis, polymyositis and inclusion body myositis are similar.

Treatment for myositis is based largely on titration of medication to the severity and response of disease manifestations. Since the cause and course of polymyositis and dermatomyositis are not fully known, we lack the information needed to make strategic interventions which will be predictably safe and successful. Accuracy in diagnosis, precision of assessment during the course of illness, and a spirit of cooperation between patient and physician are essential to allow the use of optimum therapy over the necessary time (Fig. 36.1).

DIAGNOSTIC ACCURACY

Diagnosis is based upon three criteria which characterize the presence of inflammatory myopathy: muscle dysfunction, abnormal laboratory tests (elevation of muscle enzymes; abnormal electromyography), and an abnormal muscle biopsy. Muscle dysfunction is evidenced by weakness, and, early in the course of illness, by muscle soreness and tenderness. Atrophy may occur with chronic illness. Abnormalities in laboratory tests include elevation of the serum activities of certain enzymes (e.g. creatine kinase) with electromyographic findings of myopathy and muscle irritability. Most importantly, muscle biopsy demonstrates evidence of inflammation with myonecrosis. In an individual patient, one or more of these criteria may not be demonstrable, and the treating physician must exercise skill in interpretation for diagnosis. However, since therapy may be associated with risk, it is good to place the diagnosis on as sound a foundation as possible, which generally means testing in each of these areas, including muscle biopsy.

REQUIREMENTS FOR SUCCESSFUL THERAPY
Accuracy of diagnosis
Compatible criteria History and physical findings Laboratory studies Histological findings Electrophysiological (EMG) findings
Rule out disorders of the nervous system Neuropathic disorders Lower motor neuron disease Myasthenia gravis
Rule out other causes of myopathies Metabolic Inherited Endocrine Electrolyte disorders Drug and toxin Infectious Traumatic Ischemic
Accuracy of assessment of course of illness
Muscle function
Muscle strength
Laboratory studies

Fig. 36.1 Requirements for successful therapy of myositis.

Many clinical conditions can mimic features of inflammatory muscle disease. Endocrine disorders, in particular thyroid disease, may be associated with myopathy. Hyperthyroidism may produce muscle weakness with enzyme levels which are normal or low. Hypothyroidism, on the other hand, may result in muscle aching, cramps, soreness, weakness, and, if severe, in marked elevation of levels of creatine kinase (CK). For this reason, it is worthwhile obtaining thyroid function tests in patients suspected of having myopathy.

Lyme disease, toxoplasmosis and infections caused by viruses such as influenza, coxsackie, hepatitis and HIV, may all produce myopathy which can be severe and, in certain instances, chronic. Certain disorders of the nervous system, myasthenic syndromes, and lower motor neuron diseases produce weakness with mildly elevated CK levels. Although electrolyte imbalance, especially in outpatients, is rarely a source of confusion, abnormalities in electrolytes, such as the serum potassium, may result in muscle weakness. Hypophosphatemia, which occurs in the recovery phase of acute alcoholism, produces muscle pain, necrosis, weakness, and marked enzyme elevations.

Drugs and medications also can cause myopathies which resemble myositis syndromes. Penicillamine, used in the treatment of rheumatoid arthritis (RA), may rarely cause a syndrome indistinguishable from polymyositis. The lipid lowering agents lovastatin and gemfibrozil may produce muscle necrosis and rhabdomyolysis. Diuretics also may lead to electrolyte imbalance and muscle weakness. Alcohol can produce both a chronic myopathy with weakness and atrophy as well as an acute syndrome of muscle necrosis and rhabdomyolysis. The use of illicit agents, especially cocaine, may result in a syndrome of rhabdomyolysis. All of the foregoing emphasize the need to consider many different causes of muscle dysfunction. The diagnosis of myositis requires both the fulfillment of criteria and the exclusion of other illnesses which may be potential sources of confusion.

ASSESSMENT OF DISEASE ACTIVITY

The assessment of the course of illness, after the establishment of diagnosis, represents one of the most important elements of patient management. Since medication is adjusted to clinical response, the measurement of clinical response with accuracy and precision is vital. In this regard the clinician should consider both physical and laboratory features. In patients with dermatomyositis, remission of rash may be anticipated to be a mark of disease remission. The clinician, however, should be aware that degree and severity of rash frequently may not vary with other aspects of the disease. Persistent rash can be a chronic and vexing problem even in patients otherwise doing well. For this reason it is not always possible to use rash as a guide to therapy, although in an individual patient it may be. Likewise, nailbed and periungual telangiectasia may not change in concert with other aspects of the disease [1].

Muscle weakness is the dominant manifestation of patients with myositis, and two complementary approaches should be gauged periodically to assess progress. First, and probably most important, is

FUNCTIONAL GRADING SCALE	
Activity	**Score**
1. Transfer from supine to sitting	
2. Transfer from sitting to standing	
3. Walking	
4. Stair climbing Ascending Descending	
5. Care of head and face (e.g. hair, tooth brushing)	
6. Dressing Donning jacket or buttoned shirt Donning pants	
7. Lifting objects above shoulder level (elbow extended) Light household work Heavy household work	
Total Score	
Scoring	
Cannot do	0
Requires help from a person	1
Person not needed but does with difficulty (uses aids, e.g. cane, railing, mechanical device)	2
Can do alone without difficulty	3
Maximum score	30

Fig. 36.2 Grading scale for assessment of function in patients with myositis.

assessment of function for activities of daily living (ADL). Functional scoring schemes can provide overall semiquantitative guides to disease severity. Figure 36.2 demonstrates one approach to grading function to which elements of the physical examination can be added. Note can be made of gait, heel and toe walking, the ability to rise from a low seat, to cross the legs, raise the arms and arise from the supine position. The second approach uses direct measurements of muscle strength employed repetitively over time in a quantifiable manner. Manual muscle strength testing (Fig. 36.3) has been used for this purpose. Finer gradations between scores can be interpolated to increase the sensitivity of the manual muscle assessment, but assessment may be affected by observer variation [2]. Biomechanical measures have also been employed in the clinical setting to quantify muscle strength more sensitively and with less observer subjectivity [3]. Ongoing assessment of muscle strength is an important guide to therapy.

In general, the reason for accepting the risks of therapy is to maintain or gain strength. Assays of strength and function represent the means of determining whether this goal is being achieved. In this connection, the clinician should keep certain factors in mind. Muscle weakness may result from inflammation in muscle. The inflammatory infiltrates and the products they elaborate may interfere with the efficiency of contraction and muscle function. Control and remission of inflammation as the result of medical therapy, therefore, should be expected to lead to an increase in strength and endurance. This does happen and can be documented in the clinical setting.

MANUAL MUSCLE STRENGTH TESTING GRADES	
0	No muscle contraction
1 (trace)	Palpable contraction, little or no motion
2 (poor)	Motion possible but not against gravity
3 (fair)	Motion against gravity possible
4 (good)	Motion possible against manual resistance
5 (normal)	Motion possible against considerable manual resistance

Fig. 36.3 Manual muscle strength testing grades.

However, inflammation may also lead to myofiber necrosis and replacement by connective tissue. In this case, particularly in older individuals with a limited ability to regenerate fibers, weakness is the result of myofiber loss, and strength cannot be regained by the use of medication aimed at controlling inflammation. In a practical sense it is likely that both processes (interference with function by inflammation, and loss of myofibers) occur together to produce weakness. The role of the treating physician, therefore, is to use medications to increase function to the degree possible. It may not be possible in some patients to anticipate a full return of strength. At present one cannot determine to what degree each of the two processes is responsible for weakness. The use of the muscle biopsy is not precise. Different muscles are affected to different degrees, and the biopsy represents a sample made at one place and time. However, the presence of end-stage muscle with myofiber replacement by connective tissue suggests only a limited capacity for strength recovery.

Laboratory features are also assessed in an ongoing fashion. Remission to normal of elevated serum enzyme levels is a favorable sign, and elevations in the course of follow-up may indicate disease exacerbations. However, some patients may exhibit chronically and moderately elevated serum enzyme levels without change of strength. Rarely patients may have normal levels in the presence of disease flare, as manifested by new rash and increasing weakness [4]. These aspects all support the importance of clinical evaluation based upon total assessment of disease signs, rash, function, strength, and laboratory values as they relate to the individual patient.

PREVENTION

Exacerbations and remissions often occur in the course of polymyositis and dermatomyositis, but inciting agents or events have not been identified. Therefore, specific precautions cannot be recommended. Nonetheless, attention to prevention of complications is important. Contractures, particularly at the shoulders, knees, and ankles, should be prevented whenever possible. A program of physical therapy should begin with passive range of motion exercises at disease onset and progress to strengthening maneuvers when disease remission permits. Accompanying disease manifestations, including Raynaud's phenomenon and esophageal dysmotility, may be significantly alleviated by timely preventive measures (see Chapter 35).

EDUCATION AND PSYCHOSOCIAL SUPPORT

The course of illness in patients with polymyositis and dermatomyositis may run over several years, during which time there are generally periods of exacerbations and remissions. It is common, even in patients who do well, to have an exacerbation of disease manifestations during the first or second year. This chronicity of illness with unanticipated periods of flare produces stress in both the patient and physician. Doubts and difficulties of assessment of progress lead to anxiety. In this context it is important to be able to measure progress and to keep the overall goals and course in mind. The patient should be educated to expect downturns and to remain aware of the progress already made. The physician must not allow temporary periods of frustration and anxiety to lessen a calm control of the selection of therapeutic agents.

In addition to these factors, patients will experience difficulties in coping with their life situation, jobs, and family relations. This is a time when support is required, based upon a realistic appraisal of goals and needs. Corticosteroid therapy itself also may be a contributing factor to periods of psychological change. Early in therapy, when high doses are instituted, difficulty in sleeping, lack of concentration, and mood changes are common. The patient should be educated to anticipate these changes, which are usually transient, and not to assume them to be the result of disease. Nonetheless, fear of the future, uncertainty about the ability to provide for oneself and family, and periods of clinical worsening and sleeplessness, may all combine to undermine the psychological endurance needed to continue. Here a spirit of understanding and guidance, along with the ability to supply the information necessary to allow the patient to anticipate and cope with changes in the future, are important elements in patient care. Mutual understanding and trust must exist in order to maintain a relationship which by reason of disease chronicity will be long lasting.

PHYSICAL FACTORS

Few data about exercise and the need to build up muscle to its previous level of function are available. Passive range of motion exercises should begin at disease onset and continue throughout. In general, a gentle, graded and supervised program of muscle strengthening should begin when evidence of disease activity has subsided and drug therapy is minimal. However, in patients with long-standing, treated illness with moderately elevated serum enzyme values, the need to institute an active exercise program may be met before these guidelines are satisfied. In all instances, care must be taken not to place excessive demands upon muscle which has only limited 'fitness'. Although it might be anticipated that serum enzyme levels would sharply increase with the institution of physical activity under these circumstances, this generally does not occur if the program is gentle, carefully supervised, and begins with modest goals. Contractures, particularly at the shoulders, knees, and ankles, should be prevented whenever possible. Contractures may occur rapidly in children and markedly weakened adults and present severe impediments to subsequent recovery. The need for continual reassessment and appropriate modification of a program of physical therapy from the onset of illness cannot be overemphasized. In many cases, the family and the patient may be adequate to implement this program. In others it is advisable to secure the participation of a qualified physical therapist.

Demands of the life situation must be considered so that they do not jeopardize the patient's ability to successfully cope with illness. The work environment should be evaluated, as well as the need for rest periods during the day. Given the likelihood of exacerbations and remissions over time, a flexible approach to physical activity is best. In general, an understanding relationship between patient and physician will adequately allow exploration of these factors and their modification when necessary.

Finally, it should be remembered that these general recommendations do not arise from scientific evidence but rather from a perspective based upon experience and what seems to be a sensible approach. Other views might be feasible, but whatever course is followed, assessment should be ongoing and as careful as possible, to be certain that progress is being made in the optimum manner.

PHARMACOLOGIC AGENTS

As in other areas of the management of myositis syndromes, adequately controlled observations which would allow precise judgments and recommendations are not available with respect to pharmacological agents. Nonetheless, experience and practice have established general approaches to their use in disease treatment.

Corticosteroids

Corticosteroids represent the mainstay of therapy for most patients. The usual practice is to begin treatment with daily oral medication in the range of 40–80mg/day of prednisone or its equivalent for approximately 4–6 weeks or until maximum benefit or remission of disease is achieved. The dose may then be gradually reduced with careful monitoring of clinical state and laboratory findings. An algorithm for this approach has been proposed [5]. For children, similar doses, usually expressed as 1–2mg/kg/day, are employed initially. In severe or acute situations intravenous bolus therapy has been used. Doses of 500–1000mg of methylprednisolone given daily for 3-day periods have been employed in an attempt to achieve a more rapid remission [6]. Modifications of this regimen have also been used [7]. Alternate day therapy, usually beginning with doses near 100mg prednisone orally every 2 days, has also had success [8].

Untoward effects of corticosteroid therapy have been encountered in both adults and children. Psychological changes, with sleeplessness, irritability, and emotional lability, may occur early and subside without specific treatment. In some patients, however, psychological aberrations may be so disturbing that they require reduction in the dose of corticosteroid and/or addition of other medications. Effects on bones – the development of osteoporosis and osteonecrosis (particularly of the femoral heads) – represent potentially serious problems. Skin fragility and cataract formation also may occur with chronic treatment. In addition, hypertension, exacerbation of diabetes mellitus, cardiovascular decompensation, and susceptibility to infection may become problems in certain individuals. Alopecia, hirsutism of the face, and characteristic changes in appearance related to excess corticosteroid intake may also be vexing problems. With chronic treatment the question of corticosteroid-induced muscle weakness may arise and be difficult to evaluate.

Despite these difficulties, most patients with polymyositis and dermatomyositis can usually be treated with corticosteroid alone. Careful and frequent monitoring can be used to titrate the dose of medication to the patient's need and minimize the chances of development of unwanted effects. Situations in which other agents may be considered include:

- life-threatening, progressive illness unresponsive to adequate corticosteroid therapy;
- partially responsive illness requiring doses of corticosteroids that have side effects difficult or impossible to tolerate;
- chronic illness with poor response and/or progressive deterioration;
- contraindication or inability to tolerate the use of corticosteroids.

Methotrexate

Methotrexate has been used in the treatment of patients with dermatomyositis and polymyositis for over two decades [9], and there have been several reports documenting its usefulness and effectiveness, including its corticosteroid-sparing property [10]. In most dosage protocols, methotrexate is used in conjunction with corticosteroid. Initially it was given intravenously in doses of 10–15mg/week with gradual increments up to 50mg/week. Subsequent studies have indicated intramuscular and even subcutaneous routes to be effective. With the acceptance of oral methotrexate for the treatment of RA, similar schedules have been employed for patients with myositis. Weekly oral methotrexate, in doses from 7.5–30mg, is now probably the most common approach.

Although untoward effects of methotrexate usage may be quite varied, most concern has centered on possible hepatic and pulmonary effects. Studies performed in patients with RA have indicated little or no risk of cirrhosis in patients treated with the oral weekly schedules, although some morphologic changes occur. Hepatotoxicity may also be manifested by elevation in transaminase levels. Pulmonary toxicity may be difficult to detect, especially in the early stages, since it may arise insidiously with fibrosis and modest alterations of pulmonary function. On the other hand, it may be manifested by abrupt dramatic pneumonitis with fever and cough. Bone marrow suppression (leukopenia and anemia) have been noted. Stomatitis, gastrointestinal hemorrhage, skin effects, nephropathy and reduction of host defenses against infection may be other complications of therapy.

Azathioprine

Azathioprine has also been used successfully. A controlled study demonstrated that patients treated with azathioprine and corticosteroids showed improvements in functional ability and required less prednisone for maintenance than patients treated with prednisone alone [11]. In this study, the dose was 2mg/kg/day which was continued until the concurrent prednisone dose could be reduced to less than 15mg/day. At that point, azathioprine was reduced as tolerated. For active disease, doses in the range of 150mg orally are generally used, often after gradually incremented steps. Doses may then be reduced to 50–75mg daily for maintenance after remission has been achieved. Areas of potential toxicity include bone marrow suppression, gastrointestinal intolerance, hepatotoxicity and increased susceptibility to infection.

Cyclophosphamide

Cyclophosphamide has probably been used in fewer patients than methotrexate or azathioprine. It has been used orally, and more recently intravenously. However, conflicting data have been reported with this agent, and poor results have also been noted [12]. Combined cytotoxic agents have been given to corticosteroid-resistant patients with good results [13,14].

Cyclosporin

Cyclosporin has been used successfully in small numbers of patients. Doses have ranged from 2.5–3.5mg/kg/day. In one case, improvement was observed in a child who had been treated with cyclosporin alone. However, not all observers have reported success with cyclosporin. Nephrotoxicity and the development of hypertension are among possible untoward effects [15,16].

Hydroxychloroquine

Hydroxychloroquine, 2–5mg/kg/day, has also been used concomitantly with corticosteroids in patients with dermatomyositis with improvement in both rash and muscle strength and with a decrease in the amount of prednisone therapy needed. Beneficial effects have not always been sustained, and retinal toxicity represents a potential hazard [17,18].

Other Forms of Therapy

Other forms of more specialized therapy have been used in difficult cases. These have included plasmapheresis [19], whole body radiation [20] and intravenous immunoglobulin [21]. No prospective controlled trials of these forms of therapy are available.

THE DECISION TO TREAT

Once the diagnosis has been accurately made, the critical questions for both patient and physician are when and how to treat. Pharmacologic agents are employed when there is evidence of muscle weakness and/or organ involvement (such as pulmonary disease). However, individual situations may be problematic. For example, the patient with elevated serum enzymes and little or no evidence of weakness presents a challenge. If the apparently normal strength occurs in the context of a history of loss of power, the ancillary examinations of biopsy and electromyography may be useful. Histologic evidence of marked inflammation, particularly resulting in myonecrosis, is generally a strong argument for institution of pharmacologic therapy. Similarly, a characteristically abnormal EMG and a compelling history of loss of power, despite 'normal' strength, support the institution of therapy. A second situation is that of a patient with the characteristic skin rash of dermatomyositis and only borderline findings for muscle involvement. Clinical judgment must be used to balance the risks against the possible gains. There are no absolute guidelines, but topical corticosteroid therapy may be tried to see whether the rash responds. Close monitoring is vital since rash may appear before other signs of myopathy are manifest. Indeed, six patients have been described with classic heliotrope rash (periorbital discoloration), maculopapular violaceous rash over the interphalangeal joints, and periungual telangiectasia, who did not develop clinical evidence of muscle involvement until months, or in some cases years, later [22].

COMORBID CONDITIONS AND COMPLICATIONS

The presence of comorbid conditions and/or complications makes the burden of illness more difficult to bear. In particular, cardiopulmonary status may influence the patients' abilities to perform the tasks by which strength and function are gauged. Dysphagia may reflect underlying abnormalities of deglutition which can increase the risk of aspiration and interfere with nutrition, particularly if severe.

Therapeutic agents also require careful monitoring. Electrolytes need to be assessed in the context of corticosteroids and diuretics. Cytotoxic agents raise concern about teratogenicity and the risk of later development of malignant disease, especially in the case of azathioprine and cyclophosphamide. These risks need to be weighed against the substantial overall corticosteroid-sparing effects of cytotoxic agents in many patients.

REFERENCES

1. Ganczarczyk ML, Lee P, Armstrong SK. Nailfold capillary microscopy in polymyositis and dermatomyositis. Arthritis Rheum. 1988;**31**:116–19.
2. Mendell JR, Florence J. Manual muscle testing. Muscle Nerve. 1990; S16–S20.
3. Kroll M, Otis J, Kagen L. Serum enzyme, myoglobin and muscle strength relationships in polymyositis and dermatomyositis. J Rheumatol. 1986;**13**:349–55.
4. Bohan A, Peter JB, Bowman RL, Pearson CM. A computer-assisted analysis of 153 patients with polymyositis and dermatomyositis. Medicine. 1977;**56**:255–86.
5. Oddis CV, Medsger T. Current management of polymyositis and dermatomyositis. Drugs. 1989;**37**:382–90.
6. Yanagisawa T, Sueishi M, Nawata Y, et al. Methyl prednisolone pulse therapy in dermatomyositis. Dermatologica. 1983;**167**:47–51.
7. Laxer RM, Stein LD, Petty RE. Intravenous pulse methylprednisolone treatment of juvenile dermatomyositis. Arthritis Rheum. 1987;**30**:328–34.
8. Uchino M, Araki S, Yoshida 0, Uekawa K, Nagata J. High single-dose alternate-day corticosteroid regimens in treatment of polymyositis. J Neurol. 1985;**232**:175–8.
9. Malaviya AN, Many A, Schwartz RS. Treatment of dermatomyositis with methotrexate. Lancet. 1968;**2**:485–88.
10. Metzger AL, Bohan A, Goldberg LS, Bluestone R, Pearson CM. Polymyositis and dermatomyositis: combined methotrexate and corticosteroid therapy. Ann Intern Med. 1974;**81**:182–9.
11. Bunch TW. Prednisone and azathioprine for polymyositis. Arthritis Rheum. 1981;**25**:45–8.
12. Cronin ME, Plotz PH. Current concepts in idiopathic inflammatory myopathies: polymyositis, dermatomyositis and related disorders. Ann Intern Med. 1989;**111**:143–57.
13. Tiliakos NA. Low dose cytotoxic combination therapy in intractable dermatopolymyositis. Arthritis Rheum. 1987;**30**:S14.
14. Wallace DJ, Metzger AL, White KK. Combination immunosuppressive treatment of steroid-resistant dermatomyositis/polymyositis. Arthritis Rheum. 1985;**28**:590–2.
15. Dantzig P. Juvenile dermatomyositis treated with cyclosporine. J Am Acad Dermatol. 1990;**22**:310–11.
16. Heckmatt J, Hasson N, Saunders C, et al. Cyclosporin in juvenile dermatomyositis. Lancet. 1989;**1**:1063–6.
17. Olson NY, Lindsley CB. Adjunctive use of hydroxychloroquine in childhood dermatomyositis. J Rheumatol. 1989;**16**:1545–7.
18. Woo TY, Callen JP, Voorhees JJ, et al. Cutaneous lesions of dermatomyositis are improved by hydroxychloroquine. J Am Acad Dermatol. 1984;**10**:592–600.
19. Dau PC. Plasmapheresis in idiopathic inflammatory myopathy. Arch Neurol. 1981;**38**:544–52.
20. Kelly JJ, Madoc-Jones H, Adelman LS, Andres PL, Munsat TL. Response to total body irradiation in dermatomyositis. Muscle Nerve. 1988;**11**:120–3.
21. Roifman CM, Schaeffer FM, Wachsmuth SE, Murphy G, Gelfand E. Reversal of chronic polymyositis following intravenous immune serum globulin therapy. JAMA. 1987;**258**:513–15.
22. Krain LS. Dermatomyosis in 6 patients without initial muscle involvement. Arch Dermatol. 1975;**111**:241–5.

37

OVERVIEW OF THE INFLAMMATORY VASCULAR DISEASES

Robert W Lightfoot Jr

Definition

- The vasculitides are all characterized by inflammation within or through a vessel wall, with resultant damage to blood flow and sometimes to vessel integrity.
- Involvement may include only one, or many, organ systems and vessels of predominantly one or of many types.

Clinical features

- The clinical syndromes are a result of ischemia to tissues supplied by the damaged vessels and the systemic features of fever, weight loss and anorexia accompanying widespread inflammation.

HISTORY

The appreciation of systemic vasculitis as a disease entity began early in the 19th century. In 1801 Heberden described a five-year-old boy with what was almost certainly the first case of the syndrome on which Schönlein in 1837 and Henoch in 1874 would further elaborate, and which we now know as Henoch–Schönlein purpura (HSP) [1–3]. As early as 1852, Rokitansky had described the pathologic features of polyarteritis nodosa (PAN) [4], the disease for which Kussmaul and Maier in 1866 would provide the now classical description [5].

The majority of vasculitic syndromes were described in the 20th century. The description by Osler in 1903 of another primarily vasculitic systemic disorder, systemic lupus erythematosus (SLE), created little diagnostic difficulty because the clinical syndrome was at that time clinically quite distinct from PAN and HSP. In 1908 Takayasu described the retinal ischemic findings resulting from the large vessel aortovasculitis which now carries his name [6]. In 1936 Klinger described the first case of the syndrome subsequently defined in detail by Wegener (Wegener's granulomatosus; WG). Behçet described the vasculitis bearing his name in 1937; Zeek described hypersensitivity vasculitis in 1948 [7]; and in 1951 Churg and Strauss delineated the PAN-like syndrome with eosinophilia (CSS) [8].

As the number of syndromes increased, there developed a need for a classification system to distinguish between them. In the absence of any specific diagnostic laboratory tests, most classifications stratified these diseases on the basis of the size of the typical vessel involved (Fig. 37.1), and used combinations of clinical and nonspecific laboratory abnormalities to distinguish them.

While SLE and rheumatoid arthritis (RA) are listed among the vasculitides, they are now eliminated from discussions of the dilemma of diagnosing vasculitic syndromes. Indeed, in the most recent major work on classifying the vasculitides by the American College of Rheumatology in 1990 [9], vasculitis in both SLE and RA were dropped from the statistical analysis, since they were so clearly distinguishable by clinical and serologic parameters from the other vasculitic syndromes.

Similarly, the realization that mixed cryoglobulins or monoclonal immunoglobulins could act effectively as immune complexes upon aggregation, separated the vasculitis seen in these syndromes from the larger group of idiopathic vasculitides.

In 1982 Davies *et al.* described antibodies to neutrophil cytoplasmic antigens (ANCA) in patients with segmental necrotizing glomerulonephritis [10]. Van der Woude, Nolle, Falk and others subsequently documented that one such antibody, directed against proteinase-3 in the neutrophil alpha granules, was both extremely sensitive and relatively specific for active WG [11–13].

Some authors have advocated a classification system including 'primary' and 'secondary' vasculitides [14]. 'Secondary' vasculitis refers to that form of vasculitis occurring in the presence of a disease for which there are relatively specific laboratory tests and whose pathogenesis is understood. 'Primary' vasculitis has no such associa-

STRATIFICATION OF VASCULITIS SYNDROMES

Type of vasculitis	Aorta and its branches	Large and medium-sized arteries	Medium-sized muscular arteries	Small muscular arteries	Venules, arterioles
Takayasu's arteritis	●				
Temporal arteritis	●	●			
Polyarteritis nodosa		●	●	●	
Churg–Strauss arteritis		●	●	●	
Isolated CNS vasculitis			●	●	
Wegener's granulomatosis			●	●	●
Vasculitis associated with connective tissue diseases				●	●
Leukocytoclastic vasculitis: Henoch–Schönlein purpura Hypersensitivity vasculitis Others				●	●

Fig. 37.1 Listing of the common vasculitis syndromes, stratified by size of the vessels most commonly involved.

tions. In this context, WG can now be considered 'secondary' because of the recent spate of reports on the ANCA assay. Nevertheless, for the majority of the vasculitides specific diagnostic tests are lacking. For them, diagnosis must still be based on size of vessel involved and associated nonspecific clinical and laboratory features.

PATHOGENESIS

The pathogenesis of the vasculitides has been the subject of a recent excellent review by Savage [15]. There are essentially three ways in which inflammation in blood vessels can occur:

- Direct noxious attack by an agent.
- Involvement in a process directed specifically at components in vascular tissue (e.g. anti-basement membrane disease).
- Passive involvement secondary to an inflammatory process not predominantly directed toward vascular tissue (e.g. immune complex disease).

Direct Noxious Attack by an Agent

None of the vasculitides discussed elsewhere in detail in this textbook are clear examples of this form of vasculitis. However, vasculitis in many infectious processes may be examples of this mechanism [16]. The purpura that occurs in some rickettsial infections may represent another example. Hypertensive arteritis, the cholesterol emboli syndrome and the syndrome following injection of particulates such as talc in intravenous drug abusers are other examples. However, for the vast majority of vasculitides, there is no evidence for this mechanism.

Involvement in a Process Directed Specifically at Components in Vascular Tissue

Antibodies directed against basement membrane can cause capillaritis in the lung and renal glomeruli [14]. However, cutaneous and more widespread vasculitis is not classically seen in these syndromes [14]. Antibodies directed against endothelial cells (AECA) have been identified in SLE, RA, scleroderma, Wegener's and other conditions [15]. Such antibodies have been shown to facilitate the cytotoxic potential of leukocytes against endothelial cells, as well as antibody-dependent cellular cytotoxicity. Endothelial cells which have been exposed to cytokines such as tumor necrosis factor, interleukin-1 and interferon-γ show enhanced expression of surface antigens reactive with such antibodies. AECA from children with Kawasaki syndrome, a model for polyarteritis, cause lysis of such stimulated endothelial cells. It is likely that the role of AECA in causing disease will become increasingly better defined because of the current intense interest in endothelial cell pathophysiology.

Passive Involvement Secondary to an Inflammatory Process not Predominantly Directed Toward Vascular Tissue

The greatest evidence exists for this mechanism of vascular inflammation. The model of experimentally induced acute and chronic serum sickness has been invoked as the most relevant example. When an animal is immunized intravenously with a single injection of a nonaggregated foreign antigen which has a long intravascular half-life, elimination of the antigen proceeds at a slow rate until the synthesis of antibody begins. At that point complexes of antibody with the injected antigen are formed in the circulation. As the antibody repertoire becomes broader and the overall level of antibody higher over a few days, larger complexes form, and rapid elimination of antigen in these complexes ensues, along with the activation and depletion of complement components.

Removal of these opsonized complexes occurs by several mechanisms. First, complement-containing complexes are bound to complement receptors on circulating erythrocytes, following which they are transported through the mononuclear phagocyte system (MPS). There they are stripped off the erythrocytes by phagocytic cells which internalize and destroy them. In addition, complexes not bound to erythrocytes are eliminated by interaction with the Fc and C3 receptors on fixed and circulating phagocytic cells. During this phase, immune complex vasculitis and glomerulitis occur. Eventually, antigen is eliminated, antibody predominates, and the lesions disappear. Several factors may impair rapid immune complex elimination and lead to chronic serum sickness vasculitis and death due to chronic renal or other organ failure:

- Daily repeated injections of large concentrations of antigen may induce chronic serum sickness. This may occur because the animal is put in a state of chronic antigen excess. The relatively small immune complexes that occur on the antigen excess side of the classical antigen–antibody precipitin curve are relatively poor complement fixers and are eliminated by the MPS slowly. An alternative explanation for this effect is that high concentrations of antigen render the recipient animal tolerant to all but a few of the determinants on the antigen, thus limiting the repertoire of antibodies synthesized. Because an oligovalent antigen can form only a restricted lattice complex with antibody, only small complexes can form. The same mechanism may be operative for antigens that are relatively poor immunogens *per se*, such as native DNA, which plays a major role in the immune complex nephritis of SLE.
- Complexes may form in such profusion that the cells of the MPS and complement receptors on erythrocytes are saturated and their function on cell surfaces impaired, leading to persistence of complexes in the circulation and their ultimate deposition in tissues.
- The expression of complement receptor for C3 fragments on cell surfaces may be genetically low, predisposing to poor elimination of opsonized complexes [15].
- In humans, null genes for one of the alleles of the fourth component of complement (C4) may predispose to poor elimination by the MPS [15].
- Genetic deficiencies of one of the early components of the complement system may impair immune complex processing. Such deficiencies are associated with a greater than 50% incidence of lupus-like immune complex disease [15].

In some instances, organ damage may result because the antigen in question has a particular affinity for a specific tissue. An example may be the demonstration that DNA has an affinity for the glomerular basement membrane, which could explain in part the propensity for nephritis in SLE.

The pathogenic reactants are known in only a few of the vasculitis syndromes. In essential mixed cryoglobulinemia, in the glomerular vasculitis of lupus nephritis, in the vasculitis caused by aggregating monoclonal paraproteins and in the arteritis associated with circulating hepatitis B or C surface antigen and antibody there is support for the deposition of immunoglobulin as a causative factor in the accompanying vascular wall inflammation.

In WG, proteinase-3 which is normally found in the azurophilic granules of neutrophil cytoplasm, is found on the cell surface as well. Reaction of the antineutrophil cytoplasmic antibodies against proteinase-3 (C-ANCA) with this antigen on the surface of cells has been shown to generate inflammatory mediators.

While the above mechanisms may indeed be operative in some syndromes, there is little direct pathogenic evidence in most of the vasculitides. In addition, the above does not explain the extreme variability in size of vessels involved in the different vasculitides nor the reason for the rather unique clinical and histologic features seen in some of them. For example, Churg–Strauss vasculitis is seen in chronic eosinophilic syndromes and is characterized by granulomas which are predominantly extravascular. Wegener's causes classic granulomatous vasculitis although there is no understanding of the propensity for invasive inflammatory disease of the upper respiratory structures in this syndrome.

INVESTIGATIONS AND DIFFERENTIAL DIAGNOSIS

Most patients with vasculitis syndromes present initially as diagnostic dilemmas, usually with nonspecific systemic symptoms, or evidence for unexplained malfunction in one or several organ systems, or both. It is rarely clear at the outset that a vasculitis is the cause. Differential diagnosis consists of documenting that vasculitis is indeed present, and in defining to the fullest degree possible, which of the syndromes listed in Figure 37.1 is present. This differentiation is important for the following reasons:

- Some vasculitides are benign and self-limiting; examples are Henoch-Schönlein purpura, which typically requires only symptomatic therapy in spite of widespread organ involvement, and hypersensitivity angiitis secondary to a drug, which usually responds upon withdrawal of the offending agent. While occasional drug-induced vasculitides can be life threatening, such as that caused rarely by allopurinol, to treat either HSP or drug purpura aggressively as a matter of routine would be a serious error.
- While many of the potentially lethal vasculitides are managed aggressively at the outset with a combination of high dose corticosteroids, immunosuppressive drugs and occasionally with such therapies as plasmapheresis and intravenous immunoglobulin G, some vasculitides respond poorly to this approach while responding dramatically to simpler regimens. For example, WG was universally fatal when treated with steroids alone but has now been shown to respond dramatically to cyclophosphamide in conventional 2mg/kg doses by mouth. Subacute bacterial endocarditis is a form of vasculitis which is clearly better treated with appropriate antibiotics than with the aggressive regimen above, but the diagnosis must first be suspected and appropriate studies carried out to identify the etiologic organism. Similarly, atrial myxoma may be more appropriately treated surgically.
- Since much is known regarding the pathogenesis of some vasculitides, such as SLE, establishing the diagnosis early may lead to serologic identification of those patients at greatest risk for some clinical presentations such as renal disease, thromboembolic disease, fetal loss or other complications of SLE.

The Diagnostic Algorithm

Diagnosis of the vasculitides is based on a combination of clinical, serologic, histologic and angiographic parameters. An algorithm for differential diagnosis in a patient suspected of having vasculitis is shown in Figure 37.2. A complete history and physical examination are most important, as many of the syndromes are based on clinical rather than laboratory criteria. For example, the history of eosinophilia and atopy may suggest a diagnosis of Churg–Strauss arteritis, while a history of jaw or tongue claudication is suggestive of giant cell arteritis. The specific historical and physical features that distinguish each type of vasculitis can be found in the respective chapters dealing with these syndromes in this textbook, as well as in the American College of Rheumatology study published in 1990 [9].

The next level in the algorithm involves simultaneously testing for: autoantibodies; monoclonal proteins; infection with agents known to be associated with vasculitis, such as the hepatitis and HIV viruses; evidence of complement consumption and cryoglobulins, as may occur in SLE or other connective tissue diseases, primary or secondary cryoglobulinemia or heritable abnormalities of the complement pathway. At the same time studies are done to establish the extent of organ system involvement as suggested in Figure 37.2. The serologic studies may give an immediate diagnosis. The survey of organ systems will establish the extent of involvement. A patient with cutaneous small vessel vasculitis whose serologic studies are negative and in whom there is no evidence of involvement of systems other than the skin may well be served best by cautious observation.

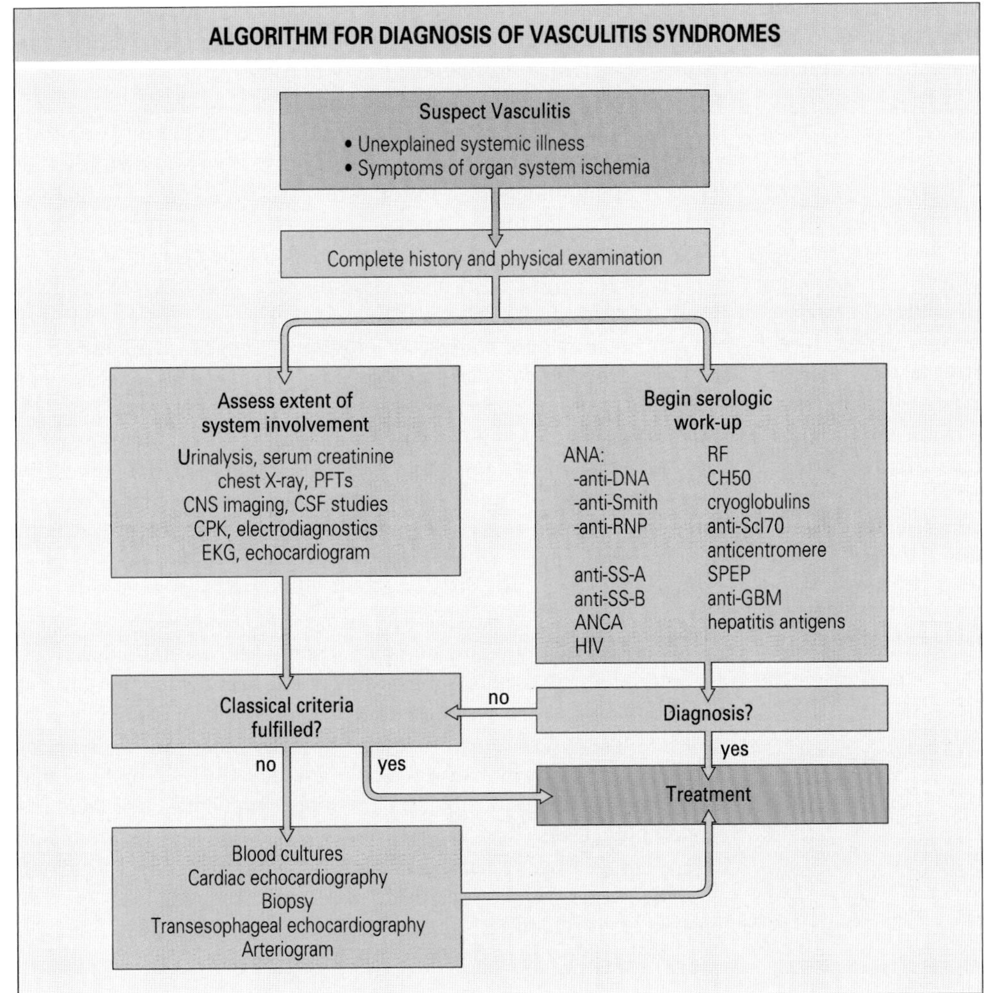

Fig. 37.2 Algorithm depicting the approach to diagnosing the vasculitis syndromes.

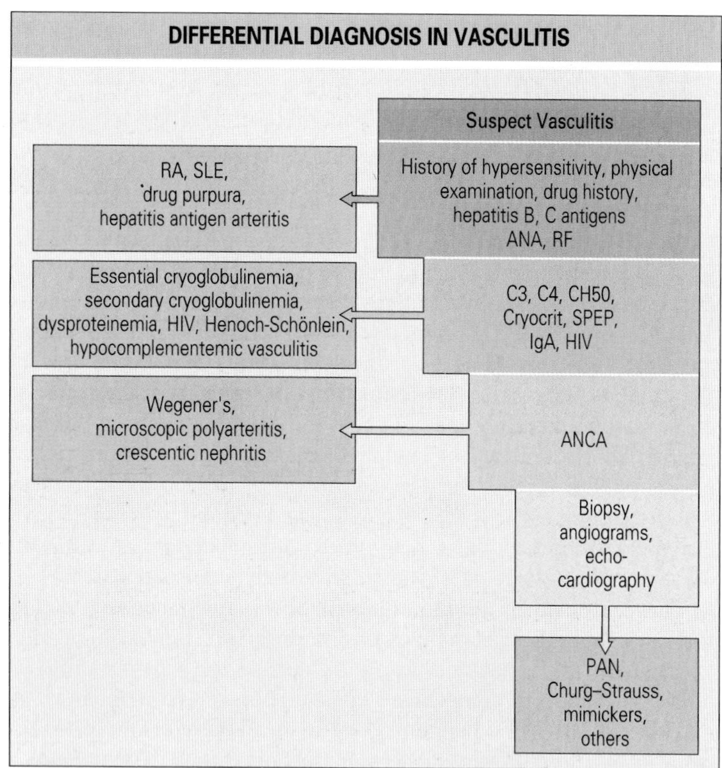

Fig. 37.3 Diagrammatic representation of the process of differential diagnosis in vasculitis. Diagnosing vasculitis amounts intellectually to stepwise sequential testing for the more easily diagnosed syndromes before resorting to the more invasive, and often less diagnostic procedures of biopsy and angiography.

The algorithm in Figure 37.2 is perhaps time consuming. If a patient is felt to have a vasculitis that is imminently life-threatening or compromising some important function such as vision or renal function, one may have to initiate therapy with steroids pending confirmation of the diagnosis. In such instances it becomes imperative to complete the algorithm, since endocarditis, myxomatous emboli and, indeed, nearly every other systemic inflammatory illness can be improved transiently with high dose steroids

Differential Diagnosis

The process of differential diagnosis of the vasculitides is represented schematically in Figure 37.3, in which each cycle of diagnostic inquiry identifies or excludes a possible diagnosis. At the final step are those syndromes for which there are no diagnostic laboratory tests, and which require documentation by biopsy or angiography, while excluding curable mimickers of vasculitis. These mimickers are listed in Figure 37.4. Angiography to detect an ulcerated atheroma is not always feasible, since the syndrome is most often seen in those patients with extensive vascular disease whose kidneys may not tolerate the dye load needed for aortography. Standard echocardiography is routinely performed in patients with atypical vasculitis to search for valvular vegetations or myxomata.

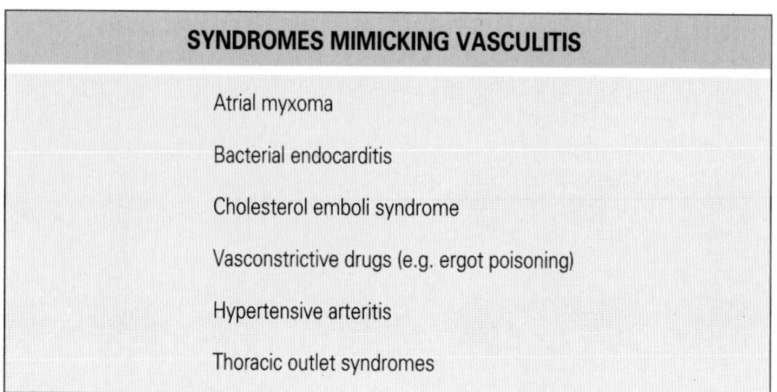

SYNDROMES MIMICKING VASCULITIS
Atrial myxoma
Bacterial endocarditis
Cholesterol emboli syndrome
Vasconstrictive drugs (e.g. ergot poisoning)
Hypertensive arteritis
Thoracic outlet syndromes

Fig. 37.4 Mimickers of vasculitis.

The author knows of several pseudovasculitis syndromes where routine echocardiography failed to show vegetations, but transesophageal echocardiography revealed them. Ulcerated aortic atheromata have also been demonstrated by the transesophageal procedure as well. This new technique should currently be considered the echocardiographic technique of choice in the differential diagnosis of vasculitis.

If the noninvasive portion of the algorithm does not provide a clear diagnosis, biopsy and angiography must be considered.

Biopsy

The yield from biopsy of a given tissue is directly proportional to the evidence for involvement of that tissue. Thus, if the only abnormality on lab testing is an elevated CPK, especially if the MM fraction is elevated, a unilateral EMG is indicated. The exam should be focused on the proximal extremity and paraspinal muscles, which are larger and more commonly involved. If electrophysiologic abnormalities are found, the same muscle group on the contralateral side should be biopsied. In this way histologic artefact from the prior EMG needle is avoided. It should be mentioned that in any chronic muscle condition, synthesis of MB CPK by the diseased muscle occurs. The clinician should not automatically assume cardiac involvement is present in patients, such as those with vasculitis, simply because of elevation of the MB fraction.

If peroneal neuropathy is seen on the EMG, a sural nerve biopsy is indicated. If temporal artery or other cranial vessel symptoms are present, temporal artery biopsy can be positive in as many as 50% of patients [17].

The skin lesions of vasculitis are often purpuric or urticarial. While biopsy of these lesions rarely reveals more than was suspected clinically, occasionally cholesterol crystals, myxomatous emboli or foreign material accompanying injection of illicitly obtained substances may be demonstrable. Therefore, skin lesions should be biopsied when the diagnosis is unclear. A punch biopsy is generally insufficient for examination of the larger dermal and subdermal vessels that are involved in syndromes such as PAN, and a surgical biopsy of skin should be obtained.

In the majority of instances, the histology on skin biopsy reveals vasculitis without specific diagnostic changes [14,17] and therefore the clinician should not expect the skin biopsy to resolve the diagnosis. One should avoid the pathologic interpretation of 'perivasculitis', since this finding is very nonspecific and can be seen in lesions as benign as self-induced bruises. Pathology in the true vasculitides listed in Figure 37.1 pervades the vessel wall.

Occasionally, no findings are present to suggest involvement of the more accessible tissues, such as skin, nerve or muscle. Biopsy of kidney, liver or lung is indicated if laboratory or radiographic studies suggest that these organs are involved. Biopsy of necrotic nasopharyngeal tissue in patients suspected of having WG has generally been of use only in ruling out neoplastic or invasive fungal disease but has not yielded confirmation of Wegener's. The recent studies of ANCA in Wegener's suggest that it will have a higher positive predictive value.

There are no histologic features that are pathognomonic of any given vasculitis, and it is therefore common, even when visceral biopsies are done, to be left without a specific diagnosis. It is for this reason that elaborate classification systems based on clinical and laboratory criteria, such as those developed recently by the American College of Rheumatology [9], have evolved. There are, nevertheless, findings that may dominate the histopathology in various vasculitides and therefore be strongly suggestive of a specific diagnosis. Some of the dominant histopathologic features of the major vasculitides are shown in Figure 37.5. In patients with no specifically diagnostic laboratory tests, a combination of the characteristics in Figures 37.1 and 37.5 may offer the only likelihood of approximating a specific diagnosis.

Angiography

Angiography is preferable to biopsy when:

- The risk with biopsy is greater than that with angiography. When brain or intestinal involvement is suggested by the clinical picture, angiography is clearly safer than open biopsy. In patients allergic to contrast agents, consideration should be given to giving allergy prophylaxis and proceeding with angiography before resorting directly to, for example, open brain biopsy. In patients with abnormal liver function tests, it is debatable whether needle liver biopsy is preferable to angiography.
- The syndrome suspected is one involving medium-sized or larger vessels. In general, the syndromes at the bottom of Figure 37.1 involve vessels too small to be seen angiographically. On the other hand, Takayasu's arteritis involves the aorta and its main branches, which are not generally accessible to biopsy but are easily demonstrable on angiograms. Similarly, when temporal artery biopsy is negative in patients with suspected giant cell arteritis, aortic arch angiography may be positive. In the computer-generated decision analysis algorithm developed by Albert [18] for diagnosis of polyarteritis, visceral angiography of the celiac, renal and mesenteric systems is preferable to blind biopsy of asymptomatic muscle nerve or kidney.

In practice, a combination of biopsy and angiographic approaches is used, weighing for each procedure the likelihood of diagnostic results, against the risks of the procedure in patients with a given *a priori* likelihood of one of the vasculitis syndromes. A unique problem in this regard is the syndrome called 'isolated vasculitis of the central nervous system'. This vasculitis is limited to the brain and spinal cord.

SUMMARY

In general, diagnosing vasculitis involves considering those diseases diagnosable by specific laboratory tests, determining the extent of organ system involvement through the history, physical exam and nonspecific laboratory tests, ruling out curable mimickers of vasculitis and resorting to a combination of biopsy and angiography to document the diagnosis and estimate prognosis. It is the clinician's responsibility for the care of such patients to document with the fullest precision the exact vasculitic syndrome present, not only to appreciate the prognostic threat, but also to guide therapy in the event that one of the major side effects of these potentially very toxic drugs occurs.

BIOPSY FINDINGS IN MAJOR VASCULITIS SYNDROMES

	Vessel size	Fibrinoid	PMNs	Lymphocytes/ Monocytes	Eosinophils	Giant cells	Granulomas	Comments
Takayasu's arteritis	aorta, main branches, pulmonary	–	++	++++†	±	++++†	++++†	During inactive stage lesions are primarily fibrotic
Giant cell arteritis	large arteries	+	rare	+++	±	++	+++	Giant cell granulomas seen in only 50%; 'skip' areas common
Polyarteritis nodosa	medium to small arteries, venules, arterioles	++++	+++	+++	+	–	rare*	Sectoral involvement; lesions in various stages
Churg–Strauss arteritis	small>medium arteries, veins, arterioles, venules	+++	+	++	++++	++	++++	Granulomas are extravascular; gastrointestinal and heart>kidney
Wegener's granulomatosis	medium-large arteries, small arteries, veins, capillaries	+++	+++	+++	+	++	+++	Almost always in lung; renal vasculitis in <50%; focal segmental glomerulitis
Behçet's syndrome	arterioles, venules>medium-sized vessels	±	+++ (early)	+++ (late)	rare	–	–	Leukocytoclasis
Hypersensitivity vasculitis	arterioles, venules> capillaries	++	+++	+++	+	–	+*	Leukocytoclasis
Henoch-Schönlein purpura	arterioles, venules> capillaries	++	++	++	rare	–	–	Leukocytoclasis

* In variants
† During active phase

Fig. 37.5 Table contrasting major biopsy findings in the major vasculitis syndromes.

REFERENCES

1. Heberden W. Commentari di morboriana-historia et curatione. London: T. Payne; 1801.
2. Schönlein J. Allegemeine und specielle Pathologie und Therapie, vol 2. Herisau: Literatur-Comptoir; 1837: 48.
3. Henoch E. Uber eine eigenthumliche Form von Purpura. Berl Klin Wochenschr. 1874;**11**:641–3.
4. Rokitansky K. Uber einige der wichtigsten Krankheiten der Arterien. Denkschr dK Akad d Wissensch. 1852;**4**:49.
5. Kussmaul A, Maier R. Uber eine bisher nicht beschreibene eigenthumliche Arterienerkrankung (Periarteritis nodosa), die mit Morbus Brightii und rapid fortschreitender allgemeiner Muskellahmung einhergeht. Dtsch Arch Klin Med. 1866;**1**:484–517.
6. Takayasu M. A case with unusual changes of the central vessels in the retina. Acta Soc Opthalmol Jpn. 1908;**12**:554–63.
7. Zeek P, Smith C, Weeter J. Studies on periarteritis nodosa. III. The differentiation between the vascular lesions of periarteritis nodosa and of hypersensitivity. Am J Pathol. 1948;**24**:889–918.
8. Churg J, Strauss L. Allergic granulomatosis, allergic angiitis and periarteritis nodosa. Am J Pathol. 1951;**27**:277–301.
9. Hunder G, Arend W, Bloch D, et al. The American College of Rheumatology 1990 criteria for the classification of vasculitis. Introduction. Arthritis Rheum. 1990;**33**:1065–7.
10. Davies D, Moran J, Niall J, et al. Segmental necrotising glomerulonephritis with antineutrophil antibody: possible arborvirus aetiology? Br Med J. 1982;**285**:606.
11. Van der Woude F, Rasmussen N, Lobatto S, et al. Autoantibodies against neutrophils and monocytes: tool for diagnosis and marker of disease activity in Wegener's granulomatosis. Lancet. 1985;**1**:425–9.
12. Falk R, Jennette J. Anti-neutrophil cytoplasm autoantibodies with specificity for myeloperoxidase in patients with systemic vasculitis and idiopathic necrotising and crescentic glomerulonephritis. N Engl J Med. 1988;**318**:1651–7.
13. Nolle B, Specks U, Ludenmann J, et al. Anticytoplasmic autoantibodies: their immunodiagnostic value in Wegener granulomatosis. Ann Intern Med. 1989;**111**:28–40.
14. Dahlberg P, Overholt E, Lockhart J. Diagnostic approach to vasculitis. In: Churg A, Churg J, eds. Systemic vasculitides. New York: Ikagu-Shoin; 1991:41–54.
15. Savage C. Pathogenesis of systemic vasculitis. In: Churg A, Churg J, eds. Systemic vasculitides. New York: Ikagu-Shoin; 1991:7–30.
16. Reinisch C, Moyer C. Animal models of vasculitis. In: Churg A, Churg J, eds. Systemic vasculitides. New York: Ikagu-Shoin; 1991:31–40.
17. Lie J. Illustrated histopathologic classification criteria for selected vasculitic syndromes. Arthritis Rheum. 1990;**33**:1074–87.
18. Albert D, Rimon D, Silverstein M. The diagnosis of polyarteritis nodosa. I. A literature-based decision analysis approach. Arthritis Rheum. 1988;**31**:1117–27.

38

POLYARTERITIS

Doyt L Conn

Definition

- Small and medium-sized artery inflammation involving the skin, kidney, peripheral nerves, muscle and gut.
- Involvement of other organs is rare.

Clinical features

- Constitutional symptoms – fever, anorexia, weight loss.
- Skin involvement – palpable purpura, infarctions, livedo reticularis.
- Arthralgia and arthritis.
- Peripheral neuropathy.
- Renal involvement – red blood cells and red blood cell casts, proteinuria, renal insufficiency.
- Gut involvement – abdominal pain, liver function abnormalities.

HISTORY

Polyarteritis, also called periarteritis and polyarteritis nodosa (PAN), is a disease of small and medium-sized arteries. The disease was first described by Kussmaul and Maier in 1866 when they reported a case of necrotizing arteritis and called it periarteritis nodosa [1]. Their patient had widespread inflammation of small and medium-sized arteries, and in some areas there were focal inflammatory exudations which gave rise to palpable nodules along the course of the arteries. Nodules are uncommon today probably because the disease is diagnosed more quickly and treated sooner.

In 1952 Zeek classified the necrotizing vasculitides into five categories based upon the clinical and pathologic findings, including the size of artery involved [2]. This classification is presently still in use. In 1970, Gocke and coworkers demonstrated hepatitis B surface (HB_s) antigen and IgM in an involved artery in a patient with PAN [3]. This demonstrated that a virus can trigger vasculitis. A number of other viruses as well as other disease processes have been shown since then to be associated with polyarteritis.

Glucocorticoids (prednisone) is the standard medication used to treat vasculitis today with its use first described in 1951 [4]. Cytotoxic agents have been used for a number of years in the management of vasculitis, but the use of cyclophosphamide (CP) was popularized by Fauci *et al.* in 1979 for the management of polyarteritis [5]. The precise role of cytotoxic agents in the management of polyarteritis is still being elucidated.

EPIDEMIOLOGY

Polyarteritis is an uncommon disease. Estimates of the annual incidence rate for PAN-type systemic vasculitis in a general population range from 4.6 per 1,000,000 in England, 9.0 per 1,000,000 in Olmsted County, Minnesota, to 77 per 1,000,000 in a hepatitis B hyperendemic Alaskan Eskimo population. Estimated annual mortality rate for PAN in New York City in the 1950s was 1.2–1.5 per 1,000,000. The disease is more common in males with a sex ratio of about 2:1. Polyarteritis is observed in children and elderly with the average age of diagnosis ranging from the mid-40s to mid-60s. It is observed in all racial groups [6].

CLASSIFICATION

Although many classification schemes have been devised for the necrotizing vasculitides, none has been entirely satisfactory for the clinician. Recently, a subcommittee of the American College of Rheumatology developed criteria for the classification of seven forms of vasculitis by analysis of data from 1000 cases collected from 48 centers [7–14]. These seven types of vasculitis included PAN, Churg–Strauss syndrome (CSS), Wegener's granulomatosis (WG), hypersensitivity vasculitis, Henoch–Schönlein purpura (HSP), giant cell arteritis and Takayasu's arteritis (TA). The criteria for each were derived by comparing findings in patients with one form of vasculitis with those from other forms of vasculitis as a group. The criteria selected in these studies were those that both identify each vasculitis and separate it from others. As a result, the full spectrum of manifestations are not included in all instances, and the criteria are not appropriate to use in diagnosis of individual patients. However, the criteria do provide a standard way to evaluate and describe patients with vasculitis in therapeutic, epidemiologic, and other studies, allowing comparisons of results from different centers.

The ACR criteria for the classification of PAN are not very helpful for the clinician because they do not take into account the fact that in order for this diagnosis to be made clinically, evidence of vascular involvement must be demonstrated by either biopsy or angiography (Fig. 38.1).

1990 CRITERIA FOR THE CLASSIFICATION OF POLYARTERITIS NODOSA

Criterion	Definition
1. Weight loss >4kg	Loss of 4kg or more of body weight since illness began, not due to dieting or other factors
2. Livedo reticularis	Mottled reticular pattern over the skin of portions of the extremities or torso
3. Testicular pain or tenderness	Pain or tenderness of the testicles, not due to infection, trauma, or other causes
4. Myalgias, weakness or polyneuropathy	Diffuse myalgias (excluding shoulder and hip girdle) or weakness of muscles or tenderness of leg muscles
5. Mononeuropathy or polyneuropathy	Development of mononeuropathy, multiple mononeuropathies, or polyneuropathy
6. Diastolic BP >90mmHg	Development of hypertension with the diastolic BP higher than 90mmHg
7. Elevated BUN or creatinine	Elevation of BUN>40mg/dl (14.3μmol/l) or creatinine >1.5mg/dl (132μmol/l), not due to dehydration or obstruction
8. Hepatitis B virus	Presence of hepatitis B surface antigen or antibody in serum
9. Arteriographic abnormality	Arteriogram showing aneurysms or occlusions of the visceral arteries, not due to arteriosclerosis, fibromuscular dysplasia, or other noninflammatory causes
10. Biopsy of small or medium-sized artery containing PMN	Histologic changes showing the presence of granulocytes or granulocytes and mononuclear leukocytes in the artery wall

Fig. 38.1 1990 criteria for the classification of polyarteritis nodosa (traditional format). For classification purposes, a patient with vasculitis shall be said to have PAN if at least 3 of these 10 criteria are present. The presence of any 3 or more criteria yields a sensitivity of 82.2% and a specificity of 86.6%. BP = blood pressure; BUN = blood urea nitrogen; PMN = polymorphonuclear neutrophils. Adapted from Lightfoot *et al.* [7].

CLINICAL MANIFESTATIONS OF POLYARTERITIS NODOSA		
Organ	Manifestation	Estimated percent prevalence
Peripheral nerve	Mononeuritis multiplex	50–70%
Kidney	Focal necrotizing glomerulonephritis	70%
Skin	Palpable purpura, infarctions, livedo	50%
Joint	Arthralgias	50%
	Arthritis	20%
Muscle	Achiness	50%
Gut	Abdominal pain, liver function abnormalities	30%
Heart	Congestive heart failure, myocardial infarction	low
Central nervous system	Seizures, CVA	low
Lung	Interstitial pneumonitis	low
Eye	Retinal hemorrhage	low
Testis	Pain	low
Temporal artery	Jaw claudication	low

Fig. 38.2 Clinical manifestations of polyarteritis nodosa.

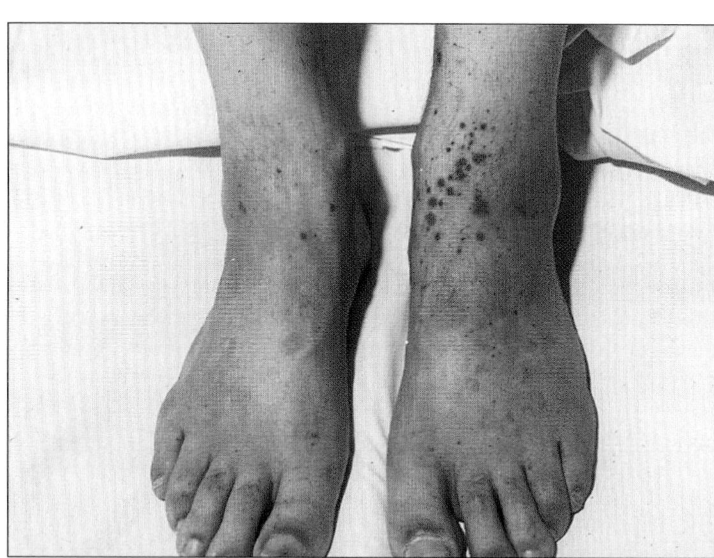

Fig. 38.3 Palpable purpura. With permission from Conn DL [46].

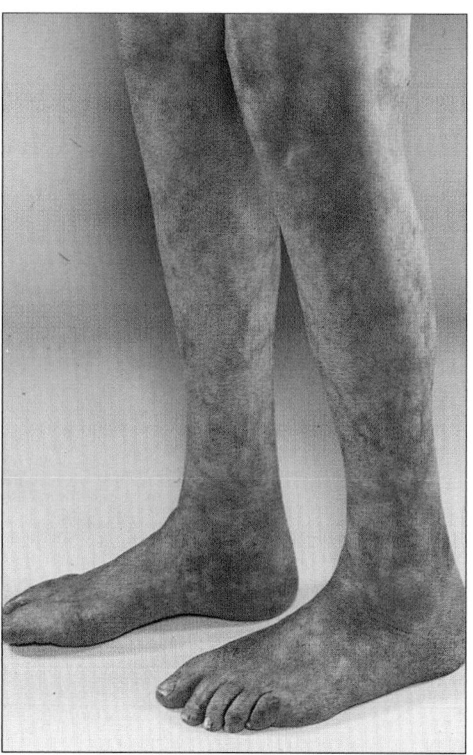

Fig. 38.4 Livedo vasculitis. With permission from Conn DL [46].

CLINICAL FEATURES

The disease may present in a variety of ways. There is a spectrum of severity from mild, limited disease to progressive disease which may be fatal (Fig. 38.2). Virtually any organ may eventually be affected. Typically, the patient experiences constitutional features of fever, malaise, weight loss, and diffuse aching along with manifestations of multisystem involvement such as a skin rash, peripheral neuropathy and an asymmetric polyarthritis. Visceral involvement, such as the kidney or gut, may present coincidentally with these features, or they may appear later. In other cases, single organ involvement may be present alone and may remain limited, including isolated involvement of the skin, peripheral nerves, and visceral organs [15,16].

Cutaneous Lesions

Cutaneous lesions include palpable purpura, infarctions, ulcerations, livedo vasculitis, and ischemic changes of the distal digits (Figs 38.3, 38.4 & 38.5). Arthralgia or arthritis is present in polyarteritis in as many as 50% of patients [17]. The patient with polyarteritis may present with, or have early in the course of the disease, a polymyalgia rheumatica syndrome. An asymmetric, episodic, nondeforming polyarthritis involving the larger joints of the lower extremity may occur in 20% of cases and is common early in the disease [18].

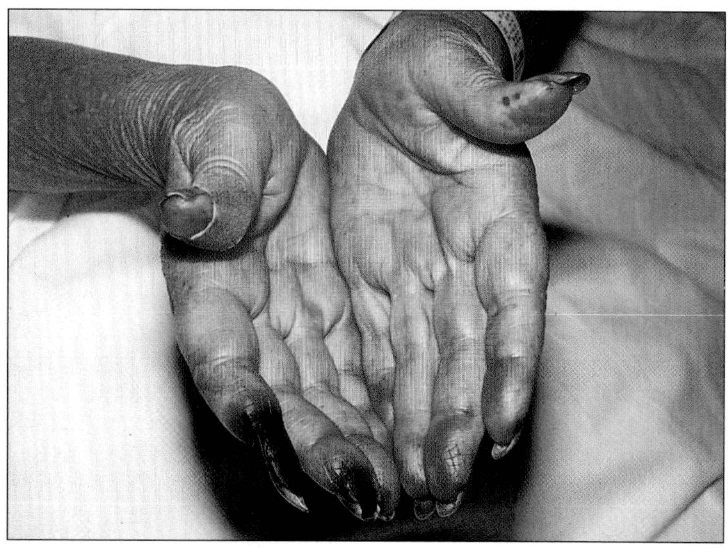

Fig. 38.5 Digital tip infarctions. With permission from Conn DL [46].

Neuropathy

Peripheral neuropathy may occur in 50–70% of cases and may be the initial manifestation [19]. The upper and lower extremities are affected with about the same frequency. The onset may be sudden, with pain and paresthesias radiating in the distribution of a peripheral nerve, followed in hours or days by a motor deficit of the same peripheral nerve. This may progress asymmetrically to involve other peripheral nerves and produce a mononeuritis multiplex or a multiple mononeuropathy. With additional nerve damage, the final result may be a symmetrical polyneuropathy involving all sensory modalities and motor functions. Less commonly, a slowly evolving distal sensory neuropathy may occur. Clinical manifestations suggestive of CNS involvement are much less common than those of peripheral nerve involvement, but the two may appear together. Features suggestive of CNS involvement are seizures and hemiparesis [20].

Renal Involvement

Clinical renal involvement occurs in about 70% of cases. Proteinuria is common and, rarely, a nephrotic syndrome may develop. Equally common is a change in urinary sediment, with red cells and red cell casts suggestive of glomerular involvement [21]. Hypertension may develop as a result of renal artery or glomerular involvement and is present in about 25% of cases [22].

Gastrointestinal Involvement

Abdominal pain is the most common gastrointestinal symptom and roughly correlates in location with the organ involved [23]. A patient may rarely present with abdominal pain due to localized gallbladder or appendiceal involvement. In cases of diffuse abdominal pain, mesenteric thrombosis must be considered. Abdominal distention may indicate mesenteric thrombosis with or without peritonitis. Hematemesis, melena, and hematochezia are caused by vasculitis of the upper or lower gastrointestinal tract. Liver involvement, although common in autopsy studies, is not as common clinically and may be associated with HB_S antigen. The only abnormality reflecting liver involvement may be an elevated level of alkaline phosphatase without elevated bilirubin or transaminase levels [24].

Cardiac and Pulmonary Involvement

Cardiac involvement is common pathologically but is recognized less often clinically. Myocardial infarction, when it occurs, is usually silent [25]. Congestive heart failure may develop as a result of coronary insufficiency or hypertension (or both).

Uncommonly, patients with polyarteritis have pulmonary involvement. Lung infiltrations may be diffuse and may precede the development of vascular involvement in other organs. However, pulmonary lesions are more common in patients whose findings fit better with granulomatous vasculitis (WG and CSS).

NONSPECIFIC CLINICAL AND LABORATORY FINDINGS IN VASCULITIS
Constitutional symptoms of fever, fatigue, anorexia, weight loss
Polymyalgia rheumatica
Nondestructive oligoarthritis
Elevated erythrocyte sedimentation rate
Anemia
Thrombocytosis
Diminished serum albumin concentration

Fig. 38.6 Nonspecific clinical and laboratory findings in vasculitis. Adapted from Conn DL [46].

Other Features

Diffuse involvement of skeletal muscle arteries may cause pain and intermittent claudication [26]. Testicular involvement is manifested by pain, but clinical involvement indicated by swelling or induration has been reported to be present in only a small percentage of patients in most series [27]. In the eye, polyarteritis may result in an exudative retinal detachment or toxic retinopathy with retinal hemorrhage or exudates [28].

Temporal artery involvement may infrequently occur in PAN and in other forms of systemic vasculitis including WG and CSS. It may be associated with jaw claudication. The pathologic picture in such cases reveals fibrinoid necrosis without giant cells [29].

Polyarteritis may be a manifestation or complication of other diseases, such as rheumatoid arthritis (RA) [30], Sjögren's syndrome [31], mixed cryoglobulinemia [32], hairy cell leukemia [33], myelodysplastic syndrome and other hematologic malignancies [34].

Laboratory Tests

Most tests are nonspecific and reflect the systemic inflammatory nature of the disease (Fig. 38.6). An elevated ESR, normochromic anemia, thrombocytosis, and diminished levels of serum albumin are usually present. Eosinophilia is generally associated with pulmonary involvement, particularly in allergic angiitis and granulomatosis (CSS).

Diminished concentrations of serum whole complement and C3 and C4 components may be associated with active disease [18] and may be present in about 25% of the cases [17]. Such cases usually have diffuse cutaneous or renal disease. Rheumatoid factor may be present. HB_S antigen has been found in 10–54% of patients, depending on the series [18,35]. In some cases the antigen is detected in the serum transiently, with serial determinations necessary to detect it.

PATHOLOGY

The pathology of polyarteritis consists of focal yet panmural, necrotizing inflammatory lesions in small and medium-sized arteries. The lesion may occur in all parts of the body but there is usually less involvement of the pulmonary and splenic arteries [2,36]. The inflammation is characterized by fibrinoid necrosis and pleomorphic cellular infiltration, with predominantly polymorphonuclear (PMN) leukocytes and variable numbers of lymphocytes and eosinophils (Fig. 38.7). The normal architecture of the vessel wall, including the elastic laminae, is disrupted. There may be thrombosis or aneurysmal dilatation at the site of the lesion. Healed areas of arteritis show proliferation of fibrous tissue and endothelial cells, which may lead

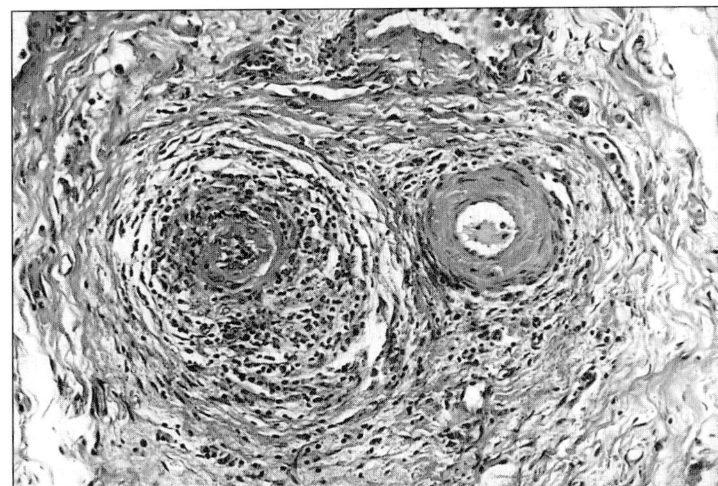

Fig. 38.7 Polyarteritis involving the gallbladder artery showing pleomorphic inflammatory cell infiltration and fibrinoid necrosis. With permission from Conn DL [46].

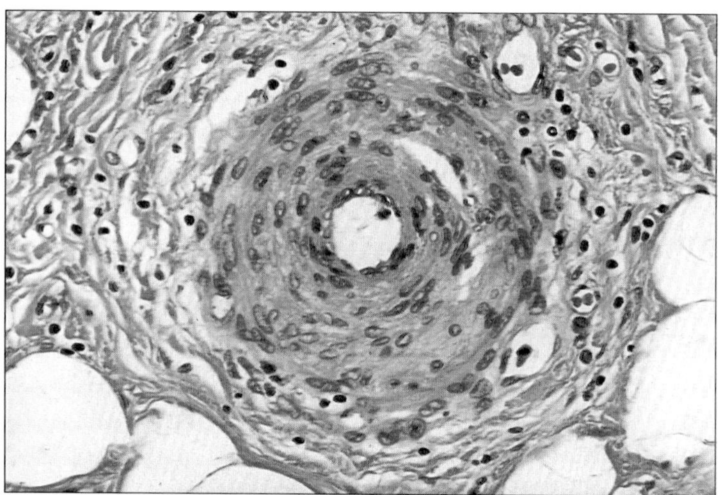

Fig. 38.8 Chronic polyarteritis with intimal proliferation and chronic fibrotic changes. With permission from Conn DL [46].

to vessel occlusion (Fig. 38.8). Lesions at all stages of progression and healing may be seen pathologically if sufficient tissue is available for study.

It is difficult to determine the frequency of involvement of various organs in polyarteritis because of the heterogeneity of patients included in most studies. The kidney may be involved in 70–80% of the patients with polyarteritis. In autopsy studies, inflammation in the arcuate and interlobar arteries and arterioles is frequently found, all in the same kidney, along with evidence of infarction [21]. Glomerulonephritis may be present in one third of cases and is usually segmental and proliferative. 'Microscopic polyarteritis' refers to involvement of small vessels and associated segmental glomerulitis.

Arteries of the gastrointestinal tract may be involved in up to 50% of cases studied by autopsy. Vessels of liver and jejunum are most commonly affected [23]. In the liver, findings include vasculitis along with aneurysms, infarctions, and hepatitis [37]. The gallbladder and appendix are involved in approximately 10% of cases in which other gut involvement is demonstrated by tissue study. Rarely, polyarteritis may manifest itself solely as involvement of the gallbladder or appendix [38,39].

Peripheral nerves may be involved in 50% of cases with polyarteritis. The vascular lesions may be widespread and may involve the entire length of an affected nerve. Small arteries, 70–200μm in diameter, located in the epineurium are affected. The arterial alterations are similar to those in other organs, and a patient may show a spectrum of pathologic change from fibrinoid necrosis in acute lesions to intimal proliferation and perivascular fibrosis in more chronic lesions. The nerve fiber degeneration that results depends upon the extent of vascular involvement. The arterial changes that occur in peripheral nerves in patients with RA, WG, and allergic angiitis and granulomatosis are indistinguishable from those changes in polyarteritis [40].

Cutaneous involvement varies from a few percent to 50% [41]. Skeletal muscle and the mesentery are involved in 30% of cases [42]. The CNS is involved in approximately 10%. Inflammation may be found in the vertebral, carotid, meningeal, cerebral and deep arteries within the brain. The heart is commonly involved in polyarteritis studied at autopsy. These findings include coronary arteritis, myocardial infarction, pericarditis, and cardiac hypertrophy [25]. Rarely, cases of isolated coronary arteritis have been described [43]. Testicular vascular involvement is common pathologically, but uncommon clinically.

PATHOGENESIS

In most cases of vasculitis the cause is not known. An immune complex mediated mechanism of disease is frequently considered. Circulating immune complexes are frequently found in systemic vasculitis and less commonly the total serum hemolytic complement is diminished [18]. Immune deposits of immunoglobulins and complement are seldom found in involved tissue in polyarteritis [44]. The antigen triggering immune complex disease is usually not known. Hepatitis B surface antigen is known to initiate an immune complex induced vasculitis in a variable percent of cases, from 10% to 55% depending upon the locale of the patient population studied [18,35].

Viruses may contribute to the pathogenesis of vasculitis either by inducing an immune complex or by directly invading the endothelial cell and altering function [45]. Recently, human immunodeficiency virus (HIV) has been associated with a polyarteritis pattern of disease. Other viruses associated with vasculitis besides hepatitis B are cytomegalovirus, hepatitis A, human T cell leukemia–lymphoma virus 1 and parvovirus [46].

Due to an alteration of the endothelial cell, or as a result of a cross-reacting mechanism, antibodies to endothelial cells may occur. Antibodies to endothelial cells, using cultured human umbilical endothelial cells as antigens, are detected in Kawasaki disease and SLE but not in polyarteritis [47,48]. When autologous monocytes are used as the antigen because of their antigenic similarity to endothelial cells, antibodies are detected in a variety of vasculitic syndromes including polyarteritis, WG and temporal arteritis [49]. The role of these antibodies is not known.

Preliminary studies indicate that there may be elevation of particular cytokines in certain vasculitic syndromes. In one study there was a marked increase in the serum interferon-α (IFN-α) and interleukin-2 (IL-2) levels and a moderate increase in the levels of tumor necrosis factor (TNF-α) and IL-1β in PAN and CSS vasculitis [50]. In patients with WG the IFN-α and IL-2 were elevated but the other cytokines were normal. The numbers in this preliminary study were small, but it is possible that there is a particular pattern of cytokine abnormalities in certain vasculitic syndromes indicating that injury of certain cell types may release a particular cytokine.

An experiment of nature has provided other possible mechanisms of injury that could lead to arteritis. Rarely, hairy cell leukemia can be complicated by polyarteritis [35]. In some of these cases, hairy cells have been found in the vasculitic lesions, but it is not known whether they contribute to the pathogenesis or are 'innocent bystanders'. However, it is possible that the hairy cells themselves are pathogenic. Studies have also shown that in some patients with hairy cell leukemia, antibodies are directed toward certain determinants on hairy cells that cross-react with endothelial cells.

Injury to the blood vessel and specifically the endothelium will alter blood vessel wall contractility. The endothelium of blood vessels in experimental animals and humans modulates the underlying smooth muscle tone by the production of a dilator substance – endothelial derived relaxing factor (EDRF)–nitric oxide [51]. A healthy and intact endothelium responds to stimulation by relaxation as a result of EDRF–nitric oxide prodution. Not only is EDRF–nitric oxide a mediator of dilation but it has an antiproliferative action on fibroblasts and smooth muscle cells. There is evidence that EDRF–nitric oxide is deficient in hypertension, atherosclerosis and diabetes mellitus [52]. Another endothelial cell-derived local vasodilator is prostacyclin. The production of prostacyclin by endothelial cells decreases with age, diabetes mellitus, atherosclerosis and presumably vasculitis [52].

Coagulation abnormalities may occur in systemic vasculitis and could influence occlusive artery changes. For example, patients with active TA have hyperfibrinogenemia and hypofibrinolytic activity [53]. Studies of hemostasis in vasculitis has been limited, but the data reported shows activation of coagulation without inhibition of clotting.

The levels of cytokines, eicosanoids, EDRF–nitric oxide, and coagulation and fibrinolytic factors have not been studied critically in any of the systemic vasculitides. However, from studies in experimental animals and in human disease it would seem reasonable to expect that the net effect of injury to the endothelial cell would

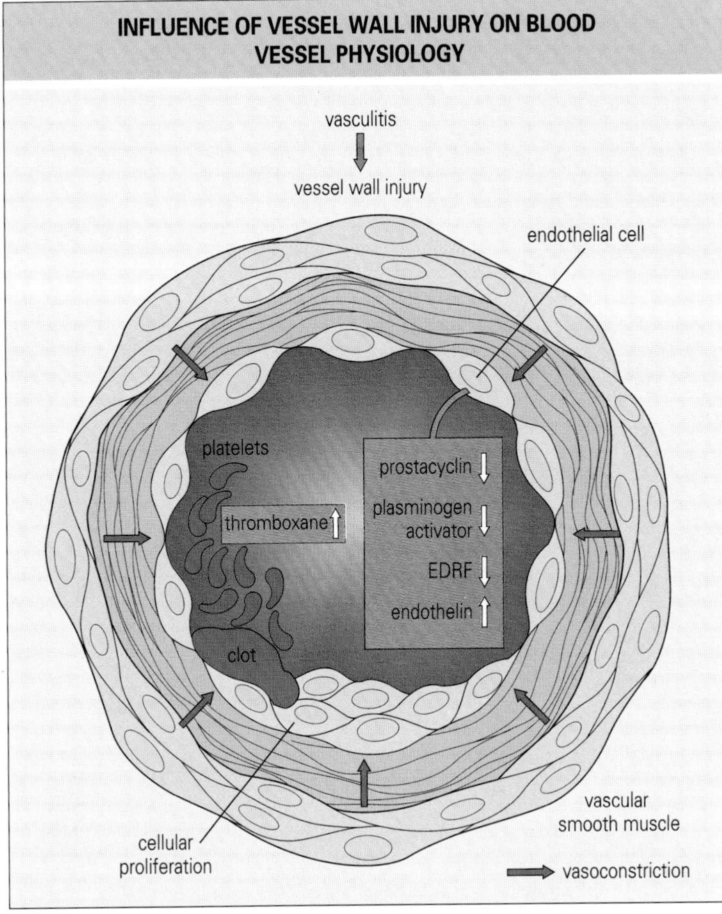

Fig. 38.9 Influence of vessel wall injury on blood vessel physiology. Adapted from Conn DL, Tompkins RB, Nichols WL [55].

result in vasoconstriction, platelet aggregation, clot formation, and the release of growth factors that could result in cellular proliferation and luminal occlusion (Fig. 38.9).

Occlusive Vasculopathy

It is likely that some of the same pathophysiologic factors that are important in the pathogenesis of atherosclerosis are also important in some cases of the systemic vasculitides, but the pathologic process in systemic vasculitis occurs more rapidly. An occlusive vasculopathy can complicate human organ transplantation by affecting allographs. Vascular endothelial cells in the allographs are targets of immunologic reactions and the end result is artery wall, intimal, and smooth muscle proliferation [54]. A common pathologic finding in polyarteritis is the occlusion of blood vessels due to clot organization and/or intimal and smooth muscle proliferation with only a few inflammatory cells present [4]. This process may be promoted by glucocorticoids [55].

DIFFERENTIAL DIAGNOSIS

Because the symptoms in polyarteritis are so diverse, the diagnosis is often difficult and delayed. However, making the diagnosis as early as possible is important because the disease may progress with time to involve vital organs, and the extent of involvement determines the outcome. Polyarteritis should be suspected in a patient with findings of fever, chills, weight loss, fatigue, and multisystem involvement. Polymyalgia rheumatica syndrome and an oligoarthritis involving large joints may be early manifestations of polyarteritis. A careful examination may reveal early cutaneous manifestations, a peripheral neuropathy or renal involvement that might provide clues to the diagnosis. The emergence of a multiple mononeuropathy is an important clue to an underlying arteritis (Fig. 38.10).

KEY CLINICAL FEATURES SUGGESTIVE OF POLYARTERITIS
Skin lesions (palpable purpura, livedo reticularis, necrotic lesions, infarcts of tips of digits)
Peripheral neuropathy (mononeuritis multiplex)
Renal sediment abnormalities

Fig. 38.10 Key clinical features suggestive of polyarteritis. Adapted from Conn DL [46].

It must be remembered that patients with septicemia, infective endocarditis, malignancy, left atrial myxoma, and atherosclerosis with large artery aneurysms and peripheral cholesterol embolization may resemble patients with polyarteritis (Fig. 38.11). In addition, patients with RA, Sjögren's syndrome, mixed cryoglobulinemia, and certain malignancies such as hairy cell leukemia may have a complicating polyarteritis.

Diagnostic algorithms have been described as guides for the diagnosis of polyarteritis [56]. However, the diagnosis of polyarteritis must be determined by sampling accessible tissue by biopsy, and if clinically involved tissue is not accessible, then a visceral angiogram should be considered. Evidence of vascular involvement is established by biopsy or angiography. The most accessible involved tissues are the skin, sural nerve, testes, and skeletal muscle. In each of these situations, small arteries should be sampled and a positive diagnosis is based on the demonstration of small vessel necrotizing arteritis. The finding of a perivascular inflammation or intimal proliferation without fibrinoid necrosis of the arterial wall should also suggest the diagnosis of polyarteritis.

Involvement of the sural nerve can be verified by electromyography. When the sural nerve biopsy is performed, an entire cross-sectional segment of the nerve must be obtained to provide sufficient material for adequate sampling of epineurial arteries. Small vessels in the dermis can be sampled by punch skin biopsies. Small arteries should be sampled by excisional biopsy of subcutaneous tissue and skeletal muscle. Up to 30–50% of 'blind' muscle biopsies may reveal arteritis. The frequency of a positive muscle biopsy specimen is probably higher when painful or stiff muscles are sampled. A testicular biopsy should be reserved for those patients with clinically involved areas of the testis indicated by pain and/or induration.

In cases with abnormalities of urine sediment or proteinuria, renal biopsy will usually reveal a focal segmental necrotizing glomerulonephritis and in about 50% of cases a small vessel vasculitis may be demonstrated [18]. However, biopsy of renal tissue is unhelpful in the differential diagnosis of vasculitis but may be diagnostically

DISEASES SIMILAR TO PAN

Disease	PAN-like features
Left atrial myxoma	Skin emboli
Cholesterol embolization	Livedo vasculitis of the feet
Infections:	
staphylococcus	Skin emboli
gonococcus	
Lyme disease	Peripheral neuropathy
Infective endocarditis	Skin lesions
	Glomerulitis
Malignancy	Skin lesions
	Constitutional features
Arterial dissections	Angiographic similarity
Ergotism	Vasospasm

Fig. 38.11 Diseases similar to PAN.

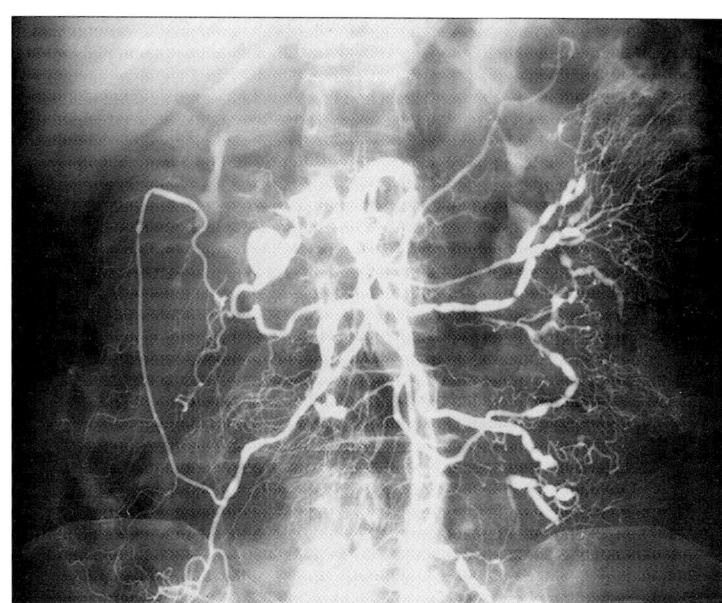

Fig. 38.12 Visceral angiogram in polyarteritis showing areas of segmental narrowing and aneuryms. With permission from Conn DL [46].

useful if no other organs are involved and no other tissue is available for sampling. Arteriography is helpful diagnostically and may provide information on prognosis. Positive findings include arterial saccular or fusiform aneurysms and narrowing or tapering of the arteries (Fig. 38.12). This procedure is most appropriate when involved organs are not available for biopsy and when there is evidence of intra-abdominal involvement including liver function abnormalities and renal sediment abnormalities. It is unusual for the angiogram to be positive in cases without obvious visceral symptoms, signs, or laboratory abnormalities. Aneurysms have been found most commonly in the kidney and liver, but also may be found in the mesenteric arteries. The lesions may disappear with improvement of the arteritis. The presence of aneurysms is associated with more severe and extensive disease [57].

PROGNOSIS

The outcome in polyarteritis is dependent upon the presence and extent of visceral and CNS involvement. Most of the deaths occur within the first year of disease (Fig. 38.13) [17,41]. Deaths occurring within the first year are usually due to uncontrolled vasculitis, frequently as a result of delay in the diagnosis of the disease or from infectious complications of treatment. Deaths occurring after one year of disease are usually either a result of complications of treatment, such as superimposed infections, or vascular deaths such as a myocardial infarction or stroke. The prognosis of untreated polyarteritis is poor and the 5-year survival is less than 15% [19]. Survival has improved with the use of glucocorticoids, and most studies reveal a 5-year survival of between 50–60%. There is no convincing evidence that a combination of glucocorticoids and cytotoxic agents results in a better outcome [17,58].

MANAGEMENT

The management of polyarteritis should be based on the extent and rate of involvement. In patients with limited and nonprogressive disease, daily or divided daily doses of prednisone will usually suffice. In patients with extensive visceral involvement and evidence of progression of disease, despite good doses of glucocorticoids, the addition of a cytotoxic agent should be used. Other modalities of treatment have been advocated in such a situation including

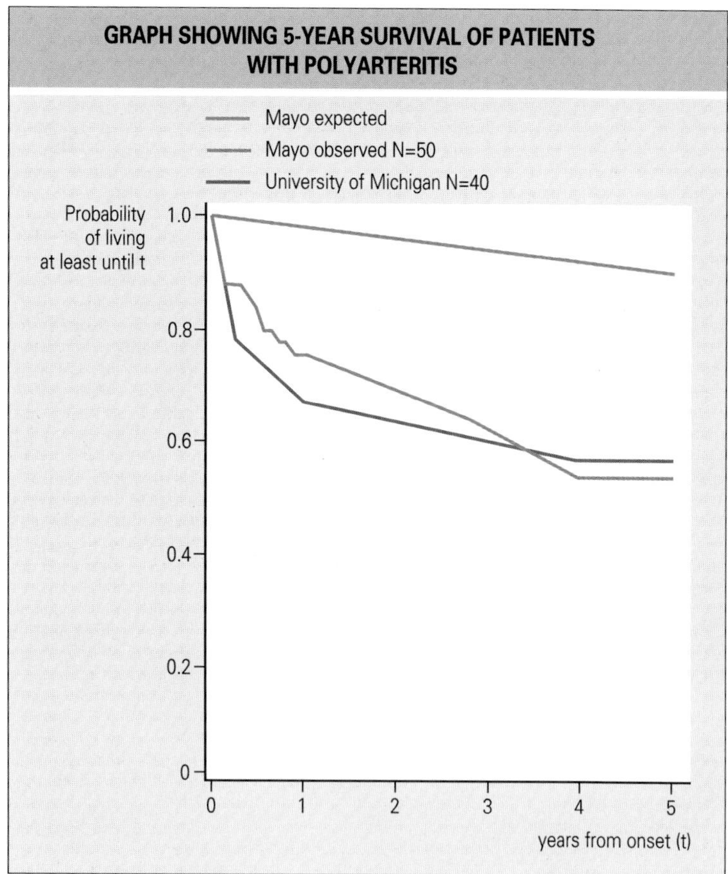

Fig. 38.13 Graph showing 5-year survival of patients with polyarteritis. Adapted from Cohen RD, Conn DL, Ilstrup DM [17] and Sack M, Cassidy JT, Bole GG [41].

azathioprine [59], intravenous (i.v.) methylprednisolone [60], i.v. methotrexate [61], and plasma exchange [62]. Cytotoxic drugs may be needed as corticosteroid-sparing agents if the disease cannot be controlled with low doses of prednisone (less than 15mg daily).

Glucocorticoids

The initial management of polyarteritis should include high doses of glucocorticoids (prednisone). The appropriate use of prednisone is important. Initially, it should be administered in a single daily dose or divided daily doses, ranging from 40 to 60mg a day. Alternate day doses have no role in the initial management (and probably not in subsequent management) of polyarteritis, because with such a regimen the patient is not treated for part of a 24-hour period and the disease may exacerbate. It is more important to control the vasculitis than to spare the hypothalamic–pituitary–adrenal axis.

In the follow-up of patients with polyarteritis, the clinical status and ESR should be monitored. As the clinical status improves and as the ESR returns to normal, tapering of the prednisone can begin. Initially, the decrements can be 5–10mg every one to two weeks. As

INDICATION FOR ADDITION OF CYTOTOXIC DRUG TO PREDNISONE IN THE MANAGEMENT OF SYSTEMIC VASCULITIS

On initial evaluation, rapidly progressive vasculitis with significant visceral involvement

Prednisone in high daily divided doses is not controlling the activity and progression of vasculitis

Prednisone dose cannot be tapered to tolerable level and still control the disease

Fig. 38.14 Indication for addition of cytotoxic drug to prednisone in the management of systemic vasculitis.

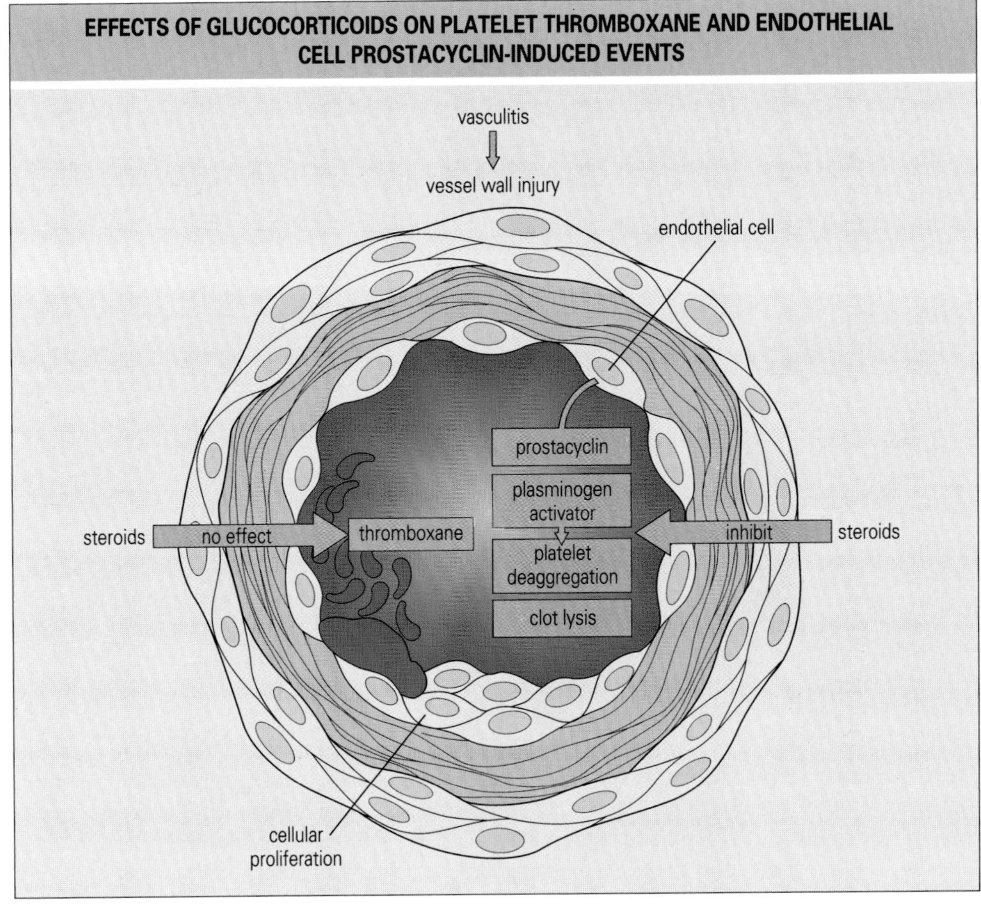

Fig. 38.15 Diagram showing the possible effects of glucocorticoids on platelet thromboxane and endothelial cell prostacyclin-induced events. Adapted from Conn DL, Tompkins RB, Nichols WL [55].

the prednisone dose becomes lower, the decrements should be less. When the total dose of prednisone is down to approximately 15mg a day, the reduction in dose should be 1mg every several weeks. Frequently the patient must be maintained on a low dose of prednisone for an indefinite period of time.

Cytotoxic Therapy

There are uncontrolled retrospective studies demonstrating the benefit of cyclophosphamide in one study [5], azathioprine in another study [59] and no added benefit of cytotoxic therapy in several other studies [58]. It is difficult to compare studies because they are retrospective and differ in patient composition, duration and severity of disease, age of the patient, the presence of other disease processes, and duration and type of treatment. Consequently, it is not possible to obtain definitive information from the literature regarding the exact role of cytotoxic drugs in the treatment of polyarteritis.

We depend on our knowledge of factors that influence outcome and balance this with the potential side effects of cytotoxic drugs. A cytotoxic drug should probably be added to prednisone in the following situations (Fig. 38.14): (i) On initial evaluation when the vasculitis is rapidly progressing involving visceral organs; (ii) prednisone in sufficient daily divided doses does not control the activity and progression of disease; and (iii) the prednisone cannot be tapered to a tolerable level and still control the disease.

When a cytotoxic drug is added, it probably should be an alkylating agent because the onset of action occurs in several weeks with these agents. Cyclophosphamide is the popular choice, but there is no reason to consider it to be more efficacious than chlorambucil. The oncogenic potential and effect on germinal cells of both drugs are equal. Otherwise, chlorambucil is less toxic. Alkylating agents are given with prednisone and with control of disease, as the prednisone dose is tapered, the alkylating drug dose will also have to be lowered (otherwise it will likely induce cytopenia). There is no published experience regarding the efficacy of pulse i.v. doses of cyclophosphamide given monthly in the treatment of polyarteritis.

Glucocorticoids and cytotoxic agents are used to treat the vascular inflammation. However, the effects of inflammation on the blood vessel wall with resulting platelet aggregation, vasoconstriction, clot formation, and cellular proliferation are important factors in determining the final vascular outcome. Modification of these factors should be considered in management. It is possible that the older patient who develops polyarteritis and has concomitant atherosclerosis may have a greater tendency to develop an occlusive vasculopathy.

Glucocorticoids are effective in controlling the inflammation, but occasionally vascular occlusion will still develop, with the glucocorticoids possibly promoting this process by permitting platelet aggregation, vasospasm, and endothelial and smooth muscle proliferation [4]. One possible explanation for this is related to the effects of glucocorticoids on arachidonic acid. It is possible that glucocorticoids inhibit endothelial cell prostacylin production to a greater extent than platelet-derived thromboxane production (Fig. 38.15) [40]. Consequently, in the management of polyarteritis, the use of an antiplatelet drug concomitantly with initiation of glucocorticoids might modify this potential vasospastic and platelet aggregating effect. (Fig. 38.16). It is not know which antiplatelet drug might be the most efficacious. It is also possible that agents directed toward inhibiting cytokines, growth factors, and cellular proliferation will

TREATMENT SCHEME

Target	Agent(s)
Inflammation	Prednisone Cytotoxic drugs Immunotherapy
Platelet–endothelial cell mechanism (vasospasm, platelet aggregation)	Antiplatelet drugs Vasodilating agents
Cellular proliferation	? Cytotoxic drugs

Fig. 38.16 Treatment scheme.

be important in the future. It is possible that an important effect of the cytotoxic drugs is to inhibit cellular proliferation and thus prevent arterial occlusion, although this mechanism has not been demonstrated. The use of vasodilating drugs (calcium channel blockers) may be important if there is significant vasospasm.

Late complications and deaths associated with polyarteritis include renal vascular hypertension, cerebrovascular disease, and coronary artery disease [17]. These vascular occlusive complications may be due to the effects of arterial inflammation, glucocorticoid augmented atherosclerosis and glucocorticoid influenced vascular occlusion. The concomitant use of antiplatelet drugs with glucocorticoid treatment might modify some of these late vascular complications.

Other Therapies

Intravenous immunoglobulin

This mode of therapy has been used successfully in Kawasaki disease to reduce the prevalence of coronary artery aneurysms [63]. It is assumed that the reduction and the prevalence of coronary aneurysms is due to a beneficial effect on the vasculitis. The use of i.v. immunoglobulin is an experimental treatment approach and if it is used in systemic vasculitis it should be used in a controlled study as has been done in Kawasaki disease.

Monoclonal antibody therapy

It is attractive to consider a more targeted therapeutic approach in polyarteritis. This type of treatment is promising in seropositive RA where certain MHC class II antigens and T-cell receptors are associated with the disease and these determinants can be targeted for treatment [64]. No such HLA marker or T-cell receptor domain has been implicated in polyarteritis. Nevertheless, a recent case study has been reported in which a patient with recalcitrant systemic necrotizing vasculitis was treated with a panlymphocyte antibody and a murine anti-CD4 monoclonal antibody which resulted in a one year remission [65]. This study should stimulate a more detailed study of associated HLA antigens, T cells and T-cell receptors in polyarteritis and perhaps a future controlled study with this type of monoclonal antibody.

CHURG–STRAUSS SYNDROME

Definition

- Small and medium-sized artery granulomatous inflammation.
- Frequently involving the skin, peripheral nerves and lungs.
- Associated with a peripheral eosinophilia.

Clinical features

- History of atopy.
- Constitutional symptoms – fever, anorexia, weight loss.
- Asthma.
- Peripheral neuropathy.
- Skin involvement – nodular lesions over pressure areas.
- Peripheral eosinophilia.

ALLERGIC ANGIITIS AND GRANULOMATOSIS (CHURG–STRAUSS SYNDROME)

The association of asthma, eosinophilia, vasculitis, and extravascular granulomas was termed allergic angiitis and granulomatosis by Churg and Strauss in 1951 [66]. These authors considered allergic factors to be important in the development of the disease. This form of vasculitis is rare, although no detailed epidemiologic analyses are available. Thirty patients with this condition were found over a 25-year period in one center [67]. The male-to-female ratio appears to be about 2:1 and the age at onset varies from 15 to 70 years, with a mean of about 38 [68]. Criteria for the classification of CSS has been established and may be used in the future for epidemiologic studies (Fig. 38.17) [10].

CLINICAL FEATURES

There may be three phases of disease. A prodromal period which may last for years (over 10 years) consisting of allergic manifestations of rhinitis, polyposis and asthma. The second phase includes peripheral blood and tissue eosinophilia with Löffler's syndrome, eosinophilic pneumonia, or eosinophilic gastroenteritis. The third phase is the systemic vasculitis. These phases may appear simultaneously. The development of fever and weight loss may herald the onset of systemic disease. At this time, chest radiographs are abnormal in approximately half the cases and show changes ranging from patchy, shifting pneumonic infiltrates (Löffler's syndrome), through massive bilateral nodular infiltrates without cavitation, to diffuse interstitial lung disease. The symptoms of asthma often subside when the vasculitis emerges.

Cutaneous lesions occur in approximately two thirds of the patients. Subcutaneous nodules are the most common skin manifestation. Petechiae, purpura, or skin infarctions may be seen. Peripheral neuropathy, usually mononeuritis multiplex, is found in the majority of patients. Cardiac involvement is common and may result in congestive heart failure. Abdominal symptoms occur in a small percentage of cases; these may be due to granulomatous vasculitis of vessels of the stomach or small bowel. Bloody diarrhea, simulating chronic ulcerative colitis, may be caused by ischemia of the mucosa of the large bowel. Granulomatous involvement of the bowel, liver, or omentum may produce a palpable mass.

Renal disease has been found to be frequent in some series and less common in others. Renal failure occurs infrequently [68]. Eosinophilic granulomatous involvement of the prostate and lower urinary tract is an unusual feature of this disease. Polyarthralgias and arthritis are uncommon. Rarely, ulceration of the cornea or CNS manifestions, such as seizures, may occur.

1990 CRITERIA FOR THE CLASSIFICATION OF CHURG–STRAUSS SYNDROME

Criterion	Definition
Asthma	History of wheezing or diffuse high-pitched rales on expiration
Eosinophilia	Eosinophilia >10% on white blood cell differential count
Mononeuropathy or polyneuropathy	Development of mononeuropathy, multiple mononeuropathies, or polyneuropathy (i.e. glove/stocking distribution) attributable to a systemic vasculitis
Pulmonary infiltrates, nonfixed	Migratory or transitory pulmonary infiltrates on radiographs (not including fixed infiltrates), attributable to a systemic vasculitis
Paranasal sinus abnormality	History of acute or chronic paranasal sinus pain or tenderness or radiographic opacification of the paranasal sinuses
Extravascular eosinophils	Biopsy including artery, arteriole, or venule, showing accumulations of eosinophils in extravascular areas

Fig. 38.17 1990 criteria for the classification of Churg–Strauss syndrome. For classification purposes, a patient with vasculitis shall be said to have CSS if at least 4 of these 6 criteria are positive. The presence of any 4 or more of the 6 criteria yields a sensitivity of 85% and a specificity of 99.7%. Adapted from Masi AT *et al.* [8].

Laboratory Tests

The characteristic laboratory abnormality is eosinophilia [66]. The eosinophilia often decreases as the patient improves or is treated. With active disease, anemia and an elevated ESR are found. Serum rheumatoid factor may be present in low titer [68]. In the few patients studied an elevated serum IgE has been found although the serum complement has been normal [18,68].

PATHOLOGY

The characteristic pathologic changes in this disease include small necrotizing granulomas as well as necrotizing vasculitis involving small arteries and venules [66]. Granulomas are typically about 1mm or more in diameter and are commonly located near small arteries or veins. They are composed of a central eosinophilic core surrounded radially by macrophages and epithelioid giant cells. Inflammatory cells are also present in the granulomas, with eosinophils predominating in the early state of development and lesser numbers being present in the healing stages. Polymorphonuclear leukocytes and lymphocytes are found in varying but smaller numbers. Macrophages and giant cells predominate in the more chronic lesions. Necrotizing vasculitis of small arteries and veins are always seen in involved tissue. Extravascular granulomas and fibrinoid necrosis may be seen in about 50% of cases.

DIAGNOSIS

The diagnosis of Churg–Strauss vasculitis is made on the basis of both clinical and pathologic features. As noted, the patient is usually middle-aged and has a history of asthma that has been present for several years. The apppearance of a systemic illness in this setting should lead the clinician to consider this diagnosis. Diagnostically helpful features are noncavitary lung infiltrates, nodular skin lesions, peripheral neuropathy, significant eosinophilia and an elevated level of serum IgE. The diagnosis may be substantiated by biopsy of the involved tissues, usually the lung or the skin, which reveals the characteristic eosinophilic necrotizing extravascular granulomas and necrotizing small vessel vasculitis.

MANAGEMENT AND OUTCOME

The treatment of choice is glucocorticoids in a dosage sufficient to control the inflammatory manifestations of the disease. An initial dosage of 40 to 60mg of prednisone per day, in divided doses, or the equivalent dosage of another glucocorticoid, is usually sufficient to control the disease. Data concerning the use of cytotoxic agents in this condition are meager.

The outlook may be better than that observed in patients with typical polyarteritis. Rose and Spencer noted that patients who had PAN with lung involvement had a less fulminating course and that approximately one third were living at the end of 1 year [69]. There were some deaths due to lung disease in this group but fewer due to renal failure than in patients without lung involvement. In a study of 30 patients with allergic angiitis and granulomatosis, Chumbley and coworkers noted a 90% 1-year survival rate and a 62% 5-year survival rate [67]. In this series, the most common cause of death was myocardial infarction, followed by congestive heart failure. Other causes of death were status asthmaticus, salmonella septicemia, ruptured aneurysm, renal failure, pneumonia, and small bowel infarction. Some of these deaths were direct complications of the glucocorticoid treatment.

REFERENCES

1. Kussmaul A, Maier R. Ueber eine bisher nicht beshriebene eigenthumliche Arterienerkrankung- (Periarteritis nodosa), die mit Morbus Brightii und rapid fortschreibtender allgemeiner Muskellahmung einhergeht. Dtsch Arch Klin Med. 1866;**1**:484–517.
2. Zeek PM. Periarteritis nodosa and other forms of necrotizing angiitis. N Engl J Med. 1953;**248**:764–72.
3. Gocke DJ, Hsu K, Morgan C, et al. Association between polyarteritis and Australian antigen. Lancet. 1970;**2**:1149–53.
4. Baggenstoss AH, Schick RM, Polley HF. The effect of cortisone on the lesions of periarteritis nodosa. Am J Pathol. 1951;**27**:537–59.
5. Fauci AS, Katz P, Haynes BF, et al. Cyclophosphamide therapy of severe systemic necrotizing vasculitis. N Engl J Med. 1979;**301**:235–8.
6. Michet CJ. Epidemiology of vasculitis. In: Rheumatic Disease Clinics of North America, chp 2. Conn DL, ed. Philadelphia: WB Saunders; 1990:261–8.
7. Lightfoot RW, Michet BA, Bloch DA, et al. The American College of Rheumatology 1990 Criteria for the Classification of Polyarteritis Nodosa. Arthritis Rheum. 1990;**33**:1088–93.
8. Masi AT, Hunder GG, Lie JT, et al. The American College of Rheumatology 1990 Criteria for the Classification of Churg–Strauss Syndrome (allergic granulomatosis and angiitis). Arthritis Rheum. 1990;**33**:1094–100.
9. Leavitt RY, Fauci AS, Bloch DA, et al. The American College of Rheumatology 1990 Criteria for the Classification of Hypersensitivity Vasculitis. Arthritis Rheum. 1990;**33**:1101–7.
10. Calabrese LH, Michel BA, Bloch DA, et al. The American College of Rheumatology 1990 Criteria for the Classification of Hypersensitivity Vasculitis. Arthritis Rheum. 1990;**33**:1108–13.
11. Mills JA, Michel BA, Bloch DA, et al. The American College of Rheumatology 1990 Criteria for the Classification of Henoch-Schönlein Purpura. Arthritis Rheum. 1990;**33**:1114–21.
12. Hunder GG, Bloch DA, Michel BA, et al. The American College of Rheumatology 1990 Criteria for the Classification of Giant Cell Arteritis. Arthritis Rheum. 1990;**33**:1122–8.
13. Arend WP, Michel BA, Bloch DA, et al. The American College of Rheumatology 1990 Criteria for the Classification of Takayasu Arteritis. Arthritis Rheum. 1990;**33**:1129–34.
14. Rich AR. The role of hypersensitivity in periarteritis nodosa: As indicated by seven cases developing during serum sickness and sulfonamide therapy. Bull Johns Hopkins Hosp. 1942;**71**:123–40.
15. Diaz-Perez JL, Winkelmann RK. Cutaneous periarteritis nodosa. Arch Dermatol. 1974;**110**:407–14.
16. Dyck PJ, Benstead TJ, Conn DL, et al. Nonsystemic vasculitic neuopathy. Brain. 1987;**110**:843–54.
17. Cohen RD, Conn DL, Ilstrup DM. Clinical features, prognosis, and response to treatment in polyarteritis. Mayo Clin Proc. 1980;**55**:146–55.
18. Conn DL, McDuffie FC, Holley KE, Schroeter AL. Immunological mechanism in systemic vasculitis. Mayo Clin Proc. 1976;**51**:511–18.
19. Frohnert PP, Sheps SG. Long-term follow-up study of periarteritis nodosa. Am J Med. 1967;**43**:8–14.
20. Ford RG, Siekert RG. Central nervous system manifestations of periarteritis nodosa. Neurology. 1965;**15**:114–22.
21. Ralston DE, Kvale WF. The renal lesions of periarteritis nodosa. Proc Mayo Clin. 1949;**24**:18–27.
22. Davson J, Ball J, Platt R. The kidney in periarteritis nodosa. Quart J Med. 1948;**17**:175–202.
23. Wold LE, Baggenstoss AH. Gastrointestinal lesions of periarteritis nodosa. Proc Mayo Clin. 1949;**24**:28–35.
24. Cowan RE, Mallinson CN, Thomas GE, et al. Polyarteritis nodosa of the liver: A report of two cases. Postgrad Med J. 1977;**53**:89–93.
25. Holsinger DR, Osmundson PJ, Edwards JE. The heart in periarteritis nodosa. Circulation. 1962;**25**:610–18.
26. Golding DN. Polyarteritis presenting with leg pains. Br Med J. 1970;**1**:277–8.
27. Roy JB, Hamblin DW, Brown CH. Periarteritis nodosa of epididymis. Urology. 1977;**10**:62–3.
28. Wise GN. Ocular periarteritis nodosa: Report of two cases. Arch Ophthalmol. 1952;**48**:1–11.
29. Morgan GJ, Harris ED Jr. Non-giant cell temporal arteritis: Three cases and a review of the literature. Arthritis Rheum. 1978;**21**:362–6.
30. Ball J. Rheumatoid arthritis and polyarteritis nodosa. Ann Rheum Dis. 1954;**13**:277–90.
31. Alexander EL, Arnett FC, Provost TT, et al. Sjögren's syndrome: Association of anti-Ro(SS-A) antibodies with vasculitis, hematologic abnormalities, and serologic hyperreactivity. Ann Intern Med. 1983;**98**:155–9.
32. Gorevic PD, Kassab HJ, Levo Y, et al. Mixed cryoglobulinemia: Clinical aspects and long-term follow-up of 40 patients. Am J Med. 1980;**69**:287–308.
33. Gabriel SE, Conn DL, Phyliky RL, et al. Vasculitis in hairy cell leukemia: Review of literature and consideration of possible pathogenic mechanisms. J Rheumatol. 1986;**13**:1167–72.
34. Mertz LE, Conn DL. Vasculitis associated with malignancy. Curr Opin Rheumatol. 1992;**4**:39–46.

35. Trepo CG, Zuckerman AR, Bird RC, et al. The role of circulating hepatitis B antigen/antibody immune complexes in the pathogenesis of vascular and hepatic manifestations in polyarteritis nodosa. J Clin Path. 1974;**27**:863–8.
36. Moskowitz RW, Baggenstoss AH, Slocumb CH. Histopathologic classification of periarteritis nodosa. A study of 56 cases confirmed at necropsy. Proc Mayo Clin. 1963;**38**:345–57.
37. Mowrey FH, Lundbeg EA. The clinical manifestations of essential polyangiitis (periarteritis nodosa), with emphasis on the hepatic manifestations. Ann Intern Med. 1954;**40**:1145–64.
38. LiVolsi VA, Perzin KH, Porter M. Polyarteritis nodosa of the gallbladder, presenting as acute cholecystitis. Gastroenterology. 1973;**65**:115–23.
39. Hall JW, Sun SC, Mackler W. Arteritis of the appendix. Arch Pathol. 1950;**40**:240–6.
40. Dyck PJ, Conn DL, Okazaki H. Necrotizing angiopathic neuropathy: Three-dimensional morphology of fiber degeneration related to sites of occluded vessels. Mayo Clin Proc. 1972;**47**:461–75.
41. Sack M, Cassidy JT, Bole GG. Prognostic factors in polyarteritis. J Rheumatol. 1975;**2**:411–20.
42. Maxeiner SR Jr, McDonald JR, Kirklin JW. Muscle biopsy in the diagnosis of periarteritis nodosa: An evaluation. Surg Clin North Am. 1952;**32**:1225–33.
43. Ahrohein JH. Isolated coronary periarteritis: Report of a case of unexpected death in a young pregnant woman. Am J Cardiol. 1977;**40**:287–90.
44. Ronco P, Verroust P, Mignon F, et al. Immunopathological studies of polyarteritis nodosa and Wegener's granulomatosis: A report of 43 patients with 51 renal biopsies. Quart J Med. 1983;**52**:141–9.
45. Friedman HM. Infection of endothelial cells by common human viruses. Rev Infect Dis. 1989;**2**(Suppl 4):700–4.
46. Conn DL. Polyarteritis. In: Rheumatic Disease Clinics of North America, chp 7. Conn DL, ed. Philadelphia: WB Saunders; 1990:341–62.
47. Baguley E, Hughes GRV. Antiendothelial cell antibodies. J Rheumatol. 1989;**16**:716–7.
48. Cines DB. Disorders associated with antibodies to endothelial cells. Rev Infect Dis. 1989: **2**(Suppl 4):S705–11.
49. Brasile L, Kremer JM, Clarke JL, et al. Identification of an autoantibody to vascular endothelial cell-specific antigens in patients with systemic vasculitis. Am J Med. 1989;**87**:74–80.
50. Grau GE, Roux-Lombard P, Gysler C, et al. Serum cytokine changes in systemic vasculitis. Immunology. 1989;**68**:196–8.
51. Palmer RMJ, Ashton DS, Moncada S. Vascular endothelial cells synthesize nitric oxide from L-arginine. Nature. 1988;**333**:664–6.
52. Vane JR, Anggard EE, Botting RM. Regulatory functions of the vascular endothelium. N Engl J Med. 1990;**323**:27–36.
53. Kanaide H, Takeshita A, Nakamura M. Etiologic aspects of coagulopathy in Takayasu's aortitis. Am Heart J. 1982;**104**:1039–45.
54. Muller-Hermelink HK, Dammrich JR. Die obliterative transplantatvasculopathie: Pathogenese und pathomechanismen. The obliterative transplant vasculopathy: Pathogenesis and pathomechanism. Verh Dtsch Ges Path. 1989;**73**:193–206.
55. Conn DL, Tompkins RB, Nichols WL. Glucocorticoids in the management of vasculitis – A double edged sword? J Rheumatol. 1988;**15**:1181–3.
56. Albert DA, Rimon D, Silverstein MC. The diagnosis of polyarteritis nodosa. I. A literature-based decision analysis approach. Arthritis Rheum. 1988;**31**:1117–27.
57. Ewald EA, Griffin D, McCuen WJ. Correlation of angiographic abnormalities with disease manifestations and disease severity in polyarteritis nodosa. J Rheumatol. 1987;**14**:952–6.
58. Guillevin L, Huong Du LT, Godeau P, et al. Clinical findings and prognosis of polyarteritis nodosa and Churg-Strauss angiitis: A study in 165 patients. Br J Rheumatol. 1988;**27**:258–64.
59. Leib ES, Restivo C, Paulus HE. Immunosuppressive and corticosteroid therapy of polyarteritis nodosa. Am J Med. 1979;**67**:941–7.
60. Neild GH, Lee HA. Methylprednisolone pulse therapy in the treatment of polyarteritis nodosa. Postgrad Med J. 1977;**53**:382–7.
61. Tannenbaum H. Combined therapy with methotrexate and prednisone in polyarteritis nodosa. Can Med Assoc J. 1980;**123**:893–4.
62. Lhote F, Guillevin L, Leon A, et al. Complications of plasma exchange in the treatment of polyarteritis nodosa and Churg–Strauss angiitis and the contribution of adjuvant immunosuppressive therapy: A randomized trial in 72 patients. Artificial Organs. 1988;**12**:27–33.
63. Newburger JW, Takahashi M, Burns JC, et al. The treatment of Kawasaki syndrome with intravenous gamma globulin. N Engl J Med. 1986;**315**:341–7.
64. Weyand CM, Goronzy JJ. Disease-associated human histocompatibility leukocyte antigen determinants in patients with seropositive rheumatoid arthritis. J Clin Invest. 1990;**85**:1051–7.
65. Mathieson PW, Cobbold SP, Hale G, et al. Monoclonal-antibody therapy in systemic vasculitis. N Engl J Med. 1990;**323**:250–4.
66. Churg J, Strauss L. Allergic granulomatosis, allergic angiitis, and periarteritis nodosa. Am J Pathol. 1951;**27**:277–301.
67. Chumbley LC, Harrison EG Jr, DeRemee RA. Allergic granulomatosis and angiitis (Churg–Strauss syndrome): Report and anlaysis of 30 cases. Mayo Clin Proc. 1977;**52**:477–84.
68. Lanham JG, Elkon KB, Pusey CD, Hughes GR. Systemic vasculitis with asthma and eosinophilia: A clinical approach to the Churg–Strauss syndrome. Medicine (Balt). 1984;**63**:65–81.
69. Rose GA, Spencer H. Polyarteritis nodosa. Quart J Med. 1957;**26**:43–81.

39

POLYMYALGIA RHEUMATICA AND GIANT CELL ARTERITIS

Brian L Hazleman

Definition

Polymyalgia Rheumatica

- A clinical syndrome of the middle aged and elderly characterized by pain and stiffness in the neck, shoulder and pelvic girdles, often accompanied by constitutional symptoms.
- The clinical response to small doses of corticosteroids can be dramatic.

Giant Cell Arteritis

- A vasculitis of unknown etiology occurring primarily in the elderly. Other terms commonly used include temporal arteritis, cranial arteritis and granulomatous arteritis.
- Early recognition and treatment can prevent blindness and other complications due to occlusion or rupture of involved arteries.

Clinical features

Polymyalgia Rheumatica

- The musculoskeletal symptoms are usually bilateral and symmetrical.
- Stiffness is usually the predominant feature; it is particularly severe after rest and may prevent the patient getting out of bed in the morning.
- Muscular pain is often diffuse and is accentuated by movement; pain at night is common.
- Muscle strength is unimpaired although the pain makes interpretation of muscle testing difficult.
- Corticosteroid treatment is usually required for at least 2 years. Most patients should be able to stop taking corticosteroids after 4–5 years.
- Systemic features include low-grade fever, fatigue, weight loss and an elevated ESR.

Giant Cell Arteritis

- There are a wide range of symptoms, but most patients have clinical findings related to involved arteries.
- Frequent features include fatigue, headaches, jaw claudication, loss of vision, scalp tenderness, polymyalgia rheumatica and aortic arch syndrome.
- Unlike other forms of vasculitis, giant cell arteritis rarely involves the skin, kidneys and lungs.
- The ESR is usually highly elevated but may be normal or only slightly increased in up to 2% of patients with active disease.

HISTORY

The earliest description of giant cell arteritis may have been in the 10th century in the Tadkwat of Ali Iba Isu, where removal of the temporal artery was recommended as treatment. Dequeker describes two paintings – Jan Van Eyck's work in the Municipal Museum, Bruges depicting the Holy Virgin with Canon Van der Paele (1436) and Pieri di Cosimo's portrait of Frasceso Gamberti (1505), now in the Rijks Museum, Amsterdam [1]. Both show signs of prominent temporal arteries and contemporary accounts document rheumatic pains, difficulty attending morning service with possible stiffness and general ill health.

No further evidence for the existence of either polymyalgia rheumatica or giant cell arteritis exists until the late 19th century, when recognizable descriptions of each were documented in opposite ends of the British Isles. In 1888 Bruce described five cases of 'severe rheumatic gout' [2]. Patients were aged from 60 to 70 years and suffered from widespread muscular and joint pains. Jonathan Hutchinson in 1890 described 'a peculiar form of thrombotic arteritis of the aged, which is sometimes productive of gangrene' [3].

For 40 years there seem to be no published reports until Horton and colleagues described the typical histologic appearances at temporal artery biopsy. In the early 1950s several authors used a variety of names to describe a similar condition adding constitutional symptoms and an elevated erythrocyte sedimentation rate (ESR) to the symptom complex, but it was Barber who suggested the present name [4]. It was not until 1963 that any cases of polymyalgia rheumatica were reported in the United States under its new name.

Several authors mentioned myalgic symptoms in early reports of temporal arteritis but Porsman first pointed out the similarity between temporal arteritis and 'arthritis of the aged'. In 1960 Paulley and Hughes reported on 67 patients, emphasizing the occurrence of 'an arthritic rheumatism' in giant cell arteritis, providing more solid clinical evidence for the relationship between polymyalgia rheumatica and giant cell arteritis [5]. Histologic support came from the work of Alestig and Barr [6], and Hamlin and colleagues [7] confirmed the coexistence of the two conditions. Those wishing to preserve the identity of the two diseases point out that arteritis is not found in many patients with polymyalgia, and that in some, central arthritis and ligamentous disease can explain the pattern of myalgia.

EPIDEMIOLOGY OF GIANT CELL ARTERITIS	
Peak age (years)	60–75
Sex distribution (F:M)	3:1
Biopsy positive	
Annual incidence (/100,000)	6.7
Annual incidence rate over 50 years of age (/100,000)	18.3
Geography	Mainly Northern Europe and Northern states of United States
Genetic associations	HLA-DR4

Fig. 39.1 Epidemiology of giant cell arteritis.

EPIDEMIOLOGY

Giant cell arteritis affects the White population almost exclusively (Fig. 39.1). Most reports originate from Northern Europe and parts of the Northern United States. However, the diseases are recognizable worldwide and there have been several reports of their occurrence in American Blacks. There is no difference in clinical findings or in the response to corticosteroids from those described in Caucasians. Both polymyalgia rheumatica and giant cell arteritis affect elderly people and are seldom diagnosed below the age of 50 years. A study of biopsy-proven giant cell arteritis diagnosed from 1950 through to 1985 in Olmsted County, Minnesota, demonstrated an average annual incidence and prevalence of 17 and 223, respectively, per 100,000 inhabitants aged 50 years or more. The age-adjusted incidence rates were approximately 3 times higher in women than in men. In addition the incidence increased in both sexes with higher age. The incidence also increased significantly during the period 1950–1985 for females but decreased in males over the same period (Fig. 39.2) [8].

The incidence rates reported from Olmsted County are similar to those in Goteborg, Sweden. Between 1970 and 1975, the incidence rate was 16.8 per 100,000 inhabitants in Sweden versus 18.3 per 100,000 in Minnesota. In a study of 284 biopsy-proven cases of giant cell arteritis collected over a 10-year period (1977–1986) in Goteborg, Nordborg and Bengtsson [9] observed an incidence rate among those aged 50 years or more of 18.3 per 100,000; for women it was 25 per 100,000 and for men 9.4 per 100,000. The reasons for this increase in incidence rate and the difference in incidence rates between the sexes are not clear. Increased awareness and improved diagnostic skill cannot be the only explanation because comparable changes in both sexes would then be expected. Also, the proportion of biopsies revealing arteritis did not change significantly in either study. The biopsy rate increased in both studies, probably reflecting an increasing number of patients presenting with symptoms compatible with giant cell arteritis. The temporal arteries and aorta of all adults who died in Malmö throughout one year were examined by Ostberg, and although active temporal arteritis was not found, evidence of previous arteritis was found in 1.7% of the 889 cases [10]. It was found that in 75% of these subjects there had been either biopsy evidence or a clinical history suggestive of temporal arteritis. This study certainly suggests that giant cell arteritis may be under-diagnosed, but further studies are required.

The variety of symptoms and lack of specificity of signs and symptoms contribute to make such studies difficult, and indeed the epidemiology of polymyalgia rheumatica has been less well defined. Silman and Currey found three cases of polymyalgia in 247 residents over 65 years in old peoples' homes and day centers. Only one case had been previously diagnosed. Kyle and colleagues, using a similar questionnaire in 656 patients over 65 years, found a prevalence of arteritis/polymyalgia of 3300/100,000 [11]. Polymyalgia has been found to account for 1.3–4.5% of the patients attending rheumatic disease clinics but clearly these figures are influenced by the type of clinical load [12].

Familial aggregation of polymyalgia rheumatica and giant cell arteritis has been reported by several workers. Liang *et al.* again emphasized this intriguing relationship [13]. In addition to their own 4 pairs of first degree relatives, they noted a further 6 pairs in the world literature occurring in a patient population of less than 500. Clustering of cases in time and space was seen in Liang's study and suggests that, in addition to a genetic predisposition, environmental factors may be important. Kyle *et al.* described a husband who developed polymyalgia rheumatica within 1 month of his wife's relapse; and Rhodes noted that nine of 11 cases seen over 6 years in a practice of 3000 lived in one small part of the same village, and of these two lived in the same house, two were neighbors and two others close friends [14].

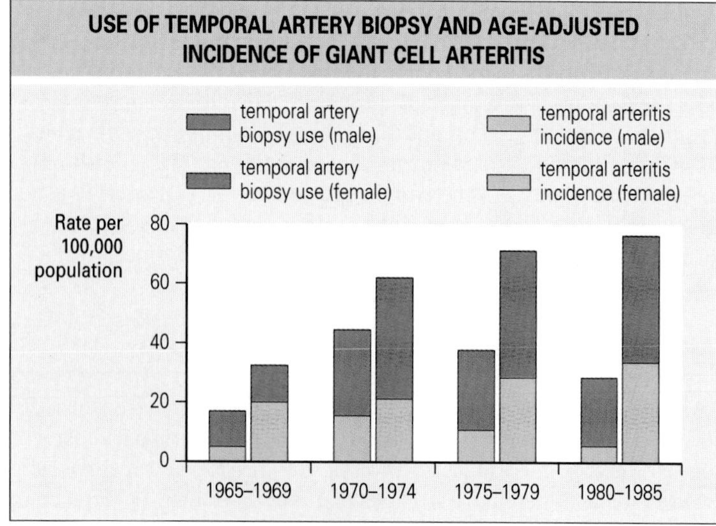

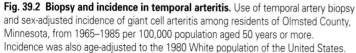

Fig. 39.2 Biopsy and incidence in temporal arteritis. Use of temporal artery biopsy and sex-adjusted incidence of giant cell arteritis among residents of Olmsted County, Minnesota, from 1965–1985 per 100,000 population aged 50 years or more. Incidence was also age-adjusted to the 1980 White population of the United States.

Immunogenetics

The increased prevalence of cases of polymyalgia rheumatica and giant cell arteritis in individuals of European background compared to other populations, and reports of multiple family cases, has suggested a genetic relationship, possibly linked to the immune system. In polymyalgia rheumatica, most studies of HLA typing have used serologic methods. Class I antigens have shown variable results which suggests that a significant relationship is unlikely. Hazleman *et al.* found that HLA-B8 was significantly more common in polymyalgia (59%) and giant cell arteritis (50%) than in arthritis (27%).

Several workers have found the frequency of the class II antigen HLA-DR4 in polymyalgia rheumatica and giant cell arteritis to be about twice that in normal controls. In some reports HLA-DR4 has been increased in polymyalgia rheumatica and not in giant cell arteritis [15]. Sakhas and colleagues have examined 44 patients with polymyalgia rheumatica of whom two had giant cell arteritis [16]. Standard techniques were used for restriction fragment length polymorphism (RFLP) analysis to determine class II antigens, the switch region of immunoglobulin μ heavy chain gene (Sμ), and T-cell antigen receptor (TcR) α/β, d chain genes, in order to identify possible genetic markers associated with this disease. As in previous studies, an increased frequency of HLA-DR4 specificity was found which was highly significant. The other analyses were negative. In addition, the number of DR4 homozygous patients was greater than expected by chance alone. The findings clearly strengthen the concept that HLA-DR4 is an important susceptibility factor for polymyalgia rheumatica and giant cell arteritis.

CLINICAL FEATURES

Age, Sex and Onset

The mean age at onset of giant cell arteritis and polymyalgia rheumatica is approximately 70 years, with a range of about 50 to more than 90 years of age. Younger patients have been reported but these are atypical. Women are affected about twice as often as men. The onset of the disease can be dramatic and some patients can give the date and hour of their first symptom. Equally, the onset can be insiduous. In most instances the symptoms have been present for weeks or months before the diagnosis is established, a mean of 6.2 months in one series [12].

Constitutional symptoms, including fever, fatigue, anorexia and weight loss and depression, are present in the majority of patients and may be an early or even an initial finding and can lead to delay in diagnosis [17]. They may be striking and suggest many different conditions. These patients may be labeled pyrexia of unknown origin (PUO) and subjected to many investigations. Giant cell arteritis was found in 15% of patients over 65 presenting with PUO. Mowat and Hazleman noted a weight loss of 3–23kg (mean 6kg) in 32 of 59 patients [12]. A hidden malignancy can mimic the symptoms of polymyalgia rheumatica but these patients do not usually respond to corticosteroids. Although at present there is no evidence to suggest that malignancy is more common in patients with polymyalgia than in other people, deterioration in health or a poor initial response to corticosteroids must always be taken seriously and a search for an occult neoplasm made. In some cases, onset is associated with recent bereavement.

Polymyalgia Rheumatica

Musculoskeletal involvement

Patients usually locate the source of their pain and stiffness to the muscles. The onset is commonest in the shoulder region and neck, with eventual involvement of the shoulder and pelvic girdles and the corresponding proximal muscle groups. Involvement of distal limb muscles is unusual. The symptoms are usually bilateral and symmetrical. Stiffness is usually the predominant feature, is particularly severe after rest, and may prevent the patient from getting out of bed in the morning. The muscular pain is often diffuse and movement accentuates the pain; pain at night is common. Muscle strength is usually unimpaired, although the pain makes interpretation of muscle testing difficult. There is tenderness of involved structures including periarticular structures such as bursae, tendons and joint capsules, although the muscle tenderness is generally not as severe as that in myositis. In late stages muscle atrophy may develop, with restriction of shoulder movement. An improvement of shoulder range is rapid with corticosteroid therapy, unlike that seen in frozen shoulder. Occasionally the painful arc sign of subacromial bursitis is present; this is important to recognize as a local injection of corticosteroid will give relief and save the patient from an increase in systemic corticosteroid dosage.

Synovitis

Polymyalgia has traditionally been viewed as a condition affecting muscles and many reports have emphasized the rarity of joint involvement. Recent emphasis has been given to a possible association between synovitis and the muscle symptoms in polymyalgia rheumatica. It has also been suggested that both axial and peripheral synovitis often occur.

Inflammatory synovitis and effusions have been noted by several authors, the reported incidence varying from 0 to 100% in various series [12]. Synovitis of the knees, wrists and sternoclavicular joints is most common, but involvement is transient and mild. Erosive changes in joints and/or sclerosis of the sacroiliac joints have been reported although they are difficult to demonstrate in the sternoclavicular joints except by tomography. Abnormal technetium pertechnetate scintigrams have shown widespread uptake over several joints, particularly shoulders, knees, wrists and hands. Abnormalities persisted after treatment.

The arthroscopic appearances are indistinguishable from rheumatoid arthritis (RA); the synovial tissue shows nonspecific inflammatory changes and the synovial fluid has the appearance of a mild inflammatory exudate. The synovitis of polymyalgia differs from that of RA in that it does not cause typical juxta-articular osteoporosis and erosions, and reports of more pronounced joint changes may be partly explained by the variable diagnostic criteria used. In view of the controversy concerning the incidence of joint involvement, Kyle *et al.* examined 56 patients for evidence of inflammatory synovitis and performed radiographs, isotope scans and thermography [18]. They found synovitis in only one patient when the disease was active and concluded that peripheral and axial synovitis was uncommon. They attributed the discrepancies in frequency of synovitis reported in various studies to differing diagnostic criteria, the definition of synovitis and difficulty in interpretation of scans and radiographs due to coexisting degenerative disease.

Giant Cell Arteritis

Headache

Headache is the most common symptom and is present in two thirds or more of patients. It usually begins early in the course of the disease and may be the presenting symptom. The pain is severe and generally localized to the temple. However, it may be occipital or be less defined and precipitated by brushing the hair. It can be severe even when the arteries are clinically normal and, conversely, may subside even though the disease remains active. The nature of the pain varies; some patients describe it as shooting and others as a more steady ache. Scalp tenderness is common, particularly around the temporal and occipital arteries, and may disturb sleep. Tender spots or nodules or even small skin infarcts may be present for several days. The vessels are thickened, tender and nodular with absent or reduced pulsation (Fig. 39.3). Occasionally they are red and clearly visible.

Ophthalmic features

Visual disturbances have been described in 25–50% of cases, although the incidence of visual loss is now regarded as much lower, about 6–10% in most series. This is probably because of earlier recognition and treatment.

There are a variety of ocular lesions which are essentially due to occlusion of the various orbital or ocular arteries (Fig. 39.4) Blindness is the most serious and irreversible feature. The visual loss is usually sudden, painless and permanent; it may vary from mistiness of vision, or involvement of a part of the visual field, to complete blindness. There is a risk of the second eye being involved if the patient is not treated aggressively. Involvement of the second eye can occur within 24 hours. Blindness may be the initial presentation of giant cell arteritis but tends to follow other symptoms by

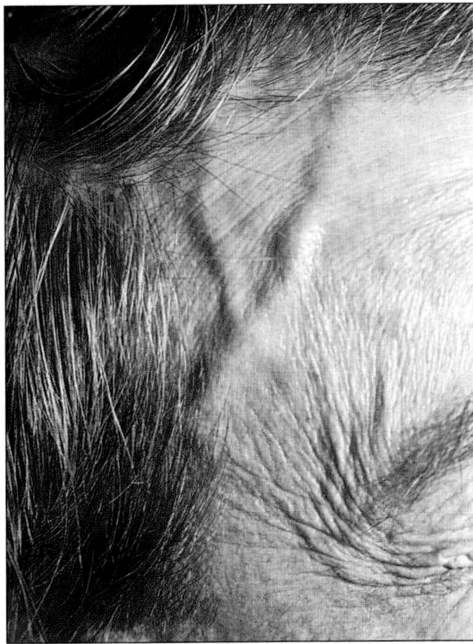

Fig. 39.3 Photograph of dilated temporal arteries in a patient with giant cell arteritis.

OCULAR LESIONS IN GIANT CELL ARTERITIS

Lesions	Feature
Optic nerve ischemic lesions:	
Anterior ischemic optic neuropathy	The commonest lesion and associated with partial or more frequently complete visual loss
Posterior ischemic optic neuropathy	Less common and may cause partial or complete visual loss
Retinal ischemic lesions:	
Central retinal artery occlusion	Leads to severe visual loss
Cilio-retinal artery occlusion	Seen occasionally and associated with anterior ischemic optic neuropathy
Choroidal infarcts	Seen rarely
Extraocular motility disorders	Seen rarely and not usually associated with visual loss
Anterior segment ischemic lesions	Seen rarely and not usually associated with visual loss
Pupillary abnormalities	Usually secondary to visual loss
Cerebral ischemic lesions	Associated visual loss is rare

Fig. 39.4 Ocular lesions in giant cell arteritis.

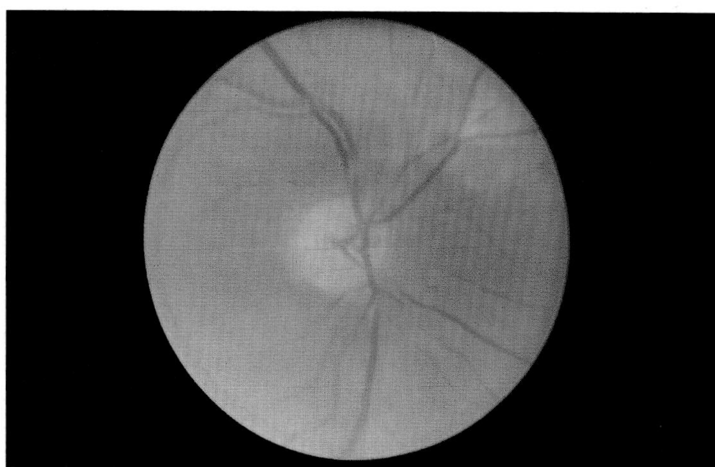

Fig. 39.5 A fundus photograph showing optic atrophy secondary to giant cell arteritis.

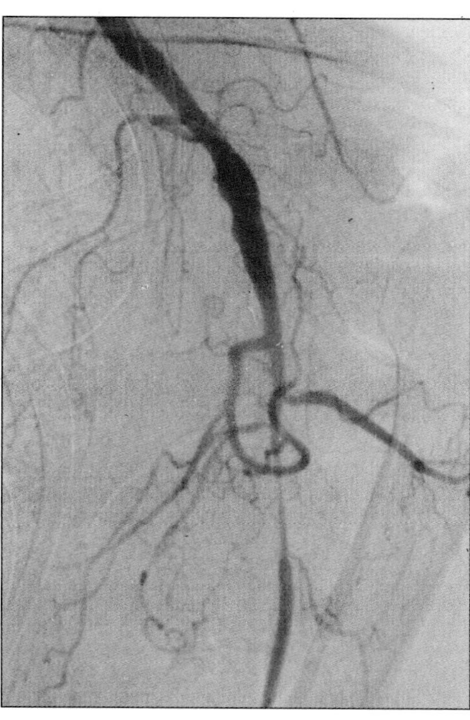

Fig. 39.6 Arteriogram showing narrowing of axillary artery in giant cell arteritis.

several weeks or months (Fig. 39.5). Visual symptoms are an ophthalmic emergency; if they are identified and treated urgently, blindness is almost entirely preventable.

Pain in the face and ear

Pain on chewing, due to claudication of the jaw muscles, occurs in up to two thirds of patients. Tingling in the tongue, loss of taste, and pain in the mouth and throat can also occur, presumably due to vascular insufficiency.

The widespread nature of the vasculitis has been previously mentioned. Clinical evidence of large artery involvement is present in 10–15% of cases (Fig. 39.6), and in some instances aortic dissection and rupture occur. Bruits are often present over large arteries and there may be tenderness, particularly over the subclavian artery. An early sign of arteritis is increased sensitivity of the carotid sinus. Light pressure will often lead to transient asystole for two or more beats so it is advisable for the patient to be lying down when examined.

Other symptoms

Less common features of giant cell arteritis include hemiparesis, peripheral neuropathy, deafness, depression and confusion. Involvement of the coronary arteries may lead to myocardial infarction. Aortic regurgitation and congestive cardiac failure may also occur. Abnormalities of thyroid and liver function are well described and will be detailed later in this chapter. An association between carpal tunnel syndrome and polymyalgia has been noted by several authors. Local corticosteroid injection and/or surgical decompression are sometimes necessary.

RELATIONSHIP BETWEEN POLYMYALGIA RHEUMATICA AND GIANT CELL ARTERITIS

Paulley and Hughes were the first to link the two conditions, suggesting that polymyalgia was a prodromal manifestation of temporal arteritis [5]. Alestig and Barr supported this observation when they found temporal arteritis in patients with polymyalgia rheumatica who had no symptoms or signs of arteritis [6]. Certainly, it is difficult to maintain a practical distinction between them by clinical or histologic criteria. Patients originally suffering from polymyalgia rheumatica have later had symptoms of cranial arteritis, and in a number of patients with typical myalgia and no symptoms from the temporal region, biopsies have shown arteritic changes. Systemic involvement is similar in groups with or without clinical and/or biopsy evidence of arteritis.

In patients with polymyalgia rheumatica who have no symptoms or signs of arteritis, positive temporal biopsies are found in 10–15%. Those wishing to preserve the identity of the two diseases base their argument on the latter figure and of the failure to find evidence of arteritis in many patients with polymyalgia followed for many years. Conversely, there are many similarities between the two conditions. The age and sex distribution is similar, the biopsy findings show an identical pattern and the laboratory features are similar, even though many are nonspecific inflammatory changes. In addition, there is similarity in the myalgia, the associated systemic features, and in the response to corticosteroid therapy.

The onset of myalgic symptoms may precede, coincide with, or follow that of the arteritic symptoms. No difference has been found between the characteristics of those myalgic patients with a positive biopsy and those with no histologic evidence of arteritis. Mild aching and stiffness may persist for months after other features of giant cell arteritis have remitted. There is little evidence to suggest that the musculoskeletal symptoms are related to vasculitis. Many patients with giant cell arteritis do not have polymyalgia rheumatica, even when large vessels are involved. In addition, the finding of joint swelling in some patients and the production of pain by the injection of 5% saline solution into the acromioclavicular, sternoclavicular and manubriosternal joints suggests that polymyalgia rheumatica in some patients may be a particular form of proximal synovitis.

INVESTIGATIONS

The ESR is usually greatly elevated and provides a useful means of monitoring treatment, although it must be appreciated that some elevation of the ESR may occur in otherwise healthy elderly people. A normal ESR is occasionally found in patients with active biopsy-proven disease [12].

Anemia, usually of a mild hypochromic type, is common and resolves without specific treatment, but a more marked normochromic anemia occasionally occurs and may be a presenting symptom [17]. Leukocyte and differential counts are generally normal; platelet counts are also usually normal but may be increased. Protein electrophoresis may show a nonspecific rise in α_2-globulin with less frequent elevation of α_1- and gammaglobulins. Quantification of acute phase proteins and α_1-antitrypsin, orosomucoid, haptoglobin and C-reactive protein (CRP) are no more helpful than the ESR in the assessment of disease activity [19].

Abnormalities of thyroid and liver function have also been well described. Thomas and Croft, in a retrospective survey of 59 cases of

DIFFERENTIAL DIAGNOSIS OF POLYMYALGIA RHEUMATICA	
Neoplastic disease	Muscle disease
Joint disease	Polymyositis
Osteoarthritis, particularly of cervical spine	Myopathy
Rheumatoid arthritis	Infections e.g. bacterial endocarditis
Connective tissue disease	Bone disease, particularly osteomyelitis
Multiple myeloma	Hypothyroidism
Leukemia	Parkinsonism
Lymphoma	Functional

Fig. 39.7 Differential diagnosis of polymyalgia rheumatica.

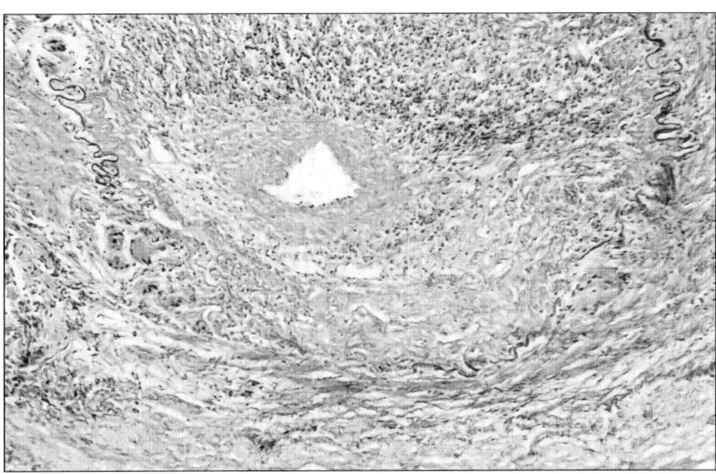

Fig. 39.8 Elastic stain of temporal artery showing disruption of elastic lamina in giant cell arteritis and narrowing of the lumen.

giant cell arteritis, found five patients with hyperthyroidism [20]. The arteritis followed the thyrotoxicosis by intervals of 4–15 years in three cases, and in two occurred simultaneously. Individual cases of hypothyroidism have also been reported. Dent and Edwards found seven cases of polymyalgia rheumatica or giant cell arteritis in 250 patients with autoimmune thyroid disease [21]. All cases occurred in women over 60, giving a prevalence of 9.3% in this age group.

Raised serum values for alkaline phosphatase were found in up to 70% of patients with polymyalgia rheumatica [12]. Bromsulfthalein retention is also often abnormal and transaminases may be mildly elevated. Liver biopsies have shown portal and intralobular inflammation with focal liver cell necrosis and small epithelioid cell granuloma. The pathologic significance of these abnormalities are unclear. Abnormal liver scans may also occur [22]. The clinical implications of these findings are important. In patients presenting with nonspecific features, the findings of abnormal liver function tests and abnormal scans may be misleading and prompt investigations for malignancy.

DIFFERENTIAL DIAGNOSIS

The diagnosis of polymyalgia rheumatica is initially one of exclusion. The differential diagnosis (Fig. 39.7) in an elderly patient with muscle pain, stiffness and a raised ESR is wide because the prodromal phases of several serious conditions can mimic it. In practice, nonspecific clinical features and the frequent absence of physical signs make diagnosis difficult.

Polymyalgia rheumatica can usually be differentiated from late-onset RA by the absence of prominent peripheral joint pain and swelling. In patients with polymyositis, the muscular weakness is the predominant factor limiting movement, whereas in polymyalgia rheumatica pain causes limited function.

The diagnosis of giant cell arteritis should be considered in any patient over the age of 50 years who has recent onset of headache, transient or sudden loss of vision, myalgia, unexplained fever or anemia or an elevated ESR. Because the symptoms and signs may vary in severity and be transient, patients must be questioned carefully about recent and current symptoms. The arteries of the head, neck and limbs should be examined for tenderness, enlargement, thrombosis and bruits. If a temporal artery biopsy is performed, a symptomatic or clinically abnormal segment of the artery should be chosen. Klein *et al.* emphasized the need for long arterial specimens if blind biopsy is to be undertaken [23]. Angiography of the temporal arteries is not usually helpful – there is no characteristic abnormality and false positives (usually due to atheroma) are not uncommon. An angiographic examination of the aortic arch and its branches may prove helpful in patients with symptoms of large artery involvement. Temporal artery biopsies need not be carried out in all patients with polymyalgia rheumatica. If clinical evidence for giant cell arteritis is absent, and if symptoms are mild and of recent onset, or conversely stable and of long duration, then the patient can be followed closely without biopsy. Blindness is uncommon in such patients.

There is usually little difficulty in separating giant cell arteritis from other forms of arteritis, because of the different distribution of lesions, histopathology, and organ involvement. However, occasionally necrotizing arteritis can involve the temporal artery.

Delay in Diagnosis

Despite a typical pattern of musculoskeletal symptoms and the presence in many of significant systemic features, there is often a considerable delay of several months before diagnosis [12,17]. Patients and physicians also tend to ascribe the symptoms to degenerative joint disease expected in an older population, or even to psychological illness. In others, the systemic features of the disease and the laboratory abnormalities can lead to diagnostic confusion and often extensive investigation.

PATHOLOGY

The histologic appearance of giant cell arteritis is one of the most distinctive of vascular disorders. The dense granulomatous inflammatory infiltrates which characterize the acute stages of the disease resemble those of Takayasu's arteritis, but the clinicopathologic features in patients with positive temporal artery biopsies are diagnostic. The arteritis is histologically a panarteritis with giant cell granuloma formation, often in close proximity to a disrupted internal elastic lamina. Large and medium-sized arteries are affected, the involvement is patchy and 'skip lesions' are often found. They were identified in 28% of patients by Klein *et al.*, and were as short as 330μm, but long portions of arteries may be involved [23]. More patients with 'skip lesions' had normal arteries to palpation but did not have a more benign disease.

The gross features are not characteristic. The vessels are enlarged and nodular and have little or no lumen. Thrombosis often develops at sites of active inflammation. Later, these areas may recanalize. The lumen is narrowed by intimal proliferation (Fig. 39.8). This is a common finding in arteries and may result from advancing age, nearby chronic inflammation or low blood flow. The adventitia is usually invaded by mononuclear and occasionally polymorphonuclear inflammatory cells, often cuffing the vasa vasorum; here fibrous proliferation is frequent. The changes in the media are dominated by the giant cells, which vary from small cells with 2–3 nuclei up to masses of 100μm containing many nuclei. Here there is invasion by mononuclear cells resembling histiocytes. Fibrinoid necrosis is infrequent. Giant cells are not seen in all sections and therefore are not required for the diagnosis if other features are compatible. The more sections that are examined in the area of arteritis, the more likely it is that giant cells will be found.

A progression of changes can be demonstrated, from the active infiltrative phase to the scarred artery with little cellular infiltrate. At first the most severe changes are centered on the internal elastic lamina, which becomes swollen and fragmented. Fragments of elastic tissue can be demonstrated within giant cells which are surrounded with plasma cell and lymphocytic infiltration (Fig. 39.9). Other electron microscopy studies have suggested altered or damaged smooth muscle cells are critical in the pathogenesis.

Corticosteroids reduce the inflammatory cell infiltrate so temporal artery biopsy should, if possible, be carried out before treatment is started. Therapy should not be delayed until a biopsy has been performed as most will be abnormal 48 hours after treatment.

Histologic changes also occur in temporal arteries with advancing age; they differ only in degree with those encountered in giant cell arteritis and it can sometimes be difficult to distinguish between them. However, an inflammatory cell infiltrate does not occur except in relationship to large plaques of atherosclerosis. The degree of intimal thickening in arteritis is usually greater, a well-developed smooth muscle layer is seen by the lumen and loss of the internal elastic lamina is considerable. The histologic changes of healed arteritis include medial chronic inflammation with ingrowth of new blood vessels, focal medial scarring and a bizarre pattern of intimal fibrosis; the latter is the most important change. The biopsy finding of healed vasculitis by no means excludes the possibility of active lesions elsewhere. Not infrequently, episodes of vasculitis are recurrent. The widespread nature of the vasculitis has been well documented, and occasionally veins are affected.

Involvement of the aorta and its branches, the abdominal vessels and the coronary arteries have all been described. Although there is a high incidence of involvement of the head and neck vessels in giant cell arteritis, it is interesting that the intracranial vessels are seldom involved. Wilkinson and Russell studied the head and neck vessels and demonstrated a close correlation between the susceptibility to arteritis and the amount of elastic tissue present in the arterial wall [24]. The highest incidence of severe involvement was noted in the superficial temporal arteries, vertebral arteries and ophthalmic and posterior ciliary arteries. The internal carotid, external carotid, and central retinal arteries were affected less frequently (Fig. 39.10). In some instances follow-up biopsy or autopsy surveys have shown persistence of mild chronic inflammation even though symptoms have resolved.

There is little to support a concept of primary muscle disease in polymyalgia rheumatica. Serum aldolase and creatine phosphokinase are normal and there is no abnormality on electromyography. Muscle biopsy has shown type II atrophy alone and there is no evidence of inflammatory changes. Histochemical examination of muscle has demonstrated some abnormalities of the motor nerve terminals and endplates, which have been interpreted as consistent with a neuropathy. However, it is generally considered that these changes are nonspecific.

Liver biopsy can show nonspecific inflammatory changes or focal liver cell necrosis. There are occasional reports of granulomata and hepatic arteritis. Synovial biopsy has shown nonspecific inflammatory changes with lymphocytic infiltration of knees, sternoclavicular joints and shoulders.

ETIOLOGY AND PATHOGENESIS

At present it is impossible to define the underlying pathologic abnormality in polymyalgia and, indeed, it may well be that there are several different mechanisms responsible for a largely similar pattern of pain. The relative homogeneity of groups of patients, and the apparent rapid clinical response to corticosteroids, does not exclude this possibility. Although the increasing incidence of giant cell arteritis and polymyalgia rheumatica after the age of 50 implies a relationship with aging, the significance of this observation is not understood.

A distinct prodromal event is often noted by patients resembling influenza or viral pneumonia. However, viral studies have produced negative results [12]. The known association of hepatitis B with polyarteritis nodosa led Bacon *et al.* to seek a similar association in polymyalgia [25]. Although hepatitis antigen was not found in any of the 12 patients tested before the commencement of corticosteroid therapy, hepatitis B surface (HB_s) antibody was found in nine cases. This finding has not been confirmed. Fessel suggested that contact with pet birds, especially parakeets, might be a factor in etiology, representing some immunological reaction to psittacosis or constituent of their food [26]. Others have been unable to support this suggestion.

Both the humoral and cellular immune systems have been implicated in pathogenesis. The latter seem the most important. Giant cell arteritis is limited to vessels with an internal elastic lamina, and electron microscopy shows fragmentation of this with mononuclear cell accumulation compatible with cell-mediated injury. Fragments of elastic tissue can be demonstrated within giant cells. Immunoglobulins and complement have also been detected in the vessel wall of patients with arteritis by immunofluorescence. Deposits have been noted both intra- and extracellularly of all immunoglobulin classes plus complement (C3), adjacent to the internal elastic lamina in

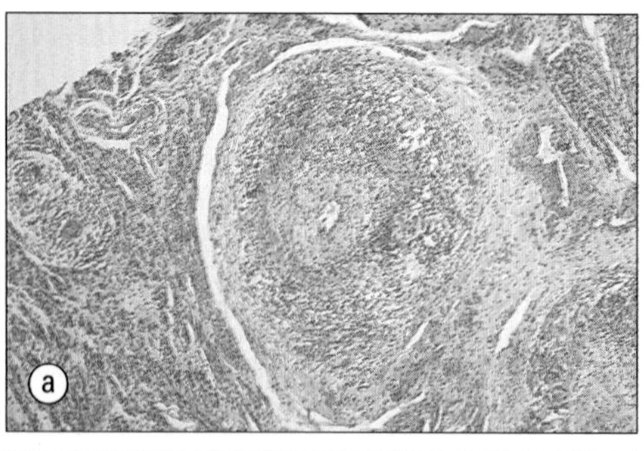

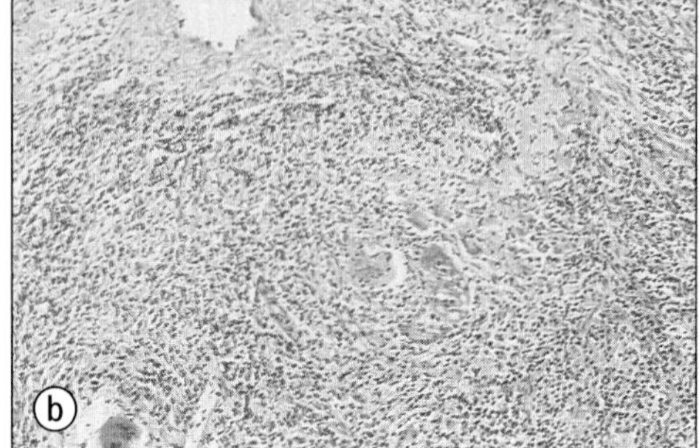

Fig. 39.9 Histology of giant cell arteritis. Low powered view of arterial wall showing infiltration by lymphocytes and plasma cells (a). High powered view showing giant cells in close relationship to elastic lamina (b).

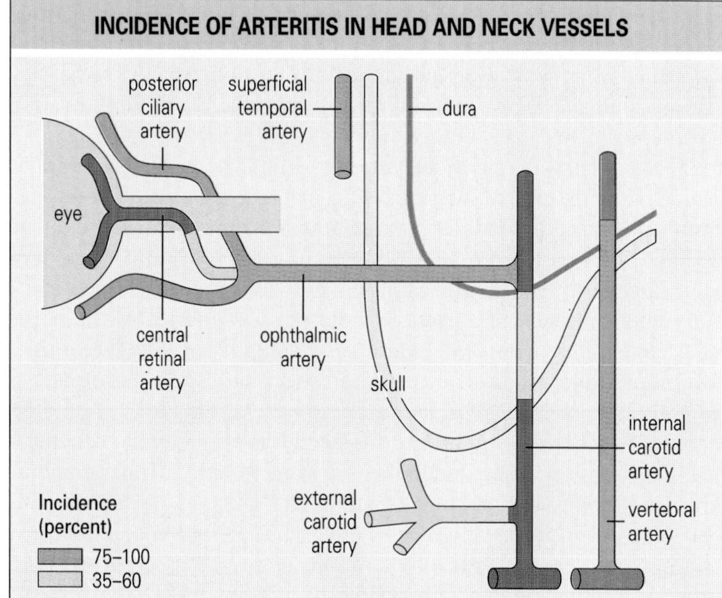

Fig. 39.10 Incidence of arteritis in pathological study of head and neck vessels.

many cases. The presence of immunoglobulin or complement within a lesion does not prove that it has been caused by hypersensitivity. Such a finding may be due to nonspecific immune complex deposition at the site of vascular injury of different cause. Using an immunoperoxidase method, Gallagher and Jones found only intracellular deposits and did not detect extracellular complement [27]. This pattern of intracytoplasmic staining for immunoglobulins would be anticipated in any chronic inflammatory reaction. It is possible that the changes reflect a nonspecific reaction to injury. Similar changes have been reported after experimental dilatation of carotid arteries in rabbits. Dasgupta and colleagues have reported antibodies against intermediate filaments in two thirds of patients at the onset of giant cell arteritis [28]. Antibodies against intermediate filaments are found in viral infections and autoimmune diseases.

Increased numbers of circulating lymphoblasts are seen in patients with active polymyalgia rheumatica and immunoglobulins are also elevated. These observations have led to the suggestion that these diseases may have an immunologic basis, perhaps an age-related autoimmune process directed against arterial wall constituents. There is no difference in in-vitro lymphocytotoxicity to arterial smooth muscle between the cells from patients with active untreated giant cell arteritis/polymyalgia rheumatica and normal controls. The lymphocytes in the arteritic lesions express the T-cell phenotype and only a few B cells are found [29]. The $CD4^+$ subset dominates over the $CD8^+$ subset in most studies and a low number of natural killer (NK) cells are seen.

Macrophages are seen in the arterial wall and the majority express HLA-DR antigen. About one quarter of the infiltrating T cells express the HLA-DR antigen, which suggests that these cells are immunologically activated. Further support for a local activation of the T cells is the finding of interleukin-2 receptors (IL-2R) on the lymphocytes from biopsy specimens [29]. The IL-2R expression on lymphocytes is not as frequent as the HLA-DR expression. The reason for this discrepancy is not known but is seen in other inflammatory lesions. They also reported interdigitating reticulum cells in 40% of patients with biopsy-proven giant cell arteritis; these were seen in patients with a shorter disease duration. It has been suggested that interdigitating reticulum cells are seen in lesions where a local stimulus for an immune response is suspected, but not in diseases due to immune complexes or degenerative processes. A selective depletion of circulating $CD8^+$ T lymphocytes in patients with giant cell arteritis has been observed in most studies [30]. No increase of HLA-DR expression has been found on circulatory $CD4^+$ T cells; this contrasts with the high incidence on the T lymphocytes in the arterial wall.

Park *et al.* found no clear correlation between the results of the three assays for immune complexes and no clear correlation between the presence of immune complexes and the ESR, graded disease activity and the presence of arteritis [31]. Using the Raji cell immunoassay, Papaioannou *et al.* found that immune complex concentrations showed a positive correlation with the ESR and gammaglobulin levels [32]. These varying results may be due to different methods of detection and of case selection.

It has been proposed that a serum toxic factor leads to endothelial breakdown and then to disruption of the internal elastic lamina. Elastin fragments are chemotactic to monocytes which have elastolytic potential and is increased in giant cell arteritis. Also, linear deposits of leukocyte elastase is found along the fragmented internal elastic lamina.

MANAGEMENT

Introduction

Corticosteroids are mandatory in the treatment of giant cell arteritis; they reduce the incidence of complications such as blindness and rapidly relieve symptoms. Nonsteroidal anti-inflammatory drugs (NSAIDs) will lessen the painful symptoms, but they do not prevent arteritic complications. The response to corticosteroids is usually dramatic and occurs within days. Corticosteroid treatment has improved the quality of life for patients, although there is no evidence that therapy reduces the duration of the disease. A fear of vascular complications in those patients with a positive biopsy often leads to the use of high doses of corticosteroids. Recent studies have emphasized the importance of adopting a cautious and individual treatment schedule and have highlighted the efficacy of lower doses of prednisolone.

Management Techniques

Initially, the corticosteroids should be given in a sufficient dosage to control the disease and then maintained at the lowest dose which will control the symptoms and lower the ESR. In giant cell arteritis, corticosteroids should preferably be given after the diagnosis has been confirmed histologically. However, where giant cell arteritis is strongly suspected, there should be no delay in starting therapy as the artery biopsy will still show inflammatory changes for several days after corticosteroids have been started and the result is unlikely to alter therapeutic decisions. If the temporal (or other) artery biopsy shows no arteritis, but the suspicion of disease is strong, corticosteroid treatment should be started. The great danger is delaying therapy as blindness may occur at any time.

There are few clinical trials to help decide on the correct initial dose. The recommended initial dose for polymyalgia rheumatica/giant cell arteritis varies from 10 to 100mg prednisolone daily. Intravenous corticosteroids are occasionally used if there are visual complications. In practice most studies report using 10–20mg prednisolone daily to treat polymyalgia and 40–60mg for giant cell arteritis because of the higher risk of arteritic complications in giant cell arteritis. Some ophthalmologists suggest an initial dose of at least 60mg as they have seen blindness occur at a lower dose. However, this has to be balanced against the potential complication of high dosage in this older age group. The initial corticosteroid dose and rate of corticosteroid tapering have been evaluated prospectively by Kyle and Hazleman [33]. They found that patients with polymyalgia relapsed frequently on an initial dose of 10mg prednisolone daily, but those taking 20mg for the first month were well controlled.

Reducing the dosage from 7.5mg to 5mg in the second month was also associated with some relapses. Patients with giant cell arteritis were treated with 40mg for 5 days and then continued on 40mg or reduced to 20mg for the first month. An initial dose of 40mg controlled symptoms in most cases, whereas giving 20mg and then reducing to 15mg/day after 4 weeks led to more relapses. There is little information on the rate of corticosteroid reduction once initial symptoms are controlled. Weekly decrements of not more than 5mg have been proposed. The reduction is more gradual when a daily dose of 10mg is reached. It is suggested that 1mg every 2–4 weeks is sufficient. These dosages are suggestions only and not to be interpreted rigidly as individual cases vary greatly. Clinical relapse may occur without a rise in ESR and the ESR may rise without corresponding symptoms. Measurement of acute phase proteins does not prove to be more helpful than the ESR in follow-up.

Rapid reduction or withdrawal of corticosteroids has been reported to contribute to deaths in patients with giant cell arteritis [34]. Thirteen of 17 deaths were felt to be due to using an inadequate dose of corticosteroids or reducing the dose too rapidly. Fortunately, complications are rare and the activity of the disease seems to decline steadily. Relapses are more likely during the initial 18 months of treatment and within 1 year of withdrawal of corticosteroids. There is no reliable method of predicting those most at risk, but arteritic relapses in patients who presented with pure polymyalgia rheumatica are unusual. Temporal artery biopsy does not seem helpful in predicting outcome.

Controversy exists over the expected duration of the disease. Most European studies within the last 20 years report that between one third and one half of the patients are able to discontinue corticosteroids after 2 years of treatment. Studies from the Mayo Clinic in the US have reported a shorter duration of disease for both polymyalgia rheumatica (11 months was the median duration of treatment and three quarters of patients had stopped taking corticosteroids by 2 years) and giant cell arteritis (most patients had stopped taking corticosteroids within 2 years). The consensus view seems to be that stopping treatment is feasible from 2 years onwards. This view is supported by recent laboratory studies by Dasgupta and colleagues [28]. They measured serum T-cell subsets before and during treatment and found a profound and selective reduction of $CD8^+$ suppressor/cytotoxic cells, which persisted for up to 1 year despite satisfactory symptomatic control and a normal ESR and CRP concentration. After 2 years of treatment $CD8^+$ cells had returned to those found in normal controls.

Patients who are unable to reduce the dosage of prednisolone because of recurring symptoms, or who develop serious corticosteroid-related side effects, pose particular problems. Azathioprine has been shown to exert a modest corticosteroid-sparing effect. There has been a recent report of the value of methotrexate in three 'coticosteroid resistant' cases of polymyalgia rheumatica/giant cell arteritis. However, one patient had an overlap connective tissue disease and another was inadequately treated initially.

The risks of relapse, particularly with arteritic complications, have to be balanced against the risks of corticosteroid-associated side effects. Between one fifth and a half of patients may experience serious side effects. A recent study suggested that if the initial dose of prednisolone is 10mg or less, and maintenance doses of less than 7.5mg are used, patients were virtually free of side effects [35]. Serious side effects are significantly related to high initial doses, maintenance doses, cumulative doses and increased duration of treatment.

Some conclusions can be drawn. The overall strategy should be to use an adequate dose of prednisolone for the first month to obtain good symptomatic control with a fall in ESR, then to aim for maintenance doses of less than 10mg after six months. The exact doses will need to be adjusted to the needs of the individual patient. A possible schedule is 15mg prednisolone/day for polymyalgia rheumatica, reducing the dose to about 7.5–10mg by 6–8 weeks. Patients with giant cell arteritis should be treated with 40mg daily for the first month unless visual symptoms persist, when higher doses (60–80 mg) may be needed. A suitable dose reduction would be to 20mg at about 8 weeks. For both conditions, gradual reduction by 1mg every 2–3 months can be attempted, with possible withdrawal of corticosteroids after 2 years. Reduction of doses of prednisolone on alternate days once doses of less than 5mg are reached makes withdrawal easier, and the addition of an NSAID at this stage may reduce some of the minor muscular symptoms that patients develop as corticosteroids are reduced. Some patients, however, find it impossible to stop taking the final 2–3mg and this level of maintenance dose is probably safe.

Summary

In summary, patients should be warned to expect treatment for at least 2 years, and most should be able to stop taking corticosteroids after 4–5 years. Monitoring for relapse should continue for 6 months to 1 year after stopping corticosteroids; thereafter patients should be asked to report back urgently if arteritic symptoms occur. The risk of this happening is small and unpredictable. A few patients may need low-dose treatment indefinitely. Polymyalgia rheumatica and giant cell arteritis are amongst the more satisfying diseases for clinicians to diagnose and treat because the unpleasant effects and serious consequences of these conditions can be almost entirely prevented by corticosteroid therapy. Unfortunately, there is no objective means of determining the prognosis in the individual and decisions concerning duration of treatment remain empirical.

REFERENCES

1. Dequeker JV. Polymyalgia rheumatica with temporal arteritis as painted by Jan Van Eyck in 1436. Can Med Assoc J. 1981;**124**:1597–8.
2. Bruce W. Senile rheumatic gout. Br Med J. 1888;**2**:811–13.
3. Hutchinson J. A peculiar form of neurotic arteritis of the aged which is sometimes productive of gangrene. Arch Surg. 1890;**1**:323–7.
4. Barber HS. Myalgic syndrome with constitutional effects. Polymyalgia rheumatica. Ann Rheum Dis. 1957;**16**:230–7.
5. Paulley JW, Hughes JP. Giant cell arteritis or arthritis of the aged. Br Med J. 1960;**2**:1562–7.
6. Alestig K, Barr J. Giant cell arteritis; biopsy study of polymyalgia rheumatica, including one case of Takayasu's disease. Lancet. 1963;**1**:1228–30.
7. Hamrin B, Jonsson N, Landberg T. Involvement of large vessels in polymyalgia arteritica. Lancet. 1965;**1**:1193–6.
8. Machedo EBV, Michet CJ, Ballard DJ, et al. Trends in incidence and clinical presentation of temporal arteritis in Olmsted County, Minnesota 1950–1985. Arthritis Rheum. 1988;**31**:745–9.
9. Nordberg E, Bengtsson BA. Epidemiology of biopsy proven giant cell arteritis. J Intern Med. 1990;**227**:233–6.
10. Ostberg G. On arteritis with special reference to polymyalgia arteritica. Acta Path Microb Scand. 1973;**237**(Suppl.):1–59.
11. Kyle V, Silverman B, Silman A, et al. Polymyalgia rheumatica/giant cell arteritis in general practice. Br Med J. 1985;**13**:385–8.
12. Mowat AG, Hazleman BL. Polymyalgia rheumatica: A clinical study with particular reference to arterial disease. J Rheumatol. 1974;**1**:190–202.
13. Liang M, Simkin PA, Hunder GG, Wilske KR, Healey LA. Familial aggregation of polymyalgia rheumatica and giant cell arteritis. Arthritis Rheum. 1974;**17**:19–24.
14. Rhodes DJ. Giant cell arteritis in general practice. J R Coll Gen Pract. 1976;**26**:237–346.
15. Cid MC, Ercilla G, Vilaseca J, et al. Polymyalgia rheumatica: a syndrome associated with HLA-DR4 antigen. Arthritis Rheum. 1988;**31**:678–82.
16. Sakhas LI, Loqueman N, Panayi GS, Myles AB, Welsh KS. Immunogenetics of polymyalgia rheumatica. Br J Rheumatol. 1990;**29**:331–4.
17. Jones JG, Hazleman BL. Polymyalgia rheumatica and giant cell arteritis – a difficult diagnosis. J R Coll Gen Pract. 1981;**31**:283–9.
18. Kyle V, Tudor J, Wraight EP, Gresham GA, Hazleman BL. Rarity of synovitis in polymyalgia rheumatica. Ann Rheum Dis. 1990;**49**:155–7.
19. Kyle V, Cawston TE, Hazleman BL. ESR and C-reactive protein in the assessment of polymyalgia rheumatica/giant cell arteritis on presentation and during follow up. Ann Rheum Dis. 1989;**48**:408–9.
20. Thomas RD, Croft DN. Thyrotoxicosis and giant cell arteritis. Br Med J. 1974;**2**:408–9.
21. Dent GR, Edwards OM. Autoimmune thyroid disease and the polymyalgia rheumatica–giant cell arteritis syndrome. Clin Endocrinol. 1978;**9**:215–19.
22. Kyle V, Wraight EP, Hazleman BL. Liver scan abnormalities in polymyalgia/giant cell arteritis. Clin Rheum. 1991;**10**:294–7
23. Klein GE, Campbell RJ, Hunder GG, Carney JA. Skip lesions in temporal arteritis. Mayo Clin Proc. 1976;**51**:504–8.
24. Wilkinson IMS, Russell RWR. Arteries of the head and neck in giant cell arteritis. A pathological study to show the pattern of arterial involvement. Arch Neurol. 1972;**27**:378–87.
25. Bacon PA, Doherty S, Zuckerman AJ. Hepatitis B antibody in polymyalgia rheumatica. Lancet. 1975;**2**:476–8.
26. Fessel WJ. Polymyalgia rheumatica, temporal arteritis and contact with birds. Lancet. 1969;**2**:1249–50.
27. Gallagher PJ, Jones K. Immunohistochemical findings in cranial arteritis. Arthritis Rheum. 1982;**25**:75–9.
28. Dasgupta B, Duke O, Kyle V, Macfarlane DG, Hazleman BL, Panayi GS. Antibodies to intermediate filaments in polymyalgia rheumatica and giant cell arteritis: a sequential study. Ann Rheum Dis. 1987;**46**:746–9.
29. Cid MC, Campo E, Ercilla G, et al. Immunohistochemical analysis of lymphoid and macrophage cell subsets and their immunologic activation markers in temporal arteritis. Influence of corticosteroid treatment. Arthritis Rheum. 1989;**32**:884–93.
30. Dasgupta B, Duke O, Timms AM, Pitzalis C, Panayi GS. Selective depletion and activation of $CD8^+$ lymphocytes from peripheral blood of patients with polymyalgia rheumatica and giant cell arteritis. Ann Rheum Dis. 1989;**48**:307–11.
31. Park JR, Jones JG, Harkiss GD, Hazleman BL. Circulatory immune complexes in polymyalgia rheumatica and giant cell arteritis. Ann Rheum Dis. 1981;**40**:360–65.
32. Papaioannou CC, Gupta RC, Hunder GG, McDuffie FC. Circulatory immune complexes in giant cell arteritis and polymyalgia rheumatica. Arthritis Rheum. 1980;**23**:1021–5.
33. Kyle V, Hazleman BL. Treatment of polymyalgia rheumatica and giant cell arteritis. I. Steroid regimes in the first 2 months. Ann Rheum Dis. 1989;**48**:658–61.
34. Nordberg E, Bengtsson BA. Death rates and causes of deaths in 284 consecutive patients with giant cell arteritis confirmed by biopsy. Br Med J 1989;**299**:549–50.
35. Kyle V, Hazleman BL. Treatment of polymyalgia rheumatica and giant cell arteritis. II. The relationship between steroid dose and steroid associated side effects. Ann Rheum Dis. 1989;**48**:662–6.

CONNECTIVE TISSUE DISORDERS

40

PRACTICAL PROBLEMS

BEHÇET'S SYNDROME

Hasan Yazici

Definition of the Problem

Behçet's syndrome is a distinct type of systemic vasculitis characterized by the development of chronic relapsing uveitis that may cause blindness, recurrent oral and/or genital ulcerations, and neurologic impairments. Patients have a peculiar hyperreactivity of the skin in response to simple trauma ('the pathergy reaction'). Criteria have been developed to help differentiate Behçet's from other forms of vascultis. Treatment of patients with Behçet's, particularly eye disease, requires the use of immunosuppressive drugs such as azathioprine or cyclosporin A.

The Typical Case

TW, a 26 year-old-man, presented with a 1-year history of recurrent oral ulcers and erythematous skin lesions of his legs and recent development of blurred vision and lower extremity thrombophlebitis. On physical examination, superficial aphthous ulcerations were noted on the surfaces of the buccal mucosa and a hypopyon was detected in the left eye (Fig. 40.1).

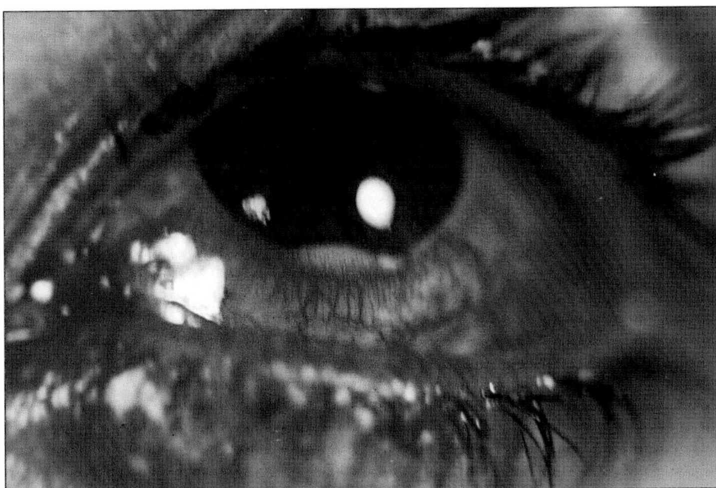

Fig. 40.1 Hypopyon uveitis. A precipitate of white cells is formed in the anterior chamber of the eye.

Diagnostic Problems

The diagnosis of Behçet's syndrome rests on the recognition of a constellation of clinical manifestations. Recently, a set of criteria for the classification of Behçet's have been proposed based on the computer analysis of clinical features from 914 cases collected worldwide (Fig. 40.2). Comparison groups of other diseases with manifestations that may be confused with Behçet's were also included in the analysis. Using recurrent aphthous ulceration as a constant feature, these criteria require the presence of two other sets of organ involvement for diagnosis. In this scheme a positive pathergy reaction (Fig. 40.3) is equivalent to involvement of an organ system.

While recognition of the syndrome may be straightforward, 'incomplete' forms of the disease with recurrent aphthae and involvement of one other organ system may present a diagnostic challenge. Although patients with Reiter's syndrome may have oral

CRITERIA FOR THE DIAGNOSIS OF BEHÇHET'S SYNDROME (INTERNATIONAL STUDY GROUP FOR BEHÇET'S DISEASE)

In the absence of other clinical explanations, patients must have:

1. Recurrent oral ulceration (aphthous or herpetiform) observed by the physician or patient recurring at least three times in one 12-month period;

and two of the following:

2. Recurrent genital ulceration.
3. Eye lesions: anterior uveitis, posterior uveitis, cells in the vitreous by slit lamp examination or retinal vasculitis observed by an ophthalmologist.
4. Skin lesions: erythema nodosum, pseudofolliculitis, papulopustular lesions or acneiform nodules in postadolescent patients not on corticosteroids.
5. Pathergy, read by a physician at 24–48 hours.

Fig. 40.2 ISG Criteria for the diagnosis of Behçet's syndrome.

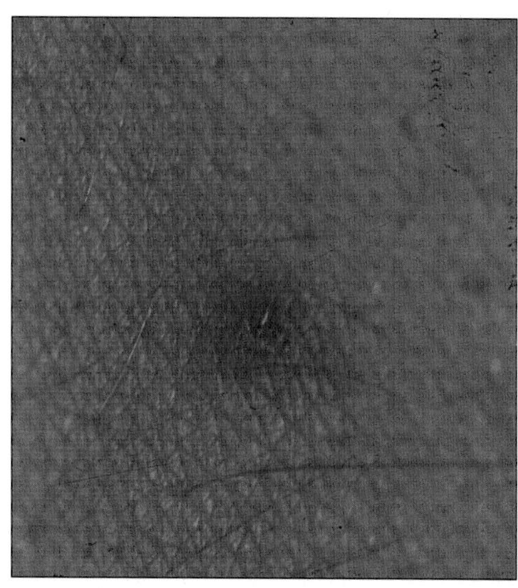

Fig. 40.3 Pathergy reaction. This phenomenon is quite unique to Behçet's syndrome.

and genital ulcers, male Behçet's patients have scrotal lesions rather than those of the glans penis typically seen in Reiter's. Furthermore, Behçet's patients do not have urethritis. Stevens–Johnson syndrome (erythema multiforme exudativum) also presents with mucocutaneous manifestations which can mimic Behçet's, but ocular involvement is usually conjunctival and corneal without chronic relapsing uveitis. Thrombophlebitis and arterial aneurysm formation is not part of Stevens-Johnson syndrome. Occasionally, a patient with inflammatory bowel disease may have associated oral ulcers, skin lesions and episcleritis which may be impossible to differentiate from Behçet's. Another diagnostic challenge is the patient with multiple sclerosis and several features of neuro-Behçet's.

Therapeutic Options

Drug management is directed at suppression of inflammation, especially during the early years of the disease. Young male patients are at increased risk for ocular complications and require aggressive medical management.

Immunosuppressants are considered to be the main line of treatment for eye involvement. Azathioprine at 2.5mg/kg/day has been shown to maintain visual acuity and to prevent the emergence of new eye disease. Therapy with azathioprine has, however, not been shown to improve compromised vision. The drug cyclosporin A is an alternative to azathioprine, and it effectively and rapidly acts to treat the eye disease in Behçet's syndrome. Nephrotoxicity, particularly at doses greater than 5mg/kg/day, the rather uniform relapses that one observes with the cessation of therapy, and the high cost of the drug often limit therapy. In addition, in cyclosporin use there is a tendency for the initial beneficial effect to dampen with continued use (i.e. after 6 months). An alternative approach is to start the treatment of acute eye disease with cyclosporin and to try to maintain the improvement with azathioprine. However, formal experience with this regimen is currently lacking. Other cytotoxic agents, such as chlorambucil and cyclophosphamide, are used but have been less well studied.

Local mydriatics should be used in the acute inflammatory stages of eye disease to prevent synechiae formation. The role of steroid eye drops is less clear. Permanent structural changes in the eye may be approached surgically (i.e. vitrectomy). Results of eye surgery are not uniformly satisfactory and care must be taken to avoid new attacks of ocular inflammation in the postoperative period.

The therapy of CNS lesions usually entails high dose glucocorticosteroids (around 60mg/day prednisone) and immunosuppressants. Gastrointestinal involvement may be managed by sulfasalazine 2–6g/day. Surgery may be required to resect segments of affected bowel in patients with severe abdominal disease or in patients with aneurysms of peripheral vessels.

There is a debate as to the role of heparin or oral anticoagulants in patients with thrombophlebitis. If the thrombi are not extensive, antiplatelet drugs (i.e. low-dose aspirin) are probably sufficient. In addition, immunosupressives are probably indicated in thrombi of large vessels, although formal evidence showing the efficacy of this approach is lacking.

Brief courses of systemic corticosteroids may be useful to shorten the duration of an attack both in the eye and in other organs. In addition, topical steroid preparations are of some benefit. However, there is no formal evidence that long-term systemic corticosteroids are effective and there is increasing concern as to their toxicity. As a consequence, large centers that treat Behçet's patients are currently using less corticosteroids. Colchicine is helpful in the treatment of erythema nodosum and arthralgias. In patients with severe cutaneous manifestations and/or systemic vasculitis, cyclophosphamide given in doses of 2–2.5mg/kg/day orally or 500–1500mg by intravenous boluses monthly is indicated. Antiviral drugs, like acyclovir and transfer factor, appear to be ineffective.

In general, for any serious organ involvement, drug treatment can be stopped after 2 years of remission. However, there are rare exceptions to this rule.

REFERENCES

O'Duffy JD. Behçet's disease. Curr Opin Rheumatol. 1994;**6**:39–43.

Ek L, Hedfors E. Behçet's disease: a review and a report of 12 cases from Sweden. Acta Derm Venereol. 1993;**73**:251–4.

Allen NB. Miscellaneous vasculitic syndromes including Behçet's disease and central nervous system vasculitis. Curr Opin Rheumatol. 1993;**5**:51–6.

Stratigos AJ, Laskaris G, Stratigos JD. Behçet's disease. Semin Neurol. 1992; **12**:346–57.

Yazici H, Barnes CG. Practical treatment recommendations for pharmacotherapy of Behçet's syndrome. Drugs 1991;**42**:796–804.

SJÖGREN'S SYNDROME

Haralampos M Moutsopoulos & Athanasios G Tzioufas

Definition of the Problem

The classic signs and symptoms of Sjögren's syndrome include enlargement of the parotid glands with mucosal dryness manifest by dry mouth (xerostomia) and dry eyes (xerophthalmia). Evaluation of patients requires the physician to determine whether the Sjögren's is of the primary or secondary form and, most importantly, to differentiate Sjögren's syndrome from a variety of other causes of salivary gland pathology. Treatment of this condition is mostly symptomatic.

The Typical Case

JT, a 60-year-old woman, presented with a 3-month history of fatigue, arthralgias and troublesome dryness of her eyes and mouth. On physical examination, prominent enlargement of her parotid glands was evident (Fig. 40.4). Laboratory studies revealed mild anemia with a hematocrit of 32%, positive rheumatoid factor and antinuclear antibody, and an erythrocyte sedimentation rate (ESR) of 60mm/hr (Westergren). A Schirmer's test was found to be abnormal (3mm wetting in 5 min) and a minor salivary gland biopsy showed marked lymphocytic infiltration of the glandular tissues.

Diagnostic Problems

Sjögren's syndrome is a slowly progressive, inflammatory autoimmune disease affecting primarily the exocrine glands. It is commonly present in patients with chronic, immune-mediated inflammatory disorders including rheumatoid arthritis, systemic lupus erythematosus, systemic sclerosis and polymyositis (secondary Sjögren's

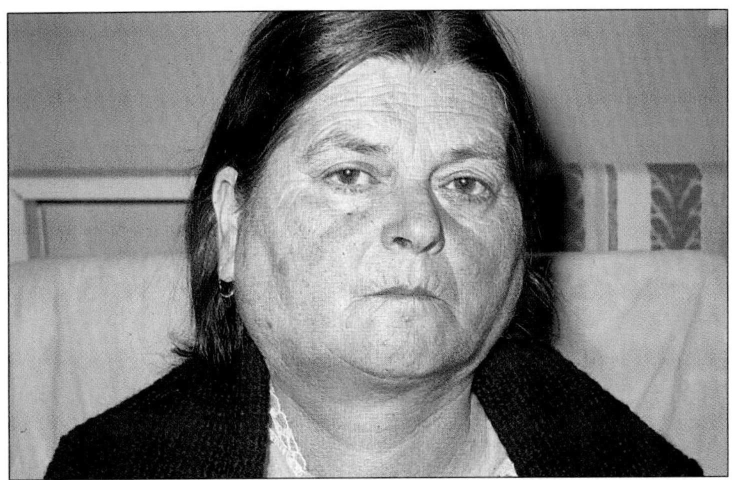

Fig. 40.4 Primary Sjögren's syndrome. Parotid gland enlargement.

syndrome). In the absence of other autoimmune disease, the syndrome is classified as primary Sjögren's syndrome. Sjögren's syndrome must be differentiated from a number of other disorders that affect the salivary glands (Fig. 40.5). Minor salivary gland biopsy serves as the cornerstone for the diagnosis and reveals focal aggregates of lymphocytes, plasma cells, and macrophages adjacent to and replacing the normal acini. Larger foci often exhibit formation of germinal centers. The predominant cells in the minor salivary gland infiltrates is the one bearing the T-helper phenotype ($CD4^+$).

A number of objective studies are helpful to determine functional impairments of ocular or oral glands. The Schirmer's tear test is used for the evaluation of tear secretion by the lacrimal glands. The test is performed with strips of filter paper 30mm in length. The strip is slipped beneath the inferior lid, with the remainder of the paper hanging out (Fig. 40.6). After 5 min the wetting length of the paper is measured. Wetting of less than 5mm/5 min is a strong indication for diminished secretion.

Keratoconjunctivitis sicca, the sequelae of decreased tear secretion, is diagnosed using Rose Bengal staining of the corneal epithelium. Rose Bengal is an aniline dye which stains the devitalized or damaged epithelium of both the cornea and conjunctiva. Slit-lamp examination after Rose Bengal staining shows a punctate or filamentary keratitis. Studies that may be done to measure salivary gland function include sialometry to determine salivary flow rates, sialography to assess anatomic changes of the salivary ducts, and scintigraphy using ^{99m}Tc pertechnetate.

Autoantibodies are commonly detected in Sjögren's patients, in particular rheumatoid factors, antinuclear antibodies, and antibodies to extractable nuclear antigens. The most common autoantibodies to cellular antigens are directed against two ribonuclear antigens known as Ro(SS-A) and La(SS-B). These autoantibodies are not specific for Sjögren's syndrome but may be found in other autoimmune diseases, especially systemic lupus. The incidence of anti-Ro(SS-A) antibodies is approximately 40–45% in Sjögren's syndrome and 25–30% in lupus. The anti-La(SS-B) antibody is detected in one-half of Sjögren's syndrome patients and 10% of lupus patients.

Therapeutic Options

The treatment of patients with Sjögren's syndrome is mainly symptomatic with the goal of keeping mucosal surfaces moist. Dry eyes should be lubricated with artificial tears as often as necessary. A variety of preparations are available that differ primarily in viscosity and preservative. The thicker, more viscous drops require less frequent application, although they can cause blurring and leave residue on the lashes. Less viscous drops require more frequent applications. Patients usually test several different preparations to determine which one is most suitable for their own individual needs. Soft contact lenses may help to protect the cornea, especially in the presence of filamentary keratitis. However, the lenses themselves require wetting, and the patients must be followed very carefully because of the increased risk of infection. Avoidance of windy and/or low humidity environments is helpful. Cigarette smoking and drugs with anticholinergic side effects, such as phenothiazines, tricyclic antidepressants, antispasmodics and anti-Parkinsonian agents, should be avoided whenever possible.

DIFFERENTIAL DIAGNOSIS OF PAROTID GLAND ENLARGEMENT
Bilateral
Viral infection (mumps, influenza, Epstein–Barr, coxsackie A, cytomegalovirus, HIV) Sjögren's syndrome Sarcoidosis Miscellaneous (diabetes mellitus, hyperlipoproteinemia, hepatic cirrhosis, chronic pancreatitis, acromegaly, gonadal hypofunction) Recurrent parotitis of childhood
Unilateral
Salivary gland neoplasm Bacterial infection Chronic sialadenitis

Fig. 40.5 Differential diagnosis of parotid gland enlargement.

Treatment of xerostomia is difficult. No single method is consistently effective, and most efforts are aimed only at palliation. Stimulation of salivary flow by sugar free, highly flavored lozenges is generally helpful. In contrast, dry food, heavy smoking and drugs with anticholinergic side effects, which further decrease the salivary flow, should be avoided. Most patients carry water, sugarless lemon drops or chewing gum. Adequate oral hygiene after meals is a prerequisite for prevention of dental disease. Topical treatment with stannous flouride enhances dental mineralization and retards damage to tooth surfaces. In cases of rapidly progressive dental disease, the flouride can be directly applied to the teeth from plastic trays that are used at night. Vaginal dryness is treated with lubricant jellies and dry skin with moisturizing lotions.

Systemic corticosteroids (0.5–1.0mg/kg/day of prednisone) and immunosuppressive drugs such as cyclophosphamide are used for severe extraglandular disease, including interstitial pneumonitis, glomerulonephritis, vasculitis and peripheral neuropathy. Sjögren's patients are at increased risk for the development of lymphoma and treatment depends on the histologic type, the location and the extension. Decisions regarding chemotherapy and/or radiation should be guided by experienced oncologists.

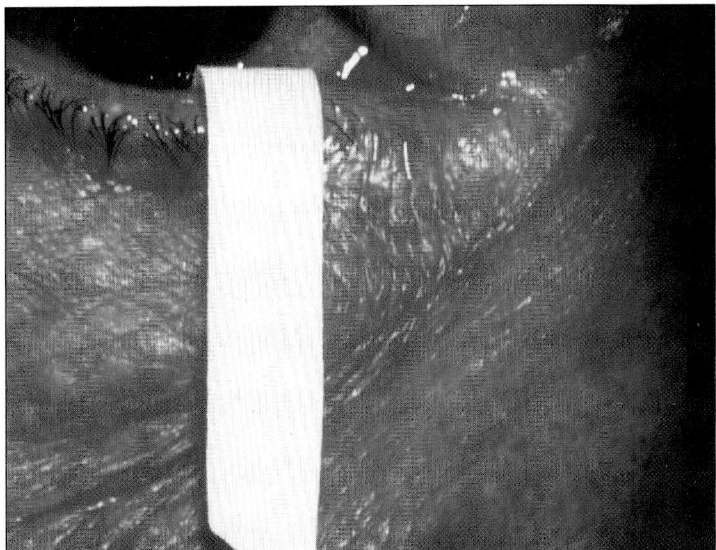

Fig. 40.6 Schirmer's test. Wetting of less than 5mm/5min of the filter paper strip is shown.

REFERENCES

Wu AJ, Fox PC. Sjögren's syndrome. Semin Dermatol. 1994;**13**:138-43.
Fox RI, Saito I. Criteria for diagnosis of Sjögren's syndrome. Rheum Dis North Am. 1994;**20**;391–407.
Atkinson JC, Wu AJ. Salivary gland dysfunction : causes, symptoms, treatment. J Am Dent Assoc. 1994;**125**:409–16.
Foster HE, Gilroy JJ, Kelly CA, Howe J, Griffiths ID. The treatment of sicca features in Sjögren's syndrome: a clinical review. Br J Rheumatol. 1994;**33**:278–82.
St Clair EW. New developments in Sjögren's syndrome. Curr Opin Rheumatol. 1993; **5**:604–12.

POSITIVE ANTINUCLEAR ANTIBODY

John H Klippel

Definition of the Problem

Patients with unexplained arthritis or systemic signs and symptoms are commonly tested for antinuclear antibodies (ANAs) to help determine if they have a 'rheumatic' or 'autoimmune' disease. The finding of an ANA, when combined with the history and clinical examination, may help to confirm a suspected diagnosis of a connective tissue disorder or be attributed to various nonrheumatologic conditions in which ANAs develop. In many patients, the symptoms and positive ANAs are judged to be part of an early, undifferentiated rheumatic syndrome in which patience and time are needed to reveal the diagnosis. In some patients, the cause of the ANA is never satisfactorily explained.

The Typical Case

PM was a 45-year-old secretary seen for a 6-month history of fatigue, intermittent fevers, and pain and stiffness in her hands that was most prominent in the morning. A family history revealed type I diabetes mellitus in her mother and a younger sister with severe lupus nephritis. On physical examination she seemed mildly depressed. Her blood pressure was 138/92 and temperature 36.8°C. The musculoskeletal examination was unremarkable save for questionable tenderness of several of the metacarpophalangeal joints; no evidence of joint effusions or synovial thickening or subcutaneous nodules was found. Laboratory studies revealed an ESR of 15mm/hour (Westergren), a negative rheumatoid factor, and a positive ANA at a titer of 1:320 in a homogeneous pattern (Fig. 40.7).

Diagnostic Problems

Although ANAs are commonly regarded as an indication of a connective tissue disorder, particularly systemic lupus erythematosus (SLE), many other causes of ANAs are recognized (Fig. 40.8). In general, patients with bona fide connective tissue disorders will have clinical signs and symptoms compatible with a distinct syndrome and a tentative diagnosis will be formulated before the results of the ANA test become available. Such patients rarely present diagnostic dilemmas; in doubtful cases, further serologic testing for disease-specific antibodies to nuclear or cytoplasmic antigens may aid in diagnosis (Fig. 40.9). Yet for many patients, the finding of a positive ANA test is unexpected and prompts a careful review of the history and physical examination to determine a cause for this result.

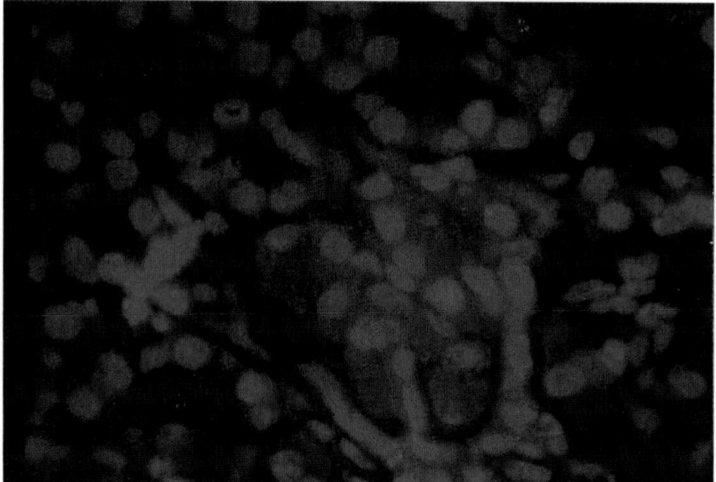

Fig. 40.7 Homogeneous antinuclear antibody immunofluorescence pattern. Courtesy of Dr N Rothfield.

Numerous studies have documented the presence of ANAs in normal, healthy people. In general, the antibody titer is low (<1:40) and of a homogeneous or diffuse pattern. The frequency increases with age – 20 to 25% of persons over the age of 60 years are ANA-positive – and is probably higher in families in which there is a patient with rheumatic illness. Surveys of asymptomatic family members of patients with lupus, Sjögren's syndrome, or scleroderma indicate that up to as many as one-half of the first-degree relatives are ANA-positive. Whether pregnancy can be associated with the development of a positive ANA is unclear. This has been reported in several studies, but not confirmed by others.

Many drugs have been shown to lead to a positive ANA. The two most common offenders, by far, are procainamide and hydralazine, and prospective studies have shown that 50–75% of patients treated with these drugs develop a positive ANA. The majority of patients with drug-induced ANAs are entirely asymptomatic. However, clinical syndromes that resemble SLE or polymyositis may develop. Typically, symptoms subside or resolve with discontinuation of the drug. However, treatment with anti-inflammatory medications, including corticosteroids, may be required in patients with severe complications. Drug-induced ANAs may persist for many months, or even years, after the offending drug is discontinued.

Antinuclear antibodies have been associated with various forms of chronic liver disease, including chronic active hepatitis, primary biliary cirrhosis and even alcoholic liver disease. In HBsAG-positive viral hepatitis, ANAs have been shown to resolve despite persistence of viral markers. Antibodies to centromere proteins have been demonstrated in patients with primary biliary cirrhosis. Presumably, such patients have a *forme fruste* of limited scleroderma (CREST syndrome). The role of ANAs in regulating the course of hepatitis or leading to extrahepatic immune complex disease is unclear. In patients with membranous glomerulonephropathy and chronic active hepatitis, acid eluates of the kidneys have been shown to contain antibodies to the ribonuclear protein U1 RNP; the antibodies are greatly concentrated compared to the serum, suggesting that they are deposited within the kidney and probably contribute in some way to renal pathology.

Antinuclear antibodies have been found in a high proportion of patients with idiopathic pulmonary fibrosis as well as the fibrotic lung changes that develop following asbestos exposure. The antibodies are detected more frequently in females and appear to correlate with duration of pulmonary findings, Raynaud's phenomenon and digital vasculitis. These findings suggest some relationship to scleroderma. Antinuclear antibodies have also been noted in patients with primary pulmonary hypertension.

Chronic infectious diseases, particularly parasitic infections, may cause ANAs. In populations in which malaria is endemic, the prevalence of positive ANA is extraordinarily high; interestingly, the specificity appears to be against single-stranded DNA. Other parasitic diseases in which ANAs have been observed include

CAUSES OF POSITIVE ANTINUCLEAR ANTIBODIES
1. Rheumatic diseases
Systemic lupus erythematosus Polymyositis Sjögren's syndrome Scleroderma Vasculitis Rheumatoid arthritis
2. Normal, healthy individuals
Females > males, prevalence increases with age Relatives of patients with rheumatic diseases ? Pregnant females
3. Drug-induced
4. Hepatic diseases
Chronic active hepatitis Primary biliary cirrhosis Alcoholic liver disease
5. Pulmonary diseases
Idiopathic pulmonary fibrosis Asbestos-induced fibrosis Primary pulmonary hypertension
6. Chronic infections
7. Malignancies
Lymphoma Leukemia Melanoma Solid tumors (ovary, breast, lung, kidney)
8. Hematologic disorders
Idiopathic thrombocytopenic purpura Autoimmune hemolytic anemia
9. Miscellaneous
Endocrine disorders (type I diabetes mellitus, Graves' disease) Neurologic diseases (multiple sclerosis) End-stage renal failure After organ transplantation

Fig. 40.8 Causes of positive antinuclear antibodies.

Trypanosoma rhodesiense, *Schistosoma japonicum* and *mansoni*, and the fluke worm *Opisthorchis viverrini*. Antinuclear antibodies have also been noted in patients with tuberculosis and leprosy. Bacterial infections with both *Salmonella* and *Klebsiella* organisms may be associated with ANAs. In the instance of *Salmonella*, idiotypic cross-reactivity, particularly between nucleic acids and the K-30 antigen, is thought to be a potential mechanism responsible for autoantibody formation. In addition, shared antigenic determinants between bacterial lipopolysaccharide and DNA-histone has been demonstrated for *Salmonella*.

Various malignancies have been reported to be associated with ANAs, including lymphomas, leukemias and solid tumors. In large granular lymphocytic leukemia, a chronic lymphocytic leukemia of T cell origin that occurs in a subset of of patients with Felty's syndrome, approximately half the patients are ANA-positive. Disappearance of the antibody has been documented in patients in

AUTOANTIBODIES HELPFUL IN THE DIAGNOSIS OF SPECIFIC RHEUMATIC DISEASES	
Disease suspected	**Autoantibody**
Systemic lupus erythematosus	Anti-dsDNA Anti-Sm Anti-Ku
Drug-induced lupus	Antihistones
Mixed connective tissue disease	Anti-RNP
Polymyositis/dermatomyositis	Anti-Jo-l (histidyl tRNA synthetase)
Scleroderma	Anti-Scl-70 (topoisomerase 1) Anticentromere
Sjögren's syndrome	Anti-Ro(SS-A) Anti-La(SS-B)
Wegener's granulomatosis	C-ANCA

Fig. 40.9 Autoantibodies helpful in the diagnosis of specific rheumatic diseases.

whom a remission is induced following chemotherapy or after resection of a solid tumor.

In patients with immune-mediated hematologic disorders such as hemolytic anemia or thrombocytopenia, an ANA typically signifies that SLE is a likely underlying disease.

The Approach to Determining the Cause of a Positive ANA

- In patients with a suspected connective tissue disorder, specific autoantibodies (e.g. anti-DNA, anti-Sm, anti-Jo-1, etc.) to help in diagnosis.
- Careful review of medications taken by the patient to exclude drug-induced ANA syndromes.
- Family history to identify ANA genetic diathesis.
- Chest examination and radiograph to detect pulmonary fibrosis or pulmonary hypertension.
- Liver enzymes and complete blood count to detect occult hepatic or hematologic disease.
- Appropriate cultures in febrile patients.

REFERENCES

Chapman JR, Charles PJ, Venables PJW, et al. Definition and clinical relevance of antibodies to nuclear ribonucleoprotein and other nuclear antigens in patients with cryptogenic fibrosing alveolitis. Am Rev Respir Dis. 1984;**130**:439–43

Kurki P, Gripenberg M, Teppo AM, Salaspuro M. Profiles of antinuclear antibodies in chronic active hepatitis, primary biliary cirrhosis and alcoholic liver disease. Liver. 1984;**4**:134–8.

Miller RA, Wener MH, Harnisch JP, Gilliland BC. The limited spectrum of antinuclear antibodies in leprosy. J Rheumatol. 1987;**14**:108–10.

Recker DP, Klippel JH. Perplexing antinuclear antibody syndrome (PANAS). In: Panush RS, ed. Postgraduate advances in rheumatology, III. Princeton: Forum Medicus; 1989:1–17.

Shoenfeld Y, Slor H, Shafir S, et al. Diversity and pattern of inheritance of autoantibodies in families with multiple cases of systemic lupus erythematosus. Ann Rheum Dis. 1992;**51**:611–18.

Solinger AM. Drug-related lupus. Clinical and etiologic considerations. Rheum Dis Clin N Am. 1988:**14**:187–202.

RENAL BIOPSY IN SYSTEMIC LUPUS ERYTHEMATOSUS

James E Balow

Definition of the Problem

Kidney disease occurs in the majority of patients with lupus. However, the legitimate indications for renal biopsy in lupus are a matter of considerable uncertainty for many clinicians. Neither an 'always' nor a 'never' approach to the renal biopsy is sound. When the clinical and noninvasive laboratory features are consonant and characteristic, renal biopsy may add little except expense and discomfort for the lupus patient. On the other hand, the rheumatology consultant is more commonly faced with situations where the natural history of lupus has been substantially modified by time and prior interventions, where clinical features are atypical and nondiagnostic, or where the renal disease activity, severity and classification are indeterminate.

Typical Cases

Case 1

A 23-year-old woman with a normal employment examination 1 year earlier presented with a 6-week history of progressive fatigue, arthralgias, pleuritis and 5kg weight gain. Edema, hypertension, hematuria, red and white cell casts, proteinuria of more than 6g/day, hypoalbuminemia and elevated cholesterol were present. Serum creatinine was 1.9mg/dl. Antinuclear and anti-DNA antibodies were present in high titers, along with low complement levels.

Case 2

A 45-year-old woman, previously in excellent health, presented with new-onset polyarthritis, Raynaud's phenomenon, cutaneous vasculitis and a large pleural effusion. Lupus serologies were diagnostic. Renal function tests, albumin and cholesterol were normal, but urinalysis showed 1.2g/day of proteinuria; microscopy showed 3–5 red blood cells per high-power field (RBC/hpf) and 1+ granular casts. One month of prednisone at 0.5mg/kg/day led to resolution of the lupus-related pleuritis. However, the low-grade urinary abnormalities and active lupus serologies persisted.

Case 3

A 23-year-old woman was referred to a rheumatologist after several years of management of lupus by a family physician. She had a 3-year history of multisystem lupus activity which was treated with variable doses of prednisone and hydroxychloroquine. During a flare of pleuropericarditis 1 year earlier, hematuria and 2+ albuminuria were noted. Serum creatinine was as high as 1.6mg/dl. No renal biopsy was performed at that time. She was treated for lupus nephritis with high-dose, daily prednisone. Her extrarenal symptoms resolved and the prednisone was tapered to 10mg/day by 9 weeks. However, the urine protein was now 1.5g/day and serum creatinine 1.4mg/dl. Urine sediment manifested low-grade activity with microscopic hematuria and occasional cellular casts; occasional broad and waxy casts being present. Serum complement was normal. Anti-DNA was present in moderate titer (no previous tests had been performed). The patient and her husband were opposed to cytotoxic drugs because of the risk of infertility, but asked the consultant to recommend the best treatment based on the prognosis of the kidney disease.

Case 4

A 23-year-old woman had a several-year history of work absenteeism due to fatigue and arthralgias. Few medical tests were performed and no diagnosis was made until she had presented recently with typical lupus facial rash. She was normotensive and had moderate pedal edema. Antinuclear and anti-DNA antibodies were present, but complement levels were normal. Urine sediment showed 5–10 RBC/hpf, 3–5 white blood cells (WBC) per hpf, moderate oval fat bodies, and granular and mixed cellular casts. Urine protein was 3.8g/day, serum albumin 2.8g/dl, cholesterol 345mg/dl and creatinine 1.4mg/dl.

Diagnostic Problems

These cases illustrate, on the one hand, the occasional patient who presents with straightforward severe lupus nephritis and, on the other hand, the challenges posed more commonly by patients in whom the clinical and laboratory features are distinctly abnormal but of relatively low grade, a prior history of nephritis is ambiguous or poorly-documented, nephritis has been substantially modified by prior treatments, or the clinical and laboratory features are compatible with more than one form of lupus nephritis.

In case 1, the clinical and laboratory parameters support a diagnosis of diffuse proliferative lupus nephritis in a patient known to have had normal findings within the previous year. Renal biopsy in a patient with the combination of classic nephritic and nephrotic syndromes is not necessary outside of a research setting.

In case 2, a renal biopsy is indicated in order to assess prognosis and the renal indications for continued or additional therapy. Had the urinary findings completely resolved on prednisone, most would argue that renal biopsy is not indicated. However, the case illustrates the more common circumstances in which definite, low-grade abnormalities exist but are an inadequate basis for classification of the type and severity of the lupus nephritis. In this case, early diffuse proliferative lupus nephritis was present (Fig. 40.10).

In case 3, the past medical history is replete with problems of interpretation. Lupus may have been present for several years. Extrarenal symptoms eclipsed and diverted the primary physician from proper evaluation of the nephritis. Under these circumstances, the consulting physician is usually unable to assess the type, severity and reversibility of the nephritis and should be reluctant to make a difficult therapeutic recommendation without a renal biopsy. In this case, renal biopsy showed a focal proliferative lupus nephritis with accumulation of substantial scarring and atrophy (Fig. 40.11).

Case 4 illustrates the difficulty in distinguishing by clinical or laboratory parameters partially treated chronic proliferative lupus nephritis from membranous lupus nephropathy. In both cases, low-grade urine sediment abnormalities and nephrotic range proteinuria can be present. Because of the difference in prognosis and the approaches to management of proliferative and membranous nephropathies, a renal biopsy is recommended to resolve such indeterminate situations. In this case, membranous nephropathy was found on renal biopsy (Fig. 40.12).

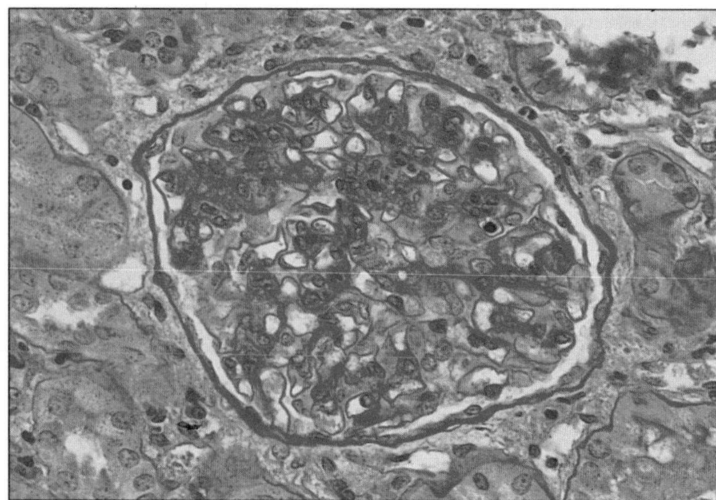

Fig. 40.10 Diffuse proliferative lupus nephritis. Glomeruli show hypercellularity and irregular capillary loop thickening (subendothelial deposits on electron microscopy).

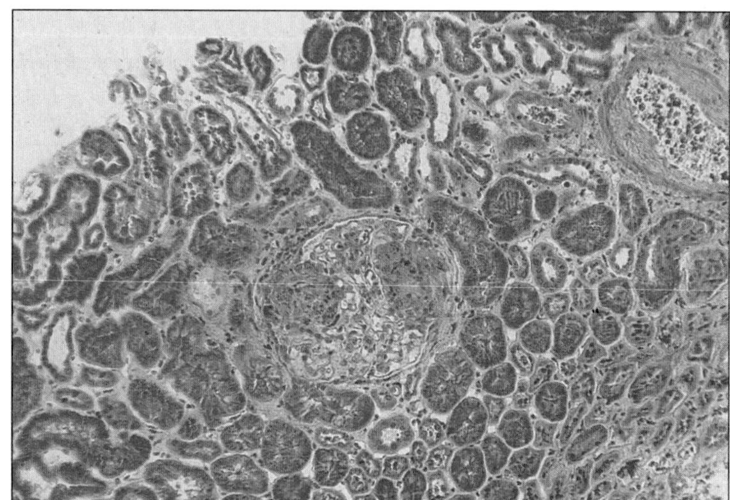

Fig. 40.11 Focal proliferative lupus nephritis. Substantial glomerular sclerosis, tubular atrophy and interstitial fibrosis are seen.

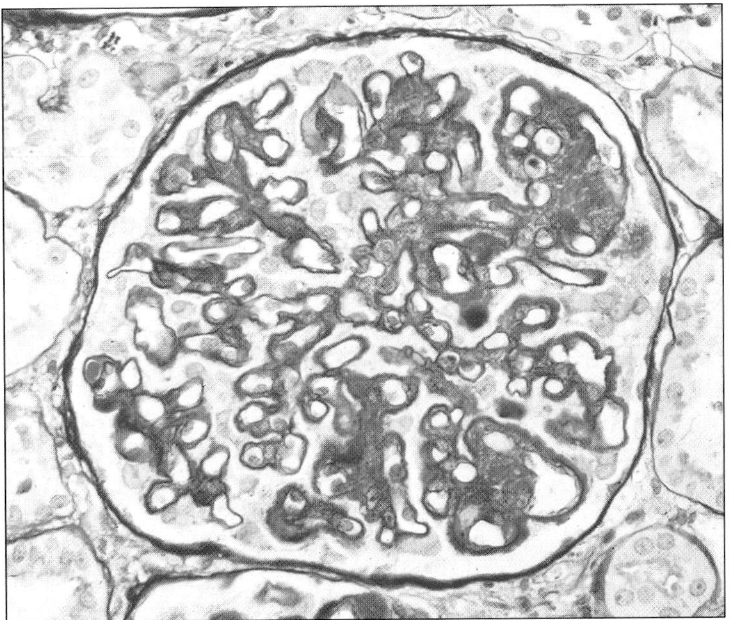

Fig. 40.12 Membranous lupus nephropathy. There is almost uniform thickening of the capillary loops (subepithelial deposits on electron microscopy). Typical mesangial expansion of lupus nephritis is evident.

INDICATIONS FOR RENAL BIOPSY IN LUPUS NEPHRITIS
Proteinuria of >1g/day
The threshold is conventionally 1–2g/day Less proteinuria does not preclude biopsy if it occurs in the context of major serologic abnormalities, especially hypocomplementemia At the other extreme, the presence of full-blown nephrotic and nephritic syndromes may make renal biopsy unnecessary
Progressive azotemia
Decreasing renal function in association with active urinary sediment is an indication for biopsy in order to assess the extent of crescents and necrosis which would warrant very aggressive therapy
Ambiguity or inconsistency of data
Lupus nephritis of indeterminate duration, severity and potential responsiveness warrants the establishment of a fresh baseline database including determination of class, activity and chronicity indices
Overlapping clinical features
Situations where clinical and laboratory data are compatible with different classes of lupus nephritis, for which different approaches to management are warranted
Redirection of therapy
Partially treated or incompletely responsive lupus nephritis for which a change in therapeutic plan is deemed appropriate

Fig. 40.13 Indications for renal biopsy in lupus nephritis.

The indications for renal biopsy are summarized in Figure 40.13.

A critically important reminder is that is imperative that an experienced physician examines the urine sediment from all patients with lupus nephritis. Errors in microscopy data from the clinical laboratory are unfortunately a frequent source of erroneous information about the status of the patient with lupus nephritis.

Conclusion

Clearly, not all of the indications for and optimal approaches to management of lupus nephritis have been determined. However, it is incumbent on the consultant to define a database with the least ambiguities, lest the patient be inappropriately overtreated or a window of therapeutic opportunity be missed.

REFERENCES

Appel GB, Cohen DJ, Pirani CL, Meltzer JI, Estes D. Long-term follow-up of patients with lupus nephritis. Am J Med. 1987;**83**:877–85.

Austin HA III, Muenz LR, Joyce KM, et al. Prognostic factors in lupus nephritis. Contribution of renal histologic data. Am J Med. 1983;**75**:382–91.

Balow JE, Austin HA III. Renal disease in systemic lupus erythematosus. Rheum Dis Clin North Am. 1988;**14**:117–33.

Esdaile JM, Levinton C, Federgreen W, Hayslett JP, Kashgarian M. The clinical and renal biopsy predictors of long-term outcome in lupus nephritis: a study of 87 patients and review of the literature. Q J Med. 1989;**72**:779–833.

Gladman DD, Urowitz MB, Cole E, Ritchie S, Chang CH, Churg J. Kidney biopsy in SLE. I. A clinical-morphologic evaluation. Q J Med. 1989;**73**:1125–33.

Nossent HC, Henzen-Logmans, Vroom TM, Berden JH, Swaak TJ. Contribution of renal biopsy data in predicting outcome in lupus nephritis. Arthritis Rheum. 1990;**33**:970–7.

OSTEONECROSIS IN SYSTEMIC LUPUS ERYTHEMATOSUS

Micha Abeles

Definition of the Problem

Osteonecrosis (avascular necrosis) of bone is the major orthopedic problem in patients with SLE. Ranging widely in reported incidence, osteonecrosis may occur in up to 52% of patients with SLE. The difference between studies in prevalence of osteonecrosis in SLE depends to a great extent on whether symptomatic rather than all patients with SLE are evaluated. The presence of osteonecrosis of the femoral head is an especially feared complication. Symptomatic patients face progressively severe pain and disability, and ultimately total hip replacement.

The Typical Case

A 26-year-old White woman presented with fever, hair loss, malaise and joint pain. Physical examination showed mild alopecia, tender proximal interphalangeal (PIP) and metacarpophalangeal (MCP) joints and a malar blush. Laboratory investigation indicated anemia, elevated anti-DNA antibodies, low C3 complement, negative VDRL, normal PT, normal urinalysis and a positive LE cell preparation. A diagnosis of SLE was made and prednisone was initiated at 60mg/day with good response.

The patient was lost to follow-up until she presented a year later with malaise, visual complaints and difficulty with thought processes. After extensive evaluation, a diagnosis of CNS involvement secondary to SLE was made. The patient was begun on prednisone 80mg/day to which she responded quickly. Six months later, while on prednisone 15mg/day, she developed fever and lethargy. Chest radiographs showed bilateral mid and lower lung field infiltrates. A diagnosis of pulmonary hemorrhage was confirmed by lung biopsy. Because of progressive respiratory distress, she was intubated and maintained on mechanical ventilation for a brief period. Methylprednisolone was increased to 100mg/day. A month after extubation the patient began to complain of pain in a variety of joints including the right shoulder, left elbow, right wrist, both hips and both knees. Radiologic investigation showed evidence of osteonecrosis in all seven joints. During the next 2 years she underwent bilateral knee and hip replacements for progressively severe pain. The shoulder, elbow and wrist became asymptomatic, and 10 years after the development of osteonecrosis, remain functional.

Diagnostic Problems

Arthritis is the most common manifestation of SLE. Approximately 90% of patients with SLE will have articular complaints at some point during the course of their disease. When present, arthritis is usually polyarticular and symmetrical, but it can be pauciarticular,

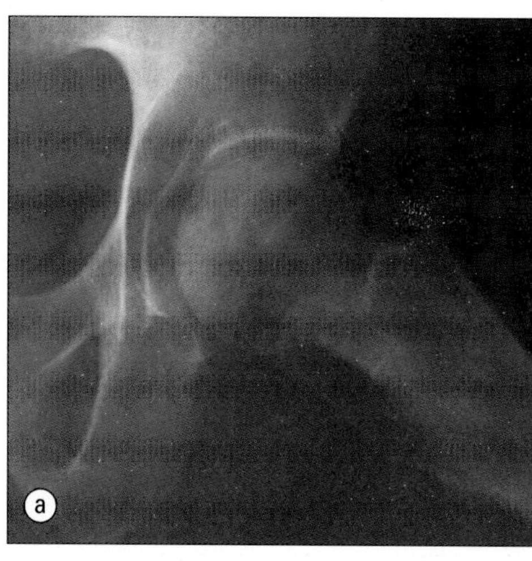

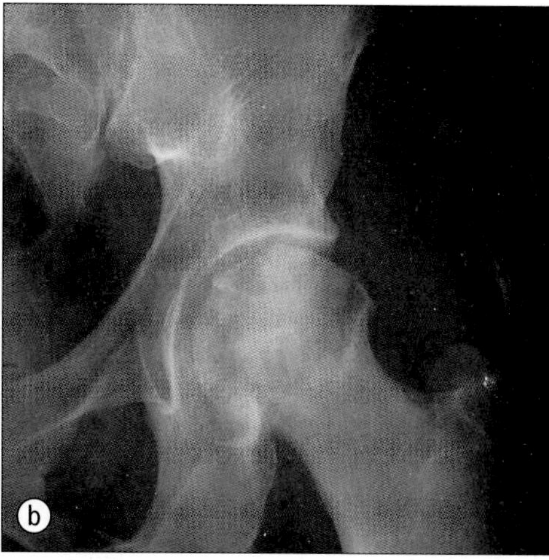

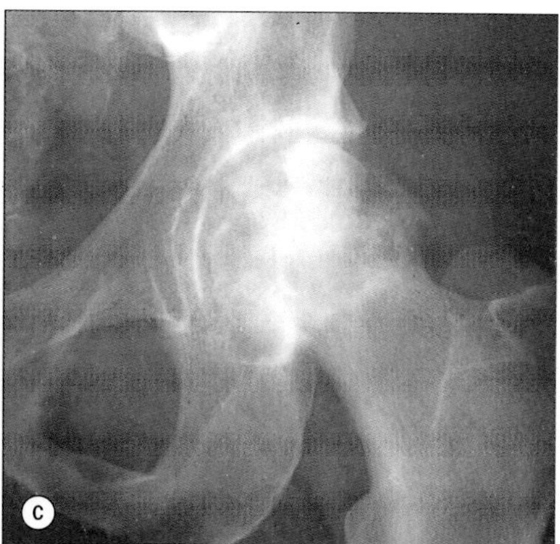

Fig. 40.14 Progressive changes of osteonecrosis of the hip in SLE. Radiographs were taken at 6-month intervals. The pathognomonic crescent sign was seen (a), followed by progressive femoral head collapse (b and c).

asymmetric and even monoarticular. Clinically, osteonecrosis also presents as a painful joint. It can be a monoarticular problem, be present in two symmetrical joints or be polyarticular. Onset can be acute or gradual, and pain can be intermittent in nature. Thus, osteonecrosis can mimic lupus arthritis. When monoarticular and acute it can also mimic septic arthritis.

A high index of suspicion for the possibility of osteonecrosis has to be maintained in any SLE patient with joint pain. This is especially true for SLE patients who have been on high doses of corticosteroids and have new-onset monoarticular or pauciarticular pain. An initial diagnostic measure should be routine radiography (Figs 40.14–40.16). If radiographs are unrevealing, additional evaluation modalities need to be considered, especially if hip pain is the problem (the femoral head is the most common target of osteonecrosis). Early osteonecrosis of the hip is also potentially treatable and thus diagnosis is paramount.

Since no single diagnostic measure is completely accurate, multiple approaches may be needed. The combination of MRI and technetium bone scan provide extremely sensitive measures to diagnose osteonecrosis (see Fig. 40.14). It is now accepted that MRI is the best noninvasive measure for diagnosing osteonecrosis. It localizes the disease, indicates the extent of involvement and is less subject to artifact. When the MRI is negative and suspicion remains high, radionuclide bone scintigraphy should be done. Although scintigraphy has been reported to give false-negative results in 10–52% of patients, a rare patient may have a positive technetium scan when the MRI is negative. The use of pinhole collimator imaging may also be occasionally positive when the MRI is negative. Invasive procedures are not routinely recommended for diagnosis. Intraosseous venography is abnormal in only 50–75% of patients, and bone marrow pressure measurements are only slightly better. Biopsy is an investigative measure and, although most specific, may be subject to sampling error. If noninvasive studies are negative and pain persists, repeat studies should be carried out within 2–4 months.

There are no helpful clinical associations with osteonecrosis apart from high corticosteroid dosage. Despite conflicting studies, neither Raynaud's phenomenon nor Cushingoid appearance serve as useful markers. Antiphospholipid antibodies may have a statistically significant association with osteonecrosis, but this relationship is not useful in diagnosis in an individual patient.

Fig. 40.15 Osteonecrosis of the shoulder in SLE. The crescent sign indicative of osteonecrosis is seen in the head of the right humerus.

Therapeutic Options

Osteonecrosis, whether associated with SLE or other entities, can only be treated primarily if it involves the femoral head. There are no data to suggest that osteonecrosis affecting other sites can be successfully treated. Agreement exists that for surgical intervention to be effective, it must be done as early as possible, before irreversible changes appear. Although there may be conflicting views as to how effective treatment is, most studies indicate that 80–90% of patients will demonstrate a progressive course to femoral head collapse and secondary osteoarthritis if no intervention is undertaken. This often results in major medical and socioeconomic costs to the patient. Thus, in a symptomatic patient, surgical intervention should be considered.

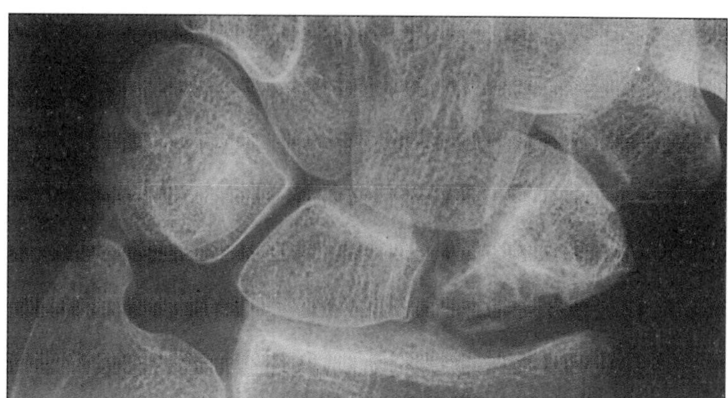

Fig. 40.16 Osteonecrosis of the scaphoid in SLE. There are lucencies and sclerosis as a result of osteonecrosis.

The most widely used early surgical treatment is core decompression. In this procedure a core from the necrotic segment of bone is surgically removed using a trephine. This procedure lowers intraosseous pressure, relieves pain, potentially stimulates vascular neogenesis, relieves ischemia and, in addition, helps to confirm the diagnosis.

All investigators agree that core decompression is most useful in stage 1 of the disease prior to routine radiologic change. Success rates for later stages (4–6) (see Figs 40.14–40.16) are extremely poor, and no intervention is recommended for these stages. Stage 3 is associated with such poor surgical results that decompression is now rarely done. Intervention for stage 2 disease is somewhat controversial because claimed success rates vary widely from well below 50% to over 50%. The use of electrical simulation with a direct current electrical stimulator has been advocated by some as a helpful adjunct to decompression. The major side effect of core decompression is fracture. With the proper surgical approach and prolonged nonweight-bearing, postoperative fractures are rare.

When osteonecrosis occurs in joints other than the hips, resting the affected joint is the only approach presently available. Splinting of the joint, if possible, should be done. If the knee or ankle is involved, an extended period of nonweight-bearing and the use of crutches is recommended, although outcome studies of such an approach are not available.

Osteonecrosis occurs months to years after a course of relatively high-dose corticosteroids or after a prolonged period of low- to moderate-dose corticosteroids. In the former situation, glucocorticosteroids have often been tapered by the time osteonecrosis is diagnosed. Whether the patient is at further risk of developing additional sites of osteonecrosis if the dose of corticosteroid is raised for a disease flare is not known. Nevertheless, it seems prudent to consider modification of the therapeutic approach in such patients. As an example, the corticosteroid dose would be raised at the time of increased disease activity, followed by the rapid addition of putative steroid-sparing agents.

Azathioprine, antimalarials, cyclophosphamide, intravenous immunoglobulins and even retinoids have been reported as useful for different aspects of the disease. These medications may ostensibly allow a more rapid tapering of corticosteroids to a lower level than otherwise possible. In the latter situation where long-term corticosteroid use is associated with osteonecrosis, a somewhat similar approach can be considered. Considering the side-effect profile of these medications, antimalarials are the initial medication of choice to add in this group.

Conclusions

- Osteonecrosis of bone is a significant cause of morbidity in SLE patients treated with corticosteroids.
- There is no helpful clinical association with osteonecrosis other than corticosteroid treatment.
- When osteonecrosis is suspected, especially when a hip is involved, extensive investigation is warranted. The initial approach is radiography of the involved joints. If this is unrevealing, then further investigation with MRI, and possibly radionuclide bone scintigraphy, should be undertaken.
- In symptomatic patients with hip pain and normal or very early radiographic changes, core decompression may be considered. Other symptomatic areas can only be treated with rest. Symptomatic joints with advanced destruction can only be treated with joint replacement.
- Asymptomatic patients in whom osteonecrosis is discovered by chance on imaging should be followed without surgical intervention.
- The dose of corticosteroid in a patient diagnosed with osteonecrosis should be adjusted according to disease activity of SLE. Steroid-sparing medications may be of help in achieving the lowest dose of steroid required in as short a time as possible.

REFERENCES

Abeles M, Urman J, Rothfield NF. Aseptic necrosis of bone in systemic lupus erythematosus: Relationship to corticosteroid therapy. Arch Int Med. 1978;**138**:750–4.

Stulberg BN, Davis AW, Bauer TW, Levine M, Easley MS. Osteonecrosis of the femoral head: A prospective randomized treatment protocol. Clin Orthop. 1991;**268**:140–51.

Warner JJ, Philip JH, Brodsky GL, Thornhill TS. Studies of nontraumatic osteonecrosis: The role of core decompression in the treatment of nontraumatic osteonecrosis of the femoral head. Clin Orthop. 1987;**225**:104–25.

Weiner ES, Abeles M. Aseptic necrosis and glucocorticosteroids in systemic lupus erythematosus: A re-evaluation. J Rheumatol. 1989;**16**:604–8.

PROBLEMS IN THE DIAGNOSIS OF RAYNAUD'S PHENOMENON

Virginia D Steen

Definition of the Problem

Raynaud's phenomenon may be a primary process present in 5% of the general population or it may be a secondary process (Fig. 40.17). Generally it is mild, requiring little intervention, but it can result in painful ulcers, loss of digits and refractory ischemia. Raynaud's phenomenon may evolve into a connective tissue disease.

The Typical Case

A 25-year-old woman presented to her family doctor with the history that her fingers had been turning blue for the past 6–12 months. After careful questioning, the doctor determined it was usually induced by emotion or cold temperature. He diagnosed Raynaud's phenomenon and reassured her that it was nothing to worry about. One year later the Raynaud's phenomenon was becoming more frequent and more severe. On referral to a rheumatologist it was determined that she smoked cigarettes and took propanolol for migraine headaches. The physical examination found no digital puffiness or swelling, periungual erythema, nailfold capillary changes, digital pitting scars, sclerodactyly or telangiectasia. Laboratory tests including complete blood count, ESR and ANA were normal or negative. She was advised to discontinue smoking, stop the propanolol and avoid excessive cold exposure.

Ten years later she returned with puffy fingers, more severe Raynaud's, a paronychia and heartburn. At this point, on examination she had puffy fingers, sclerodactyly, a digital ulcer on the tip of the right second finger, digital pitting scars and a few telangiectasias on her fingers and face. Her laboratory investigations now showed a positive anticentromere antibody and a cine-esophagram confirmed distal esophageal hypomotility. She was started on long-acting nifedipine 30mg daily and instructed to soak her finger in warm antiseptic water twice a day, air-dry it, place antibiotic ointment on the ulcer and cover it with a bandage. She was given an antireflux program.

The patient returned 1 week later. Her finger was much more swollen, erythematous and purulent, and her heartburn was more severe. She began antibiotics and an H_2-blocker.

Diagnostic Problems

Finding a cause for Raynaud's phenomenon requires a knowledge of the patient's occupational, smoking and drug history (Fig. 40.18).

CLASSIFICATION OF RAYNAUD'S PHENOMENON
1. Primary – at least 2 years of symptoms with no apparent associated disease
2. Connective tissue disease
Systemic sclerosis with diffuse or limited cutaneous scleroderma Systemic lupus erythematosus Polymyositis/dermatomyositis Rheumatoid arthritis Overlaps
3. Occupation and trauma
Vibration, percussion Injury – crutch pressure
4. Thoracic outlet
Cervical rib Shoulder-girdle compression syndromes
5. Occlusive arterial disease
Accelerated atherosclerosis Berger's disease – thromboangiitis obliterans Thrombosis or embolism
6. Drugs or toxic substances
β-Blockers Ergot Oral contraceptives Bleomycin Polyvinyl chloride
7. Reflex sympathetic dystrophy
8. Hyperviscosity of the blood
Cryoglobulin Polycythemia Paraproteinemia

Fig. 40.17 Classification of Raynaud's phenomenon.

Information about the use of vibration tools (jackhammers, etc.), trauma (falls, crutches), amount of smoking and the use of drugs (β-blockers, ergot and oral contraceptives) may be very helpful. An examination should search for any abnormal findings but should particularly focus on the hands. A careful evaluation for decreased pulses, arthritis, swollen fingers, tendon friction rubs, nailfold capillary abnormalities (Fig. 40.19), telangiectasias, digital ulcers or digital pitting scars is very important (Fig. 40.20). Laboratory studies should include a blood count, ESR, liver function tests, serum protein electrophoresis, cryoglobulins and cholesterol, as well as ANA, anticentromere antibody and anti-Scl-70 antibody.

Patients with new onset of Raynaud's phenomenon have the greatest risk of having or developing another illness. Within the first 2 years after onset, as many as 60% of such patients will develop a connective tissue disease. Among the connective tissue diseases, systemic sclerosis has the highest frequency of Raynaud's (95%) and, as a consequence, is the most likely connective tissue disease to develop in patients with new-onset Raynaud's. Puffy, swollen hands or legs, arthralgias, carpal tunnel syndrome, tendon friction rubs, nailfold capillary abnormalities, a positive ANA or anti-Scl-70 (antitopoisomerase) antibody are findings that are strongly suggestive of early diffuse scleroderma.

After many years of 'primary' Raynaud's phenomenon, a much smaller percentage of patients (around 5%) will subsequently develop a connective tissue disease, and almost all of them will develop systemic sclerosis with limited scleroderma (CREST syndrome). Heartburn, puffy fingers, digital ulcers, digital pitting scars, abnormal nailfold capillaries, telangiectasias and an anticentromere antibody are often found in patients with undiagnosed limited scleroderma. At a later stage, when there are typical cutaneous findings of systemic sclerosis, a positive anticentromere antibody, pulmonary fibrosis on chest radiography or distal esophagus dysmotility can confirm the diagnosis. Raynaud's phenomenon is also present in approximately 20% of patients with SLE and polymyositis or dermatomyositis.

EVALUATION OF A PATIENT WITH RAYNAUD'S PHENOMENON			
History	Symptoms	Examination	Laboratory
Occupation	Rash	Peripheral pulses, bruits	Complete blood counts
Trauma	Arthralgias	Digital ulcers, digital pitting scars	Erythrocyte sedimentation rate
Smoking	Carpal tunnel	Nailfold capillary abnormalities	Cryoglobulins, protein electrophoresis
Drugs	Fatigue, fever, weakness	Puffy fingers, tendon friction rubs	Antinuclear antibody, anticentromere antibody, anti-Scl-70 antibody

Fig. 40.18 Evaluation of a patient with Raynaud's phenomenon.

Therapeutic Options

Mild uncomplicated Raynaud's phenomenon is usually relatively easy to control (Fig. 40.21). The most important instruction to the patient is complete abstinence from any smoking. It must be made clear that continuation of smoking could lead to digital loss. Any

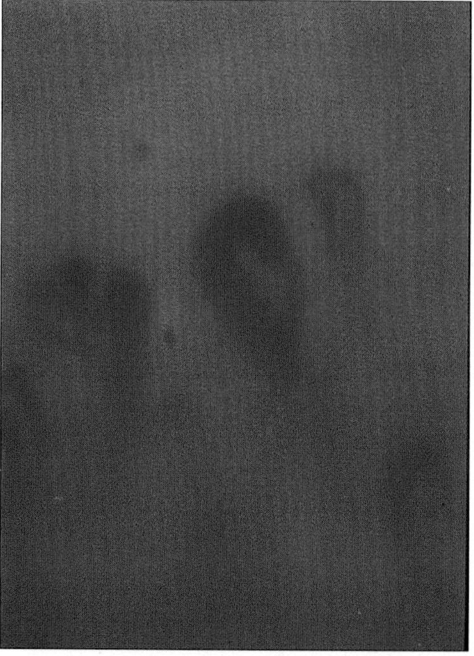

Fig. 40.19 Dilated nailfold capillary loops in Raynaud's phenomenon. Dilatation and dropout of capillaries might suggest eventual evolution to connective tissue disease.

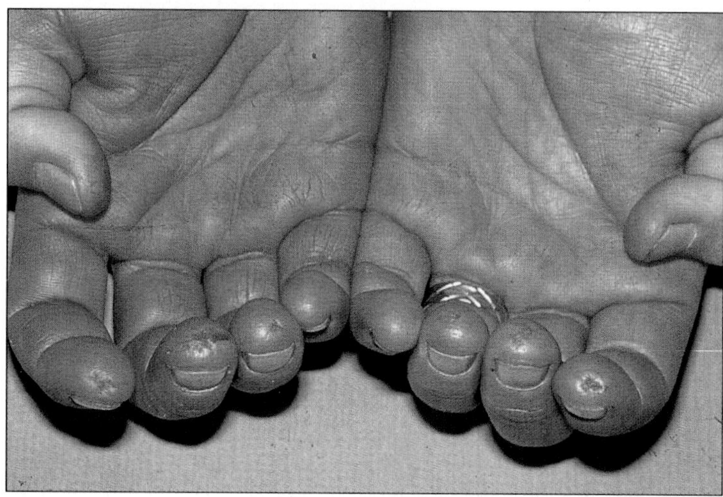

Fig. 40.20 Digital pitting scars and ulcers associated with complicated Raynaud's phenomenon and commonly seen in systemic sclerosis. These lesions are one of the main criteria for systemic sclerosis. Sclerodactyly and pulmonary interstitial fibrosis are the other two, and diagnosis of systemic sclerosis requires two of the three findings.

TREATMENT OF RAYNAUD'S PHENOMENON	
Mild	Complete abstinence from smoking Keep entire body warm (not just hands) Avoid cold exposure, particularly winter sports
Moderate	Nifedipine Prazoin Topical nitroglycerin
Digital ulcers	Maximal doses of calcium channel blockers 'Occlusive' dressing: soak in antiseptic liquid, air dry, apply antibiotic ointment, bandage
Acute ischemia	Sympathetic blocks Prostaglandin E_1 or prostacyclin (when available) Microvascular surgery Digital sympathectomy
Gangrenous, infected ulcers	Antibiotics Adequate pain control Surgical debridement Amputation (last resort)

Fig. 40.21 Treatment of Raynaud's phenomenon.

offending drugs should be discontinued if possible. Avoidance of the cold and abrupt changes in temperature is necessary.

Use of insulated gloves and hand warmers, and avoidance of outdoor winter sports and of air-conditioned public areas, are often helpful. An acceptable workplace environment may be a particular problem, and patients may have to make specific arrangements with employers.

If these simple measures are inadequate, institution of nifedipine 30mg (up to 90mg) daily is helpful. Use of the long-acting preparation is better tolerated but may be less effective than the three times a day dose. If fluid retention, light-headedness or heartburn occurs then any of the other calcium-channel blockers can be tried. Alternatively, a mild diuretic may alleviate edema, and an H_2-receptor blocker may counteract the increased reflux that nifedipine causes by decreasing the lower esophageal sphincter muscle tone. Prazosin and topical nitroglycerin have been helpful for some patients.

When digital ulcers appear, they are extremely painful and usually take weeks or months to completely heal. Maximum doses of calcium-channel blockers should be used. Patients often find a heating pad on their arm or hand is helpful. An 'occlusive' dressing, which promotes wound healing as well as preventing minor trauma, can be simply applied. The finger with the ulcer is soaked in tepid antiseptic liquid, for example half-strength hydrogen peroxide, twice a day to soften or loosen the crust or eschar. After air-drying, an antibiotic ointment is placed on the ulcer alone, avoiding the surrounding tissue. It is then covered with a bandage. Duoderm, an occlusive dressing, can be used on uninfected ulcers. Ketanserin, an antiserotonin agent, is particularly helpful in healing ulcers.

An acutely ischemic finger that threatens to become gangrenous requires more aggressive treatment. Sympathetic blocks, an arteriogram searching for a lesion amenable to microvascular hand surgery, intra-arterial phentolamine or prostaglandin E_1, intravenous prostacyclin or digital sympathectomy may be required in an effort to maintain blood flow to the finger. Arteriograms in systemic sclerosis usually show an impressive paucity of digital vessels, but primary Raynaud's may look similar when vasospasm is present.

Increasing pain, erythema, swelling or purulence suggest that the ulcer has become infected. Cultures usually demonstrate *Staphylococcus,* so dicloxicillin or cephalosporins are usually effective. Infected or gangrenous digits may require surgical debridement or amputation. The latter should be avoided until there is evidence of how much of the digit is viable, so that a single procedure can be done.

Pain control is an important part of the therapy of ischemic digital ulcers because pain can lead to additional vasospasm and more ischemia. At times, narcotic pain medication may be necessary to control symptoms adequately. Raynaud's phenomenon and resulting digital ischemia are often difficult to manage and each patient's response to therapy is different. If one approach is ineffective, an alternative should be tried.

REFERENCES

Belch JJF. Raynaud's phenomenon: its relevance to scleroderma. Ann Rheum Dis. 1991;**50**:839–45.

Cardelli MB, Kleinsmith DM. Raynaud's phenomenon and diseases. Med Clin North Am. 1989;**73**:1127–41.

Clifford PC, Martin MFR, Sheddon MF, Kirby JD, Baird RN, Dieppe PA. Treatment of vasospastic disease with prostaglandin E1. Br Med J. 1980;**281**:1031–4.

Gerbracht DD, Steen VD, Ziegler GL, Medsger TA Jr, Rodnan GP. Evolution of primary Raynaud's phenomenon (Raynaud's disease) to connective tissue disease. Arthritis Rheum. 1985;**28**:87–92.

Jay D, Coffman MD, Clement DL, et al. International study of ketanserin in Raynaud's phenomenon. Am J Med. 1989;87:264–8.

Rodeeheffer RJ, Rommer JA, Wigley F, Smith CR. Controlled double-blind trial of nifedipine in the treatment of Raynaud's phenomenon. N Engl J Med. 1983;**308**:880–3.

Yardumian DA, Isenberg DA, Rustin M, et al. Successful treatment of Raynaud's syndrome with iloprost, a chemically stable prostacyclin analogue. Br J Rheumatol. 1988;**27**:220–6.

SCLERODERMA RENAL CRISIS

Virginia D Steen

Definition of the Problem

Scleroderma renal crisis has gone from being a virtually untreatable complication to being one that can often be treated with little or no residual renal dysfunction. However, it is imperative that the diagnosis and treatment of renal crisis is made at the first opportunity. Angiotensin-converting enzyme (ACE) inhibitors must be aggressively used to prevent permanent renal damage.

The Typical Case

CD was a 34-year-old woman with a 6-month history of Raynaud's phenomenon, polyarthralgias and swollen fingers. On examination, her blood pressure was 110/70mmHg and tendon friction rubs were present in her ankles. Her hands and legs were very edematous and she had skin thickening to her elbows. A diagnosis of systemic sclerosis with early diffuse scleroderma was made and she was started on D-penicillamine. Three months later, at a routine visit, her blood pressure was 140/90mmHg and skin thickening had progressed to the mid upper arm. A hematocrit of 30% (previously 36%), a platelet count of 85,000/mm^3 and a urinalysis with 1+ protein and 5–10 red blood cells per high-power field were found. Given the possibility of D-penicillamine toxicity she was told to stop the D-penicillamine. Two weeks later she began to feel poorly, developed shortness of breath and was admitted to the hospital. Blood pressure was still 140/90mmHg, but the hematocrit was now 20%, platelet count 40,000/mm^3 and serum creatinine 4.1mg/dl. A reticulocyte count was 18% and microangiopathic hemolysis was noted on the smear. Congestive heart failure and hemoptysis led to intubation and respiratory support. Scleroderma renal crisis was diagnosed and an ACE inhibitor was started. Over the next 2 days her blood pressure remained around 130/80mmHg but renal function deteriorated further. The decline was felt to be from the ACE inhibitor, which was discontinued; when further deterioration in

FACTORS ASSOCIATED WITH SCLERODERMA RENAL CRISIS	
Predictive of SRC	Not predictive of SRC
Early disease Diffuse scleroderma Rapid progression of skin thickening New anemia New cardiac events pericardial effusion congestive heart failure Possibly high-dose steroids (normotensive)	Blood pressure Urinalysis Serum creatinine Plasma renin activity Pathologic abnormalities in renal blood vessels Anti-Scl-70 (in diffuse scleroderma patients)

Fig. 40.22 Factors associated with scleroderma renal crisis (SRC).

FEATURES OF SCLERODERMA RENAL CRISIS
Accelerated arterial hypertension – more than 170/130mmHg in 30%; normotensive renal crisis in 11%
Rapidly progressive renal failure – creatinine increases daily
Plasma renin activity increased – 90%of cases are greater than twice normal
Microangiopathic hemolytic anemia, and thrombocytopenia in almost 50% of patients
Congestive heart failure and asymptomatic pericardial effusions – common
Dyspnea, headache, funduscopic changes, seizures, abnormal urinalysis – variable in occurrence

Fig. 40.23 Features of scleroderma renal crisis.

renal function occurred, the ACE inhibitor was restarted but she progressed to renal failure requiring hemodialysis.

Over the next 9 months, she continued to take an ACE inhibitor, maintaining a normal blood pressure. At that point, she began to make urine, renal function improved and she was able to discontinue dialysis 1 year after the initial diagnosis of renal crisis. Her present creatinine is 2.4mg/dl.

Diagnostic Problems

Patients with rapidly progressive diffuse scleroderma early in their disease course are at greatest risk for renal crisis (Fig. 40.22). In addition, new anemia or heart disease may predict the development of renal crisis, but in patients with diffuse scleroderma, the presence of anti-Scl-70 (antitopoisomerase) antibody does not. Patients with longstanding diffuse scleroderma can develop this problem, but it occurs much less frequently. Less than 1% of patients with limited scleroderma develop typical renal crisis.

Patients with early diffuse scleroderma should be carefully educated that the symptoms of headache, visual changes, worsening fatigue, shortness of breath or malaise may indicate kidney involvement. They are encouraged to use a home blood-pressure cuff and to take their blood pressure weekly or at times when they have symptoms. They should be taught what their normal blood pressure is and what level they should be concerned about: a borderline elevated blood pressure for one person may actually be unacceptably high for someone who is normally 110/70mmHg. The diagnosis of renal crisis is fairly easy when malignant hypertension, microangiopathic hemolytic anemia, and azotemia are all present in a patient with early diffuse scleroderma (Fig. 40.23). However, many patients do not have microangiopathic hemolytic anemia, and early in the course azotemia may not be present. In 11% of patients with renal crisis, the blood pressure remains in normal range. The diagnosis of normotensive renal crisis depends on the presence of a microangiopathic peripheral blood smear, elevated plasma renin activity and azotemia. There are some patients who have such early disease that they have not yet developed diffuse skin changes. Some may not even have Raynaud's phenomenon. The diagnosis of systemic sclerosis and renal crisis in such patients is very difficult. Diffusely swollen hands or lower extremities, carpal tunnel syndrome, tendon friction rubs, nailfold capillary abnormalities and the presence of anti-Scl-70 could all support the diagnosis of scleroderma.

It is interesting that in the case described the microangiopathic hemolytic anemia and thrombocytopenia were seen on a routine D-penicillamine toxicity check but were not recognized as suggesting renal crisis. Any new anemia or thrombocytopenia, even if there are obvious explanations, should prompt further evaluation for impending renal crisis. The most important factor is early recognition and diagnosis, so that early intervention can occur.

Therapy

Treatment with an ACE inhibitor for scleroderma renal crisis should be started as soon as the diagnosis is made (Fig. 40.24). Prior to the availability of this family of drugs, renal crisis almost always resulted in renal failure and/or death. The blood pressure could rarely be controlled with other agents. Plasmapheresis, steroids and immunosuppressives have no effect and can only aggravate the illness via infections, further hypertension or access problems. Institution of ACE inhibitors and rapid control of blood pressure, preferably within the first 3 days, is extremely important to preserve renal function. Renal function often deteriorates after starting ACE inhibitors even though the blood pressure has normalized. Although this deterioration could be attributed to the ACE inhibitors, generally this reaction does not occur in scleroderma patients. Continuation of the ACE inhibitors is the best chance the patient has for recovery.

Short-acting ACE inhibitors provide more flexibility in dosing changes, especially in initial attempts to normalize the blood pressure. Longer acting ACE inhibitors can easily be substituted for patient convenience or in the case of allergic reactions. Other antihypertensive agents may be added when ACE inhibitors are inadequate to control the blood pressure. In normotensive renal crisis, the highest ACE inhibitor dose that maintains normal blood pressure should be used.

Supportive care, including transfusions and treatment for congestive heart failure, is often necessary. Hemodialysis and peritoneal dialysis can be adequately performed, although vascular access and peritoneal clearance may be problems. Renal transplants are well tolerated. However, half of the patients who stay on dialysis for at least 3 months are able to completely discontinue dialysis 5–18 months later if they continue on an ACE inhibitor. Thus, a hopeful attitude can be used with these patients and transplant plans should be held off at least a year. Older age in men, a serum creatinine greater than 3mg/dl at the time of the initiation of an ACE inhibitor, control of blood pressure taking more than 3 days and congestive heart failure are all factors that are associated with a poor outcome.

There are no studies yet to determine if 'prophylactic' ACE inhibitors are helpful in preventing renal crisis. Hypotension should

MANAGEMENT OF SCLERODERMA RENAL CRISIS
Early diagnosis and treatment
Angiotensin-converting enzyme (ACE) inhibitors Normalize blood pressure
Continue ACE inhibitors even if renal dysfunction progresses
Dialysis (hemodialysis and peritoneal dialysis) if needed Steroids and plasmapheresis are *not* indicated
50% of patients requiring 3 months of dialysis can discontinue dialysis in ≤18 months

Fig. 40.24 Management of scleroderma renal crisis.

be avoided as it may actually precipitate renal crisis. Any hint of hypertension, even if not associated with any other findings, should be treated with ACE inhibitors, particularly in patients at high risk of developing renal crisis. Recognizing the presence of scleroderma renal crisis and aggressively treating it with ACE inhibitors saves lives and can prevent renal failure.

REFERENCES

Helfrich DJ, Banner B, Steen VD, Medsger TA Jr. Renal failure in normotensive patients with systemic sclerosis. Arthritis Rheum. 1989;**32**:1128–34.

Steen VD, Medsger TA Jr, Osial TA Jr, Ziegler GL, Shapiro AP, Rodnan GP. Factors predicting the development of renal involvement in progressive systemic sclerosis. Am J Med. 1984;**76**:779–86.

Steen VD, Costantino JP, Shapiro AP, Medsger TA Jr. Outcome of renal crisis in systemic sclerosis: relation to availability of converting enzyme (ACE) inhibitors. Ann Intern Med. 1990;**113**:352–7.

Steen VD, Medsger TA Jr. Scleroderma renal crisis. In: Furst D, ed. Management of critically ill patients with rheumatologic and immunologic diseases. New York: Marcel Dekker Inc.;1993.

PROXIMAL WEAKNESS OF UNKNOWN ETIOLOGY

Robert L Wortmann

Definition of the Problem

Proximal muscle weakness is the cardinal manifestation of a muscle disease. Sometimes this form of weakness is the sole complaint. In some instances, weakness is associated with other symptoms of myopathic processes, including exercise intolerance, premature fatigue, myalgia, or postexertional aches and cramps. Occasionally, these latter problems bring the patient to the physician and the weakness is discerned only on careful examination. Regardless of the presentation, the causes of this problem should be investigated.

The Typical Case

A 28-year-old male presented with a chief complaint of weakness in his arms and legs that had developed and become gradually more severe over 4 months. He was still able to work as a custodian, but was having increasing difficulty with activities that required him to work with his arms lifted or extended and with climbing stairs. He had little trouble walking on level ground and had no difficulty using his hands. A thorough review of systems was not helpful. He had no systemic symptoms such as fever, malaise or weight loss. Significantly, he had had no skin rash, sicca symptoms, mucosal ulcers, hoarseness, difficulty swallowing, cough, hemoptysis, chest pain, heartburn, diarrhea, dark or wine-colored urine, symptoms of synovitis, seizures, diplopia, paresthesias, or fasciculations. He was using no drugs, medications or nutritional supplements. He had no known allergies. He was a moderate beer drinker. His past medical history revealed no previous hospitalizations, surgery or injuries. He had no children and was not aware of similar problems or muscle disease in relatives. His physical examination was entirely normal except for minimal symmetric weakness of the shoulder and pelvic girdle musculature. There was no atrophy or fasciculation. The cranial nerves were intact, sensation was normal and reflexes were equal.

Normal laboratory results included a sedimentation rate, complete blood count, urinalysis, creatinine, sodium, potassium, calcium, phosphorus, magnesium, thyroid function studies, serum glutamic oxaloacetic transminase (SGOT), lactate dehydrogenase (LDH), and aldolase. The ANA test was negative and the creatine phosphokinase (CPK) minimally elevated at 265 units (normal is less than 200 units). An electrodiagnostic evaluation performed on the right side of the body revealed normal nerve conduction velocities. Electromyography (EMG) showed normal insertional activity and no spontaneous activity. Some motor unit potentials in the deltoid, trapezius and quadriceps had reduced amplitude and short duration. These findings were interpreted to be consistent with a mild, nonspecific myopathic process.

Histology of muscle obtained using the percutaneous needle technique from the left vastus lateralis revealed no evidence of inflammation or fiber necrosis. There was, however, some variation in fiber size. The biopsy was interpreted as showing a nonspecific abnormality.

Diagnostic Problems

The problems of evaluating patients with proximal muscle weakness are two-fold. First, the list of possible causes is so long (Fig. 40.25). Second, the tests available to search for the cause are nonspecific in nature and are, by themselves, rarely diagnostic. However, if one appreciates the wide variety of potential causes and uses the tests available in a systematic fashion, then a diagnosis is usually obtained.

History

A thorough history may be the most useful means of making the diagnosis. This is true for any clinical situation, but must be emphasized for this particular problem because of the numerous diagnostic possibilities in a case of proximal muscle weakness. For example, a history of photosensitivity, mouth ulcers or pleurisy might indicate lupus, or a history of abdominal cramping or diarrhea might point toward a disease that causes malabsorption and an

POTENTIAL CAUSES OF PROXIMAL MUSCLE WEAKNESS

Collagen–vascular	Neurologic
Polymyositis Dermatomyositis Inclusion body myositis Polymyalgia rheumatica Temporal arteritis Systemic lupus erythematosus Scleroderma Sjögren's syndrome Mixed connective tissue disease Polyarteritis nodosa Rheumatoid arthritis Wegener's granulomatosis	Myasthenia gravis Amyotropic lateral sclerosis Muscular dystrophy Guillain–Barré syndrome Periodic paralysis
	Toxic (drug-related)
	Alcohol Chloroquine Clofibrate Cocaine Colchicine Corticosteroids Lovastatin Penicillamine Zidovudine (AZT)
Metabolic (primary)	
Glycogen storage disease (McArdle's disease) Lipid storage disease (carnitine deficiency) Myoadenylate deaminase deficiency Mitochondrial myopathies	
	Cancer-related
	Carcinomatous neuromyopathy Microembolization Myositis Eaton–Lambert syndrome Carcinoid
Metabolic (endocrine/nutritional)	**Infectious**
Any cause of abnormal electrolytes (elevated or decreased sodium, potassium, calcium, phosphorus, or magnesium) Hypo- or hyperthyroidism Cushing's syndrome Addison's disease Aldosteronism Uremia Hepatic failure Porphyria	Viruses (influenza, coxsackie) Toxoplasmosis *Trichinella* *Rickettsia* Bacterial toxins (staphylococcal, streptococcal, clostridial)

Fig. 40.25 Potential causes of proximal muscle weakness.

electrolyte imbalance. If, on the other hand, the etiology of the weakness is not clear on initial evaluation, it is critical to repeat a detailed system review, medication history and social history. Information concerning alcohol use or a complaint previously considered unimportant may prove critical.

Physical examination

Even when the abnormalities on physical examination are insufficient to make a specific diagnosis, they may help determine whether the cause of the weakness is the result of a disorder of muscle function (myopathic) or a problem involving nerve function (neuropathic). Myopathic conditions, including the inflammatory diseases of muscle, typically affect proximal muscles in a symmetric distribution. Shoulder and hip girdles are weak, but distal strength is normal. The remainder of the neurologic examination is normal. In contrast, neuropathic processes may cause distal as well as proximal weakness, may be asymmetric, and may be associated with other neurologic changes, such as abnormal reflexes, abnormal sensation, rigidity or fasciculation. Inclusion body myositis provides an exception to this basic rule. Individuals with that inflammatory disease of muscle may have neuropathic as well as myopathic findings. The physical examination should also be used to determine the severity of weakness as objectively as possible. This establishes a baseline, and serial assessments can then be used to determine disease progression or response to therapy.

Laboratory studies

High CPK levels are not diagnostically specific and a normal CPK does not rule out muscle pathology. The majority of elevated serum CPK levels result from muscle necrosis or leaking membranes. Inflammatory or hypoxic injury, blunt trauma and sharp trauma (intramuscular injections, EMG needle insertion, muscle biopsy) are well-recognized causes of high CPK levels. Isometric and aerobic exercise can also produce elevated CPK levels, especially in poorly conditioned individuals. Furthermore, morphine, benzodiazepine and barbiturate use may elevate the serum CPK levels by retarding the elimination of the enzyme from the circulation. Racial differences are found for the normal values of CPK, with healthy asymptomatic Black males having higher levels than Whites or Hispanics. Thus, an isolated CPK value should be interpreted with caution, because spurious elevations may result from physical exertion, muscle trauma, intramuscular injection, EMG testing or the use of certain medications.

Measurements of serum electrolytes is essential in the work-up of muscle weakness because any process that increases or decreases the concentrations of sodium, potassium, calcium, phosphorus or magnesium can cause this problem. Fasting concentrations of pyruvate and lactate may be useful if one suspects certain mitochondrial myopathies.

Circulating autoantibodies can be detected in the serum in a large number of patients with inflammatory myopathies. ANA testing may be positive at low titers in about half the patients with polymyositis, 60% of children with childhood dermatomyositis, and the majority of patients with an associated collagen vascular disease. In the latter cases, patients may also have autoantibodies more specific for those diseases. For example, anti-Sm, and anti-dsDNA antibodies are present in SLE; anti-Ro/La antibodies in Sjögren's syndrome; anti-Scl-70 and anticentromere antibodies in scleroderma and CREST syndrome; and anti-RNP in mixed connective tissue disease.

Electromyography

The characteristic findings in myopathic disorders include individual motor unit potentials (MUPs) of decreased duration and smaller amplitude and increased numbers of polyphasic potentials. Inflammatory myopathies cause changes that tend to be scattered in distribution and variable in character, but most prominent in the proximal muscles and paraspinal muscles. Earlier in the disease, low- amplitude MUPs of short duration and spontaneous fibrillation potentials are observed. The spontaneous fibrillations often fire at a slower rate than those seen in neuropathic disorders. Over time, MUPs tend to become more polyphasic and more 'positive waves' are present within the fibrillation potentials.

The EMG features of primary metabolic myopathies are quite variable. Many patients may, in fact, have relatively normal studies. Patients with McArdle's disease (myophosphorylase deficiency) or carnitine deficiency may have so-called 'myopathic' MUPs and some fibrillations, occasionally limited to the paraspinal muscles. Neuropathic disorders are characterized by denervation and reinnervation. These processes result in spontaneous activity, including fibrillation potential and positive waves, and polyphasic MUPs of large amplitude and long duration. Biphasic MUPs of large amplitude and small duration are produced by denervated motor units, whereas polyphasic MUPs of long duration result from asynchronous firing of scattered reinnervated fibers.

Forearm ischemic exercise test

The forearm ischemic exercise test (Fig. 40.26) is used in screening for various metabolic myopathies, including the recognized glycogen storage diseases (except acid maltase deficiency) and myoadenylate deaminase deficiency. Although these diseases are rare, the primary metabolic myopathies must be considered in the case of muscle weakness of unknown etiology. The normal response to forearm ischemic exercise is at least a three-fold rise over baseline for lactate and ammonia. In individuals with a glycogen storage disease, the ammonia level normally increases but lactate levels remain at baseline. On the other hand, in myoadenylate deaminase deficiency, lactate levels increase but ammonia levels do not. The forearm ischemic exercise test is an effective screening test provided the patient exercises vigorously. A submaximal exercise effort, whether due to pain, weakness or malingering, can cause a false-positive result. Therefore, failure to generate lactate or ammonia after ischemic exercise does not assure the diagnosis of the particular enzyme deficiency. Any abnormal result should be confirmed with the appropriate enzyme analysis.

Muscle biopsy

Tissue examination is invaluable in assessing myopathic conditions. Unfortunately, a specific diagnosis can be made only in cases of an enzyme deficiency state. Too often the histologic changes are simply too nonspecific. One should not expect the pathologist to solve difficult clinical problems. Four types of evaluation can be performed on skeletal muscle: histology, histochemistry, electron microscopy, and assays of enzyme activities or other constituents. These studies

FOREARM ISCHEMIC EXERCISE TESTING
Venous blood for lactate and ammonia is drawn from the nondominant arm without use of a tourniquet
Sphygmomanometer cuff is inflated to 20–30mmHg above systolic pressure around dominant upper arm
Dominant hand and forearm exercise vigorously by repeatedly squeezing ball or grip strength device every 1–2s for 2 min*
Cuff is deflated and blood samples for lactate and ammonia are drawn from dominant arm 2 min later
*Many normal people can only exercise for 90s under these conditions if they give a maximum effort This exercise may cause pain or discomfort that is relieved immediately by removal of the cuff

Fig. 40.26 Forearm ischemic exercise testing.

should be employed in a logical sequence designed for each patient. They should not be ordered in a 'shotgun' fashion hoping to find 'something'. The technique for the biopsy depends upon which tests are to be done. If histology only is required, a percutaneous needle biopsy may prove satisfactory. On the other hand, if all four evaluations are desired, an open technique is preferred.

The site of the biopsy should be selected carefully. A proximal muscle is preferred for the evaluation of myopathic problems. Ideally the area selected should be actively involved with the process, but the most severely involved area should be avoided. Severely damaged muscle is often too necrotic or scarred for meaningful interpretation. An EMG is usually helpful in localizing the site for biopsy. However, EMG needles can traumatize the muscle. Since the distribution of most myopathies is symmetric, it is best to perform the electromyography on one side of the body and take the biopsy from the identified site on the opposite side. Infiltration of the muscle with local anesthesia must also be avoided.

Hematoxylin and eosin and modified Gomori's trichrome stains are used for most histology. A wide variety of stains are used for histochemistry. Fiber type specificity and distribution can be determined using ATPase stains. Succinic dehydrogenase and NADH are oxidative enzymes and may be useful for identifying mitochondrial myopathies. Periodic acid–Schiff stains for glycogen and oil red O stains for lipid. Staining with these reagents may be increased in the respective storage diseases. However, abnormal accumulation of glycogen or lipid is not specific for storage diseases. Enzyme deficiency states may be identified with appropriate histochemical stains but are best diagnosed by subjecting the tissue protein to assays for the specific enzyme activity. Ultrastructural analysis by electron microscopy is clearly more sensitive than light microscopy for identifying abnormal glycogen or lipid deposition. This technique will also show characteristic changes in cases of inclusion body myositis, and increased numbers or altered morphology of mitochondria in mitochrondrial myopathies.

Conclusion

Proximal muscle weakness can be a difficult problem to deal with until its etiology is determined. Recognition of the nonspecificity of serum CPK levels, EMG findings and biopsy results is important in the approach to this problem. Sometimes the etiology of the weakness is quite elusive. This may be because it is caused by a rare, poorly appreciated disease or by one that evolves very slowly. Careful and repeated evaluation using the tools available to assess skeletal muscle function should eventually provide a diagnosis.

REFERENCES

Engel AG, Banker BQ. General approaches to muscle diseases. In: Engel AG, Banker BQ, eds. Myology. 1E. New York: McGraw-Hill; 1986:811–1151.

Kagen LJ. Approach to the patient with myopathy. Bull Rheum Dis. 1983;**33**:1–8.

Knochel JP. Neuromuscular manifestations of electrolyte disorders. Am J Med. 1982;**72**:521–35.

Wolf PL. Abnormalities in serum enzymes in skeletal muscle diseases. Am J Clin Pathol. 1991;**95**:402–7.

Wortmann RL. Inflammatory diseases of muscle. In: Kelley W, Harris E, Ruddy S, Sledge C, eds. Textbook of rheumatology. 4E. Philadelphia: WB Saunders; 1993:1159–88.

Wortmann RL. Metabolic diseases of muscle. In: McCarty D, Koopman W, eds. Arthritis and allied conditions. 12E. Philadelphia: Lea & Febiger; 1993:1895–1912.

POLYMYOSITIS AND MALIGNANCY

Harry Spiera

Definition of the Problem

In the initial evaluation of a patient with polymyositis/dermatomyositis, the physician must decide the extent of the evaluation to search for an occult neoplasm. Patients with dermatomyositis and, to a lesser extent, polymyositis have a higher incidence of malignancy than expected in the general population. As a result of this, many clinicians have considered it as part of the work-up of patients with polymyositis/dermatomyositis, to search for an occult neoplasm.

The Typical Case

A 36-year-old woman, who was previously in good health, complained of the onset of fatigue, aching in her joints, and difficulty rising from a chair, climbing stairs and getting out of a bathtub. She had trouble combing her hair and difficulty in initiating the swallowing mechanism, with food occasionally 'going down the wrong pipe'. There had been no joint swelling, Raynaud's phenomenon or fever. Her appetite was poor, and she had no bowel or urinary problems. She had noted a rash on her face, chest wall and hands.

On physical examination, the blood pressure was 118/78. The pulse was 86/min and regular and the temperature was 36.9°C. There was an erythematous rash in the V-area of her neck, over the extensor surfaces of her elbows and knees, and there were Gottron's patches over her knuckles. There was no heliotrope. There was muscle weakness involving the neck flexors and extensors, the shoulder, and hip girdles, with atrophy of the upper arms and thighs. There was no synovitis. There was some capillary dilatation and drop-out about the nail beds. There was also periungual erythema. The rest of the physical examination, including careful examination of the breasts and a pelvic and rectal examination, revealed no abnormalities.

Laboratory examination revealed a normal, complete blood count. The ESR was 42mm/hour (Westergren), the CPK was 7800 units, of which 100% was MM, and the aldolase was 24.5 units. The SGOT was 76 and the SGPT 98 units. The rest of the biochemical tests, including bilirubin and alkaline phosphatase, were normal. The rheumatoid factor was negative. The ANA was positive, with a titer of 1:80 with a speckled pattern. The anti-RNP was negative. Examination of the stool on three separate occasions revealed no evidence of blood. Urinalysis was negative for protein. There were 0–1 white blood cells per high-power field, but no red blood cells. A chest radiograph was normal.

An EMG showed an increase in the insertional activity of the muscle with numerous fibrillation potentials and positive sharp waves at rest. The motor units showed decreased amplitude and duration and increased polyphasic potentials.

Muscle biopsy performed on the side of the body where an EMG was not done revealed an infiltrate of lymphocytes and plasma cells in the muscle, and perimysial tissues with an occasional polymorphonuclear leukocyte. There was necrosis of muscle fibers with phagocytosis and regeneration.

The Diagnostic Problem

The typical picture of dermatomyositis is muscle weakness and a characteristic skin rash, with laboratory findings consistent with muscle destruction, and both electrodiagnostic studies and muscle biopsy confirming the findings of dermatomyositis. The routine chest radiograph is normal, stool examination for occult blood is negative, breast and pelvic examination reveal no abnormalities, and urinalysis is negative. The question is whether such a patient, in addition to being started on treatment for dermatomyositis, should be subjected to a careful search for a tumor.

Personal experiences have prompted me to undertake further investigations. I have seen a patient with a presentation similar to the one described, who had a hypernephroma that was totally asymptomatic and had no associated hematuria. Another young patient with a normal chest radiograph was found on CT scan of the chest to have Hodgkin's disease, and another had carcinoma of the colon, though her stool examinations for blood were negative. Another young woman, who did not have a mammogram as part of an initial evaluation, developed an inflammatory carcinoma within a few months of the onset of her rapidly progressive dermatomyositis. There are many more such observations, both in my personal experience and in the medical literature.

It is therefore my practice to investigate such a patient for occult malignancy. In addition to the routine examinations previously noted, I would advocate CT scan of the chest and abdomen, a barium enema, an upper-gastrointestinal tract series, as well as a sonogram of the pelvis and a mammogram. The total cost of these studies amounts to approximately US$2000 (1993 values). It would seem that this expenditure in a disease that has a low prevalence would be justified if in even only a small proportion could carcinoma be found at a curable stage. To date, no prospective study has been done comparing patients in whom a search for neoplasm is done and those in whom a search is not done.

Criticisms of the past studies indicating a relationship between polymyositis/dermatomyositis and malignancy have been related to the small size of the study groups and the lack of uniform criteria for the diagnosis of polymyositis/dermatomyositis. To some extent, this has been resolved by results of a study from Sweden, in which 788 patients hospitalized for polymyositis/dermatomyositis were analyzed. In this study, it was demonstrated that patients with polymyositis had a somewhat higher risk of cancer than the general population. Patients with dermatomyositis, however, had a substantially increased risk of cancer that was indeed accompanied by an increased mortality from cancer.

Conclusions

All patients with dermatomyositis/polymyositis should undergo a work-up for neoplasia, with only the following exceptions:

- children, in whom cancer is infrequent;
- patients in whom polymyositis complicates SLE, scleroderma, mixed connective tissue disease or rheumatoid arthritis, as no increased incidence of malignancy has been found in these patients.

REFERENCES

Barnes B. Dermatomyositis and malignancy: a review of the literature. Ann Intern Med. 1976;**84**:68–76.

Schulman P, Kerr LD, Spiera H. A re-examination of the relationship between myositis and malignancy. J Rheumatol. 1991;**18**:1689–92.

Sigurgeirsson B, Lindelof B, Edhag O, Allander E. Risk of cancer in patients with dermatomyositis or polymyositis: a population based study. N Engl J Med. 1992;**326**:363–7.

MONONEURITIS MULTIPLEX

David B Hellmann

Definition of the Problem

Mononeuritis multiplex is a distinctive peripheral neuropathy characterized by acute damage first to one named nerve root, and then, one at a time, to one or more other nerve roots. The usual cause is nerve infarction resulting from widespread destruction of epineural arterioles by vasculitis, diabetes or other conditions (Fig. 40.27). Mononeuritis multiplex develops in nearly two-thirds of patients with polyarteritis nodosa (PAN), and in a significant minority of patients with SLE or rheumatoid arthritis (RA). When systemic vasculitis causes mononeuritis multiplex, the patient almost always has some other systemic signs or symptoms, such as weight loss, fever or arthralgia. Indeed, the combination of mononeuritis multiplex and any other systemic feature is often one of the earliest and most specific bedside clues that a patient has systemic vasculitis.

CAUSES OF MONONEURITIS MULTIPLEX
Common
Diabetes Multiple compressions Connective tissue diseases (e.g. systemic lupus erythematosus, rheumatoid arthritis Sjögren's syndrome, scleroderma, cryoglobulinemia, sarcoidosis) Systemic vasculitis (e.g. polyarteritis nodosa with or without hepatitis B, Wegener's granulomatosis, lymphomatoid granulomatosis, giant cell arteritis) Nonsystemic vasculitic neuropathy
Rare
Infectious diseases (e.g. hepatitis A, Lyme disease, acquired immunodeficiency syndrome, trichinosis, leprosy, *Mycoplasma pneumoniae*, malaria, leptospirosis) Malignancy paraneoplastic syndrome with carcinoma, angioimmunoblastic lymphadenopathy Other hypereosinophilic syndrome cholesterol embolization graft-versus-host disease morphea jellyfish stings

Fig. 40.27 Causes of mononeuritis multiplex.

The Typical Case

Six months ago, JP, a previously healthy 67-year-old man, developed a tingling sensation over the dorsum of the left foot. Over the next three weeks he noted left foot drop, right foot numbness, fever, malaise, polymyalgia and polyarthralgia. Two months later he noted painful paresthesia and weakness, first in the left hand and then in the right. Subsequently, he lost 10kg, stumbled frequently because of the foot drop, dropped tools because his grip had weakened, and slept fitfully because of fever and painful paresthesia.

He appeared chronically ill, with a blood pressure of 172/104mmHg and a temperature of 38.6°C. He had livedo reticularis over the thighs and wasting of the interosseous muscles of the left hand and the thenar muscles of the right hand. He was unable to dorsiflex the left foot. He had decreased pin-prick sensation over the dorsum of the left foot, the plantar aspect of the right foot, the palmar aspect of the 4th and 5th fingers of the left hand, and the palmar aspect of the first three fingers of the right hand. The hematocrit was 27%, the ESR 121mm/hour, the serum creatinine 2.1mg/dl, and the urinalysis showed 2+ protein, and 5–10 RBC/hpf (×400) with red blood cell casts. A test for hepatitis B surface antigen was positive. Electroneurologic testing revealed an axonal neuropathy involving the left peroneal, right tibial, left ulnar and right median nerves. A renal arteriogram showing microaneurysms in the renal and hepatic circulation confirmed PAN.

With prednisone, cyclophosphamide and physical therapy, the patient felt better, his fever resolved and he gained weight. Three months later, the neurologic deficits in the hands had resolved, and those in the feet had improved.

Diagnostic Problems

How does the physician diagnose mononeuritis multiplex?

The key is recognizing that the patient's symptoms and deficits developed sequentially and in the distribution of named nerve roots. With most other peripheral neuropathies, deficits begin in both hands or both feet simultaneously. With mononeuritis multiplex, however, the deficits develop in one nerve at a time. The patient described above was typical in noting that the left foot was affected weeks before the right.

Deep muscle discomfort in the proximal portion of the extremity may herald by hours or a day the onset of more distal deficits, which reach maximal severity over hours to a few days. Because of the abrupt and painful onset, many patients will recall the day or the week the neuropathy began. Virtually all patients will have sensory abnormalities, chiefly painful paresthesia. A third will also have motor deficits, which can range from mild weakness (e.g. decreased hand grip) to complete loss of movement (e.g. foot drop). Hyperesthesia is often so marked that the patient cannot tolerate having the affected area touched.

Although the lesions can occur anywhere in the peripheral nervous system, the favored sites are the lower extremities (40% of cases), the upper extremities (30%) or both (20%). Given the predilection for the peroneal, tibial, median and ulnar nerves (Fig. 40.28), deficits are usually more marked distally than proximally. Thoracic or cranial nerve root involvement is less common. Characteristically, the lesions are asymmetric. Even late in the course, when the deficits may be bilateral, asymmetry of the lesions is still detectable. The patient described, for example, eventually had bilateral hand involvement but his symptoms involved different areas (nerves) of each hand. Thus, neurologic symptoms that develop sequentially and distribute themselves asymmetrically strongly suggest that a patient has mononeuritis multiplex.

The clinical diagnosis of mononeuritis multiplex can be supported by nerve conduction and electromyographic studies demonstrating a multifocal axonal neuropathy. Even when the diagnosis is certain on clinical grounds, the electrical studies help document the severity of the neuropathy, and provide a baseline for future comparison.

Does the patient with mononeuritis multiplex have a rheumatic disease?

Although mononeuritis multiplex can be caused by many disorders (see Fig. 40.27), once diabetes and trauma are excluded, the vast majority of cases have one of three causes:

- a systemic connective tissue diseases such as SLE or RA which, although not primarily vasculitic in nature, can be complicated by vasculitis;
- a systemic vasculitic disorder such as PAN, Wegener's granulomatosis (WG) or lymphomatoid granulomatosis;
- nonsystemic vasculitic neuropathy.

In patients with a connective tissue disease such as RA or SLE, mononeuritis multiplex is usually a late complication, beginning months to years after the underlying disease is diagnosed. The emergence of mononeuritis multiplex in these patients indicates that they have developed a polyarteritis-like vasculitis. These patients usually have other signs of vasculitis, such as digital gangrene, leg ulcers or abdominal ischemia.

In patients with systemic vasculitis, mononeuritis multiplex occurs early, usually before the diagnosis of the vasculitis is established. Almost all patients with a systemic vasculitis and mononeuritis multiplex have other systemic symptoms or signs such as weight loss, fever or arthralgia. A previously healthy individual who develops mononeuritis multiplex and other systemic symptoms probably has a systemic vasculitis.

Approximately one-third of the patients with mononeuritis multiplex have no identifiable systemic disease, but do have biopsy evidence of an ischemic neuropathy. Consequently, these patients are believed to have a nonsystemic vasculitic neuropathy. 'Vasculopathic' might be more accurate than 'vasculitic', since perivascular inflammation is much more common on nerve biopsy than transmural vessel inflammation with necrosis. Whatever its name, this disorder is distinct. Unlike patients with systemic necrotizing vasculitis, patients with nonsystemic vasculitic neuropathy have no systemic symptoms, however subtle; they have no physical findings beyond the neurologic examination and their blood tests are normal. The neuropathy often progresses slowly, and in up to a third of patients it improves spontaneously. Although potentially disabling, it does not affect survival. Even after years or decades of observation, patients show no evidence of developing a multisystem disease. The exact cause of this vasculopathic neuropathy remains obscure.

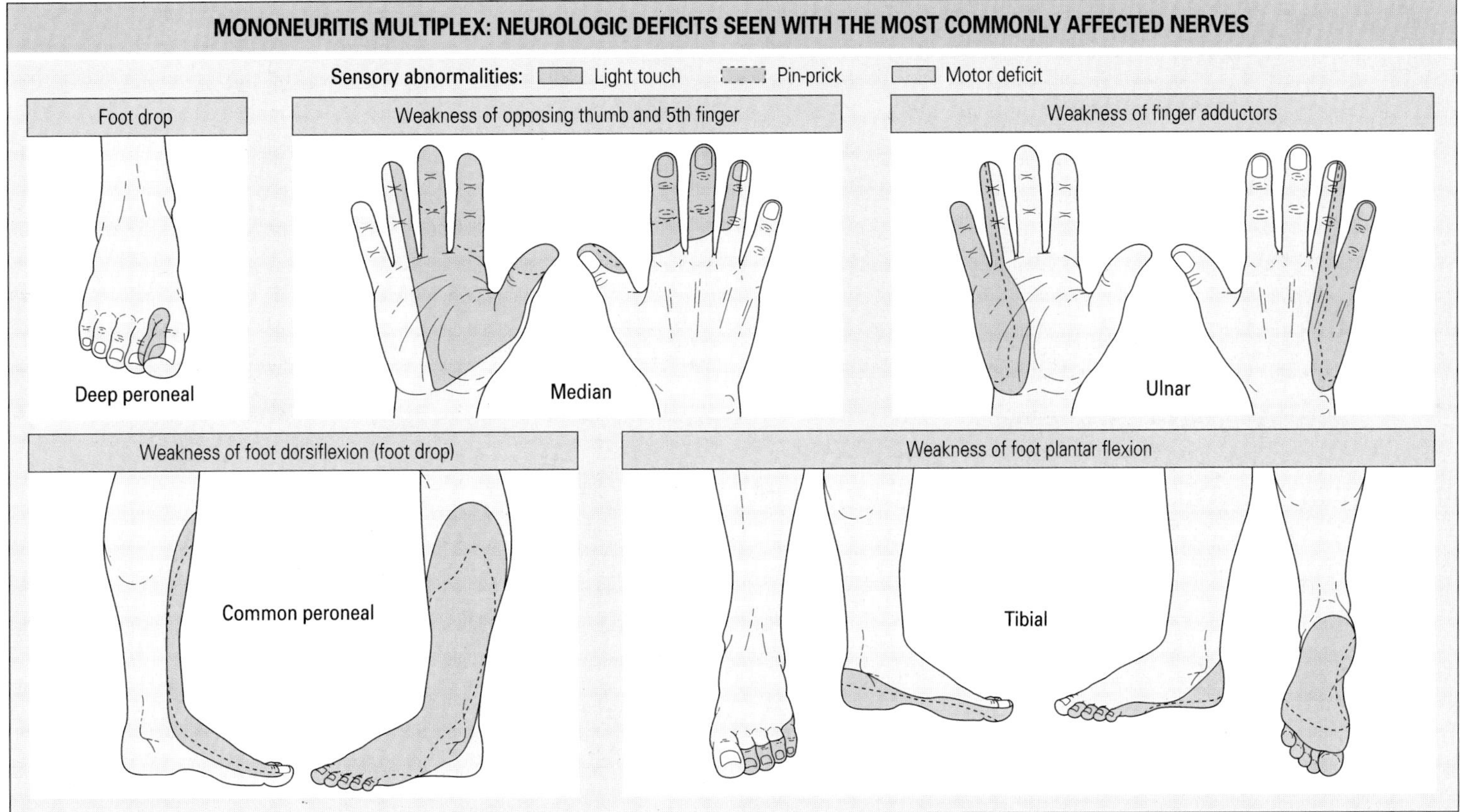

Fig. 40.28 Deficits seen with the most commonly affected nerves in mononeuritis multiplex. Shaded areas indicate regions of sensory abnormalities typically found with mononeuritis multiplex affecting the median, ulnar, common peroneal, and tibial nerves. Examples of associated motor deficits are also given.

The scope and the yield of the laboratory evaluation of a patient with newly discovered mononeuritis multiplex are dictated largely by the initial history and physical examination (Fig. 40.29). For example, patients who have well-established SLE and develop mononeuritis multiplex along with vasculitic damage in other organs will not need extensive diagnostic testing. Previously healthy patients, who experience a nearly simultaneous onset of mononeuritis multiplex with other systemic symptoms, usually have a systemic vasculitis, such as polyarteritis, WG, giant cell arteritis or cryoglobulinemia. These patients will benefit most from laboratory studies directed to these disorders: ESR, urinalysis, chest radiograph, liver function tests, hepatitis B antibodies, cryoglobulins, serum and urine immunoelectrophoresis, antineutrophil cytoplasmic antibodies (ANCA) and human immunodeficiency virus (HIV) antibody. In these patients, if electrophysiologic testing of the sural nerve is abnormal, the nerve biopsy will often (60%) demonstrate vasculitis. Sural nerve biopsy need not be done if biopsy or angiography of another site is even more likely to secure the diagnosis. In the remaining patients who have mononeuritis multiplex without any other symptoms or findings, the laboratory investigation regardless of extent is usually negative. Nerve biopsy in these individuals will show vasculopathy limited to the peripheral nerves.

Therapeutic Options

Treatment for mononeuritis multiplex is determined by the cause. A patient found to have an underlying rheumatic disease should be treated for that disease. Thus, a patient with mononeuritis multiplex and WG should be treated in the same way as any other patient with active WG, i.e. with prednisone and cyclophosphamide. If mononeuritis multiplex first develops, as it sometimes does, shortly after initiation of immunosuppressive therapy for active vasculitis in other organ systems, the treatment need not be judged a failure. In the absence of any other new organ damage, the mononeuritis multiplex in these cases probably represents thrombosis of epineural vessels damaged by previous, and not necessarily ongoing, inflammation. Deciding how to treat mononeuritis multiplex complicating polyarteritis associated with HIV infection is agonizing: the danger of traditional immunosuppressive therapy is apparent, and the value of intravenous γ-globulin or cyclosporin is unknown. In patients with RA or SLE, mononeuritis multiplex indicates a superimposed systemic vasculitis that may warrant aggressive therapy with immunosuppressive drugs, such as cyclophosphamide.

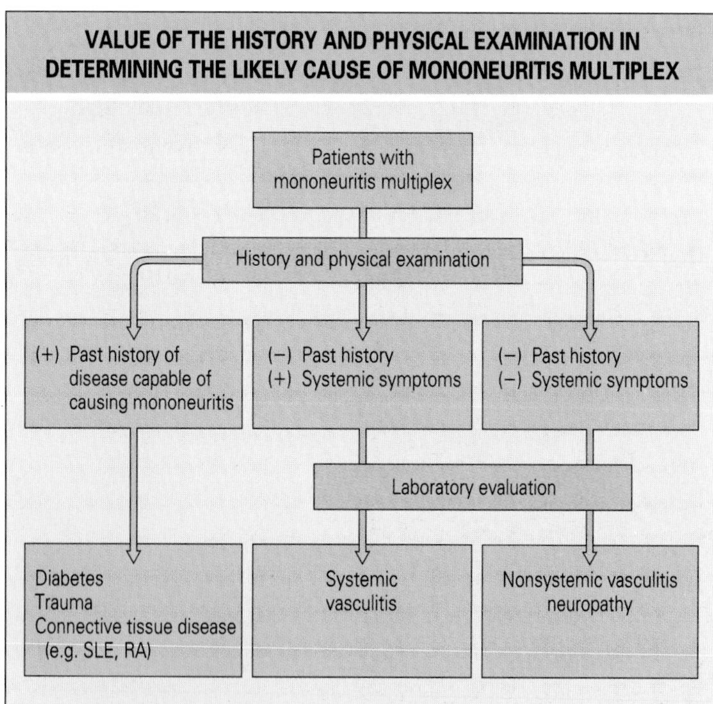

Fig. 40.29 Value of the history and physical examination in determining the likely cause of mononeuritis multiplex.

About three-quarters of the patients with mononeuritis multiplex and a rheumatic disease will improve with treatment. Patients usually start improving after 6 weeks of therapy and reach maximum benefit by 6–18 months. Because shorter nerves heal faster than longer ones, the hands improve before the feet.

Therapeutic choices are even more difficult in patients with nonsystemic vasculitic neuropathy of the peripheral nerves. These patients' comparatively benign course argues against aggressive therapy. However, uncontrolled studies involving small numbers of these patients suggest that they will benefit from treatment with prednisone alone or prednisone plus an immunosuppressive drug such as azathioprine. Treatment decisions must, therefore, be individualized and influenced by the severity of the mononeuritis multiplex, the rapidity of neurologic worsening, and the risks of prednisone or immunosuppressive therapy.

All patients with mononeuritis multiplex need supportive therapy for effective rehabilitation. Severely affected patients will require prolonged in-patient rehabilitation. Physical and occupational therapists should be consulted early to help prevent contracture, assist in building strength, and design splints or devices needed to improve mobility and functioning. Painful paresthesia may respond to low doses of amitriptyline.

Conclusions

- The diagnosis of mononeuritis multiplex is based on recognizing that the patient's symptoms and deficits developed one at a time and in the distribution of named nerve roots.
- Once diabetes and trauma are excluded, most cases of mononeuritis multiplex are caused by systemic connective tissue diseases such as SLE or RA, systemic vasculitic disorders such as PAN, or nonsystemic vasculitic neuropathy.
- The combination of mononeuritis multiplex and any other systemic symptom or sign is one of the most specific clues that the patient has systemic vasculitis.
- In patients with SLE or RA, mononeuritis multiplex is a late complication, whereas in patients with systemic vasculitis, mononeuritis multiplex occurs early.
- The treatment of mononeuritis multiplex is dictated by the underlying disease.

REFERENCES

Chang RW, Bell CL, Hallett M. Clinical characteristics and prognosis of vasculitic mononeuropathy multiplex. Arch Neurol. 1984;**41**:618–21.

Dyck PJ, Conn DL, Okazaki H. Necrotizing angiopathic neuropathy: Three-dimensional morphology of fiber degeneration related to sites of occluded vessels. Mayo Clin Proc. 1972;**47**:461–75.

Dyck PJ, Benstead TJ, Conn DL, Stevens JC, Windebank AJ, Low PA. Nonsystemic vasculitic neuropathy. Brain. 1987;**110**:843–54.

Hellmann DB, Laing TJ, Petri M, Whiting-O'Keefe Q, Parry GJ. Mononeuritis multiplex: The yield of evaluations for occult rheumatic diseases. Medicine. 1988;**67**:145–53.

Guillevin L, Du LTH, Godeau P, Jais P, Wechsler B. Clinical findings and prognosis of polyarteritis nodosa and Churg–Strauss angiitis: a study of 165 patients. Br J Rheumatol. 1988;**27**:258–64.

Kissel JT, Slivka AP, Warmolts JR, Mendell JR. The clinical spectrum of necrotizing angiopathy of the peripheral nervous system. Ann Neurol. 1985;**18**:251–7.

FLARE OF POLYMYALGIA RHEUMATICA WITH CORTICOSTEROID TAPER

Mark H Arnold & Leslie Schreiber

Definition of the Problem

Polymyalgia rheumatica (PMR) is a common inflammatory disease of the elderly.

As the diagnosis of PMR is principally clinical, differentiation from soft tissue syndromes such as shoulder capsulitis may be difficult (Fig. 40.30). In patients with established PMR, as treatment is tapered and withdrawn, an exacerbation of symptoms may occur. It is important to establish whether symptoms involving the head/neck and shoulder girdle musculature truly represent a disease exacerbation or the emergence of other pathology.

The Typical Case

A 67-year-old woman with classical PMR (abrupt onset of symmetrical shoulder girdle pain and stiffness in association with a normochromic, normocytic anemia with hemoglobin of 10.3g/l, and elevated Westergren ESR (72mm/hour) responded initially to prednisolone 15mg/day. Three months later, she re-presented with neck pain when the dose of prednisolone was reduced to 8mg/day. The pain was not accompanied by early morning stiffness or diurnal variation. There had been some discomfort involving the left posterior shoulder, without sensory disturbance or paresthesiae in the arm.

Physical examination revealed normal posture of the neck and shoulder girdle musculature, without wasting. Active neck movements were restricted by pain, particularly with extension and lateral flexion of the cervical spine to the left. Compression of the neck in this position worsened the level of discomfort. There was no other bony tenderness, neurovascular assessment of the upper limbs was normal, and both shoulders were found to have a full and pain-free passive and active range of movement. The general examination was normal. The ESR was 24mm/hour and the hemoglobin was normal (13.3g/l). Cervical radiographs revealed widespread neurocentral and zygapophyseal joint degenerative changes with mild compromise of neuroforaminae (see Fig. 40.31).

Because physical examination was able to reproduce the pain with axial loading of the cervical spine, and there was no evidence of the restricted shoulder-girdle motion that would be expected in recurrent PMR (especially if the patient is examined in the morning), the history and clinical findings were in fact suggestive of mechanical spinal pain, and conventional treatment was employed.

Diagnostic Problems

When the pattern of neck pain is asymmetric and not accompanied by a return of morning stiffness and constitutional symptoms, this is more suggestive of referred somatic pain from the cervical spine rather than PMR. In the case described, there were no symptoms to suggest a radicular pattern of pain due to impingement of cervical nerve roots. In the case of inflammatory symptoms, one expects a gradual rather than sudden return of symptoms, and symmetric stiffness of a similar pattern to the patient's original pain.

The patient must be closely questioned regarding scalp tenderness, visual disturbances, jaw, tongue and upper limb claudication symptoms, because biopsy-proven giant cell arteritis (GCA) complicating PMR occurs in 15% of cases, and may present at atypical sites. Occipital pain occurring in patients with PMR may occasionally represent occult giant cell arteritis, even in the setting of a normal ESR.

Other disorders, including herpes zoster, may develop in elderly patients treated with corticosteroids and cause significant pain prior to vesicle formation. Scalp tenderness should be sought, and palpation of the temporal arteries and assessment of patency and ocular fundoscopy should be performed to assess for the possibility of GCA. Bony metastatic disease and multiple myeloma should be excluded at the time of initial presentation.

Laboratory results in this setting may not be of great help. The ESR and other acute-phase reactants may remain normal in up to 50% of patients, despite disease exacerbation. Recent work suggests that reduced circulating CD8 lymphocyte levels may be helpful in both the diagnosis and assessment of disease activity (reduced levels characterizing active disease), but the sensitivity and specificity of this test is yet to be determined. Radiographs of the cervical spine may be of little practical help in assessment. Bone scintigraphy is unnecessary unless occult metastatic disease is suspected.

DISORDERS TO EXCLUDE IN DIAGNOSIS AND ASSESSMENT OF POLYMYALGIA RHEUMATICA
Rheumatic diseases
Cervical and lumber spondylosis Rotator cuff syndromes and frozen shoulder Soft tissue rheumatism Polymyalgic presentation of rheumatoid arthritis Fibromyalgia Polymyositis Vasculitis (including giant cell arthritis)
Neurologic conditions
Parkinson's disease Stiff-man syndrome Cervical radiculopathy
General medical and metabolic conditions
Hyperthyroidism Metabolic bone disease Myeloma Metastatic disease

Fig. 40.30 Disorders to be excluded in the diagnosis and subsequent assessment of polymyalgia rheumatica.

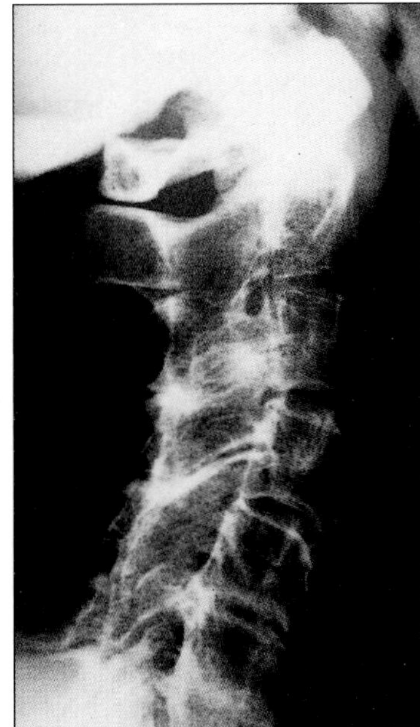

Fig. 40.31 Extensive age-related cervical spondylosis.

Therapy

In recurrence of PMR, if the patient fails to respond to physical therapies and analgesics over the course of 3–4 weeks, then it may be appropriate to increase the dosage of oral corticosteroids to the dosage level which controlled symptoms prior to the current exacerbation. It is not appropriate, in the first instance, to use dramatically higher dosages, as this increases the risk of cumulative corticosteroid related side effects.

The commonest therapeutic mistake is to commence with too high an initial dose of corticosteroids and reduce too rapidly. There is no universally accepted protocol to guide the clinician. Therapy with 15mg prednisone/prednisolone daily should be commenced and this dose continued for 2–3 weeks, ensuring that the patient experiences the expected response, then reducing by weekly decrements of lmg to l0mg/day. The dose is then reduced by lmg each 4 weeks until the 'therapeutic window' of recurrent symptoms is reached.

If it is not possible to reduce the dosage to 7mg/day or less after 6 months, then the addition of an oral NSAID may be helpful. The minority of patients will require the addition of an immunosuppressive agent such as azathioprine or methotrexate for a steroid sparing effect, although there have been no controlled studies evaluating this approach.

Conclusions

In patients with PMR who develop recurrent symptoms as the dose of corticosteroid is reduced, it is essential to exclude other causes of regional pain. This avoids unnecessarily protracted treatment with high doses of corticosteroids. As with the diagnosis of this disease, reassessment is based on clinical criteria, recognizing the concurrence of other common causes of regional pain in this age group and vigilance for the development of GCA.

REFERENCES

Elling H, Elling P. Decreased level of suppressor/cytotoxic T cell (OKT8) in polymyalgia rheumatica and giant cell arteritis: relation to disease activity. J Rheumatol. 1985;**12**:306–9.

Fitzcharles MA, Esdaile JM. Atypical presentations of polymyalgia rheumatica. Arthritis Rheum. 1990;**33**:403–6.

Jundt JW, Mock D. Temporal arteritis with normal erythrocyte sedimentation rates presenting as occipital neuralgia. Arthritis Rheum. 1991;**34**:217–19.

Kyle V, Hazleman BL. Treatment of polymyalgia rheumatica and giant cell arteritis. 1. Steroid regimens in the first two months. Ann Rheum Dis. 1989;**48**:658–61.

Kyle V, Hazleman BL. Treatment of polymyalgia rheumatic and giant cell arteritis. 2. Relation between steroid dose and steroid associated side effects. Ann Rheum Dis. 1989;**48**:662–6.

Kyle V, Cawston TE, Hazleman BL. Erythrocyte sedimentation rate and C reactive protein in the assessment of polymyalgia/giant cell arteritis on presentation and during follow up. Ann Rheum Dis. 1989;**48**:667–71.

INDEX

Common abbreviations: AS (Ankylosing spondylitis); OA (Osteoarthritis); PA (Psoriatic arthritis); PyA (Pyrophosphate arthropathy); RA (Rheumatoid arthritis); ReA (Reactive arthritis); SA (Septic arthritis); SLE (Systemic lupus erythematosus)

C

D

Common abbreviations: AS (Ankylosing spondylitis); OA (Osteoarthritis); PA (Psoriatic arthritis); PyA (Pyrophosphate arthropathy); RA (Rheumatoid arthritis); ReA (Reactive arthritis); SA (Septic arthritis); SLE (Systemic lupus erythematosus)

Common abbreviations: AS (Ankylosing spondylitis); OA (Osteoarthritis); PA (Psoriatic arthritis); PyA (Pyrophosphate arthropathy); RA (Rheumatoid arthritis); ReA (Reactive arthritis); SA (Septic arthritis); SLE (Systemic lupus erythematosus)

Common abbreviations: AS (Ankylosing spondylitis); OA (Osteoarthritis); PA (Psoriatic arthritis); PyA (Pyrophosphate arthropathy); RA (Rheumatoid arthritis); ReA (Reactive arthritis); SA (Septic arthritis); SLE (Systemic lupus erythematosus)

Common abbreviations: AS (Ankylosing spondylitis); OA (Osteoarthritis); PA (Psoriatic arthritis); PyA (Pyrophosphate arthropathy); RA (Rheumatoid arthritis); ReA (Reactive arthritis); SA (Septic arthritis); SLE (Systemic lupus erythematosus)

Common abbreviations: AS (Ankylosing spondylitis); OA (Osteoarthritis); PA (Psoriatic arthritis); PyA (Pyrophosphate arthropathy); RA (Rheumatoid arthritis); ReA (Reactive arthritis); SA (Septic arthritis); SLE (Systemic lupus erythematosus)

Common abbreviations: AS (Ankylosing spondylitis); OA (Osteoarthritis); PA (Psoriatic arthritis); PyA (Pyrophosphate arthropathy); RA (Rheumatoid arthritis); ReA (Reactive arthritis); SA (Septic arthritis); SLE (Systemic lupus erythematosus)

Common abbreviations: AS (Ankylosing spondylitis); OA (Osteoarthritis); PA (Psoriatic arthritis); PyA (Pyrophosphate arthropathy); RA (Rheumatoid arthritis); ReA (Reactive arthritis); SA (Septic arthritis); SLE (Systemic lupus erythematosus)

T

Common abbreviations: AS (Ankylosing spondylitis); OA (Osteoarthritis); PA (Psoriatic arthritis); PyA (Pyrophosphate arthropathy); RA (Rheumatoid arthritis); ReA (Reactive arthritis); SA (Septic arthritis); SLE (Systemic lupus erythematosus)

U

V

W

X

Y

Z

Common abbreviations: AS (Ankylosing spondylitis); OA (Osteoarthritis); PA (Psoriatic arthritis); PyA (Pyrophosphate arthropathy); RA (Rheumatoid arthritis); ReA (Reactive arthritis); SA (Septic arthritis); SLE (Systemic lupus erythematosus)